AO Manual of Fracture Management

Michael Wagner, Robert Frigg

Internal Fixators

Concepts and Cases using LCP and LISS

AO Manual of Fracture Management

Michael Wagner, Robert Frigg

Internal Fixators

Concepts and Cases using LCP and LISS

800 illustrations, 2280 pictures and x-rays
117 step-by-step case descriptions

Thieme

Illustrations: tadpole GmbH, CH-8048 Zürich
DVD-ROM programming: interaktion GmbH, CH-8330 Pfäffikon

Library of Congress Cataloging-in-Publication Data is available from the publisher.

Hazards
Great care has been taken to maintain the accuracy of the information contained in this publication. However, the publisher, and/or the distributor, and/or the editors, and/or the authors cannot be held responsible for errors or any consequences arising from the use of the information contained in this publication. Contributions published under the name of individual authors are statements and opinions solely of said authors and not of the publisher, and/or the distributor, and/or the AO Group.
The products, procedures, and therapies described in this work are hazardous and are therefore only to be applied by certified and trained medical professionals in environments specially designed for such procedures. No suggested test or procedure should be carried out unless, in the user's professional judgment, its risk is justified. Whoever applies products, procedures, and therapies shown or described in this work will do this at their own risk. Because of rapid advances in the medical sciences, AO recommends that independent verification of diagnosis, therapies, drugs, dosages, and operation methods should be made before any action is taken.
Although all advertising material which may be inserted into the work is expected to conform to ethical (medical) standards, inclusion in this publication does not constitute a guarantee or endorsement by the publisher regarding quality or value of such product or of the claims made of it by its manufacturer.

Distribution by Georg Thieme Verlag, Rüdigerstrasse 14, DE-70469 Stuttgart and
Thieme New York, 333 Seventh Avenue, New York, NY 10001, USA

ISBN-10: 3-13-143551-8 (GTV)
ISBN-13: 978-3-13-143551-4 (GTV)
ISBN-10: 1-58890-486-5 (TNY)
ISBN-13: 978-1-58890-486-7 (TNY)

Table of contents

Concepts

Cases

Forewords

Thomas P Rüedi

For almost 40 years AO compression plate fixation providing absolute stability—as introduced by Maurice Müller—was the gold standard in operative fracture treatment. In the 1980s the locking intramedullary nail opened up new perspectives for the stabilization of diaphyseal fractures. As an internal splint this device provides relative stability, which allows rapid fracture healing with abundant callus formation. Perren and Tepic showed in the early nineties that, thanks to locking head screws (LHS) providing angular stability, the longitudinal stabilizer, eg, a plate could be kept at a distance from the bone similar to the external fixator and without interfering with periosteal or cortical vascularity. This innovative, quite different and biologically gentle as well as less invasive fixation principle was called "internal fixation". Clinically, it was applied as the PC-Fix (point contact fixator) and LISS (less invasive stabilization system).

The actual breakthrough for the new internal fixator principle occurred however, when Michael Wagner as clinician, together with the engineer Robert Frigg, designed and developed the so-called "combination hole". The idea and new design of the screw hole—a combination of the dynamic compression unit for standard cortex screws with a threaded hole for the LHS—could be introduced in any of the existing plates and required only a few additional instruments. The new and very versatile locking compression plate system—LCP—with its three different possibilities of applications and functions found immediately wide acceptance and has revolutionized operative fracture fixation in a similar way to the original compression plate and twenty years later the interlocking intramedullary nail.

It seemed therefore logical that Michael Wagner should also pioneer the collection of LCP and LISS cases for a book that addresses not only the basic principles, attributes, and different applications of the new implants but also highlights the pearls and pitfalls of the internal fixators in the clinic. Together with the contributions of other enthusiastic but also critical users the authors share experiences with these devices and gives valuable, practical recommendations to newcomers. The best stabilization system is of little use if the vascularity of the soft as well as hard tissues are not carefully respected. An entire chapter has therefore been dedicated to the most difficult and demanding challenges of any fracture treatment—the fracture reduction.

The editors, Michael Wagner and Robert Frigg, and the co-authors have to be complimented for a most comprehensive and attractive book on the clinical applications of the new internal fixator principles with the LISS and LCP, which are introducing interesting possibilities and opportunities especially in articular fractures as well as providing new hopes for severely osteoporotic patients.

The team at AO Publishing has again displayed its ability to produce, together with Thieme Verlag, a most attractive book that will find numerous readers and thereby help to improve patient care.

Thomas P Rüedi, MD, FACS
Founding Member of the AO Foundation
Davos, April 2006

Stephan M Perren

Fracture treatment has undergone a fascinating evolution. Early in the last century the main goal of treatment was to reach solid union. Then stable fixation and functional postoperative treatment successfully eliminated fracture disease. Now we can take advantage of restoring function while inducing prompt and safe healing and reducing the risk of biological complications.

In the early days the excessive external immobilization of the neighboring articulations too often resulted in damage to the articulations and even worse to the soft tissues and blood supply. In my own "pre AO" experience I observed a high incidence of what was later called fracture disease (Sudeck's or reflex dystrophy). Swelling, pain, patchy bone loss, and stiff articulations were accepted as the natural consequence of fracture. It is interesting to note that each generation was (and is!) blinded by the "state-of-the-art".

In the late fifties the visionary Maurice E Müller and his colleagues effected a worldwide change in the fight against fracture disease. They studied and advocated precise reduction and compression fixation so that fracture healing could take place in a mechanically neutral environment. Dystrophy became a very rare incident and fracture healing showed a fascinating histology: direct healing. The price paid for focusing on mechanical advantages was that this approach did not induce early healing and so implants could not be removed earlier than one to two years postoperatively. This was not a major problem in view of the fact that the implants were mechanically protecting the fracture. Still, the observation of late union was a strong indicator that there was room for improvement. Considerable damage to the soft tissues and blood supply to bone in the hands of the less experienced resulted in complications due to a disregard for biology.

The promoters of stable internal fixation had to face harsh criticism, mainly focused on the complications of such treatment like infections and refractures. A close collaboration including clinical input, documentation, biomechanical research, and basic development allowed the AO to overcome these difficulties by defining the principles of treatment and offering thorough teaching.

From the outset less stable fixation like the more flexible version of the intramedullary nail and also external fixators, both resulting in indirect healing, were integral parts of the AO technology. But it took a long time to amalgamate observations of biological reactions to the more flexible techniques and observations relating to compression plating. As always, some ideas were not new; we mention the basic contributions to compression technology by Lambotte and Danis and those of Küntscher to nailing. Still, to bring a new method to bear on a large scale not only requires innovative and sound ideas and ingenious individual surgical skill, but also an integrated approach to improvement and teaching to allow others to achieve similar results.

In the late eighties while studying the potential of internal fixators the team of the AO Research Institute came across a more flexible plate fixation that took advantage of locked screws. The point contact fixator (PC-Fix), which is the proof of concept of the internal fixator, was born. Animal studies showed an astonishing early solid bridging of the fractures (10 weeks) and good local resistance to infection. Furthermore, the opportunity to take advantage of monocortical threaded bolts was demonstrated. Clinical studies with exceptionally high follow-up showed low complication rates in respect to infection (Norbert P Haas, Alberto Fernandez). History repeats itself as a rule: again there were pioneers:

Boitzy, Weber, and Heitemeyer (bridge plating) and we also pay tribute to Granowski (Zespol fixator). It took 40 years from the first bridge plates and nearly twenty years from successful use of the PC-Fix for the advantages of the internal fixator to be generally accepted. The difference between "me too" and leadership is rooted in basic insight and early commitment.

A new era started with great respect to biology: the era of the internal fixator. Insistence on precise reduction was replaced by restricting the aim of surgery to adequate alignment to restore the original relative positions of the two joint bearing surfaces of the long bone. Approximate alignment without touching the intermediate fragments became acceptable. The main ingredients for successful internal fixator technology still are sufficient stability for early functional treatment and, now, sufficient instability for the induction of prompt healing. The strain theory allowed definition of the degree of instability which is tolerated and the degree which induces healing.

When the bone is dead and/or infected as a result of the accident (and hopefully not of the surgery) there is a clear indication for good reduction and absolute stability and similarly precise reduction and absolute stability is a requirement for intraarticular fractures!

Living bone is able to react once it is given the chance to do so. Creating the proper biological and mechanical environment is the prerequisite. The future will show whether additional stimulation offers an advantage for fresh fractures. One may question whether stimulation will be tolerated without causing damage in desperate clinical cases such as chronic and infected nonunions. Let's not forget that it took supernatural power to revive Lazarus, in other words, I think that stimulating nearly dead cells is equally challenging.

Without perfect closure of the fracture gap it is now possible to follow the repair process within the gap radiologically. We can now pinpoint those cases that require the long-term presence of the implant to avoid refracture. Some of the ob-servations of delayed healing are not an indication of less satisfactory healing, but they are a consequence of improved visualization.

While the LISS is a further refinement of the PC-Fix, the LCP combines a stripped version of both the LC-DCP and PC-Fix with a threaded conical locking system to reduce jamming at removal. The LCP offers a convenient way of making the transition from conventional compression techniques to the internal fixator. As the two principles of plate screws, namely, screws that press the plate to the bone and those that keeping the plate elevated are incompatible, it is advisable to exercise discipline and not to mix these principles in the same bone fragment. This is also a challenge for teaching.

In view of the basic changes brought about by the internal fixator, it is of great merit that the initial chapter of this book discusses the basics of the principles. Michael Wagner has undertaken with success the task of explaining the practical aspects of the basic concepts.

The book may be understood as a technical manual but, far more, it is offering a basic understanding. This is an important aspect in view of the fact that the implant reflects only the mechanical aspect of the realization of the internal fixator philosophy; balancing biology against pure mechanics involves the implants and the surgeons. The statement of Girdlestone "rather gardening than replacement" is up-to-date.

The second chapter of the book deals with basic clinical aspects; namely reduction of the fracture as a prerequisite to successful internal fixation. When reading this chapter one is tempted to add to Girdlestone with "rather elegant surgical technique than brute force".

The chapters on LISS and LCP are actually technical manuals, "how to do it". With great care the sequential steps of the internal fixation, the special characteristics of the implants and, for instance, the importance of large span bridging and attention to screw leverage using long plates are explained.

The last chapter addresses the possible errors, "what not to do" and special procedures if difficulties arise.

I hope the reader enjoys this comprehensive book—this "first shot" as much as I have done.

Stephan M Perren, Prof. Dr. med. D.Sc. (h.c.)
Davos, April 2006

Contributors

Editor

Michael Wagner, Univ.-Prof. Dr. med.
Facharzt für Unfallchirurgie und Sporttraumatlogie
Wilhelminenspital
Montleartstrasse 37
AT-1160 Wien

Robert Frigg
Chief Technology Officer
Synthes Bettlach
Güterstrasse 5
CH-2544 Bettlach

Coeditors

Richard Buckley, MD, FRCS(c)
University of Calgary
Foothills Medical Center
1403-29 Street N.W.
CA-Calgary AB T2N 2T9

Emanuel Gautier, PD Dr. med.
Hôpital Cantonal Fribourg
Clinique de chirurgie orthopédique
CH-1708 Fribourg

Michael Schütz, Prof. Dr. med.
Princess Alexandra Hospital (PAH)
2 George Street
GPO Box 2434
AU-Brisbane 4001

Christoph Sommer, Dr. med.
Kantonspital Chur
Loëstrasse 170
CH-7000 Chur

Authors

Martin Altmann
Synthes Bettlach
Güterstrasse 5
CH-2544 Bettlach

Reto Babst, Prof. Dr. med.
Kantonsspital Luzern
Unfallchirurgie
Spitalstrasse
CH-6000 Luzern 16

Hermann Bail, PD Dr. med.
Klinik für Unfall- und Wiederherstellungschirurgie
Campus Virchow - Klinikum (CVK)
Augustenburgerplatz 1
DE-13353 Berlin

Peter Brunner
Synthes Bettlach
Güterstrasse 5
CH-2544 Bettlach

Ulf Culemann, Dr. med.
Klinik für Unfall-, Hand- und Wiederherstellungschirurgie
Universitätsklinikum des Saarlandes
Kirrberger Strasse
DE-66421 Homburg/Saar

Christopher G Finkemeier, MD
5897 Granite Hills Drive
US-Granite Bay CA 95746

André Frenk, Dr.
Synthes Bettlach
Güterstrasse 5
CH-2544 Bettlach

Michael J Gardner, MD
Cornell University Medical College
Hospital for Special Surgery
535 East 70th Street
US-New York NY 10021

Christoph W Geel, MD, FACS
Suny Upstate Medical University
Health Science Center
Orthopaedic Trauma
550 Harrison Centre, Ste 100
US-Syracuse NY 13202

Andreas Gruner, Dr. med.
Unfallchirurgische Klinik
Städtisches Klinikum Braunschweig
Holwedestrasse 16
DE-38118 Braunschweig

Norbert P Haas, Univ.-Prof. Dr. med.
Klinik für Unfall- und Wiederherstellungschirurgie
Campus Virchow - Klinikum (CVK)
Augustenburgerplatz 1
DE-13353 Berlin

David L Helfet, MD, MBCHB
Cornell University Medical College
Hospital for Special Surgery
535 East 70th Street
US-New York NY 10021

Authors (cont)

Thomas Hockertz, Dr. med.
Unfallchirurgische Klinik
Städtisches Klinikum Braunschweig
Holwedestrasse 16
DE-38118 Braunschweig

Keita Ito, Prof., MD, ScD
AO Research Institute
Clavadelerstrasse 8
CH-7270 Davos Platz

Roland P Jakob, Prof. Dr. med.
Hôpital Cantonal Fribourg
Clinique de chirurgie orthopédique
CH-1708 Fribourg

Georges Kohut, Dr. med.
Hôpital Cantonal Fribourg
Clinique de chirurgie orthopédique
CH-1708 Fribourg

Philip J Kregor, MD
Vanderbilt Orthopaedic Institute
Medical Center East
South Tower, Suite 4200
US-Nashville TN 37232-8774

Christian Krettek, Prof. Dr. med.
Hannover Medical School (MHH)
Carl-Neuberg-Str. 1
DE-30625 Hannover

Frankie Leung, MD, FRCS
Queen Mary Hospital
Pok Fu Lam
HK-Hong Kong

Wilson Li, MD
Department of Orthopaedics
and Traumatology
Queen Elizabeth Hospital
30, Gascoigne Road
HK-Kowloon, Hong Kong

Dean G Lorich, MD
Cornell University Medical College
Hospital for Special Surgery
535 East 70th Street
US-New York NY 10021

Marc Lottenbach, Dr. med.
Hôpital Cantonal Fribourg
Clinique de chirurgie orthopédique
CH-1708 Fribourg

Ingo Melcher, Dr. med.
Klinik für Unfall- und
Wiederherstellungschirurgie
Campus Virchow - Klinikum (CVK)
Augustenburgerplatz 1
DE-13353 Berlin

Erika J Mitchell, MD
Vanderbilt Orthopaedic Institute
Medical Center East
South Tower, Suite 4200
US-Nashville TN 37232-8774

Thomas Neubauer, Dr. med.
Unfallchirurgie
Wilhelminenspital
Montleartstrasse 37
AT-1160 Wien

Stephan M Perren, Prof. Dr. med.
D.Sc. (h.c.)
Senior Scientific Advisor
Dischmastrasse 22
CH-7260 Davos Dorf

Michael Plecko, MD
Unfallkrankenhaus Graz
Göstingersstrasse 24
AT-8021 Graz

Tim Pohlemann, Prof. Dr. med.
Klinik für Unfall,- Hand- und
Wiederherstellungschirurgie
Universitätsklinikum des Saarlandes
Kirrberger Strasse
DE-66421 Homburg

Heinrich Reilmann, Prof. Dr. med.
Unfallchirurgische Klinik
Städtisches Klinikum Braunschweig
Holwedestrasse 16
DE-38118 Braunschweig

Daniel A Rikli, Dr. med.
Unfallchirurgie
Kantonsspital Luzern
Spitalstrasse
CH-6000 Luzern 16

Thomas P Rüedi, Prof. Dr. med., FACS
AO International
Clavadelerstrasse 8
CH-7270 Davos Platz

Authors (cont)

Christian Ryf, MD
Clinic for Surgery and Orthopaedics
Davos Hospital
Promenade 4
CH-7270 Davos Platz

Klaus-D Schaser, Dr. med.
Klinik für Unfall- und
Wiederherstellungschirurgie
Campus Virchow - Klinikum (CVK)
Augustenburgerplatz 1
DE-13353 Berlin

Robert Schavan, Dipl.-Ing.
Barschbleek 8
DE-47877 Willich

James P Stannard, MD
University of Alabama at
Birmingham
Division of Orthopaedic Surgery
950-B Faculty Office Tower
510 20th Street South
US-Birmingham AL 35294-3409

Michael D Stover, MD
Loyola University Medical Center
Department of Orthopaedic Surgery
2160 South 1st Avenue
US-Maywood IL 60153

Gabriele Streicher, Dr. med.
Unfallchirurgische Klinik
Städtisches Klinikum Braunschweig
Holwedestrasse 16
DE-38118 Braunschweig

Norbert Südkamp, Prof. Dr. med.
Universitätsklinik Freiburg i.Br.
Klinik für Unfall- und
Wiederherstellungschirurgie
Hugstetterstrasse 55
DE-79106 Freiburg i.Br.

Hobie D Summers, MD
Loyola University Medical Center
Department of Orthopaedic Surgery
2160 South 1st Avenue
US-Maywood IL 60153

Ronald J van Heerwaarden, MD, PhD
Sint Maartenskliniek
Hengstdal 3
NL-6522 JV Nijmegen

Hans Zwipp, Prof. Dr. med.
Universitätsklinikum
Carl Gustav Carus
Klinik für Unfall- und
Wiederherstellungschirurgie
Fetscherstrasse 74
DE-01307 Dresden

Introduction

Michael Wagner

From the very outset, the goal of the Arbeitsgemeinschaft für Osteosynthese (AO) has been to improve the treatment of fractures and their sequelae. The AO proposed this by restoring integrity to the broken bone and providing the patient with early and pain-free restoration of function. The emphasis has never been solely on bone union, but has always included restoration of function—as implied in the AO's motto "Life is movement, and movement is life."

"Fracture disease" was an obstacle to healing and mobility, and its symptoms often emerged after prolonged external splinting, immobilization in traction—consisting of chronic edema, soft-tissue atrophy, severe osteoporosis, thinning of the articular cartilage, severe joint stiffness, and sometimes chronic regional pain syndromes. Fracture disease prevented patients from starting active exercise at an early stage and delayed the return of function after bone healing. The innovative techniques introduced by the AO to combat this condition had to meet high demands. Fracture reduction had to be anatomical, and the fixation had to be stable enough to eliminate pain and allow functional rehabilitation of the limb without the risks of secondary displacement, delayed union, nonunion, or deformity. The stability produced by the compression method of fracture osteosynthesis met these requirements; it was possible to start rehabilitation immediately after the operation, and most plaster immobilization techniques became outdated.

The issues that have played an important role in stimulating progress have been,

1) differentiating between the biological requirements of articular and long bone fractures;
2) greater recognition of the importance of the type and timing of treatment;
3) specific assessment of injury to the soft-tissue envelope;
4) and attention to the patient's individual functional and physiological requirements.

It is now accepted that absolute stability is mandatory only for joint fractures and some related fractures—and then only when it can be achieved without damage to the blood supply and soft tissues. Fixation of the diaphysis should always take account of length, alignment, and rotation of the limb, and the methods of choice are splinting with an intramedullary nail or an internal fixator to promote union through callus formation.

If plate osteosynthesis is required, techniques of minimal access and fixation are able to minimize insult to the blood supply to the bone fragments and adjacent soft tissue. The fixation of articular fractures requires anatomical reduction and absolute stability to enhance the healing of articular cartilage and make early motion possible so that good ultimate function will ensue. The current principle of preserving the blood supply needs to be applied at every stage of fracture management—from initial planning to consolidation. The choice of strategy and implant depends on the biological and functional demands of the fracture and should be compatible with them.

Anatomy, stability, biology, and mobilization are still the four fundamental AO principles today. However, the implications of these principles have changed in response to the findings constantly emerging from scientific investigations and clinical observations. Progressive changes in approaches and methods have been based on continuing laboratory and clinical research, with new discoveries leading to the development of many new implants and instruments. The strategy of fracture fixation with different principles, methods and techniques of internal and external fixation are dynamic, and further advances will continue to be made.

The AO principles

AO principles THEN

- Fracture reduction and fixation to restore anatomical relationships.
- Stability through fixation with compression or splinting, as required by the fracture pattern and the injury.
- Preservation of the blood supply to the soft tissues and bone through careful handling and gentle reduction techniques.
- Early and safe mobilization of the area being treated and of the patient as a whole.

These concise principles still embody the AO philosophy of patient care. In today's approach, the emphasis is still very much on the fact that maintaining the blood supply to the soft tissues and bone is the most important aspect of fracture care—so that the principles could also be restated as follows:

AO principles NOW

- Atraumatic reduction and fixation techniques are mandatory. Reduction of long bones need not be anatomical, but instead should demonstrate axial alignment with respect to length and torsion in the diaphysis and metaphysis. Anatomical reduction is mandatory for intraarticular fractures to restore joint congruency.
- Appropriate stability of the construct has to be established. Joint surfaces require anatomical reduction with absolute stability; the majority of diaphyseal fractures can be treated with methods that provide relative stability (eg, intramedullary or extramedullary splinting).
- Atraumatic soft-tissue technique should be used with appropriate surgical approaches.
- Early active mobilization of the patient is expected as the fixation construct is stable enough to allow postoperative functional care.

A comprehensive classification of long bones has helped make treatment outcomes predictable. Neither the principles nor the approaches have changed, but definitions have become more refined in relation to the different methods and techniques of fracture fixation.

The revolution is continuing today—the principles remain the same, but the methods and techniques are continually developing and implants are being modified and newly invented. Today, the AO develops sophisticated scientific and technological instrument sets that lend themselves to applications that go beyond fracture treatment. This includes the treatment of complications related to fracture care, and more recently the treatment of degenerative diseases, deformations, and defects, the problems that are becoming increasingly prevalent in the aging population (such as osteoporosis).

There has been a progressive evolution in nailing and plating:

Nailing

- From conventional to locked intramedullary nailing, and
- from reamed to unreamed nailing.

Plating

- From very stable (absolutely stable) fixation to flexible (relatively stable) fixation, and
- from compression plate fixation to locked internal fixation.

The AO principles

AO principles THEN	Influences through clinical experiences and experimental investigations	AO principles NOW
1. Anatomical, precise reduction	Applied science concerning: – bone healings, – blood supply through soft tissue and bone, – biological shortcomings of ORIF in multifragmentary shaft fractures lead to a new way of thinking. As a consequence, indirect reduction techniques were developed	Fracture reduction and fixation to restore anatomical relationships. Reductions need not be anatomical but only axially aligned in the diaphysis and the metaphysis. Anatomical reduction is required for intraarticular reductions. The principles of articular fracture care: - atraumatic anatomical reduction of the articular surfaces, - stable fixation of the articular fragments, and - metaphyseal reconstruction with bone grafting and buttressing apply today as they did at the beginning.
2. Rigid fixation, absolute stability	The most notable change in the treatment of diaphyseal fractures has been the shift from the mechanical to the biological aspects of internal fixation. The preservation of the viability and integrity of the soft-tissue envelope of the metaphysis has been recognized as the key to success. Today the dominant theme in the fixation of fractures of the diaphysis is the biology of bone and the preservation of the blood supply to bony fragments, and no longer the quest for absolute stability. Major changes have occurred in the timing of the different steps of metaphyseal reconstruction, as well as in the fixation methods and techniques. The comprehensive classification of long bones has helped predict treatment and outcome.	Stabilization with different grades of stability, from high (absolute stability) to low (relative stability). Appropriate construct stability. Stability by compression or splinting, as the fracture pattern and the injury require. The joint surfaces require anatomical reduction with absolute stability. The majority of diaphyseal fractures are treated with relative stability methods (eg, intramedullary or extramedullary splinting).
3. Preserving blood supply	The present concept still emphasizes that the blood supply through the soft tissues and bone is the most important aspect in fracture care: – atraumatic soft tissue technique through the appropriate surgical approaches, – atraumatic reduction and fixation techniques are mandatory, – implants with new bone- implant interface.	Preservation of the blood supply to soft tissues and bone by careful handling and gentle reduction techniques and a newly designed bone-implant interface.
4. Early protective motion for rehabilitation because pain was abolished and union assured		Early and safe mobilization of the part and the patient. Early active motion can also be carried out because splint fixation is stable enough to allow postoperative functional care.

Progressive evolution is the result of a long-term collaboration between the AO Research Institute (ARI), the AO Development Institute (ADI), and the Synthes manufacturers. This manual provides details of the principles and techniques involved in internal fixation using the recently developed less invasive stabilization system (LISS) and the locking compression plate (LCP). Future developments will need to address the shortcomings of the current techniques and equipment and to assess the side effects of new techniques, as well as ways of promoting healing in cases of chronically infected, atrophic nonunion. The techniques of internal fixation will also need to be further simplified to improve both safety and ease of handling, benefiting the treating surgeon and the patient.

Suggestions for further reading

Müller ME, Allgöwer M, Willenegger H (1965) Technique of internal fixation of fractures. Heidelberg: Springer-Verlag.

Müller ME, Allgöwer M, Willenegger H (1979) Manual of internal fixation. Heidelberg: Springer-Verlag.

Perren SM (2002) Evolution of the internal fixation of long bone fractures. The scientific basis of biological internal fixation: choosing a new balance between stability and biology. *J Bone Joint Surg Br*; 84(8):1093–1110.

Schatzker J (1998) M.E. Müller—on his 80th Birthday. *AO Dialogue*; 11(1):7–12.

Schenk R, Willenegger H (1964) [On the histology of primary bone healing.] *Langenbecks Arch Klin Chir Ver Dtsch Z Chir*; 308:440–452.

Acknowledgments

This book represents a logical step in publications from the AO. It is some years since the development of internal fixators and initial clinical experience has now been gained so that the time has come to meet the need for a book on this subject. As we become more sensitive to the specific requirements of adult learning, an important insight has been to recognize the educational value of a case-based learning program. In the light of this, we have devised an approach to describing the management of fractures that is based on a series of clinical cases submitted by different authors worldwide.

The editors would like to acknowledge and express their thanks to all the colleagues who contributed their texts and clinical cases. Their names are given in the following list:

We wish to express our full appreciation to our coeditors, Richard Buckley, Emanuel Gautier, Michael Schütz, and Christoph Sommer, who played an essential role in the production of this manual on LISS and LCP by writing, reviewing and refining the contributions. We thank them for taking on this great responsibility and giving their valuable time to this project.

Martin Altmann (Concepts)
Reto Babst (6.1.3, 6.3, 6.3.3, 6.3.4, 9.2.6, 9.2.7)
Hermann Bail (10.3.8)
Peter Brunner (Concepts)
Ulf Culemann (8.1.3, 8.1.4)
Christopher G Finkemeier (5.1.1, 5.2.2)
André Frenk (Concepts)
Michael J Gardner (6.1.4, 6.3.2, 7.2.4, 7.3.3, 9.1.2, 10.1.1, 10.3.5)
Emanuel Gautier (7.2.2, 8.1.1, 8.1.5, 9.1, 9.1.6, 9.2.1, 9.3.5)
Christopher W Geel (7.1, 7.1.4, 10.1.8, 10.3.4)
Andreas Gruner (7.1.6, 8.1.2, 9.2.4, 9.2.8, 9.3.2, 9.3.8, 10.1.6, 10.1.9, 10.2.12, 10.3.2, 10.3.9)
Norbert P Haas (10.3.1, 10.3.8,
David L Helfet (6.1.4, 6.3.2, 7.2.4, 7.3.3, 9.1.2, 10.1.1, 10.3.5)
Thomas Hockertz (7.1.6, 8.1.2, 9.2.4, 9.2.8, 9.3.2, 9.3.8, 10.1.6,10.1.9, 10.2.12, 10.3.2, 10.3.9)
Keita Ito (Concepts)
Roland P Jakob (9.1.6)
Georges Kohut (7.2.2)
Philip J Kregor (9.1.3, 9.1.4, 9.3.7, 9.3.9)
Christian Krettek (Concepts)
Frankie Leung (6.1.7, 10.2.4)
Wilson Li (6.1.2)
Dean G Lorich (6.1.4, 6.3.2, 7.2.4, 7.3.3, 9.1.2, 10.1.1, 10.3.5)
Marc Lottenbach (9.2.1)
Ingo Melcher (10.3.1)
Erika J Mitchell (9.1.3, 9.1.4)
Thomas Neubauer (Concepts)
Stephan M Perren (Foreword)
Michael Plecko (6.1, 6.1.8, 6.3.1, 7.1.2)
Tim Pohlemann (8.1, 8.1.3, 8.1.4)
Heinrich Reilmann (7.1.6, 8.1.2, 9.2.4, 9.2.8, 9.3.2, 9.3.8, 10.1.6, 10.1.9, 10.2.12, 10.3.2, 10.3.9)
Daniel A Rikli (7.3, 7.3.1, 7.3.5, 7.3.6)
Thomas P Rüedi (Foreword, 7.2, 10.2, 10.3)
Christian Ryf (6.1.9, 7.1.2, 7.3.2, 10.1.4, 10.2.11, 10.2.13, 10.3.1)
Klaus-D Schaser (10.3.1)
Robert Schavan (Concepts)
Michael Schütz (6.3.5, 7.1.1, 7.1.3, 9.2.3, 9.3, 9.3.6, 10.1.7)
Christoph Sommer (5.1, 5.1.4, 5.1.5, 5.2, 5.2.1, 6.1.1, 6.2, 6.2.2, 6.2.3, 6.2.4, 6.2.5, 6.2.6, 7.1.5, 9.3.3, 9.3.4, 10.1.2, 10.1.3, 10.1.5, 10.1.11, 10.2.6, 10.2.7, 10.2.8, 10.2.10, 10.3.3, 10.3.6)
James P Stannard (6.1.5)
Michael D Stover (10.3.7)
Gabriele Streicher (7.1.6, 8.1.2, 9.2.4, 9.2.8, 9.3.2, 9.3.8, 10.1.6, 10.1.9, 10.2.12, 10.3.2, 10.3.9)
Norbert Südkamp (6.1.6)
Hobie D Summers (10.3.7)
Ronald van Heerwaarden (9.3.10)
Michael Wagner (5.1.2, 5.1.3, 6.2.1, 6.2.7, 7.2.1, 7.2.3, 7.3.4, 9.1.1, 9.1.5, 9.2, 9.2.2, 9.2.5, 9.2.9, 9.3.1, 10.1, 10.1.10, 10.2.1, 10.2.2, 10.2.3, 10.2.5, 10.2.8, 10.2.9, 10.2.14, 10.2.15, 10.2.16, 10.3.10, 10.3.11)
Hans Zwipp (11)

In addition, we give a special acknowledgment to Stephan M Perren for his reviews and his foreword, to Thomas P Rüedi for supporting the project and for his foreword, to Chris L Colton for revising the extensive glossary, and to Chris G Moran for ensuring the high quality of a whole range of impressive illustrations of the surgical approaches.

Apart from the contributors and coeditors, a number of people have contributed to the production of this publication. To mention them by name is only a very small token of thanks for much hard work. Hanna Jufer and her team of illustrators reliably produced high quality drawings on schedule that fully meet our expectations. Design and layout work was initiated by Sandro Isler, whereby we benefited from his vast experience.

The creation and production of a work of this magnitude has required the dedication of a number of collaborators from AO Publishing and AO International. These include Miriam Uhlmann, who was solely responsible for coordinating the project and all those involved, and for ensuring the detailed processing of the contributions, Roger Kistler, who had the task of adjusting and finalizing the overall layout, and Doris Straub Piccirillo, Urs Rüetschi, and Andy Weymann for their specialist input and valuable support.

The time and effort invested in this project has led to a most rewarding result.

Michael Wagner, Robert Frigg

Concepts

Concepts

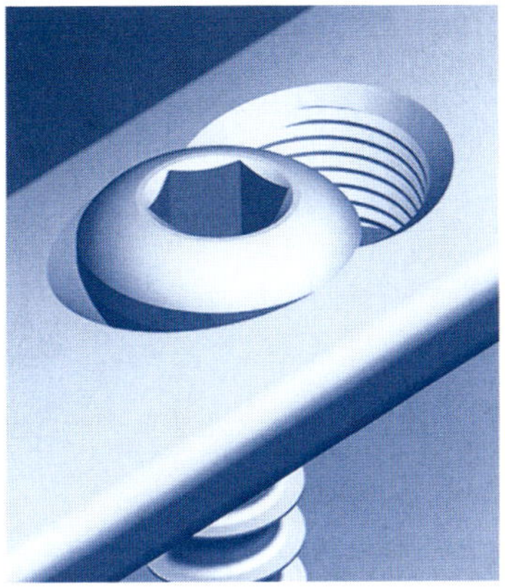

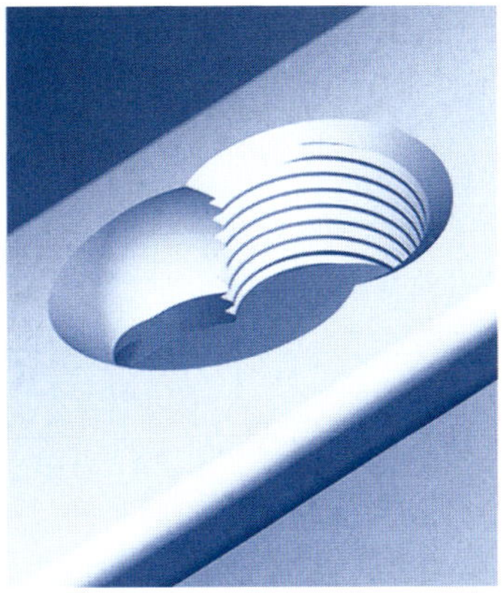

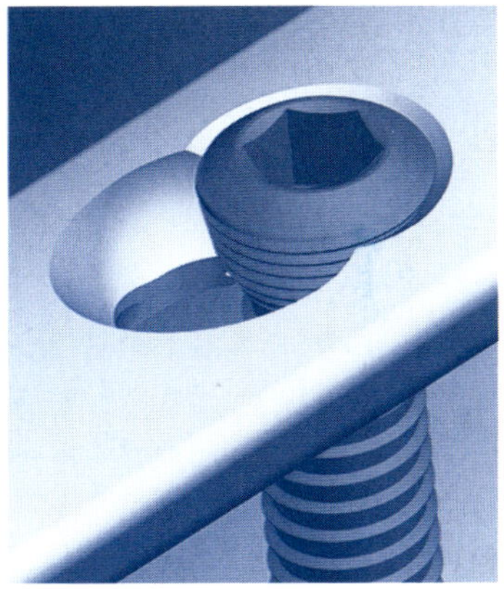

1 Background and methodological principles

1 Background and methodological principles

1 Osteosynthesis

The goals of fracture care are to achieve union, alignment, and function.

The general indications for fracture fixation are:

- To save life or limb.
- To reconstruct displaced articular fractures.
- To prevent deformity.
- To promote union when this is delayed.
- Improved function following early motion.

The most obvious indication for operative and functional treatment is an intraarticular fracture where displacement will result in loss of function. Certain diaphyseal fractures require internal fixation: the forearm because it is a "joint" and the femur because immobilization of the injured thigh musculature will lead to a stiff, weakened leg.

Fixation of an unstable pelvic fracture, with hemodynamic instability, may be life saving. In addition, stabilization of multiple long-bone fractures may reduce mortality in patients with polytrauma.

Limb saving is another major indication. With vascular and neurological injury, the bone must be stabilized to protect the repaired structures. In open fractures, stabilization will support the soft-tissues healing.

To assure union and prevent deformity is another major reason for internal fixation. The inabilities to reduce a fracture, or maintain reduction, are indications for internal fixation.

Fractures at high risk of not healing are also ideal for surgery. Finally, internal fixation is also used in bone reconstruction for nonunion and malunion.

1.1 Treatment of diaphyseal fractures: background and concepts

Historically, internal fixation has been used as a last resort to achieve fracture union. Union has always been important and function has been a lesser concern. However, this approach to fracture treatment often sacrificed function leaving a stiff and poorly functioning extremity. At the beginning of AO history almost each fracture was stabilized with the compression method after open direct anatomical reduction. However, a problem arose: The blood supply to bone was neglected as the endeavor for perfect anatomical reduction resulted in increased tissue trauma. The perception that stable fixation was necessary led to significant damage to blood supply, increasing the rate of nonunion, infection, and failure.

The development of locked intramedullary nailing confirmed that a multifragmentary diaphyseal fracture did not necessitate an anatomical reduction. With general alignment and relative stability, union could occur rapidly. This led to the development of indirect reduction techniques: If the soft tissues were protected and biological, diaphyseal fixation techniques were used, the fracture would heal with acceptable alignment and function. Ganz, Mast, and Jakob reintroduced indirect reduction methods and biological fracture fixation solutions, eg, bridge plating (Boitzy, Weber).

Research continued on bone and its blood supply. An understanding of healing in different mechanical situations led to the strain theory of Perren. Modifications of implants to provide more stability and early function, while maintaining blood supply to the bone, such as the LC-DCP, LISS, and locking compression plates (LCP) were developed.

Current concepts still emphasize the utmost importance of blood supply to the soft tissues and bones in fracture care. The AO Principles have not changed other than that the treatment of diaphyseal and metaphyseal fractures have been refined and defined with regard to mechanics, biology, and techniques:

1. Atraumatic soft-tissue technique through appropriate surgical approaches.
2. Atraumatic reduction and fixation techniques are mandatory. Reduction need not be anatomical but axial alignment is essential (in the diaphysis and the metaphysis).
3. Appropriate construct stability. The majority of diaphyseal fractures are treated with relative stability techniques.
4. Early active motion can be carried out because fixation is stable enough to allow functional aftercare.

Precise anatomical reduction of the diaphysis in the femur, tibia, and humerus is not necessary. Function is not diminished as long as length, rotation, and axial alignment are restored. The radius and the ulna are exceptions to this rule. Pronation and supination, as well as normal elbow and wrist function, depend upon the preservation of the normal anatomical shape and relationships of the two bones. Anatomical reduction of these two bones is mandatory, and stability should be achieved with an appropriate technique.

In the following sequences some important technological innovations and conceptual changes of fracture fixation are discussed.

Locked intramedullary nailing

The development of this technique showed that diaphyseal fractures do not require precise anatomical reduction, but only correct alignment and relatively stable fixation (with intramedullary splinting of the fracture zone). This resulted in rapid union through callus formation (indirect bone healing). This led to the view that indirect reduction techniques can be used to spare the soft tissues and that flexible biological fixation techniques can be used successfully in diaphysis [1, 2].

With the emphasis today on the preservation of the blood supply to the bones and soft tissues, the locked intramedullary nail has become the implant of choice for the fixation of diaphyseal fractures [3]. Locked nailing can be performed by a minimally invasive approach. Although multifragmentary fractures used to be a contraindication to nonlocked nailing, they are currently the principal indication for the use of a locked intramedullary nail. Locked nailing has also made it possible to stabilize fractures in the proximal and distal thirds of the diaphysis, as well as to treat subtrochanteric fractures with involvement of the lesser trochanter and ipsilateral fractures of the shaft and neck of the femur [4, 5]. The new generation of locked nails extends the indications towards the proximal and distal ends of the diaphysis.

From direct to indirect reduction

Interfragmentary compression requires predominantely open direct anatomical reduction. It has been recognized that direct manipulation of bone fragments, as was usual during internal fixation procedures, was a major cause of devitalization of the bone fragments [6] (see chapter 2; Tab 2-1). In order to minimize damage to the vascularization of the osseous tissue and the surrounding soft tissues, indirect reduction techniques have become popular with open reduction and internal fixation. This approach was advocated by Mast and colleagues [7] who introduced indirect reduction methods and biological solutions such as bridge plating for diaphyseal fracture fixation.

One example of an indirect reduction method is the distraction of fragments using a distractor, an external fixator, a plate, or traction applied to a limb. The fragments are reduced using ligamentotaxis (Tab 1-1) [8–10], minimizing the extent to which they are manipulated and preserving their blood supply.

Tab 1-1

Ligamentotaxis

Ligamentotaxis is the principle of molding fracture fragments into alignment as a result of tension applied to a fracture by the surrounding intact soft tissues.

Preservation of the blood supply

Historically, the most notable development in the treatment of diaphyseal fractures has been a shift away from the mechanical aspects of internal fixation toward the biological aspects. The focus in the fixation of diaphyseal fractures today is on the biology of the bone and on preserving the blood supply to the bone fragments. A quest for absolute stability is no longer the primary aim [2, 11].

Limits of compression plating: "stress protection"

It was observed in earlier clinical and laboratory studies that the cortex under the fixation plate became excessively porous due to a marked increase in the number of haversian canals [12]. This phenomenon was explained by Wolff's law of bone remodeling (Tab 1-2), and it became known as "stress protection." However, on investigating the biological effects of conventional compression plates on the underlying cortex, Perren and colleagues [13] made the important discovery that plates interfere significantly with the blood supply to the underlying cortex. The "stress protection" hypothesis was thus found to be mistaken. This led to the development of limited contact plates later to noncontact plates.

Tab 1-2

Wolff's law

Bones develop the structure best suited to resisting the forces acting on them. Any changes in either the form or function of a bone are followed by specific changes in its internal architecture and secondary alterations in its external shape—changes usually involving responses to alterations in weight-bearing stresses (form follows function). This applies only to long lasting unloading.

Wave plate and bridge plate

Imaginative thinking led to the development of the wave plate [14] and the bridge plate [15, 16]. The basic idea is to leave the fracture zone and its fragments undisturbed, by fixing the plate to the intact part of the bone on the proximal and distal sides of the fracture zone.

There are two advantages when a wave plate is used to bridge a comminuted fracture area. Firstly, when a plate is applied at a distance from the bone, it allows better perfusion of the repair tissue—with the benefits of better leverage and mechanical support from the repair tissue [17]. Secondly, when the plate spans an extended fracture area, there is more uniform deformation of the inner part of the plate that is not fixed to the bone—preventing the development of sites of excessive deformation that could lead to fatigue failure.

The technique of bridge plating (splinting method with plates) was developed to help prevent devitalization of fragments in multifragmentary fractures [6, 18]. The fracture is first reduced by means of indirect reduction. The fragmentation zone is then bridged with a plate that is fixed to the main proximal and distal fragments. This maintains length, rotation, and axial alignment. This type of internal fixation is a form of splinting. It is not absolutely stable, and union occurs through callus formation. This plating technique is mainly indicated for the fixation of multifragmentary fractures. If a simple transverse or oblique fracture is closely reduced and plated, then absolute stability has to be achieved using interfragmentary compression; otherwise failure is likely to follow due to excessive strain at the fracture site. Clinical experience with locked plates has shown that close indirect reduction and splinting of simple fracture is possible and leads to indirect fracture healing but sometimes to a delayed bone healing.

Tab 1-3 **Milestones in plate development**

Year	Product	Inventor	Description	Fixation method	Technique
1961	Formplates/T-plates		– Cancellous bone screws in the metaphyseal area	Compression	ORIF
1962/1963	Round hole plate	Müller ME [19]	– Conical holes, screws with conical heads – Removable compression device	Compression	ORIF
1963	Semi-tubular plate	Müller ME [20]	– Self-compressing plate (elongated plate holes) – Eccentric screws for interfragmentary compression	Compression	ORIF
1969	Dynamic compression plate (DCP)	Perren SM [21, 22]	– Compression cylinder at one end of the elongated plate hole (DCU) – Head of the screw is spherically undercut – Screw angulation	Compression	ORIF
1980		Brunner CF, Weber BG	– Transverse undercuts	Compression	ORIF
1981/1982		Brunner CF, Weber BG [14, 17]	– Wave plate	Splinting	
		Mast JW, Ganz R, Jakob R [18, 19]	– Concept of "indirect reduction"		
		Ganz R, Rüedi TP	– "bio-logical" plating	Splinting	less invasive
1985		Heitemeyer U, Hierholzer G [16]	– Bridging plate	Splinting	
1990	LC-DCP	Perren SM [23]	– Self-compression plate with limited contact – Undercuts – Screw angulations – Smooth plate bending – Eccentric screws	Compression or splinting	ORIF or open, less invasive
1992	PC-Fix	Tepic S, Perren SM [24]	– Point-contact-plate – Angular stable screws	Splinting, locked splinting	open, less invasive
			– Concept of submuscular plating	Splinting with conventional plates	MIPPO
1994	LISS	Frigg R, Schavan R	– LHS with threaded conical screw head – Noncontact plate – Angular stable locking head screws	Locked splinting	MIPO
2001	LCP	Wagner M, Frigg R, Schavan R	– Combination hole	Compression and locked splinting possible	ORIF or MIPO

Bone grafting

The techniques of indirect reduction and bridge plating have made bone grafting unnecessary in multifragmentary diaphyseal and metaphyseal fractures [6]. Bone grafting is now largely reserved for metaphyseal defects in articular fractures and for open fractures with bone loss.

Plates with limited bone contact

Plates having a smaller surface area in contact with the bone, even when they are thicker and more rigid, were found to cause less interference to the blood supply of bone [25]. A smaller surface contact area with the bone also leads to less intense osteoporosis than where plates which are thinner and more elastic but have a larger surface contact area with the bone. The porosis appeared to be directly related to the amount of necrosis occurring below the plate (Gautier). This observation led to the development of plates that ensure limited contact between the bone and implant, such as the limited-contact dynamic compression plate (LC-DCP).

Biological internal fixation

This approach represents the culmination of recent research, following fundamental revision of the principles of fracture fixation and conceptual and technological innovations [3, 26] (Tab 1-3). There is now a better understanding of the way in which fractures heal, and the all-important role played by the soft tissues has been recognized. As our understanding of the ways in which bones and implants interact has also improved, the importance of maintaining the vital balance between stabilization and biological function has been grasped, and biological internal fixation has been developed in order to take this into account. The principle of biological internal fixation consists of minimizing the biological damage caused by indirect reduction, the surgical approach, and by contact between the implant and the bone [2, 27]. Minimizing such damage can be achieved, but it implies less precise reduction and a less stable, more flexible fixation.

More than 100 years ago, Lane (1856–1938) first advocated the manipulation of tissues using special instruments and a "no-touch technique," as he realized that bone healing depended as much on the condition of the soft tissues as on optimal mechanical conditions. Today's concept of biological internal fixation is based on achieving a balance between stability and biological integrity. The principle of biological internal fixation consists of minimizing the biological damage caused by the surgical approach and reduction technique by anchoring the implant only in the main fragments. The minimization of trauma is achieved at the expense of less precise reduction and less stable fixation (Tab 1-4).

Indirect reduction and pure internal splinting (based on the principle of relative stability) help keep bone fragments vital. Indirect bone healing leads to early and reliable solid union. This approach can be successful whenever the accident has not resulted in complete avascularity in the bone fragments. Still complete avascularity require fracture fixation with absolute stability.

Biological internal fixation with different implant systems Tab 1-4

Implant	Method of fracture fixation	
	Position of splint	
external fixator	external	locked splinting
locked nail	internal intramedullary	locked splinting
locked internal fixator	internal extramedullary	locked splinting

Tab 1-4 Biological internal fixation with the method of locked splinting using three different implant systems according to the principle of fracture fixation with relative stability.

Three main conventional techniques are available to achieve biological internal fixation: 1) splinting stabilization with external fixators; 2) splinting stabilization with intramedullary locked nails; and 3) the use of plates as pure splints—ie, without the additional lag screw effect.

1. With external fixators, the transcutaneous infection route offsets the positive effects of minimizing implant–bone contact and flexible fixation.
2. Using an intramedullary nail allows a minimally invasive percutaneous approach, but the advantages of this are somewhat offset by the extensive damage caused to the intramedullary circulation, as well as local and general intravascular thrombosis due to tissue damage and possible fat intravasation caused by the high intramedullary pressure during reaming and insertion of the nail.
3. Splinting the fracture zone with a plate. The pioneering technique today is the locked internal fixator (locked noncontact plate) applied using a minimally invasive technique. Research and development in this area are ongoing, and further modifications and improvements with this method can be expected in the near future.

From absolute to relative stability

The method of compression fixation using lag screws and conventional plates (based on the principle of absolute stability) has therefore been supplemented by the method of splinting (based on the principle of relative stability), taking advantage of pure splint fixation with a plate [6]. The latter method provides flexible fixation that stimulates callus formation and consequently promotes early solid union.

The less invasive stabilization system (LISS) and locking compression plate with locking head screws (LCP with LHS) now incorporate the methodological principles of locked internal extramedullary splinting [28]. LISS and LCP with LHS resemble plates but act biomechanically as locked splints or fixators—locked internal fixators (LIF).

1.2 Treatment of articular fractures

The principles of the treatment of articular fractures are the same today as they have always been:

- Atraumatic anatomical reduction of the articular surfaces
- Stable fixation of the intraarticular fragments
- Reconstruction of the metaphysis with bone grafting and buttressing by bone grafting and buttress plate
- Functional postoperative treatment without immobilization

What has changed is the sequence of the different steps of metaphyseal reconstruction.

Intraarticular reconstruction must be undertaken as early as possible and with the least possible trauma to the tissues. Any delay leads to permanent deformity, as the articular fragments unite rapidly and defy later attempts at reduction. Intraarticular cartilage does not remodel [29]. Any residual incongruity becomes permanent and can lead to posttraumatic arthritis. In contrast, the diaphysis and metaphysis have a tremendous capacity for remodeling and any residual deformities can be relatively easily corrected by osteotomy.

The timing of articular and metaphyseal reconstruction and the techniques used are vital therefore. It has been recognized that preserving the viability and integrity of the soft-tissue envelope of the metaphysis is the key to success. External fixation is therefore often used as a temporary measure, to establish the length and alignment of the metaphysis, with definitive reconstruction being delayed for 2–3 weeks until the soft-tissue envelope has recovered [30, 31]. If the articular fragment or articular bone block is small and does not provide any purchase for an external fixator, then the joint is bridged temporarily to provide the necessary immobilization.

Whether final reconstruction is carried out as a primary procedure or as a delayed procedure, every possible step is taken to minimize damage to the blood supply to the soft tissue and bone. The measures required for this include indirect reduction, minimal exposure, and percutaneous screw fixation of the fragments. Buttressing is still important in preventing axial deformity, but buttressing techniques are now designed to minimize soft-tissue trauma. Buttressing can now be achieved by plating, by using an angular stable plate-screw construct such as a blade plate.

1.3 The patient and the injury

General and local factors affecting management decisions

It is important to identify the patient factors that will effect treatment, to look at the preoperative risk factors, and to identify other factors of the injury that may change the treatment plan. Patient assessment is best done through the preoperative history and physical examination as well as by various investigations that are required to determine the health of the patient and the presence of blood born pathogens. Informed consent must include a discussion of the expectations of treatment between the patient and the surgeon.

The injury itself has both systemic and fracture-associated effects. The systemic effects involve the multiple trauma patients. Fracture-associated concerns are soft-tissue injury, particularly a crush syndrome or fractures causing fat embolism, or vascular and nerve injury. The role of the soft tissue in healing, infection, and function is important and influences the timing and type of fixation. The treatment objectives of the soft-tissue injury are first to maintain tissue perfusion, to prevent necrosis, to avoid infection, and to prevent further damage of any soft tissue. This is best done by stabilizing the soft tissues to promote healing and function and ultimately to promote bone union. This is accomplished by skeletal stabilization, which decreases the injury inflammatory response and bacterial spread while increasing perfusion and promoting wound repair. The choice of fixation technique is based upon the principle that insult to biology is to be minimized while mechanical stability must allow early function. Thus, a balance must be achieved between the amount of surgical biological insult necessary to achieve stabilization, the degree of instability and the mechanical stability necessary to allow early function and to induce callus to achieve union.

Timing

Fracture surgery is emergency, urgent, or elective. Emergency surgery is immediate for life and limb-threatening problems. Where as urgent surgery occurs within 12 hours, elective can usually be booked leisurely after 24 hours and is a planned intervention with the optimized patient and surgeon.

Patient preparation will be determined by the particular nature of the injury and patient condition. Elective surgery will allow a proper case history to be completed to determine comorbidities and assessment of risks in order to optimize the outcome. An optimal plan for fracture care should exist including plans for appropriate postoperative care determined with the patient. Patients who require urgent surgery can usually be optimized, as most of this surgery is done to prevent complications such as infection in open fractures by debridement but patient understanding of the severity and consequences of the injury will be limited.

The final aspect is emergency surgery, and this is time-dependent based on the injuries present such as hemorrhage, vascular insufficiency, head injury, or other associated injuries requiring emergency life-saving intervention. It may be to save a life or a limb and little can delay it, but may also be at a point where the whole concept of limb salvage is impossible due to the fact that the patient is too ill and requires expedient surgery. This is a specific example where orthopedic trauma care supersedes fracture care thus modifying it in relation to the patient condition. This is the multiply injured patient.

Injury assessment and conditions will modify any treatment as evidenced by the multiply injured patient, but preoperative plan and tactic must include the patient and the associated injury as well as the fracture.

Ultimately the timing of surgery is not determined by the fracture but by the patient's physiological condition and soft-tissue injury. The preoperative plan allows the surgeon to go through the proposed operative fixation procedure, and so to identify potential problems before they occur. It is a visualization of the process and techniques that may be necessary to perform the reduction and fixation.

2 Concepts of fracture fixation

The theoretical principles underlying fracture fixation are the establishment of the concept of stability—absolute or relative stability meaning maximal or less mechanical stability after the osteosynthesis. The two methods applied in order to achieve these goals are compression (static or dynamic) or splinting (locked or unlocked). A variety of techniques and implant technologies are applied in the steps required to carry out these methods (Tab 1-5).

The present section describes the principles and methods of fracture fixation, compression and splinting, and bone healing, and the reaction of bone to implants. Chapter 2 describes the general techniques used for reduction and their relation to different types of fixation. Chapter 3 describes the specific techniques and procedures used for the less invasive stabilization system (LISS) and locking compression plate (LCP) technologies and the handling of the implants and instruments involved.

2.1 Principles: absolute versus relative stability

There are two main principles involved in fracture fixation—absolute stability and relative stability. Absolute stability is best achieved through interfragmental compression using the lag-screw technique. In certain situations absolute stability is achieved by plate compression. Regardless of the technique selected, the surgeon will need to obtain an anatomical reduction which restores structural continuity of the bone and provides stable fixation allowing partial weight bearing and early muscle rehabilitation of the extremity. Relative stability implies a more flexible atraumatic stabilization procedure that has the advantage of preserving blood supply [2]. The corresponding techniques can therefore be referred to as "biological internal fixation" (Tab 1-4).

The two principles of fracture fixation result from the concept of stability (Fig 1-1).

The term "stability" is used here in accordance with its meaning in clinical practice—ie, referring to the extent to which

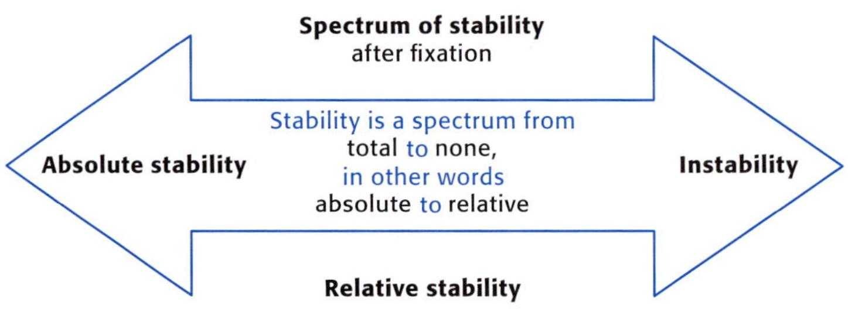

Fig 1-1 Spectrum of stability.

load-dependent displacement between the fracture surfaces is possible. If the fractured surfaces are compressed in accordance with the principle of absolute stability, then only minimal displacement between the fragments can occur. By contrast, if the fracture zone is splinted using implants that do not exert compressive forces, relative displacement can be proportional to the load applied and in inverse proportion to the rigidity of the splinting device which bridges the fracture.

Different concepts of fracture fixation

Principle of fracture fixation = grade of stabilization	Method			Technique and implants function	Bone healing
Absolute stability = high	**Compression**			Lag screw (conventional screw)	**Direct**
		Static[1]		Lag screw and protection plate	
				Compression plate	
				Tension band	
		Dynamic[2]		Tension band plate	
				Buttress plate[6]	
	Splinting		External splinting	External fixator	
			Intramedullary splinting	Intramedullary nail	
		Locked[3]	Internal extramedullary splinting	Bridging with standard plate	
				Bridging with locked internal fixator	
			External splinting	Conservative fracture treatment (cast, traction)	
		Unlocked[4]	Intramedullary splinting[5]	Elastic nail	
Relative stability = low				K-wire	**Indirect**

[1] Fracture under compression-implant under tension.
[2] Compression under function.
[3] Locked splinting with control of length, alignment, and rotation.
[4] Splinting with limited control of length, alignment, and rotation.
[5] Can be changed to dynamic compression in case of a dynamically locked nail or dynamic external fixator.
[6] Using an angular stable plate–screw construct (ie, LISS or LCP with LHS) as buttress plate, the plate acts as a blade plate. Occasionally a buttress plate may be considered as a splint.

Tab 1-5 Different concepts of fracture fixation.

Definitions

Stability is defined as the degree of displacement between fracture fragments.

Rigidity is defined as the physical properties of the implant or the ability of the implant to counter deformation. However, a rigid implant may be applied to a fractured bone in a way that is providing poor stability, ie, instability.

Stability after osteosynthesis is a spectrum from minimal to absolute. Where there is no motion between the fracture fragments, under load absolute stability exists. The second condition; relative stability, is where there is some motion between the fracture fragments. The amount of stability between fracture fragments is also determined by the degree of impaction between the fragments. This will produce intimate contact and restore structural continuity to the bone, thus restoring the load-bearing capacity to the bone (implant-bone construct shares the stresses). However, the degree of stability varies depending upon the bone contact or methodology. Healing is possible in this variable stability situation as demonstrated in the strain theory of Perren.

Strain theory

According to the strain theory, for a given amount of displacement, the width of the gap determines the resulting deformation (strain) of the repair tissue. When the strain exceeds the elongation at rupture of the tissue concerned the tissue is disrupted or cannot be produced. If this situation occurs repetitively at the fracture site, these cells are constantly destroyed and never remodel the fracture site but are ultimately reabsorbed. If there is a larger gap which many of these similar cells now traverse, a similar amount of motion, or even greater, will allow each of these cells to expand. Because there are more cells in the gap they are able to absorb more displacement, remain within their own strain levels, and not become disrupted. The larger the gap, the better the chance that secondary bone healing will occur. There are tissue-specific strain tolerances throughout the process of bone union beginning with granulation tissue which has a 100% strain level, down to lamellar bone which only has a 2% strain level and can be very easily disrupted. Depending on the phase of fracture healing and the degree of fracture stability present, union may or may not occur. Assuming that there is an adequate blood supply, the given stability of the fracture fixation will determine the type of healing and also the implant fatigue and failure thereof if appropriate stability is not chosen. Inversly low strain (large defect) will not induce bone formation.

To summarize, bone union depends on respecting the capacity of the soft tissues to maintain vascular supply to the bone, on the reduction of the fracture, and on applying the technique which provides the necessary stability for union to occur. Absolute stability means lack of displacement and demands anatomical reduction and interfragmentary compression, while relative stability permits the fracture fragments to move within their defined amount of strain and is achieved with an axial aligned reduction splinting.

Elastic, reversible versus plastic, irreversible deformation

Absolute stability means that there is no displacement of, or no relevant displacement or movement between, the fragments under a physiological load.

Internal fixation techniques based on the principle of relative stability are achieved using elastic flexible splinting. Flexible fracture fixation refers to a fixation that is elastic under load. Elastic indicates that a certain amount of deformation of the mechanical construct which occur under a specific (permitted) load. When the loading cycle is completed, the implants will return to their original form when unloaded—reversible deformation.

An overload situation may lead to plastic irreversible deformation of the implant. Plastic deformation refers to permanent displacement and, therefore, secondary dislocation of the fracture = malalignment.

Elastic and stable only differ in the point of view of the observer: elastic techniques are aimed at reversible (that is, elastic) deformation; stable techniques are understood in terms of the displacement of fragments—absolutely stable meaning absolutely no displacement; relatively stable meaning a certain amount of displacement that returns to the initial state after completion of the load cycle; and unstable, which is associated with permanent displacement, that is, secondary dislocation.

Absolute stability

The principle of absolute stability means that the compressed fracture surfaces do not displace under load. This requires an anatomical precise reduction and interfragmental compression. Compression is achieved through preload and friction on the fracture surface and healing is by direct bone union.

The features/requirements of absolute stability include:

- Precise anatomical (mostly open, direct; unfrequent percutaneous, direct) reduction.
- Stable fracture fixation (compression method).
- Preshaping the plate to match the anatomy of the bone.
- Compression caused by preloading of the bone and a certain amount of deformation in the fracture gap.
- Best achieved by lag screw and/or compression plates.
- Preloading of the lag screw to 2500 N.
- Axial preloading of the compression screws.
- The reduced bone fragments form part of the construct and carry load. The bone is the component that bears the main load.
- Elimination of relative motion between the bone fragments.
- Prevention of elongation and deformation of the repair tissue, especially in the fracture gap.
- Remodeling of the haversian system.
- Direct bone healing (osteonal remodeling) of cortical and cancellous bone; also of stably fixed necrotic bone.
- Absolute stability can also be achieved more theoretically by using an external fixator.
- High stability can be achieved by compression under function using the tension band technique.

The disadvantage of techniques involving this methodological principle is that they are associated with bone devitalization.

Relative stability

The principle of relative stability is defined as displacement between fracture fragments that is compatible with fracture healing. This motion is below the critical strain level of repair tissue as determined by the strain theory. Relative stability requires indirect healing and callus. Relative stability is dependent upon connecting a splint usually that is less rigid than bone, by a coupling device such as locking head screws or threaded bolts. These splints reduce, but do not abolish, fracture motion so pain is reduced and active muscle rehabilitation is practical. The types of splints available are locked intramedullary nails, either reamed or unreamed, bridge plates, or external fixation devices. Occasionally a buttress plate may be considered as a splint. All of these splints have in common, the fact that they bridge a defect in the bone that is not able to resist a load.

The features of relative stability include:

- Elastic fixation after indirect closed reduction, providing biologically optimal conditions. Elastic deformation of the implants occurs. The effects of resorption at the ends of the bone fragment are positive (demonstrating good blood supply) and the fracture gap enlarges. The fracture then consolidates with exuberant callus.

- Indirect healing of bone. Healing occurs because of preservation of biological function (and rapid restoration of blood perfusion).

2.2 Methods: compression versus splinting

The two basic methods used for internal fracture fixation are compression—the conventional screw/plating technique applying interfragmentary compression, in which the aim is absolute stability; and splinting—the biological internal fixation method in which the locked intramedullary nail, the external fixator, or the internal fixator spans the fracture zone and the aim is to achieve relative stability [2, 6].

Compression

Compression is a safe method of achieving highly stable fixation that is suitable for simple fracture patterns in any segment of the bone. In practice, the aim of this method is to achieve precise anatomic reduction of the fragments, stable fixation, and early rehabilitation that protects function. This leads to direct bone healing. Static compression can be achieved using the lag screw technique and/or the conventional compression plating technique. For large and/or dense bones compression plate fixation achieves absolute stability but the fragments have to be in contact remote to the plate by prebending the plate. It should be noted that despite applying absolute stability by compression and prebending, the compression is maintained only if it is greater than functional distraction applied. The friction produced will resist shear as long as the shear force is less than friction. Static compression can be also achieved by applying an external fixator with compression.

Dynamic compression

Dynamic compression can be achieved using the tension band technique, by tension band plating or buttress plating (occasionally a buttress plate may be considered as a splint). This variant of stability is the application of dynamic compression or mobilizing the physiological forces of muscle or the anatomy of eccentrically loaded bones with a functional load. In this situation the implant is applied to the tension or convex side and the tensile force is transformed by the implant to dynamic compression on the opposite side to the implant. If the load is directly applied over the fracture, compression occurs. If that load is displaced eccentrically, compression will occur on the concave side and tension on the convex side. By simply adding a tension band, this force is neutralized, but it is also important to ensure that there is an intact buttress opposite the tension cortex.

Splinting

Splinting is a more flexible method of fixation intended for use in treating multifragmentary fractures in the metadiaphyseal and diaphyseal regions of a long bone. This principle of relatively stable fracture fixation can be implemented by applying external splints such as the external fixator, or internal splints such as locked nails, bridging plates, or locked internal fixators. Relative stability depends on connecting a splint usually less rigid than bone by a coupling device such as screws. These splints reduce, but do not abolish, fracture motion so pain is reduced and active muscle rehabilitation is practical. All of these splints have in common the fact that they bridge a defect in the bone which is not able to carry a load. In order to function, splints must be coupled to the bone or limb segment.

Locked splinting

External fixators, locked nails, and locked internal fixators are locked splints. Factors that affect the stability of any splint are the size of the implant giving it strength, the position of the implant to the bone, position of its coupling to the bone and the fracture pattern. The closer the implant position to the intramedullary position the stronger it is, and weakest the further away it is. The position of the coupling devices will also control stability in all splints; the most stable being the near–far position and the least stable being far–far. A multifragmentary fracture or a complex fracture are suited best fracture patterns for pure splinting as they have small amounts of strain across the multiple and large gap. Relative stability leads to indirect bone healing. The implants span the fracture zone after indirect closed reduction and preserve the anatomical axis, length, and rotation of the fractured bone until consolidation occurs. The implant is the component that bears the main load until early callus shears the load.

One complication of a nongliding locked splint is seen in the situation where a plate is applied to the bone without adequate stability or compression at the interface between the two fracture fragments. Motion occurs—the fracture reabsorbs—motion continues to occur and because the implant maintains distraction and cannot allow the fracture to collapse to a stable position, it will loosen and fail. With a locked nail this may occur but it can be converted very easily to a gliding splint by removal of one of the locking couplings and allowing the fracture to undergo compression and return to its position of stability.

Tab 1-6 **Indications for compression vs splinting method using plates**

	Compression[1]	Splinting[2]
Simple fractures:		
diaphyseal	+	+/–
metaphyseal	+	+/–
Multifragmentary fractures:		
diaphyseal	–	+
metaphyseal	–	+
Osteotomies	+	+
Articular fractures	+	–
Fractures in porotic bones	+/–	+

+ = yes; – = no; +/– = under discussion and only in specific situation
[1] ie, lag screw and/or conventional plating technique.
[2] ie, minimally invasive plate osteosynthesis with locked internal fixators.

Indications

The indications for using the either conventional plating technique (compression method) or biological internal fixation using a plate (the splinting method with the plate spanning the fracture zone) differ (Tab 1-6) according to fracture location, fracture type, soft-tissue conditions, and quality and vascularity of the bone. If the blood supply to the fracture is severely damaged and the bone is necrotic, recovery may take many months. Conventional compression fixation then allows for protected internal remodeling over a long period. Situations of avascularity require long-term absolute stability. However, if the blood supply is good or can be restored, then it makes sense to take advantage of the additional potential of bone biology, and splinting is considered to be the method of choice. The two principles of stabilization—absolute and relative stability—and both methods—interfragmentary compression and splinting—are incompatible in the same fracture site.

2.3 Bone healing

Properties and reaction of bone to fracture and implants

Bone is strongest in compression because the apatite, or mineral phase, resists best compression. However, bone will tear apart because of the weakness of collagen fibers in tension. Cancellous bone is similar to cortical bone but less force is required to disrupt it. Bone is like a stiff spring in that it will respond by shortening and taking up force applied to it. Implants change the deformability and the contribution to stiffness.

Blood supply

Bone blood flow is a two-way system. The normal blood supply to cortical diaphyseal bone is through a nutrient medullary artery that supplies the inner 2/3 of the cortex-endosteal vessels while the periosteal vessels supply the outer 1/3 of the cortex. These periosteal vessels reach the bone through fascial and muscular attachments to bone. The metaphysis has a rich blood supply from the numerous vessels in soft-tissue attachments. In both areas significant internal anastomotic channels exist between the periosteal and endosteal vessels resulting in blood flow in either direction; inside–out or outside–in. Internally, the endosteal vessels branch off into radial arterioles that enter into the osteon formed by the osteoblast as they form bone. Thus cortical bone shows a very complex structure which allows capillaries to develop in the haversian canals and links the endosteal flow to the periosteal flow. Following fracture this complex vascular arrangement is disrupted. The soft tissues may be damaged by the accident, transportation, and surgeon, leading to periosteal loss and then surgery will lead to further devascularization.

Fracture

When bone is mechanically overloaded, it fractures. A fracture results in significant soft-tissue damage through cavitations around the bone ends which causes the fracture ends to lose their blood supply. The reaction of bone and adjacent soft tissue to the fracture stimulates bone healing to restore the original bony integrity. This is based upon living pluripotential cells, which are locally available or transported by the blood supply of the soft tissue. The surgeon is responsible for providing the appropriate mechanical environment to facilitate healing, as well as assuring maintenance of alignment by splinting or fracture fixation.

The total amount of injury caused to the bone and surrounding soft tissues is the sum of the injuries caused by the trauma, transport, and surgery. The surgical injury consists of the damage caused by the reduction, plus the approach, plus fixation of the fracture plus implant contact. The amount of iatrogenic damage can be reduced by modifying the surgical technique—eg, the way in which the soft tissues are handled and the techniques used for reduction and fixation (insertion and choice of implant and bone–implant interface).

Primary biological effects of implants

Fracture fixations result in varying degrees of stability, primarily a function of the implant and its application. A stable but flexibly fixed fracture may become visibly displaced in an elastic fashion (by as much as 20% of the gap width) during loading. An absolutely stable fracture does not displace, even microscopically. The degree of stability provided has an important effect on the type of bone healing that occurs. Flexible fixation results in micromotion, which induces exuberant callus clearly visible on x-rays, while stable fixation diminishes this. Here lies the relevance of mechanobiology to osteosynthesis.

Depending on the mechanical environment, bone will heal in two ways. Absolute stability leads to direct healing, and flexible fixation leads to indirect bone healing [6].

Direct bone healing

Direct bone healing is a biological process of osteonal bone remodeling [32]. This bypasses callus formation (indirect healing) and is, in essence, contact healing between two avascular bone surfaces. Remodeling occurs where there is contact. Although there is a qualitative correspondence between the basic aspects of healing in cortical and cancellous bone, the volume-surface ratio differs, and the speed and reliability of healing are therefore generally better in cancellous bone [33]. Only minor changes can be observed radiographically. In absolutely stable fixation, callus formation is only minimally visible, if at all. During the first few days after surgery, there is minimal activity in the bone near the fracture. The hematoma is then resorbed or transformed into repair tissue, or both. The swelling subsides, and the surgical wound heals. After a few weeks, the haversian system starts remodeling the bone internally [34]. At the same time, gaps between imperfectly fitting fragment surfaces begin to fill with lamellar bone that is orientated along the gap plane. During the subsequent weeks, cutting cones reach the fracture and cross it wherever there is bone contact or the gap is minute [35], producing a multiple microbridging effect through newly formed osteons that cross the gap. Gap healing results from the development of granulation tissue in the small gaps which then matures into lamella and cortical bone. This process is not faster than contact healing and callus is not seen. The fracture gap will not widen unless there is a instability.

Indirect bone healing

Indirect bone healing requires granulation tissue and callus precursors, and is the normal mechanism of bone healing. As callus forms and matures the callus mass stiffens and fracture stability will improve. The callus increases the diameter of the bone at the fracture site and improves the mechanical leverage. This allows for effective bone healing which can be facilitated by splinting (eg, a simple cast).

Indirect bone healing is very similar to the process of embryological bone development and includes both intramembranous and endochondral ossification. In diaphyseal fractures, it is characterized by the formation of a callus [32], the healing process which can be divided into four stages: inflammation, soft callus, hard callus, and remodeling [36, 37].

- Inflammation starts soon after the fracture occurs and lasts until fibrous tissue, cartilage, or bone formation begins (1–7 days after fracture). Initially, a hematoma forms, along with inflammatory exudate from ruptured blood vessels. Accompanied by soft-tissue injury and platelet degranulation, released cytokines initiate the inflammatory response. The hematoma is gradually replaced by granulation tissue. Osteoclasts begin to remove necrotic bone at the fragment ends.
- Soft callus. Eventually, pain and swelling decrease and soft callus is formed, approximately 2–3 weeks after the fracture. The fragments are no longer able to move freely, and there is sufficient stability to prevent shortening, but not angulation. Progenitor cells from the periosteum and endosteum become osteoblasts. Intramembranous appositional bone growth, away from the fracture gap, starts to form a cuff of woven bone subperiosteally and endosteally. Ingrowth of blood vessels into the callus follows the pattern of bone growth. Closer to the fracture gap, mesenchymal progenitor cells proliferate and migrate through the callus, differentiating into fibroblasts or chondrocytes, each producing its characteristic extracellular matrix [38].
- Hard callus. When the fracture ends are linked together by soft callus, the hard callus develops until the fragments are firmly united by new bone (3–4 months). As intramembranous ossification continues at the periosteum, cartilage within the gap is converted into rigid calcified tissue by endochondral ossification. Bony callus growth begins in areas remote from the fracture that are mechanically idle, and slowly progresses toward the gap. The initial osseous bridge is formed externally or within the medullary canal away from the cortex. Then, through endochondral ossification, the soft tissue in the gap is converted.
- Mechanics of fracture callus. Fracture callus of mineralized cartilage occurs between bone ends and is called "gap callus"; along the medullary cavity (medullary callus) and on the outer cortex (periosteal callus). The importance of callus is to provide initial stability the fracture ends so that osteogenesis can occur. The stiffness generated must resist bending and torsional forces. This stiffness is minimal in the early phase and fracture immobilization or internal fixation is thus employed. If absolute stability is provided by implants, then there is no stimulation for the callus process, and healing is by "primary" intention, ie, gap callus healing. In this case, the consolidation process is essentially bypassed in the remodeling phase.

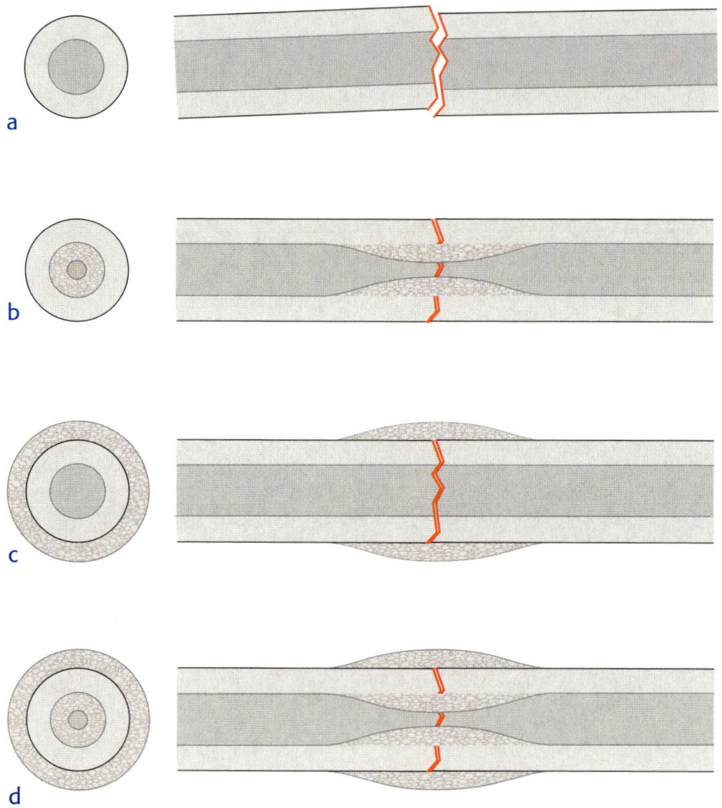

Fig 1-2a–d Callus formation in fractured bones provides resistance against bending forces. Abundant callus formation increases the resistance.

a Acute fracture.

b Medullary callus.

c Periosteal callus.

d Medullary and periosteal callus.

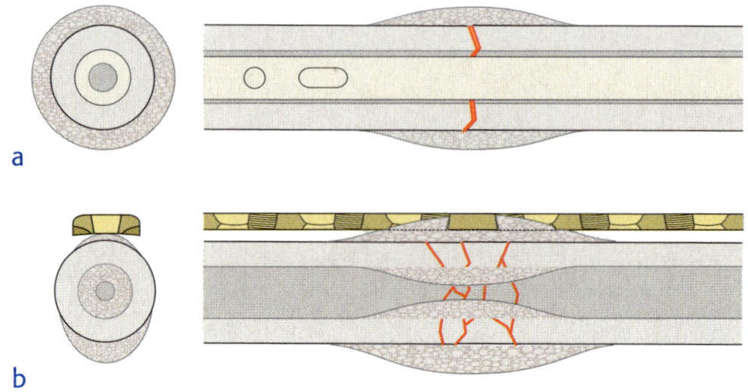

Fig 1-3a–b Callus formation with implants.

a The presence of the nail inhibits callus formation in the endosteum.

b Periosteal callus is formed on the side opposite to the plate. In case of a noncontact plate there is callus formation also beneath the plate.

In indirect fracture healing, the weakest callus is gap callus generated between well-reduced fracture ends. Medullary callus provides some resistance to bending moments. It is periosteal or extracortical callus that is most effective in providing bending forces, and bending and torsional resistance which is proportional to the 4th power of the radii of the bone cross-section through the callus mass. With intramedullary devices, one is able to see large extracortical callus, while medullary callus is minimal owing to the presence of the nail. With plate osteosynthesis, there is abundant medullary callus. Periosteal callus also forms on the side opposite to the plate, especially on the compression side of the bone (Fig 1-2; Fig 1-3).

- Remodeling. Remodeling starts once the fracture has solidly united with woven bone. Woven bone is then slowly replaced by lamellar bone through surface erosions and haversian remodeling. This process can take from a few months up to several years. It lasts until the bone has completely returned to its original morphology, including restoration of the medullary canal [39].
- Fracture healing in cancellous bone. In contrast to indirect healing in cortical bone, healing in cancellous bone occurs without the formation of a significant callus. After the inflammatory stage, bone formation is dominated by intramembranous ossification [33, 40]—probably due to the tremendous angiogenic potential of trabecular bone, as well as the often more stable fixation that is used for

metaphyseal fractures. In unusual cases with substantial interfragmentary motion, intermediary soft tissue may form in the gap, but this is usually fibrous tissue that is soon replaced by bone.

Secondary biological effects of implants

Foreign-body membrane. A foreign-body membrane builds up around any implant, depending on the material and its surface. After capsulectomy of the hip joint and total hip replacement, for example, a new capsule develops [41]. Stainless-steel implants trigger a stronger reaction than titanium. Experimental evidence suggests that absence of the membrane may be instrumental in providing protection against pathogens [42].

Remodeling. Simultaneous resorption and formation of cortical bone through haversian remodeling always occurs after any trauma to bone or in the vicinity of bone. The trauma can also be iatrogenic—eg, after internal fixation. The traces of such remodeling remain long after implantation, and probably for as long as the implant is present. Sequestration of bony islands may occasionally result from this excessive remodeling activity [43].

Role of the periosteal blood supply

Medullary blood supply is important to the diaphysis for bone healing; an intramedullary nailing disrupts this source. Periosteal blood flow alone cannot reach the endosteum and endosteal callus may be inhibited. Any bone necrosis that occurs as a consequence of the trauma is beyond the surgeon's control, but it is useful to understand its consequences. Iatrogenic bone necrosis is the result of the surgical approach to bone, the manipulations required to reduce the fracture, and any procedures preparatory to implant insertion and fixation—eg, medullary reaming, periosteal stripping, or endosteal perforation. Plate fixation preserves the medullary and metaphyseal vessels as well a periosteal vessels on the opposite side of the "footprint" caused by the plate.

Impairment of the blood supply to the periosteum at the plate–bone interface also causes porosity of the underlying bone. For this reason, the LCP and the LC-DCP have a trapezoidal cross-section and lateral undercuts that reduce the contact area and facilitate the removal.

The internal fixator (ie, noncontact plates) aims to preserve blood flow under the plate by minimizing contact with the bone. Much of the vascular supply to the callus area is derived from the surrounding soft tissue. Callus perfusion is of the utmost importance and may determine the outcome of healing. Bone can only form when supported by a vascular network, and cartilage will persist in the absence of sufficient perfusion. However, this angiogenic response is sensitive to both the method of treatment and the induced mechanical conditions.

- The vascular response appears to be greater after more flexible fixation, possibly due to larger amounts of osseous callus [2].
- Large tissue strains caused by instability reduce the blood supply, especially in the fracture gap [32].

Surgical handling and bone vitality

Vascular supply. The medullary blood vessels can be injured by drilling or screw insertion, or both. In stable conditions, the axial blood flow recovers rapidly [12, 44, 45]. Multiple screws crossing the medullary canal can affect the regional vascular pattern and cause abnormal remodeling of the endosteum. In addition, the presence of a number of aligned screws in a single cortex impairs the normal perfusion of the cortical bone. Monocortical screws only affect one cortex and possibly also the central medullary blood flow.

Thermal necrosis. It has been shown in vitro that drilling generates heat that is locally incompatible with vital biological structures [44]. In addition, repeated drilling can increase heat necrosis in bone. Drill bits have to be kept sharp and must be replaced if they become blunt; the same applies to self-drilling, self-tapping locking head screws. Irrigation and cooling during drilling procedures are important for minimizing of heat.

Local resistance to infection and necrosis

Another consideration is the implant material. Titanium is more biologically inert and vessels will grow right up to the plate edge. Stainless steel may be less effective as blood supply is reduced near the plate—a potentially avascular area for bacteria and a dead space allowing bacterial grows without defense.

Earlier research demonstrated the effect of stability on susceptibility to infection [46, 47]. Contact with the implant causes periosteal necrosis. Since necrosis impedes infection resistance, the bone–implant contact should be restricted [2, 12]. Infection can spread along an extended contiguous area of necrosis.

Local resistance to infection was studied experimentally using human pathogenic *Staphylococcus aureus* in simulated internal fixation in the rabbit tibia [35]. The study investigated the effect of the design, material, and application of the implant in relation to the number of colony-forming units required to produce an infection. The efficacy of dead space (slotted versus solid nail), the implant material (steel versus titanium versus degradable polymer), the application (reaming, approach) and the design of the implant in minimizing the occurrence of necrosis were evaluated. The overall difference in infection between the groups with an implanted steel DCP, with surface contact, and those with a titanium PC-Fix, with point contact, represented a ratio of 1:450.

Point contact alone therefore reduces the risk of large-scale necrosis. It may well be that the foreign-body effect, which was thought to reduce resistance to infection, is due less to the foreign material and more to tissue necrosis and dead space.

Refracture and necrosis-induced remodeling

What happens to the bone if implants create necrosis? The necrosis probably stimulates remodeling in the adjacent bone. The bone is remodeled as the necrotic bone is removed (the porotic stage) and is replaced by normal bone. This takes a minimum of three months and is usually complete by one to two years.

Necrosis immediately underneath an implant may also be related to refracture. Although necrotic bone is roughly similar in strength to living bone, the biological response elicited may weaken the bone [48]. Necrosis of the bone immediately underneath an implant will result in internal remodeling, resulting in porous and weakened bone that is susceptible to repeat fracture. This effect is even more harmful when, in the conventional technique, the plates are placed at the side of the bone, where functional loading produces tension. After removal of the plate, the local delay in healing caused by the avascular necrotic bone can act as a stress factor and result in repeat fracture due to traction induced by bending.

3 Mechanical aspects of plate and screw fixation

3.1 General considerations

One of the objectives of internal fixation is to restore bone integrity. The plate (implant) serves to bear the load from one fragment to the other, helping the bone carry out its mechanical function and temporarily taking on this function itself. Mechanically every plate works as a splint. Load transfer from the bone to the plate occurs by friction (in the case of plate fixation with cortex screws exerting pressure between plate and bone) and/or locking of the LHS in the thread of the plate hole by load transfer from bone through the locked screw head to the plate, to restore immediately the load-bearing capacity allowing functional postoperative treatment (in the case of the locked internal fixator) (Tab 1-7; Fig 1-4).

Tab 1-7 **Biomechanical aspects of plate and screw fixation**

Fixation method	Fracture configuration after reduction	Fixation technique	Screw type
Compression (static or dynamic)	Simple fracture type > full contact between the main fragments	Lag screw and protection plate	Cortex screw as lag screw; cortex screws [1] in neutral position or LHS [2] as plate screws
		Compression plate (and lag screw)	Cortex screws in eccentric position or axial compression with a tension device and cortex screws [1] in neutral position or LHS [2] as plate screws
		Tension band plate	Plate position important support vis-à-vis support is important, cortex screws in neutral position or LHS [2]
		Buttress plate	cortex screws [1] in neutral position or LHS [2] as plate screws
Splinting	Multifragmentary fracture > partial or no contact between the main fragments	Bridge plating or locked internal fixator	Cortex screws [1] in neutral position LHS [2]
	Simple fracture type (in exceptional cases) > full or partial contact between the main fragments	Bridge plating or locked internal fixator	Cortex screws [1] in neutral position as plate screws or LHS [2]

LHS = locking head screw(s).

Bone quality: [1] Normal, [2] Poor, also for technical reason: no primary loss of reduction, accurate shaping of the plate is not needed, MIPO easier.

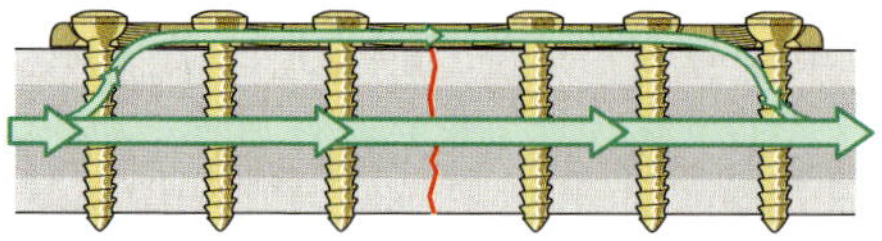

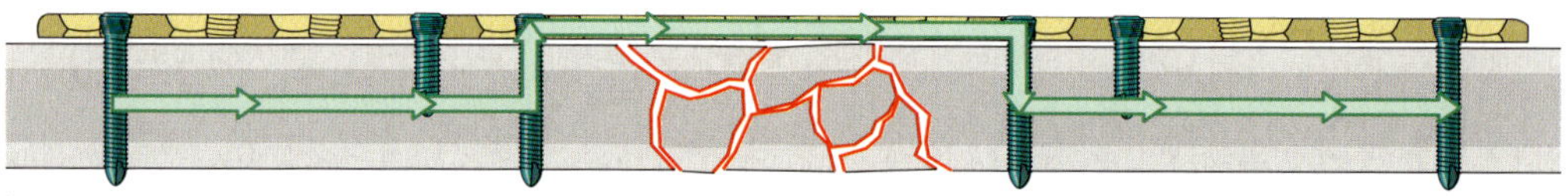

Fig 1-4a–b Load transfer from bone to splint.
a Plate and cortex screws (compression).
b Plate and locking head screws.

3.2 Plates and screws as compression tools

Conventional screws (compression screws) serve to compress a fracture (ie, interfragmentary compression) and/or fix the plate onto the bone to achieve friction between the implant and the bone and compression along the long axial axis of the bone. Cortex screws or cancellous bone screws can be used, depending on the type of bone in the anatomic region concerned. A screw applied as a lag screw crosses a fracture line and is used to create a compression force between the two bone fragments. The amount of compression that can be achieved depends on the diameter of the screw and on the bone density and mass (Fig 1-5).

The screws fix the plate to the bone. Tightening the screws presses the plate onto the surface of the bone, thus exerting a compression force. Stability of this kind of plate osteosynthesis depends on the amount of friction produced between the plate and the bone (Fig 1-4a). If the forces exerted on the bone (the load applied by the patient during movement) exceed the friction limit, relative shearing displacement will occur between the plate and the bone, causing a loss of reduction between the bone fragments or loosening of the screw, or both.

Fracture fragments cannot be compressed solely by attaching a plate with compression screws. If axial compression is the aim of the treatment, it is necessary to use a plate equipped with what are known as dynamic compression holes—a dynamic compression plate (DCP) or a limited-contact dynamic compression plate (LC-DCP). On the longitudinal axis of the plate, these dynamic compression holes have an oval shape and what is known as a dynamic compression unit (DCU) and the spherical gliding principle. The DCU is incorporated in DCP and LC-DCP. When the compression screws are inserted eccentrically into the end of the oval hole far from the fracture, the lower spherical part of the screw head meets the dynamic compression incline of the compression hole. Tightening the screw displaces the plate, and consequently the bone segment to be fixed, in the direction of the fracture. This displacement will continue until the screw head is fully inserted into the plate hole, thus pressing the plate firmly onto the bone and compressing the fracture site (Fig 1-6). Additional fracture compression can be applied by inserting a lag screw through the plate and across the fracture line

Anatomical reduction and a sufficient area of bone contact at the fracture site are prerequisites for compression plating; in addition, good quality of bone is necessary to allow the screw to press the plate toward the bone. If these prerequisites are met, absolute stability can be achieved in the fracture fixation. The benefit of absolutely stable fracture fixation is that the bone forms part of the construct. The function of the im-

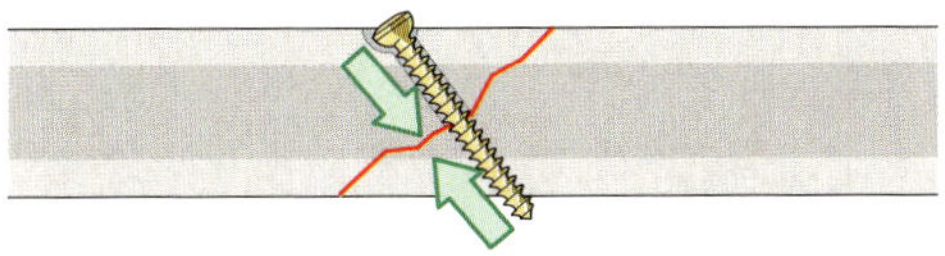

Fig 1-5 Lag screw effect using a fully threaded screw. Gliding hole in the near cortex, threaded hole in the far cortex.

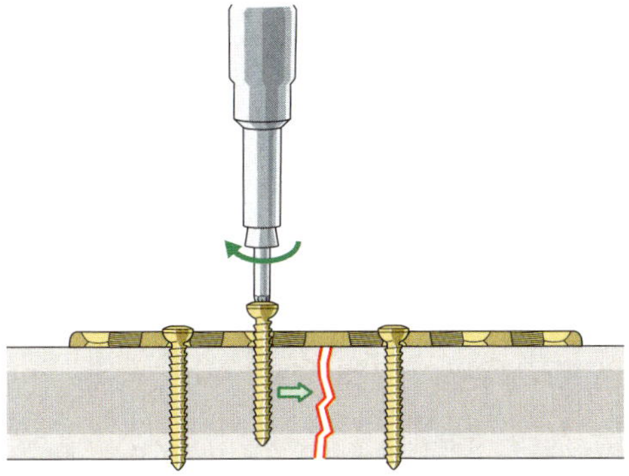

Fig 1-6 Interfragmentary compression with plating and eccentric seating of the screw (see also Fig 1-9; Fig 1-10).

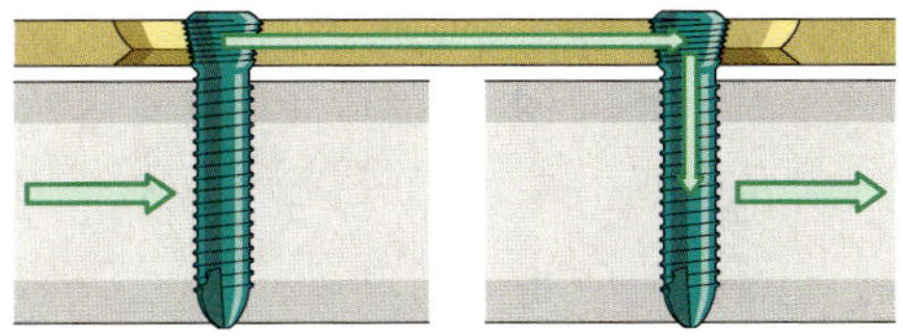

Fig | Animation 1-7 The load is transferred directly from one segment to the ather.

Animation 1-7

plant is to maintain the reduction between bone fragments while loads are transferred directly from one bone segment to another (Fig | Animation 1-7).

The disadvantage of compression plate fixation is that it requires anatomic fracture reduction. Depending on the fracture pattern and the anatomic region, it is often only possible to achieve precise reduction by extensive soft-tissue dissection under direct vision. This procedure can damage the blood supply to the fracture fragments, resulting in negative effects on fracture healing [2, 6]. In clinical practice, anatomical fracture reduction is only possible for simple fractures with a small number of fragments. Precise reduction in multifragmentary fractures is obsolete.

Another side effect of carrying out osteosynthesis using compression plates is the early bone porosis observed at the plate–bone interface [2]. A reduction in the bone mass can be seen in the early phases following fixation of compression plates. This is an effect of the pressure of the plate upon the bone, which damages the periosteum and thus disturbs vascularity and perfusion in the bone. Depending upon the severity of the injury, the vascularization of the bone may already be so restricted that additional extensive surgical trauma may reduce the potential for biological healing and increase the risk of delayed union or infection.

Different techniques for compression plating

The aim of applying plates that compress the fracture fragments is to achieve optimal approximation between the fragments. Levels of friction are developed that allow the bone to share the load. Compression cannot be seen and is difficult to produce and assess clinically. Approximation of and preload between the fragments result from the interaction between the plate and removable devices or plate screws. Strictly speaking, these should be termed "adaptation plates" rather than "compression plates."

Removable tension and compression devices

These devices are anchored firmly to the bone above the proximal or below the distal margin of the plate and are aligned with the plate (Fig 1-8). The device is linked to the plate so that axial distraction and precise fragment reduction can be achieved with the tensioning device in distraction mode. In compression mode, the fragments can again be brought into contact with each other to achieve interfragmentary compression.

Application of these devices generally requires a more extensive surgical approach. On the other hand, they make it possible to close larger fracture gaps or osteotomies. These devices can also be used for careful and controlled indirect reduction of impacted fractures [7] or to open up wedge osteotomies.

Dynamic compression plates

Dynamic compression plates compress bone by using the edge of the plate hole to cam the screw sideways during the insertion and tightening procedure (Fig 1-9). Variable slopes have been engineered to optimize this displacement effect. The dynamic compression unit (DCU) is put to the hole from the DCP, LC-DCP, and LCP. The screw is seated at the upper end of the inclined surface of the plate hole (and is therefore referred to as an "eccentric screw"), leading to various degrees of preloading of the plate in tension. This type of screw is also known as a "plate-tensioning screw," and the effect is known as "compression by the plate" [49].

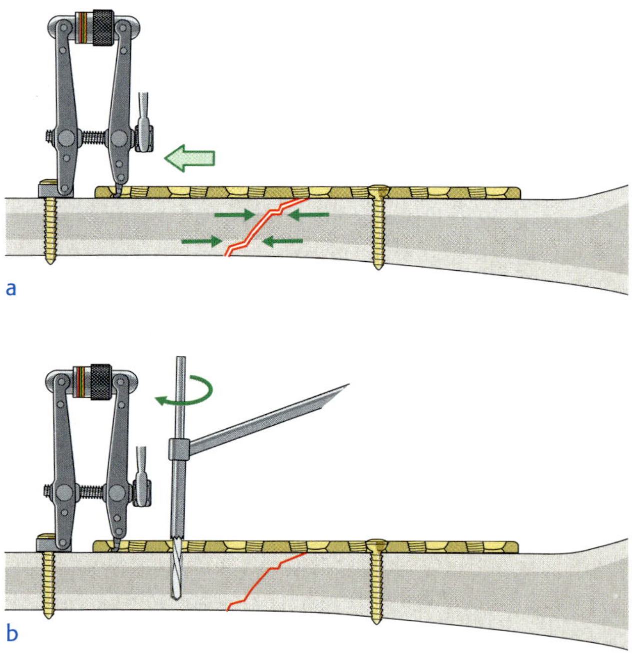

Fig 1-8a–b In oblique fractures, the articulating tension device has to be applied in such a way that the loose fragments lock into the corner formed by the opposite fracture surface and the plate if compression is produced.

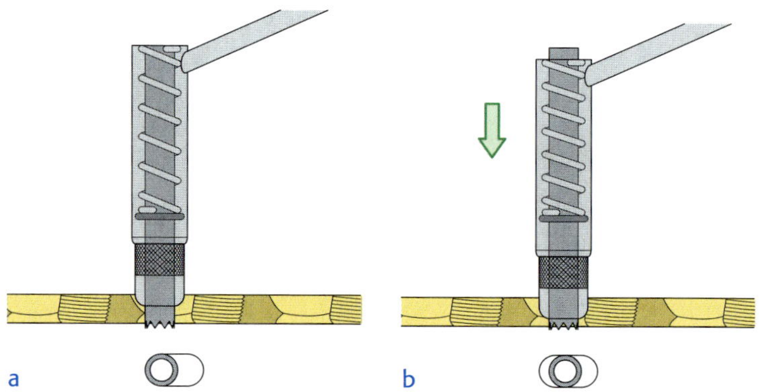

Fig 1-9a–b Application of the universal drill guide.
a Eccentric position.
b Neutral position.

Compression based on the elastic recoil of the plate

For optimal fitting, plates can be contoured to fit the surface of the bone. This is a prerequisite for conventional compression plating technique. To achieve compression on both cortices, a straight plate can be bent so that it arches across the fracture site and has no contact with the bone surface in that region. When tension is applied, the overbent plate is straightened again, leading to compression of the opposite cortex and thereby enhancing stability. Special instruments are available for prebending and contouring plates. However, it should be noted that a certain lack of overall control limits the efficacy and reliability of this procedure in clinical practice (Fig 1-10).

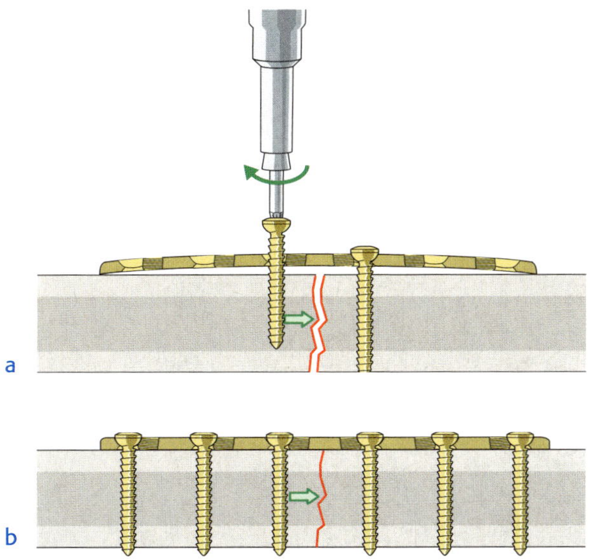

Fig 1-10a–b If the plate is slightly prebent before being applied, compression on both cortices can be achieved.

Axial compression by tensioning the plate (tension band principle)

In a few locations on the skeleton, the long bones are exposed to more or less constant asymmetrical functional loading. Plates or wires that work according to the tension band principle and carry tensile force will ensure that the bone can optimally resist compressive loading. Cortical bone itself is able to bear a considerable amount of static compression loading without harm. The plate does not need to be rigid and can be very thin (Fig 1-11).

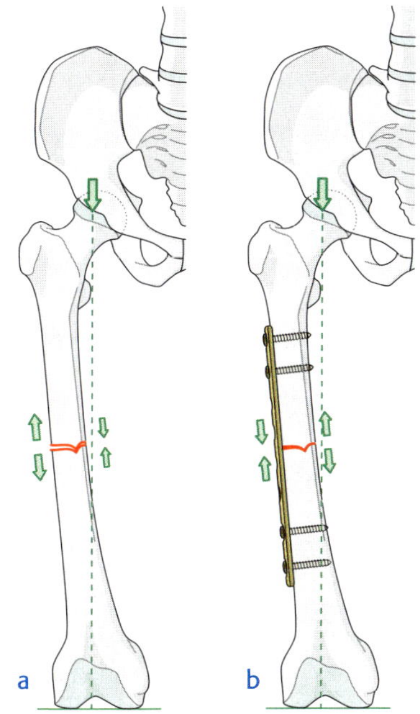

Fig 1-11a–b When applied to the tension side of the bone, a plate acts as a dynamic tension band.

- a With vertical pressure, the curved femur creates a tension force laterally and a compression force medially.
- b A plate positioned on the side of the tensile force neutralizes it at the fracture site, provided there is a cortical contact opposite to the plate.

3.3 The plate as a splint

Bridging plate fixation (DCP, LC-DCP, LCP with cortex and cancellous bone screws)

Treatment using long plates to bridge the fracture zone is known as bridging-plate osteosynthesis (Fig 1-12). In contrast to internal fixation after precise reduction with a compression plate, the bone does not contribute to the mechanical stabilization of the fracture, or only contributes to it partially. The bridging plate fixation reduces but do not abolish displacement between fracture fragments so pain is reduced and active muscle rehabilitation is practical. Whenever possible, the soft-tissue envelope in the fracture zone is left untouched intraoperatively. As mentioned above, the underlying principle here is that lower stability after fracture fixation (some movement at the fracture site, elastic fixation—principle of relative stability) will be more than adequately compensated for by the preservation of the soft tissues and the blood supply. At the same time, micromotion in the fracture zone promotes indirect healing through callus formation [32].

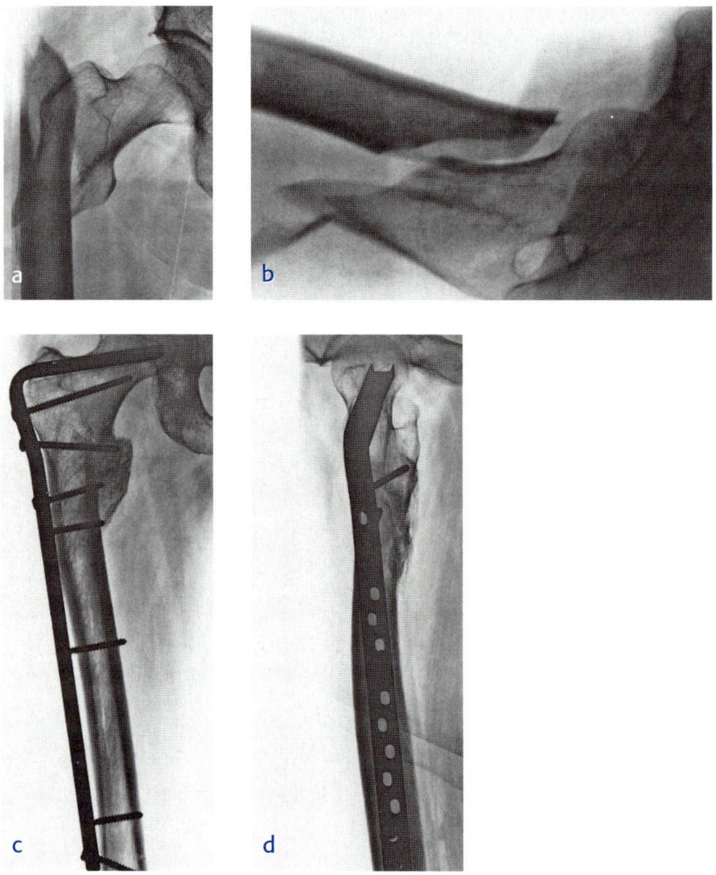

Fig 1-12a–d Biological internal fixation.
- a Preoperative AP x-ray of the injury.
- b Preoperative axial x-ray of the injury.
- c AP x-ray 6 months postoperatively.
- d Axial x-ray 6 months postoperatively.

Splinting with a conventional plate and screws—bridge plating: The spint/plate is fixed to each main fragment of the bone with compression screws, the shape of the plate has to be adapted to the bone so that the plate fixation screws can press the plate onto the surface of the bone of each main fragment. If the shape of the plate and bone do not match, the primary reduction/alignment of the fracture will be lost. Also the periosteal blood supply is disturbed. A disadvantage of bridging fixation at the metaphysis is that screw retention is poor in the cancellous bone in this area, particularly in elderly people with osteoporosis. This becomes apparent intraoperatively if screws are over tightened even slightly, and is also seen postoperatively in the form of screw loosening, with a resulting secondary loss of reduction.

Locked internal fixators (LISS, LCP) with locking head screws

The implant consists of a plate-like device and locking head screws which together act as an internal fixator (Fig 1-4b; Fig | Animation 1-13). An internal fixator is a construct where the screws (bolts, pins), which are the main load-transferring elements, are locked in the plate (or frame). The forces are transferred from the bone to the fixator across the screw necks. No compression of the plate onto the bone is required to achieve stability. Therefore the blood supply of the bone under the plate is preserved since no (or only little) contact between the plate and the bone is needed (noncontact plate).

The locking head screws of the internal fixator are actually more like threaded bolts. The bolts maintains the relative position between the body of the fixator (ie, plate) and the bone. Locking head screws are screws that are locked into a special plate hole during tightening. This gives the screw axial and angular stability relative to the plate (which serves as an internal fixator) [50]. Fracture fixation using a locked internal fixator does not depend significantly on the quality of the bone or the anatomical region of anchorage. In contrast to the compression screw, this screw–plate construct does not require friction between the plate and the bone to achieve stable fixation of the plate to the bone. The screw head is designed to lock into the plate hole, and it is therefore not necessary for the plate to be adapted precisely to the shape of the bone. The position of the plate relative to the bone remains unchanged during tightening of the locking head screws. When this locked internal fixator (LIF) construct has to bear the patient's weight, the force is transferred from one bone segment to another via the plate–screw construct. Unlike compression screws, locking head screws are more subject to bending loads than to tensile ones (Fig | Animation 1-13). Locking head screws are angular and axially stable and only radially preloaded [51].

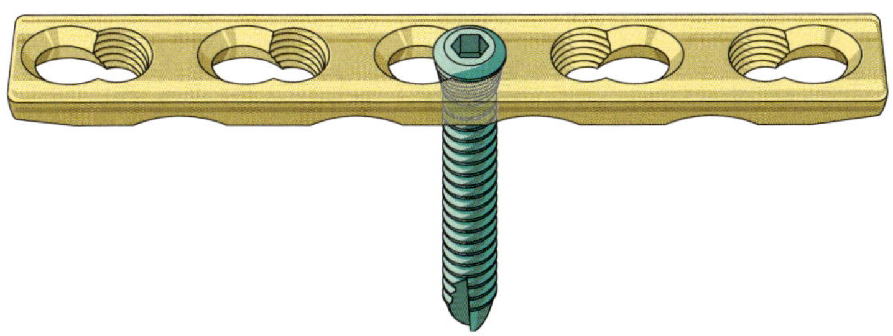

Animation 1-13

Fig | Animation 1-13 Plates (internal fixators) with locking head screws.

Optimized plate anchorage with divergent or convergent locking head screws

The benefits of locking head screws with angular stability are comparable with those of other implants that demonstrate angular stability, such as angled-blade plates. These advantages prevent the component that is anchored into the bone (the blade or screw) from toggling relative to the longitudinal carrier (the plate), thereby avoiding the loss of fracture reduction (Fig 1-14).

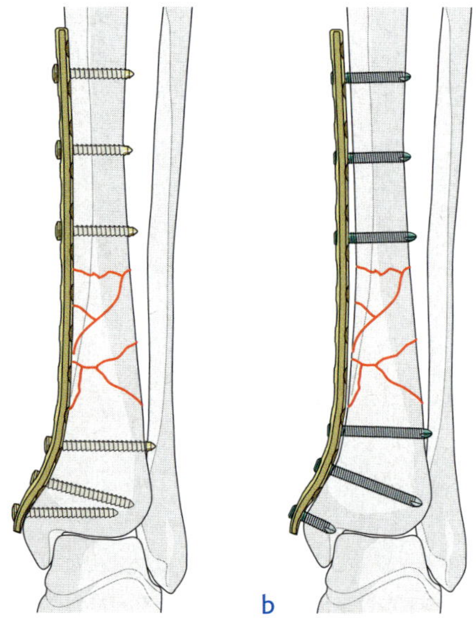

Fig 1-14a–b

a Bridging the fracture zone with a long plate. The bridging plate is only fixed to the main fragments proximally and distally. Fixation with conventional screws presses the plate against the bone, and the shape of the plate has to be adapted to the bone.

b Locked internal fixator: LHS are angular and axial stable. No compression of the plate onto the bone is required to achieve stabilitiy.

The plate hole is threaded to mate with the screw thread and ensure a locking connection, but this does not increase the purely axial pull-out resistance of the locking head screws. If the maximum pull-out resistance is exceeded, the screw will tear out a bone cylinder the size of the screw diameter (Video 1-1). When locking head screws are inserted into a bone segment at divergent angles to one another, their combined pull-out force can be increased several times. Unlike diverging compression screws, locking head screws cannot align themselves in parallel under traction and therefore create a larger area of resistance. The design of the LISS plate and the anatomically preshaped LCPs shows screw holes in divergent angles.

Video 1-1

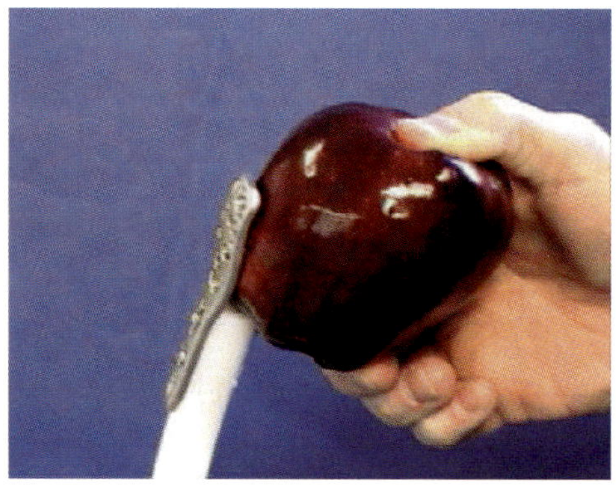

Video 1-1 Pull-out resistance demonstrated in an apple model.

Locking head screws and plate as a single, intrinsically stable construct

Unlike conventional plate and compression screw systems, plates secured with locking head screws function as a fixation unit. The construct works as a "mono block fixation". Compression screws can loosen independently of one another, often resulting in sequential screw loosening. Locking head screws are anchored into both the plate and the bone creating a single fixation construct that is extremely stable and performs well in porotic bone (Fig 1-15).

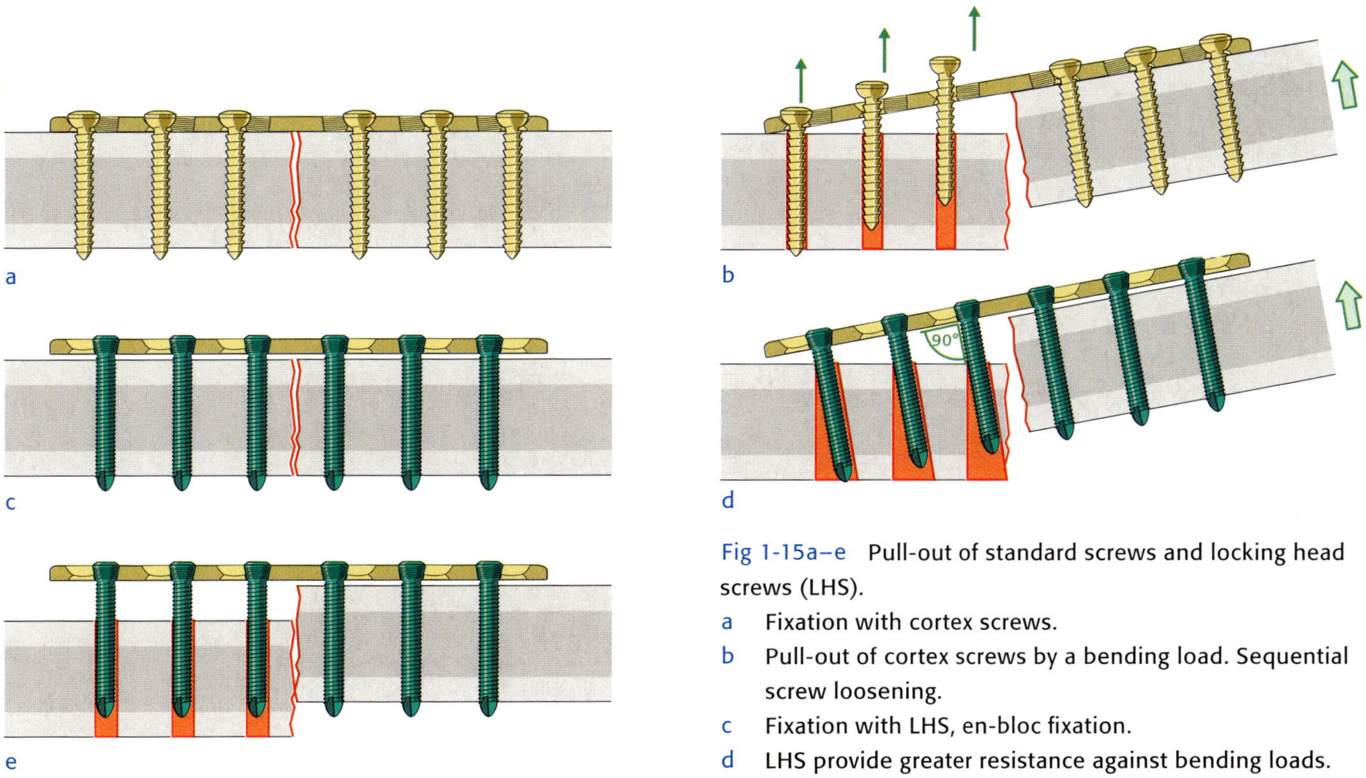

Fig 1-15a–e Pull-out of standard screws and locking head screws (LHS).

- a Fixation with cortex screws.
- b Pull-out of cortex screws by a bending load. Sequential screw loosening.
- c Fixation with LHS, en-bloc fixation.
- d LHS provide greater resistance against bending loads.
- e Pull-out of LHS with axial loading

Requirements for flexible fixation

Elastic flexible fixation can only be achieved without interfragmentary compression. A splint is a rigid structure that reduces, but does not eliminate elastic displacement of fragments during loading. The effect of the size of the implant on its structural bending rigidity is important. A practical way of achieving flexibility is to reduce the size of the metal implant. A combination of a more compliant metal such as titanium and a thinner implant is usually preferred.

The optimal conditions for splinting depend on the length of the lever provided by the plate on each side of the fracture site. For bones such as the femur and tibia that are exposed to large bending forces, long plates with a small number of screws should be considered. The number of plate screws is far less important than their position within the plate. The placement of screws at each end of the plate ensures that the full plate length will contribute to the fracture fixation. The distance between the two screws closest to the fracture in each fragment (the working length) determines the elasticity of the fracture fixation and, more importantly for the implant, also determines the distribution of the induced deformation when load is applied to the construct. If the induced implant deformation is expressed as closure and reopening of the fracture gap over a distance limited by bone abutment (ie, distance controlled deformation), then a greater distance between the two screws on either side and closest to the fracture line will offer a more uniform load transference and will reduce the risk of plastic deformation in what would otherwise be an overstressed, short plate segment.

Clinical experience has shown that an elastic bridge with three unoccupied screw holes spanning the fracture line helps distribute the induced stress over an adequate plate length.

In cases in which the deformation is not limited by the size of the fracture gap—for example, in highly multifragmentary and extensive fracture patterns in which bone abutment will not occur under loading (ie, load controlled deformation)—the maximal elastic deformation of the splint has to be reduced by adjusting the number and pattern (ie, position) of screw insertions, by applying a plaster cast, limiting weight bearing, or other appropriate means (eg, additional temporary external fixator).

Since torsional strength is mainly restricted by the number of screws, fractures of the humerus and radius which are exposed to large torsional forces should be stabilized with a plate that has a large number of screws on either side of the fracture zone. Additional screws placed between the two most peripheral screws and the two screws closest to the fracture will increase the anchorage of the plate in the bone, even in porotic bone.

4 Development of internal fixators

The concept of the locked internal fixator is a technology that takes care of the preservation of biology. It aims at simple and safe handling, at optimizing biological conditions for soft and hard tissues, and at being universally applicable. The device used resembles a plate but functions like a fixator that is fully implanted. The procedure supports biological internal fixation, that is a type of internal fixation giving priority to biology over mechanics [52]. As experience was gained with submuscular and subcutaneous plate fixation, it became clear that the surgeon required improved implants and instruments for the procedure.

4.1 History of internal fixators

Development and rationale behind locked internal fixators (LIFs)

The Zespol system (Fig 1-17), the first plate which functioned as a fixator for stabilizing long bones, was developed in the 1970s in Poland [53]. Toward the end of the 1980s, AO started to examine internal fixator systems as a further development of their plates. Another comparable device is the so-called "Schuhli" designed by Jeffrey Mast. Here the main body linking locked screws consists of a standard internal fixation plate. Its screws are held in a rigid position using a washer on the side of the plate facing the bone. This has two effects: one, the screws are locked; two, the plate body is elevated from the bone surface. The key to these internal fixators is the locking mechanism of the screw in the implant, which provides angular stability. This technical detail means that there is no need to induce compression forces at the bone surface to stabilize the bone–implant construct. The lack of compression improves fracture healing and the locking head screws obtain excellent anchorage even in osteoporotic bone. This turns a plate into an internal fixator. It functions mechanically as an external fixator, but is implanted below the skin (Fig | Animation 1-16). This method of internal extramedullary locked splinting, which reduces mobility at the fracture site but does not eliminate it, is designed to keep the bone fragments vital.

The clinical success of this type of treatment was astonishing: indirect healing resulted in early and reliable solid union. At the same time, the severity of complications declined, as there was a shift away from biological complications after compression plate osteosynthesis, due to necrosis with sequestration of bone and soft tissues, toward rare complications resulting from inadequate mechanical stability [6, 27].

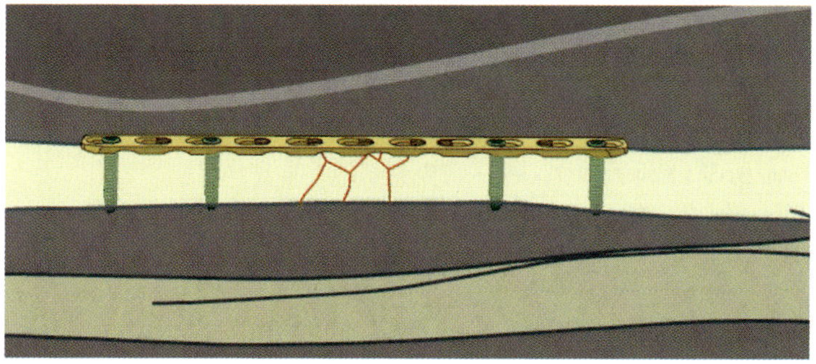

Animation 1-16

Fig | Animation 1-16 From the external fixator to the internal fixator.

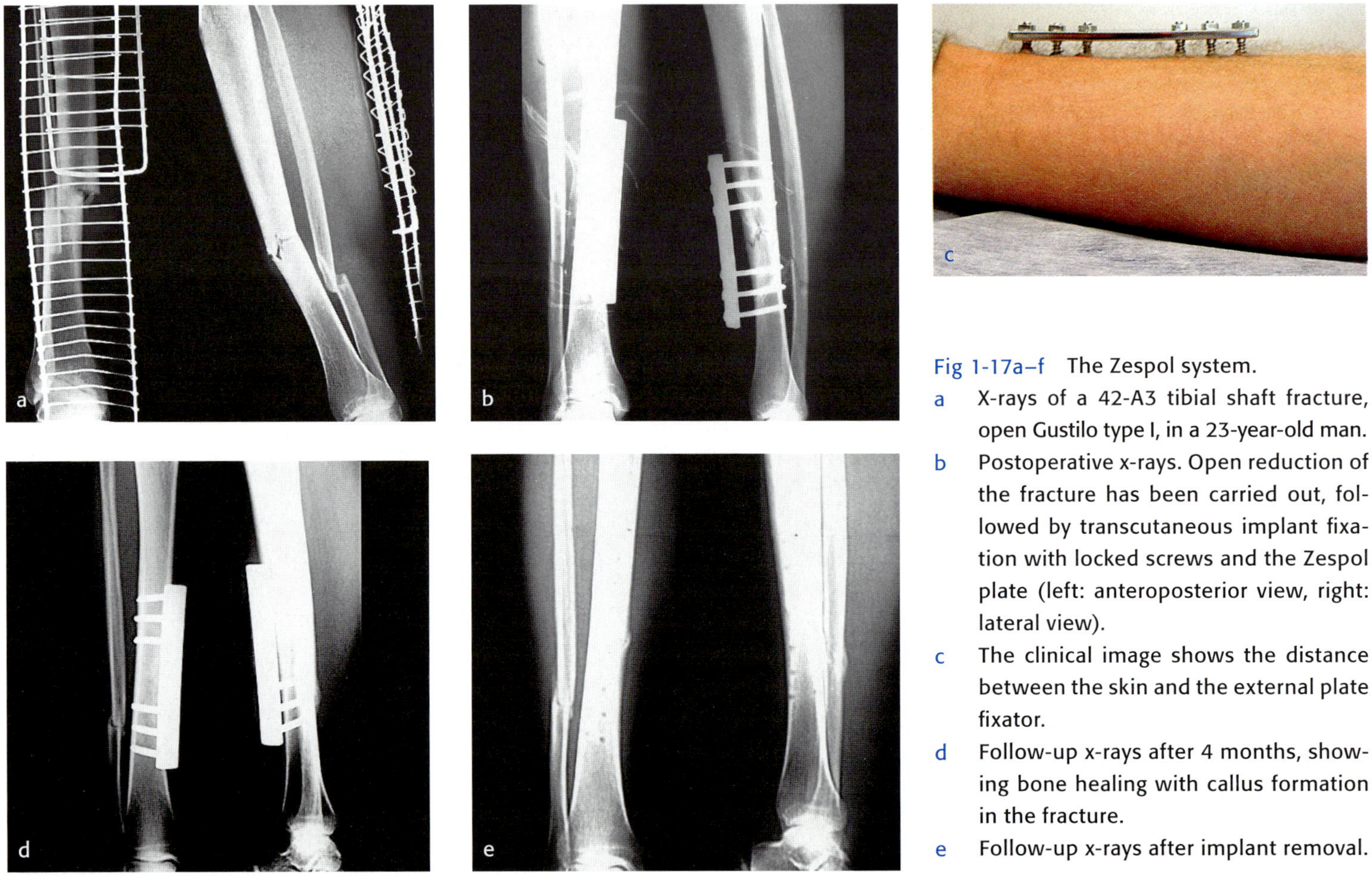

Fig 1-17a–f The Zespol system.

- a X-rays of a 42-A3 tibial shaft fracture, open Gustilo type I, in a 23-year-old man.
- b Postoperative x-rays. Open reduction of the fracture has been carried out, followed by transcutaneous implant fixation with locked screws and the Zespol plate (left: anteroposterior view, right: lateral view).
- c The clinical image shows the distance between the skin and the external plate fixator.
- d Follow-up x-rays after 4 months, showing bone healing with callus formation in the fracture.
- e Follow-up x-rays after implant removal.

The point contact fixator (PC-Fix)

The point contact fixator (PC-Fix) was developed in a joint venture by the AO Research Institute (ARI) and the AO Development Institute (ADI). This implant has minimal contact with the bone and is secured by monocortically inserted screws. The tapered head of the screw ensures that it lodges firmly in the plate hole and provides the required angular stability. Minimal contact between the plate and the bone is still necessary to ensure axial stability. Like the limited-contact dynamic compression plate (LC-DCP), the PC-Fix was shown to disrupt the underlying blood supply significantly less than the dynamic compression plate [54] (Fig 1-18). The monocortical screws appear to damage the endosteal blood supply less than conventional bicortical screws.

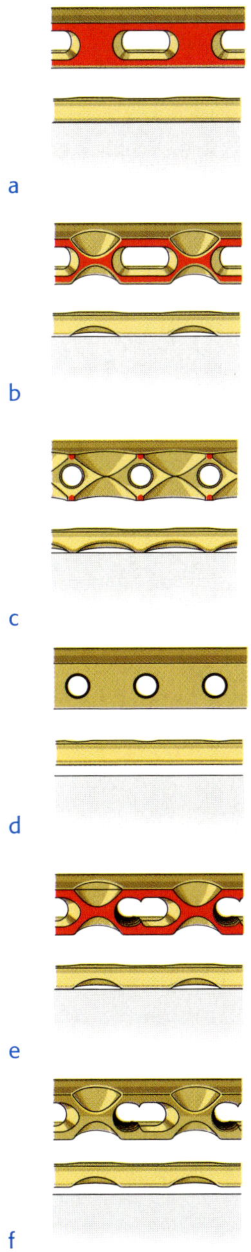

Fig 1-18a–f The undersurfaces of the plates. The area in contact with bone is shown in red.

a DCP
b LC-DCP
c PC-Fix
d LISS (noncontact plate)
e LCP with cortex screws
f LCP with locking head screws (noncontact plate)

Healing was accelerated with the PC-Fix, so that it was possible to remove it after only 3 months. Local infection resistance was improved—750 times more *Staphylococcus aureus* were required to produce the same incidence of infection with the PC-Fix as with a dynamic compression plate [55, 56]. These advantages were partly due to minimal implant contact and partly due to the switch from stainless steel to titanium.

The PC-Fix became the parent technology for the less invasive stabilization system (LISS) [57] and the locking compression plate (LCP) [58], with the latter implant providing both technologies in a more familiar plate design than that of the PC-Fix internal fixator.

From PC-Fix to LISS and LCP

The point contact fixator (PC-Fix) was the first type of plate fixator in which angular stability was achieved by establishing a conical connection between the screw heads and screw holes. However, the tapered screw–plate connection does not provide axial anchorage of the screw into the plate, so that point contact between the plate and the bone is still required to achieve stability. A new type of thread connection between the screw head and screw hole, resulting in angular and axial stability, was therefore developed so that no contact at all is required for stability. The screw simply functions as a Schanz screw.

4.2 Locking head screws (LHS)

Development of the LHS

Angular stable implants and especially angular stable non-contact plates are called locked internal fixators (LIF). Their distinguishing mechanical feature lies mainly in the fact that stability is not achieved by friction between the undersurface of the plate and the bone, with all the associated disadvantages, but rather by connecting elements between the extramedullary load carrier and the main fragments of the bone. The stable connection of the pins, blades or bolts/screws to the load carrier facilitates the mechanical bridging of the fracture zone without creating friction between the load carrier and the bone. This mechanical concept is similar to external fixator.

The figures (Fig 1-19) show that a locking head screw is subjected mainly to bending forces and shearing stresses that occur at the neck of the screw. Since the physiological loading of the bone runs perpendicular to the screw axis, the screw design had to be adapted to the new mechanical conditions. For this reason, a symmetrical thread with a coarser thread pitch, a 0.5 mm larger outer diameter and a 1.3 mm larger core diameter was chosen. These modifications have the following mechanical advantages. Increasing the projection area by 40% permits the distribution of the application forces to a larger bone area. This has definite advantages, especially for areas of cancellous bone in the vicinity of the joint. Due to the larger core diameter the screw tolerates 100% more shear stress and 200% more bending, whereby the incidence of screw failure is clearly reduced (Fig 1-20a).

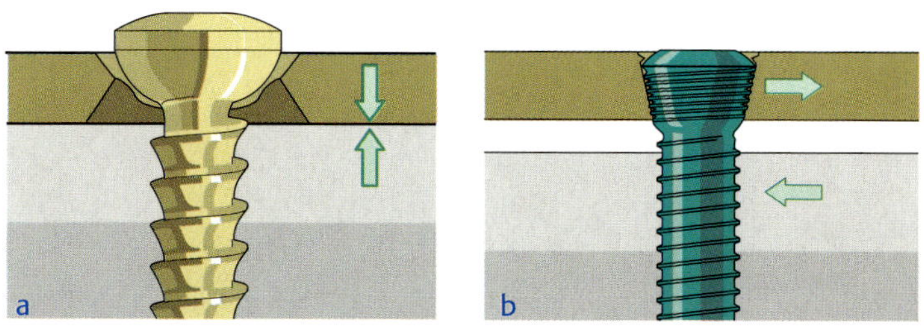

Fig 1-19a–b

a Force distribution of a plate osteosynthesis without angular stability: The screw tightening moment leads to surface pressure between the plate and bone. The friction thus created in the plate–bone contact zone stabilizes the bone fragment in relation to the load carrier. This system only becomes statically secure after bicortical screw fixation

b Typical distribution of forces for a LIF osteosynthesis with angular stability: This configuration is statically secure with only monocortical fixation since the locking head screw (LHS) is anchored in a mechanically stable manner in the load carrier

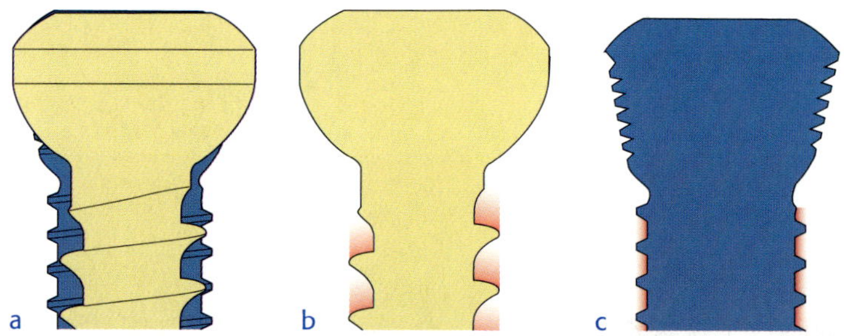

Fig 1-20a–c

a Schematic representation of both types of thread. The shaded area indicates the larger projection area.

b Surface pressure between the thread flanks and the bone (red zone) results from the axial preload arising from the insertion torque of the screw.

c Radial preload occurs when the pilot hole is smaller than the core diameter of the screw. Surface pressure in this case occurs between the screw core and the bone (red zone).

A further modification relates to the so-called preload of the screw. There is differentiation between axial and radial preload (Fig 1-20b–c).

If a conventional cortex or cancellous bone screw is inserted into the bone and tightened, axial preload of the threads to the bone will be achieved. This procedure prevents the micromovements that can lead to bone resorption and, consequently, to screw loosening. Since locking head screws are tightened not in the bone but in the plate, no axial preload will occur within the bone. The locking head screws cannot be overtightened even in poor bone structures. Nevertheless, a so-called press-fit technique, as used for pin-type connections, is applied to prevent harmful micromovements (Fig 1-21).

Further investigations have shown, however, that application in screw-bone connections can only succeed if predrilling is done very precisely as thc amount of misfit should not exceed 2% due to the elongation at yield of cortical bone. The additional request from the clinicians for a self-drilling screw came at just the right time in the development schedule. It is in fact possible to achieve radial preload in a one-step technique using a self-drilling screw. Since the success of a fixed-angle stabilization concept depends very much on the connection to the bone, a great deal of detailed work went into the development of the screws. For instance, the connecting element to the bone does not just have to be self-drilling, have a symmetrical thread, and be capable of radial preload, but drilling performance and temperature change during insertion are also of great importance for the quality of the bone–screw interface. As a result, a special test that could measure the relevant parameters was designed for the development of the screw geometry (Tab 1-8, Tab 1-9).

Optical evaluation of the bone thread also showed that the interplay between drill and thread cutting geometry is of great importance for the quality of the thread. Screws with a coarser thread pitch and a sharper drill tip perform particularly well in bone regions with a very thick cortex.

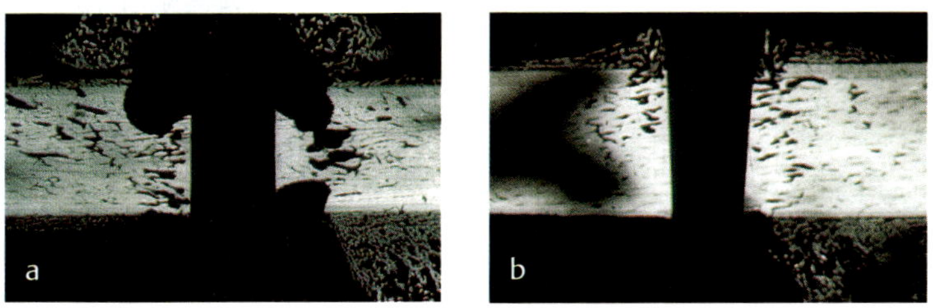

Fig 1-21a–b
a Microradiograph after insertion of a smooth pin without preload. Extensive bone resorption after 6 weeks.
b Microradiograph after insertion of a smooth pin with 0.1 mm radial preload. Minimal bone resorption after 6 weeks.

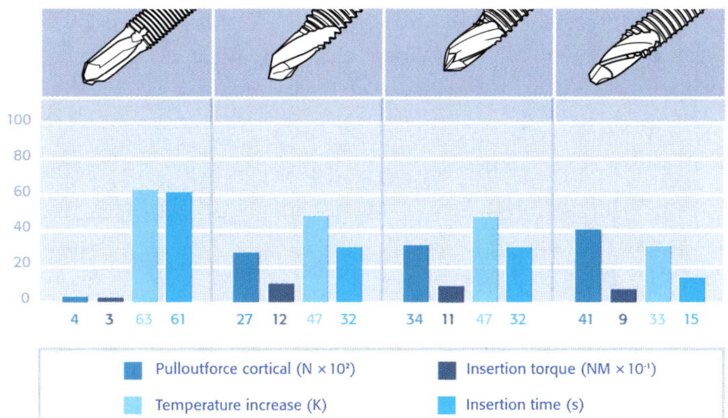

Tab 1-8 Development stages of the LHS: The drilling performance and pull-out force can be increased and temperature increase could be reduced by gradual modification of the geometry of the drill and the thread.

Video 1-3

Video 1-4

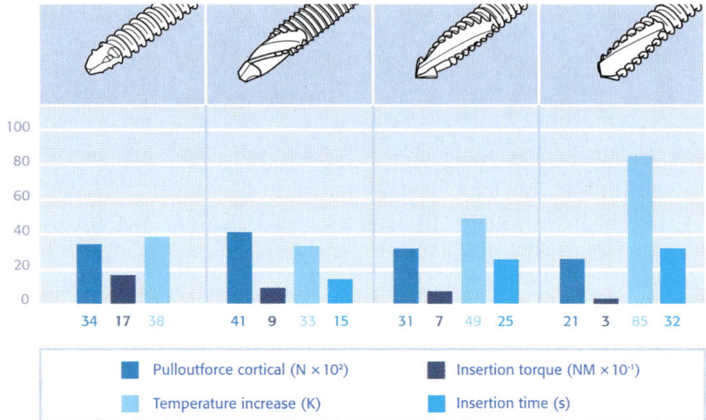

Tab 1-9 **Final comparative testing against existing screws showed the clear superiority of the new screw geometry.**

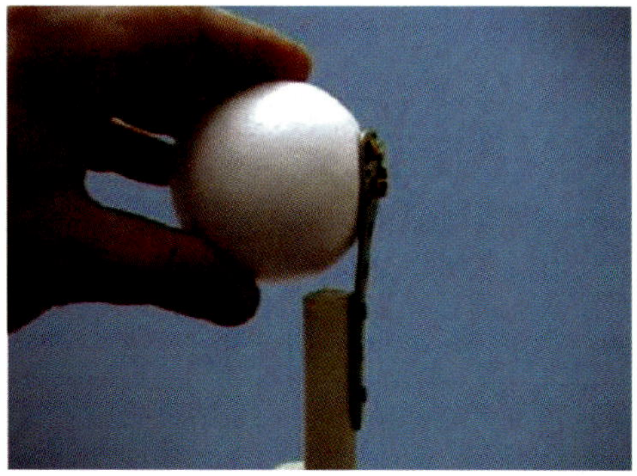

Video 1-3, Video 1-4 **Standard plate pull-out, LCP pull-out.**

In mechanical testing it was not only proven that the newly developed self-drilling, locking head screw with an optimized drill tip offered superior performance at the bone–screw interface when compared with conventional self-drilling screws but, in biomechanical testing, it was also shown that the symmetrical thread performed optimally in both cortical and cancellous bone. The results of comparative testing of a 5 mm screw with AO thread and an LHS with symmetrical flat thread on pairs of human femora clearly showed that the higher thread flanks for the same outer diameter of the screw did not lead to higher axial pull-out values. However, the superiority remains apparent due to the larger projection area and for situations of physiological loading perpendicular to the screw axis.

All tests only refer to a single screw. The advantages of angular stability become far clearer for a system comprising several screws in a plate. In a plate–screw configuration with nonlocking screws, conventional screws are stand-alone screws, sequential loosening of the screws occurs when force is applied. The lack of angular stability permits each screw to align along the axis of force. This leads to gradual loosening with pullout of the individual screws. In the case of fixed-angle application, en bloc fixation is achieved. The LHS can no longer be regarded as a stand-alone screw and the fixed-angle connection between the plate and the screw head prevents screw orientation along the axis of force. Pull-out can only occur en bloc (Video 1-4).

The effect of en-bloc fixation can be reinforced by convergent or divergent positioning of the screws, an approach applied chiefly in metaphyseal areas. Several screws inserted in convergent or divergent positions and in fixed-angle technique achieve such a high level of stability that failure can only be due to pullout of the entire system or to plate failure.

Major advantages of the LHS

Locked screws provide better anchorage both in elastic bridging fixation and in absolutely stable fixation, thus offering important advantages in the treatment of fractures in osteoporotic bone. The improved stability achieved by locking facilitates the dependable application of monocortical screws in the region of the diaphysis. The blood supply to the medullary cavity is preserved. No structural bone loss of the opposite cortex. In terms of application technique, monocortical screws are of particular advantage in blind, minimally invasive percutaneous osteosynthesis (MIPO). "Bicortical" (ie, as long as possible) locking screws offer improved stability in the epiphyseal and metaphyseal regions of the bone.

Advantages of angular stable plate systems

Anchorage of the screw in the plate hole means that the bone thread can no longer be stripped during insertion. The primary anchorage of the screw in the bone is therefore ensured even in poor quality bone.

Compression between plate and bone is unnecessary (noncontact plate). For this reason, the periosteal blood supply under the plate remains intact so that cortical bone necrosis, as described in connection with conventional plates, will not occur. This may contribute to the lower susceptibility to infection that has been observed in relation to application of an internal fixator.

The fixed-angle connection between the screw and the plate clearly offers improved long-term stability when bending and torsional forces are applied. LHS are also axially stable. It is scarcely possible for the plate to pull out of the bone because the screws cannot be sequentially loaded or pulled out due to tilting in the plate hole. Likewise, there is little opportunity for secondary tilting of a short joint block since this is effectively prevented by the fixed-angle anchorage of the screw in the plate (no secondary loss of reduction).

Since the bone is not "pulled towards" the plate during tightening of the screws, the procedure for minimally invasive plate osteosynthesis (MIPO) is greatly facilitated. The plate no longer needs to be anatomically contoured, which would hardly be possible in a closed procedure (MIPO) since surgical exposure of the bone surfaces is not required for most of the relevant regions. If the shape of the plate does not exactly match the bone surface and conventional screws are chosen, the fracture fragments are restored to their correct spatial alignment by the process of screw tightening. This effect is desirable if persistent axial deformity needs to be corrected by reduction to the plate. The effect is undesirable if there is any risk that the fragments will dislocate during tightening of standard screws because the plate has been poorly contoured. In this case, loss of reduction can be avoided by the insertion of locking head, fixed-angle screws.

Intraoperative contouring of the plate is not necessary for the application to specific bone regions of anatomically preformed plate systems with locking head screws. This in turn facilitates minimally invasive application and is also an advantage in all open procedures.

The development of the LISS for the distal femur and the proximal tibia (1995 and 1997, respectively) created the first generation of preformed fixed-angle systems. Integrated into these systems is an attachable aiming device that facilitates the insertion of the screws along the entire length of the plate, whereby self-drilling, self-tapping locking head screws can be inserted percutaneously in a single step via stab incisions. Since the development of the LCP (2000) additional preformed systems for the proximal and distal humerus, the distal radius, the proximal and distal femur, as well as for the proximal and distal tibia have been developed and are consistently proving their value in clinical application.

4.3 The less invasive stabilization system (LISS)

The different steps in the development of plating techniques is the less invasive stabilization system (LISS); the techniques and procedures involved are described in detail in chapter 3. The less invasive stabilization system (LISS) for the management of distal femoral fractures and proximal tibial fractures makes it possible to use a minimally invasive surgical technique, applying the principle of fracture fixation with relative stability.

The LISS for the distal femur (LISS-DF) and the proximal lateral tibia (LISS-PLT) are implants that act as splints. The LISS acts mechanically as an internal fixator (Fig 1-22)—it is a 100% locked internal fixator, because only locking head screws (LHS) are used. The LISS is designed for percutaneous insertion. A less invasive approach is also possible. A closed, indirect reduction and a pure splinting of the fracture zone is important. Internal fracture fixation with locked fixators is a new technology in which the aim is to preserve biological conditions.

The LISS approach is based on using anatomically shaped buttress plates that are anchored with self-drilling and self-tapping monocortical locking head screws. The screws are connected to the plate by a thread on the outer surface of the screw head and a mating thread on the inner surface of the plate hole. The angular stability between the screws and the plate no longer requires any compression between the plate and the bone to ensure secure anchorage. The LISS is a noncontact plate. Each self-drilling, self-tapping screw represents a new, sharp drill bit for drilling, a sharp tap to cut the thread, after which the screw follows into the precisely prepared hole. The monocortical, self-drilling screws lock into the plate and fasten the proximal and distal main fragments after indirect reduction has been carried out. Due to the locking design, the LHS used do not need to obtain purchase in the second cortex and can easily be inserted percutaneously and by self-drilling. This produces a better bone–plate construct as compared to the use of standard screws. The stability of the bone–implant construct results from the angular stability of the plate–screw interface rather than from the friction generated between the plate and bone, as with conventional implants. This has mechanical advantages and avoids problems related to the bone–implant interface, such as the "windshield-wiper" effect.

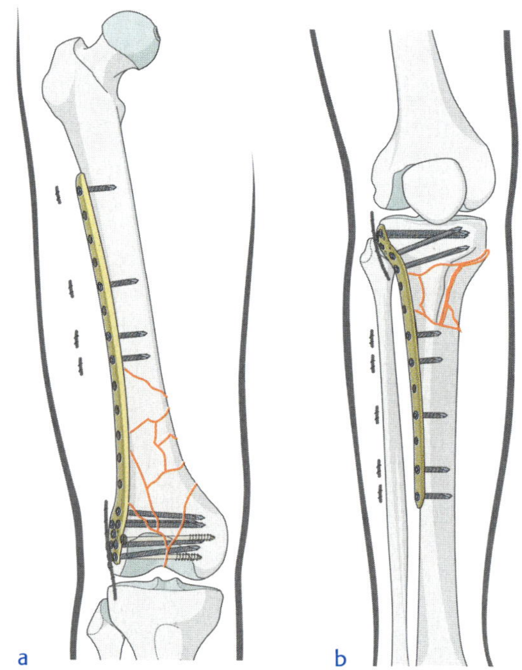

Fig 1-22a–b The less invasive stabilization system.
a LISS-DF.
b LISS-PLT.

The LISS is an anatomically preshaped internal fixator that can be inserted percutaneously by means of an adaptable insertion guide. In combination with a trocar assembly, the handle also serves as an aiming instrument for exact percutaneous placement of the self-drilling, self-tapping LHS. Based on extensive anatomical studies, the orientation of the individual screws is predetermined and cannot be changed. The reason for this is the angular stable screw–plate connection that is achieved with the outer thread of the screw head and the inner thread of the plate hole; this does not allow variable orientation of the screw.

The LISS-DF and LISS-PLT procedures described in the present manual have been in clinical use since 1997. Several studies and a large number of articles have been published on the procedures since then, reporting both the biomechanical and clinical advantages. The published data show that LISS is a valuable treatment option for fractures of the distal femur [26, 59–74] and the proximal tibia [60–74].

4.4 The locking compression plate (LCP)

The LISS was originally designed as a device that would provide angular stability and would only accommodate locking head screws; all of the plate holes are threaded. However, clinicians found that this technology was too restrictive in some cases and that an all-purpose implant system would offer greater flexibility. Research and development work in this area—with multidisciplinary collaboration among clinicians, researchers, developers, and manufacturers—ultimately led to the concept of a combination hole, which has been incorporated into the most recent type of plate, the locking compression plate—LCP.

As experience with internal fixator developed, the need arose for a single plate system that would allow the surgeon more choices [75]. Preoperatively or intraoperatively, the surgeon could choose whether or not to use conventional screws, locking head screws, or a combination of the two screw types. This led to the development of the locking compression plate (LCP), featuring combination holes (described in detail in chapter 3).

The combination hole

The LCP combination hole (Fig 1-23) allows internal fixation to be achieved by inserting either conventional screws (into the unthreaded part of the hole) or locking head screws with angular stability (into the threaded part of the figure-of-eight hole). The LHS can only be inserted at right angles to the plate. The LCP hole also makes it possible to insert different screw types into the same plate, so that the surgeon is able to choose the type depending on intraoperative requirements. In retrospect, combining two completely different anchorage techniques into a single implant was a logical approach and a straightforward, practical solution.

Two versions of the LCP with combination hole are available: a 4.5/5.0 large-fragment version, a 3.5 small-fragment and a 2.4 and 2.0 version. Special plates are also available for many anatomical regions, . These LCP is anatomically preshaped to fit the average shape of specific bones and can be inserted using open or minimally invasive techniques.

Despite the advantages of locked internal fixators, there is still a need for the anatomical reconstruction and absolute stability that are provided by conventional plates and screws. Appropriate indications for the latter include intraarticular fractures, osteotomies, complex bone reconstruction procedures, pseudarthroses, as well as fractures with traumatic damage to the blood supply. With the LCP, the surgeon has two plating methods to choose from and is able to select the more appropriate of the two techniques.

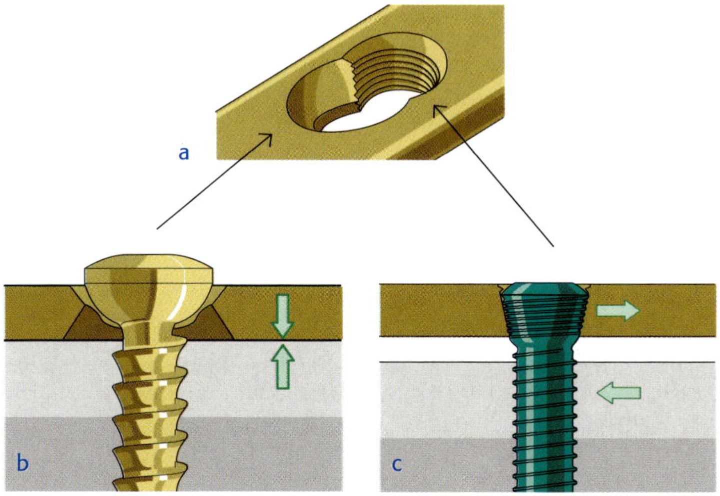

Fig 1-23a–c **Locking compression plate with combination hole.**

a **LCP combination hole combining two proven elements.**

b **One half of the hole has the design of the DC/LC-DCP (dynamic compression unit: DCU) for conventional screws.**

c **The other half is conical and threaded to accept the matching thread of the locking head screw providing angular stability.**

The option of using the LCP, either as a compression plate or as an internal fixator, provides ideal plate anchorage that can be adapted to requirements in each individual case. This significantly extends the range of indications in minimally invasive plate osteosynthesis.

Using the LCP, the surgeon is free to select the best treatment method—ie, either the compression method or locked splinting method—to bridge the fracture zone in the individual patient. Plate length and the type, amount, and position of screws used dictate the fracture fixation method and technique and have to be chosen according to the fracture situation (Tab 1-4). The LCP is in accordance with the latest plating techniques (MIPO), the aim of which is to achieve the smallest possible surgical incisions, to preserve the blood supply to the bone and adjacent soft tissues, and to ensure a minimal bone–implant interface [52].

5 Methods and techniques in plate osteosynthesis

5.1 Plate osteosynthesis today and future developments

Plates and screws are versatile implants for different methods and techniques of fracture fixation. Potentially, all types of fracture could be fixed with plates and screws. In general, fracture fixation with plates and screws produces satisfactory results. An understanding of the forces involved makes it possible to aim for low-strain osteosynthesis. Complications are usually related to surgical technique and there is a risk of damage to bone and soft tissue. This is usually associated with an increased risk of infection, nonunion, or implant failure. Thermal necrosis at the drill holes is often underestimated.

There are still good indications for the conventional plating technique: articular fractures (with buttress plating) and simple diaphyseal and metaphyseal fractures (compression or protection plating). Anatomical reduction of the fracture has always been the goal in the conventional plating technique, but, over time, the technique of bridging plate osteosynthesis was developed for multifragmentary shaft fractures—a technique that, by reducing vascular damage in the bone, allows healing with callus formation, as seen after locked nailing. Since the damage to the soft tissues and the blood supply is less extensive, faster fracture healing can be achieved.

The more recent locked internal fixators involving LISS and LCP using LHS consist of plate and screw systems in which the screws are locked into the plate. The locking process minimizes the compressive forces exerted on the bone by the plate. This method of screw–plate fixation means that the plate does not have to touch the bone at all, which is particularly advantageous for minimally invasive plate osteosynthesis (MIPO). With these new screws, precise anatomical contouring of a plate is no longer necessary and the plate does not have to be pressed onto the bone to achieve stability. This prevents intraoperatively primary displacement of the fracture caused by inexact contouring of a plate. The LISS plates are preshaped to match the average anatomical form of the relevant site and do not require further intraoperative alteration. The basic locked internal fixator technique aims to achieve flexible elastic fixation to stimulate spontaneous healing, including the induction of callus formation.

It is now accepted that the pursuit of absolute stability, which was originally thought to be necessary for almost all fractures, is mandatory only for joints and certain joint-related fractures (ie, fractures of the radius and ulna), and then only when it can be achieved without damage to the blood supply and soft tissues. At the diaphysis, length, alignment, and rotation must always be respected. When fixation is required, splinting by nail insertion or application of an internal fixator is usually preferable and leads to union by callus formation. Even when the clinical situation favors the use of a plate, proper planning and the current techniques for minimal access and fixation will reduce the degree of insult to the blood supply to the bone fragments and soft tissues.

Simple diaphyseal fractures and multifragmentary, more complex fractures react differently to conventional compression plating and to splinting by nailing or bridging with a locked internal fixator. If compression plating is used in simple fractures, absolute stability must be achieved. In contrast, splinting can be used to treat all multifragmentary fractures. A diaphyseal fracture in the forearm, where long bone morphology is combined with quasiarticular functions, requires special consideration. Intraarticular fractures require anatomical reduction and absolute stability to facilitate the healing of articular cartilage and make early motion possible, which is essential for good ultimate function.

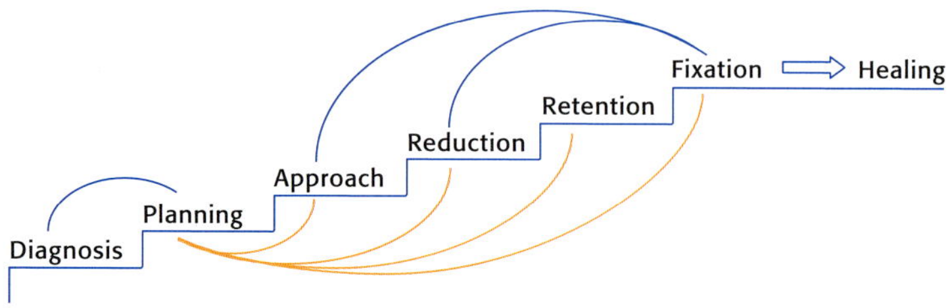

Fig 1-24 **Correlation and interaction between the steps of surgery.**

The imperatives of soft-tissue care, originally expressed in the principle of preserving the blood supply to the bone, need to be addressed in every phase of fracture management. A clear understanding of the roles of direct and indirect reduction, together with informed assessment of how the fracture pattern and soft-tissue injuries relate to each other, will lead to adequate preoperative planning and correct decisions on treatment strategy and technique (Fig 1-24).

Future developments

To obtain the greatest benefits from the principles of biological internal fixation and minimally invasive plate osteosynthesis (MIPO), simple methods are needed to allow reduction of the metaphyseal end fragments. As in locked nailing, biological internal fixation only requires reduction of the main fragments in which the articular surfaces are present. The required method would allow reduction and temporary maintenance of the main fragments in the correct three-dimensional position in relation to bending, torsion, and length. This would make MIPO simple. These aims may be within the reach of simple mechanical methods on computer-aided technology.

A method of assessing the viability of the bone before, or at least during, surgery would also be helpful for selecting the method of stabilization and improving the prognosis. It is difficult to judge whether bone is viable. It is important to know this, as a combination of necrotic bone and elastic fixation can cause problems. Internal fixators are at a disadvantage here since indirect bone healing is not possible. Further studies are needed on the precise threshold conditions for strain in relation to amplitude and timing.

Stabilizing fractures in patients with osteoporosis is a priority, and fracture implants that allow loading to be monitored in vivo would be helpful. The threshold conditions for flexible fixation—ie, the limits of strain in clinical conditions—need to be analyzed further.

In animal studies, the technique of internal fixation with point contact fixators has been shown to reduce the incidence of infection and to facilitate early solid union **[56]**. The advantages of biological internal fixation are the simplicity of handling, the prompt contribution to healing made by the bone, and resistance to infection and possibly repeat fracture.

5.2 Compression method—conventional plating technique

The LCP is a versatile implant and can be used for both methods of fracture fixation—compression and splinting method and also in different techniques (Tab 1-15).

The compression method of fracture fixation, aiming for absolute stability, involves open reduction and internal fixation (ORIF) using plates and cortex and/or cancellous bone screws. This approach, the principles of which are outlined above, became established as a standard and successful technique for treating bone fractures (Fig 1-25). The success of the technique depends on the precision of the reduction and the degree of stabilization. Wide surgical exposure is necessary to achieve reduction, and soft tissues were often stripped from fracture fragments.

Different concepts of fracture fixation

Principle of fixation = grade of stabilization	Method			Technique and implant's function	Bone healing
Absolute stability = high	**Compression**			Lag screw (conventional screw)	**Direct**
		Static[1]		Lag screw and protection plate (DCP, LC-DCP, LCP)	
				Compression plate (DCP, LC-DCP, LCP)	
				Tension band	
		Dynamic[2]		Tension band plate (DCP, LC-DCP, LCP)	
				Buttress plate[6] (DCP, LC-DCP, LCP and conventional screw)	
	Splinting		External splinting	External fixator	
			Intramedullary splinting	Intramedullary nail	
		Locked[3]	Internal extramedullary splinting	Bridging with conventional plate (DCP, LC-DCP, LCP and conventional screw)	
				Bridging with locked internal fixator (LISS, LCP and LHS)	
			External splinting	Conservative fracture treatment (cast, traction)	
		Unlocked[4]	Intramedullary splinting[5]	Elastic nail	
Relative stability = low				K-wire	**Indirect**

Possible with LCP

[1] Fracture under compression—implant under tension.
[2] Compression under function.
[3] Locked splinting with control of length, alignment, and rotation.
[4] Splinting with limited control of length, alignment, and rotation.
[5] Can be changed to dynamic compression in case of a dynamically locked nail or dynamic external fixator.
[6] Using an angular stable plate-screw construct (ie, LISS or LCP with LHS) as buttress plate, the plate acts as a blade plate. Occasionally a buttress plate may be considered as a splint.

Tab 1-10 Different conceps of fracture fixation (possibilities for using LCP).

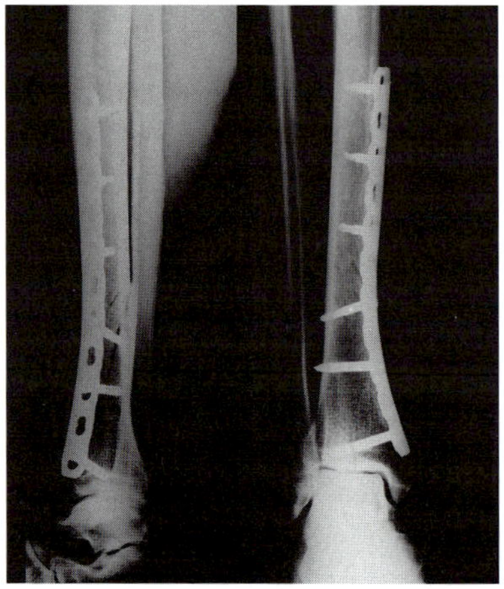

Fig 1-25 The conventional plating technique using the compression method.

Advantages

- Restoration of the precise anatomy and early function.
- Stable internal fixation—interfragmentary compression (lag screw and/or plates).
- Lag screw—the best technique to achieve interfragmentary compression.
- Angulation of screws.
- The reduced bone fragments shares the load.
- Early mobilization and early function.

Prerequisites

- Open (in the most cases), direct reduction to achieve precise alignement and full contact of the fragments.
- Extensive open surgical approach to the bone—for reduction, insertion, and fixation of the plate.
- Stable internal fixation, interfragmentary compression.
- No motion between the fracture fragments—absolute stability.
- Preshaping of the plate to match the anatomy of the bone.
- Pretensioning (overbending) of the compression plate in order to achieve stable fixation-elastic recoil of the plate.
- Bicortical insertion of the screws.
- Compression between the implant and the bone.
- Stability results from friction between the plate and the bone and/or a preloaded lag screw.
- Good bone quality (sufficient screw holding).

Shortcomings and disadvantages

- In multifragmentary shaft fractures, precise anatomical reduction is often not possible without a substantial risk of iatrogenic soft-tissue trauma.
- Compression of the periosteum disturbs the blood supply to the bone and leads to bone necrosis beneath the plate.
- Primary loss of reduction due to imprecise contouring of a plate leads to malalignment (ie, displacement of the fragments while fixing the plate with compression screws)
- Compression screws can be overtightened.
- Compression screws are preloaded.
- Secondary loss of reduction (loosening of screws) leads to malalignment and instability.
- Osteoporosis (insufficient screw holding).
- Repeat fractures tend to occur (due to necrotic bone under the plate and bicortical screw holes).

With experience, it became increasingly evident that there was a biological price to pay for precise reduction and absolutely stable fixation. Handling and even cleaning of the bone fragments before and during reduction was likely to result in dead bone that might only revascularize slowly and require long-term protection.

5.3 Splinting method

Splinting with standard plates and cortex screws

New methods involving minimal risk were therefore developed to accelerate bone regeneration and bone healing in difficult fractures. Whereas anatomical reduction of the fracture was the goal in the conventional plating technique, the aim in bridging plate osteosynthesis for multifragmentary shaft fractures is to reduce vascular damage to the bone. The use of indirect reduction, as advocated by Mast and colleagues [7], was intended to take advantage of the soft-tissue attachments, which align the bone fragments spontaneously when traction is applied to the main fragments.

Advantages

- Internal fixation with preservation of biological integrity.
- Closed indirect reduction.
- Minimization of biological damage due to the surgical approach and reduction technique, and by anchoring the implant only in the main fragments.
- Flexible (less stable) fixation that stimulates callus formation, facilitating early solid union.

Prerequisites

- Indirect closed reduction without exposure of the fracture.
- Smaller insertion and incisions only for the implant fixation.
- Elastic bridging of the fracture zone with a conventional plate and cortex screws.
- The use of long plates as pure splints—ie, without the additional lag screw effect.
- Fixation of long implants to the proximal and distal main fragments only.
- The plate has to be preshaped to the anatomy of the bone.
- In general, bicortical cortex screws are used to achieve sufficient friction between the plate and the bone in the proximal and distal main fragment.
- Relative stability (elastic fixation) promotes callus formation.
- The bone and soft tissue are still alive and/or can recover after the accident, transportation, and surgical approach.

Less experienced surgeons can also use this technique with an open, but less invasive approach. The fracture zone remains untouched.

Shortcomings and disadvantages

- Closed reduction and the intraoperative control of alignment are not easy.
- Minimally invasive plate application and fixation using a conventional plate is not easy.
- Standard screws inserted bicortically are used to achieve sufficient friction between the plate and the main fragments.
- The plate has to be accurately preshaped to the anatomy of the bone for the main fragments.

Locked splinting with locked internal fixators

The newly developed locked internal fixators used in the LISS and LCP are based on the principles of biological internal fixation and minimally invasive plate osteosynthesis (MIPO) (Fig 1-26). The MIPO approach and bridge plating is possible with conventional plates, but there are additional advantages if the MIPO technique is combined with the use of a locked internal fixator—there is no need for precise contouring of the plate, drilling, measuring, or tapping, because self-drilling, self-tapping monocortical LHS are used. These screws lend themselves optimally to monocortical fixation, in which case it is not necessary to select the length of the screw precisely and a protruding screw tip is not able to damage or irritate the soft tissues, tendons, or muscles.

Only small incisions are necessary to insert the plate with the MIPO technique—with benefits including not only improved

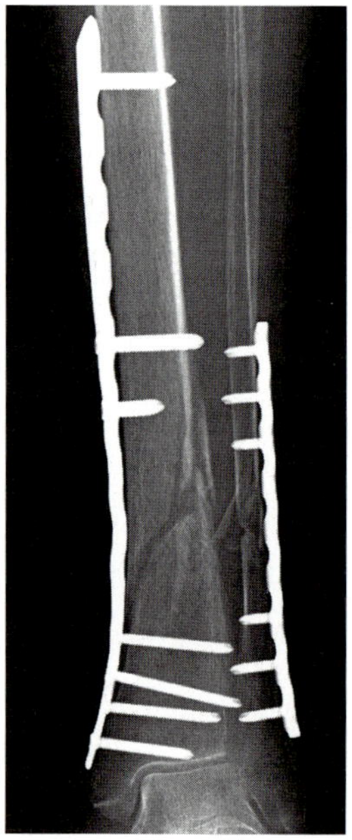

Fig 1-26 LCP as LIF using the splinting method.

cosmetic results, but above all protection of the fracture zone. "The skin protects the fracture zone from the surgeon." [Christoph Sommer].

The technology developed for the blind insertion and application of internal fixators can also be used with open approaches. The open approach, using an aiming device, can help the surgeon become accustomed to the more demanding technique of aligning the internal splint. The locked monocortical screws require alignment of the implant and the bone axis within comparatively narrow limits. Open procedures can be used for initial training in the techniques.

Also using LCP with LHS as locked internal fixator (locked splinting method) in the MIPO technique has many technical and biological advantages.

Advantages

- Biological internal fixation avoids the need for precise reduction, especially of the intermediate fragments, and takes advantage of indirect reduction.
- The aim of indirect reduction is to align the proximal and distal main fragments. This avoids exposure of the individual bone fragments.
- Submuscular/subcutaneous slide insertion techniques are possible.
- Minimization of biological damage caused by the surgical approach, the reduction, and at the implant–bone interface (MIPO). This is achieved at the expense of precise reduction and stable fixation.
- Flexible elastic fixation to stimulate spontaneous healing, including the induction of callus formation.
- Locked internal fixators are noncontact plates; no compression of the plate onto the bone is required.
- There is no need for shaping when using LISS or anatomically preshaped LCP.
- Optimal predefined screw placement and screw orientation based on anatomical studies, facilitates the application of anatomically preshaped LISS and LCP plates.
- There is no need for exact preshaping of the LCP to match the bone anatomy.
- There is no need for drilling, measuring, or tapping, since self-drilling, self-tapping monocortical LHS are used.
- Preservation of all blood supply to the bone including periosteal blood supply.
- Locking the screw into the plate ensures angular, as well as axial, stability and eliminates any unwanted movement of the screw.
- There is a reduced risk of secondary loss of reduction.
- The technique works well in osteoporotic bone.
- For treatment of multifragmentary, complex fractures.
- MIPO is easier using locked noncontact plates.
- There is improved local resistance to infection.
- Less risk of refracture

Prerequisites

- Indirect closed reduction without exposure of the fracture.
- Small incisions for insertion of the implants.
- Implants that have minimal bone contact (eg, LISS and LCP). The internal fixators are slightly raised above the bone surface to eliminate any mismatch between the preshaped implant and the anatomy of the bone.
- Elastic bridging of the fracture zone (principle of relative stability stimulates callus formation).
- Plates/fixators are used as pure splints—ie, without the additional lag screw effect.
- Self-drilling, self-tapping locking head screws can be used for monocortical insertion; self-tapping locking head screws can be used for monocortical or bicortical insertion.
- In LISS alone, a geometrical correlation has to be achieved between the aiming device and the plate for closed application.

Less experienced surgeons can also use this technique with an open, but less invasive approach. The fracture zone remains untouched.

Shortcomings and disadvantages

- The stability of the fracture fixation depends on the rigidity of the construct.
- Closed reduction and intraoperative control of alignment are not easy.
- Minimally invasive plate application and fixation are not easy.
- With the predetermined screw orientation, possible difficulties can arise when inserting a locking head screw in nonanatomically preshaped LCPs (penetration of articular surface).
- Reduction toward the plate can only be achieved with special instruments or bumps or standard screws.
- Excessive demands on the system: the bone is not carrying any load because it has not been precisely reduced.
- Delayed healing in the diaphyseal region when the medullary and/or periosteal blood supply to the interrupted bone fragments following the injury are deperiosted , and through iatrogenic additional disturbance of the blood supply to the bone and soft tissue, (wrong reduction and fixation).

6 Minimally invasive plate osteosynthesis (MIPO)

The timing and technique of intervention is crucial to respecting the important role of the soft tissue in bone healing. Minimally invasive surgery helps to reduce the iatrogenic trauma. Damage to tissue in the injury zone is the major factor for the occurrence of complications such as bone devitalization, infection, delayed union, and nonunion.

For minimally invasive surgery (MIS) in fracture care, the terms minimally invasive osteosynthesis (MIO) or minimally invasive plate osteosynthesis (MIPO) are used.

Minimally invasive osteosynthesis for joint fractures requires a soft-tissue window which is large enough to achieve a precise anatomical reduction. After anatomical reduction the principle of absolute stability is applied using the compression method.

Tab 1-11 **Definition of MIPO**

Definition of MIPO
Access to the bone through soft tissue windows (not only small skin incisions but also careful gentle handling of deep layers of the soft tissue).
Minimal trauma to the soft tissue and the bone by indirect reduction.
Minimal additional trauma at the fracture site when direct reduction is necessary.
Reduction tools which cause „small footprints".
Implants with adequate bone-implant interface: – Noncontact plates, angular stable screws, – Monocortical screw fixation – Optimized screw placement according to the anatomical region

MIPO for shaft fractures include indirect closed or percutaneous direct reduction and a soft-tissue window away from the fracture site, large enough for implant insertion and to see and to palpate the plate and the bone.

Reduction

Another principle of MIPO is to reduce the trauma to the soft tissue and to the bone by indirect reduction. For diaphyseal fractures the restoration of the length, axis, and rotation is needed. Small individual fracture fragments need not to be anatomically reduced. Only the correct position of the adjacent joints is important. For indirect reduction maneuvers the following equipment is used: manual traction, traction table, large distractor, external fixator, push–pull forceps.

Some times direct reduction maneuvers are necessary. When direct reduction is necessary use tools with "small foot prints" percutaneously, close to the fracture. The percutaneous use of a pointed reduction clamp, collinear reduction forceps or reduction handles/joysticks help to minimize the additional trauma at the fracture site.

Indications for direct percutaneous fracture reduction are simple articular fractures, simple metaphyseal and diaphyseal fractures.

Fixation

Multifragmentary fractures of the diaphyseal or metaphysical zone are fixed by the locked splinting method. The fracture zone is bridged with a locked internal fixator.

Simple fracture type of the shaft or metaphysis can be treated by the compression method. Reduction tools with small foot prints and locked noncontact plates to protect percutaneous lag screws help to reduce the iatrogenic trauma.

Alternatively simple shaft fractures can be fixed after reduction by the splinting method without lag screw.

Disadvantages of MIPO

- Difficulties in indirect closed reduction
- Increased C-arm exposure
- Malunion
- Pseudoarthrosis through diastases
- Delayed union with flexible fixation in simple fractures

Advantages of MIPO

- Faster bone healing
- Reduced infection rate, no or less need for bone graft
- Less postoperative pain (small incisions)
- Faster rehabilitation (less soft-tissue trauma)
- More aesthetic result

Benefits of minimally invasive techniques with locked plates

It was originally argued that the tunneling required to achieve blind insertion of the plate would result in the same amount of damage as with the open surgical approach. However, studies conducted by Krettek's group on the effect of ligating the perforating arteries, for example, during open surgical procedures for femoral fractures disproved this argument [76, 77]. Although MIPO techniques can be used with plates and compression screws, the advantages of the technique using locked splints and monocortical self-drilling screws are greater.

In surgical approaches involving access through contused areas of skin in which stability is required, the minimally invasive approach offers considerable advantages.

The mechanical benefits of these systems (ie, locked noncontact plates) are as follows. There is no need for precise anatomical preshaping of the plate—a procedure which is in any case hardly possible with blind minimally invasive techniques. LCP used as internal fixator with LHS are noncontact plates. This feature considerably facilitates the MIPO procedure. The preshaped plates supplied by the manufacturer are based on measurements of the average shape required, using computed-tomography data and cadaver bones. Since the plate does not need to be pressed onto the bone when it is being used as an internal fixator, minor variations in the bone will result in areas of plate stand-off from the bone. Anatomically preshaped LCP are available for certain metaphyseal areas (the proximal and distal humerus, olecranon, distal radius, distal femur, and proximal and distal tibia), and LISS devices are available for the treatment of fractures of the distal femur and the proximal lateral tibia. An additional advantage of the anatomically preshaped plates is that they make it possible to insert the screw in an appropriate direction to suit the anatomical conditions, allowing optimal anchorage. The guiding blocks help ensure the correct axial insertion of the drill sleeves and locking head screws. If required, standard screws can be inserted before the guiding block is positioned.

Anatomically preshaped plates
Strong demands for anatomically preshaped plates
Advantages for anatomically preshaped plates:
– No intraoperative shaping of the plate required – Plate helps achieving the anatomical reduction – Aiming blocks to insert the locking head screws – Clear indications for a given implant – Defined placement for a given implant – Clear rules of how to use the given implant – Optimized screw placement according to the anatomical region

Tab 1-12

Table 1-12 Advantages of anatomically preshaped plates.

With regard to application technique, monocortical screws are advantageous in the blind MIPO technique. If the surgeon is familiar with the insertion of self-drilling, selft-tapping screws, preparatory predrilling and measurement of screw length may not be necessary. The self-drilling, self-tapping and self-tapping locking head screws can be inserted initially using a power tool. Only the final fixation needs to be carried out with a torque screwdriver. Short monocortical locking head screws are used in the diaphysis.

The angular stability of the screw–plate system provides significantly improved long-term resistance to external bending and torsional forces. The plate is unlikely to pull out of the bone, as the screws are incapable of toggling, sliding, or becoming dislodged. The screw cannot be overtightened, as its thread mates with that of the plate hole. In addition, the angular and axial stability of the screws prevents secondary tilting of a short joint fragment (so that there is no secondary loss of reduction). The locking head screw will always gain purchase in the bone, even in cases of poor bone quality; divergent and convergent insertion of adjacent locking head screws provides better fixation in osteoporotic bone **[78–80]**. Examples are shown in Fig 1-27.

Locked internal fixators such as LISS and LCP with LHS also provide important biological benefits. The improved stability allows reliable application of monocortical screws in the diaphyseal area. Monocortical screws cause less interference with blood flow. Locking the screw into the plate ensures both angular and axial stability without compression of the plate onto the bone. The intramedullary circulation is conserved; and the far cortex and adjacent soft tissues are protected from damage, as has been confirmed by biomechanical investigations and reports of clinical outcomes. However, bicortical anchorage is recommended in situations with a thin cortex or osteoporotic bone, and in the treatment of humeral shaft frac-

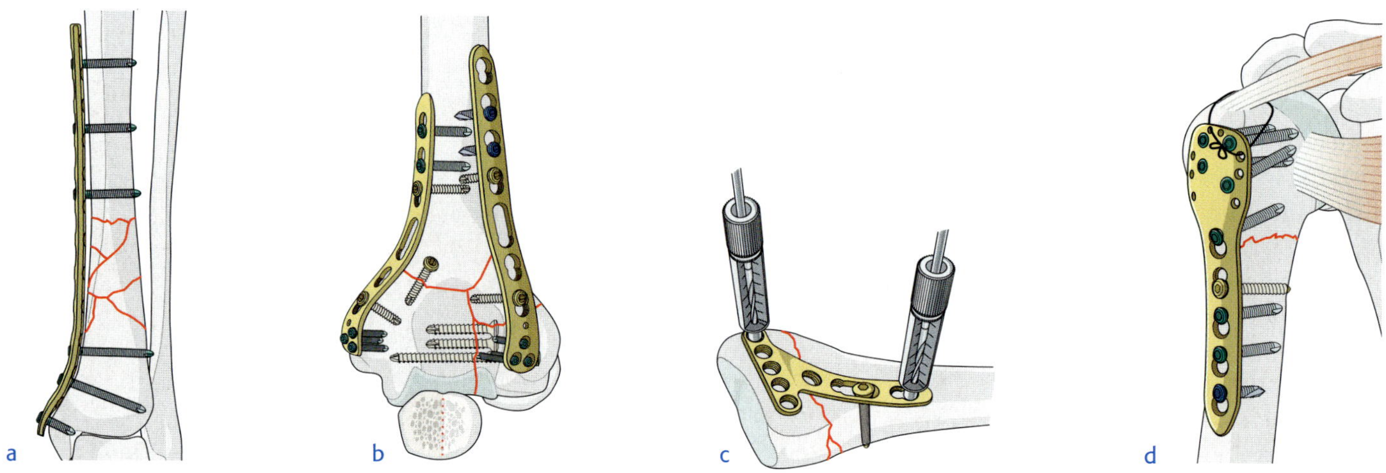

Fig 1-27a–d Examples of anatomically preshaped plates.

a LCP metaphyseal plate 3.5/4.5/5.0, for distal tibia.

b LCP distal humerus plate (DHP).

c LCP distal radius plate 2.4.

d Locking proximal humerus plate (LPHP).

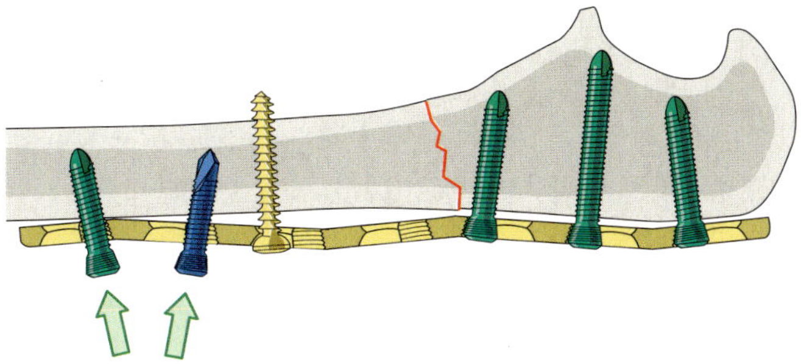

Fig 1-28 The pull-out resistance of the whole construct can be improved by bending the plate into a wave-like form, so that the screws can be inserted divergently and convergently.

tures (bones that are prone to high torsional forces). Bicortical anchorage is advantageous when fixation of a short main fragment allows the screws to be placed close to each other and for technical reasons in bones with a small diameter (ie, ulnar and radial shaft). The insertion of a bicortical LHS is recommended whenever a standard screw has been inserted intraoperatively into a combination hole for the purpose of temporary reduction. In situations with malalignment of the plate in the longitudinal axis of the bone, a monocortical screw will be insufficient to maintain the reduction, and a bicortical screw is therefore suggested. In the metaphysis, the use of the longest possible monocortical or bicortical locking head screws is recommended.

Internal fixators with few monocortically inserted LHS also demonstrate fewer repeat fractures after removal of the implant; the implants can be removed earlier due to rapid bone consolidation. Earlier plate removal due to rapid bone consolidation was showed in animal testing under controlled situation. In the clinical situation, time to bone consolidation is influenced by the initial and surgical trauma; and there are no changes to the bone structure under the plate.

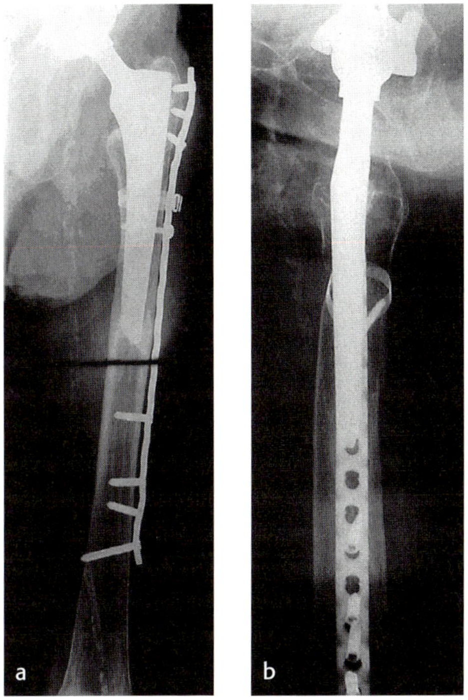

Fig 1-29a–b Treatment of a periprosthetic fracture with a 4.5/5.0 locking compression plate (LCP) and cerclage wire. There is wave-shaped prebending of the distal part of the plate to accommodate severe osteoporosis and prevent loosening of the plate. The locking head screws are inserted divergently and convergently into the waved part of the plate to improve screw anchorage.

Advantages

In summary, the new systems (ie, locked noncontact plates) offer clinicians the following advantages:

- The locked internal fixator is a stable system consisting of a plate and locked screws. The stability of the fracture fixation depends on the stiffness of the construct. There is no need to press the plate onto the bone, and the blood supply to the bone is preserved. Locking the screw into the plate to ensure angular as well as axial stability eliminates the possibility of intraoperative overtightening.
- The screw is incapable of toggling, sliding, or becoming dislodged, substantially reducing the risk of postoperative secondary loss of reduction.
- Fixation by placing multiple screws with angular stability in the epiphyseal and metaphyseal fragments make it possible to treat many fractures where therapy was not possible with previous fixation devices.
- There is improved stability in multifragmentary, complex fractures with loss of a medial/l ateral buttress or bone loss.
- The locked screw–plate interface provides angular stability, which avoids subsidence in the metaphyseal areas. It also allows medial or lateral fixation, usually without reconstructing the opposite medial or lateral buttress (without double plating), and without the use of a primary bone graft.
- There is no need to contour the plate precisely to the anatomy, which greatly facilitates the (MIPO) surgical procedure. Since stability does not rely on compression between the plate and the bone, the plate does not have to be anatomically contoured. This is especially true for the metaphyseal areas, in which the shape of the bone can be quite complex.
- There is no primary loss of reduction.
- The new systems offer an improved biological environment that promotes healing. Locked internal fixators do not compress the periosteal blood supply and consequently cause less interference with the fracture hematoma and fracture healing. The elastic fixation of a locked internal fixator acts more like an intramedullary nail or external fixator, allowing bone healing with callus formation.
- Improved fixation and biology may lead to better clinical outcomes and faster healing.
- The systems provide better fixation in osteoporotic bones, especially in the epiphyseal and metaphyseal areas. In osteoporotic bone, LHS are more highly resistant to bending and torsional forces, with less pullout of the screw. LHS cannot be overtightened in porotic bone.
- Divergently or convergently locked screws improve the pull-out resistance of the whole construct—for example, using anatomically preshaped plates or a plate bent into slight but continuous or multiple undulations (known as a multiple-wave plate; see Fig 1-28; Fig 1-29).
- The plate–bone interface is not loaded along the screw axis and the tendency for the thread to strip in the bone is reduced. The locking head screws have a higher core diameter to resist cantilever and bending forces at the screw–cortex interface. Screws with angular stability are not subject to the toggling ("windshield-wiper" effect) seen with standard screws.
- These systems do not, or very rarely, require primary bone grafting.

Indications

The common indications for the use of LISS and LCP/LHS for internal fixation are as follows:

- Epiphyseal and metaphyseal fractures: short articular block, minimal bone mass for anchorage, angular stability.

Situations in which the MIPO technique is indicated and possible

- Since accurate contouring of the plate is neither possible nor necessary when locking head screws are used, there is no loss of initial reduction. The LISS and LCP are also recommended in the diaphyseal area if they can be used with

the MIPO technique and if intramedullary locked splinting (locked nail) is not possible.
- Fractures with severe soft-tissue injuries.
- Fractures in osteoporotic bones. Since there is better resistance to bending and torsional forces and less pullout of the screw–plate construct, no stripping of the bone thread during insertion of the screw (no overtightening of the screw is possible).
- Diaphyseal and metaphyseal fractures in children.

The clinical application of LISS and LCP is currently considered advantageous in cases of unavoidable surgery for distal radial fractures close to the joints, distal humeral fractures, elbow dislocation fractures, proximal upper arm fractures, distal femoral fractures, tibial plateau fractures, and proximal and distal tibial fractures including pilon fractures. The procedure is also highly beneficial for stabilizing osteotomies and also in tumor surgery.

7 Bibliography

1. **Brug E, Winckler S** (1991) [A return to callus healing using dynamic osteosynthesis procedures. Principles, indications, complications, x-ray diagnosis of interlocking nailing and dynamic monofixators in comparison with conventional bone plates]. *Radiologe;* 31(4):165–171.
2. **Perren SM** (2002) Evolution of the internal fixation of long bone fractures. The scientific basis of biological internal fixation: choosing a new balance between stability and biology. *J Bone Joint Surg Br;* 84(8):1093–1110.
3. **Tulic G, Bumbasirevic M, Dulic B, et al** (2003) [Principles and new methods of flexible fixation of fractures of long bones]. *Acta Chir Iugosl;* 50(2):105–113.
4. **Wu LD, Wu QH, Yan SG, et al** (2004) Treatment of ipsilateral hip and femoral shaft fractures with reconstructive intramedullary interlocking nail. *Chin J Traumatol;* 7(1):7–12.
5. **Miedel R, Ponzer S, Tornkvist H, et al** (2005) The standard Gamma nail or the Medoff sliding plate for unstable trochanteric and subtrochanteric fractures. A randomised, controlled trial. *J Bone Joint Surg Br;* 87(1):68–75.
6. **Leunig M, Hertel R, Siebenrock KA, et al** (2000) The evolution of indirect reduction techniques for the treatment of fractures. *Clin Orthop Relat Res;* 375:7–14.
7. **Mast J, Jakob R, Ganz R** (1989) Planning and reduction technique in fracture surgery. Heidelber: Springer.
8. **Vidal J, Buscayret C, Fischbach C, et al** (1977) [New method of treatment of comminuted fractures of the lower end of the radius: "ligamentary taxis"]. *Acta Orthop Belg;* 43(6):781–789.
9. **Vidal J** (1979) Treatment of articular fractures by "ligamentotaxis" with external fixation., in Brooker HS andEdward CC: External fixation: current state of the art. Baltimore, Williams and Wilkins.
10. **Rüedi TP, Sommer C, Leutenegger A** (1998) New techniques in indirect reduction of long bone fractures. *Clin Orthop Relat Res;* 347:27–34.
11. **Collinge CA, Sanders RW** (2000) Percutaneous plating in the lower extremity. *J Am Acad Orthop Surg;* 8(4):211–216.
12. **Matter P, Brennwald J, Perren SM** (1974) [Biological reaction of bones to osteosynthesis plates]. *Helv Chir Acta;* 0Suppl12:1–44.
13. **Perren SM, Cordey J, Rahn BA, et al** (1988) Early temporary porosis of bone induced by internal fixation implants. A reaction to necrosis, not to stress protection? *Clin Orthop Relat Res;* 232:139–151.
14. **Brunner C, Weber BG** (1982) Special techniques in internal fixation. Berlin: Springer-Verlag.
15. **Müller KH, Witzel U** (1984) [A bridgeplate for osteosynthesis of osseous shaft defects of the femur caused by failure of plate osteosynthesis]. *Unfallheilkunde;* 87(6):237–246.
16. **Heitemeyer U, Hierholzer G** (1985) [Bridging osteosynthesis in closed compound fractures of the femur shaft]. *Aktuelle Traumatol;* 15:205–209.
17. **Blatter G, Weber BG** (1990) Wave plate osteosynthesis as a salvage procedure. *Arch Orthop Trauma Surg;* 109(6):330–333.
18. **Schatzker J** (1998) Fractures of the distal femur revisited. *Clin Orthop Relat Res;* 347:43–56.
19. **Müller ME** (1962) [Surgical treatment of coxarthrosis.] *Schweiz Med Wochenschr;* 17;92:1476–1480.
20. **Müller ME** (1963) Internal fixation for fresh fractures and for non-union. *Proc R Soc Med;* 56:455–460.
21. **Allgöwer M, Ehrsam R, Ganz R, et al** (1969) Clinical experience with a new compression plate „DCP". *Acta Orthop Scand Suppl;* 125:45–61.
22. **Perren SM, Russenberger M, Steinemann S, et al** (1969) A dynamic compression plate. *Acta Orthop Scand Suppl;* 125:31–41.
23. **Perren SM, Klaue K, Pohler O, et al** (1990) The limited contact dynamic compression plate (LC-DCP). *Arch Orthop Trauma Surg;* 109(6):304–310.
24. **Tepic S, Remiger AR, Morikawa K, et al** (1997) Strength recovery in fractured sheep tibia treated with a plate or an internal fixator: an experimental study with a two-year follow-up. *J Orthop Trauma;* 11(1):14–23.

25. **Klaue K, Fengels I,Perren SM** (2000) Long-term effects of plate osteosynthesis: comparison of four different plates. *Injury;* 31(Suppl2):B51–62.
26. **Schütz M, Schäfer M, Bail H, et al** (2005) [New osteosynthesis techniques for the treatment of distal femoral fractures]. *Zentralbl Chir;* 130(4):307–313.
27. **Krettek C, Müller M, Miclau T** (2001) Evolution of minimally invasive plate osteosynthesis (MIPO) in the femur. *Injury;* 32(Suppl3):SC14–23.
28. **Schütz M, Südkamp NP** (2003) Revolution in plate osteosynthesis: new internal fixator systems. *J Orthop Sci;* 8(2):252–258.
29. **Hayes DW Jr, Brower RL, John KJ** (2001) Articular cartilage. Anatomy, injury, and repair. *Clin Podiatr Med Surg;* 18(1):35–53.
30. **Haidukewych GJ** (2002) Temporary external fixation for the management of complex intra- and periarticular fractures of the lower extremity. *J Orthop Trauma;* 16(9):678–685.
31. **McAuliffe JA** (2005) Combined internal and external fixation of distal radius fractures. *Hand Clin;* 21(3):395–406.
32. **Goodship AE, Cunningham JL, Kenwright J** (1998) Strain rate and timing of stimulation in mechanical modulation of fracture healing. *Clin Orthop Relat Res;* 355Suppl:S105–115.
33. **Uhthoff HK, Rahn BA** (1981) Healing patterns of metaphyseal fractures. *Clin Orthop Relat Res;* 160:295–303.
34. **Schenk R, Willenegger H** (1963) [on the Histological Picture of So-Called Primary Healing of Pressure Osteosynthesis in Experimental Osteotomies in the Dog.]. *Experientia;* 19:593–595.
35. **Rahn BA, Gallinaro P, Baltensperger A, et al** (1971) Primary bone healing. An experimental study in the rabbit. *J Bone Joint Surg Am;* 53(4):783–786.
36. **Klaushofer K, Peterlik M** (1994) [Pathophysiology of fracture healing]. *Radiologe;* 34(12):709–714.
37. **Remedios A** (1999) Bone and bone healing. *Vet Clin North Am Small Anim Pract;* 29(5):1029–1044.
38. **Sarmiento A, Latta LL** (1995) *Functional fracture bracing: tibia, humerus, and ulna.* Berlin Heidelberg New York: Springer-Verlag.
39. **Carter DR, Beaupre GS, Giori NJ, et al** (1998) Mechanobiology of skeletal regeneration. *Clin Orthop Relat Res;* 355Suppl:S41–55.
40. **Athanasiou KA, Zhu C, Lanctot DR, et al** (2000) Fundamentals of biomechanics in tissue engineering of bone. *Tissue Eng;* 6(4):361–381.
41. **Ingham E, Fisher J** (2005) The role of macrophages in osteolysis of total joint replacement. *Biomaterials;* 26(11):1271–286.
42. **Ungersbock A, Pohler O, Perren SM** (1994) Evaluation of the soft tissue interface at titanium implants with different surface treatments: experimental study on rabbits. *Biomed Mater Eng;* 4(4):317–325.
43. **Perren SM** (1979) Physical and biological aspects of fracture healing with special reference to internal fixation. *Clin Orthop Relat Res;* 138:175–196.
44. **Rhinelander FW** (1974) The normal circulation of bone and its response to surgical intervention. *J Biomed Mater Res;* 8(1):87–90.
45. **Farouk O, Krettek C, Miclau T, et al** (1997) Minimally invasive plate osteosynthesis and vascularity: preliminary results of a cadaver injection study. *Injury;* 28(Suppl1):A7–12.
46. **O'Meara PM** (1992) Management of open fractures. *Orthop Rev;* 21(10):1177–1185.
47. **Schmidt AH, Swiontkowski MF** (2000) Pathophysiology of infections after internal fixation of fractures. *J Am Acad Orthop Surg;* 8(5):285–291.
48. **Stürmer KM** (1996) [Pathophysiology of disrupted bone healing]. *Orthopäde;* 25(5):386–393.
49. **Cordey J, Blümlein H, Ziegler W, et al** (1976) [Study of the behavior in the course of time of the holding power of cortical screws in vivo]. *Acta Orthop Belg;* 42Suppl1:75–87.
50. **Egol KA, Kubiak EN, Fulkerson E, et al** (2004) Biomechanics of locked plates and screws. *J Orthop Trauma;* 18(8):488–493.
51. **Kääb MJ, Frenk A, Schmeling A, et al** (2004) Locked internal fixator: sensitivity of screw/plate stability to the correct insertion angle of the screw. *J Orthop Trauma;* 18(8):483–487.
52. **Wagner M** (2003) General principles for the clinical use of the LCP. *Injury;* 34(Suppl2):B31–42.

53. **Granowski R, Ramotowski W, Kaminski E, et al** (1984) ["Zespol"—a new type of osteosynthesis. I. An internal self-compressing stabilizer of bone fragments]. *Chir Narzadow Ruchu Ortop Pol;* 49(4):301–305.
54. **Eijer H, Hauke C, Arens S, et al** (2001) PC-Fix and local infection resistance--influence of implant design on postoperative infection development, clinical and experimental results. *Injury;* 32(Suppl2):B38–43.
55. **Arens S, Eijer H, Schlegel U, et al** (1999) Influence of the design for fixation implants on local infection: experimental study of dynamic compression plates versus point contact fixators in rabbits. *J Orthop Trauma;* 13(7):470–476.
56. **Johansson A, Lindgren JU, Nord CE, et al** (1999) Material and design in haematogenous implant-associated infections in a rabbit model. *Injury;* 30(10):651–657.
57. **Frigg R, Appenzeller A, Christensen R, et al** (2001) The development of the distal femur less invasive stabilization system (LISS). *Injury;* 32:SC24–31.
58. **Wagner M, Frenk A, Frigg R,** (2004) New concepts for bone fracture treatment and the locking compression plate. *Surg Technol Int;* 12:271–7.
59. **Gosling T, Schandelmaier P, Müller M, et al** (2005) Single lateral locked screw plating of bicondylar tibial plateau fractures. *Clin Orthop Relat Res;* 439:207–214.
60. **Wong MK, Leung F, Chow SP** (2005) Treatment of distal femoral fractures in the elderly using a less-invasive plating technique. *Int Orthop;* 29(2):117–120.
61. **Kregor PJ, Stannard JA, Zlowodzki M, et al** (2004) Treatment of distal femur fractures using the less invasive stabilization system: surgical experience and early clinical results in 103 fractures. *J Orthop Trauma;* 18(8):509–520.
62. **Fankhauser F, Gruber G, Schippinger G, et al** (2004) Minimal-invasive treatment of distal femoral fractures with the LISS (Less Invasive Stabilization System): a prospective study of 30 fractures with a follow up of 20 months. *Acta Orthop Scand;* 75(1):56–60.
63. **Hahn U, Prokop A, Jubel A, et al** (2002) [LISS versus condylar plate]. *Kongressbd Dtsch Ges Chir Kongr;* 119:498–504.
64. **Markmiller M, Konrad G, Südkamp N** (2004) Femur-LISS and distal femoral nail for fixation of distal femoral fractures: are there differences in outcome and complications? *Clin Orthop Relat Res;* 426:252–257.
65. **Ricci WM, Rudzki JR, Borrelli J Jr** (2004) Treatment of complex proximal tibia fractures with the less invasive skeletal stabilization system. *J Orthop Trauma;* 18(8):521–527.
66. **Ricci AR, Yue JJ, Taffet R, et al** (2004) Less Invasive Stabilization System for treatment of distal femur fractures. *Am J Orthop;* 33(5):250–255.
67. **Schütz M, Müller M, Krettek C, et al** (2001) Minimally invasive fracture stabilization of distal femoral fractures with the LISS: a prospective multicenter study. Results of a clinical study with special emphasis on difficult cases. *Injury;* 32(Suppl3):SC48–54.
68. **Schütz M, Haas NP** (2001) [LISS—internal plate fixator]. *Kongressbd Dtsch Ges Chir Kongr;* 118:375–379.
69. **Syed AA, Agarwal M, Giannoudis PV, et al** (2004) Distal femoral fractures: long-term outcome following stabilisation with the LISS. *Injury;* 35(6):599–607.
70. **Weight M, Collinge C** (2004) Early results of the less invasive stabilization system for mechanically unstable fractures of the distal femur (AO/OTA types A2, A3, C2, and C3). *J Orthop Trauma;* 18(8):503–508.
71. **Cole PA, Zlowodzki M, Kregor PJ** (2004) Treatment of proximal tibia fractures using the less invasive stabilization system: surgical experience and early clinical results in 77 fractures. *J Orthop Trauma;* 18(8):528–535.
72. **Schütz M, Kääb MJ, Haas N** (2003) Stabilization of proximal tibial fractures with the LIS-System: early clinical experience in Berlin. *Injury;* 34(Suppl1):A30–35.
73. **Stannard JP, Wilson TC, Volgas DA, et al** (2003) Fracture stabilization of proximal tibial fractures with the proximal tibial LISS: early experience in Birmingham, Alabama (USA). *Injury;* 34(Suppl1):A36–42.

74. **Stannard JP, Wilson TC, Volgas DA, et al** (2004) The less invasive stabilization system in the treatment of complex fractures of the tibial plateau: short-term results. *J Orthop Trauma;* 18(8):552–558.
75. **Frigg R** (2003) Development of the Locking Compression Plate. *Injury;* 34(Suppl1):B6–10.
76. **Krettek C, Schandelmaier P, Miclau T, et al** (1997) Minimally invasive percutaneous plate osteosynthesis (MIPPO) using the DCS in proximal and distal femoral fractures. *Injury;* 28(Suppl1): A20–30.
77. **Farouk O, Krettek C, Miclau T, et al** (1999) Minimally invasive plate osteosynthesis: does percutaneous plating disrupt femoral blood supply less than the traditional technique? *J Orthop Trauma;* 13(6):401–406.
78. **Sommer C,Gautier E** (2003) [Relevance and advantages of new angular stable screw-plate systems for diaphyseal fractures (locking compression plate versus intramedullary nail]. *.Ther Umsch;* 60:751–756.
79. **Ring D, Kloen P, Kadzielski J, et al** (2004) Locking compression plates for osteoporotic nonunions of the diaphyseal humerus. *Clin Orthop Relat Res;* 425:50–54.
80. **Korner J, Lill H, Müller LP, et al** (2003) The LCP-concept in the operative treatment of distal humerus fractures--biological, biomechanical and surgical aspects. *Injury;* 34(Suppl2):B20–30.

2 Surgical reduction techniques

2 Surgical reduction techniques

The first step in the management of any displaced fracture is to determine whether reduction is to be surgical or nonsurgical. Reduction can be carried out as a closed or open procedure.

Reduction is the act of restoring the anatomically correct position of the fragments, including the process of reconstructing cancellous bone by relieving impaction. Reduction thus reverses the process that created the fracture displacement during the injury. Logically, this requires the application of forces and moments in directions opposite to those which produced the fracture. Preliminary analysis of the displacement of fragments and of the deformation and impaction of bone provides the basis for planning the tactical steps necessary. This applies to all methods, whether they are nonsurgical, surgical, closed, or open **[1]**.

Displacement in diaphyseal and metaphyseal bones is clinically easily detected using conventional x-rays taken in at least two planes perpendicular to each other. In the metaphysis and epiphysis, oblique views, often supplemented by computed tomography with multiplanar reconstruction, may be necessary to fully assess fragmentation, fragment displacement, deformation, and impaction.

Careful analysis of the site and extent of bone deformation, as well as of the direction and degree of displacement, is the basis for selecting the most appropriate approach and reduction technique and for choosing a suitable implant or fixation device.

When a fracture occurs, shortening of the limb takes place, and this has to be overcome by longitudinal pulling (traction). If necessary, the fracture fragments have to be disengaged, either by recreating the deformity or by rotation. The fracture fragments are manipulated into the correct position by aligning them along the longitudinal axis and correcting their rotation. These principles of manipulative reduction can be carried out using direct and indirect techniques. The method of reduction chosen has to spare the soft tissues surrounding the fracture as much as possible. This is important to achieve bony union, prevent infection, and restore function. Reduction manipulation is central to the art of fracture surgery (method and technique of fracture fixation).

The reduction techniques used have to be gentle and atraumatic. They need to preserve any remaining vascularity, since an adequate tissue response is a prerequisite for healing. Adequate blood supply to the repair tissues is crucial. Bone healing will be delayed or will cease if one or both of the following factors are impaired: mechanical conditions at the fracture (strain) and the remaining capacity of the affected tissue for a biological response.

Accuracy of the reduction at joint level, and the stability achieved by the implants, are mechanical prerequisites for the biological response—ie, the type of healing achieved. In turn, the healing process is influenced by any additional surgical damage to the bone and the surrounding soft-tissue envelope which occurs during the process of reduction and fixation (exposure and implant positioning and fixation to the bone).

1 Aim of reduction

The aim of reduction in diaphyseal and metaphyseal bone is to restore the correct alignment of the epiphyses. Whether the fracture between the main fragments is simple, multifragmentary, segmental, or shows bone loss, the aim of reduction is to reduce the epiphyses into correct relationship to each other. This means restoring the bone to its original length, axis, and rotation. In the articular segment, anatomical reduction of the joint surfaces, with elevation of impacted areas, is mandatory to prevent posttraumatic osteoarthrosis

[1–3]. In addition, correct spatial orientation of the epiphysis with respect to the diaphysis should be achieved, to avoid limb malalignment. Ideally, no residual displacement should be tolerated. However, a widely accepted convention regards any form of reduction as being acceptable in which residual displacement is less than half the thickness of the articular cartilage. It can be that during surgery it is occasionally not possible to achieve an even better reduction of a given joint without additional risks as are involved in a second surgical approach, prolonging the operation. Less than perfect reduction sometimes has to be accepted in order to preserve the adjacent anatomical structures. Fracture of the articular surface is often accompanied by irreparable damage to the cartilage due to impaction at the time of injury [4].

2 Different types of surgical reduction

There are two fundamentally different techniques for fracture reduction—direct and indirect. The term "direct reduction" implies that the reduction of the fracture fragments is achieved by applying forces and moments directly in the vicinity of the fracture zone—the fracture fragments can be manipulated directly. Indirect reduction means that the forces and moments act away from the fracture. Reduction is accomplished using instruments or implants introduced distant to the fracture zone, or through minimal incisions. Both reduction techniques—direct and indirect—can be performed as open, percutaneous, or closed procedures. (Tab 2-1; Tab 2-2).

Tab 2-1 **Direct versus indirect reduction**

	Direct reduction Reduction of the fracture fragments is achieved by applying forces and moments directly in the vicinity of the fracture zone—the fracture fragments can be manipulated directly.	**Indirect reduction** Indirect reduction means that the forces and moments acting away from the fracture are used to manipulate and finally reduce the fracture, by a limited open exposure.
Definition	*Open direct reduction* The fracture lines are exposed surgically, and the bone fragments are reduced under direct vision and with instruments directly applied to each fragment, usually near the fracture site. *Percutaneous direct reduction* The fracture lines are not exposed surgically. Reduction instruments are applied through stab incisions.	*Indirect closed reduction* The fracture lines are not directly exposed and visualized, and the fracture area remains covered by the surrounding tissues. Reduction is carried out with instruments or implants that are introduced away from the fracture zone. *Open indirect reduction* Open but only limited exposure of the fracture.
Control of reduction	Easy, with direct visualization. With an image intensifier when the percutaneous direct reduction technique is used.	With an image intensifier, or by clinical assessment of the alignment.
Indications	Articular fractures, simple metaphyseal/diaphyseal fractures, forearm fractures.	Multifragmentary metaphyseal and diaphyseal fractures.
Pearls	In the articular segment, anatomical and precise reduction of the joint surface, with elevation of the impacted areas, is mandatory in order to avoid post-traumatic osteoarthrosis.	

Tab 2-1 **Direct versus indirect reduction (cont)**

	Direct reduction	Indirect reduction
Pearls (cont)	In simple diaphyseal fracture patterns, direct reduction is technically straightforward and the results are easy to check. With precise local approximation of the two main fragments, the length and axial and rotational alignment of the bone itself are reestablished. Biologically, surgical exposure in easy fracture situations of this type should not add substantial vascular damage to the bone or soft tissues. However, this can only be achieved if the surgery is carried out carefully, with meticulous soft-tissue handling and with limited epiperiosteal exposure of the bone.	In the diaphysis and metaphysis, correct alignment of the two main fragments carrying the joint surfaces is important. The aim is to restore the overall length of the bone as precisely as possible, as well as the axial and rotational alignment. In biological terms, indirect reduction techniques offer enormous advantages, as they only cause minimal additional surgical damage to tissues that have already been traumatized by the fracture. All instruments required for reduction are introduced away from the fracture zone, only compromising the tissue perfusion in an area in which trauma has not already disturbed the blood supply.
Pitfalls	In more complex diaphyseal fractures, the classical approach used in direct reduction techniques may lead to misguided attempts to expose and fix each individual fragment. In this process, the surgeon would devascularize each of the fragments in sequence. The repeated use of bone clamps and other reduction tools or implants may completely devitalize the fragments in the multifragmentary area, with potentially disastrous consequences for the healing process, including delayed union, nonunion, infection, or implant failure. It is only with a thorough understanding of the biology of bone and soft tissues and an awareness of poor results obtained after excessive devascularization that the surgeon is able to avoid failures after open reduction and internal fixation.	In practice, correct reduction using indirect techniques is much more difficult to achieve. It requires accurate assessment of the soft-tissue lesion, an understanding of the fracture pattern, and meticulous preoperative planning. In addition, the actual process of reduction is more demanding and requires the use of an image intensifier or intraoperative radiography.
Principle of fracture fixation	Absolute stability	Relative stability
Method of fracture fixation	Compression method—requiring precise, accurate reduction. Stability of the fixation depends on compression producing friction between and preload (elastic deformation) of the fragment ends.	Splinting method—stability of the fixation depends on the rigidity of the splint and its anchorage to bone.
Techniques	Lag screw (usually) Lag screw and protection plate Compression plate Buttress plate Tension band, tension plate	Minimally invasive osteosynthesis (MIO), ie: Intramedullary nailing Elastic nailing External fixator Splinting with conventional plates Bridging the fracture zone with a locked internal fixator (LISS and LHS, LCP and LHS) Minimally invasive plate osteosynthesis (MIPO) technique.
Surgical approach	Open, for reduction and implant placement and fixation. Length of approach corresponds to the length of the implant used. In case of a simple fracture type a direct percutaneous reduction with a minimally invasive approach is possible. Since there is no direct visualization of the fracture site to confirm the reduction directly, an image intensifier must be used to monitor the result of the reduction. Sometimes a combination of closed indirect reduction maneuver with manual traction and a percutaneous direct reduction maneuver with pointed reduction forceps or collinear reduction clamp is the best way for atraumatic reduction.	Length of approach corresponds to the section of the implant used. Only incisions for implant insertion, outside of the fracture area (plate and screws; nails and locking bolts).

Tab 2-2 **Different types of reduction**

Reduction type	Approach	Placement of instruments or forces	Reduction control	Visualization and surgical devascularization	Difficulty of reduction control
Direct	Open	Close to the fracture	Direct view		
Direct	Percutaneous	Close to the fracture	No direct visualization, image intensifier, x-rays, clinical check		
Indirect	Limited open	Distant to the fracture	Limited visualization, image intensifier		
Indirect	Closed	Distant to the fracture	No direct visualization: x-rays, image intensifier, clinical check		

2.1 Factors influencing the choice of type of reduction

The choice of the reduction method depends on the bone, the pattern and location of the fracture, and the extent of associated soft-tissue injury. The goal in fracture surgery is always to preserve the viability of bone by minimizing surgical trauma to periosseous muscle and to the fascial attachments that provide the bone with its vascular supply. As these tissues are connected to the bone fragments, applying longitudinal tension causes the fragments to align themselves. The surgeon has to decide whether traction should be applied manually by an assistant, using the traction table or distractor, or via a plate, using the indirect reduction technique. If the traction table or distractor is used, the precise positioning of the traction or fixation pins should be selected. If open reduction is planned, the surgeon should consider which special forceps and clamps will be necessary to achieve and temporarily hold the reduction. The surgeon also has to decide whether an image intensifier, serial x-rays, or 3-D CT scans will be necessary to guide and control the reduction procedure and implant insertion.

Several points are to be considered:

- Soft tissues
- Fracture configuration
- Fracture location
- Control of reduction (clinical, optical, radiographical)

In moderate-energy fractures, the periosteum is torn, but the muscle and interosseous membrane may be intact and can guide the reduction into place. In high-energy fractures, only the skin may be intact. Normally the main fragments can easily be reduced by traction. But intercalated fragments do not automatically reduce because of the loss of soft-tissue connections. Low-energy fractures are often associated with partial intact periosteum creating a good soft-tissue hinge useful during the process of reduction.

The fracture configuration most suitable for indirect reduction is a complex multifragmentary fracture, while the simpler fractures are usually more suitable for direct open or direct percutaneous fracture reductions. For a simple fracture type and a situation where precise reduction is not required, indirect closed reduction is also an option.

In the diaphysis and metaphysis, axial alignment in the frontal and sagittal planes is required. It is important to correct rotation in the horizontal plane as well as translation and length changes. Anatomical reduction of the fragments is therefore not necessary, but anatomical alignment of the limb segment is mandatory.

Joint involvement may sometimes require an additional direct approach. In articular fractures, the anatomical reduction of the articular surface is mandatory and there is no place for indirect reductions in restoring joint congruity, unless the fractures have some soft-tissue attachments. Depressed joint fragments have no soft-tissue attachments; no matter how much traction is applied, the fracture will not reduce without a direct reduction.

Since percutaneous direct or closed indirect reduction limits visualization of the fracture site, there is no means of confirming the reduction directly. The best way of overcoming this limitation is to use an image intensifier to monitor the result of the reduction.

The surgical incisions and exposures used are related to the reduction methods. Several principles must be observed. Firstly, incisions need to be both straight and long enough to release tension during retraction. Secondly, no incision should be made over subcutaneous bones or in skin areas showing important contusion and soft-tissue damage. Thirdly, no subcutaneous flaps should be created. After advancing below the deep fascia, thick fascial–cutaneous flaps can be developed if necessary, to expose the fracture for reduction and stabilization. Finally, working systematically through the fracture sites is very important to ensure that no further damage occurs.

Preoperative planning will determine the type of reduction, the forces which need to be overcome, and the positioning of the reduction device. The preoperative plan can be modified depending on the surgical incision required to achieve implant placement or reduction. Indirect reduction can be successfully accomplished using a radiolucent operating table and image intensifier as visual aids.

2.2 Direct open reduction

Complete pharmacological relaxation is necessary for reduction of femoral and tibial shaft fractures.

The term "direct open reduction" implies that the fracture area is exposed surgically or is already wide open. All maneuvers are seen and monitored under direct vision (Fig 2-1). This kind of reduction technique is easier than indirect reduction and the reduction can be more precise. The fragments are grasped by surgical instruments rather than by hand. Reduction of the fracture fragments is achieved by applying forces and moments directly in the vicinity of the fracture zone.

Direct reduction has been defined as direct repositioning of the bone fragments under direct vision, with instruments being directly applied to each fragment, usually near the fracture site. To allow access, it may be necessary to strip muscles from the fragments, particularly those that are adjacent to the implant, and this may require extraperiosteal exposure of the fracture site. The fracture is then reduced by traction, either manual or using a distractor, an external fixator, or a traction table. A temporary fixation device such as a clamp or K-wire is applied, and fixation then follows, usually with a plate-independent lag screw or a lag screw inserted into a plate to achieve interfragmentary compression and to maintain the reduction. The extent of the dissection is limited by the use of pointed retractors, pointed reduction forceps, or temporary cerclage.

In simple diaphyseal fracture patterns, direct open reduction is technically straightforward, and the result is easy to control. With precise local approximation of the two main fragments, the length and axial and rotational alignment of the bone itself are reestablished. Biologically, the surgical exposure should not cause additional substantial vascular damage to the bone or soft tissues in easy fracture situations such as this. However, this is only possible if the surgery is carried out carefully, with meticulous soft-tissue handling and limited epiperiosteal exposure of the bone [5, 6]. Open reduction is carried out to reduce a displaced fracture and to apply an implant to stabilize the reduction. When attention focuses on the implant and the reduction, soft tissues are often neglected, unnecessarily sacrificing the healing potential of the soft tissues.

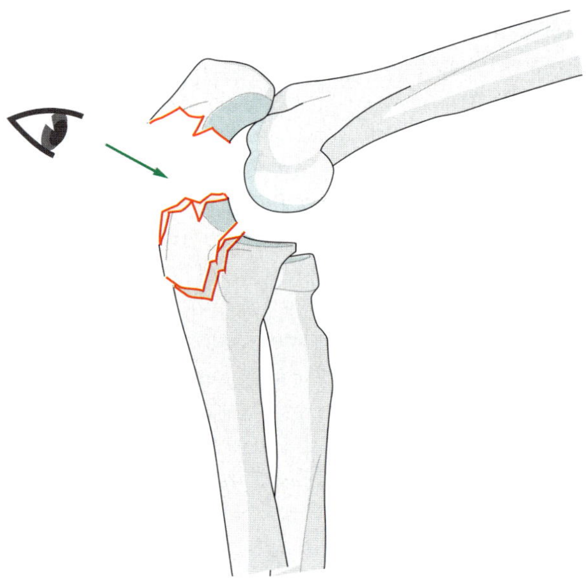

Fig 2-1 Reduction under direct vision (open, direct reduction).

2.3 Direct percutaneous reduction

In case of a simple fracture type, a direct percutaneous reduction with a minimally invasive approach is possible. Since there is no direct visualization of the fracture site to confirm reduction directly, an image intensifier must be used to monitor the result of the reduction.

Sometimes a combination of a closed indirect reduction maneuver with manual traction and a percutaneous direct reduction maneuver with pointed reduction forceps or a collinear reduction clamp is the best way for atraumatic reduction. This is true for simple shaft, as well as articular, fractures. Simple oblique or spiral fractures can be reduced with the help of a pointed reduction forceps or pelvic reduction forceps working through small stab incisions for each branch of the forceps. The collinear reduction clamp is an alternative tool. A simple split fracture of the joint can be reduced by manual traction and/or direct, percutaneous manipulation with a joy stick, later fixed with a pelvic reduction forceps or with the collinear reduction clamp (Fig 2-2).

In more complex diaphyseal fractures, conventional direct reduction techniques may lead to misguided attempts to expose and fix each individual fragment—with each fragment being devascularized in sequence. Repeated use of bone clamps and other reduction tools or implants may completely devitalize the fragments in a multifragmentary area, with disastrous consequences for the healing process, including delayed union, nonunion, infection, or implant failure. Only a good understanding of bone and soft-tissue biology and an awareness of poor results observed after excessive devascularization can help the surgeon avoid such failures following open reduction and internal fixation [7].

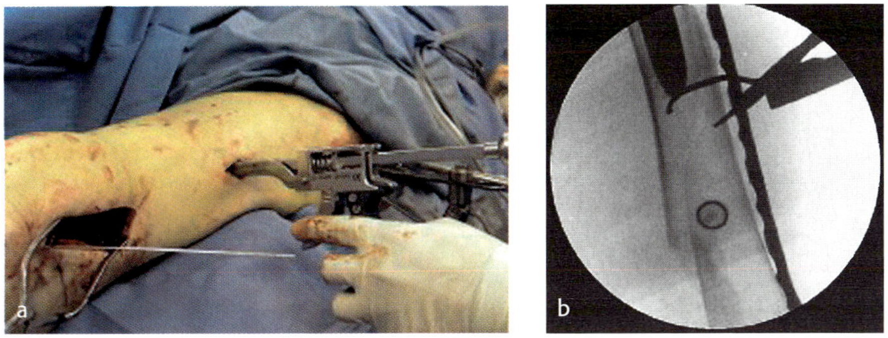

Fig 2-2a–b Direct percutaneous reduction with a collinear reduction clamp.

2.4 Indirect reduction, open or closed

Reduction is achieved by using instruments or implants introduced away from the fracture zone, or through minimal incisions. Some specific implants, such as the intramedullary nail or an anatomically preshaped plate, act both as a reduction tool and as a stabilization system.

There are two different types of indirect reduction—open and closed. Open indirect reduction involves an open approach, but with indirect reduction maneuvers and a "no-touch" technique. The term "closed indirect reduction" implies that the fracture lines are not directly exposed or visible and that the fracture zone remains covered by the surrounding soft tissues.

In practice, correct reduction is much more difficult to achieve using indirect techniques. It requires accurate assessment of the soft-tissue lesion, an understanding of the fracture pattern, and meticulous preoperative planning. In addition, the actual reduction procedure is more demanding and requires the use of an image intensifier or intraoperative radiography for reduction control. In biological terms, however, indirect reduction techniques offer enormous advantages, since only minimal additional surgical damage is caused to tissues already traumatized by the fracture. All instruments required for reduction are introduced away from the fracture zone, so that tissue perfusion is only compromised in an area not already disturbed by trauma.

Most of the instruments and implants available can be used for either technique of fracture reduction, and surgical success in preserving the biology of the tissues does not depend on the specific instrument or implant used for the reduction.

2.5 Open indirect reduction

Indirect reduction involves "blind" repositioning of the bone fragments using some form of distraction, achieved by manual traction, an instrument, or implant, so that soft tissues around the fracture site are minimally disturbed (Fig 2-3). The mechanics of the reduction procedure are the same—traction to correct shortening, and unlocking the fracture to correct translation and rotation. The technique of indirect reduction requires exposure to apply the reduction devices, but not to visualize the fracture. The reduction devices are usually remote, particularly if it is possible to use the distraction device. Temporary fixation is usually part of the reduction technique, followed by definitive fixation by splinting using intramedullary nails, bridging plates, locked internal fixators, or external fixators.

Numerous aids are available for indirect reduction—implants, distractors, clamps, or any combination of these. For example, in an interference plate reduction on an oblique fracture, the plate pushes the fracture upward along oblique incline, thus reducing it indirectly. Only one side of the fracture needs to be exposed. This antiglide or interference technique can be used for simple oblique fractures. More commonly, however, distraction is applied through a series of different devices such as a distractor, push-pull techniques with plates, traction tables, or other types of traction device.

To achieve reduction, traction is normally applied along the long axis of the limb. This can only work if the fragments are still connected to some soft tissue. Traction can be applied manually, with the aid of a traction table, or using a distractor. The traction table has the disadvantage that traction has

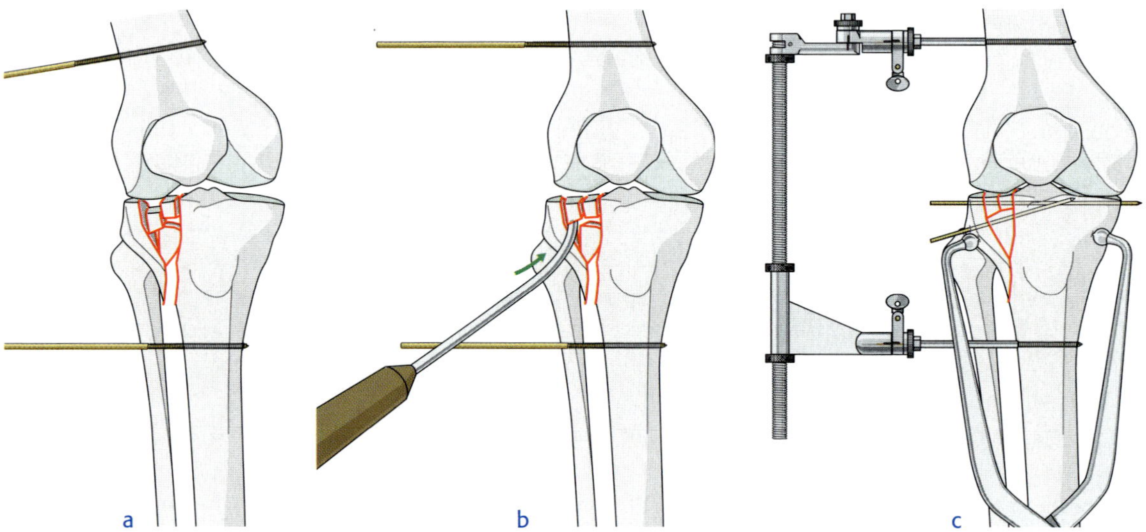

Fig 2-3a–c Open direct fracture reduction.

a–b Indirect reduction of lateral 41-B3 fracture with large distractor. The impacted articular surface must be elevated with a pusher through the fracture.

c Compression using the pelvic reduction forceps and preliminary fixation with K-wires.

to be applied across at least one joint. It is not possible for the surgeon to move the limb, and the surgical approach is frequently compromised. The distractor, applied directly to the main fragments, allows the limb to be manipulated during surgery. Angular or rotational corrections are difficult to carry out when the distractor is subject to loading, and the construct may be cumbersome. As there is an inherent tendency for naturally curved bone to be straightened by the distraction procedure, the eccentric force produced by a unilaterally mounted distractor may produce additional deformity.

2.6 Closed indirect reduction

Biological fracture fixation (see Tab 1-1) is used usually after some form of indirect reduction. Locked nails, locked internal fixators, and external fixators are used for this purpose. Biological fracture fixation means the combination of a closed indirect reduction technique and the use of implant producing low additional implant-inherent vascular damage to bone and soft tissues.

External fixators, locked nails, and locked internal fixators are used for this purpose—all of them not relying on bone-implant contact for load transfer. The fixation is elastic, with relative stability (see Tab 1-5).

The goal of indirect reduction is to achieve preliminary alignment of a fractured bone, either before any attempt of internal fixation is made or in conjunction with a fixation device. The mechanical principle underlying indirect reduction is distraction, and this applies equally to diaphyseal and metaphyseal bone. The muscle envelope surrounding the diaphysis of most long bones provides a logical rationale for indirect reduction, since controlled pulling on the muscle and periosteal attachments of any single fragment will tend to align it in the desired direction. In addition, a muscle envelope under distraction exerts concentric pressure towards the shaft, easing the fragments into place. The same also applies to metaphyseal and epiphyseal bone segments, although the distraction required to align the fragments is transferred not so much via muscle attachments as through capsular tissues, ligaments, and (less often) tendons. This phenomenon, which is regularly observed in nonsurgical fracture management, is referred to as "ligamentotaxis" (see Tab 1-1). Similarly, traction applied to an entire limb using a traction table produces indirect reduction at a fracture focus. However, applying an implant or large distractor to a single bone helps control reduction more effectively and also allows subtile adjustments to be made. If feasible, indirect reduction techniques with a distractor (Fig 2-4) or external fixator and plate can be combined. Other instruments and tools for indirect reduction, such as plates, in conjunction with the articulated tension device and bone spreaders, are described below.

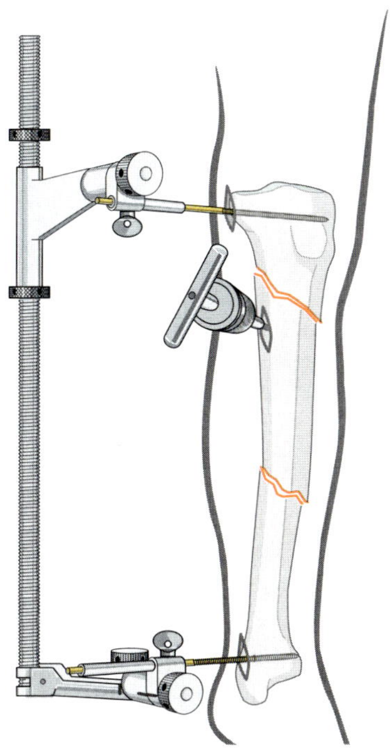

Fig 2-4 **Indirect fragment manipulation with the large distractor.**

2.7 Reduction and fixation of metaphyseal and diaphyseal fractures

- Diaphyseal fractures can be reduced directly or indirectly; independently of the technique, any reduction maneuver should be as gentle as possible to the soft tissues and periosteum surrounding the fracture in order to preserve the existing blood supply. Fixation techniques most often used in the treatment of diaphyseal fractures are intramedullary nailing, plating (with either the compression or splinting method), and external fixation.
- A minimally invasive approach after closed indirect reduction is used to insert intramedullary nails. Locked intramedullary nails allow multifragmentary fractures to be fixed at the correct length in case of at least partial contact between the main fragments. Intramedullary nails are internal splints that are load-sharing and allow early weight bearing. As they allow a certain degree of movement at the fracture site, their use is associated with callus formation and early bone union.
- Plates and screws may be a good option for shaft fractures that extend to the metaphyseal area or into a joint. They can be inserted either by an open, less invasive, or minimally invasive approach after direct or indirect reduction techniques.
- In simple fractures that are easily reduced anatomically, the conventional interfragmentary lag screw, combined with a protection plate, remains an excellent means of fixation.
- Plating of complex, multifragmentary diaphyseal fractures should be carried out with minimally invasive techniques, using indirect reduction and the locked splinting method, bridging the fracture zone with an internal fixator, and leaving the fracture focus untouched.
- External fixators are still the gold standard in cases of severe soft-tissue injury, and in parts of the world where nails and plates are more difficult to obtain and risks are involved for logistical and technical reasons, such as the unavailability of image intensification. However, fracture healing may be delayed, and pin-track problems (infection, loosening) are common. External fixators are therefore not a popular choice for definitive fixation, and a change of method is often considered either once the soft-tissue problem is solved or in combination with a plastic reconstruction of the soft-tissue envelope.

2.8 Reduction and fixation of articular fractures

- Intraarticular fractures generally require open, direct, and precise reduction, with stable fixation. Only simple or nondisplaced intraarticular fractures can be reduced in a closed manner with image intensification control. All fracture surfaces have to be thoroughly cleaned of hematoma and any early callus. At this stage, loose osteochondral fragments can be removed from the wound, but impacted fragments should not yet be elevated from the underlying cancellous beds. Regardless of their size, all intraarticular fragments should initially be retained as keys to the final reduction. If there is inadequate stability, the large distractor or an external fixator can be used to maintain distraction and axial alignment and to allow a degree of indirect reduction of fracture fragments. The intact joint surfaces and the opposing articular surfaces are used to assess the reduction of displaced or impacted intraarticular fragments. Approaching the fracture via a window created in the metaphyseal cortex, central, depressed fragments can be elevated and reduced. Impacted osteochondral fragments should be elevated from the underlying metaphyseal bone along with an adequate block of cancellous bone using an osteotome or elevator. This technique maintains the connection between the subchondral cortical bone and its underlying cancellous bone, facilitating possible future fixation.
- Although free cartilage or osteochondral fragments without cancellous bone support could be helpful in position-

ing major intraarticular fragments, it would be difficult to fix and maintain their position later if their long-term viability is questionable. They are therefore discarded after they have been used for reduction control of major fragments. Bone defects remaining within the metaphysis are filled with an autogenous cancellous or corticocancellous graft to provide early support for the articular surface and to stimulate reconstitution of metaphyseal bone. Cortical reduction and soft-tissue attachments can guide the reduction of peripheral fracture fragments and their associated articular surfaces. Pointed reduction forceps and K-wires are used to hold the fracture temporarily in position while the accuracy of reduction is confirmed.

- Special circumstances can necessitate deviation from the usual reconstruction protocol. In simple fractures with a single large fragment that has split away from the joint and which is causing instability, closed reduction can be carried out in the operating room. Using image intensification, the reduction can be confirmed and is followed by stabilization of the fracture using guide wires and cannulated screws. In the presence of intraarticular and metaphyseal fragmentation (C3 injuries), there are no parts of the articular surface that are in continuity with the metaphysis. Regularly the first step is reconstruction of the epiphysis (articular fracture), followed by reduction of the joint block to the dia-metaphysis as a second step. Sometimes, the order of the steps of reduction has to be reversed and first the metaphysis is reduced to the diaphysis to anatomical landmarks for epiphyseal reduction and reconstruction.
- Direct inspection of the joint surface, either arthroscopically or through arthrotomy, serves to evaluate the reduction of the cartilaginous surfaces. Intraoperative image intensification or radiography provides information on the bone reduction. Fixation of the intraarticular portion can be completed when reduction is satisfactory.
- Lag screw fixation causes compression between the cancellous surfaces and results in stable fixation of the fragment. Care needs to be taken not to overcompress these fragments. If there are multiple small fragments, reduction of the fracture and support for the small fragments can be maintained with fully threaded position screws to hold the fragments in place without compression. In this case, absolute stability may not be obtained due to the small areas of contact between the fragments.

3 Instruments and techniques

The most important mechanism for reducing a fracture is traction, which is normally applied along the long axis of the limb. In the case of a multifragmentary intraarticular fracture, traction across a joint may be able to reduce fragments by ligamentotaxis (see Tab 1-1). Traction can be applied manually, by means of a traction table, a distractor, or an external fixator.

3.1 Reduction instruments

- **Traction tables.** The widely used traction table has the disadvantage that tracttion is usually applied across at least one joint. The limb cannot be moved by the surgeon, and the surgical approach is frequently compromised (Fig 2-5).
- **Small reduction table.** The small reduction table has the advantage that traction and angular or rotational corrections are applied directly to the main fragments.
- **Distractor.** Applied directly to the main fragments, the distractor makes it possible to maneuver the limb during surgery. Angular or rotational corrections are difficult or even impossible with the distractor under axial load, and the construct may be cumbersome. As there is an inher-

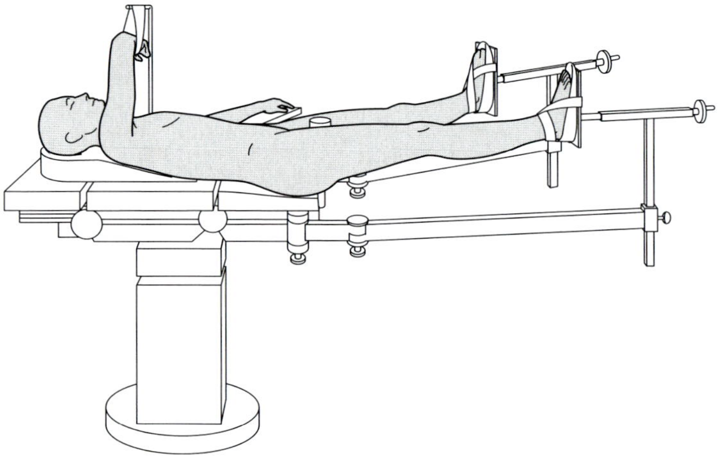

Fig 2-5 Traction table.

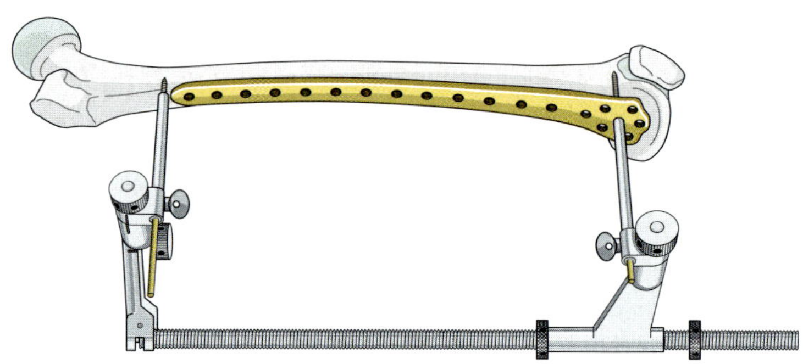

Fig 2-6 LISS distractor.

ent tendency for curved bones to straighten during the distraction procedure, the eccentric force produced by the unilaterally mounted distractor may produce additional deformity (see Fig 2-4).

- **LISS distractor.** The LISS distractor (Fig 2-6) is the combination of the large distractor with the LISS-DF plate. One bolt of the distractor fixes the plate through a plate hole to the distal femur. The other bolt is fixed onto the proximal femur. The LISS distractor allows a controlled application of force (distraction and/or compression) by the reduction maneuver. This makes reduction possible against the plate before final fixation of the LISS plate [8].
- **External fixator.** The external fixator can be used for indirect reduction, but gentle lengthening is more difficult than with the distractor. When traction is applied across a joint (Fig 2-7), ligaments and soft tissues around the fracture area can help achieve reduction through ligamentotaxis (see Tab 1-1) or soft-tissue taxis, respectively. The main fields of application for this device are multifragmentary metaphyseal/epiphyseal fracture, where the condition of the soft tissue or fracture fragmentation does not allow the use of open or direct reduction and stabilization techniques.

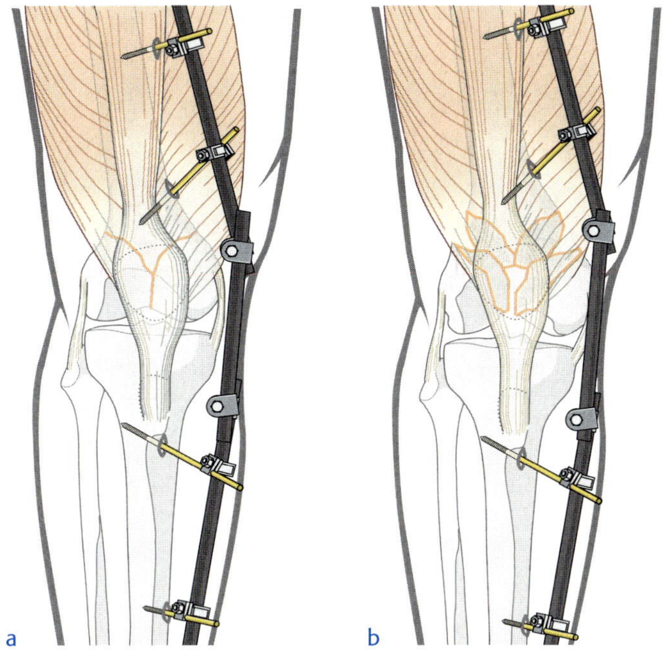

Fig 2-7a–b Joint-bridging external fixator.

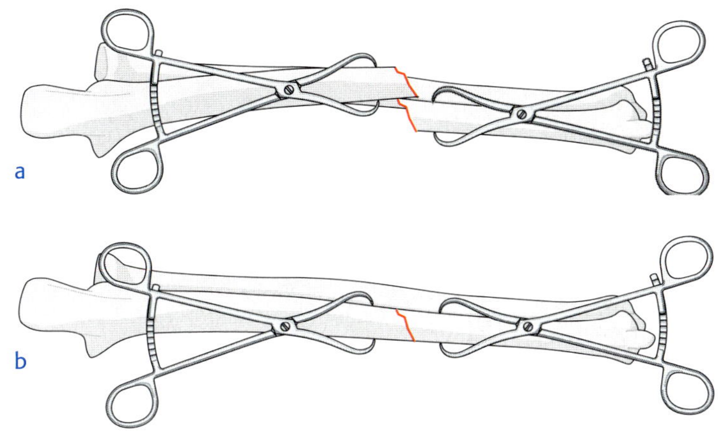

Fig 2-8a–b Direct manual reduction using two pointed reduction forceps.

a Each main fragment is held with a pointed reduction forceps.

b Lengthening is achieved by manual traction while correct rotation and axial alignment can be controlled with the forceps.

3.2 Reduction forceps

- **Pointed reduction forceps** (Weber forceps). The pointed reduction forceps is the first choice as a reduction tool, as it is gentle to the periosteal sleeve and can be used for direct and indirect reduction. Good grip, no slip of the clamp (Fig 2-8).
- **Reduction forceps, serrated jaws**. Due to the angulation of the jaws easier introduction through the second and third window of an ilioinguinal approach and possibility for its use through the greater sciatic notch onto the quadrilateral surface through the Kocher-Langenbeck approach.
- **Bone holding forceps, self-centering** (Verbrugge forceps). The main function of this forceps is to hold a plate to the diaphyseal bone. Due to its specific design, it allows considerable circumferential exposure of the bone, as its pointed end has to reach completely around the bone.

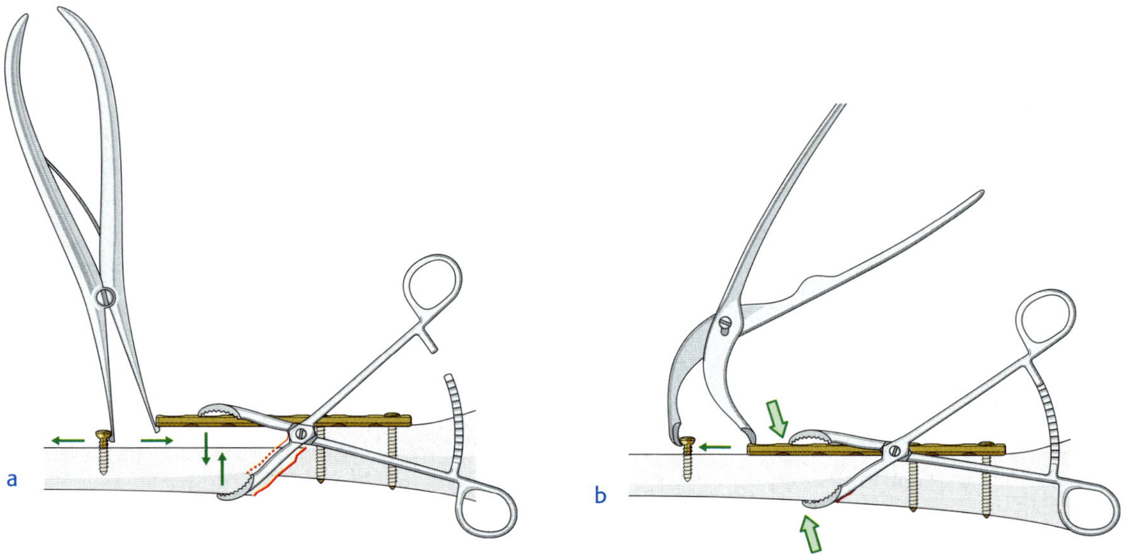

Fig 2-9a–b Push-pull technique.

a The bone spreader, placed between the end of a plate and an independent screw, can be used to distract or push apart the fracture fragments.

b Thereafter, and suing the same independent screw, interfragmentary compression can be obtained by pulling the plate end towards the screw with a small Verbrugge clamps.

- **Bone spreader.** This device can be used for distraction if it is placed between the end of a plate and an independent screw 1 cm from the end of the plate ("push-pull technique") (Fig 2-9).
- **Collinear reduction clamp.** The collinear reduction clamp allows axial reduction of bone fragments through a small skin incision via the axial sliding mechanism on its forceps (Fig 2-10).
- **Pelvic reduction forceps with pointed ball tips** ("King Tong" and "Queen Tong" forceps), symmetrical and asymmetrical. These reduction forceps are mainly used to reduce pelvic ring lesions or acetabular fractures (Fig 2-11).
- **Pelvic reduction forceps** (Farabeuf forceps). The Farabeuf forceps is designed to grasp screw heads inserted on either side of a fracture line (3.5 mm or 4.5 mm screws) (Fig 2-12). Manipulation of the forceps allows compression and also permits limited manipulations in two different planes. However, distraction of the fracture gap is not possible.

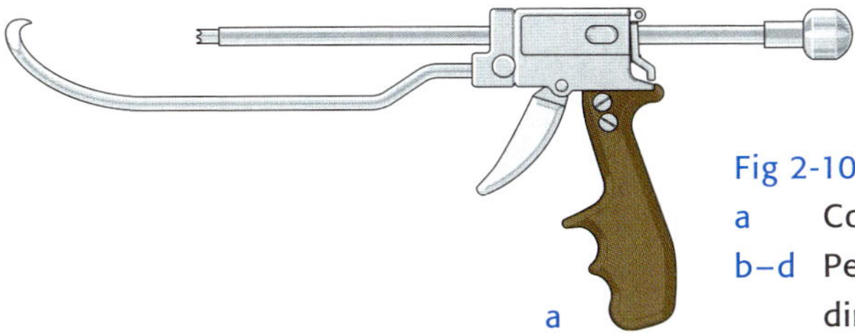

Fig 2-10a–d
a Collinear reduction clamp.
b–d Periprosthetic 32-A1 fracture. Final reduction is achieved directly using the collinear reduction clamp.

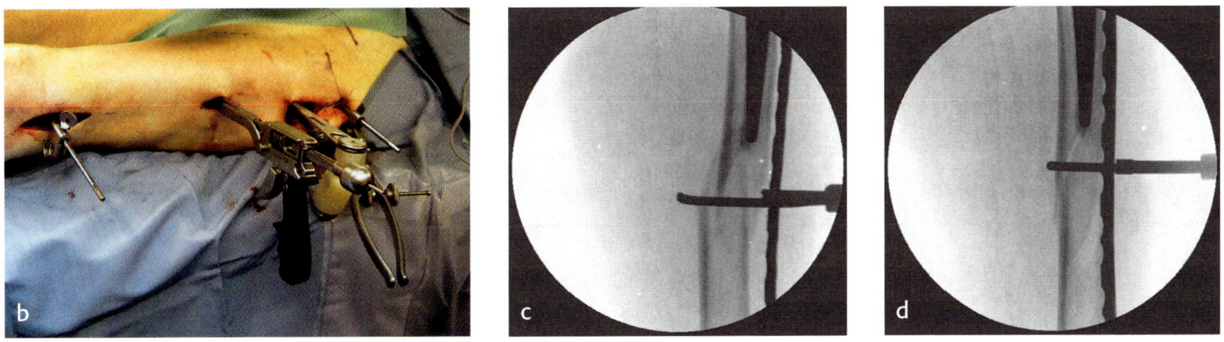

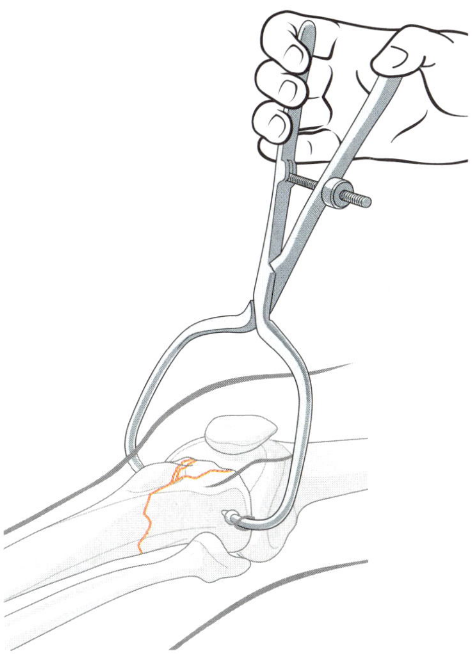

Fig 2-11 Indirect reduction using forceps with ball points.

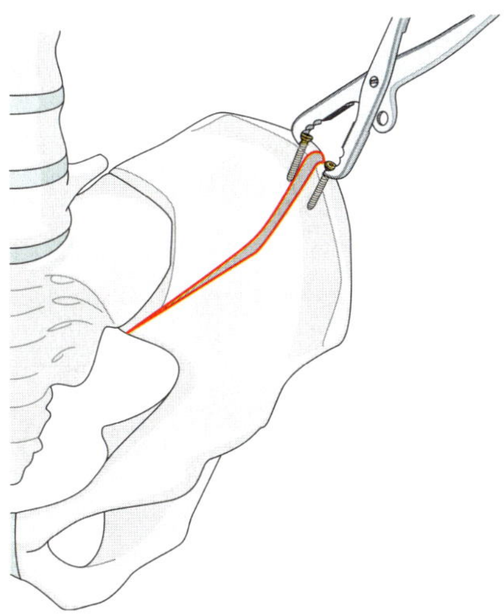

Fig 2-12 The Farabeuf forceps is mainly used for fracture reduction of the pelvic ring in the area of the iliac crest or the SI joint. It is anchored on both sides of the fracture with either 3.5 or 4.5 mm cortex screws. The forceps is helpful only to reduce a side-to-side displacement or to close a fracture gap. Distraction is not possible.

- **Pelvic reduction forceps** (Jungbluth forceps). This is fixed onto both fragments with a 4.5 mm or 3.5 mm cortex screw, allowing the fragments to be moved and reduced in three planes (distraction and compression, as well as lateral displacement in two planes) (Fig 2-13).

3.3 Other instruments, tricks, and hints useful for reduction

- **Hohmann retractor.** In cortical bone, the small-tipped Hohmann retractor can be used as a lever or pusher to achieve reduction (Fig 2-14).
- **Ball spike with pointed ball tip, bone impactor, bone hook.** Fracture reduction in one direction can be carried out by instruments that are designed to push or pull. Using the ball spike, fragments can be pushed firmly into the right position. Through a cannulated version of the ball spike a K-wire for temporary fragment fixation is helpful. The K-wire can also be used to insert a cannulated screw.
- **Joystick reduction.** In manipulation of large bony fragments a Schanz screw can be inserted as a joystick. Large threaded pins with holders are also being devised. The insertion of a Schanz screw into the pelvic ischium is a technique commonly used for manipulation of the posterior column of the acetabulum (in case of a posterior column, transverse, or T-shaped fracture). The open or percutaneous insertion of threaded or unthreaded K-wires allows manipulation of bone fragments with or without direct visualization. The technique is mainly used in intraarticular fractures of the distal radius and proximal humerus [3, 9] (Fig 2-15).
- **Reduction handle, toothed,** to gain and maintain stable intraoperative fixation of fracture (Fig 2-16).

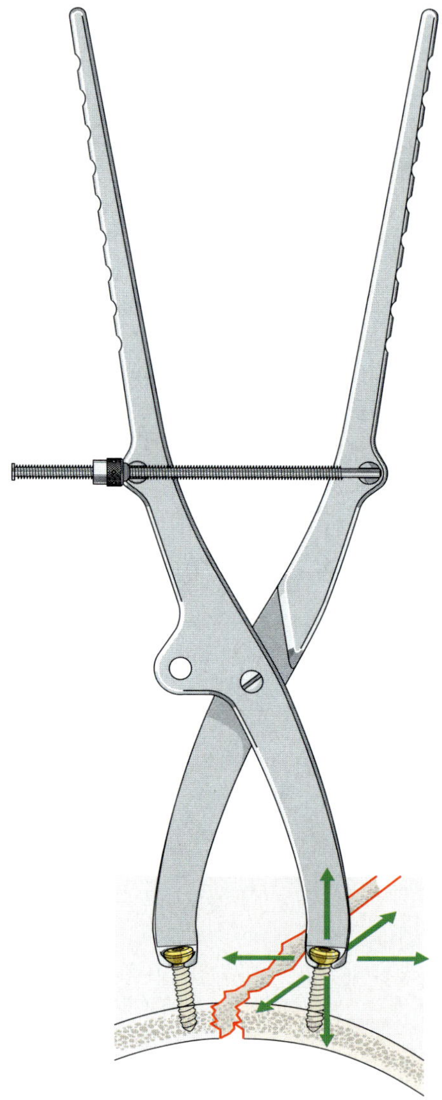

Fig 2-13 The Jungbluth forceps is fixed to fragments with 4.5 mm cortex screws. This firm connection allows translational reduction maneuvers in all three planes.

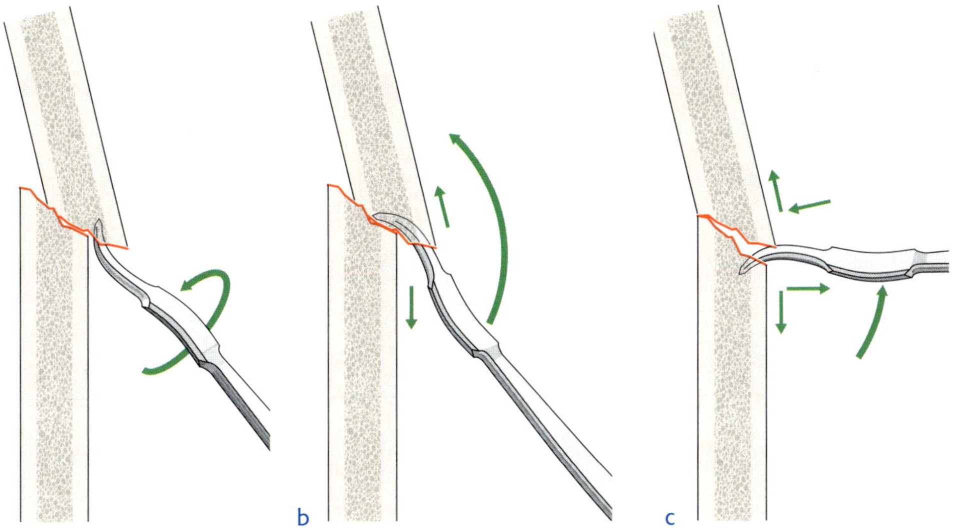

a b c

Fig 2-14a–c Diaphyseal reduction with the small Hohmann retractor. In cortical bone the tip of the Hohmann retractor is placed between the two fragments. By turning and bending the retractor handle the fragments can be disengaged and reduced. Another turn is usually required to remove the Hohmann retractor.

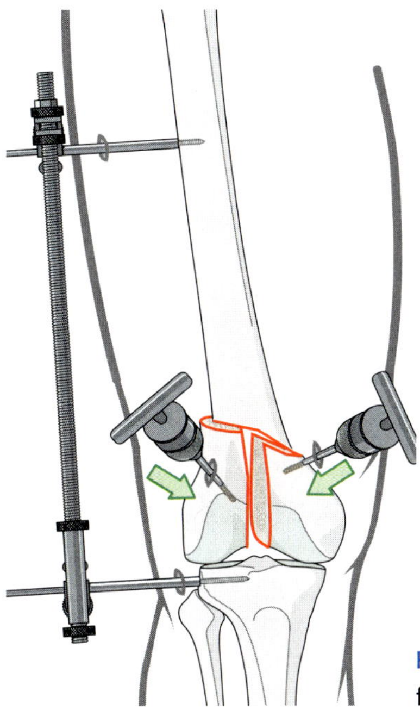

Fig 2-15 The joystick technique may also be used to control rotation of the femoral diaphysis when reducing a supracondylar fracture.

- **Kapandji reduction.** With a K-wire inserted through the fracture gap, the radiostyloid fragment of a distal radial fracture can be manipulated and rotated in a fashion similar to the technique with the Homann retractor. Definitive stabilization is achieved by completing the insertion of the K-wire into the opposite cortex of the bone.
- **Temporary and definitive cerclage.** Temporary cerclage can be helpful in reducing a multifragmentary fracture (mainly butterfly fragments or type B spiral fragments) in the diaphysis. The technique has the disadvantage that it involves temporary circumferential denuding of the bone during application of the wire [2]. Reduction and fixation with wires has attracted increasing interest in the treatment of periprosthetic fractures in elderly patients [10] because it is a low-energy trauma with low soft-tissue compromise.

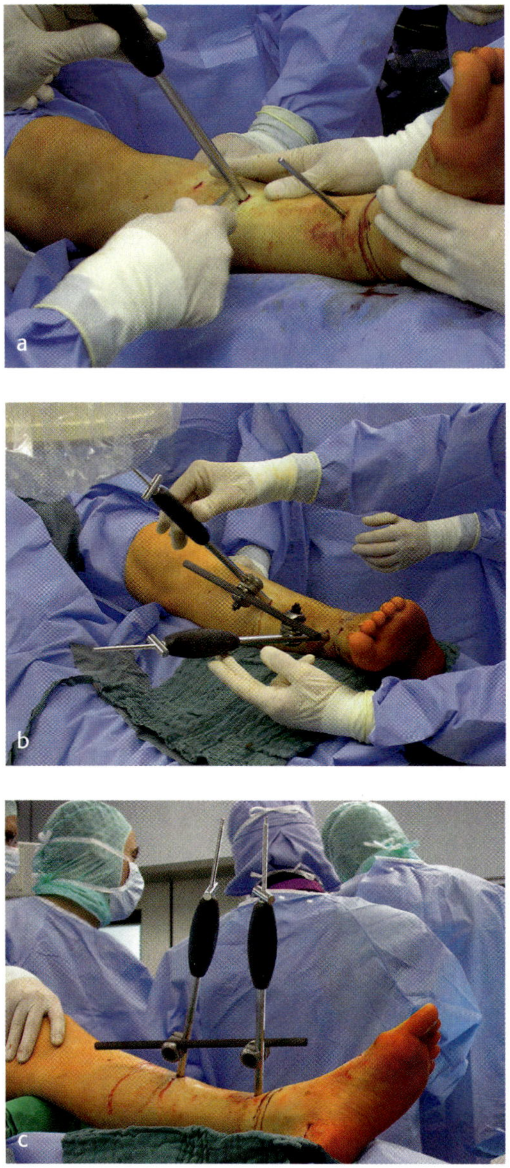

Fig 2-16a–c Reduction with the toothed reduction handles.

a Insertion of the threaded rod and attachment of the reduction handle.

b Applying large combination clamps and a carbon fiber rod without tightening the construct. Reduce the fragments.

c Tighten the combination clamps to temporarily hold the reduction.

3.4 Reduction with the help of implants (reduction onto an implant)

Ideally, an implant should contribute both to the reduction and stabilization of a fracture. Reduction can be achieved using an implant by interfering with the bone.

- **Reduction onto a plate** (see chapter 3). Fractures of any relatively straight portion of the diaphysis can be reduced using a plate that acts as a splint to restore alignment before definitive fixation. Distracting the fracture increases the tension in the soft tissues, which tends to realign the fragments into their original position. The push-pull technique using a bone spreader and the Verbrugge clamp (push-pull clamp) is an elegant and often used method of distracting and reducing a fracture—for example, in forearm bones or in delayed surgery for a malleolar fracture (Fig 2-17).
- **Antiglide plate.** Another simple and gentle reduction mechanism uses the plate for antiglide purposes [11]. Applying a properly contoured plate to one fragment of an oblique metaphyseal fracture results in automatically reducing the opposite fragment. This technique corrects small displacements and angulation while maintaining stability as the reduction takes place (Fig 2-18).
- **Angled blade plate.** When an angled blade plate is correctly inserted into the proximal or distal epiphyseal/metaphyseal segment of the femur, its shape will bring the diaphyseal segment into anatomical alignment. The blade of the plate is first inserted into the proximal or distal end fragment. The shaft is then reduced to the side plate, with the Verbrugge clamp being used to hold the two together. Fine-tuning of the reduction can be achieved with the push–pull technique using the articulated tension device (Fig 2-19) [1,2].

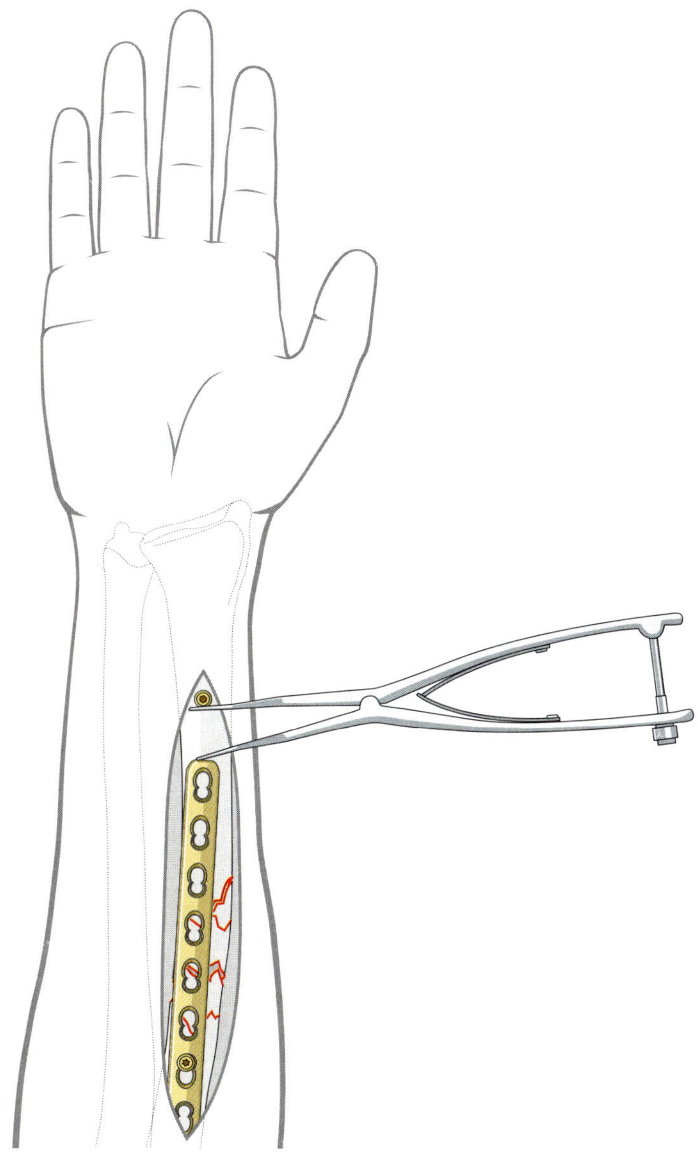

Fig 2-17 Open, but indirect reduction with a bone spreader and a plate.

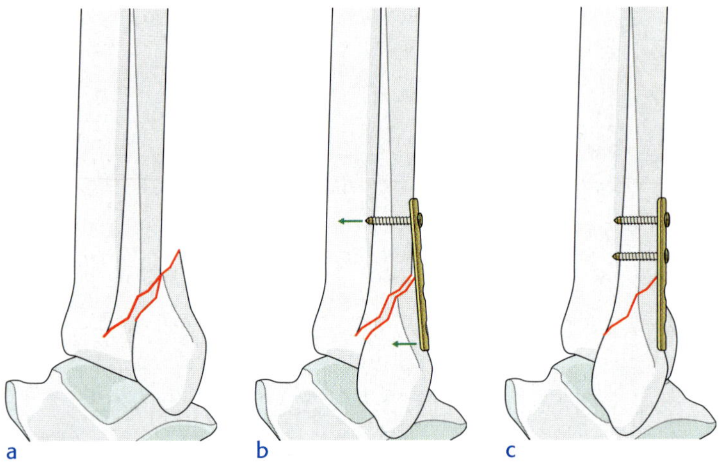

Fig 2-18a–c Indirect reduction with a plate in buttress mode.

a Posteriorly displaced fracture (type B) of the lateral malloelus.

b Fixation of a 4-hole or 5 hole one-third tubular plate posteriorly onto the proximal fragment.

c Tightening of the screw forces the distal fragment to glide distally and anteriorly along the oblique fracture plane into the correct position, where it is firmly locked by the plate.

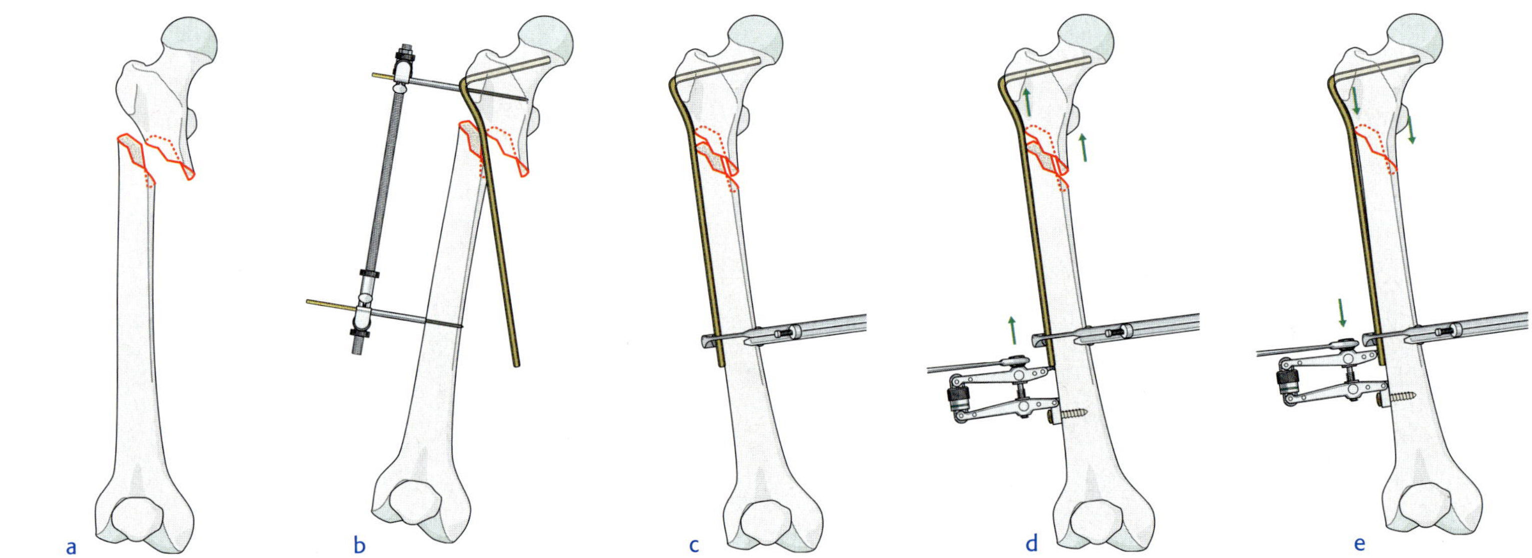

Fig 2-19a–e Reduction with the help of the condylar blade plate.

a Displacement of a proximal femur fracture with the proximal fragment in adduction and flexion.

b Introduction of the 95°angled blade plate (= condylar blade plate) and distraction of the fracture with the large distractor.

c Provisional fixation with a reduction forceps distally.

d Use of the articulating tension device to distract the fracture and to allow complete reduction proximally.

e By reversion of the small hook, the tension device is used for interfragmentary compression.

- **Reduction screw.** A cortex screw can be used to reduce the bone segment onto the plate or to reduce a severely displaced butterfly fragment.
- **Special instruments for locked internal fixators**—less invasive stabilization system (LISS), locking compression plate (LCP), anatomically preshaped LCP. The goals of reduction with the new generation of implants are the same as they were with the conventional standard plates. However, these implants appear to be more difficult to apply, particularly if they are used as internal fixators with submuscular or subcutaneous insertion in combination with indirect reduction techniques. In this type of situation, the diaphyseal fracture has to be reduced first using a distraction device temporarily maintaining the correct alignment of the bone. Anatomically preshaped LISS- and LCP plates are then inserted without additional contouring. Non anatomically preshaped plates should be approximately contoured according the anatomical location, to avoid undesired disturbance of covering soft tissue. The implant is then inserted and fixed to the bone with locking head screws. The implant is then inserted without preshaping and fixed to the bone with locking head screws. Only a few instruments are available to help the surgeon accomplish this difficult task. One of these is the "whirlybird" instrument, which allows correction of varus and valgus deformities with a LISS in position [12] (Fig 2-20; Fig | Animation 2-21). Anatomically preshaped plates (LISS, special LCP) make the reduction maneuver easier and can be fixed onto the metaphyseal fracture fragment first.

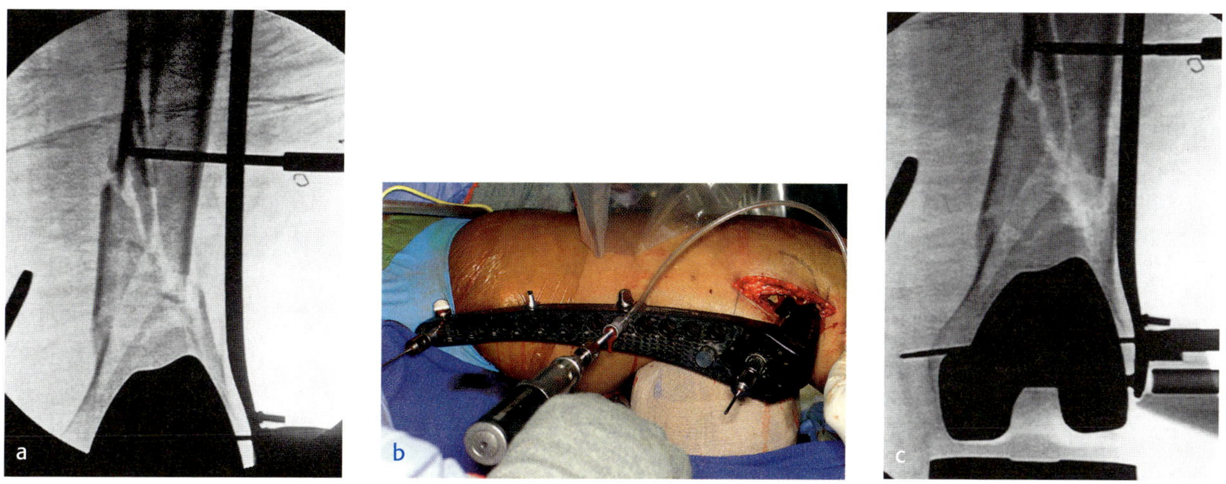

Fig 2-20a–c Pulling device ("whirlybird").
Correction of varus and valgus deformities with a LISS plate in position.

Animation 2-21

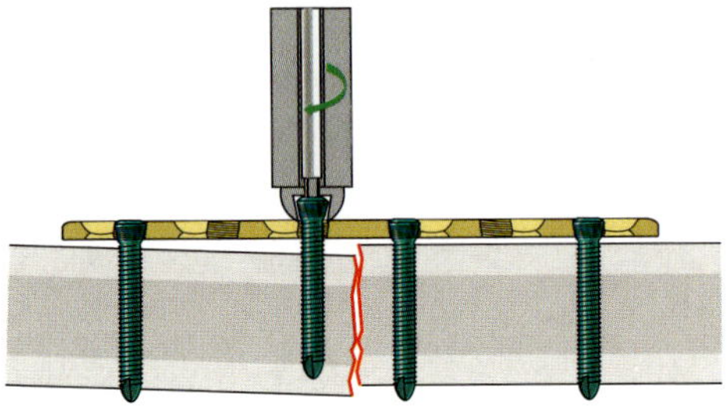

Fig | Animation 2-21 "Whirlybird".

- **Fine-tuning.** Using LHS, the screw driver and the screw holding sleeve allows correction of varus and valgus deformities and reduction onto the plate.

3.5 Minimally invasive reduction

There are two different principles of reduction for minimally invasive plate osteosynthesis (MIPO). The first principle is indirect reduction which implies traction along the axis of the limb and the help of the soft tissues for the reduction maneuver (ligamentotaxis). The second principle is direct reduction which means that the reduction is achieved close to the fracture and percutaneously.

Direct fracture reduction for MIPO

Hazards:

- Exposure can be too wide
- Excessive periosteal stripping

Aids for direct reduction:

- Towel
- Joystick
- Hohmann retractor
- Plate
- Screw
- Collinear reduction clamp
- Pointed reduction forceps
- Cerclage wire

Indication:

- Articular fractures
- Simple metaphyseal fractures
- Irreducible fractures
- Osteotomies, nonunions

Goals for direct fracture reduction for MIPO:

- Anatomical reconstruction
- Absolute stability by rigid fixation

Indirect fracture reduction for MIPO

Indication:

- Diaphyseal fractures

Goals for indirect fracture reduction for MIPO:

- Restoration of length, axis, and rotation
- Correct position of the adjacent joints
- Individual fracture fragments need not be anatomically reduced

Aids for indirect reduction:

- Manual traction
- Large distractor
- Push-pull forceps
- Traction table
- External fixator

4 Assessment of reduction

Once a fracture has been reduced using either direct or indirect techniques, it has to be checked. There are various ways of doing this, including direct visualization, palpation (digital or instrumental), clinical observation, radiography, image intensification, indirect vision using an arthroscope or an endoscope, or with a computer-guided or computer-assisted system. Some of these techniques are more reliable than others; however, much depends on their availability.

The small indentations or landmarks that are present in every fracture line have to be noted if the fracture focus is visible. If a fracture surface cannot be directly visualized but can be reached with the fingertip, palpation may be helpful—for example, of the quadrilateral surface in the pelvis to check the reduction of an acetabular fracture. This can also be carried out with an appropriate instrument to evaluate the accuracy of reduction of an articular surface—for example, in a tibial plateau fracture. Clinical assessment of reduction and rotational alignment may be difficult and unreliable, but it is often necessary, particularly in closed intramedullary nailing or MIPO in case of shaft fracture of the leg.

Whenever possible, intraoperative checking of the fracture reduction and fixation should be carried out using image intensification or radiography in two planes.

4.1 Intraoperative techniques for checking alignment

Length. Restoring length in a simple fracture is usually uncomplicated. The individual fracture configuration will offer some guide in assessing length. The surgeon can math the geometry of fracture fragments and make sure they are in the same level. In the case of complex fractures the risk of obtaining an incorrect length is much higher. Preoperative measurement of the appropriate implant lenght (intramedullary nail) of the unaffected side is useful and this reading will serve as a guideline to the surgeon.

The surgeon can compare reduction with the unaffected side during surgery. Such comparison can only be possible if the patient is lying supine. The contralateral femoral length is measured taking the femoral head and the lateral femoral condyle as reference and marking the length on the measuring device using a clip. The injured side is measured identically and the length discrepancy can be easily determined. When a ram with a handle is used, the limb length can be adjusted continuously in both directions. The length of the tibia is much easier to evaluate than that of the femur, and clinical methods are usually sufficient. In some cases the reduced simple fibula fracture is helpful.

Frontal–sagittal plane. In simple midshaft fractures of the femur and tibia, frontal and sagittal plane alignment is usually not a problem. While CCD (caput-collum-diaphysis) angles can be measured and checked by image intensification, the evaluation of the correct weight-bearing axis is usually more difficult, especially in complex, multifragmentary, or metaphyseal fractures. But the use of a straight implant on a more or less straight portion of the diaphysis makes alignment easier.

The cable technique (Fig 2-22) considerably facilitates intraoperative assessment of axial alignment in the frontal plane. With the patella facing anteriorly, the centers of the femoral head and of the ankle joint are marked under image intensification either on the skin or the surgical drapes. The long cable of the electrocautery is then spanned between these two points, with the image intensifier centered on the knee joint. Varus/valgus alignment can now be determined using the projection of the cable. Sagittal alignment is determined using a lateral x-ray.

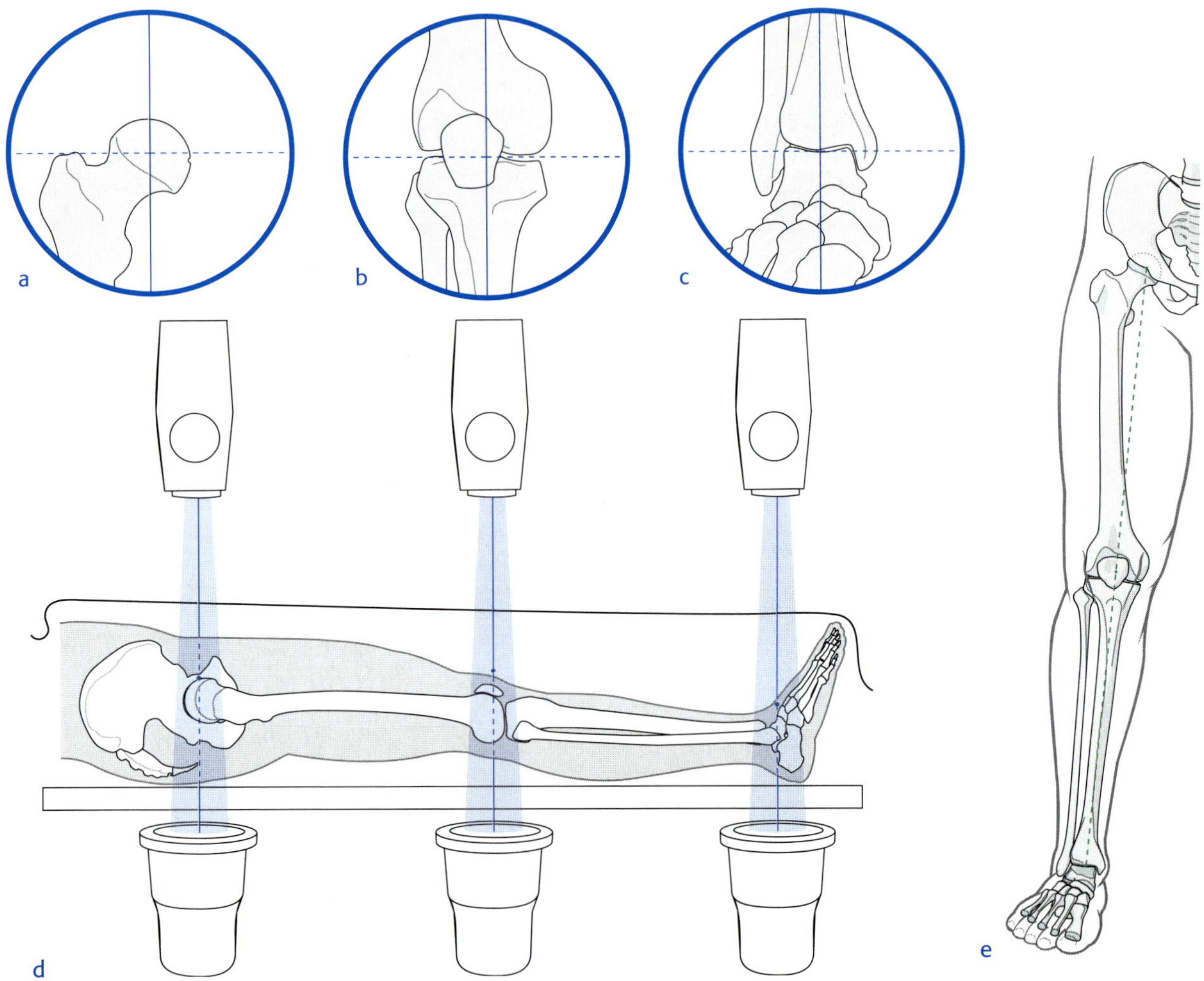

Fig 2-22a–e The cable technique considerably facilitates intraoperative assessment of axial alignment in the frontal plane.

- a With the image intensifier beam strictly vertical, the center of the femoral head is centered on the screen. A pen then marks the center of the femoral head on the patient's skin.
- b When the knee joint is viewed the cable should run centrally. Any deviation of the projected cautery cable from the center of the joint indicates the axial deviation in the frontal plane.
- c In a similar way the center of the ankle joint is marked. An assistant now spans the cable of the electrocaution between these two landmarks.
- d View from lateral.
- e Cautery cord spans from the center of the femoral head to the center of the ankle joint.

Rotation. There are several methods for intraoperative assessment of the rotation of nailed or bridged fractures of the femur and the tibia. Clinical assessment is not very precise and depends on the positions of the patient and the leg during surgery. Preoperatively, the rotation of the intact limb is established, with the knee and the hip flexed at 90°. Intraoperatively, after nailing and temporary locking of the fractured bone, the rotation is checked again. In the tibia, rotation should be checked with the knee in flexion and the foot dorsiflexed. However, in addition to comparisons of the position of the feet, the range and symmetry of foot rotation also have to be taken into account. Rotation control after reduction and fixation: using a lateral x-ray of the knee joint and an AP of the ankle joint.

Several signs are available to assist radiographic assessment of femoral rotation. These include the lesser trochanter sign, the cortical step sign, and the bone diameter sign:

- **Lesser trochanter sign.** (Fig 2-23) The radiographic contour of the lesser trochanter relative to the proximal femoral shaft depends on the rotation of the bone. Preoperatively, the shape of the lesser trochanter of the uninjured

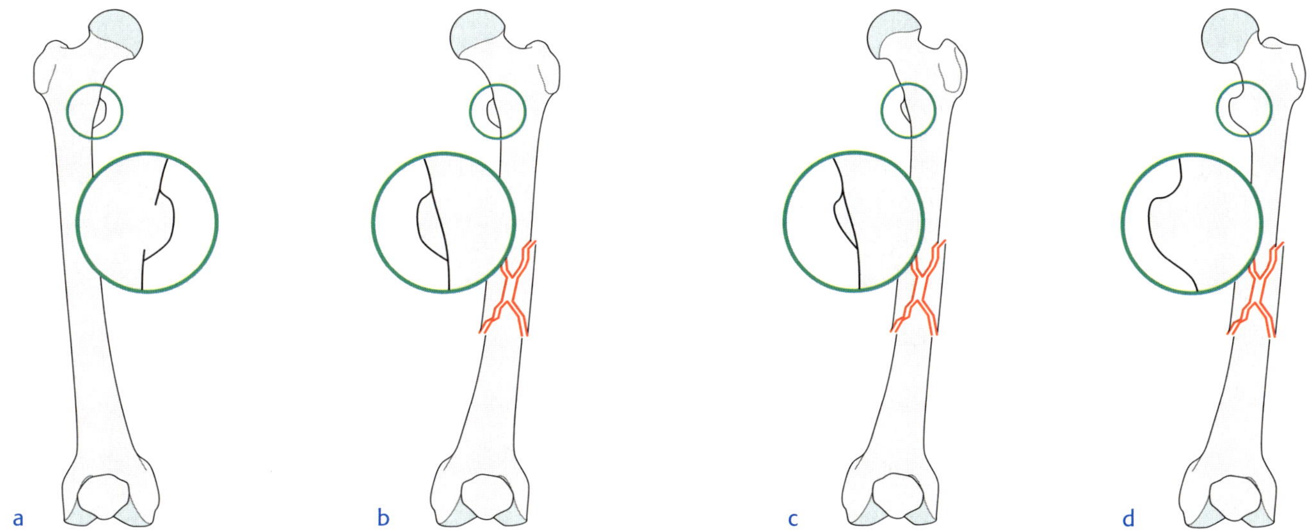

Fig 2-23a–d Intraoperative radiological assessment of rotation, with comparison of the shape of the lesser traochanter with the contraletarl side (lesser trochanter shape sign).

a Before positioning the patient, the shape of the lesser trochanter of the intact opposite side (patella facing anteriorly) is stored in the image intensifier.

b After distal locking and the patella facing anteriorly, the proximal fragment is rotated until the shape of the lesser trochanter matches the one of the intact side already stored.

c In cases of external malrotation the lesser trochanter is smaller and partially hidden behind the proximal femoral shaft.

d In cases of internal malrotation the lesser trochanter appears enlarged.

jured limb is stored as a digital image. The hip, with the patella facing in an anterior direction, is analyzed and the image stored in the image intensifier. Before proximal locking, with the patella still facing forward, the proximal fragment can be rotated around the nail using a Schanz screw until the shape of the lesser trochanter appears to be symmetrical with that on the stored image from the uninjured side. In the case of an external malrotation, the lesser trochanter is smaller because it is partially hidden by the femoral shaft. With internal malrotation, however, the lesser trochanter looks larger.

- **Cortical step sign.** (Fig 2-24) In transverse or short oblique fractures, the correct rotation can be judged by the thickness of the cortices of the proximal and distal main fragments.
- **Bone diameter sign.** (Fig 2-25) This is helpful at levels at which the bone diameter is oval rather than round. In cases of malrotation, the transverse diameters of the proximal and distal fragments are projected with different diameters. However, all these signs are not very accurate. Rotational malalignment of less than 10°–15° are not detectable with either one of the three methods.

4.2 Computer-assisted reduction

The most recent developments include the use of computer-guided systems to assist placement of instruments and implants and to localize bone fragments three-dimensionally. These systems are based on direct intraoperative imaging with an image intensifier or preoperative computed tomography. Anatomical landmarks on the proximal and distal side of the fracture zone can provide a basis for calculating residual displacement (translational or rotational) using specific mathematical algorithms [13, 14]. In the future, semi-automatic reduction of long-bone fractures at least can be envisaged.

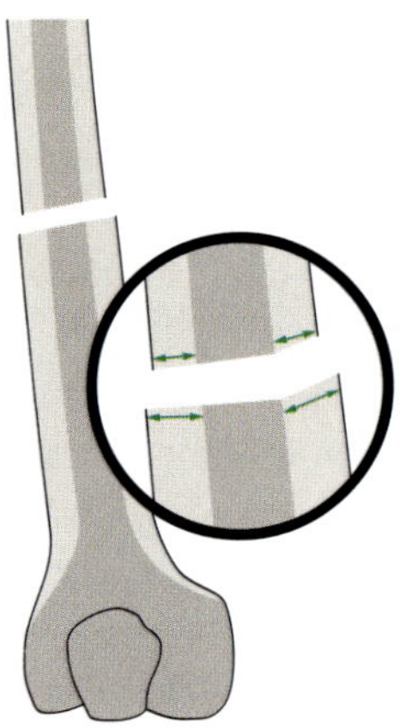

Fig 2-24 **Cortical step sign. In the presence of a considerable rotational deformity, this can be diagnosed by the different thickness of the cortices.**

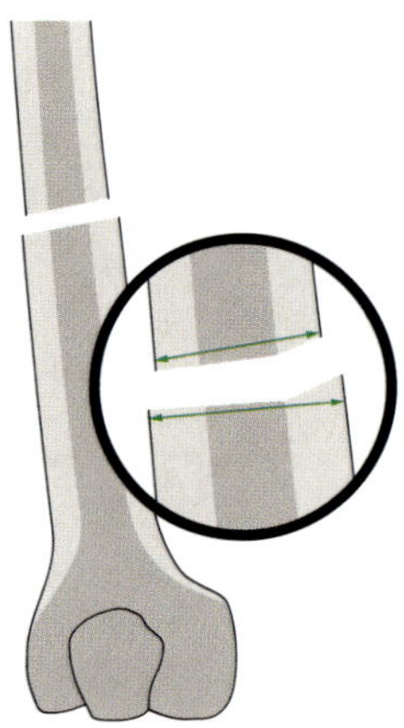

Fig 2-25 **Diameter difference sign. This sign is positive at levels where the bone cross-section is oval rather than round. With malrotation, the diameters of proximal and distal main fragments appear to be of different sizes.**

5 Conclusions

Reduction technique is extremely important. Reduction needs to take into account both the soft tissues and the fracture configuration and should not compromise the healing process. This is the first step in determining surgical strategy. A sense of balance needs to be maintained based on the injury, location, and fracture. The words "correct" and "anatomical" now refer to reduction techniques that are mechanically adequate and minimally harmful to the soft tissues. Thorough planning and adaptation of the technique to the given individual situation is essential in all cases.

6 Bibliography

1. **Mast J, Jakob R, Ganz R** (1989) *Planning and Reduction Technique in Fracture Surgery*. 1st ed. Berlin Heidelberg New York: Springer-Verlag.
2. **Müller ME, Allgöwer M, Schneider R, et al** (1990) *Manual of Internal Fixation*. 3rd ed. Berlin Heidelberg New York: Springer-Verlag.
3. **Schatzker J, Tile M** (1987) *The Rationale of Operative Fracture Care*. 3rd ed. Berlin Heidelberg New York: Springer-Verlag.
4. **Marsh JL, Buckwalter J, Gelberman R, et al** (2002) Articular fractures: does anatomical reduction really change the result? *J Bone Joint Surg Am*; 84(7):1259–1271.
5. **Leunig M, Hertel R, Siebenrock KA, et al** (2000) The evolution of indirect reduction techniques for the treatment of fractures. *Clin Orthop Relat Res*; (375):7–14.
6. **Ruedi T, Sommer C, Leutenegger A** (1998) New techniques in indirect reduction of long bone fractures. *Clin Orthop Relat Res*; (347):27–34.
7. **Gautier E, Perren SM, Ganz R** (1992) Principles of internal fixation. *Curr Orthop*; 6:220–232.
8. **Babst R, Hehli M, Regazzoni P** (2001) [LISS tractor. Combination of the "less invasive stabilization system" (LISS) with the AO distractor for distal femur and proximal tibial fractures.] *Unfallchirurg*; 104(6):530–535.
9. **Heim U, Pfeiffer KM** (1988) *Internal Fixation of Small Fractures*. 3rd ed. Berlin Heidelberg New York: Springer-Verlag.
10. **Mouhsine E, Garofalo R, Borens O, et al** (2004) Cable fixation and early total hip arthroplasty in the treatment of acetabular fractures in elderly patients. *J Arthroplasty*; 19(3):344–348.
11. **Weber BG** (1981) *Special Techniques in Internal Fixation*. Berlin Heidelberg New York: Springer Verlag.
12. **Cole PA, Zlowodzki M, Kregor PJ** (2003) Less Invasive Stabilization System (LISS) for fractures of the proximal tibia: indications, surgical technique and preliminary results of the UMC Clinical Trial. *Injury*; 34(Suppl 1):16–29.
13. **Hüfner T, Pohlemann T, Tarte S, et al** (2002) Computer-assisted fracture reduction of pelvic ring fractures: an in vitro study. *Clin Orthop Relat Res*; (399):231–239.
14. **Messmer P** (2001) Computergestützte dreidimensionale Osteosyntheseplanung und -simulation auf der Grundlage zweidimensionaler Röntgenbilder und ihre Bedeutung für die Ausbildung. Habilitation Universität Basel.

3 Techniques and procedures in LISS and LCP

3 Techniques and procedures in LISS and LCP

1 The less invasive stabilization system (LISS)

1.1 Implants and instruments

Although the less invasive stabilization system (LISS) may appear to be quite complex (see chapter 1), it actually requires very few instruments. These have been specially designed for the system and are not available in the standard instrument sets for plates and screws.

The system consists of instruments required to join the fixator and the insertion guide together. These include the stabilization bolt, fixation bolt, and drill sleeve. The other instruments have been designed to facilitate the temporary positioning of the fixator, the adjustment of its position, and reduction before the first screws are inserted to attach the fixator to the bone. These include K-wires that can be inserted through the insertion guide and the aiming device for K-wires.

LISS plate

The LISS plate is designed for the distal lateral femur aspect (LISS-DF) and the proximal lateral tibia (LISS-PLT) and acts as an anatomically shaped buttress plate anchored with self-drilling, self-tapping, monocortical locking head screws. The screws are connected with the plate by a thread on the outer edge of the screw head and on the inner edge of the plate hole. The LISS is an anatomically preshaped internal fixator that can be inserted percutaneously by means of an adaptable insertion guide. The LISS is as a true internal fixator since longer constructs are applied than in conventional plating. The LISS-DF and the LISS-PLT are available in three lengths (5, 9, or 13 holes), right and left version. With the development of the LCP combination hole there are also two anatomically preshaped LCP-DF and LCP-PLT available (Fig 3-1).

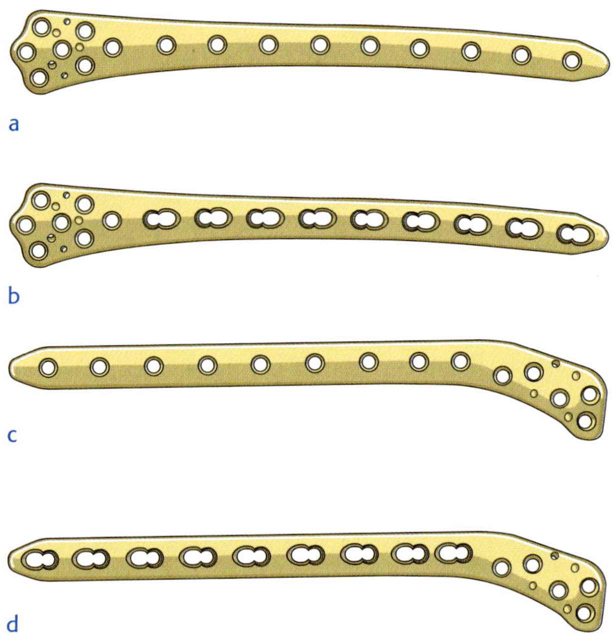

Fig 3-1a–d Different types of internal fixators for the distal femur and the proximal lateral tibia.

- a LISS-DF plate
- b LCP-DF plate
- c LISS-PLT plate
- d LCP-PLT plate

Locking head screws (LHS)

There are only self-drilling, self-tapping LHS in the LISS set (see chapter 1). In case of osteoporotic bone with very thin cortex, bicortical self-tapping locking head screws from the LCP 4.5/5.0 set can be used to fix the LISS to the shaft fragment (Fig 3-2a–c).

Self-tapping periprosthetic locking head screws

It became apparent during development of the LISS that the self-drilling locking head screw, with its long drill tip, could not be used in the area of the prosthetic shaft in the treatment of periprosthetic fractures. Consequently, a self-tapping locking head screw that provides adequate stability even in very thin cortical bone above the level of the prosthesis was developed. As these screws require predrilling, a 4.3 mm drill and drill guide were designed for the purpose (Fig 3-2d). The drill guide can be screwed into the holes of the fixator to ensure precise predrilling.

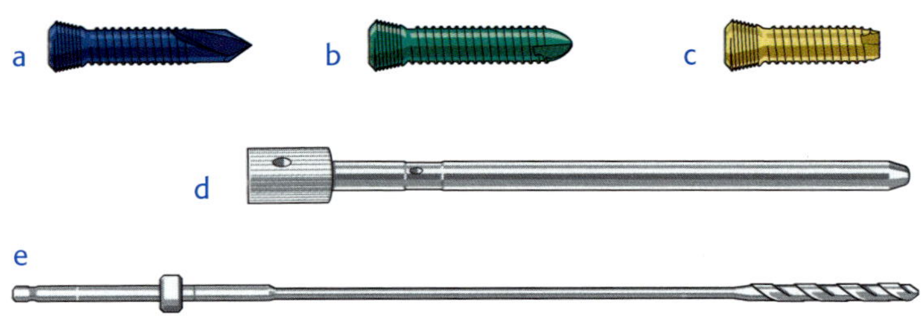

Fig 3-2a–e Different types of locking head screws.
a Self-drilling, self-tapping locking head screw.
b Self-tapping locking head screw.
c Periprosthetic locking head screw.
d–e Drill guide and 4.3 mm drill for periprosthetic LHS.

Insertion guide

The guide used to insert and position the implant consists of two parts: an aluminum part with a three-point connection to the fixator and a radiopaque carbon-reinforced polyetheretherketone (PEEK) attachment (Fig 3-3).

Aiming device

The aiming device for the K-wires positioned at the proximal end of the fixator is shown in Fig 3-4a. Proximal and distal placement and adjustment of the fixator position can be car-

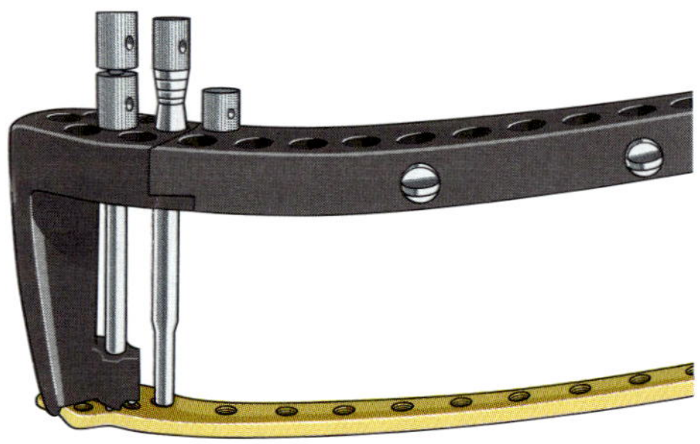

Fig 3-3 The two-part radiopaque insertion guide for the LISS-DF implant, with the fixation bolt, drill sleeve, and stabilization bolt.

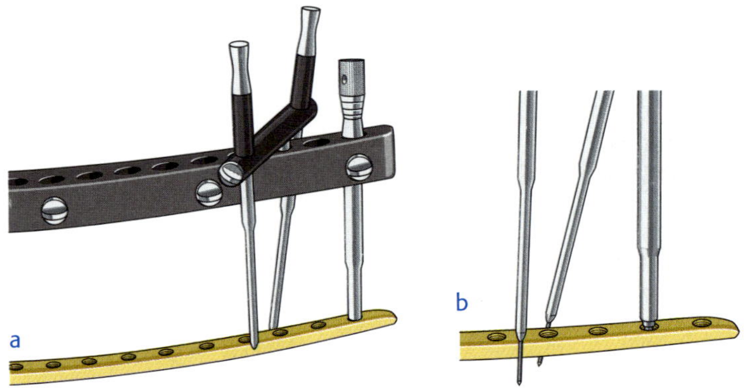

Fig 3-4a–b Aiming device for K-wires.
a The aiming device is centered by the help of the insertion guide.
b Temporary fixation of the LISS with K-wires.

ried out after removal of the K-wire sleeves and the aiming device. At the same time, the lateral K-wires prevent the internal fixator from migrating into the sagittal plane. Once the correct position has been determined, the fixator can be locked temporarily with a K-wire through the fixation bolt or the stabilization bolt (Fig 3-4b).

Pulling device ("whirlybird")

Fracture reduction often has to be fine-tuned during the LISS procedure. The pulling device allows fine adjustment of the angulation and translation of fragments in the frontal plane (Fig 3-5).

However, that is not its only application.It is also recommended for insertion of the very first screw, as the bone is capable of migrating medially during the first screw insertion. If the pulling device is used in an adjacent hole, then the fixator is attached to the bone and migration is prevented.

Drill sleeve

The development of the self-drilling Schanz screw showed that it was possible to design self-drilling screws that would generate no more heat during insertion than that generated by a new, sharp drill bit. A hot drill bit is removed from the bone once the hole has been drilled, whereas the self-drilling screw is left in the bone. In standard open procedures, drills can be irrigated, but this is not possible in minimally invasive percutaneous procedures. So a special water-cooled drill sleeve was developed for use during blind percutaneous insertion of the screws, to conduct heat away from the drilling site. The drill sleeve consists of a standard syringe and infusion set and is used together with a special power screwdriver shaft that directs cooling sterile saline to the screw–bone interface (Fig 3-6).

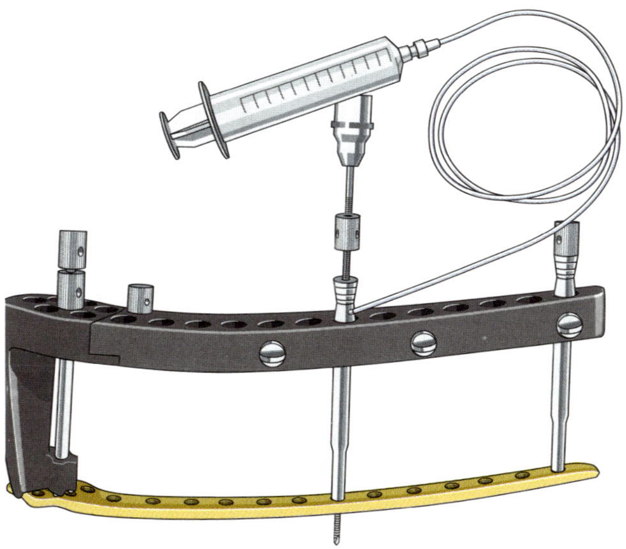

Fig 3-5 Use of the pulling device through the drill sleve. The drill sleeve is connected to a syringe with an infusion tube to ensure cooling of the self-drilling pulling device.

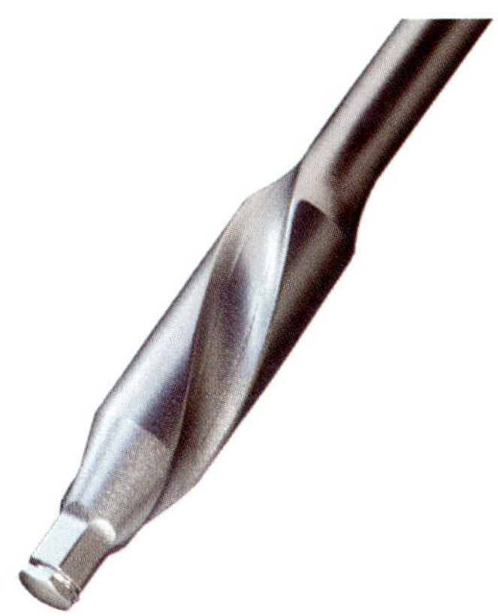

Fig 3-6 Special power screwdriver that directs cooling sterile saline to the screw-bone interface.

To prevent the drill sleeve from spinning and entangling the infusion line, the drill sleeve was designed to mate over a short distance with a matching square section in the insertion guide. In addition, the end of the hexagonal screwdriver shaft has a small retaining ring or bolt that prevents the screw from falling into the drill sleeve during insertion. This is very important, since the self-drilling screws can only be inserted by machine and not manually. Inadequate linkage between the hexagonal recess of the screw and the screwdriver shaft could damage the recess in the screw head.

Torque-limiting hexagonal screwdriver

The connection between the screw head and the fixator is very important for the long-term stability of the whole construct. However, this requires minimum tightening moment of the screw in the fixator while at the same time the connection has to be protected against over tightening. A torque-limiting hexagonal screwdriver was therefore specially designed that disengages at a defined moment of 4.0 Nm—ensuring adequate tightening moment while simultaneously protecting the system against over tightening (Fig 3-7). All of the locking head screws have to be tightened with the torque-limiting screwdriver. Tightening the screws with a power-driven device should always be avoided.

Animation 2-21

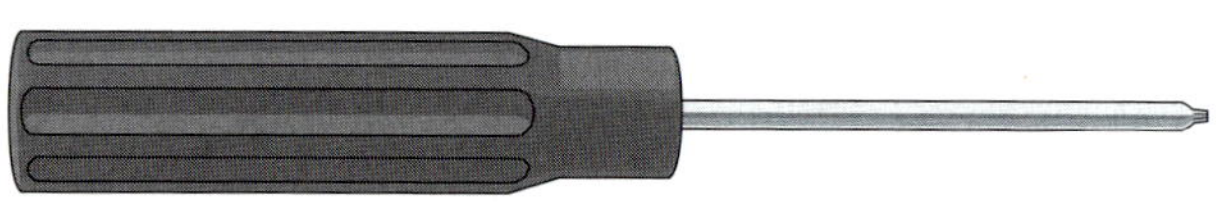

Fig 3-7 The torque-limiting hexagonal screwdriver ensures adequate tightening.

Aids in reduction and LISS fixation

A number of complementary concepts are helpful in closed reduction techniques (see chapter 2). These include:

- **Early intervention.** Fractures are addressed as soon as possible. If shattered, high-energy fractures are not stabilized within the first 24 hours, an external bridging of the fracture zone is applied to maintain the length of the fractured limb.
- **Muscle relaxation by chemical paralysis.** Complete clinical paralysis of the patient is necessary.
- **Supracondylar towel rolls.** Supracondylar towel rolls (bumps) are placed in the area posterior to the supracondylar region. The towel rolls are helpful for reduction of the hyperextension of the distal femoral fragment that is commonly seen. In addition, the towel roll acts as a fulcrum for the vector force of manual traction. Relatively small adjustments in the size and/or location of the towel rolls can have a marked effect on correction of the fracture in the sagittal plane.
- **Manual traction.** Forceful manual traction is helpful for establishing length and rotation and may facilitate varus/valgus correction. Manual traction is applied to the ankle region with a force vector that is directed posteriorly. With the towel rolls being used as a fulcrum, manual traction facilitates reduction of the hyperextension deformity of the distal femoral condyle.
- **Schanz screw inserted into the femoral condyle.** Particularly when there is a very short distal femoral segment, correction of the hyperextension deformity may be difficult. In such cases it is helpful to use an anterior-to-posterior Schanz screw or reduction handles as a joystick to derotate the distal fragment into the proper reduction.
- **Pulling device** ("whirlybird") (see Fig 3-5, and Fig | Animation 2-21). The pulling device is a self-drilling, self-tapping screw that can be drilled through a drill sleeve into the diaphyseal cortex, either in the distal or the proximal region. Screwing a knurled nut onto the LISS pulling de-

vice will actually approximate the cortex (ie, fragment) to the LISS fixator. The device can therefore be used to make small corrections in varus/valgus deformities. More than one pulling device can be used to achieve small translation corrections of the proximal segment. Placement of the pulling device can be likened to clamp placement, as it stabilizes the reduction during insertion of the self-drilling, self-tapping screws.

- **Mallet.** A mallet is occasionally necessary to push medially on an adducted and/or flexed proximal fragment. It can also be used on the distal fragment to correct excess valgus (see case 9.3.7).
- **Large distractor or external fixator.** The large distractor or external fixator can be useful in achieving and maintaining metaphyseal and diaphyseal reduction. However, its use may make fine adjustments in fracture reduction difficult.
- **LISS distractor.** The LISS distractor is the combination of the large distractor with the LISS-DF plate. One bolt of the distractor fixes the plate through a plate hole to the distal femur. The other bolt is fixed onto the proximal femur. The LISS distractor allows a controlled application of force (distraction and/or compression) by the reduction maneuver. This makes reduction possible against the plate before final fixation of the LISS plate. Modification of the well-known LISS technique by integrating the distractor into the LISS plate to simplify reduction and to provide temporary retention of the fracture has the potential to reduce the fluoroscopy exposure, the operation time, the rate of malalignments, and the learning curve for this MIPO technique.
- **Small reduction table.** The small reduction table facilitates fine adjustments to fracture reduction.
- **Collinear reduction clamp or large pelvic reduction forceps.** Both clamps and forceps are often used for reduction maneuver in MIPO technique.

1.2 Less invasive stabilization system for the distal femur (LISS-DF)

Indications

The indications for LISS in the distal femur include all extraarticular (supracondylar, distal shaft) and articular fractures [1] that cannot be treated with screws alone—for example, Müller AO Classification 33-A1–A3 and 33-C1–C3 fractures of the distal femur (Tab 3-1) [2]. The LISS technique is advantageous in severe articular fractures [3], as it allows free placement of lag screws and does not additionally disrupt the condylar complex after reconstruction. It preserves the soft tissues in the metaphyseal and diaphyseal regions as a result of minimally invasive insertion and closed reduction [1, 4, 5]. LISS also makes it possible to stabilize fractures where implants are already in situ—eg, total knee replacements [6]—whether they have a medullary stem or not. Since screws can be inserted into all seven distal screw holes, the LISS offers a high degree of stability and reliability in osteoporotic bone [7–11].

Indications for LISS-DF in femoral fractures
Supracondylar fractures (33-A1–A3)
Articular fractures (33-C1–C3)
Distal shaft fractures (32-B1–B3 and 32-C1–C3 if nailing is not possible)
Periprosthetic fractures (distal to hip prosthesis or proximal to knee prosthesis)
Repeated fracture with implants in place
Fractures in osteoporotic bone
Pathological fractures

Tab 3-1

No other implant currently available has such a wide range of applications. There are certain cases for which LISS provides a unique solution, especially when the distal articular block of the femur is short. These include: multiplane, complex distal articular injuries, especially with a short distal segment, osteoporotic fractures, and fractures above total knee arthoplasties.

Timing

Surgical stabilization of distal femoral fractures should only be carried out by a surgeon with adequate understanding of the fracture, a suitable surgical team, and stable patient conditions. If these conditions are not available, then particularly in the case of high-energy, highly displaced fractures, an external joint bridging fixator can provide an excellent temporary device with which to stabilize the limb, maintain limb length, and minimize movement at the fracture site, which generally aggravates soft-tissue swelling. External fixator pins placed at a significant distance from the knee joint (eg, in the proximal femur and distal tibia) will not compromise the future surgical site for the supracondylar femoral fracture.

Radiography and computed tomography

AP, lateral, and oblique x-rays are mandatory before preoperative planning for stabilizing the fracture. Poor-quality AP and lateral x-rays, especially when the leg is shortened are often insufficient for adequate identification of significant articular pathology. X-rays under traction give additional information. In cases of complex multiplane articular fractures, axial computed tomography (CT) with frontal and sagittal plane reconstructions may be helpful in planning the reduction and surgical stabilization.

In fractures with a complex multifragmentary metaphyseal zone, an AP x-ray of the contralateral unimpacted femur is very helpful for preoperative planning.

Patient positioning

If possible leg length and rotational profile of the contralateral extremity is examined preoperatively, to ascertain the correct rotational profile of the distal femur. With the patient in supine position, surgical intervention is best carried out on a completely radiolucent table that allows complete imaging of the lower leg. The leg should be freely movable. Appropriate padding is placed under the uninvolved limb, which is then secured. The contralateral leg can be placed in an obstetric leg holder. Preparation and draping should allow complete exposure of the proximal femur and hip region, especially if the longer 13-hole LISS plate is to be used. The knee joint line should be placed slightly distal to the hinged part of the table to allow flexion of the knee during surgery. Excessive traction and a fully extended knee should be avoided; the force of the gastrocnemius would draw the distal fragment into recurvature. This not only makes reduction of the fracture difficult, but also endangers the popliteal artery and vein. In very short distal fragments, it is recommended to flex the lower leg to approximately 60°. This also reduces the traction force of the gastrocnemius. Intraoperative image intensifier control is necessary.

Approaches

The surgical procedure essentially depends whether or not an articular fracture requires open reduction. In nonarticular fractures (Müller AO Classification A1–A3) and fractures with simple articular involvement (Müller AO Classification C1 and C2), a lateral approach to the distal femur is used (Fig 3-8). A lateral parapatellar approach is preferable for multiplane articular involvement, medial-based intercondylar splits, additional Hoffa fractures, and separate intercondylar notch fragments. The surgeon utilizes the approach required to view the articular surface, and traditional lag screw fixation of the articular surface is performed (Fig 3-9).

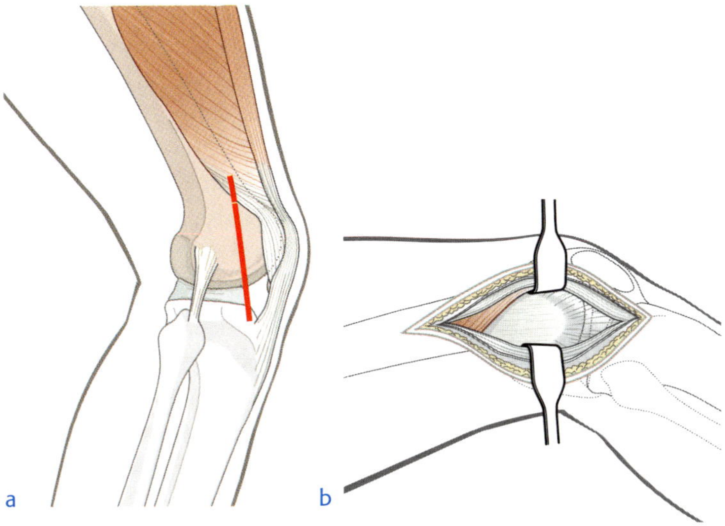

Fig 3-8a–b The lateral approach for insertion of the LISS-DF.

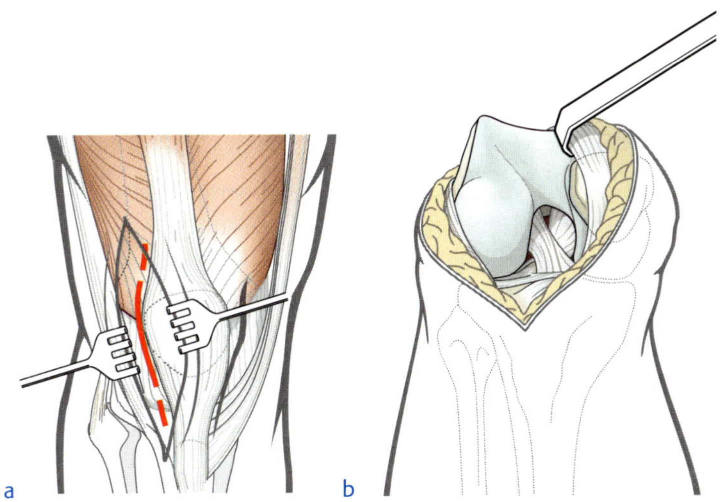

Fig 3-9a–b The lateral parapatellar approach for insertion of the LISS-DF. A medial dislocation of the patella ensures an optimal overview of the articulation.

The patient is placed in the supine position. For purely extraarticular fractures of the distal femur, a lateral incision approximately 8 cm long is made from Gerdy's tubercle and extended in a proximal direction to expose the lower margin of the vastus lateralis. If there is any doubt, a lateral image intensifier image may be helpful. The skin incision should be made in exact prolongation of the shaft. The skin and subcutaneous tissue are divided by sharp dissection. The iliotibial tract is split in the direction of its fibers. No attempt is made to visualize the metaphyseal component of the fracture. Although the joint capsule need not be opened in cases of nonarticular fracture, visualization or palpation of the anterior aspect of the lateral femoral condyle may be helpful for correct positioning of the LISS fixator on the distal femoral condyle. This approach is only appropriate for extraarticular and completely undisplaced articular fractures. It is not adequate for controlling even small displacements of articular fractures.

For all displaced articular fractures of the distal femur (not only complex ones), a lateral parapatellar approach (including a medial dislocation of the patella) should be selected that ensures an optimal overview of the articulation. The joint capsule can then be divided in line with the split in the iliotibial ligament. LISS fixation in displaced articular fractures begins with direct visualization and stable internal fixation of the articular surface. Priority is always given to precise anatomical reconstruction of the articular surface.

Strategy for fracture reduction and fixation

Articular fracture reduction and fixation. Traditional reduction and fixation of the articular surface is performed first. Reduction aids for the articular surface that may be helpful include:

- Schanz screws or reduction handles in the medial and lateral femoral condyles, for use as joysticks during reduction of the intercondylar fracture.

- Reduction forceps with points (Weber forceps), or pelvic reduction forceps, pelvic reduction forceps with pointed ball tips, a collinear reduction clamp that presses the lateral and medial femoral condylar blocks together.
- K-wires for temporary insertion to maintain the reduction of the articular blocks until definitive lag screw fixation is achieved.
- Dental picks, which can be helpful for fine manipulation of articular segments.

After reduction of the articular surface, multiple 3.5 mm cortex lag screws and 4.0 mm or 4.5 mm cannulated lag screws are inserted in a lateral to medial direction for fixation of any intercondylar fractures, or in an anterior to posterior direction for fixation of Hoffa fractures. For fixation of small osteochondral fragments in the intercondylar notch, 2.7 mm lag screws can also be used. Attention can now be given to reduction and fixation of the metaphyseal and diaphyseal component of the fractures by implantation of the LISS. This starts with temporary closed indirect reduction and retention of the articular block on the shaft, with limb length and the correct axial and rotational alignment being taken into account. Application of a distractor or external fixator may be useful for this surgical step, but is not absolutely necessary. An experienced LISS user can carry out immediate indirect reduction, taking full advantage of the anatomically precontoured implants.

Closed reduction is carried out on the metaphyseal and diaphyseal component of the fracture, followed by submuscular fixation using LISS fixation. The LISS is inserted on the distal femur under the vastus lateralis muscle in the epiperiostal space and is advanced in a proximal direction. Attention must be given to correct positioning of the LISS fixator in the condylar area, and particularly on the femoral shaft. K-wires are used to fix this position and are inserted through the insertion guide, and the self-drilling, self-tapping locking head screws are mounted in the trocar assemblies. Clinical experience has shown that the use of long implants fixed with specific locking head screws is advantageous, as it leads to good distribution of strain across both implant and bone. It is preferable to use monocortical locking head screws in the shaft area and long locking head screws in the metaphyseal zone. As a rule, four screws should be securely inserted into the shaft and five or six screws into the condylar block.

Step-by-step surgical sequence for LISS-DF fixation

A well-defined step-by-step process is used for LISS-DF fixation after articular fracture reduction and fixation.

Step 1: preoperative selection of the implants

The preoperative x-ray planning template (Fig 3-10) is used to determine the length of the LISS plate and the position of the screws. It should be noted that all template images are enlarged by 10% to account for average radiograph magnification. However, magnification may vary.

Preoperative screw-length selection using an AP x-ray. To select the proper screw length for the condyle, take a preoperative x-ray with calibrator and select the screw lengths using Tab 3-2.

- Take an AP x-ray of the distal femur.
- Place the x-ray calibrator medially or laterally at the height of the condyle.

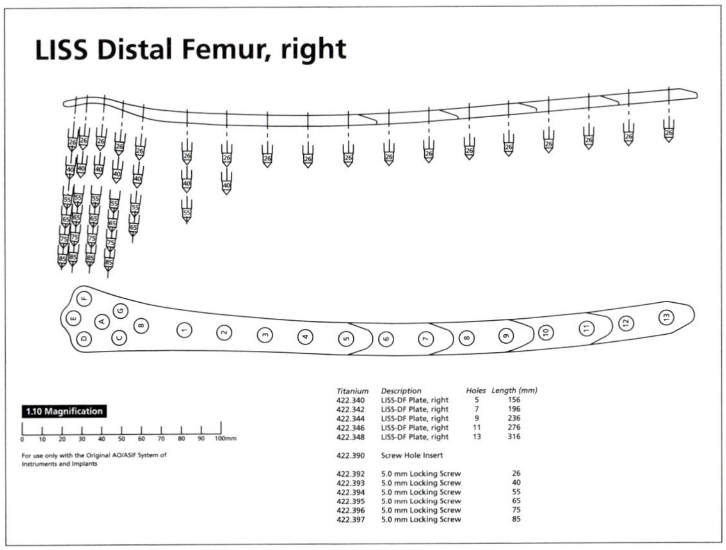

Fig 3-10 X-ray planning template for determining the length of the LISS plate and the position of the screws.

- Measure the width of the x-ray calibrator (XRC) on the radiograph.
- Measure the maximum condyle width (MCW) on the radiograph.
- Determine the real condyle width (RCW).
- Check the appropriate condyle size in Tab 3-2.
- Read off the corresponding screw length for screw holes A to G. Positions A to G are indicated on the preoperative planning template and on the LISS-DF insertion guide.

Alternatively a measuring device with a 2.0 mm K-wire 280 mm long, placed through the guide sleeve can be used.

For shaft fixation short monocortical 18 mm or 26 mm long locking head screws calculated on the x-ray are used.

Femoral condyle width (mm)	Holes A	B	C	D	E	F	G
60–80	65	40	40	55	65	65	55
81–87	75	40	55	65	75	75	65
88–95	75	55	65	65	75	75	75
96–110	85	65	75	75	75	85	85

Tab 3-2 Lengths of LHS for LISS.

Step 2: assembling the insertion instruments (Fig 3-11)

- Connect the two parts of the insertion guide.
- Insert the fixation bolt into hole A of the insertion guide.
- Place the insertion guide on the LISS three-point locking mechanism.
- Insert the fixation bolt into the LISS and tighten it slightly using the pin wrench.
- Thread the nut of the fixation bolt in the direction of the insertion guide and tighten it slightly with the pin wrench.
- For more stable fixation of the LISS to the insertion guide during insertion, introduce a second stabilization bolt with the drill sleeve into hole B (and thread it into the LISS).

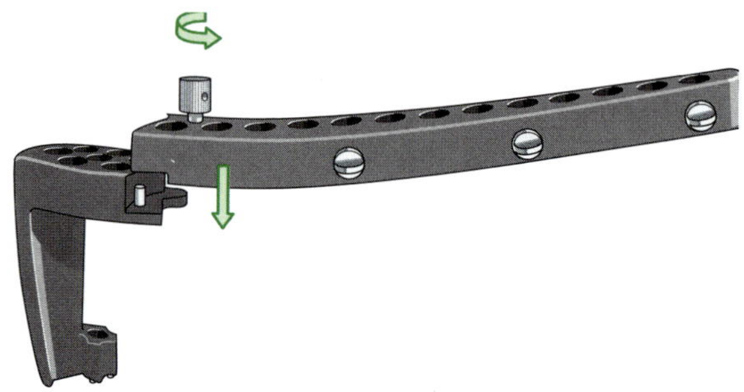

a

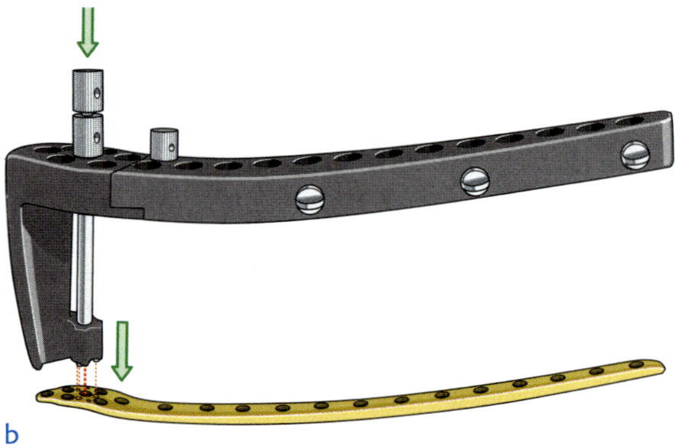

b

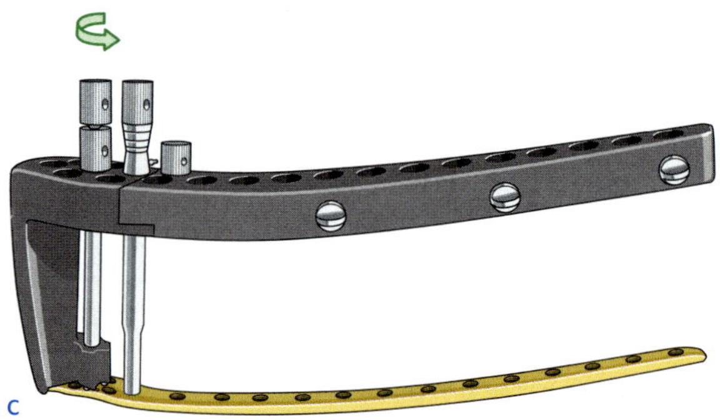

c

Fig 3-11a–c Assembling the insertion instruments with the LISS-DF.

Step 3: provisional fracture reduction

Before the LISS fixator is inserted, manual traction is applied, the supracondylar towel rolls are put in place, and the fracture reduction is visualized on both AP and lateral x-rays. The surgeon can then note specific conditions such as hyperextension of the distal femoral condyle, flexion and/or adduction of the proximal femoral shaft, and/or valgus of the distal femoral condyles. Adjustments can then be made in the position and/or size of the supracondylar towel rolls and the vector force direction of manual traction, and deformities can be corrected by careful blows or pushing with the large mallet. Note: practice and check the reduction-specific maneuver as part of the preoperative preparation. Although the LISS insertion guide is radiolucent, better visualization of the fracture reduction is obtained before LISS insertion.

Step 4: LISS insertion (Fig 3-12)

The assembled insertion guide is used to insert the LISS plate between the vastus lateralis muscle and the periosteum (= epiperiosteal space).

The LISS fixator is inserted either through the anterolateral incision or through the lateral parapatellar approach. The fixator is precontoured to accommodate the anterior curvature of the femur.

The LISS plate is slid proximally, ensuring that its proximal end remains in constant contact with the bone. The distal end of the fixator is positioned against the lateral condyle. To identify the correct position, the LISS plate is moved proximally and then back distally until the plate fits the condyle. If the proximal end of the insertion guide and the soft tissues impair insertion of the plate, it is possible to remove the radiolucent proximal part of the handle for insertion.

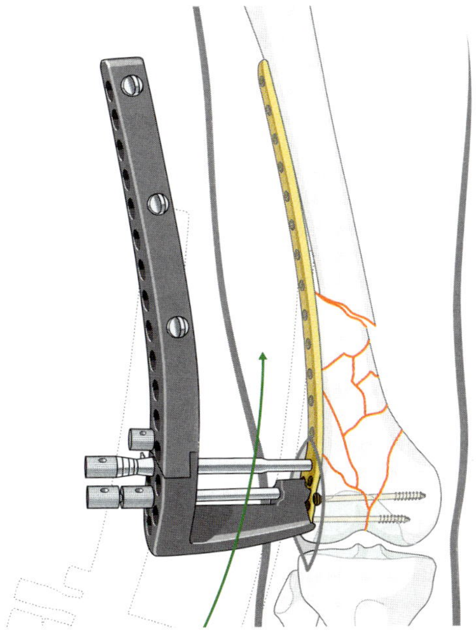

Fig 3-12 LISS insertion.

This step can be carried out under brief line image intensification, and the following techniques are helpful here:

- Noting the tactile sensation of the proximal tip of the fixator or the lateral cortex.
- Alternatively, a small incision at the proximal end of the LISS may make it easier to position the LISS relative to the proximal fragment. The position can be checked both by palpation and by vision (see also step 5 and Fig 3-13). Two Hohmann retractors can keep the implant centered on the midlateral aspect of the femur.
- Assessing the position of the insertion guide relative to the lateral aspect of the thigh.

A common tendency is to direct the fixator posteriorly; due to its weight, the insertion guide tends to tilt dorsally. If the insertion guide points parallel to the floor with the patient in the supine position, it means that the fixator is externally rotated and is no longer lying flat up against the lateral condyle. The fixation bolt has to be oriented parallel to the patellofemoral joint. Consequently, the insertion guide shows an internal rotation of about 10°. This occurrence is also visible on the AP view with an image intensifier. The fixator has to lie flat up against the condyle to ensure optimal fitting on the bone. Close positioning of the distal portion of the LISS to the lateral aspect of the condyle to avoid postoperative irritation of the iliotibial fracture.

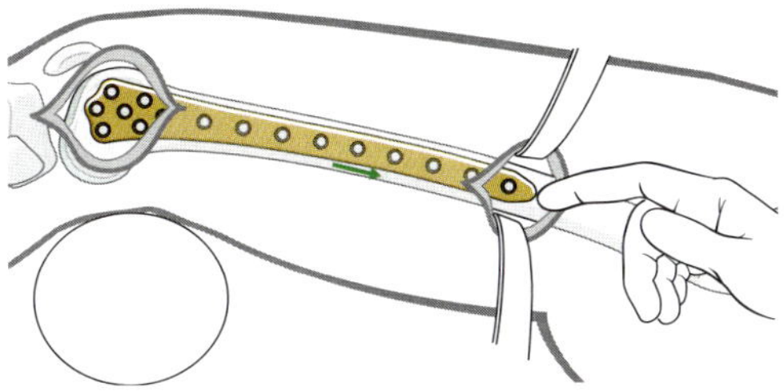

Fig 3-13 Checking the plate position by palpation and by vision.

Step 5: connecting the proximal connecting bolt (Fig 3-14)

Through an incision over either hole 5, 9, or 13, a proximal connecting bolt is screwed into the proximal end of the fixator. This creates a fixed parallelogram that facilitates further manipulation of the fixator on the midlateral aspect of the femur and ensures precise percutaneous placement of the screws through the trocars.

- Once the LISS is properly aligned with the bone, the drill sleeve and stabilization bolt are removed from hole B. The trocar is inserted through the drill sleeve in the most proximal hole of the plate. A stab incision is made, and the drill sleeve and trocar are pushed down to the LISS plate. Correct positioning of the proximal part of the LISS plate on the bone is checked, either using a K-wire or direct palpation. The position of the drill sleeve is secured with the lateral screw on the insertion guide. The trocar is replaced by the stabilization bolt. To close the frame, the stabilization bolt is threaded into the LISS plate.
- It should be noted that once the bolt has been inserted, it will be difficult to change the position of the plate–guide assembly, due to the soft tissues around the stabilization bolt.

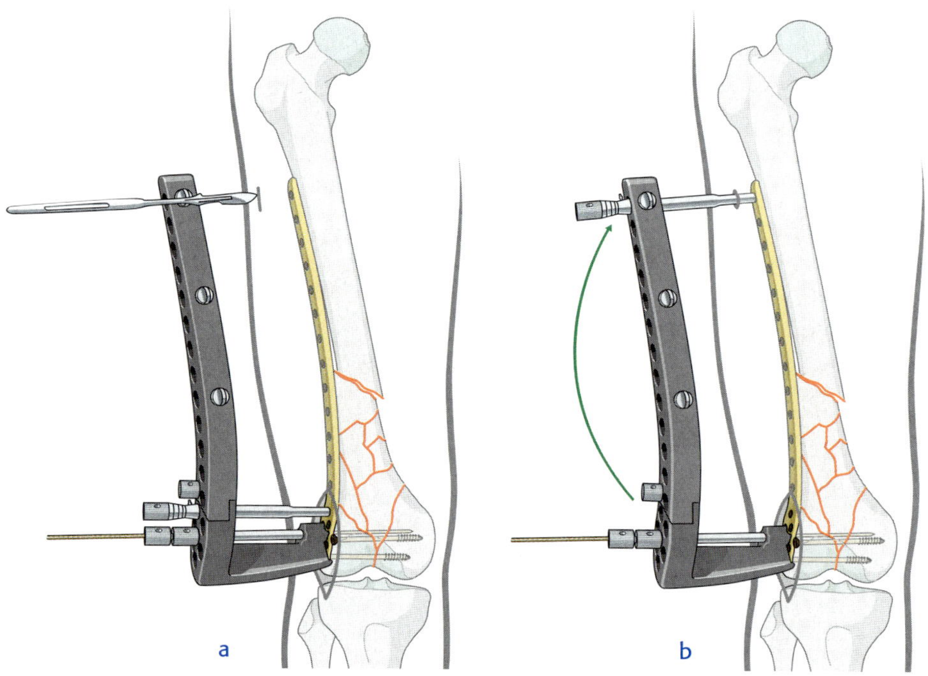

Fig 3-14a–b Connecting the proximal connecting bolt.

a Incision

b Insertion of connecting bolt

Step 6: establishing appropriate placement of the LISS fixator on the distal femoral condyle (Fig 3-15)

The LISS fixator is precontoured and should sit well on the distal femur. Several comments are helpful in establishing whether it is correctly placed:

- The fixator usually lies approximately 1.0–1.5 cm posterior to the most anterior aspect of the distal femoral condyle and approximately 1.0–1.5 cm cranial to the distal femoral condyle (Fig 3-15a). Correct placement of the fixator is often helped by pushing the fixator proximally and then allowing the LISS fixator to settle distally onto the normal flank of the femoral condyles. As the lateral cortex slopes at approximately 10–15°, the insertion guide is usually raised approximately 10–15° from the horizontal plane of the floor (Fig 3-15b). Counterpressure is exerted on the medial aspect of the distal femoral condylar region, the hand directing the insertion guide is raised approximately 10–15°, and the guide wire is then placed through drill sleeve A. This guide wire should then be parallel to the joint surface of the distal articular surface if a distal femoral valgus malalignment of 5° is identified. Small adjustments to this relationship can be made later in the sequence, as noted below.

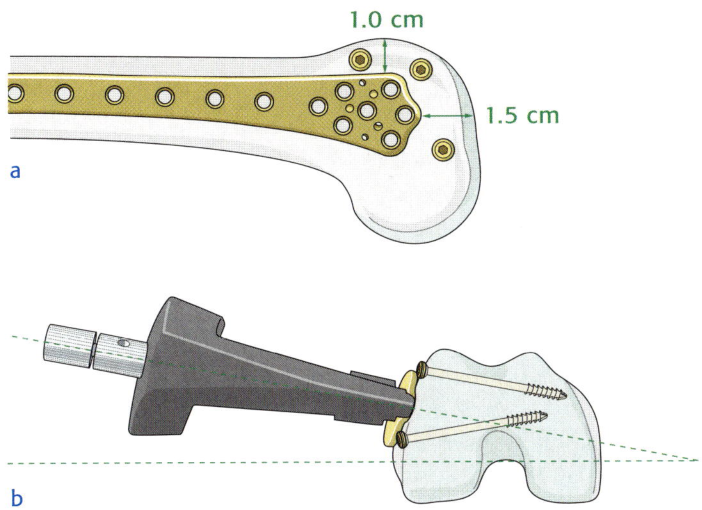

Fig 3-15a–b Establishing appropriate placement of the LISS fixator on the distal femoral condyle.

a The positioning of the lag screw has to respect the placement of the LISS. The LISS-DF lays posterior to the anterior aspect of the lateral condyle and 1.0–1.5 cm cranial to the joint surface.

b The distal part of the fixator lays on the lateral cortex of the condyle.

Step 7: checking the rotation and length of the reduction

A check is made at this point using image intensification in the AP plane to ensure that the proper length has been restored to the injured extremity. At this time, the rotational profile of the limb is also assessed, with assessment of the AP image, evaluation of the skin lines in the distal femoral region, and awareness that the foot should be externally rotated by 10–15°.

Step 8: preliminary LISS fixation (Fig 3-16)

If the length and rotation are correct, then the proximal guide wire can be inserted after it has been verified that the fixator is on the midlateral aspect of the femur and laying a proper rotational relationship. Assessing the location of the proximal aspect of the fixator may be facilitated by making a larger incision (approximately 4–5 cm) over the proximal three screw holes (either holes 11, 12, and 13 in a 13-hole fixator or holes 7, 8, and 9 in a 9-hole fixator (see Fig 3-13)). The incision is carried down in a longitudinal manner through the iliotibial ligament and the vastus lateralis so that direct palpation of the fixator and assessment of its relationship to the lateral cortex is possible. Lateral image intensification can also be used to assess placement of the fixator on the midlateral aspect of the femur. It is extremely important to establish correct placement, in order to ensure proper proximal insertion of the monocortical locking head screws. After the proper length and rotation are ensured, and appropriate positioning of the proximal aspect of the fixator on the midlateral femur has been established, the proximal guide wire can be placed. It is still possible at this point to correct the sagittal plane alignment, as noted below. Small corrections of the adduction of the proximal fragment or of the varus/valgus alignment of the distal femoral condyle are possible.

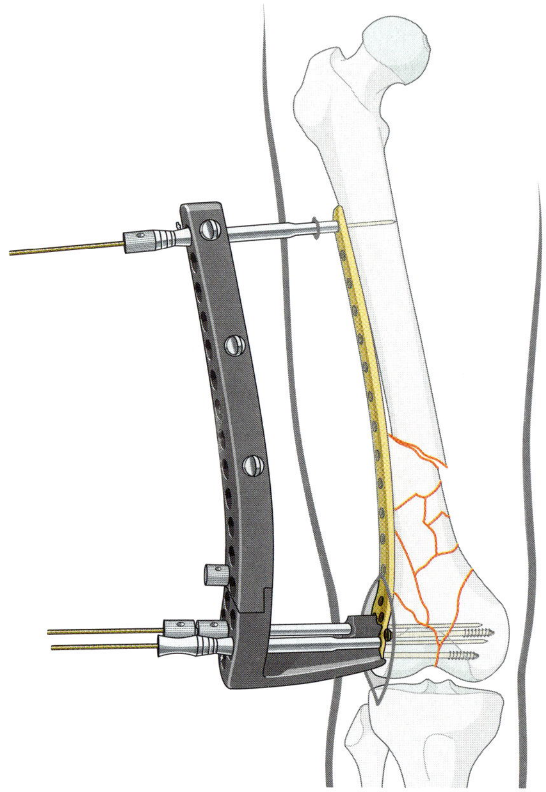

Fig 3-16 Preliminary LISS fixation. The guide wire through drill sleeve A should be parallel to the joint surface.

For preliminary fixation of the internal fixator, 2.0 mm K-wires are inserted through the fixation and stabilization bolts. The position of the LISS plate and length of the reduced injured limb are carefully checked. Alternatively, the aiming device for K-wires can be used to insert the wires on the anterior and posterior side of the fixator (see Fig 3-4a–b).

Once the reduction has been successfully completed and the LISS plate has been positioned correctly, the locking head screws can be inserted.

Step 9: placement of screws in the distal femoral block (Fig 3-17)

At this point, reassessment is made of the common hyperextension and excess valgus deformities of the distal femoral condylar block. Hyperextension is corrected by repositioning the supracondylar towel rolls, changing the direction of manual traction, and by manual pressure or by joystick control of the distal femoral block. The usual excessive valgus can be corrected using one of a variety of techniques:

- The force vector of the pull of manual traction can be altered.
- A pulling device can be placed in the proximal aspect of the distal femoral condyle. This allows correction of approximately 1–5° of excessive valgus.
- A large reduction forceps or collinear reduction clamp, with one arm placed on the proximal aspect of the distal medial femoral condyle and the other either on the fixator or the insertion guide, can be used to correct excessive valgus. It must be recognized that this will result in slight disturbance of the parallel position of the fixation in relation to the screw insertion guide. However, its use may be necessary when dealing with extremely osteoporotic bone, in which use of the pulling device can be limited by screw pullout.

After correct placement of the fixator on the distal femoral block has been achieved and following appropriate correction of any deformity, several LHS can be placed distally. All LHS are placed under saline cooling; during insertion—especially of the first LHS—the fixator is "pushed" against the distal femoral condyles, the hand is raised, and counterpressure is applied on the opposite medial aspect of the distal femoral region.

- Insertion of the self-drilling, self-tapping locking head screws. Screw placement depends on the type of fracture. The positions of the LHS should be chosen in accordance with the established biomechanical principles for internal fixation.
- The length of the condylar screws required can be calculated from Tab 3-2. It is also possible to use the measuring device with a 2.0 mm K-wire, 280 mm long, placed through the guide sleeve. Using image intensification, the K-wire is pushed to the desired depth, leaving at least 5 mm between the tip of the K-wire and the medial cortex. The screw length is measured over the K-wire using the measuring device for K-wires (Fig 3-17), leaving the guide sleeve in place, and rounded down to the nearest screw length. This will ensure that the tip of the locking head screw will not protrude through the medial cortex.

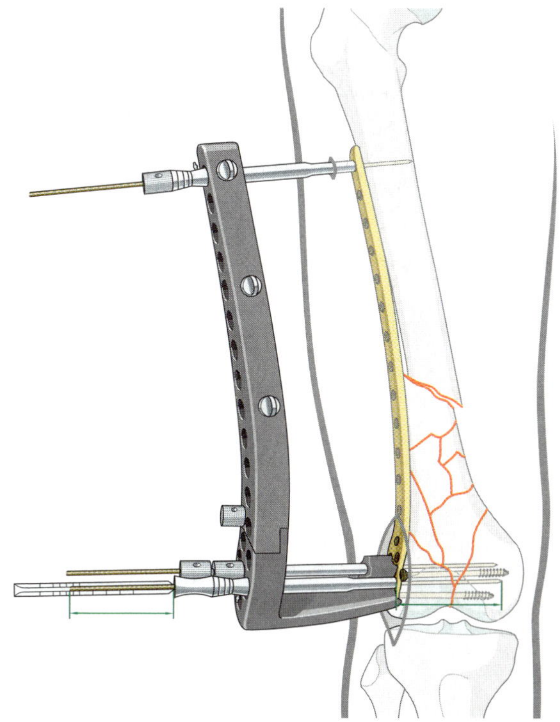

Fig 3-17 Measuring of the length with K-wire using the measuring device for K-wires.

Step 9: placement of screws in the distal femoral block (Fig 3-18) (cont)

- Battery-driven or compressed-air tools are used to insert the self-drilling, self-tapping locking head screws. Note: the torque-limiting screwdriver should be used for the final tightening (Fig 3-18).
- To provide the best interface between LHS and bone and prevent medial migration of the bone, the power tool should be used without high axial forces (3–5 kg).
- To prevent heat necrosis, it is important to cool the screw with saline solution through the drill sleeve during the drilling procedure (Fig 3-18).
- It should be noted that once the initial LHS has been inserted into each main fragment, length and rotation are defined. Antecurvatum and recurvatum deformities can still be manipulated relatively well, but there is only limited scope for correcting varus/valgus deformities.

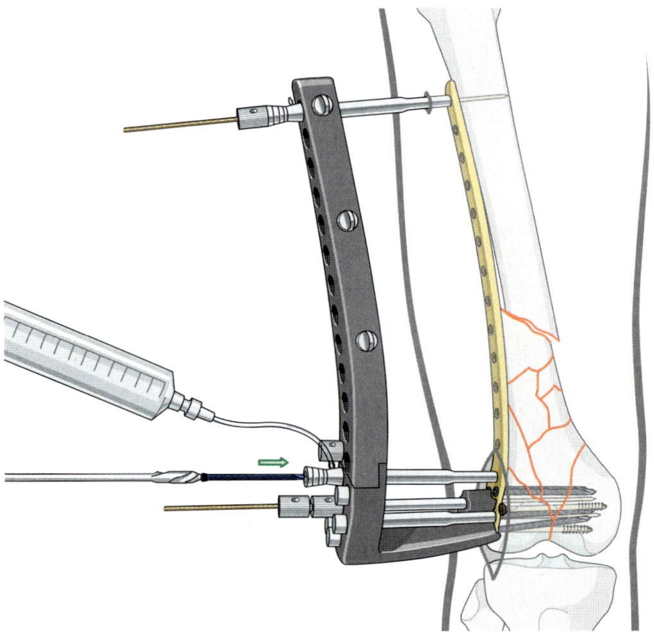

Fig 3-18 Insertion of LHS in the articular block. To prevent heat necrosis it is important to cool the screws with saline solution through the drill sleeve during the drilling procedure.

- It is therefore recommended that the first LHS should be inserted into the distal fragment. The distal LHS should be placed parallel to the knee joint.
- If a LHS has to be removed and reinserted, it should be done with the manual screwdriver, not the power tool.
- The LHS are advanced into the bone until the second guide of the screwdriver sinks into the drill sleeve. The torque-limiting screwdriver should be used for final tightening until clicking occurs at 4 Nm. It should be checked that the screw head is completely seated in the LISS plate.
- Both the screwdriver shaft and the torque-limiting screwdriver are equipped with a self-holding mechanism. Slight pressure should be used to ensure that the screwdriver shaft penetrates the socket of the screw head on pick-up.
- If the screwdriver is difficult to remove after insertion, it should be disconnected from the power tool and the drill sleeve should be removed. After the screwdriver has been reconnected to the power tool, the screwdriver is withdrawn from the screw.
- A standard 4.5 mm cortex screw can be used through the fixator if required. It should be noted, however, that the 4.5 mm cortex screw cannot be inserted through drill sleeve hole A, which serves to lock the insertion guide to the implant. This hole can therefore not be used to insert a screw while the fixation bolt is attached. If a screw is required in hole A, the fixation bolt should be removed—with the stabilization bolt still in place—and refixed in an adjacent hole that is available. Once the self-drilling, self-tapping LHS have been placed, the free-hand method can be used to insert the screw in hole A. The direction given by the fixation bolt before removal can be used, or else another plate and screw can be used to determine the correct direction for insertion.

Step 10: appropriate reduction of the proximal femoral shaft with LHS fixation (Fig 3-19)

At this point, the fixator is in an appropriate relationship to the distal femoral condyle, length and rotation have been maintained—both through continued gentle manual traction and through the proximal guide wire—and it has been established that some manual pressure may have to be placed on the anterior distal aspect of the proximal fragment, or that there is a need to correct an adduction deformity of the proximal fragment. These corrections can now be made, potentially with the help of one or two pulling devices ("whirlybird devices") (Fig 3-19a–b). Proximal LHS are then inserted. A LHS is often placed in holes next to the pulling device in order to reduce stress.

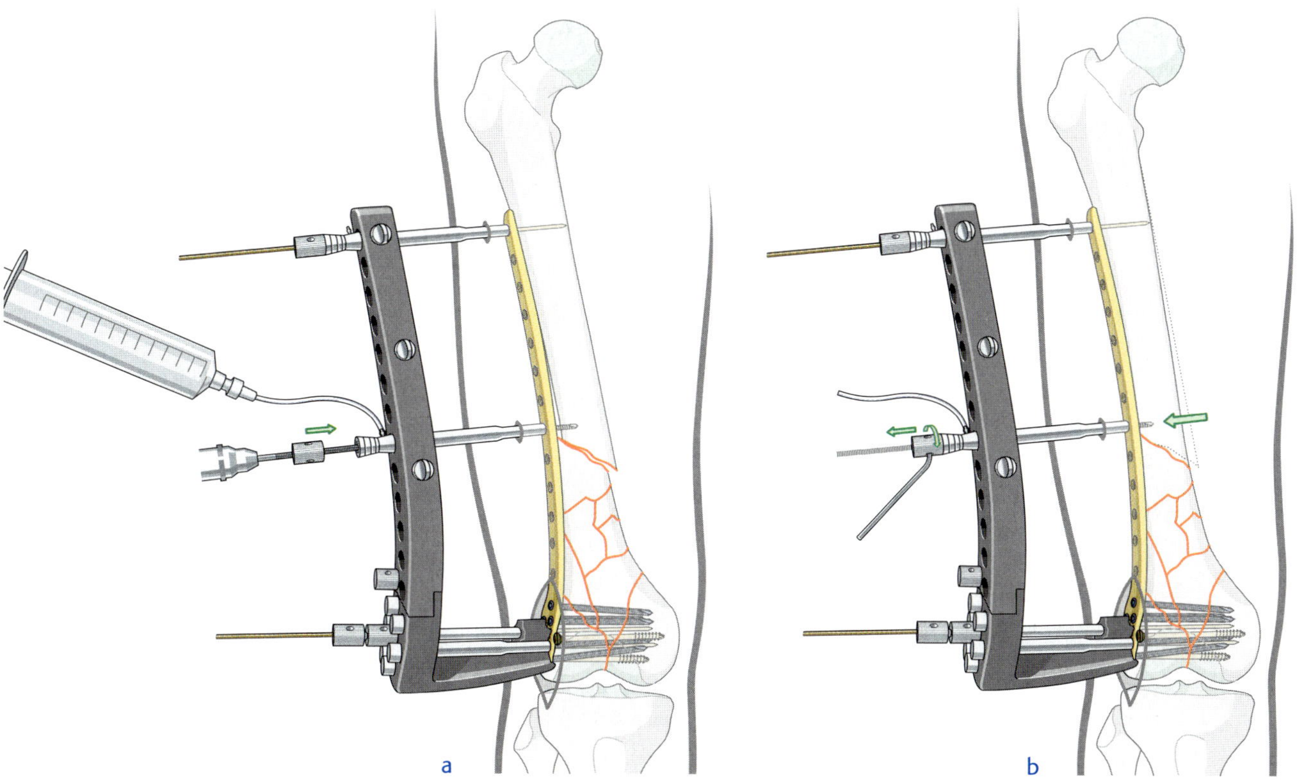

Fig 3-19a–e The pulling device ("whirlybird") can provide fine adjustments to reduction.

a It is utilized to correct slight adduction deformity of the proximal femur, and to ensure that the proximal femur does not displace during screw insertion.

b Slight improvement of the reduction of the diaphyseal component of the fracture is accomplished utilizing a pulling device.

Step 10: appropriate reduction of the proximal femoral shaft with LHS fixation (Fig 3-19) (cont)

LHS with a length of 26 mm are used in the diaphyseal region. If the cortex is very thick, predrilling can be carried out using the pulling device or special locking head screws 35 mm long with a long drilling tip.

Insertion of the initial LHS tends to push the bone medially, particularly in cases of dense bone and/or unstable reductions. The pulling device helps solve this problem. The pulling device, without the knurled nut, is inserted through the drill sleeve into the neighboring hole of the first permanent LHS. The power tool is stopped before the entire screw length of the pulling device has been inserted. The power tool is removed. Screwing the knurled nut onto the pulling device allows the bone to be pulled toward the LISS plate. Since the tip of this instrument has a diameter of 4.0 mm, replacing it with a 5.0 mm LHS still ensures good purchase in the bone.

While the pulling device is being inserted, it is important to monitor the advancement of the screw tip carefully. The power tool must be stopped before the pulling device is seated on the plate. Failure to do so may result in stripping the thread in the bone. Note: In case of osteoporotic bone with very thin cortex bicortical self-tapping LHS can be used to fix the LISS to the shaft fragment.

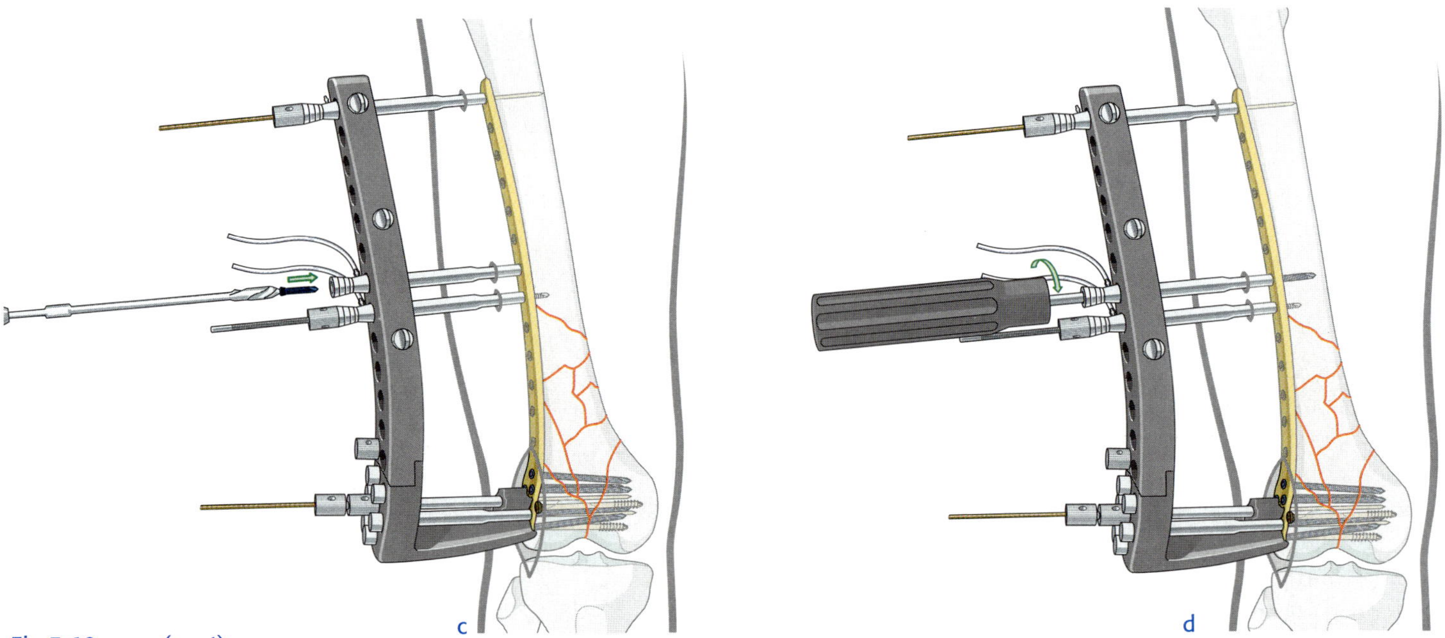

Fig 3-19a–e (cont)

c The pulling device helps to prevent pushing the bone medially during insertion of the initial LHS. The pulling device is inserted through the drill sleeve into the neighboring hole of the first permanent LHS.

d The torque-limiting screwdriver should be used for final tightening.

Step 10: appropriate reduction of the proximal femoral shaft with LHS fixation (Fig 3-19) (cont)

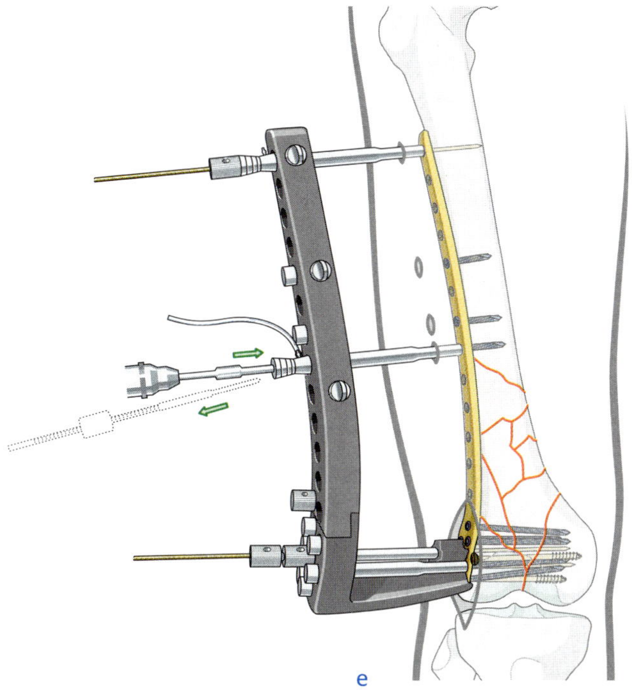

e

Fig 3-19a–e (cont)

e Since the tip of the pulling device has a diameter 4.0 mm replacing it with a 5.0 mm LHS still ensures good purchase in the bone.

Step 11: additional screw placement

Additional LHS are subsequently placed both proximally and distally. In general, a total of five proximal and five distal LHS are placed. In cases of severe osteoporosis, six proximal and six distal LHS can be used. Biocortical self-tapping LHS for shaft fixation in server osteoporosis is recommended.

In simple fracture types the screws close to the fracture line have to stay away from the fracture in the proximal and distal fragment especially when there is a gap after reduction in order to leave a screw-free zone above the fracture. In a multifragmentary fracture the screws should be placed in the main fragment as close as possible to the fracture zone so that the working length of the internal fixator is not too long and therefore not too elastic. Leave 2–3 plate holes unused to avoid stress concentration in the implant.

In multifragmentary fractures no screws are used in the fracture zone. Three to four plate holes at the fracture zone should stay without screws.

In this case the screws in both main fragments should be as close as possible to the fracture zone. The distance between these screws determine the elasticity of the fixator.

Step 12: placement of the most proximal LHS, removal of the insertion guide, and placement of the "A" distal femoral LHS (Fig 3-20)

The proximal connection bolt can be removed and the most proximal LHS inserted into the fixator. The insertion guide is then disconnected from the fixator. If desired, a LHS or a screw hole inserter can be inserted into the A distal femoral screw position.

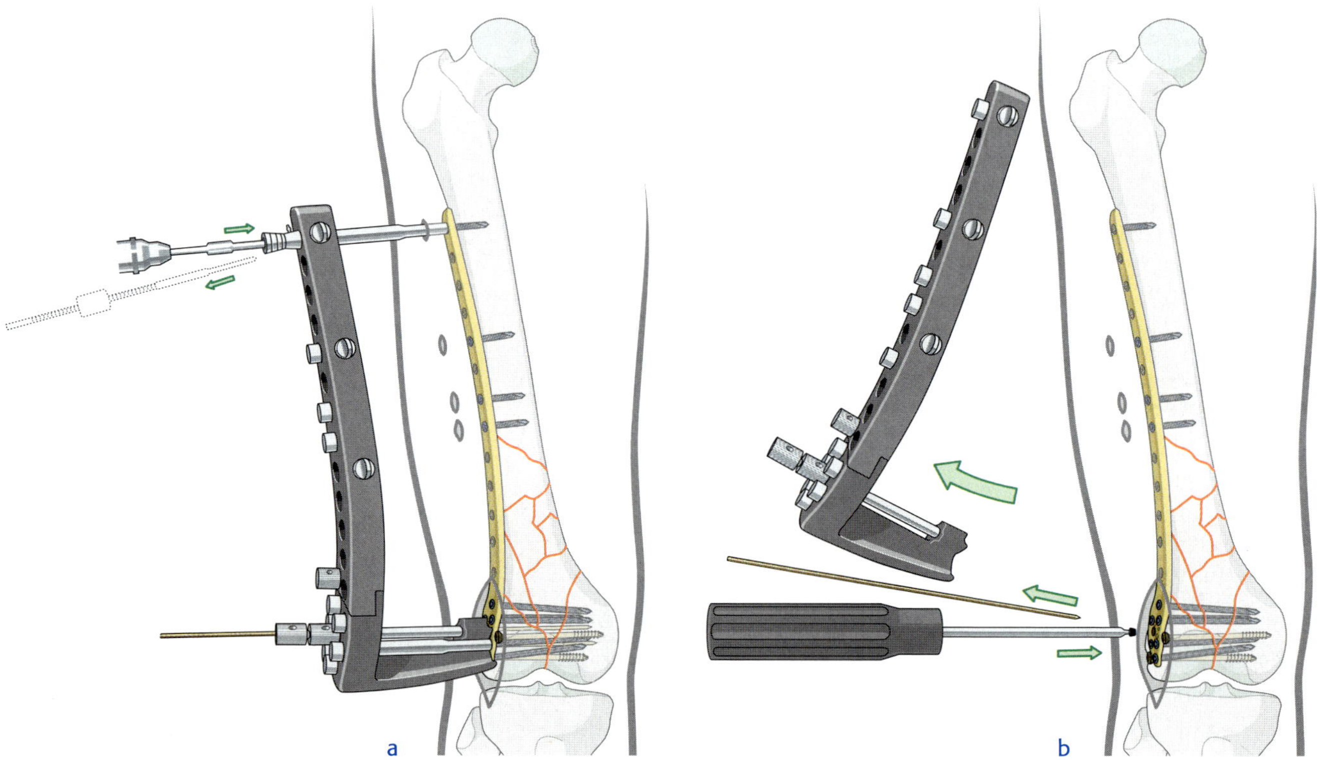

Fig 3-20a–b

a Removal of the proximal connection bolt and insertion of the most proximal LHS.

b Disconnect the insertion guide from the internal fixator. Optionally an LHS or a screw hole inserter can be inserted into hole A to keep the hole free from bone ingrowth.

Step 13: intraoperative assessment of fracture reduction and stability after fixation

Length, alignment, and rotation should be clinically checked. The knee is taken through a full range of gentle motion to ensure appropriate fracture fixation. Fracture reduction and fracture fixation are then assessed using AP, lateral, and oblique x-rays. Specific questions to be answered in this assessment include:

1 Is there any sagittal plane deformity? How satisfactory is the valgus/varus alignment? The cable method is recommended for checking the alignment of the limb (see chapter 2—4.1).
2 Is there significant hyperextension of the distal femoral condyles?
3 Length, alignment, and rotation should also be checked clinically.
4 How satisfactory is the placement of the fixator on the midlateral aspect of the femoral shaft?
5 How satisfactory is the placement of the LISS fixator on the lateral aspect of the distal femoral condyle?
6 Are all of the screws really placed monocortically into the bone, or are some positioned too far anteriorly or posteriorly?
7 Are any of the distal LHS in the patellar groove or intercondylar notch? (Although rare, this can occur with distal malrotation or excessive anterior or posterior positioning of the fixator.) This can be assessed intraoperatively and by image intensification with the intercondylar notch view.
8 It should be checked that self-drilling, self-tapping locking head screws have not perforated the medial cortex.

Step 14: wound closure (Fig 3-21).

All of the wounds are copiously irrigated. The joint capsule is closed using absorbable sutures, as is the iliotibial ligament (both proximal and distal incisions). The skin and subcutaneous tissue are closed in the routine manner (Fig 3-21).

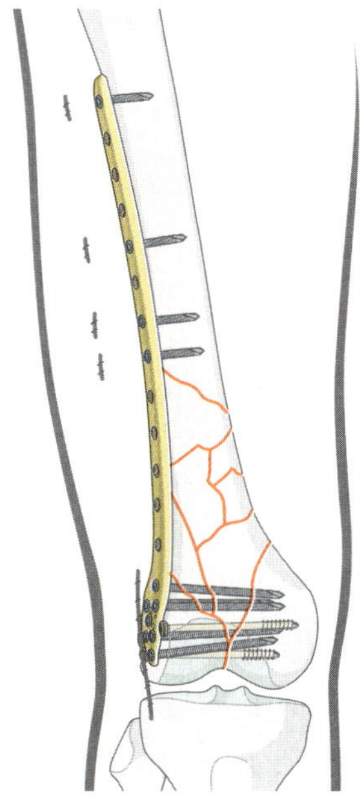

Fig 3-21 Position of the LISS after definitive osteosynthesis and wound closure.

LCP-DF

LCP-DF can be applied in the same way as LISS but also in a more invasive approach without insertion guide. For proper distal screw placement a smaller guiding block can be used. To find the correct position of the LCP-DF on the lateral aspect of the proximal femur shaft a small incision is used to palpate or to see the proximal end of the plate. Contrary to the LISS-DF the LCP-DF has combination holes so the surgeon can use angulated cortex screws.

Tab 3-3 **LISS-DF and LCP-DF cases**

Case	Classification	Implant used	Page
Spiral wedge femoral shaft fracture	32-B1	LISS-DF, 13 holes	521
Complex spiral femoral shaft fracture	32-C1	LISS-DF, 13 holes	531
Simple spiral femoral shaft fracture, implant failure	32-A1	LISS-DF, 13 holes	535
Simple spiral femoral shaft fracture, periprosthetic	32-A1	LISS-DF, 13 holes	547
Femoral shaft fracture, periprosthetic	32-A1	LISS-DF, 13 holes	551
Extraarticular distal femoral fracture	33-A2	LCP-DF, 9 holes	556
Supracondylar femoral fracture with joint involvement	33-C2	LISS-DF, 9 holes	569
Intraarticular distal femoral fracture	33-C2	LISS-DF, 13 holes	573
Complete articular multifragmentary distal femoral fracture	33-C3	LISS-DF, 13 holes	583
Open complete articular multifragmentary distal femoral fracture	33-C3	LISS-DF, 9 holes	587
Open complete intraarticular multifragmentary distal femoral fracture	33-C3	LISS-DF, 13 holes	593
Periprosthetic distal femoral fracture with implanted total knee endoprosthesis	33-A2	LISS-DF, 5 holes	601
Bilateral open supracondylar femoral fractures above total knee arthroplasty	33-A3	LISS-DF, 13 holes	605
Double osteotomy for valgus leg deformity due to lateral compartment knee osteoarthritis		LISS-DF, 5 holes	611

1.3 Less invasive stabilization system for the proximal lateral tibia (LISS-PLT)

Indications

The indications for LISS in the proximal lateral tibia include fractures of the proximal shaft, the metaphysis, and intraarticular fractures in which treatment with screws alone is not possible [4] (Tab 3-4). The principle of angular stable screw fixation gives the LISS-PLT system distinct biomechanical advantages over comparable devices for similar indications [7]. Once the system has been applied to the lateral aspect of the tibia, it prevents varus collapse in metaphyseal and diaphyseal fractures and in fractures of the tibial plateau with medial condyle involvement. This means that the LISS-PLT can also be used in the treatment of proximal tibial fractures that involve both the lateral and medial condyles—Müller AO Classification type 41-A2, A3, C1, C2, C3, and all proximal type 42 fractures [2]. In the Schatzker Classification for tibial plateau fractures, the indications include Schatzker type V and VI fractures [12].

The LISS fixator is not specifically indicated for isolated fractures of the tibial diaphysis in the mid-third, but is quite useful for segmental shaft fractures involving the proximal half of the tibia and for ipsilateral diaphyseal and bicondylar tibial plateau fractures. Other less common conditions in which the LISS-PLT has been used include pathological lesions with impending fracture of the proximal tibia, and periprosthetic fractures, and fractures in osteoporotic bone.

Tab 3-4

Indications for LISS-PLT in proximal tibial fractures
Metaphyseal fractures (multifragmentary)
Proximal shaft fractures (multifragmentary, not nailable)
Segmental shaft fractures (not nailable)
Articular fractures (41-A2, A3, C1, C2, C3)
Fractures in osteoporotic bone
Pathological fractures
Periprosthetic fractures

Timing

The LISS-PLT may not always be the procedure of choice for primary treatment. In cases in which there is severe soft-tissue damage in the region of the fracture or fractures, it may not be advisable to carry out a single-stage procedure to insert an angular stable internal fixator. In these situations, temporary fracture fixation with an external fixator can provide stability for the skeletal injury and soft tissues until definitive management is possible. This prevents further soft-tissue compromise and alleviates swelling. The timing of the conversion procedure in a two-staged technique is critical for promoting healing in these high-risk injuries.

X-ray and computed tomography

See chapter 1.2.

Patient positioning

The patient should be placed in the supine position on a radiolucent table. The leg should be freely movable. The contralateral leg can be placed in an obstetric leg holder. It is important to ensure that both lateral and AP image intensification of the proximal tibia can be obtained in this position. Bumps made with towel rolls can be used to flex the knee into the appropriate position (see chapter 1.2).

Step-by-step surgical sequence for LISS-PLT fixation

Step 1: preoperative selection of the implants

AP and lateral x-rays of the injured limb are used; x-rays of the other extremity may be useful for comparison. The preoperative x-ray planning template (Fig 3-22) is used to determine the length of the LISS plate and the position of the screws. Both template images are enlarged by 10% to account for average radiograph magnification. However, magnification may vary. Clinical experience has shown that the use of long implants fixed with locking head screws is advantageous, as it results in good distribution of the strain across both the implant and bone. It should be noted that the screws in holes A and C point toward the articular surface of the knee. In hole A, the tip of a 40 mm long locking head screw will lie approximately at the same level as the top of the plate. In hole C, the tip of a 75 mm long locking head screw will lie approximately at the same level as the top of the plate. It is preferable to use monocortical locking head screws in the shaft area and long locking head screws in the metaphyseal zone.

The screws in the tibial shaft will normally be self-drilling, self-tapping locking head screws 26 mm or 18 mm long. In cases of osteoporosis with soft bone and thin cortex, bicortically inserted self-tapping locking head screws (from the 4.5/5.0 LCP set) are recommended. As a rule, four locking head screws should be securely inserted into the shaft and five or six locking head screws into the condylar block. Preoperative planning of the use of plate independent lag screws should take place if necessary.

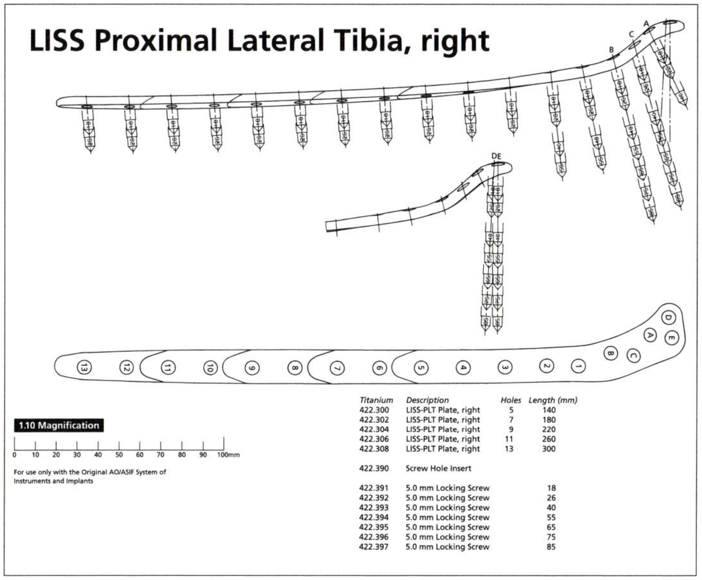

Fig 3-22 X-ray planning template for determine the length of the LISS-PLT plate and the position of the screw.

Step 2: incisions (Fig 3-23)

Depending on the need, it is possible to make either a curved (hockey-stick) or a straight skin incision from Gerdy's tubercle about 5 cm in distal direction. Approximately 0.5 cm from the tibial ridge, the anterior tibial muscle is detached from the bone and retracted, and the LISS is inserted into the space between the periosteum and the muscle. To allow correct positioning of the proximal part of the LISS, it is important to dissect the muscle attachment site adequately.

For complex articular fractures, an anterolateral arthrotomy that provides good control of the reduction may be preferable. An additional medial, or posteromedial, or posterior approach (Fig 3-23c) is used for some bicondylar fractures. An additional incision on the distal end is possible when the long 13-hole LISS-PLT plate is being used.

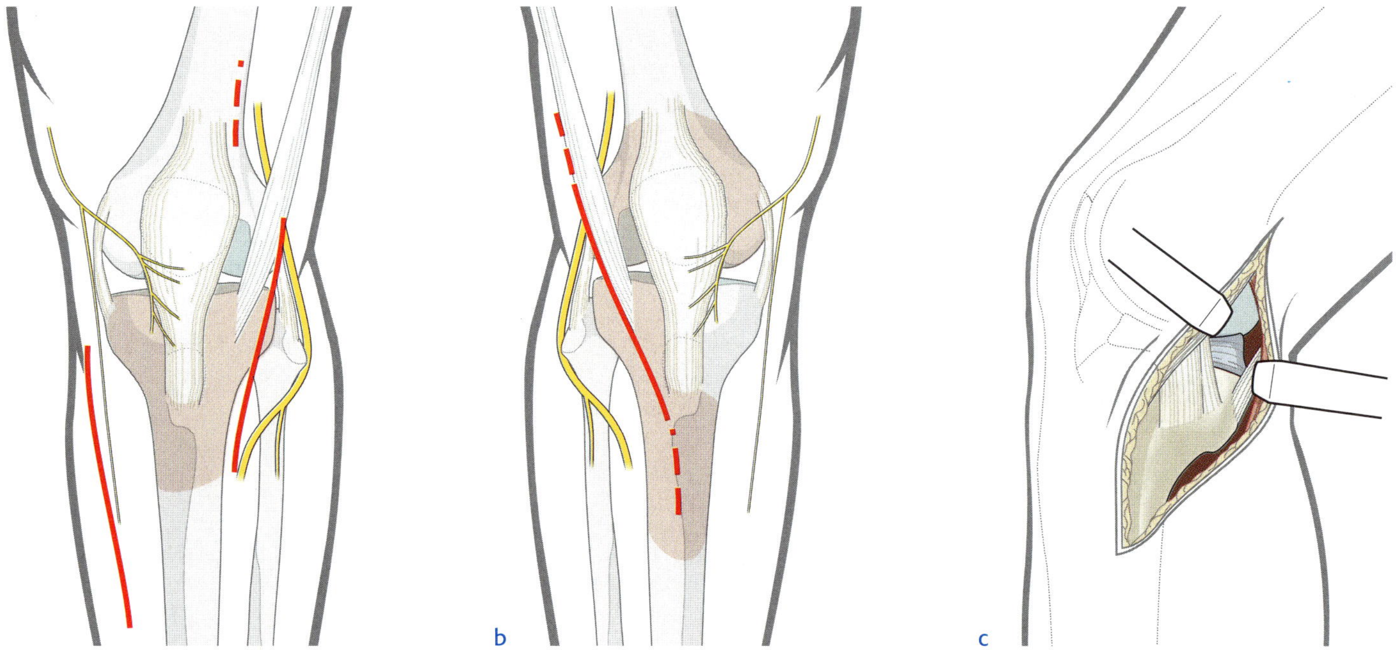

a b c

Fig 3-23a–c Incisions for LISS-PLT.

a Lateral approach to the tibial head. For displaced articular fractures a more extended approach is necessary.

b–c For some bicondylar tibial head fractures an additional medial or posteromedial approach is necessary.

Step 3: reduction and stabilization of the intraarticular fracture

The exact anatomical reconstruction of articular surfaces must always take priority. In the case of fractures of the tibial plateau, a lateral arthrotomy should be carried out as appropriate for the specific fracture characteristics in each case. Alternatively, an arthroscopically controlled reduction of the articular surface is sometimes possible. If the fracture is intraarticular, the whole joint should first be reconstructed and stabilized. Lag screws are used to achieve interfragmentary compression between the articular fragments using cannulated cortex screws. Care should be taken to ensure that these additional screws do not collide with the locking head screws inserted through the insertion guide. Figure 3-24 shows the possible zone for plate independent lateral lag screws in the lateral condyle. Once the joint surface has been reconstructed, temporary reduction of the articular block on the shaft can be achieved, taking into account the restoration of limb length and correction of the axial and rotational alignment. It may be helpful to use a distractor or external fixator for this surgical step, but it is not absolutely necessary. An experienced LISS user can carry out indirect reduction as the primary procedure, taking full advantage of the anatomically precontoured implants.

Some displaced medial plateau fractures initially require medial reduction and stabilization with a small posteromedial antiglide plate.

Reduction of the metaphyseal fracture. The fracture can be aligned manually by traction, with a temporary knee-bridging external fixator or with a distractor. Intraoperative x-ray or image intensifier assessment is recommended to check reduction. Indirect reduction is preferable in the metaphysis and shaft area. However, care has to be taken to ensure that the length, rotation, and axial alignment of the main fragments are correct. The reduction then has to be securely held to allow the reduced fragments to be bridged with the LISS fixator.

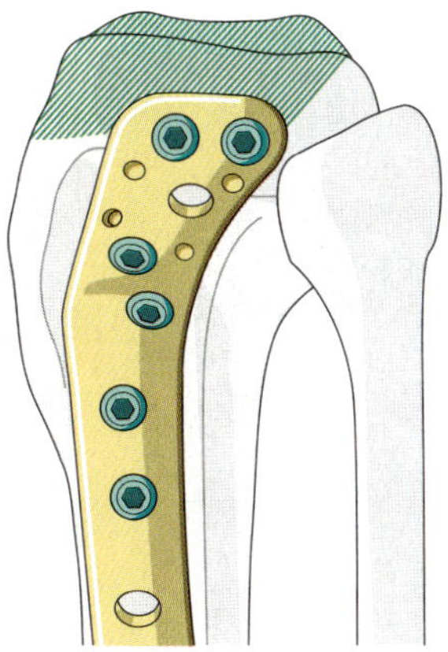

Fig 3-24 Possible zone for insertion of lateral lag screws in the tibial condyle.

Step 4: assembly of the insertion instruments (Fig 3-25)

The two parts of the insertion guide are connected. The fixation bolt is inserted through hole A of the insertion guide. The insertion guide is placed on the LISS three-point locking mechanism. The fixation bolt is then threaded into the LISS. The nut of the fixation bolt is threaded and tightened slightly with the pin wrench.

For more stable fixation of the LISS to the insertion guide during insertion, the stabilization bolt can be introduced with the drill sleeve through hole C and threaded into the LISS.

To prevent tissue ingrowth and facilitate implant removal, it is possible to close the unoccupied screw holes can be closed using a screw hole insert before the LISS plate is inserted.

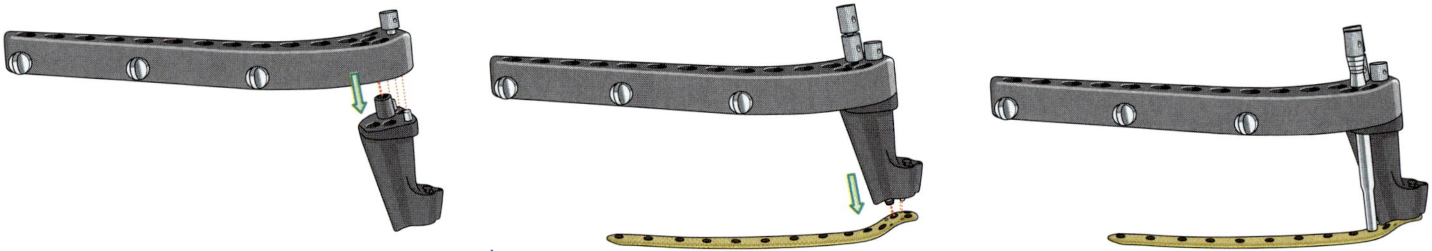

a b c

Fig 3-25a–c Assembly of the insertion instruments.

Step 5: LISS insertion (Fig 3-26)

The internal fixator is inserted between the anterior tibial muscle and the periosteum in the epiperiosteal space. The LISS plate is slid in the distal direction, with its distal end in constant contact with the bone. The proximal end of the fixator is positioned against the lateral condyle. The correct position of the LISS on the condyle is carefully identified.

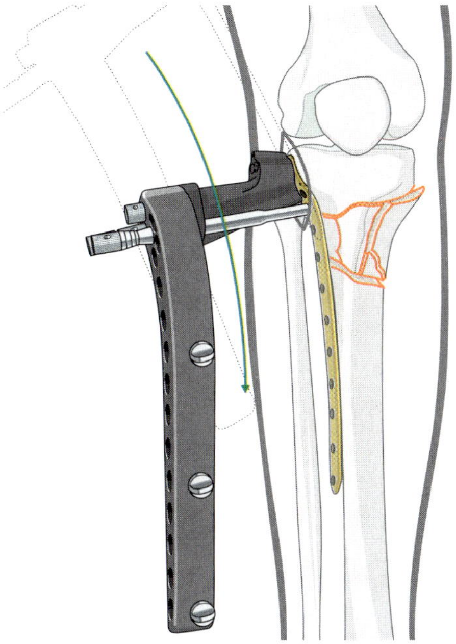

Fig 3-26 Insertion of the LISS-PLT.

Step 6: checking the position of the LISS-PLT (Fig 3-27)

A check is carried out to ensure correct positioning of the LISS—distally on the anterolateral side of the tibia and proximally on the lateral condyle. The internal fixator must be lying flat against the condyle (Fig 3-27). Due to its weight, the insertion guide has a tendency to tilt dorsally. If it is difficult to identify the correct position of the LISS on the condyle, the proximal soft tissues can be further released by enlarging the opening.

The LHS in hole D is angulated toward the posterior side of the medial condyle. Excessive internal rotation of the insertion guide has therefore also has to be prevented, as this screw might endanger the popliteal artery.

Correct positioning of the distal part of the plate is checked either with the image intensifier or through direct palpation.

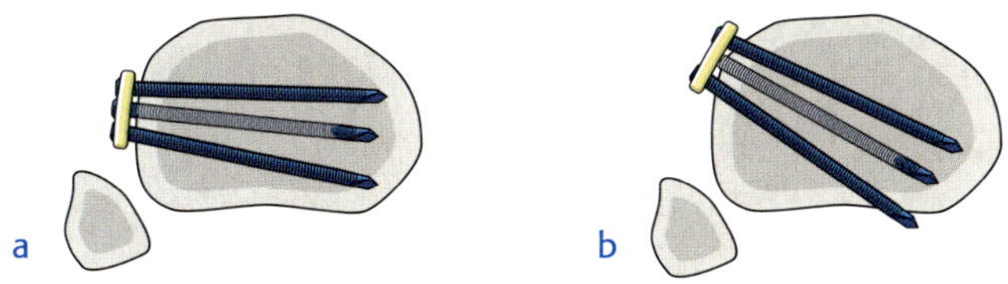

Fig 3-27a–b Position of the LISS fixator.

a Correct position of the LISS-PLT. The screw in hole D aimes to the posteromedial corner of the condyle.

b Excessive internal relation of the insertion guide results in a wrong position of the LISS. The LHS in hole D might then endanger the popliteal artery.

Step 7: building a frame (Fig 3-28)

Once the LISS is properly aligned with the bone, the drill sleeve and stabilization bolt are removed from hole C. The trocar is inserted into the drill sleeve through the most distal hole on the plate (5, 9, or 13). A stab incision is made (Fig 3-28a), and the drill sleeve and trocar are inserted down to the LISS plate.

If a 13-hole LISS plate is being used, careful soft-tissue dissection has to be carried out down to the plate before inserting the trocar and drill sleeve, in order to visualize the superficial fibular nerve.

The position of the drill sleeve is secured with the fixation screw on the insertion guide. The trocar is replaced with the stabilization bolt (Fig 3-28b). The stabilization bolt is threaded into the LISS plate to close the frame.

It should be noted that once the bolt has been inserted, it becomes difficult to change the position of the plate–guide assembly, due to the soft tissues around the stabilization bolt.

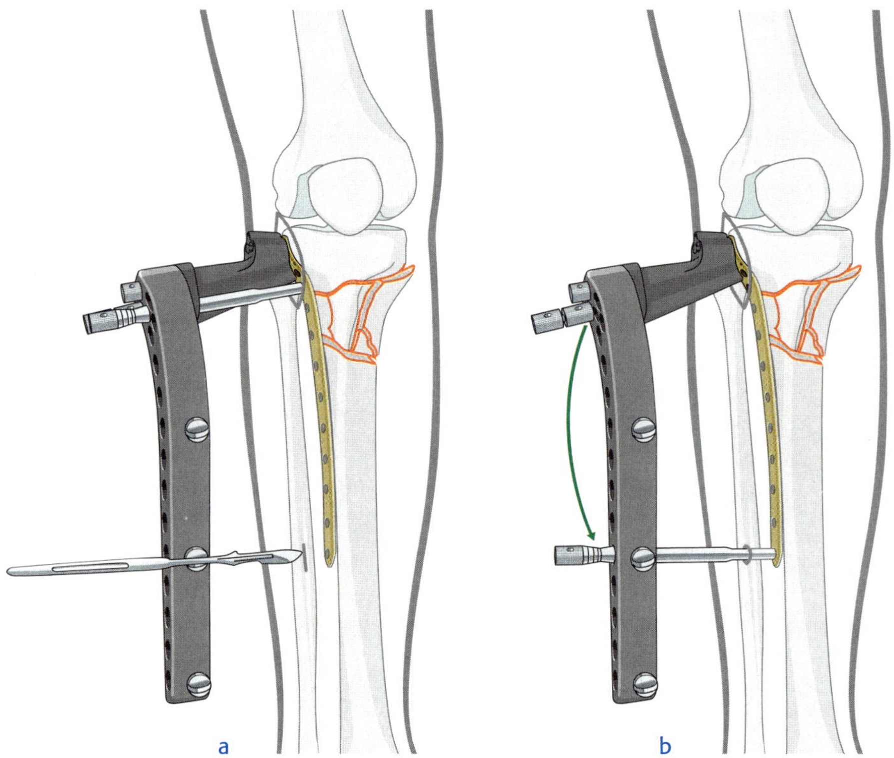

Fig 3-28a–b Building a frame.

a Make a small incision over the most distal hole.

b Remove the drill sleeve and the stabilization bolt from hole C. Insert the trocar in the drill sleeve through the most distal hole of the plate.

Step 8: preliminary fixation of the LISS-PLT (Fig 3-29)

For preliminary fixation of the internal fixator, 2.0 mm K-wires are inserted through the most proximal K-wire hole on the insertion guide (guided only through the aluminum foot part of the insertion guide) and through the stabilization bolt in the most distal hole of the LISS.

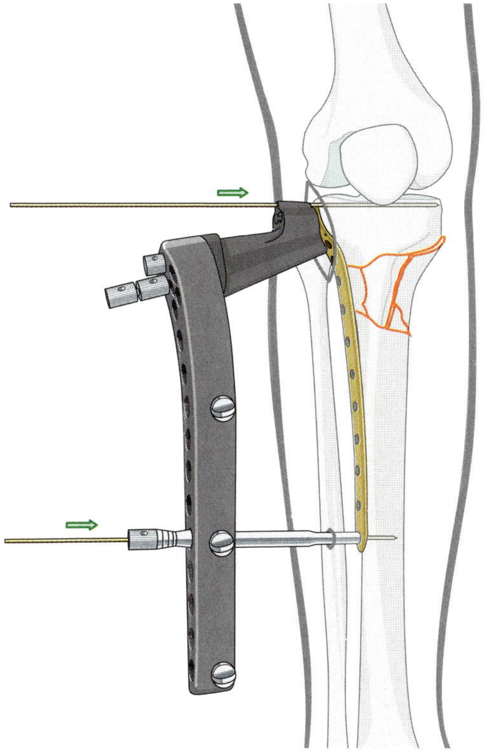

Fig 3-29 Preliminary fixation of the LISS plate with two K-wires.

Step 9: checking the reduction and positioning of the LISS-PLT

The position of the LISS and the reduction (length, alignment, and rotation) of the injured limb are carefully checked. When the reduction has been successfully completed and the internal fixator is in the correct position, the initial LHS can be placed.

Step 10: screw placement (Fig 3-30) (see also the notes on screw placement with the LISS-DF device above)

Screw placement depends on the type of fracture. The positions of the LHS should be chosen in accordance with the established biomechanical principles for internal fixation. The LHS should be inserted remote from the fracture gap in the main fragments. At least four LHS should be used per fracture side. Three to four plate holes at the fracture zone should stay without screws.

- It should be noted that once the initial LHS has been inserted into each main fragment, length and rotation are defined. Antecurvatum and recurvatum deformities can still be adjusted within narrow limits. For this reason, it is recommended to start inserting the first LHS in the proximal fragment.
- If a screw has to be removed and reinserted, the hand torque-limiting screwdriver should be used and not the power tool.
- The length of the condylar LHS required can be calculated from Table 3-2. It is also possible to use the measuring device with a 2.0 mm K-wire (Fig 3-30a), 280 mm long, placed through the centering sleeve in the drill sleeve. Using image intensification, the K-wire is pushed to the desired depth, leaving at least 5 mm between the tip of the K-wire and the medial cortex. The screw length is measured over the K-wire using the measuring device for K-wires, leaving the guide sleeve in place, and rounded down to the nearest screw length. This will ensure that the tip of the screw will not protrude through the medial cortex.
- To improve visualization of the condyle, the drill sleeves for the two most proximal holes (holes D and E) are guided through the aluminum foot part of the insertion guide only. To prevent rotation of the drill sleeve, it is therefore necessary to hold it with two fingers during insertion or removal of the K-wire, as well as during insertion or removal of the two most proximal screws (Fig 3-30b).

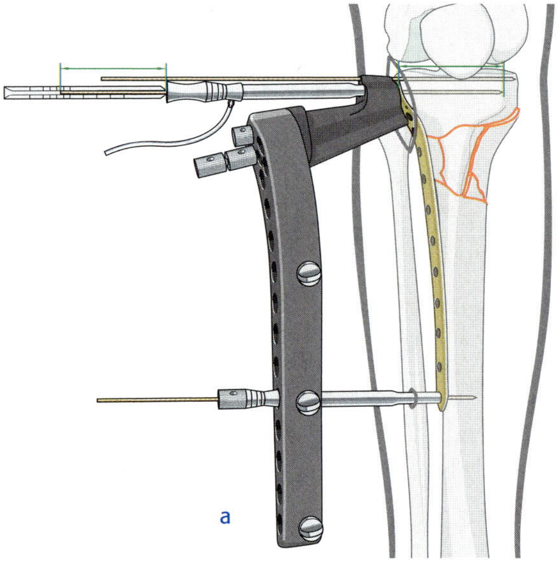

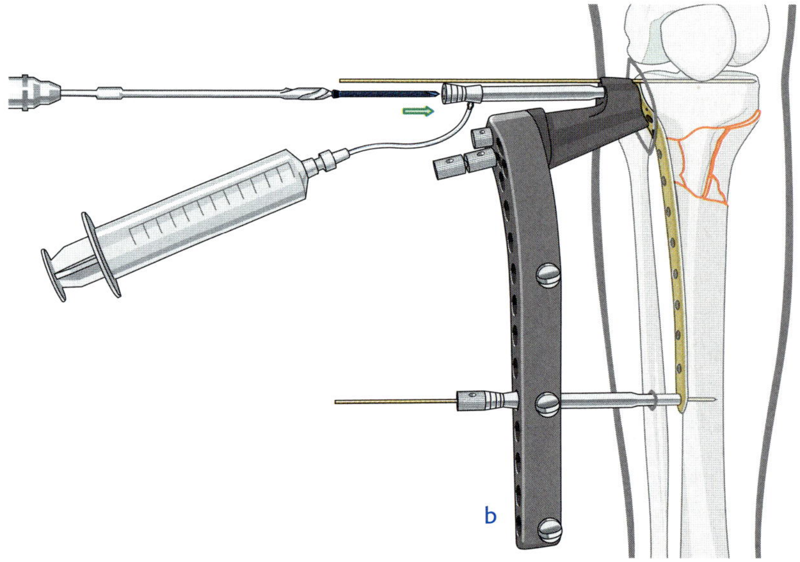

Fig 3-30a–e Screw placement.

a Measuring of the length with a K-wire using the measuring device for K-wires.

b Insertion of LHS in the articular block.

Step 10: screw placement (Fig 3-30) (cont)

- The image intensifier should be oriented obliquely to allow accurate visualization of the point at which the K-wire exits anteromedially or posteromedially.
- 26 mm or 18 mm LHS should be used in the shaft region (Fig 3-30c).
- Initially, a stab incision is made and the trocar is inserted through the drill sleeve.
- If a 13-hole LISS plate is being used, careful soft-tissue dissection has to be carried out down to the plate for holes 10 to 13 before inserting the trocar and drill sleeve, in order to visualize the superficial fibular nerve. Alternatively, blunt dissection from ventral to dorsal can also be carried out.
- Battery-driven or compressed-air tools are used to insert the self-drilling, self-tapping LHS, as only these tools provide the required drill speed. Note: For the final tightening the torque-limiting screwdriver has to be used.
- It is also important to cool the locking head screws with saline solution through the drill sleeve during the drilling procedure, to prevent thermal necrosis. The insertion sleeves have a side nipple to allow irrigation. Use standard tubing and syringes with saline solution.
- Both the screwdriver shaft and the torque-limiting screwdriver are equipped with a self-holding mechanism. Slight pressure should be used to ensure that the screwdriver shaft penetrates the socket of the screw head on pick-up.
- The screws should be advanced into the bone until the bulge of the screwdriver disappears in the drill sleeve. The torque-limiting screwdriver is used for final tightening until clicking occurs at 4 Nm (Fig 3-30d). It should be checked that the screw head is sitting completely in the LISS plate. Soft tissue entrapped between the screw head and the plate can prevent the screw head from being flush with the plate. In such cases, a long hexagonal screwdriver from the pelvic instrument set can be used to complete the tightening.

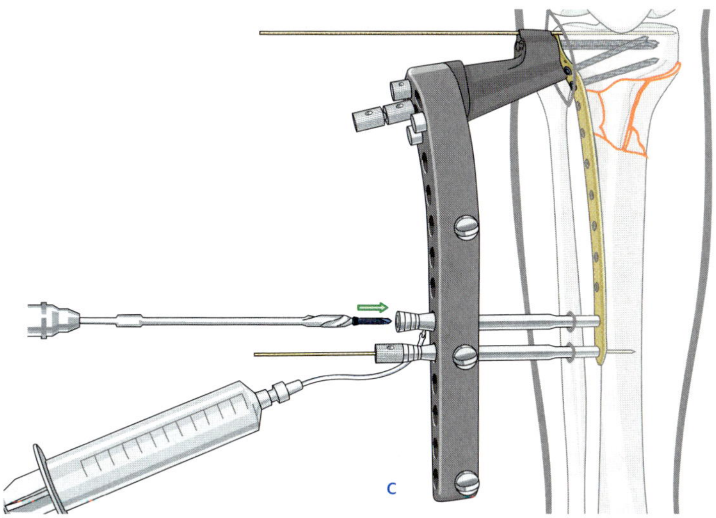
c

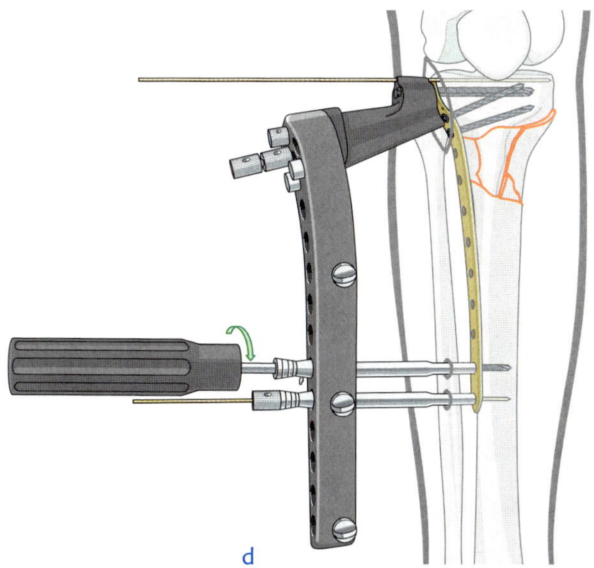
d

Fig 3-30a–e (cont) Screw placement.
c Insertion of the first distal LHS after checking proper position.
d For final tightening the torque-limiting screwdriver has to be used.

Step 10: screw placement (Fig 3-30) (cont)

- The most distal LHS on the fixator should be inserted last (Fig 3-30e), just before removal of the insertion guide, in order to ensure the stability of the construct. The stabilization bolt is then removed and the screw is inserted through the drill sleeve.
- If the LHS is difficult to insert or stops advancing before locking to the plate, then it may be necessary to remove the screw and clean entrapped bone from the cutting flutes using a K-wire. The screw can be reused if the hexagonal socket has not been damaged. If the cortex is very thick, the pulling device can be used for predrilling. Alternatively a special LHS with a longer drill bit can be used.
- If the screwdriver is difficult to remove after insertion, it should be disconnected from the power tool and the drill sleeve should be removed. After the screwdriver is reconnected to the power tool, the screwdriver is withdrawn from the screw.
- A standard 4.5 mm cortex screw can be used through the fixator if required. However, it should be noted that the 4.5 mm cortex screw cannot be inserted through drill sleeve hole A, which serves to lock the insertion guide to the implant. This hole can therefore not be used to insert a LHS while the fixation bolt is attached. If a screw is required in hole A, the fixation bolt should be removed—with the stabilization bolt still in place—and refixed in an adjacent hole that is available. The drill sleeve is placed in hole A and the appropriate screw is inserted. If all the locking head screws have been placed, the free-hand method can be used to insert the LHS in hole A. The direction given by the fixation bolt before removal can be used, or else another plate and screw can be used to determine the correct direction for insertion.

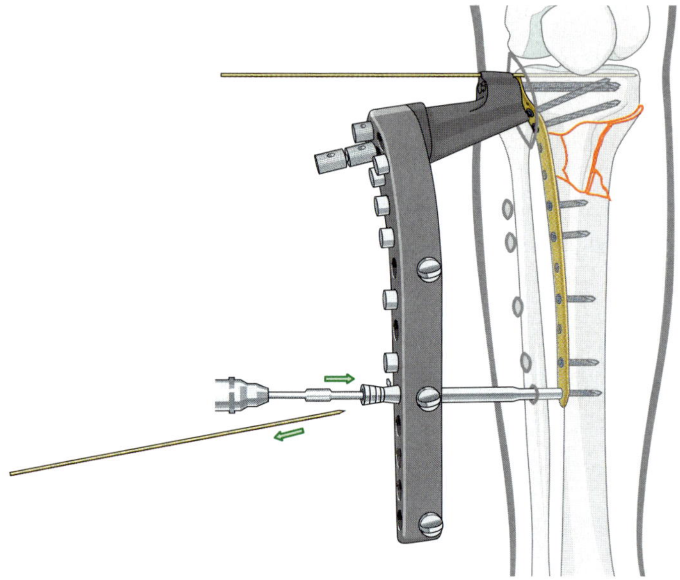

Fig 3-30a–e (cont) Screw placement.
e Removal of the K-wire and insertion of a LHS in the most distal plate hole.

Step 11: removal of the insertion guide, and placement of the "A" proximal tibial LHS (Fig 3-31)

The insertion guide is then disconnected from the fixator. If desired, a LHS or a screw hole inserter can be inserted into the "A" proximal tibial screw position. (Fig 3-31)

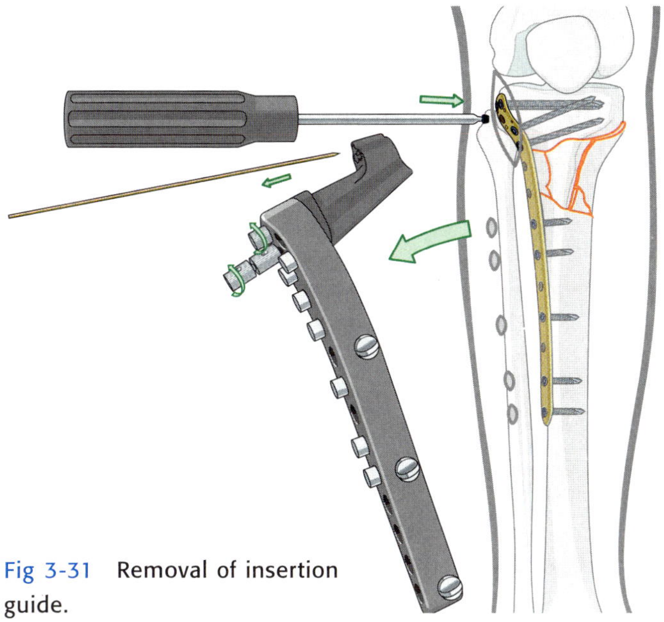

Fig 3-31 Removal of insertion guide.

Step 12: Intraoperative assessement of fracture reduction and stability after fixation

Length, alignment, and rotation should be clinically checked. The knee is taken through a full gentle range of motion to ensure appropriate fracture fixation. Fracture reduction and fracture fixation are then assessed using AP, lateral, and oblique x-rays. Specific questions to be answered in this assessment include:

1. Is there any sagittal plane deformity? How satisfactory is the valgus/varus alignment? The cable method is recommended for checking the alignment of the limb (see chapter 2—4.1).
2. Length, alignment, and rotation should also be checked clinically.
3. How satisfactory is the placement of the fixator on the mid-lateral aspect of the tibia?
4. How satisfactory is the placement of the LISS fixator on the lateral aspect of the tibial condyle?
5. Are all of the screws really placed monocortically into the bone, or are some positioned too far anteriorly or posteriorly?
6. Are any of the LHS in the popliteal fossa and endanger the popliteal artery? (Although rare, this can occur with excessive anterior and internal rolated or posterior positioning of the fixator.) This can be assessed intraoperatively and by image intensification.
7. It should be checked that self-drilling, self-tapping locking head screws have not perforated the medial cortex.

Step 13: wound closure (Fig 3-32)

See chapter 1.2.

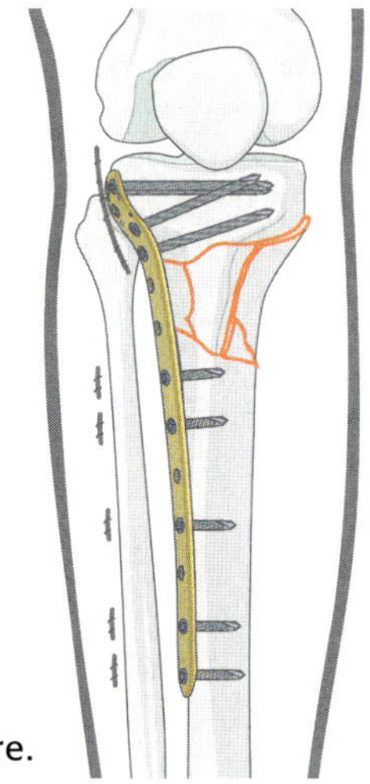

Fig 3-32 Position of the LISS-PLT after definitive osteosynthesis and wound closure.

LCP-PLT

LCP-PLT can be used in the same way as a LISS-PLT but in a more invasive approach without insertion guide. For proper proximal screw placement a smaller guiding block can be used. To find the correct position of the LCP-PLT on the aspect of the lateral distal tibia a small incision is used to palpate or to see the proximal end of the plate. Contrary to the LISS-PLT the LCP-PLT has combination holes so the surgeon can use angulated cortex screws.

Tab 3-5 **LISS-PLT cases**

Case	Classification	Implant used	Page
Tibial plateau fracture; and spiral wedge proximal tibial shaft fracture	41-B3; 42-B1	LISS-PLT, 13 holes	633
Partial articular proximal tibial fracture with split-depression	41-B3	LISS-PLT, 5 holes	645
Complete articular proximal tibial fracture with long spiral fracture of the shaft	41-C1; 42-A2	LISS-PLT, 13 holes	657
Simple articular fracture proximal tibial with metaphyseal comminution	41-C2	LISS-PLT, 13 holes	661
Articular multifragmentary proximal tibial fracture	41-C3	LISS-PLT, 13 holes	669
Open complex irregular tibial and fibular shaft fracture	42-C3	LISS-PLT, 13 holes	759

Approaches

A lateral approach to the tibial head is recommended for the treatment of extraarticular fractures of the proximal tibia. Access along the proximal contour of the tibia should be extended in a medial direction to detach the anterior tibial muscle close to the bone, with part of the muscle fascia on the bone being left intact to ensure easier refixation of the muscle. For more severely displaced articular fractures more extended approaches are necessary (see step 2).

Strategy for fracture reduction and fixation

A further consideration when planning the surgical procedure is whether or not there is an intraarticular fracture that requires open reduction. Fracture reduction and fixation proceed in two distinct steps, with reduction of the intraarticular fracture being carried out first. Anatomical reduction and internal fixation with compression screws are mandatory in articular fractures. The second step is the closed, indirect reduction of the metaphyseal fracture and fixation by locked splinting method.

1.4 Postoperative treatment

Postoperative treatment follows the same principles as in conventional internal fixation procedures and basically consists of functional treatment with free mobilization of the knee joint and partial weight bearing. Mobilization of the patient and limb is started immediately after the operation. The operated limb may be rested on a continuous passive motion machine as soon as the patient returns to the ward. Toe-touch weight bearing starts immediately. Progressive weight bearing depends on the specific fracture situation (additional articular fracture) commences when significant callus formation in the supracondylar region becomes apparent, or as soon as the healing of other ipsilateral injuries allows. Hinged knee braces are not used. Physical rehabilitation should be started immediately postoperatively, including range-of-motion exercises. Restrictions may be appropriate in special cases.

1.5 Implant removal

The implant should only be removed after complete consolidation of the fracture. The sequence of removal procedures is the reverse of the implantation process [13]. An incision is initially made in the path of the old scar for the insertion guide, and the insertion guide is mounted. To facilitate application of the insertion guide during implant removal, hole A has to be closed with a screw hole inserter if a screw has not been inserted into this hole while the first operation.

Stab incisions are made. The cleaning tool helps clean the hexagonal recess in the screw head. The torque-limiting hexagonal screwdriver is used to remove the LHS manually. Removal of the LHS is completed with a power tool.

When removing a 13-hole LISS plate, careful soft-tissue dissection has to be carried out down to the plate before inserting the trocar and drill sleeve, in order to visualize the superficial fibular nerve.

After all of the LHS have been removed, the LISS plate is removed. If the plate is still stuck after all of the LHS have been removed, the insertion guide should be removed first, and only the fixation bolt should be used for subsequent loosening of the LISS.

1.6 Implant-specific problems and complications

(See chapter 4) One of the complications specific to LISS-DF is proximal screw pullout. Possible predisposing factors for this include failure to place the LISS-DF on the shaft laterally, and possibly incorrect rotation, which causes tangential placement of the screws in the shaft cortex so that the screws only gain purchase in a small section close to the tip of the screw. Pullout occurs typically after approximately 6–8 weeks—ie, as soon as the patient increases weight bearing.

If the plate is lying too far anteriorly or posteriorly, the screws will not be centered in the medullary canal, so that the screws do not have adequate purchase (Fig 3-33).

Bending and twisting of the LISS plate is not allowed, as this results in misalignment between the holes on the insertion guide and the corresponding plate holes.

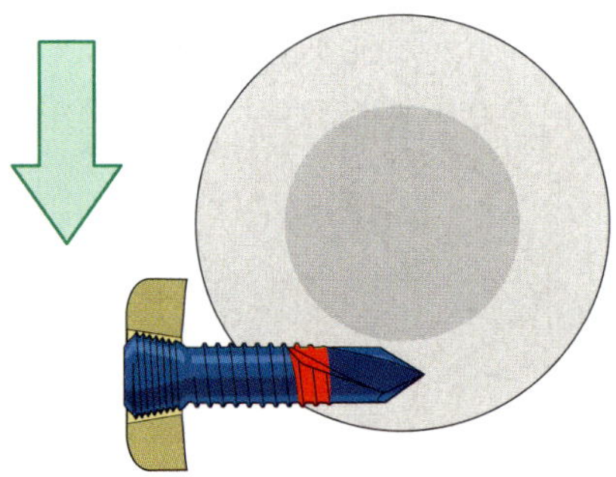

Fig 3-33 The fixator is often misplaced slightly anterior or posterior to the midshaft of the proximal femur. If this happens in conventional plating, one can simply then drill either anteriorly or posteriorly. This is not possible with LISS fixation, as the screws enter perpendicular to the surface of the plate. If the fixator is slightly off center from the midlateral aspect of the femur or if it is slightly rotated, the screws will not obtain adequate purchase in the cortex.

1.7 Clinical results

Since the introduction of the first anatomically contoured locking plate systems for fractures involving the knee in 1997, most publications have reported on the excellent results achieved even for extremely complex distal femoral and proximal tibial fractures. However, technical difficulties during its application and negative effects on the healing process were also observed.

The union rate was 93% with a 3% infection rate. Most importantly, the problem of varus collapse of the distal femoral block has been addressed. Biomechanically, the LISS has tested superior to the blade plate and the retrograde intramedullary nail for fixation of supracondylar femoral fractures in osteoporotic bone. This has also been seen clinically, with no secondary loosening of distal fixation or varus collaps. It is a relatively elastic implant so whenever an osteoporotic fracture fixation construct is loaded by the patient, the implant can elastically deform rather than cause destruction at the bone-screw interface.

Additional clinical studies found in the literature evaluating the LISS-DF: [14–21].

Additional clinical studies found in the literature evaluating the LISS-PLT: [22–30].

2 The locking compression plate (LCP)

With its newly designed combination hole, the LCP makes it possible to implement the principles of both compression and splinting for fracture stabilization in the same implant [31] (see chapter 1, for a discussion of compression versus splinting). The development of the LCP is outlined in chapter 1.

The following considerations are important when deciding whether or not to use the LCP:

- Clinical factors:
  - Fracture location and configuration
  - Soft-tissue condition
  - Patient's general condition (multiple trauma, Injury Severity Score, Glasgow Coma Scale)
- Other factors:
  - Indications for other implants: is an intramedullary nail suitable for shaft fractures in long bones?
  - Borderline indications for intramedullary nails: metaphyseal zone, size of the medullary canal, etc.
  - Presence of other implants
  - Availability of implants (eg, LCP), instruments, and intraoperative imaging
  - Surgeon's personal experience and preference

The biomechanical principles and various techniques for using LCP in various indications are summarized in Tabs 1-6 and 1-7.

2.1 Implants and instruments

Selecting the plate

The standard LCP has the same cross-section and mechanical properties as the corresponding LC-DCP. The same type of implant can therefore be chosen for specific bone segments and fracture configurations (Tab 3-6). There are large and small fragment standard LCP available.

Special plates are available for the epiphyseal and metaphyseal area of long bones. These differ from the standard LCP in that the plate segment close to the joint has a thinner cross section, leading to less interference with the usually thin soft-tissue envelope and allowing the insertion of screws one size smaller close to the joint than in the diaphyseal area (LCP metaphyseal 3.5/4.5/5.0 and LCP metaphyseal 3.5). This type of plate can be used more or less universally close to joints.

Anatomically preshaped plates are also available for different anatomical areas: proximal humerus, distal humerus, olecranon, distal radius, proximal femur, distal femur, proximal tibia, distal tibia, pilon, and calcaneus. These have the advantage that intraoperative shaping of the plate is no longer needed, with screw insertion being facilitated with the use of guiding blocks (Tab 1-12). Specific LCP for opening and closing wedge osteotomies of the distal femur and the proximal tibia are also available.

Tab 3-6 **Select the appropriate locking compression plate (LCP)**

Implant	Indication
LCP 4.5/5.0, broad	• Metaphyseal/diaphyseal fracture of the femur and humerus • Nonunion of the tibia/humerus
LCP 4.5/5.0, narrow	• Metaphyseal/diaphyseal fracture of the tibia • Metaphyseal/diaphyseal fracture of the humerus in small women • Anterior and posterior pelvic ring segment • Anterior sacroiliac joint plating • Posterior ilio-iliac plating • Symphysis pubis
LCP metaphyseal plate 3.5/4.5/5.0	• Metaphyseal/diaphyseal fractures of the distal tibia with a short distal fragment • Tibial plateau fracture • Metaphyseal/diaphyseal fractures of the proximal and distal humerus
LCP reconstruction plate 4.5/5.0	• No clear indication
LCP T- and L-plate 4.5/5.0	• Epiphyseal/metaphyseal fractures of the proximal tibia • Unicondylar fracture of the distal femur
LCP 3.5	• Metaphyseal/diaphyseal fractures of the forearm • Epiphyseal/metaphyseal fractures of the proximal or distal humerus • Clavicular fractures • Tibial plateau fractures • Malleolar fractures (type C) • Sacral fractures
LCP metaphyseal plate 3.5	• Epiphyseal/metaphyseal fractures of the distal humerus, distal radius, and olecranon
LCP reconstruction plate 3.5	• Epiphyseal/metaphyseal fractures of the distal humerus, symphysis pubis, acetabular fractures
One-third tubular plate	• Malleolar fractures (type A, B, C)
Anatomically preshaped plates	• Specific region for which the plate is designed

Selecting the screw type

Five different types of screws can be used with the LCP. Careful analysis of the intended function is required to ensure optimal use of the different types (Tab 3-7) [32, 33].

- Cortex screw, self-tapping cortex screw, cortex shaft screw.
- Cancellous bone screw, partially or fully threaded. The partially threaded cancellous bone screws are cancellous shaft screws.
- Self-drilling, self-tapping locking head screw (for monocortical use only).
- Self-tapping locking head screw (for mono- or bicortical use).

Tab 3-7 **Select the correct screw type**

Type of screw	Bone segment	Function of screw	Anchorage
Cancellous bone screw • partially (ie, cancellous shaft screw) or • fully threaded	Epiphysis Metaphysis	Free, plate-independent lag screw [1] Plate lagging screw [1] Plate fixation screw	As long as possible
Cortex screw , self-tapping cortex screw	Diaphysis Epiphysis Metaphysis	Free, plate-independent lag screw Plate lagging screw Plate fixation screw Position screw Reduction screw	Monocortical or bicortical
Cortex shaft screw partially threaded	Diaphysis	Free, plate-independent lag screw Plate lagging screw	Monocortical
Self-tapping locking head screw	Diaphysis Epiphysis Metaphysis	Plate fixation screw Plate dependent position screw	Monocortical or bicortical (in metaphysis and epiphysis as long as possible)
Self-drilling, self-tapping locking head screw	Diaphysis	Plate fixation screw	Monocortical

[1] Only partially threaded cancellous screws can be used as lag screws.

Tab 3-8 **Different functions and rules of screws**

Function	Type of screw	Effect	Prerequirements
Lag screw • free, plate-independent • plate lagging screw	Cortex screw [1] cortex shaft screw [2] cancellous shaft screw [2]	Interfragmentary compression	Gliding hole, threaded hole for a fully threaded screw or a partially threaded screw
Eccentric screw = compression screw	Cortex and self-tapping cortex screw Cancellous bone screw	Interfragmentary compression	Dynamic compression unit (DCU) and hemispheric screwhead of conventional screw
Plate fixation	Cortex and self-tapping cortex screws Cancellous bone screw Self-tapping locking head screws (LHS)	Friction between bone a plate Locking	For conventional screws good bone quality prebending of the plate
Position screw • free, plate-independent • through a plate hole	Cortex and self-tapping cortex screws Cancellous bone screws, fully threaded Self-tapping LHS, only plate-dependent	Hold the relative position between two fragments	
Reduction screw	Cortex screw self-tapping cortex LHS/fine tuning	Reduction onto the plate, Reduction of a butterfly fragment	No interfragmentary compression LHS, screwdriver, screw holding sleeve

Self-tapping screws are not recommended to use as lag screws. [2] Partially threaded.

The following factors are critical for the appropriate choice of screw:

- The mechanical principle of fixation required:
  - Locked splinting method to achieve the principle of relative stability versus interfragmentary compression method to achieve the principle of absolute stability.
  - Locked internal fixator versus standard plating technique
  - Plate fixation on the bone with LHS (noncontact plate) or (compression, friction) with standard screws
  - Technique of reduction and plate insertion.
  - Minimally invasive plate osteosynthesis (MIPO) technique versus open reduction and internal fixation (ORIF).
  - Epiphyseal/metaphyseal area versus diaphyseal area.

Cancellous bone screw and cortex screw. Cancellous bone screws or cortex screws can be used as lag screws, plate dependent lag screw or position screws, either alone (plate-independent), or through a plate hole. In combination with a plate these screws are also used as eccentric compression screws or as plate fixation screws. Their use is recommended when the screw has to be inserted at an angle in case of axial malalignment between the bone and plate axis, or to avoid screw penetration into a joint; when interfragmentary compression with eccentric screw insertion or a lag screw is required; or with a bridge plating technique with good bone quality. Cancellous bone screws or cortex screws are also used for reduction of a fragment onto the plate. These screws are usually anchored in both cortices; monocortical screw insertion is only carried out exceptionally.

Cancellous bone screws or cortex screws have the advantages that the screws can be angulated inside the plate hole, making it possible to reduce fragments onto the plate. Their disadvantage is that they compromise the blood supply to the bone cortex, due to the need for direct contact between the plate and the bone to allow load transmission by a friction force.

Locking head screws. All LHS provide angular and axial stability inside the plate hole. They act more like a bolt than a screw, and there is a complete absence of axial preloading inside the screw during its insertion. Under functional loading they are loaded in bending and in axial load depending on the external loading condition. LHS cannot be used as lag screws.

The advantages of LHS include improved anchorage in bone due to the slight increase in the outer screw diameter and altered loading conditions. On the biological side, they also have the advantage of requiring no contact between the plate and bone, thus protecting the periostal blood supply to the bone. The lack of angulation inside the plate can be a disadvantage in the epiphyseal bone segment.

A disadvantage is that the surgeon may completely lose the feel for the quality of the bone during screw insertion and tightening, when the screw head engages in the conical-threaded plate hole. Percutaneous insertion of short monocortical LHS in the diaphyseal area is critical at the end of the plate, when there is some malalignment between the long bone axis and the plate. In these situations, anchorage is not obtained with a short screw, despite the surgical sensation that there is good tightening (Fig 3-34). Technically, the problem can be solved either by inserting a long self-tapping LHS or by using an angulated cortex or cancellous bone screw (Fig 3-35). The problem can be avoided at an early stage of the procedure by using the drill bit to center the screw and feel the bone cortex before the monocortical self-drilling, self-tapping LHS is inserted. Alternatively, a small incision can be made at the plate end and the position of the plate can be assessed on the lateral side of the bone by manual palpation and by vision.

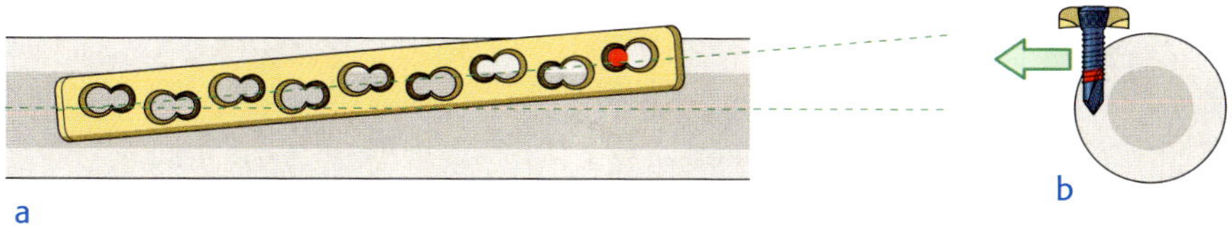

Fig 3-34a–b
- a Malalignment between the bone axis and plate leads to an eccentric plate position.
- b At the far end of the plate, a monocortical locking head screw will not anchor in the bone in these conditions.

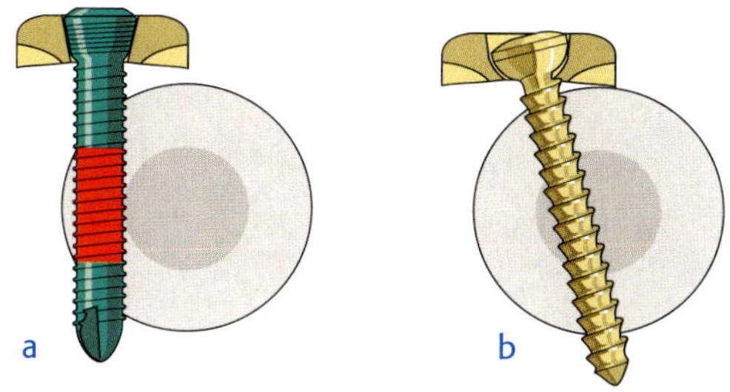

Fig 3-35a–b Screw insertion in an eccentric plate position. To overcome the problem of insufficient anchorage of a monocortical self-drilling, self-tapping screw when the plate is positioned eccentrically, it is recommended either to insert (a) a long bicortical self-tapping screw or (b) a cortex screw that allows angulation in the plate hole.

Two different types of LHS are available—self-drilling and self-tapping, or self-tapping.

Self-drilling, self-tapping LHS. Self-drilling, self-tapping LHS are used only as monocortical screws in the diaphyseal segment of bone when excellent bone quality is present. The cutting tip of the screw prevents destruction of the bone thread in the near cortex when there is a narrow medullary cavity, because the screw tip is able to penetrate into the opposite cortex (Fig 3-36) (see chapter 4). When a self-drilling, self-tapping LHS is anchored in both cortices, the drilling unit protrudes well into the soft tissues, with a potential risk of damage to neurovascular structures behind (Fig 3-37).

Setting a self-drilling, self-tapping LHS percutaneously, using a freehand technique (without using an aiming device) sometimes results in an imperfect centering of the screw tip in the plate hole and in insufficient anchorage of the head inside the plate hole due to angulation of the LHS.

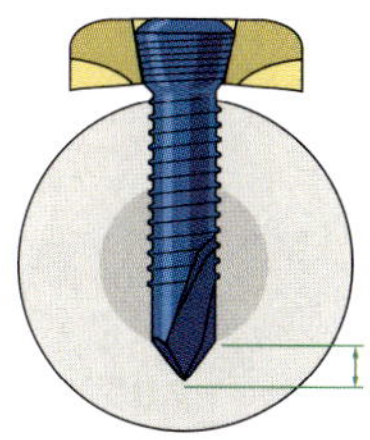

Fig 3-36 Self-drilling, self-tapping locking head screws should only be used in the diaphyseal bone segment and only as monocortical screws. The cutting tip of the screw presents destruction of the bone thread in the near cortex when there is a narrow medullary cavity.

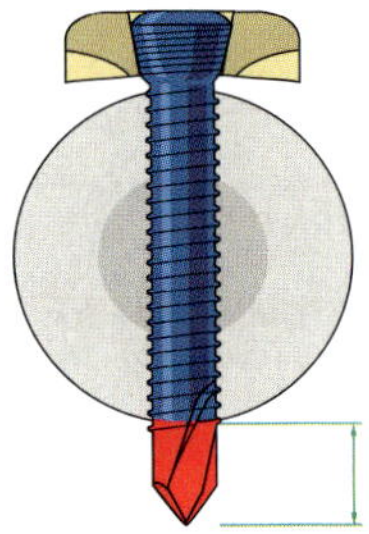

Fig 3-37 Protrusion length of self-drilling, self-tapping screws. Due to the length of the self-drilling unit the tip of the screw protrudes from the bone when it is anchored with the screw thread in both cortices. Self-drilling, self-tapping locking head screws should only be used as monocortical screws, to prevent damage to the soft tissues opposite the plate.

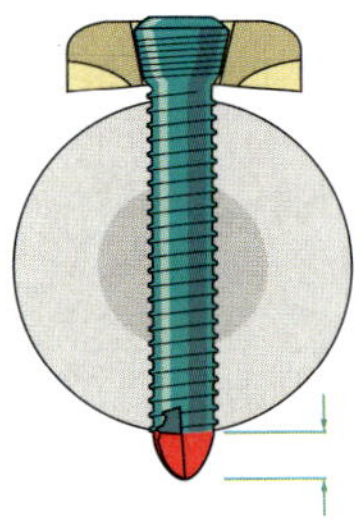

Fig 3-38 In order to gain purchase in both cortices, the self-tapping screw has to protrude from the bone. However, due to the relatively smooth screw tip, no damage to the neurovascular structures opposite the plate occurs.

Self-tapping LHS. Self-tapping LHS are used in the epiphyseal, metaphyseal, and diaphyseal segments of the bone when the insertion of bicortical LHS or the longest possible LHS is planned. Since a self-tapping LHS does not have a cutting tip, the tip is blunt (Fig 3-38). To provide good anchorage of the screw threads in both cortices, the self-tapping LHS should protrude slightly beyond the far cortex.

Self-tapping LHS require predrilling through the threaded drill sleeve. Used correctly, the mono- or bicortical self-tapping LHS is always perpendicular in the center of the threaded, conical part of the combination hole.

In the presence of osteoporosis, the bone cortex is usually thin. In these conditions, the working length of a monocortical LHS is short, so that poor anchorage is obtained even with locking head screws (Fig 3-39). This problem can lead to complete loss of screw anchorage, resulting in instability of

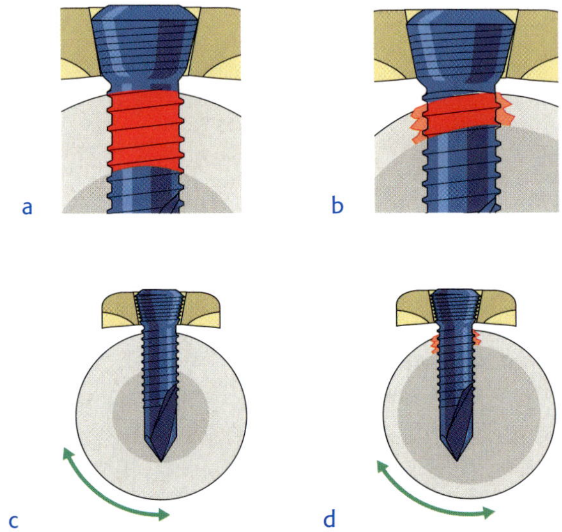

Fig 3-39a–d The working length of monocortical screws depends on the thickness of the bone cortex.

- a In normal bone, this working length is sufficient.
- b In osteoporotic bone, by contrast, the cortex is usually very thin, so that the working length of a monocortical screw is insufficient. This difference in working length is important when osteoporotic bones such as the humerus have to be stabilized.
- c In normal bone, the length of anchorage of the screw thread is sufficient enough to withstand rotational displacement.
- d When there is osteoporosis, the working length is very short due to the thin cortex, and under torque the bone thread will quickly wear out, leading to secondary displacement and instability.

the fixation—a common situation in bones that are mainly subjected to torsional loading (eg, humerus). The use of bicortical self-tapping LHS is recommended in all segments for all osteoporosis-associated fractures. This approach improves the working length and avoids potential problems at the interface between the screw thread and the bone (Fig 3-40).

Even the shortest monocortical self-tapping LHS will destroy the bone thread if the screw tip touches the opposite cortex before the screw head has locked into the plate hole. If this occurs, the monocortical LHS should be replaced with a bicortical self-tapping LHS, which will ensure anchorage in the opposite cortex (Fig 3-41). To avoid the problem of bone thread destruction the measuring of the correct length of the screw after drilling is important.

In bones with a small diameter the problem can be avoided at an early stage of the procedure by drilling both cortices (eg, bones with small diameter as forearm or fibula).

Monocortical or bicortical LHS. Monocortical LHS can only be used in the diaphyseal segment of long bones when the bone quality is normal, when the cortex is thick enough to allow anchorage of the screw with a sufficient working length of the thread, and when the specific bone has a low loading level in torque.

Bicortical LHS are recommended in the following situations: weak osteoporotic bone; thin bone cortex that does not provide a sufficient working length for the screw; high torque loading in the plated bone segment; a short main fragment that only allows a limited number of screws; in bones with small diameter; when a cortex screw used for reduction is replaced by an LHS; and destruction of the bone thread in the near cortex due to incorrect insertion of the LHS.

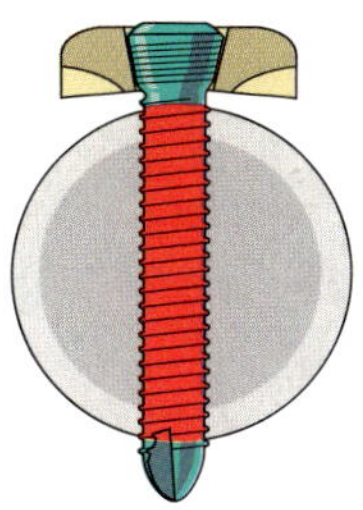

Fig 3-40 Improvement of the working length. In osteoporotic bone with a very thin cortex, the standard use of bicortical screws is recommended, as the longer working length leads to a much better torque resistance.

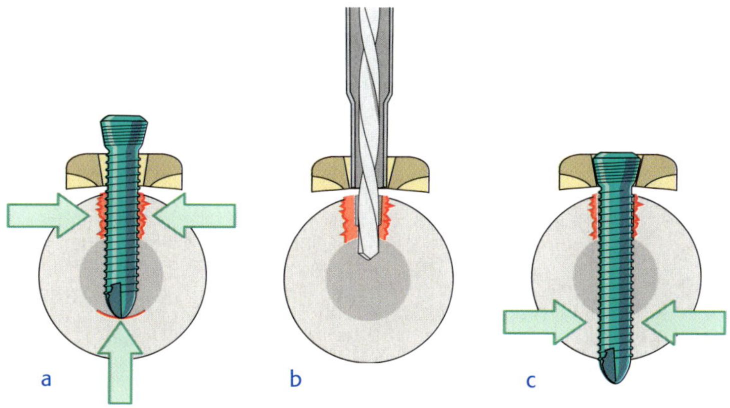

Fig 3-41a–c
- a Danger of insertion of monocortical self-tapping LHS. In bones with a small diameter, the tip of the screw can contact the opposite bone cortex before the screw head has engaged in the thread of the plate hole. This leads to the destruction of the bone thread in the near cortex and complete loss of anchorage of the screw.
- b The situation can be resolved by using a threaded drill sleeve the opposite cortex is drilled in the correct axis.
- c Inserting a self-tapping bicortical LHS to obtain anchorage in the opposite cortex.

Positioning the implant

The standard positions used for the LC-DCP can also be used for positioning the LCP. Its function as an locked internal fixator or as protection plate fixed with locking head screws has not yet led to a modification of the standard approaches. When the LCP is used as an internal fixator, it can be placed on any bone surface that can be conveniently approached even with a minimally invasive plate osteosynthesis technique.

Length of the implant (Tab 3-9; Figs 3-42, 3-43)

The choice of the appropriate length of the LCP (and of all plates) is one of the most important steps in internal fixation. It depends on the fracture pattern and the method and mechanical principle being used for fixation. In intramedullary nailing, there is no question regarding the length of the nail, which is more or less equal to the complete length of the fractured bone from one epiphysis to the other.

Tab 3-9 **Guidelines for plate fixation in simple and multifragmentary fractures**

	Simple fracture	Simple fracture	Multifragmentary fracture
Biomechanical principle	Interfragmentary compression (splinting in exceptional cases)	Splinting in exceptional cases without lag screw	Splinting
Reduction technique	Mainly direct	Indirect or percutaneous direct [1]	Preferably indirect
Insertion	At least partly open	Open, less invasive, MIPO	Closed, minimally invasive
Shaping of the plate	Has to be fitted to bone surface	Accurate shaping not needed with LHS	Accurate shaping not required with LHS
Plate span ratio $= \frac{\text{plate length}}{\text{fracture length}}$	$> \frac{8-10}{1}$	$> \frac{2-3}{1}$	$> \frac{2-3}{1}$
Screw type	• Cortex screws in eccentric position for compression • Cortex screw in neutral position or LHS for plate fixation	• Cortex screws or LHS in good bone • LHS in poor bone and with MIPO technique	• Cortex screws or LHS in good bone • LHS in poor bone and with MIPO technique
Monocortical/bicortical screws	• Cortex screws: bicortical	• Cortex screws: bicortical	• Cortex screws: bicortical
LHS in the diaphysis	• Self-drilling/self-tapping monocortical or self-tapping bicortical	• Self-drilling/self-tapping monocortical or self-tapping mono or bicortical	• Self-drilling/self-tapping monocortical or self-tapping mono or bicortical
LHS in the epiphysis/metaphysis	• Self-tapping bicortical	• Self-tapping bicortical	• Self-tapping bicortical
Plate screw density (see text)	≤ 0.4–0.3	≤ 0.5–0.4	≤ 0.5–0.4
Screws per main fragment (n)	≥ 3; 2 exceptionally	≥ 3; 2 exceptionally	≥ 3; 2 exceptionally
Cortices per main fragment (n)	3–5	≥ 4	≥ 4
Screw position	Short middle segment without screws	Middle segment without screws also without lag screws	Long middle segment without screws
Empty plate holes over the fracture	0–3	≤ 2	≥ 3

[1] Splinting of simple fractures should respect the biomechanical rules according to the strain theory.

Effects of plate length on screw loading

The length of the plate and the position of the screws affect the loading conditions of the screws. The "end-of-fragment" screws are the ones that are critically and maximally loaded, and should be considered separately from the other plate screws. Each bending moment is the product of a force and a distance; the force can be reduced under a given bending moment by increasing the length or leverage. Thus, the longer the plate, the smaller the pull-out force acting on the screws—an effect that is purely due to the improvement of the plate leverage acting on the screws (Fig 3-42a–d). This applies both to standard screws and locking head screws.

Longer plates reduce the stress in the plate as well as to the screws. From the mechanical point of view, it is therefore better to use very long plates. When the LCP is applied as an internal fixator with locking head screws, screw loading mainly occurs with bending and not with pullout. All of the screws are loaded simultaneously, and failure at the interface between the screw thread and the bone may be less frequent. Nevertheless, the working length of an internal fixator should also be kept long and well-spaced. With indirect reduction, minimally invasive insertion, and the LCP fixation with LHS, no biological disadvantages have been observed with long implants.

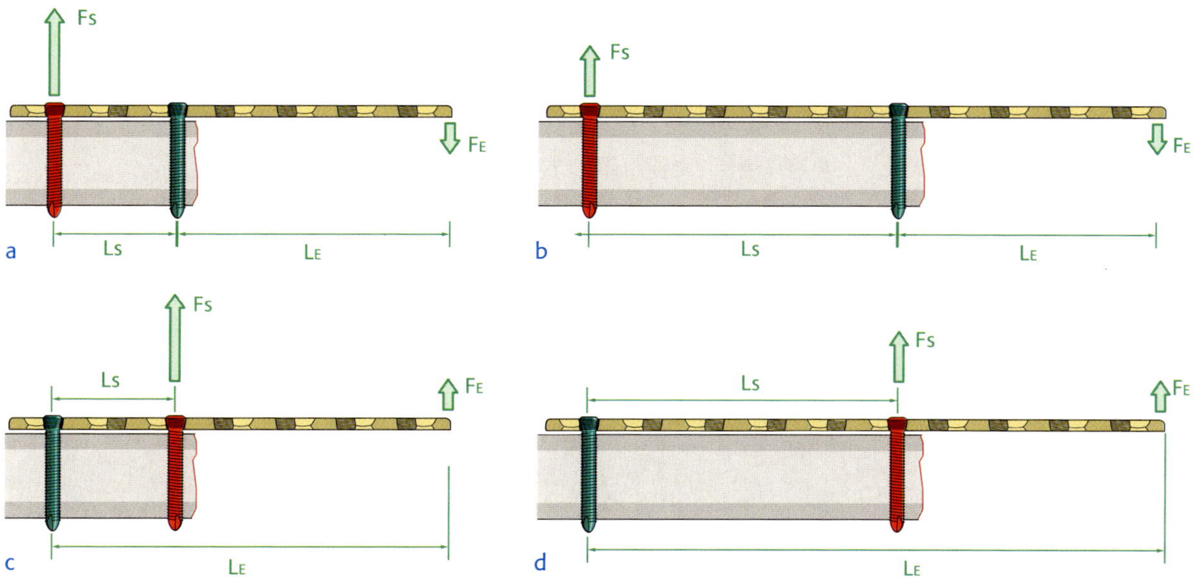

Fig 3-42a–d Pull-out force on screws and working leverage of the plate. When a relatively short plate is used, the screw loading is relatively high due to the short working leverage of the screws in both directions of a bending moment (a, c). Using a longer plate increases the working leverage for each screw. Under a given bending moment, the pull-out force of the screws is therefore reduced (b, d).

F_E External force creating a bending moment on the plate.
L_E Lever arm of the external force.
F_S Pull-out force of the screw.
L_S Lever arm of the screw.

Effect of plate length and screw position on plate loading

Bending a plate over a short segment enhances the local strain on the implant. Bending it over a longer segment and limiting the deformation by intercalated bone fragments reduces the local strain (ie, stress distribution) and provides protection against fatigue failure of the implant (Fig 3-43).

In compression plating, after precise reduction of a simple fracture, with the plate and the bone both sharing the load, the two middle plate screws can be inserted as closely as possible to the fracture site, with the peripheral screws inserted at each end of the plate. In simple fractures without precise reduction—leaving a gap and splinting the fracture, leave two to three plate holes without screws to avoid stress concentration at a small plate segment. In a multifragmentary diaphyseal fracture bridged with an internal fixator as a nongliding splint, the long distance between the two screws adjacent to the fracture is determined by the fracture zone. This result in less elastic deformation of the plate and the interfragmentary tissues [5,6].

For practical use there are some basic rules:

1 Length of plate: first determine the fracture length, then chose the plate length three times the fracture length.
2 Number of screws and position of screws: few screws but position precisely planned, only 50% of plate holes occupied with screws.

The placement and position of the screws is more important than the number of screws.

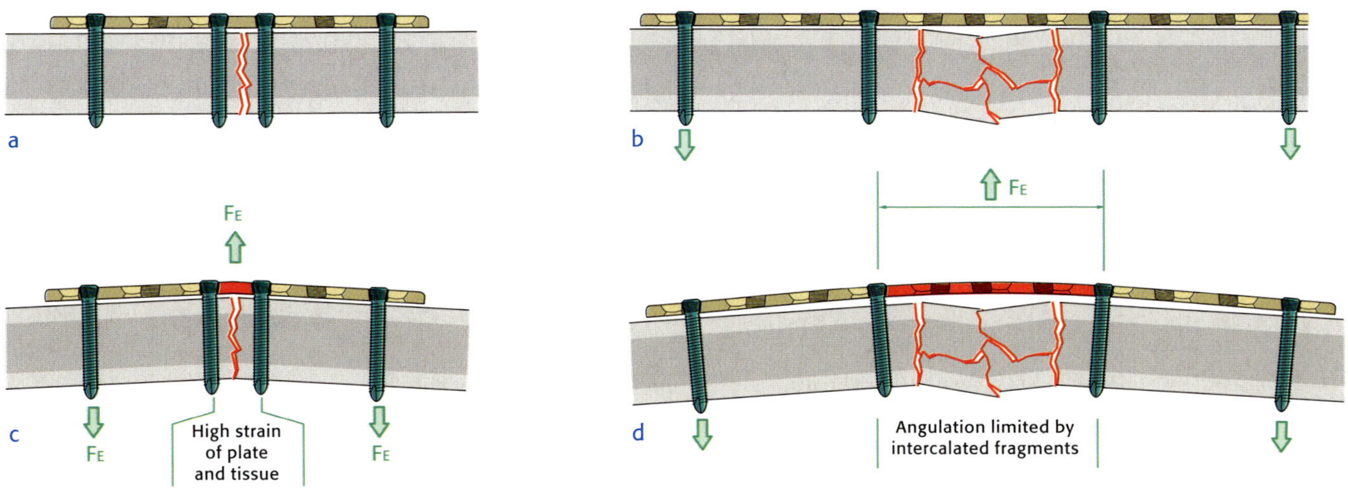

Fig 3-43a–d Plate strain in three-point bending. Depending on the degree, bending moment leads to reversible deformation (ie, reversible angulation) of the implant. When the segment to be bent is short (a), the relative deformation (strain) is high and the implant is liable to undergo fatigue failure quite soon. Where the plate spans a longer area of a multifragmentary fracture (b, d), the same bending moment leads to less stress concentration of the plate when the intercalated fragments are squeezed between the main fragments. The deformation is distributed over a longer distance, leading to low implant strain and higher resistance against fatigue failure.

F_E External force creating a bending moment on the plate.

The external fixator also bridges almost the entire length of the bone. In contrast, the length of the plate has continued to be a matter of controversy for some time. In the past, a short (often too short) plate was often chosen to avoid a long skin incision and extensive soft-tissue dissection. With the newer techniques of indirect reduction, with subcutaneous or submuscular insertion of the implant and the locked splinting method to bridge the fracture zone, the plate length can be increased without additional soft-tissue dissection. Little or no additional biological damage is caused, and the plate length can be adapted to the mechanical requirements of the specific fracture. From the mechanical point of view, plate loading and screw loading should be kept as low as possible to avoid fatigue failure of the plate due to cyclic loading, or pullout of the screws due to excessive single overloading.

Three segments of the plate can be distinguished: the middle segment at the fracture site between the two innermost screws, and the proximal and distal plate segments anchoring the implant onto the proximal and distal main fragments. The length of the plate and the positioning of the screws influence the loading conditions in the plate and screws. The length of the middle plate segment and the method of spanning the fracture are responsible for the biological response of fracture healing (indirect healing, direct healing, or failure to heal) (Fig 3-44).

The ideal length for the internal fixator can be determined using two values: the plate span ratio and the plate screw density [34]. The plate span ratio is the ratio of plate length to overall fracture length. Experience has shown that the plate span ratio should be greater than 2:1 or 3:1 in multifragmentary fractures and greater than 8:1, 9:1, or 10:1 in simple fractures. The plate screw density is the proportion of the number of screws inserted to the number of plate holes. Values below 0.5 to 0.4 are recommended, indicating that fewer than half of the plate holes are occupied by screws.

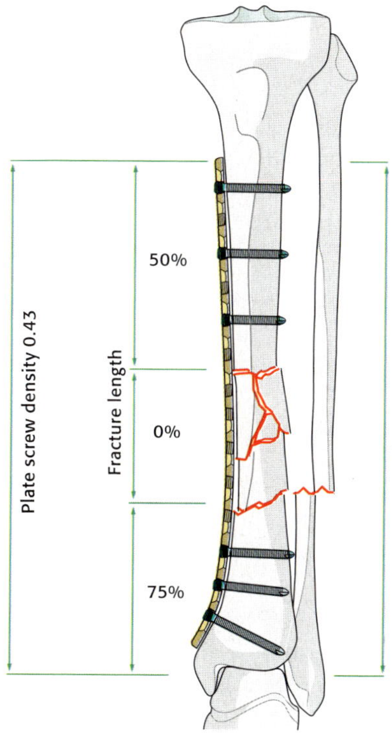

Fig 3-44 Importance of the plate-span ratio and plate-screw density in bridge plating technique. The schematic drawing shows a mechanically sound fixation of a multifragmentary diaphyseal fracture in the lower leg. The ratio between the length of the plate and the length of the fracture is known as the plate–span ratio. In this case, the ratio is high enough—ie, approximately 3, indicating that the plate is three times longer than the overall fracture area. The plate–screw density is shown for all the three bone segments. The proximal main fragment has a plate–screw density of 0.5 (three out of six holes occupied); the segment over the fracture has a density of 0 (none out of four holes occupied); and the distal main fragment has a density of 0.75 (three out of four holes occupied holes). The higher plate–screw density in the distal main fragment has to be accepted, since for anatomical reasons there is no way of reducing it. The overall plate-screw density for the construct in this example is 0.43 (six screws in a 14-hole plate).

Number of screws (Tabs 3-8, 3-9)

Earlier AO guidelines recommending specific numbers of screws, and monocortical or bicortical in each fragment should no longer be the only decisive factors when anchoring a plate in the main fragments. For adequate stabilization, it is much more important to insert few screws with high plate leverage to reduce the load on the screws.

From a purely mechanical point of view, two monocortical locking head screws in each main fragment in the shaft area are the minimum requirement for keeping the construct stable. However, this type of construct will fail if one screw breaks due to overloading or if the interface between the bone cortex and the screw thread develops bone resorption and loosening (screw pullout). The use of two bicortical screws in each fragment does not improves the situation in relation to screw fatigue failure, but it does enhance the working length of the screw and thus improve the anchorage at the interface between the screw thread and the bone. Even when the surgeon ensures that all of the screws are inserted correctly, this type of construct can only be used in healthy bone. For safety reasons, a minimum of three screws per main fragment is recommended in all other cases.

When fractures are being fixed in the epiphyseal and metaphyseal areas, neither the length of the plate nor the number of screws should be chosen on the basis of mechanical considerations alone. The longest possible LHS are recommended but penetration of articular surface must be avoided. The local anatomy and the length of the epiphyseal and/or metaphyseal fragment are also relevant in the decision. In these cases, the use of a metaphyseal plate or anatomically preshaped plates is recommended to achieve balanced fixation, with load bearing being distributed equally between the proximal and distal plate segments anchored in the two main fragments.

2.2 LCP in conventional compression plating

In some fracture situations, the LCP with combination holes can be used with a conventional plating technique—ie, fracture fixation using the compression method based on the principle of achieving absolute stability and direct bone healing. The surgical technique and instruments here are similar to those in conventional plating with DCP or LC-DCP.

Indications

- Simple fractures of the diaphysis and metaphysis: cases in which precise anatomical reduction is necessary for the functional outcome; simple transverse or oblique fractures with little soft-tissue compromise and good bone quality (compression plating or protection plating in combination with a lag screw or tension band fixation).
- Intraarticular fractures (buttress plate).
- Delayed union or nonunion.
- Closed-wedge osteotomies.
- Complete avascularity of the bone fragments.

The following conditions have to be met for the use of the compression method:

- Precise reduction of the fragments—in most cases requiring open, direct reduction.
- Precise anatomical preshaping of the plate (if the protection plate is to be fixed with cortex screws).
- Good bone quality, to ensure adequate anchorage of cortex or cancellous bone screws.
- Minor soft-tissue damage.

Technique

The method of interfragmentary compression can be achieved using the following approaches:

- Compression plate for axial compression (in transverse fractures).
- Lag screw and protection plate (in oblique fractures).
- Tension band principle using a plate.
- Buttress plate and lag screw.

Axial compression. After open and direct precise anatomical reduction of the fracture and preshaping of the plate, interfragmentary compression is applied using the eccentric cortex screw option in the dynamic compression unit (DCU) of the LCP combination hole (Fig 3-45). Fracture compression can also be applied using a tensioning device (Fig 3-46). Osteosynthesis is then completed with cortex screws inserted in the neutral position.

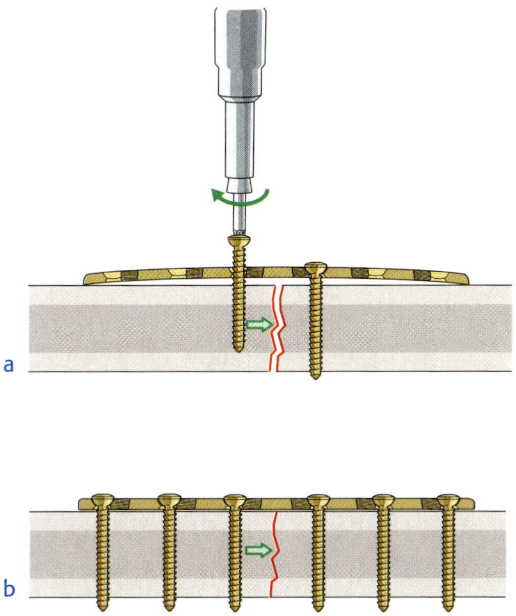

Fig 3-45a–b Interfragmentary compression.

a Interfragmentary compression is applied using a eccentric cortex screw. In order to apply compression forces on the vis-à-vis cortex bending of the plate is necessary.

b Osteosynthesis is then completed with the insertion of cortex screws in the neutral position.

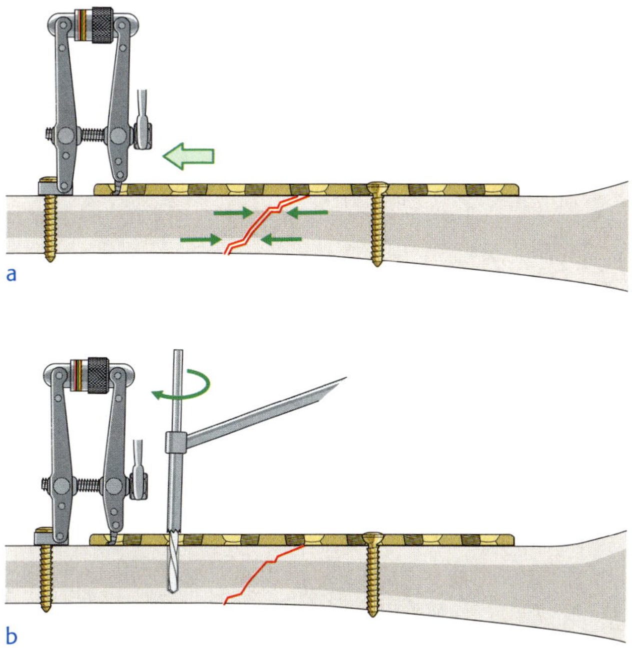

Fig 3-46a–b Interfragmentary compression using a tensioning device.

If different screws are combined in compression plating, the cortex screws should be inserted in the middle part of the plate in their eccentric positions first, to achieve fracture compression (Fig 3-47). As a modification, the LCP can initially be fixed to one of the main fragments with one or two LHS. Subsequently, compression can be applied by inserting one eccentric screw into the other fragment, or by applying the tensioning device (Fig 3-48; Fig 3-49). Osteosynthesis is then completed with locking head screws.

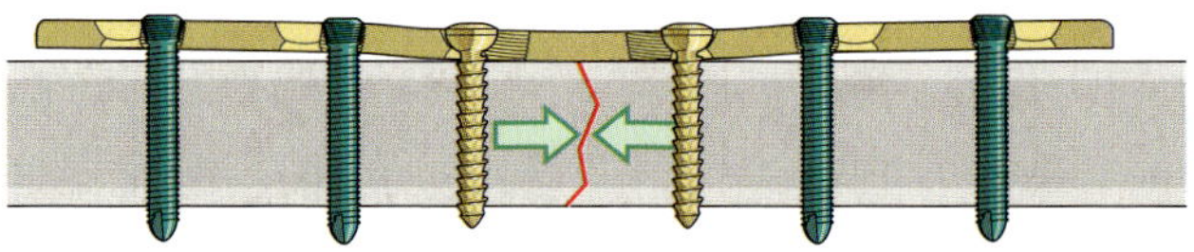

Fig 3-47 Interfragmentary compression using dynamic compression unit. If different screws are combined, the cortex screws should be inserted in the middle part of the plate in eccentric position first. In a second step the LHS are inserted. Only in the zone where cortex screws are used there is compression between the plate and the bone with additional disturbance of the periostal blood supply possible.

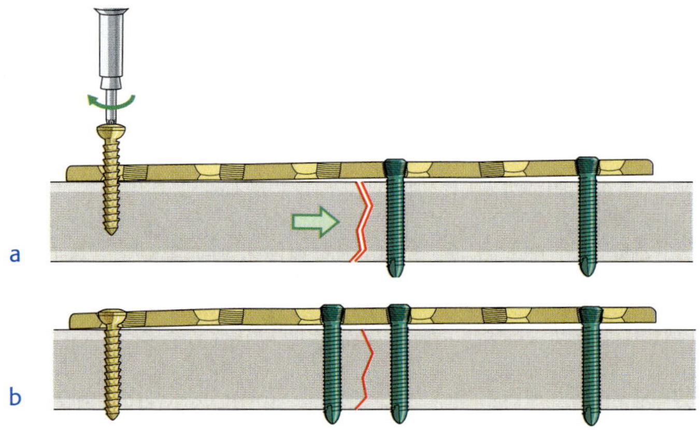

Fig 3-48a–b

a After reduction of this fracture the plate is fixed with LHS to one fragment. Then an eccentric cortex screw is inserted in the dynamic compression part of the combination hole at the other end of the plate.

b Finally stabilization with an additional LHS. No compression to the periosteum in the fracture zone. Interfragmentary compression plating using dynamic compression unit.

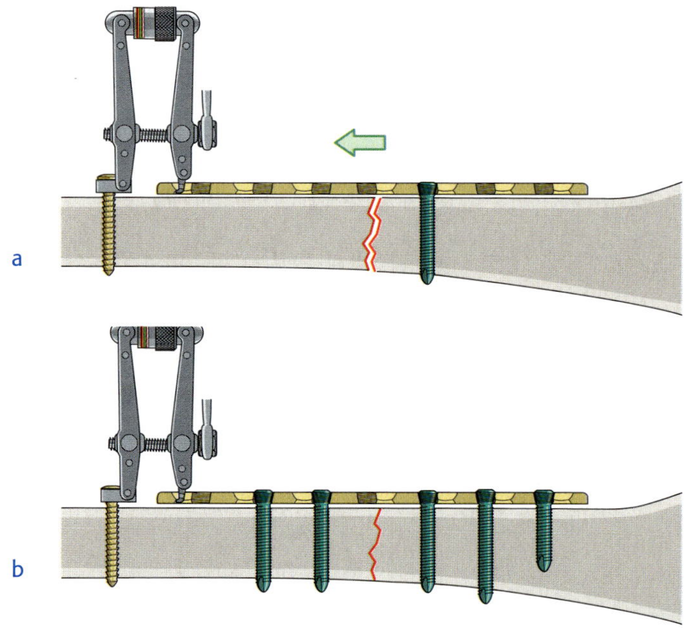

Fig 3-49a–b In osteoporotic bone subsequently compression can be applied by a tensioning device.

Lag screw and protection plate. Interfragmentary compression of a simple fracture in the metaphyseal or diaphyseal segment, or of an intraarticular fracture, can also be accomplished using a lag screw inserted through the plate. In comparison with independent lag screws positioned away from the plate, this approach presents the following advantages and difficulties:

- The plate acts like a large washer.
- A wide range of inclinations of the lag screw in the plate hole are required for optimal function.
- Inserting a lag screw into a plate hole: The position of the protection plate is given by correct placement of the lag screw through the fracture line.
- Compression of the plate onto the bone by the lag screw.
- Additional cortex screws are used to increase the friction between plate and bone.

If there is good bone quality and an open approach is possible so that accurate plate contouring can be carried out, then cortex or cancellous bone screws can be inserted. This protection plate construct helps protect the fractured bone from bending and torsional forces.

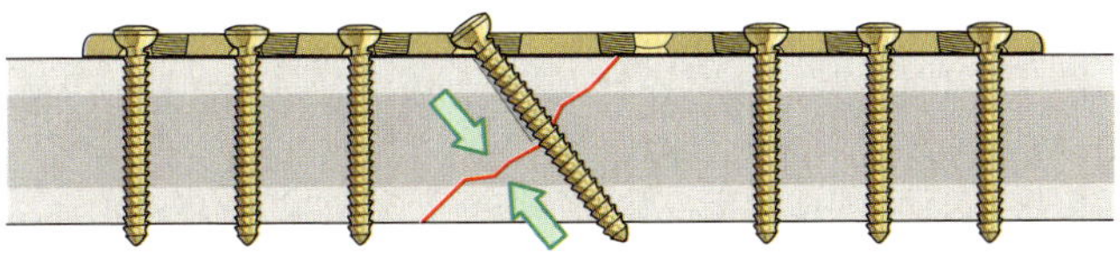

Fig 3-50 Conventional plating technique: Lag screw through the plate hole requires a precise positioning of the plate to allow the correct direction of the lag screw. Fixation of the protection plate with cortex screws requires precise adaptation of the implant to the bone and good bone quality.

Conventional compression plating requires precise adaptation of the implant to the bone in order to maintain precise reduction; the screws apply a compressive preload at the interface between the plate and the bone, and the fragments are pulled towards the implant (Fig 3-50). Using the LCP with cortex or cancellous bone screws therefore requires accurate shaping of the plate in the same way as with a conventional LC-DCP. Imperfect shaping of the plate leads to a mismatch between plate and bone surface resulting in primary loss of reduction when tightening the cortex or cancellous bone screws. If LHS are inserted to support the reduction and compression being maintained by the lag screws, no uncontrollable forces due to pressure of the plate on the bone surface will be created. This way the risk of primary reduction loss is eliminated. Locking head screws are preferred also in osteoporotic bone, thus increasing fixation stability (Fig 3-51b).

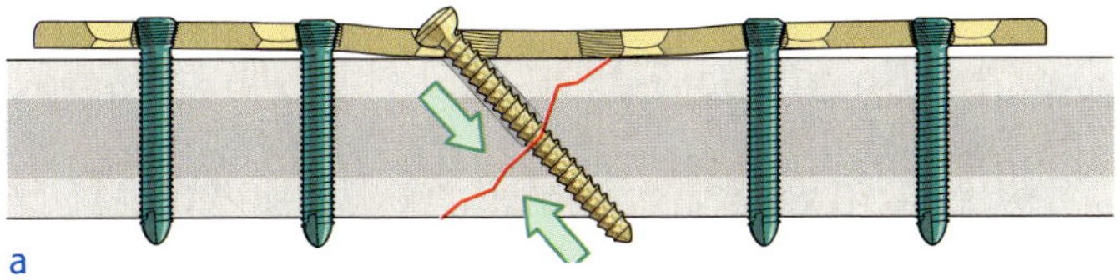

a

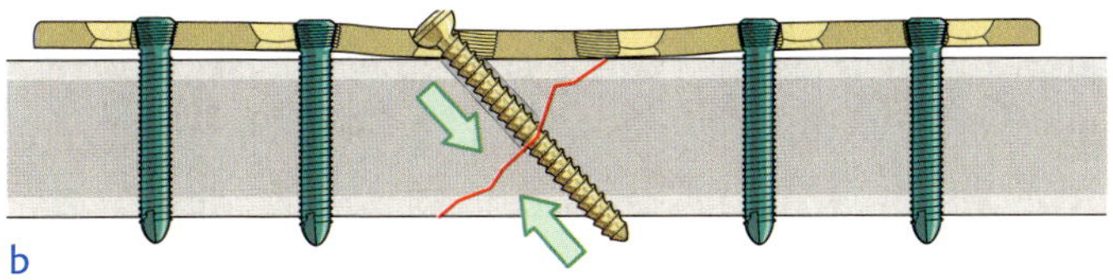

b

Fig 3-51a–b Lag screw and fixation of the protection plate with LHS. In case of osteoporosis the fixation of the protection plate with LHS gives a better hold of the screws. No uncontrolled forces due to pressure of the plate on the bone surface will be created.

a Normal bone quality.

b Osteoporotic bone.

The lag screw can also be placed independently from the plate, with a protection plate being fixed with locking head screws (Fig 3-52). To find the correct place and angulation of a free, plate independent lag screw is easier than using a lag screw in a plate hole. The positioning of the protection plate (without a plate independent lag screw) is easy and not dictated by the lag screw and fracture plane. The use of a noncontact plate, fixed with LHS respects the periosteal blood supply. There is no risk of a primary loss of reduction. This technique is much easier as a lag screw through a plate hole.

Butress plate. In a metaphyseal/epiphyseal shear or split fracture, fixation with lag screws alone may not be sufficient. The interfragmentary compression with lag screws should therefore be combined with a plate with buttress or antiglide function. To prevent any sliding of the plate LHS should be used.

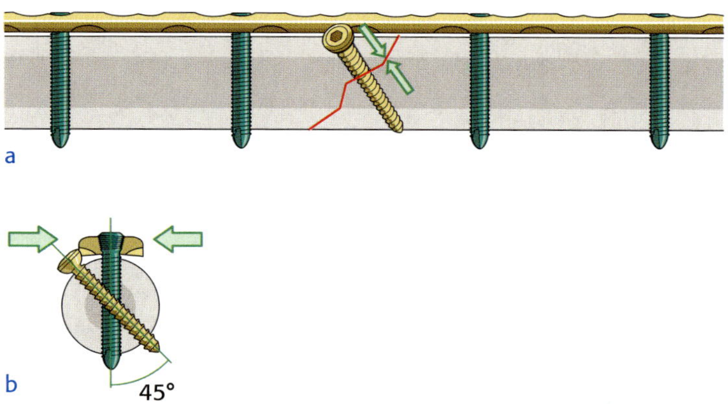

Fig 3-52a–b Protection plate with independent lag screw.

2.3 LCP with splinting

Bridge plating can be carried out with both standard screws and locking head screws. The method of bridging the fracture zone with conventional plates and cortex screws, using a no-touch technique combined with indirect reduction, was a great step forward when it was first introduced; only the main fragments were fixed to the plate. With conventional screws, it had been necessary to preshape the plate to fit the main fragments. With the combination hole of the LCP it is possible to use both cortex screws and LHS in healthy bone. In osteoporotic bone only LHS should be used for increased plate fixation (Fig 3-53).

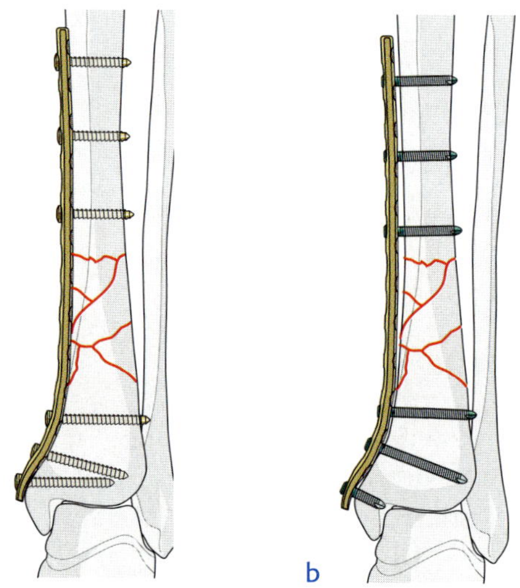

Fig 3-53a–b

a Bridging the fracture zone with conventional plate and cortex screws.

b Bridging the fracture zone with LCP and LHS in osteoporotic bone. The locked internal fixator has no or only limited contact to the bone surface.

LHS are preferable for bridge plating procedures, as it is easier to carry out the MIPO technique with LHS because there is no need to preshape the plate and there is no pull of fragment onto the plate resulting in primary loss of reduction. In addition, there is little or no disturbance to the periosteal blood supply. LHS can transmit more load to the plate/fixator. In splinting the plate/fixator has to withstand more load. Technically, the locked splinting method (pure splinting) can be carried out either using an open approach or with the MIPO technique and indirect, closed reduction.

Splinting the fracture zone is an elastic fixation with relative stability; the displacement of the fracture ends under load must be reversible. This elastic fixation allows pain-free mobility but simultaneously induces bone formation (callus), a precondition of relative stability of fixation is that the bone fragments are vital.

Indications

The LCP is used as a locked internal fixator to bridge the fracture zone with a less invasive or MIPO technique—ie, the locked splinting method with an internal fixator, based on the principle of relative stability—in the following cases:

- Multifragmentary fractures of the diaphysis and metaphysis.
- Simple fractures of the diaphysis and metaphysis (in cases where approximate reduction is adequate for the functional outcome, although it is important to strictly observe the biomechanical principles of strain tolerance).
- Fractures in problem zones where there are relative contraindications to intramedullary nailing—eg, shaft fractures with anomalies of the medullary morphology; fractures in children and adolescents with wide-open epiphyses; shaft fractures in patients with multiple injuries.
- Open-wedge osteotomies (eg, in the proximal tibia).
- Periprosthetic fractures.
- Other implants in situ.
- Secondary fractures or redislocation, instability after intramedullary nailing.
- Delayed conversion from an external fixator to the definitive internal fixation.
- Tumor surgery.
- LCP as external fixator in emergency situations.
- LCP as external fixator in problematic fractures such as open fractures which are severely contaminated or infected with high possibility of chronic osteomyelitis. This is a simple technique and the acceptance of the patient is better. But there are some disadvantages: The fracture has to be reduced before LCP fixation and there is no chance for a secondary correction like in external fixator. The transcutaneous fixation of the LCP has the risk of screw/pin infection.

Example cases for this indication are shown in section 2.6 of this chapter.

Technique

There are two prerequisites for using the LCP as a locked internal fixator:

- The locked bridging internal fixator has to be long—the longer the plate, the better.
- The space between the locking head screws in each main fragment and in relation to the fracture zone has to be adequate.

Locking a screw into the fixator increases stability and avoids the risk of primary dislocation of fragment towards the plate by tightening the screws and decreases the risk of for secondary fracture displacement due to toggling of the screw inside the plate hole. The advantages of using locking head screws are that in the shaft area the screw length can be reduced to a monocortical size and that self-drilling, self-tapping screws can be used that remove the need for length measurement. In healthy bones, monocortical LHS are adequate, but at least three screws should be inserted into each main fragment on either side of the fracture. In osteoporotic bone, it is strongly recommended that at least three LHS should be inserted into each main fragment on either side of the fracture, and that at least one or two of these LHS should be inserted bicortically.

Bicortical insertion of LHS is recommended in the following conditions:

- Osteoporosis
- Thin cortex
- High torsional forces during rehabilitation and physical therapy
- Short main fragment
- Small medullary diameter
- When a cortex screw was used for reduction through the same plate hole
- Destruction of the bone thread in the near cortex due to incorrect insertion of the LHS

It is important to avoid stress concentrations at the fracture site, and this can be achieved by leaving two or three plate holes without screws in the fracture zone (Fig 3-54) Distribution of stress is important to the internal fixator technique in order to avoid stress concentration and implant failures.

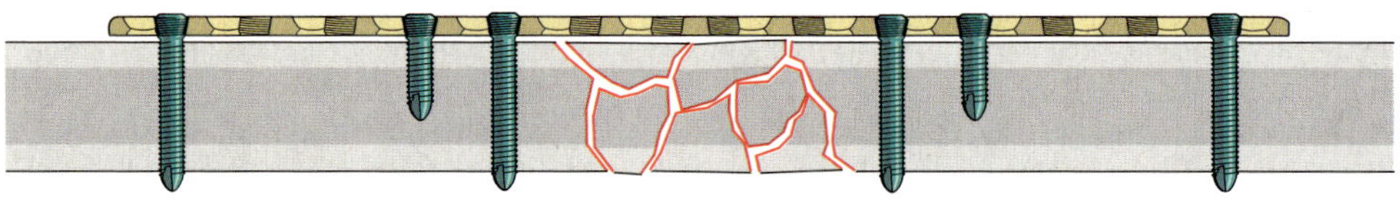

Fig 3-54 **Prerequisites for using the LCP as a locked internal fixator: long plate/fixator; adaquate space between the LHS in each main fragment. Avoid stress concentration while leaving out three or four plate holes without screws in the fracture zone.**

2.4 LCP with a combination of the two methods

The compression method and splinting method should only be used in combination in situations in which the bone has been fractured in two different places. In this condition (two different fractures), the two biomechanical principles—absolute stability through interfragmentary compression and relative stability by splinting with an internal fixator—are combined in one single bone with one LCP.

A combination of the two different methods—compression and splinting is only possible in situations in which the bone is fractured in two different places.

Indications

- Segmental fractures with two different fracture patterns (one simple and one multifragmentary). In these cases, conventional interfragmentary compression is used to stabilize the simple fracture, while splinting with an internal fixator stabilizes the multifragmentary fracture area.
- Intraarticular fractures with a multifragmented extension into the diaphysis.

In these cases, the anatomical reduction and interfragmentary lag screw compression of the articular component is combined with a bridging fixation from the reconstructed joint block to the diaphysis.

Example cases for this indication are shown in section 2.6 of this chapter.

2.5 Combinations of different screws

It is possible to combine the two plating fixation techniques—simultaneously applying compression with conventional screws and locking head screw fixation using a single plate—and this can be valuable, depending on the indication or situation. It is important to be familiar with the different features of both techniques. Probably the most frequent use of a combination technique will be for treating fractures adjacent to the joint, with locking head screws being used to fix the fragment close to the joint and standard screws being used to apply axial compression between the metaphysis and the diaphysis in a simple fracture type (individual blade plate).

The splinting method can be carried out with an internal fixator and an additional reduction screw (reducing the plate onto the bone or reducing a displaced fragment) or positioning screw. In addition, the conventional screw–plating technique (the compression method) can be used, but with fixation of the protection plate using locking head screws.

Articular fractures treated with lag screws and a buttress plate fixed with LHS.

2.6 Case examples

Plate osteosynthesis

LCP can be used for plate osteosynthesis when there is poor bone quality (osteoporosis) [35–37], independently of the specific fracture configuration and fixation principle (including periprosthetic fractures).

Fractures close the joint

Fractures close to the joint or extending into the joint, such as multifragmentary metaphyseal fractures, are borderline indications for intramedullary nailing, but good indications for screw–plate systems with angular stability [4, 35, 37] (Fig 3-58).

Multifragmentary fracture and severe soft-tissue injury

The LCP is also indicated for fractures associated with serious soft-tissue defects and multifragmentary fractures of the shaft that require bridging for restoration of the correct length and axial and torsional alignment [4, 38].

In the next section you find typical case examples how the LCP can be used in different ways. The first cases are examples for the compression method according to the principle of absolute stability of fracture fixation. Also different techniques and different plate functions are shown.

The second group of cases deals with the method of locked internal extramedullary splinting to achieve relative stability.

Finally, some few cases are presented with two fractures in one bone. In such situations there is the necessity to use the LCP for the compression and splinting method at the same time.

Case examples with the compression method

Simple radial shaft fracture—22-A1

- Principle of fracture fixation: absolute stability
- Method of fracture fixation: compression
- Technique: open, direct precise reduction
- Fixation: plate independent lag screw and protection plate
- Function of the LCP: protection plate
- Fixation of the LCP with LHS (ie, noncontact plate)

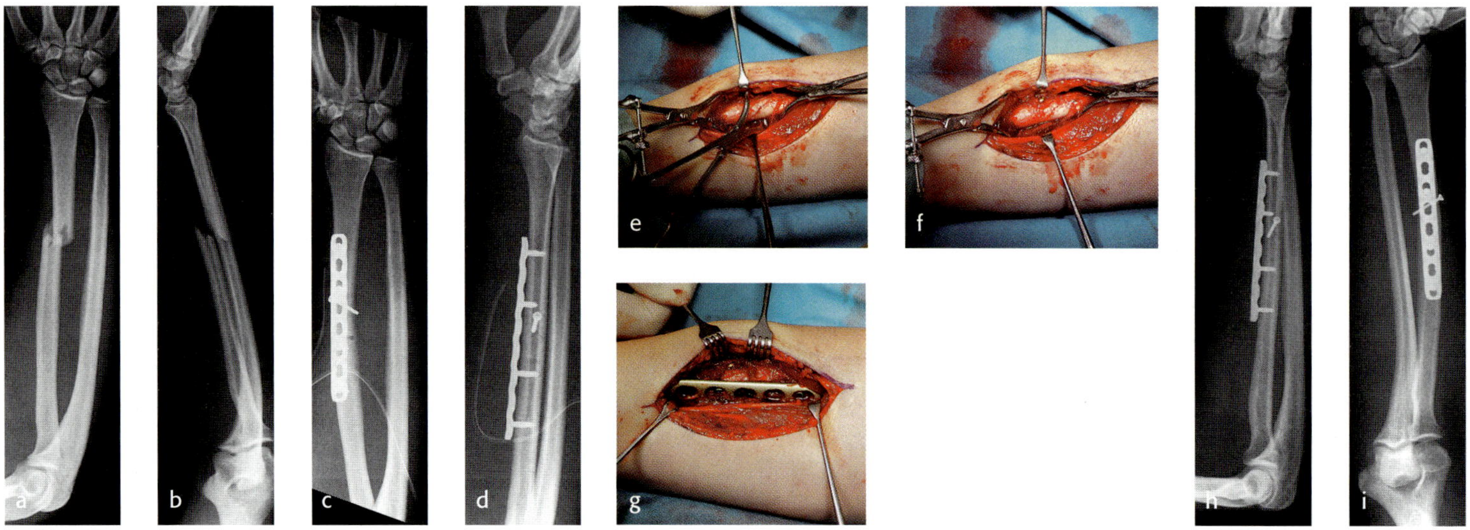

Fig 3-57a–i 25-year-old man fell on the street and sustained a simple forearm shaft fracture.

a–b AP and lateral view.

c–d Postoperative x-rays, AP and lateral view. Stable fixation with a plate independent lag screw and a LCP 3.5 as protection plate fixed with LHS. Compression method—principle of absolute stability allows functional postoperative treatment.

e–g Intraoperative pictures; open direct reduction, plate independent lag screw, protection plate fixation with LHS (noncontact plate).

h–i AP and axial view 5 months after operation, bone healing.

Simple split fracture of the tibial head—41-B1

- Principle of fracture fixation: absolute stability
- Method of fracture fixation: compression
- Technique: open, direct precise reduction
- Fixation: plate dependent lag screw and buttress plate
- Function of the LCP: buttress plate
- Fixation of the LCP with angular stable LHS (ie, partially noncontact plate)
- Articular fracture as indication using a LCP as buttress plate.

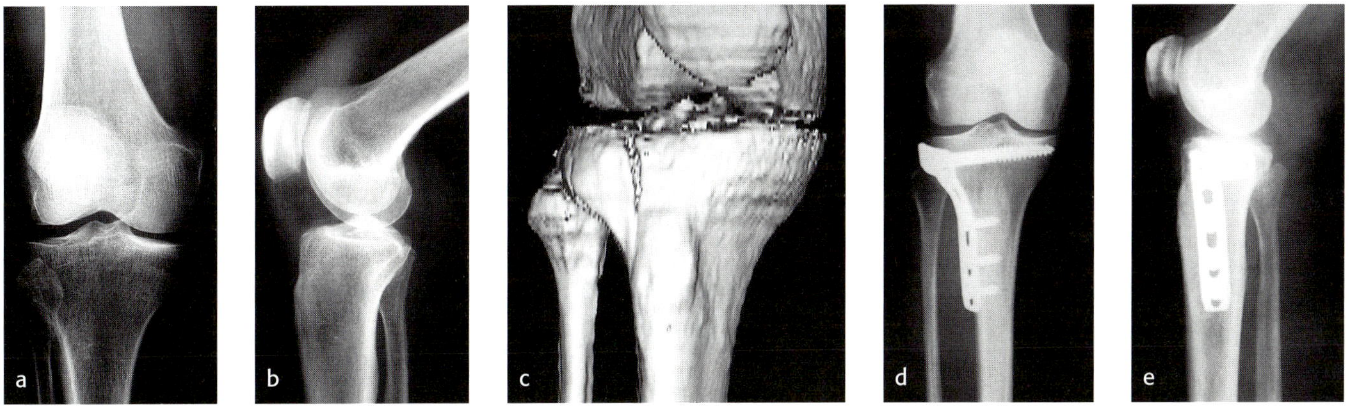

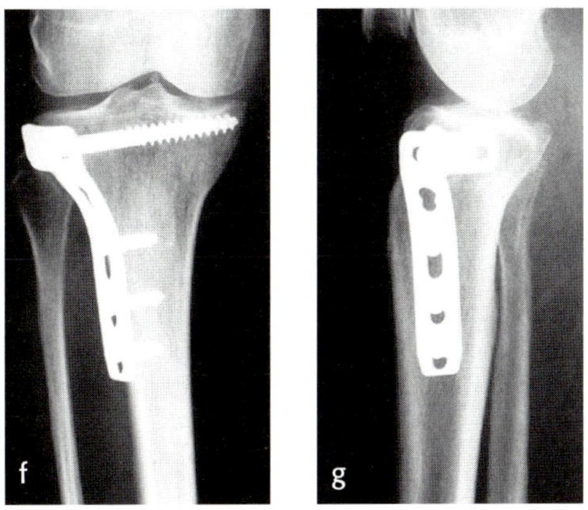

Fig 3-58a–g 60-year-old man fell on the street and sustained a split fracture of the tibial head.

a–b AP and lateral view.

c CT scan frontal plane.

d–e AP and lateral view postoperative x-rays.

f–g Follow-up x-rays after 6 weeks.

Complete articular multifragmentary proximal tibial fracture—41-C3

- Principle of fracture fixation: absolute stability
- Method of fracture fixation: compression
- Technique: open and percutaneous, direct precise reduction; MIPO, percutaneous lag screw
- Fixation: plate independent lag screws and buttress plate
- Function of the LCP: buttress plate
- Fixation of the LCP with angel stable LHS (ie, noncontact plate, blade plate)

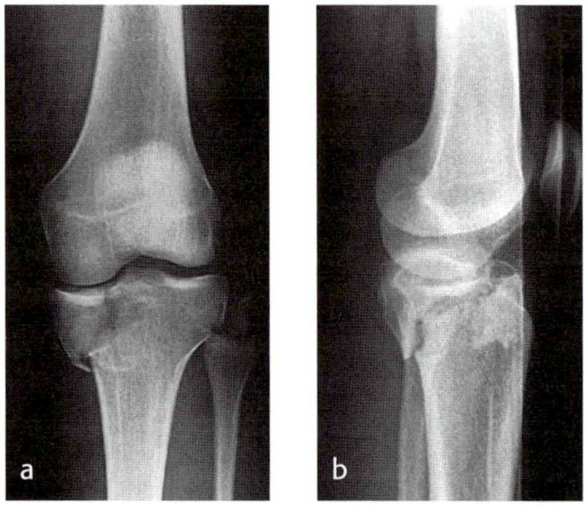

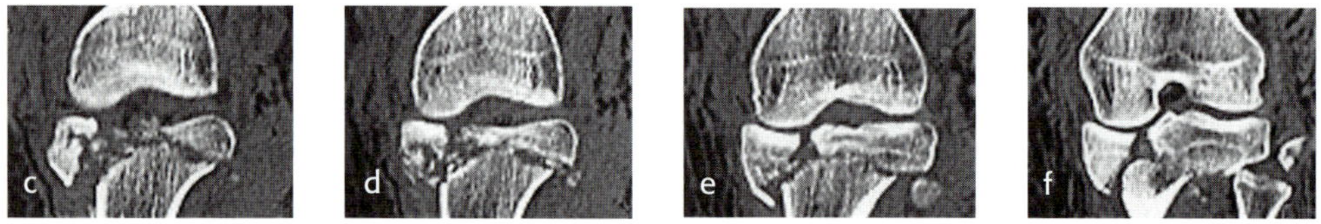

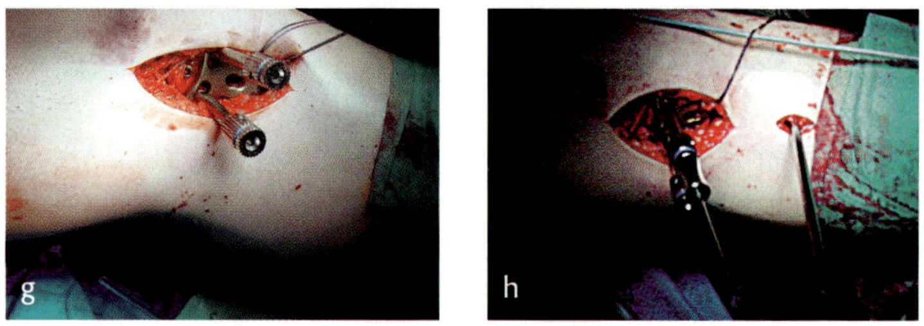

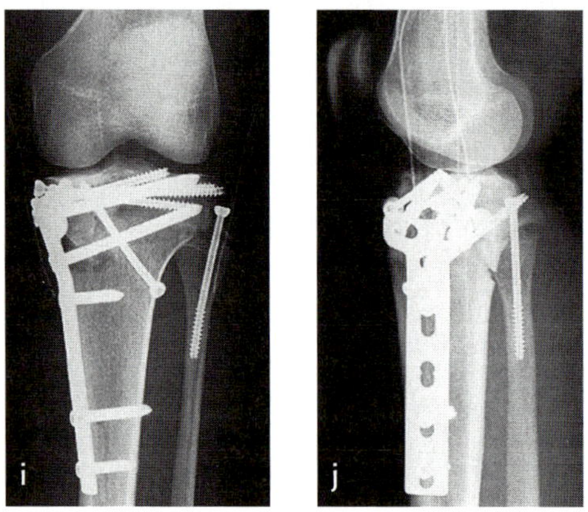

Fig 3-59a–p A 21-year-old female suffered a fracture of the tibial head due to a riding accident.

a–b Preoperative x-rays.

c–f CT scans of the multifragmentary intraarticular fracture. Using the MIPO technique, a tibial LCP was inserted subcutaneously from the medial aspect.

h An additional incision was made to insert locking head screws.

i–j Postoperative images. Fracture stabilization has taken place with lag screws and medial slide insertion of a 5-hole T-plate. The osseous avulsion of the fibular collateral ligament was treated by tension-band plating and a lag screw.

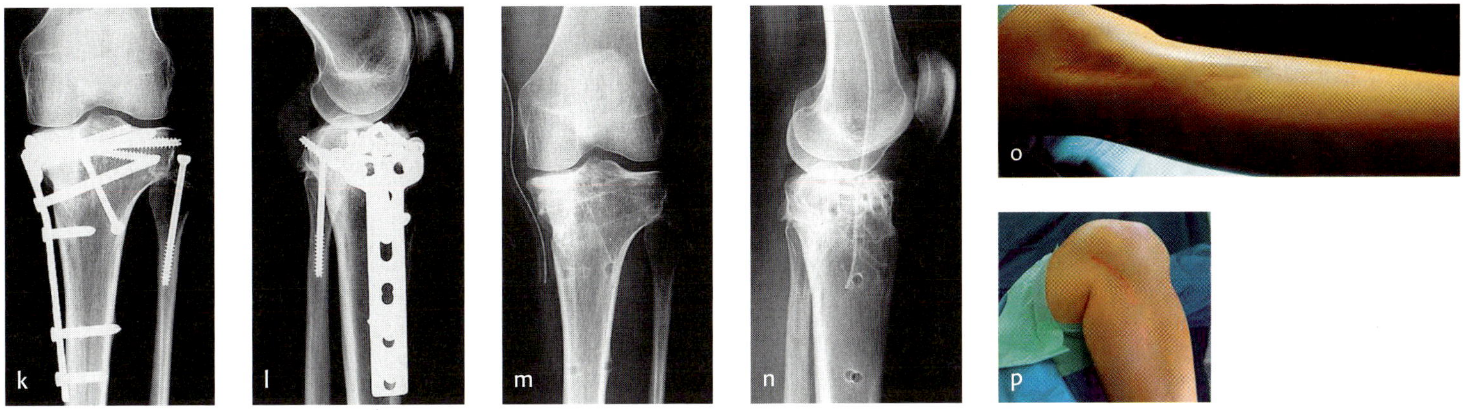

Fig 3-59a–p (cont)
k–l X-rays after 1 year.
m–n X-rays after implant removal.
o–p On completion of the treatment, the patient had free function, no pain, and only minor scars.

Nonunion of a subcapital humeral fracture

- Principle of nonunion fixation: absolute stability
- Method of nonunion fixation: compression
- Technique: open, direct reduction and with a reduction screw
- Fixation: compression plate (eccentric cortex screw) after reduction with a plate dependent reduction screw (fully threaded cancellous bone screw)
- Function of the LCP: compression plate and tension band plate
- Fixation of the LCP in the humeral head with angular stable LHS (ie, blade plate), in the shaft with LHS after interfragmentary compression with the eccentric cortex screw.
- Delayed union or nonunion are often an indication for compression plate fixation method.

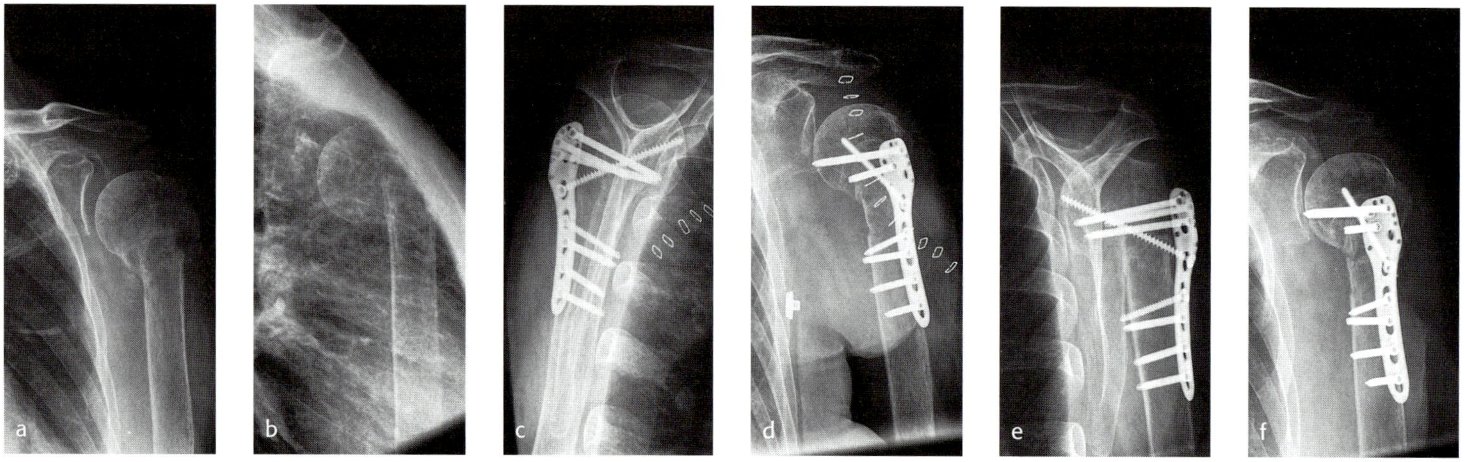

Fig 3-60a–f 79-year-old woman with nonunion of a subcapital humeral fracture.

a–b Nonunion of a subcapital humeral fracture after conservative treatment.

c–d Stable fixation with a LPHP, compression method allows functional postoperative treatment.

e–f AP and axial view 6 weeks after operation, bone healing.

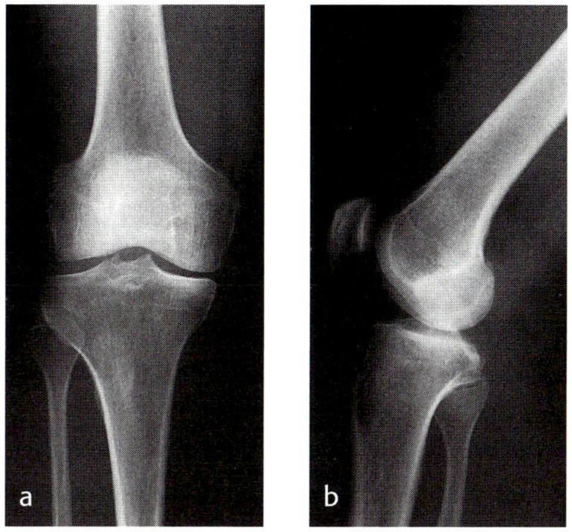

Closed wedge osteotomy

- A good indication for plate fixation with the compression method is a closed wedge osteotomy.
- Principle of closed wedge osteotomy fixation: absolute stability
- Method of closed wedge osteotomy fixation: compression
- Technique: open, direct reduction by manual closing of the osteotomy gap after removal of the bony wedge and also with a temporary reduction screw and compression with this eccentric placed screw (ie, intraoperative working screw).
- Fixation: compression plate (compression with an eccentric cortex screw, after interfragmentary compression this screw was removed and changed to a LHS)
- Function of the LCP: compression plate
- Fixation of the LCP with LHS (ie, noncontact blade plate)

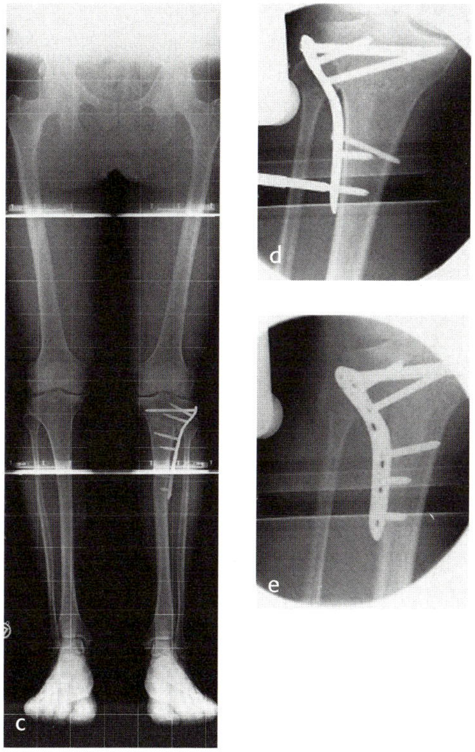

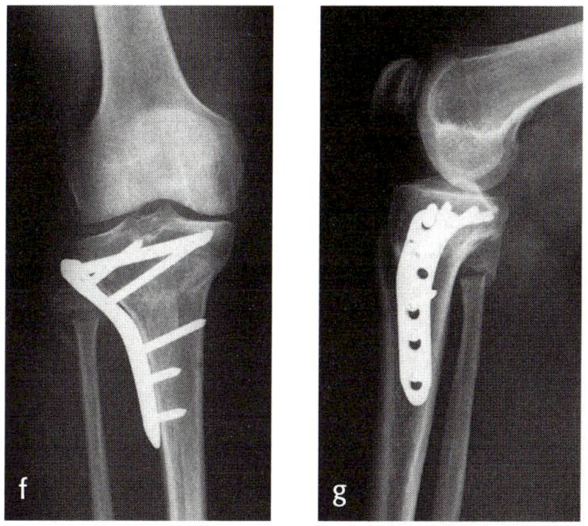

Fig 3-61a–g 72-year-old man.

a–b Varus arthritis right knee.

c Long axis shows the varus malalignment of the right leg. On the left knee the same operation already was some years before.

d–e Intraoperative x-ray. The osteotomy gap is closed by means of a cortex screw (ie, reduction screw) and the distal part of a TomoFix tibial head plate, lateral tibia is fixed with monocortical locking head screws.

f–g AP and lateral view 7 weeks postoperative stable situation immediate weight bearing after the operation.

Case examples with the splinting method

Tibial shaft fracture, periprosthetic—42-B1

- Principle of fracture fixation: relative stability
- Method of fracture fixation: locked internal extramedullary splinting
- Technique: MIPO; closed, indirect reduction
- Fixation: bridging the fracture zone with a locked internal fixator
- Function of the LCP: pure splint, locked internal fixator
- Fixation of the LCP with LHS
- Periprosthetic fractures are good indication for plate fixation with LCP and LHS using MIPO technique.

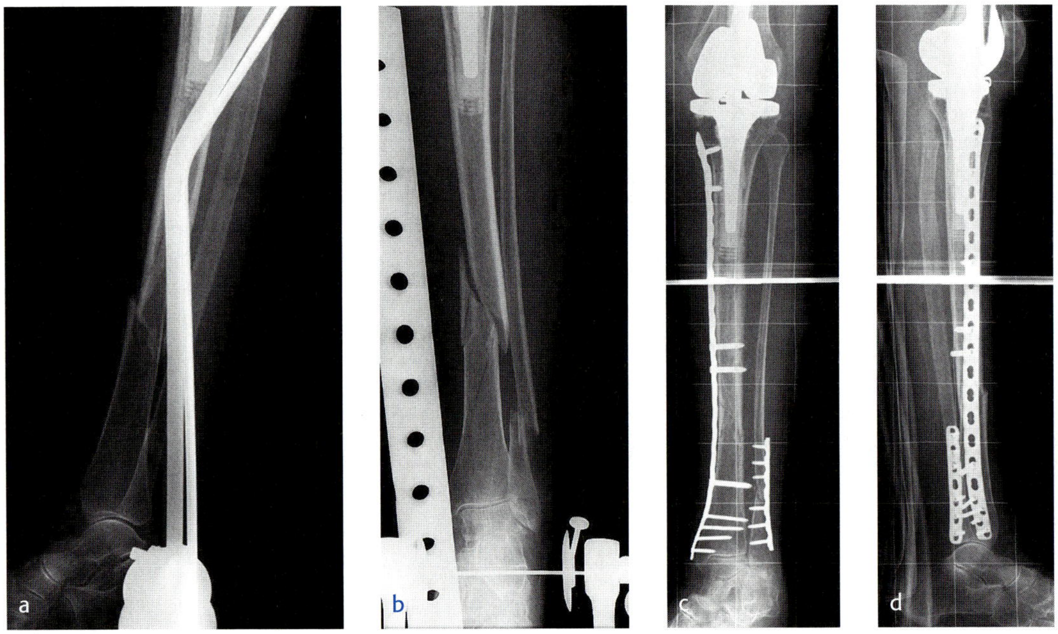

Fig 3-62a–d 76-year-old woman fell in the bathroom and sustained a periprosthetic tibial shaft fracture.

a–b Preoperative AP and lateral view.

c–d Postoperative AP and lateral view; closed reduction and locked splinting with a LCP metaphyseal plate in MIPO technique. Open reduction and compression plate fixation of the fibula fracture.

Simple spiral tibial shaft fracture in a child—42-A1

- Principle of fracture fixation: relative stability
- Method of fracture fixation: locked internal extramedullary splinting
- Technique: MIPO; closed, indirect reduction
- Fixation: bridging the fracture zone with a locked internal fixator
- Function of the LCP: pure splint, locked internal fixator
- Fixation of the LCP with LHS

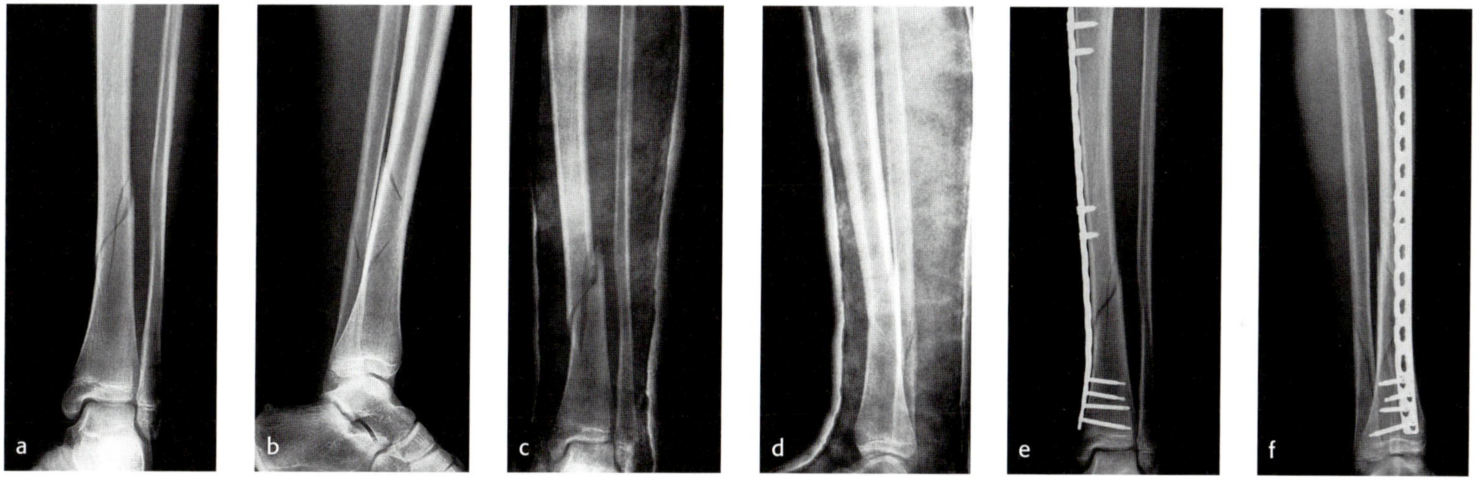

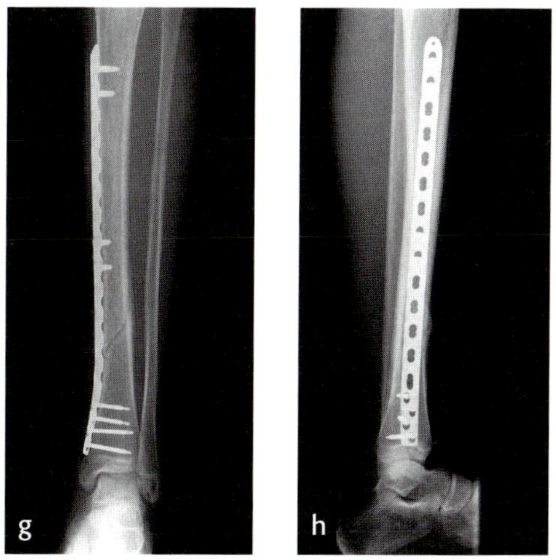

Fig 3-63a–n 15-year-old boy fell while ice skating and sustained a fracture of the tibial shaft.

a–b AP and lateral view.

c–d Unsuccessful conservative treatment.

e–f Operative stabilization in MIPO technique splinting with a metaphyseal LCP.

g–h After 2 months callus formation on the lateral side.

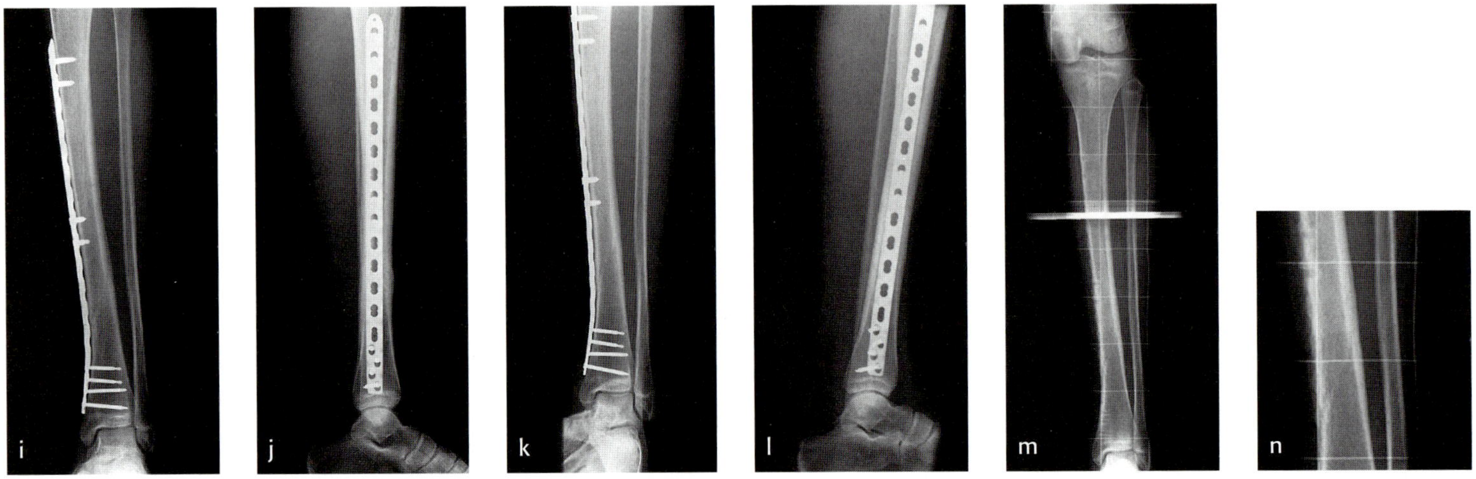

Fig 3-63a-n (cont)

i–j After 4 months complete healing.

k–l After 9 months the fracture.

m X-ray after implant removal shows periostal and endostal bone healing of the fracture and also a periostal callus formation under the plate (noncontact plate with undercuts).

n Detail, periostal callus formation under the plate (noncontact plate with undercuts).

Osteolysis of the femur, imminent fracture, palliatve splinting of the osteolysis zone

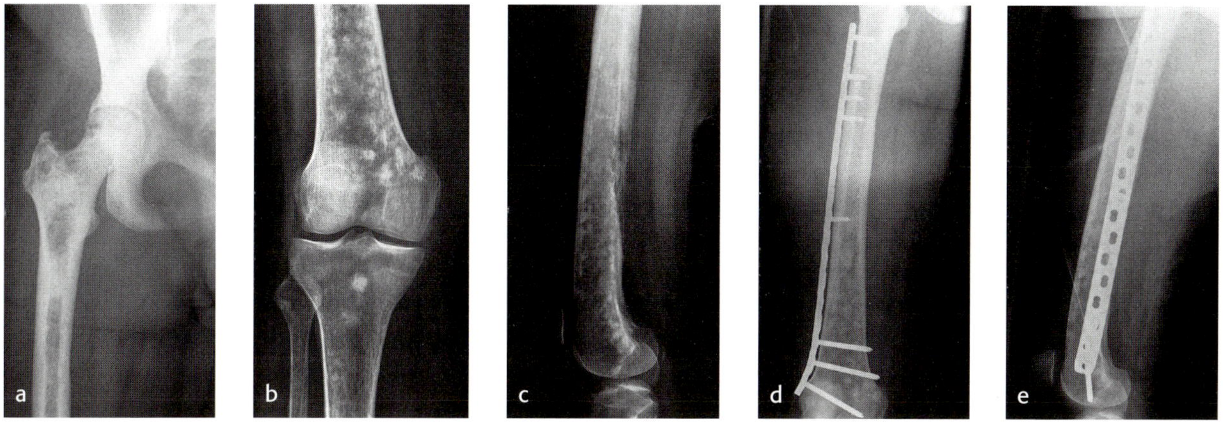

Fig 3-64a–e 46-year-old woman, without trauma.
a–c AP and lateral view.
d–e Palliative Stabilisation; MIPO, bridging the ostelysis zone. Mobilization with full weight bearing.

Medial open wedge high tibial osteotomy, varus gonarthrosis, splinting of the open wedge osteotomy

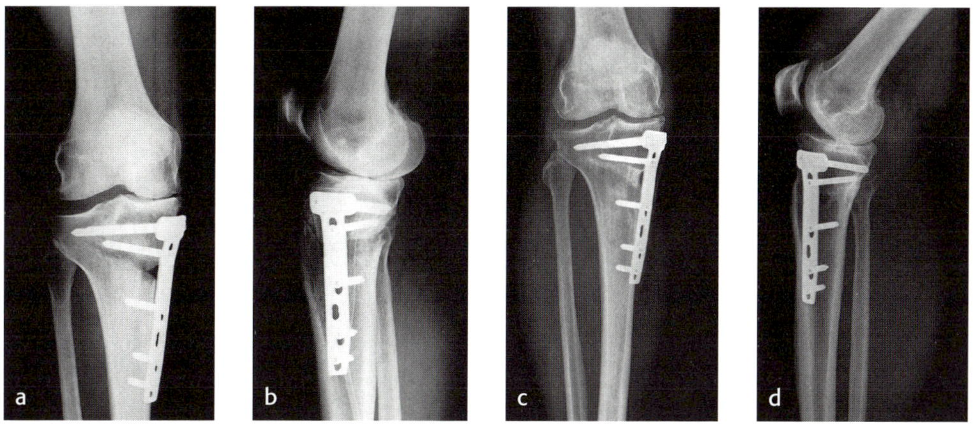

Fig 3-65a–d 50-year-old man.
a–b Angular stable fixation after biplanar osteotomy on the medial proximal tibia.
c–d Bone healing without bone graft or bone substitute.

Segmental tibial shaft fracture/LCP as external fixator

Rare indication

- Principle of fracture fixation: relative stability
- Method of fracture fixation: locked external splinting
- Technique: transcutaneous fixation of the LCP with LHS; closed, indirect reduction
- Fixation: bridging the fracture zone with an external fixator (LCP with transcutaneous LHS)
- Function of the LCP: pure splint, locked external fixator
- Fixation of the LCP with transcutaneous LHS.

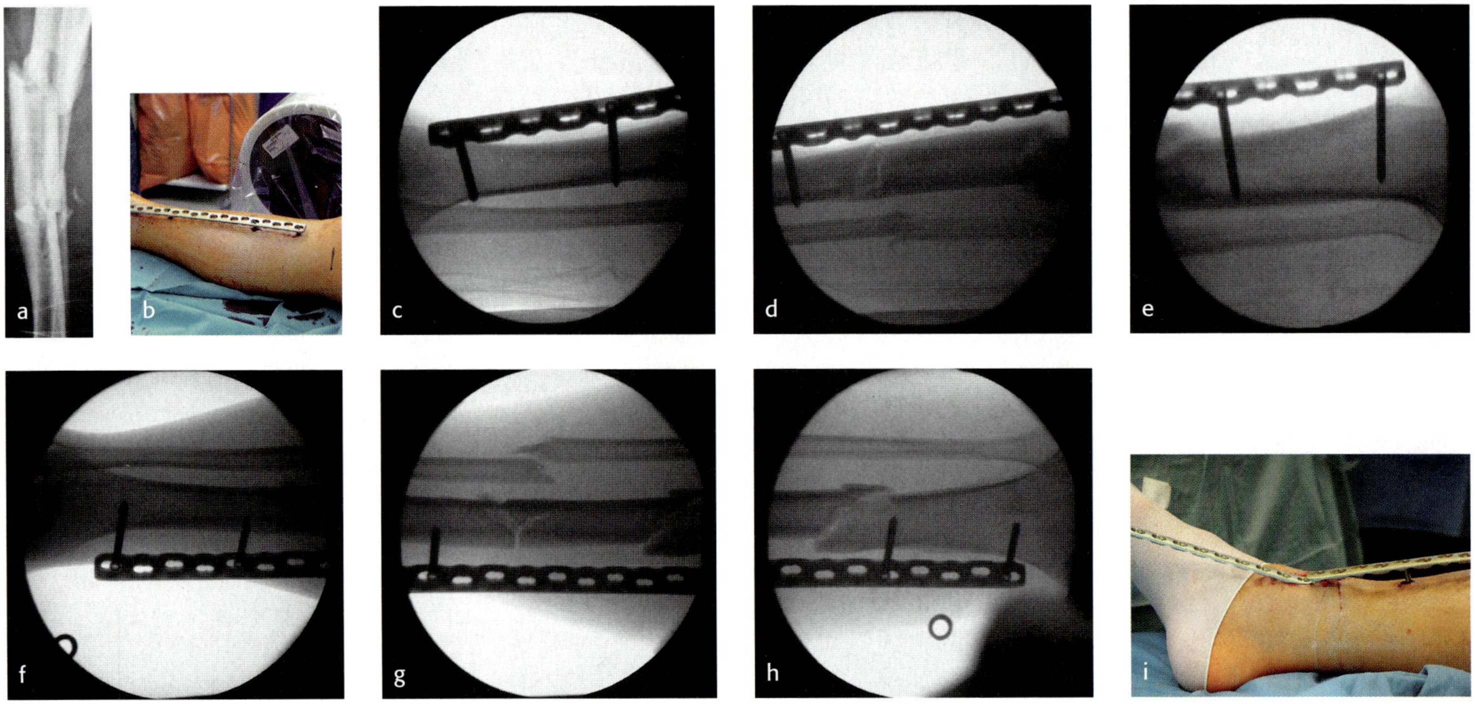

Fig 3-66a–i 58-year-old female pedestrian was struck by a car and sustained multiples injuries.

a Injury x-ray.

b–h Transcutaneous fixation of a broad LCP as external fixator. Intraoperative pictures show the fixation of the LCP with two locking head screws on each main fragment.

i Second operation: insertion of a small LCP from distal to proximal MIPO with a locked internal fixator.

Case examples with two fractures in one bone

In such situations there is the possibility/necessity to use the LCP for the compression and the splinting method at the same time.

Complete articular simple (1), metaphyseal multifragmentary (2) proximal tibial fracture—41-C2

- Principle of fracture fixation: absolute stability for the articular fracture (1) and relative stability for the metaphyseal multifragmentary fracture (2)
- Method of fracture fixation: interfragmentary compression for the articular fracture (1) and locked internal extramedullary splinting for the metaphyseal multifragmentary fracture (2)
- Technique: MIPO and lag screws
- Reduction: Direct, percutaneous for the articular fracture (1) and closed, indirect reduction for the metaphyseal multifragmentary fracture (2)
- Fixation: lag screws for the articular fracture bridging the metaphyseal fracture zone with a locked internal fixator
- Function of the LCP: pure splint, locked internal fixator
- Fixation of the LCP with LHS

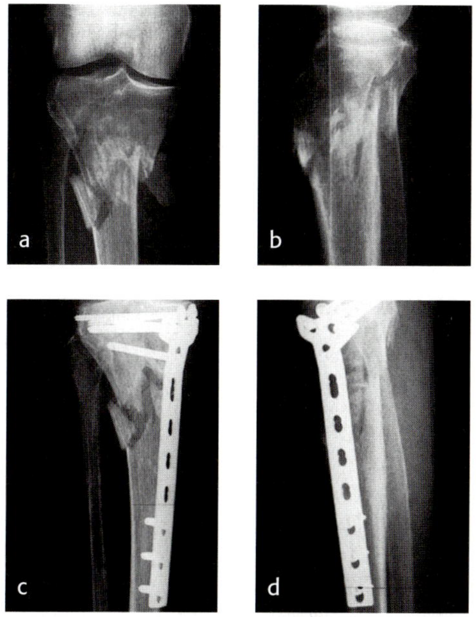

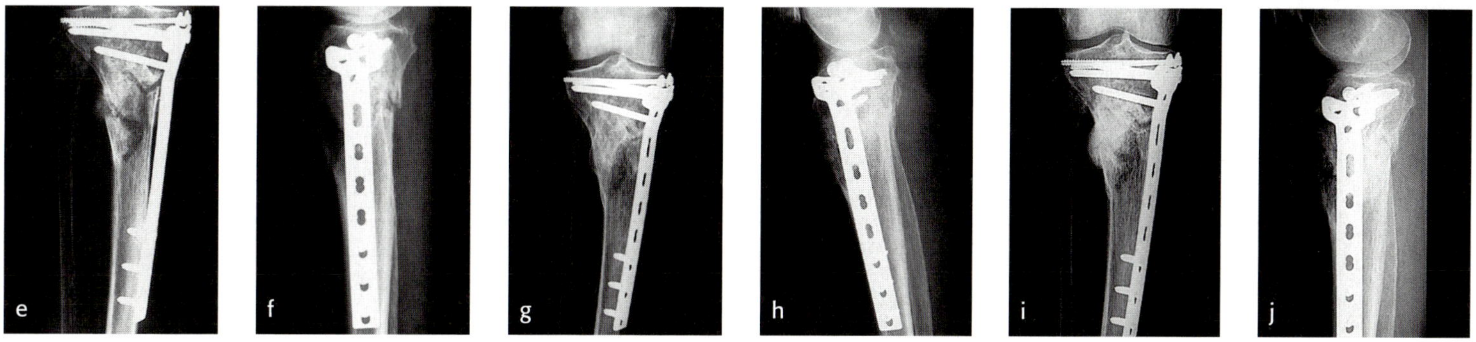

Fig 3-67a–j An 83-year-old female was knocked down by a car and sustained multiple injuries. She was suffering from severe osteoporosis.

a–b Preoperative x-rays. There is a multifragmentary fracture of the proximal tibia (41-C2) and severe soft-tissue injury on the lateral side of the tibia.

c–d After closed reduction of the articular fracture, fixation with two 4.5 mm cannulated lag screws with metal washers was carried out. The multifragmentary metaphyseal fracture zone was then bridged with an 8-hole 4.5/5.5 tibial LCP after closed reduction. The isolated medial and anterior bone fragments were left untouched.

e–f Postoperative x-rays 4 weeks later. Callus formation has started.

g–h X-rays after 4 months: bone consolidation can be seen.

i–j Findings at the 1-year follow-up examination.

42-C3 multifragmentary fracture of the proximal tibial shaft (1) with avulsion fracture of the tibial tuberosity (2)

- Principle of fracture fixation: relative stability for the multifragmentary fracture (1) and absolute stability for the simple avulsion fracture (2)
- Method of fracture fixation: locked internal extramedullary splinting (1) and compression (2 = avulsion fracture)
- Technique: MIPO; closed, indirect reduction (1), percutaneous, direct (2).
- Fixation: bridging the fracture zone with a locked internal fixator (1) and interfragmentary compression with lag screw (2).
- Function of the LCP: pure splint, locked internal fixator
- Fixation of the LCP with LHS

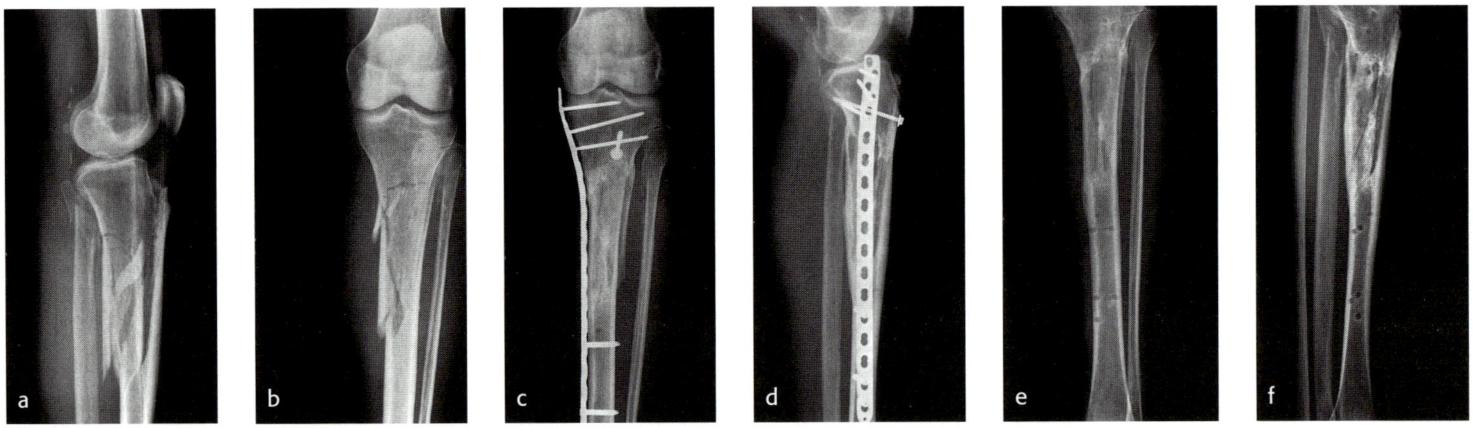

Fig 3-68a–f 63-year-old man fell on the street.

a–b AP and lateral view.

c–d X-rays after 20 month after fixation with a metaphyseal LCP additional lag screw fixation of the avulsion fracture of the tibial tuberosity. Indirect bone healing

e–f X-rays after implant removal.

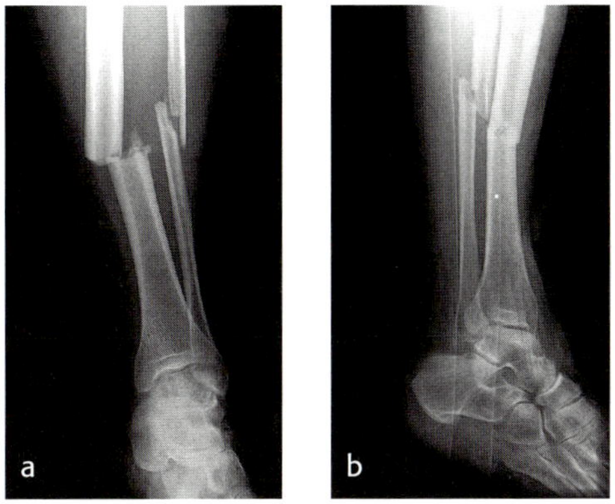

Segmental proximal tibial fracture (1) and open complex segmental tibial shaft fracture (2)—42-C2

- Principle of fracture fixation: absolute stability for the simple, proximal fracture (1) and relative stability for the shaft fracture (2)
- Method of fracture fixation: interfragmentary compression for the proximal, simple, metaphyseal fracture (1) and locked internal extramedullary splinting for the shaft fracture (2)
- Technique: MIPO and lag screws
- Reduction: Direct, percutaneous for the simple fracture (1) and closed, indirect reduction for the shaft fracture (2)
- Fixation: lag screws and protection plate for the simple fracture (1) and bridging the shaft fracture with a locked internal fixator (2)
- Function of the LCP: protection plate and locked internal fixator
- Fixation of the LCP with LHS

Fig 3-69a–k 50-year-old man with ski injury; open tibial shaft fracture Gustilo type II.

a–b Injury x-rays, AP and lateral view. Segmentale proximal tibial fracture with simple fracture pattern, distally with small comminution and soft-tissue injury.

c–e Percutaneous inserted plate, compression, method with lag screw and protection plate for the proximal simple fracture; distal fracture locked splinting.

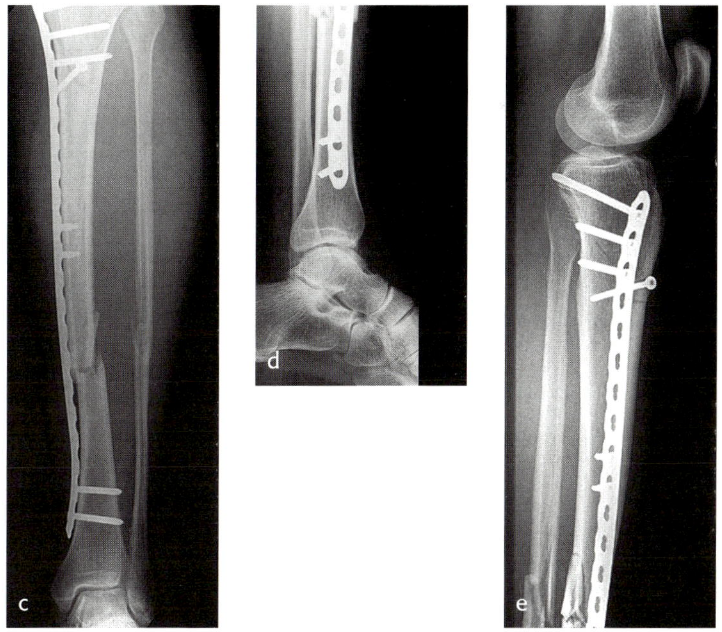

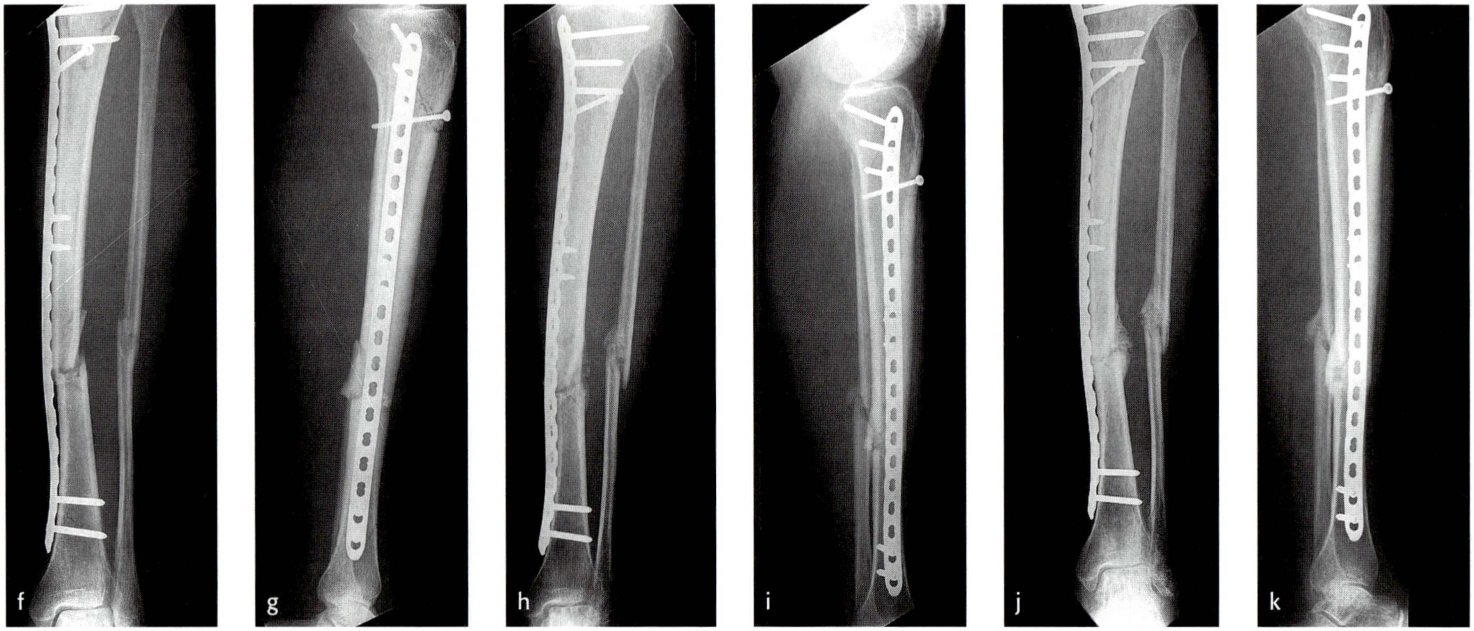

Fig 3-69a–k (cont)

f–g Follow-up x-rays after 3 months, AP and lateral view.

h–i Follow-up x-rays after 6 months, AP and lateral view.

j–k AP and lateral x-rays showing bone healing after 8 months.

2.7 Clinical results

The following are recent clinical studies on the use of LCP: [36, 39–42]

3 Bibliography

1. **Schütz M, Schäfer M, Bail H, et al** (2005) [New osteosynthesis techniques for the treatment of distal femoral fractures]. *Zentralbl Chir*; 130:307–13.
2. **Müller ME, Nazarian S, Koch P, et al** (1990) *The comprehensive classification of fractures of long bones*. Berlin Heidelberg New York: Springer Verlag.
3. **Schütz M, Müller M, Regazzoni P, et al** (2005) Use of the less invasive stabilization system (LISS) in patients with distal femoral (AO33) fractures: a prospective multicenter study. *Arch Orthop Trauma Surg*; 125:102–108.
4. **Messmer P, Regazzoni P, Gross T** (2003) [New stabilization techniques for fixation of proximal tibial fractures (LISS/LCP)]. *Ther Umsch*; 60(12):762–767.
5. **Schütz M, Müller M, Kääb M, et al** (2003) Less invasive stabilization system (LISS) in the treatment of distal femoral fractures. *Acta Chir Orthop Traumatol Cech*; 70(2):74–78.
6. **Kolb W, Guhlmann H, Friedel R, et al** (2003) [Fixation of periprosthetic femur fractures with the less invasive stabilization system (LISS)—a new minimally invasive treatment with locked fixed-angle screws]. *Zentralbl Chir*; 128(1):53–59.
7. **Schütz M, Südkamp NP** (2003) Revolution in plate osteosynthesis: new internal fixator systems. *J Orthop Sci*; 8(2):252–258.
8. **Schandelmaier P, Partenheimer A, Koenemann B, et al** (2001) Distal femoral fractures and LISS stabilization. *Injury*; 32Suppl3:SC55–63.
9. **Wick M, Müller EJ, Kutscha-Lissberg F, et al** (2004) [Periprosthetic supracondylar femoral fractures: LISS or retrograde intramedullary nailing? Problems with the use of minimally invasive technique]. *Unfallchirurg*; 107(3):181–188.
10. **Wong MK, Leung F, Chow SP** (2005) Treatment of distal femoral fractures in the elderly using a less-invasive plating technique. *Int Orthop*; 29(2):117–120.
11. **Zlowodzki M, Williamson S, Cole PA, et al** (2004) Biomechanical evaluation of the less invasive stabilization system, angled blade plate, and retrograde intramedullary nail for the internal fixation of distal femur fractures. *J Orthop Trauma*; 18(8):494–502.
12. **Schatzker J, McBroom R, Bruce D** (1979) The tibial plateau fracture. The Toronto experience 1968–1975. *Clin Orthop Relat Res*; 138:94–104.
13. **Georgiadis GM, Gove NK, Smith AD, et al** (2004) Removal of the less invasive stabilization system. *J Orthop Trauma*; 18(8):562–564.
14. **Fankhauser F, Gruber G, Schippinger G,et al** (2004) Minimal-invasive treatment of distal femoral fractures with the LISS (Less Invasive Stabilization System): a prospective study of 30 fractures with a follow up of 20 months. *Acta Orthop Scand*; 75(1):56–60.
15. **Kregor PJ, Stannard JA, Zlowodzki M, et al** (2004) Treatment of distal femur fractures using the less invasive stabilization system: surgical experience and early clinical results in 103 fractures. *J Orthop Trauma*; 18(8):509–520.
16. **Markmiller M, Konrad G, Südkamp N** (2004) Femur-LISS and distal femoral nail for fixation of distal femoral fractures: are there differences in outcome and complications? *Clin Orthop Relat Res*; 426:252–257.
17. **Ricci AR, Yue JJ, Taffet R, et al** (2004) Less Invasive Stabilization System for treatment of distal femur fractures. *Am J Orthop*; 33(5):250–255.
18. **Schütz M, Haas NP** (2001) [LISS—internal plate fixator]. *Kongressbd Dtsch Ges Chir Kongr*; 118:375–379. German.

19. **Schütz M, Müller M, Krettek C, et al** (2001) Minimally invasive fracture stabilization of distal femoral fractures with the LISS: a prospective multicenter study. Results of a clinical study with special emphasis on difficult cases. *Injury*; 32Suppl3:SC48–54.
20. **Syed AA, Agarwal M, Giannoudis PV, et al** (2004) Distal femoral fractures: long-term outcome following stabilisation with the LISS. *Injury*; 35(6):599–607.
21. **Weight M, Collinge C** (2004) Early results of the less invasive stabilization system for mechanically unstable fractures of the distal femur (AO/OTA types A2, A3, C2, and C3). *J Orthop Trauma*; 18(8):503–508.
22. **Gosling T, Schandelmaier P, Müller M, et al** (2005) Single lateral locked screw plating of bicondylar tibial plateau fractures. *Clin Orthop Relat Res*; 439:207–214.
23. **Lysholm J, Gillquist J** (1982) Evaluation of knee ligament surgery results with special emphasis on use of a scoring scale. *Am J Sports Me*; 10(3): 150–154.
24. **Rasmussen PS** (1973) Tibial condylar fractures. Impairment of knee joint stability as an indication for surgical treatment. *J Bone Joint Surg Am*; 55(7):1331–1350.
25. **Hahn U, Prokop A, Jubel A, et al** (2002) [LISS versus condylar plate]. *Kongressbd Dtsch Ges Chir Kongr*; 119:498–504.
26. **Ricci WM, Rudzki JR, Borrelli J, Jr** (2004) Treatment of complex proximal tibia fractures with the less invasive skeletal stabilization system. *J Orthop Trauma*; 18(8):521–527.
27. **Cole PA, Zlowodzki M, Kregor PJ** (2004) Treatment of proximal tibia fractures using the less invasive stabilization system: surgical experience and early clinical results in 77 fractures. *J Orthop Trauma*; 18(8):528–535.
28. **Schütz M, Kääb MJ, Haas N** (2003) Stabilization of proximal tibial fractures with the LIS-System: early clinical experience in Berlin. *Injury*; 34Suppl1: A30–35.
29. **Stannard JP, Wilson TC, Volgas DA, et al** (2003) Fracture stabilization of proximal tibial fractures with the proximal tibial LISS: early experience in Birmingham, Alabama (USA). *Injury*; 34Suppl1:A36–42.
30. **Stannard JP, Wilson TC, Volgas DA, et al** (2004) The less invasive stabilization system in the treatment of complex fractures of the tibial plateau: short-term results. *J Orthop Trauma*; 18(8):552–558.
31. **Frigg R** (2003) Development of the Locking Compression Plate. *Injury*; 34Suppl1: B6–10.
32. **Ellis T, Bourgeault CA, Kyle RF** (2001) Screw position affects dynamic compression plate strain in an in vitro fracture model. *J Orthop Trauma*; 15(5):333–337.
33. **Field JR, Tornkvist H, Hearn TC, et al** (1999) The influence of screw omission on construction stiffness and bone surface strain in the application of bone plates to cadaveric bone. *Injury*; 30(9):591–598.
34. **Rozbruch SR, Müller U, Gautier E, et al** (1998) The evolution of femoral shaft plating technique. *Clin Orthop Relat Res*; 354:195–208.
35. **Sommer C, Gautier E** (2003) [Relevance and advantages of new angular stable screw-plate systems for diaphyseal fractures (locking compression plate versus intramedullary nail]. *Ther Umsch*; 60:751–756.
36. **Ring D, Kloen P, Kadzielski J, et al** (2004) Locking compression plates for osteoporotic nonunions of the diaphyseal humerus. *Clin Orthop Relat Res*; 425:50–54.
37. **Korner J, Lill H, Müller LP, et al** (2003) The LCP-concept in the operative treatment of distal humerus fractures—biological, biomechanical and surgical aspects. *Injury*; 34Suppl2:B20–30.
38. **Wagner M** (2003) General principles for the clinical use of the LCP. *Injury*; 34Suppl2: B31–42.

39. **Fankhauser F, Boldin C, Schippinger G, et al** (2005) A new locking plate for unstable fractures of the proximal humerus. *Clin Orthop Relat Res*; 430:176–181.
40. **Imatani J, Noda T, Morito Y, et al** (2005) Minimally invasive plate osteosynthesis for comminuted fractures of the metaphysis of the radius. *J Hand Surg [Br]*; 30(2):220–225.
41. **Schütz M, Kolbeck S, Spranger A, et al** (2003) [Palmar plating with the locking compression plate for dorsally displaced fractures of the distal radius--first clinical experiences]. *Zentralbl Chir*; 128(12):997–1002.
42. **Sommer C, Gautier E, Müller M, et al** (2003) First clinical results of the Locking Compression Plate (LCP). *Injury*; 34Suppl2:B43–54.

4 Pitfalls and complications

4 Pitfalls and complications

1 Implant-related problems

Bending of the locking compression plate. It is possible to bend the LCP 3.5 and 4.5/5.0, straight and narrow (Fig 4-1). Severe bending of the plate leads to deformation of the thread-bearing part of the combination hole, making the hole incapable of holding a locking head screw.

Solution: Leave a plate hole of this type without screw or use only cortex or cancellous bone screws.

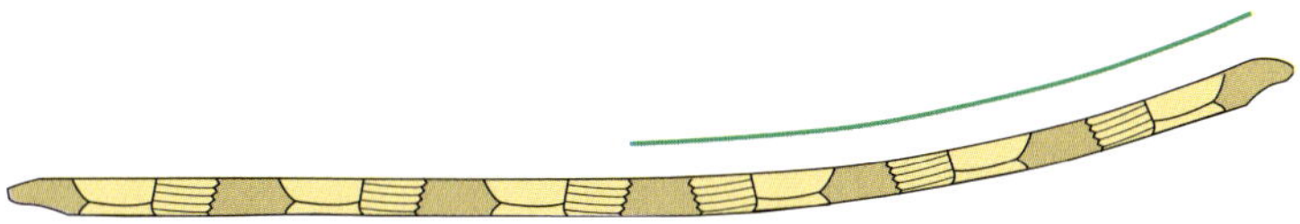

Fig 4-1 The LCP has an even stiffness without the risk of buckling at the screw holes.

Joint perforation. Locking head screws can only be inserted into the plate hole in the thread axis, so the direction is predetermined; attention should be given to avoid possible joint perforation (Fig 4-2a).

Solution: The correct length of screw should be measured and checked using image intensification. The risk of joint perforation is also reduced using metaphyseal or anatomical preshaped plates (Fig 4-2b–e).

Screw jamming and problems during implant removal. See technical errors.

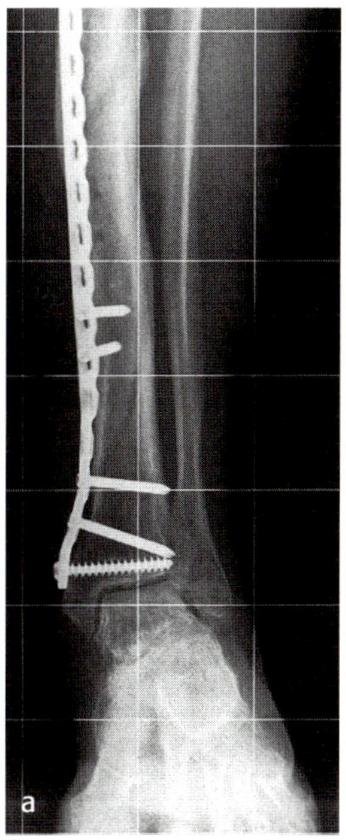

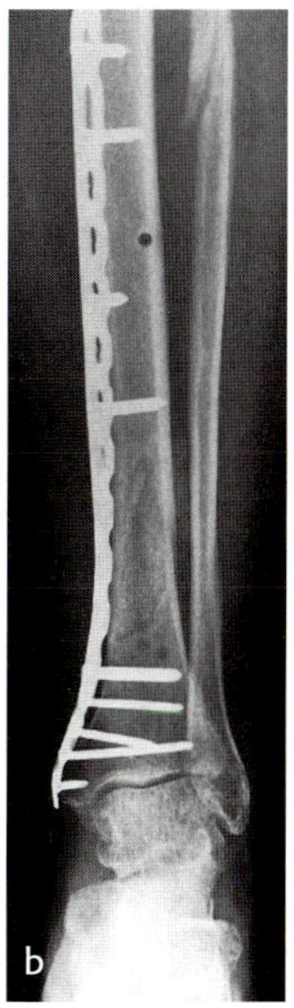

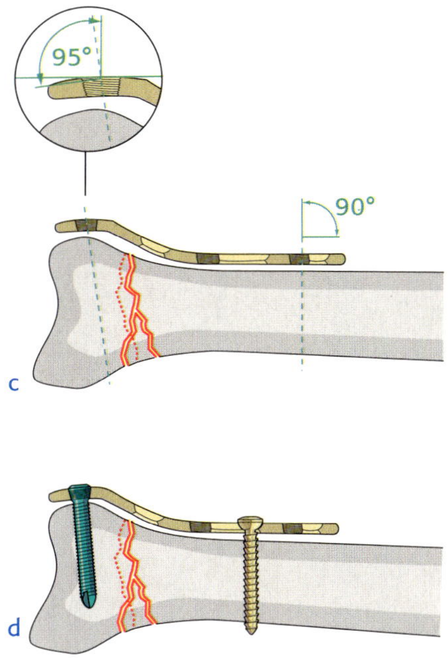

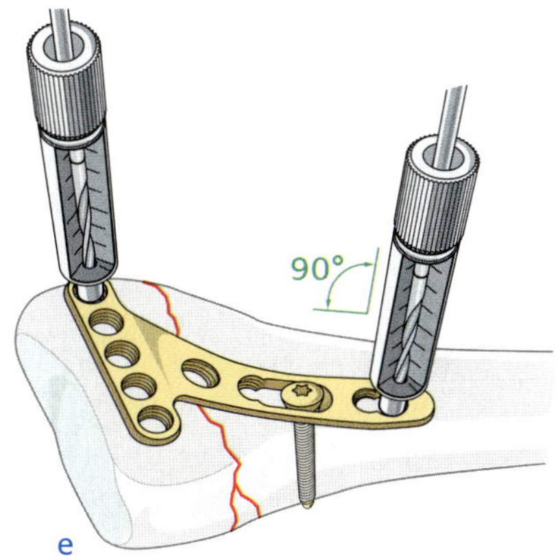

Fig 4-2a–e Joint perforation.

a To avoid joint perforation a cortex or cancellous bone screw with free angulation is inserted in the most distal combination hole.

b–e In anatomical precontoured plates the direction of the LHS is predetermined to avoid a possible joint perforation. To find the perpendicular seat of the screw the threaded drill sleeves should be used.

Lack of feedback when tightening locking head screws. Tightening locking head screws will always lead to a stable interface between screw and plate even without any bone contact. There is also no qualitative feedback for the surgeon regarding the bone quality.
Solution: It is very important to check the position of the plate before insertion of the locking head screws.

Helicopter effect. In order to tighten the first LHS, the opposite end of the plate must be firmly stabilized with holding forceps, a K-wire, a screw, or a drill bit; otherwise it can turn with the screw during the locking procedure and cause damage of the soft tissues (Fig 4-3). The same applies to the procedure for extraction of the last LHS during implant removal.

2 Technical errors

2.1 Incorrect fixation of the LCP/LISS

Problem of screw length. Monocortical inserted self-tapping LHS must not be too long, and the screw tip must not touch the opposing cortical bone, as this could lead to pull-out of the bone thread (Fig 4-4a). A self-drilling, self-tapping LHS should never be used bicortically, as the sharp cutting screw tip damages the soft tissue (Fig 4-4b). Removal of self-drilling, self-tapping screws which are too long can be difficult, due to bone growth into the drill flutes if the tip of the screw ends in the opposite cortex (Fig 4-4c).

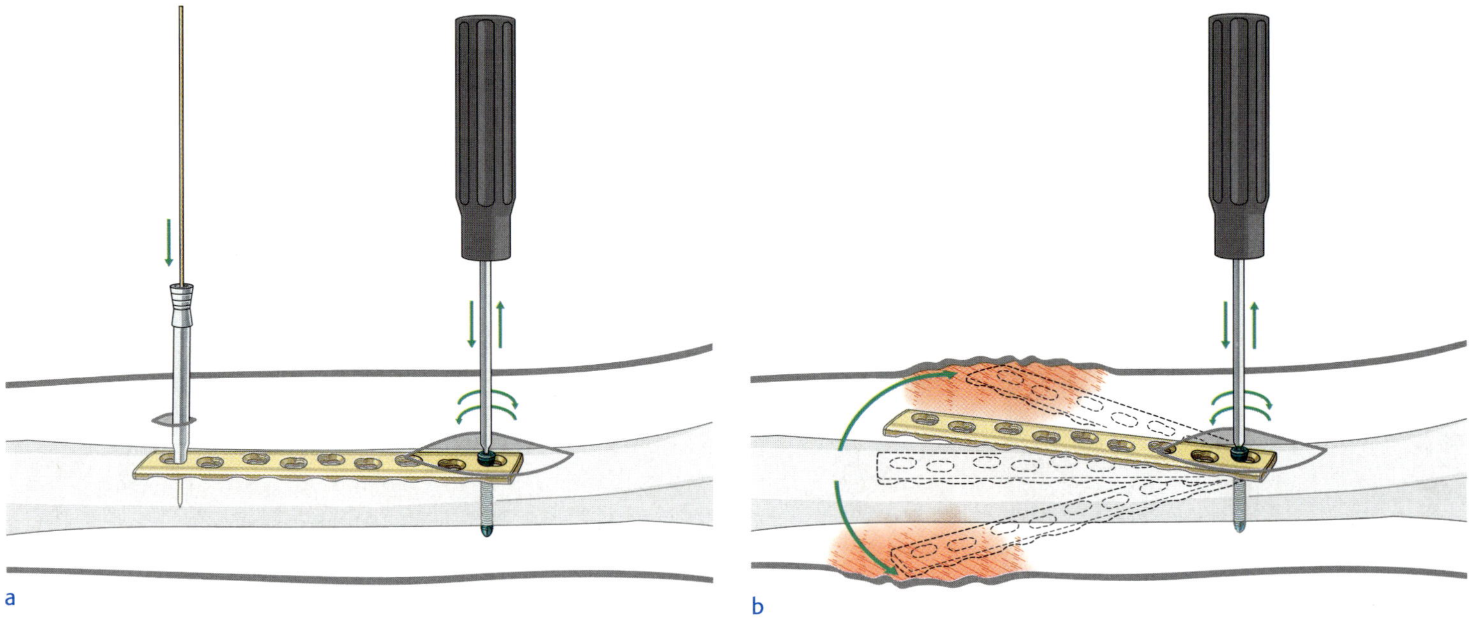

Fig 4-3a–b Temporary stabilization opposite to the first inserted LHS prevents the plate from rotating and causing damage to the surrounding soft tissue.

Solution: The proper length of a self-drilling, self-tapping monocortical screw has to be calculated with the help of x-rays. The length of a self-tapping screw can always be measured by depth gauge.

Screw jamming. Each LHS must be tightened using the appropriate torque-limiting screwdriver. (Fig 4-5)
Solution: Never tighten a LHS using a power tool.

Screw loosening can occur due to incorrect insertion technique. Screw loosening is mainly due to incorrect tightening of the locking head screws.
Solution: Using the threaded drill sleeve, drill and measure the correct length and insert the screw in a 90° perpendicular direction.

Incorrect direction of locking head screws. This problem can occur when the LHS are wrongly seated in an incorrect direction.
Solution: Whenever possible, a protective threaded drill sleeve should be used for predrilling to prevent the screw from being placed in the wrong direction.

Fatigue failure of a fixation construct due to stress concentration in simple diaphyseal fractures. This problem is usually seen in incorrect fixations in which the plate has insufficient elasticity and where the screws are placed too close to the fracture gap. Insufficient reduction and inadequate fixation (ie, wrong position of screws) of a simple diaphyseal fracture can lead to early breakage of the plate or to nonunion (Fig 4-6a-h).
Solution: To avoid stress concentration of the plate, in simple diaphyseal fractures, leave two to three plate holes unused over the fracture zone in order to make it possible for energy to be absorbed over a longer area of the implant (Fig 4-6i).

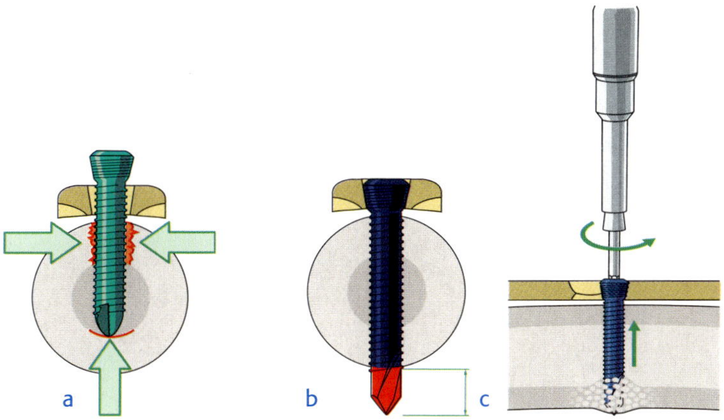

Fig 4-4a–c Problem of screw length.

- a Monocortical self-tapping LHS must not touch the opposite cortex, as this could lead to pullout.
- b Self-drilling, self-tapping LHS should never be used bicortically, as the shaprt tip damages the soft tissue.
- c When the tip of the self-drilling, self-tapping screw ends in the opposite cortex, screw removal can be difficult due to bony ingrowth into the drill flutes.

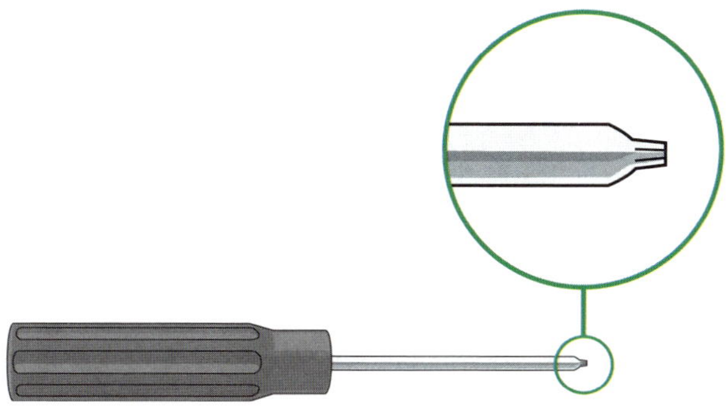

Fig 4-5 Each LHS must be tightened using the appropriate torque-limiting screwdriver. The calibration of this screwdriver for the 4.5/5.0 mm LHS is 4.0 Nm, for the 3.5 mm LHS 1.5 Nm.

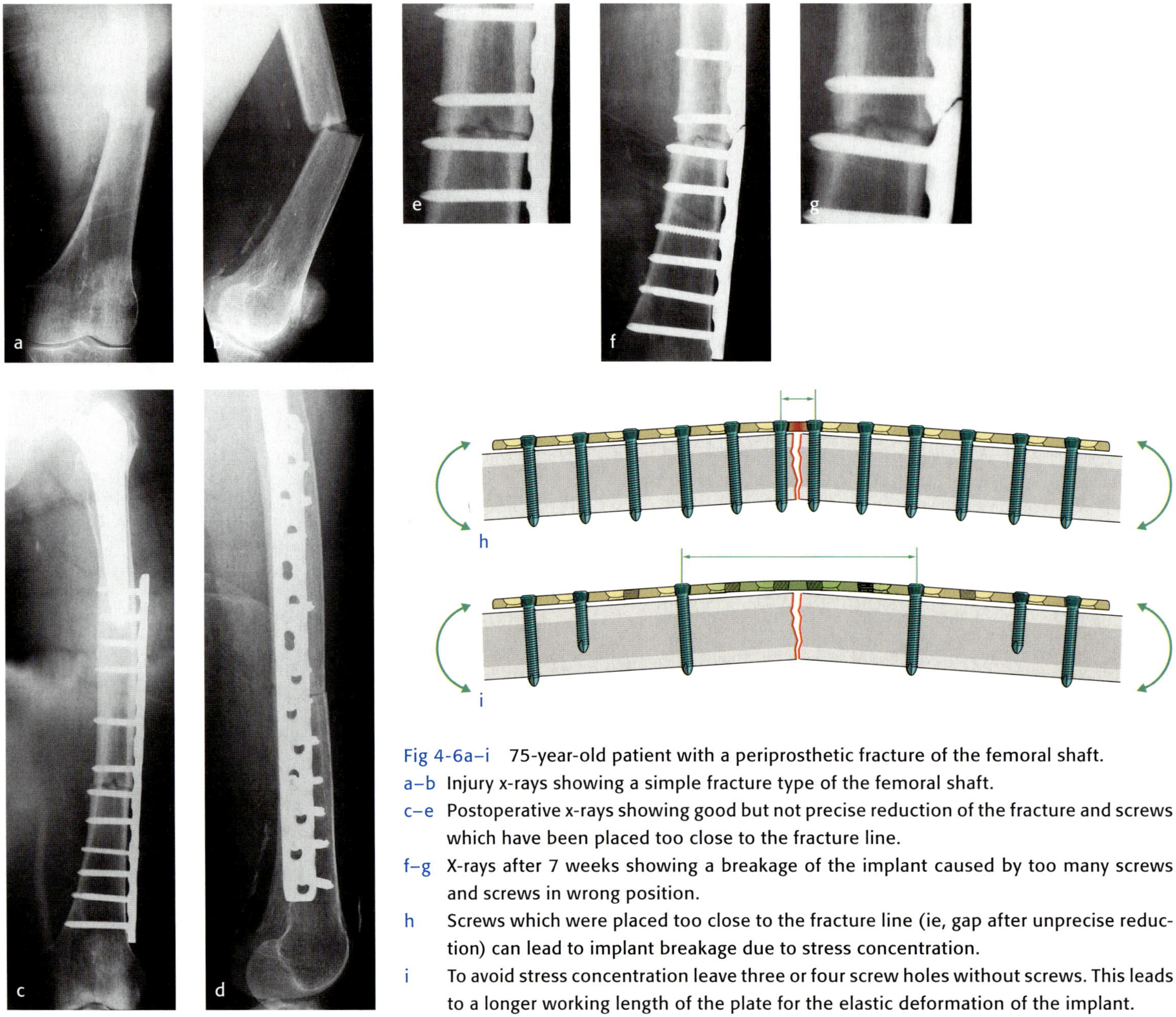

Fig 4-6a–i 75-year-old patient with a periprosthetic fracture of the femoral shaft.

a–b Injury x-rays showing a simple fracture type of the femoral shaft.

c–e Postoperative x-rays showing good but not precise reduction of the fracture and screws which have been placed too close to the fracture line.

f–g X-rays after 7 weeks showing a breakage of the implant caused by too many screws and screws in wrong position.

h Screws which were placed too close to the fracture line (ie, gap after unprecise reduction) can lead to implant breakage due to stress concentration.

i To avoid stress concentration leave three or four screw holes without screws. This leads to a longer working length of the plate for the elastic deformation of the implant.

Loss of fixation construct in a main bone segment. This type of failure is seen in cases in which the screw–bone interface has been subjected to excessive stress.

Solution: The rigidity of the whole construct has to be reduced in order to decrease the stress on the interface (Fig 4-7). This can be achieved by using longer plates (ie, a longer bridging element). Bicortical screws used to anchor a plate in a bone with a thin cortex will increase the holding strength against torsional forces (eg, in an osteoporotic humeral shaft) or pullout (eg, femoral shaft).

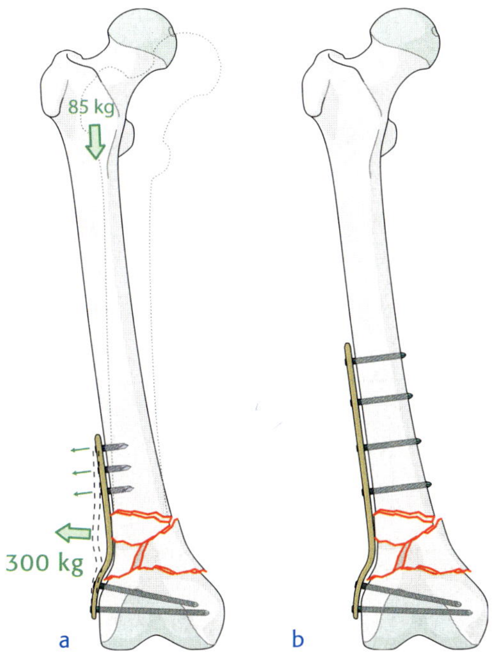

Fig 4-7a–b Loss of fixation construct in a main bone segment

a The elastic deformation of the plate under physical load acts like a bow. This leads to pullout of the construction from the bone.

b Using longer plates and bicortical screws reduce the stress on the screw-bone interface and increases the holding strength.

- If there are too few screws, the plate may pull out. Three to four screws in each main fragment are recommended depending on indication. Avoid a short plate with only two or three monocortical LHS (Fig 4-8).
- Inadequate plate fixation can occur despite the use of an adequate number of locking head screws. LHS can become misplaced due to placement off-center of the plate (ie, can be locked into the plate even if the bone has only been partially penetrated or completely missed) (see Tab 3-9).
- If the wrong screws are selected, eg, monocortical LHS in the humeral shaft or osteoporotic bone, the plate may pull out.

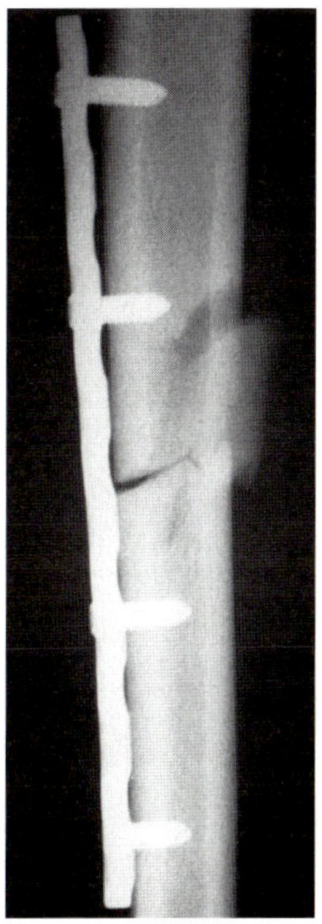

Fig 4-8 Wrong fixation with a too short plate, too few and monocortically inserted screws in the humeral shaft.

- If the plate is fixed to a main fragment under tension, ie, elastic deformation of the plate, the plate will be able to pull out. Reduction of the plate to the bone after fixation with LHS to the two main fragments is impossible and leads to pullout of the plate (Fig 9a–b).
  Solution: Never reduce a plate to the bone under high tension. The plate must be aligned and approximately preshaped to the bone anatomy after reduction.

Loosening of LHS despite the use of a torque-limiting screwdriver. This type of failure can only arise if the LHS has been inserted off-axis relative to the LCP hole. The insertion axis of the locking head screws is defined by the LCP hole axis. In most straight LCP plates, the locking hole axis is perpendicular to the plate surface. In all anatomically preshaped plates, the axis of the hole is predefined for optimal screw placement in the given anatomical region. This optimization ensures the best anchorage of the plate by maximizing the possible number of screws and working length of the plate and by reducing the risk of anatomical misplacement and collision of screws (Fig 4-10).

Solution: Use the aiming block/device for anatomical preshaped LCP or the threaded drill sleeves for standard LCP to insert the LHS.

Inserting LHS in a tense, thick cortex. By inserting a self-drilling, self-tapping LHS, the torque-limiting screwdriver may unlock before the screw head is locked in the plate hole because of the high resistance of the thick cortex.
Solution: Check the proper position of the LHS screw head in the plate using the image intensifier.

LHS placed in the compression unit of the combination hole. Misplacement of a locking head screw can occur if the plate hole cannot be visualized (eg, in minimally invasive procedures).
Solution: Use of the threaded drill sleeve to identify the threaded portion of the combination hole can reduce the risk of misplacement (Fig 4-11).

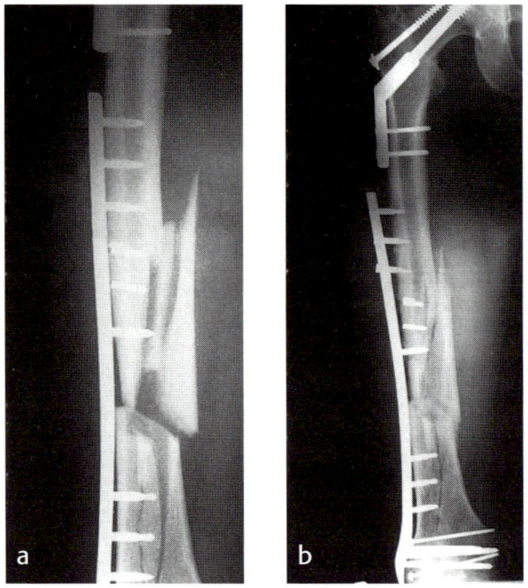

Fig 4-9a–b

a In treating a complex, floating knee injury, the LISS-DF was reduced onto the shaft fragment with a strong traction force because the reduction pathway was too large. If one observes the implant carefully, one can see that this has actually led to the deformation of the extremely rigid LISS (the proximal section bends against the shaft). In addition, two broken threads from the pulling devices are proof of a certain level of force used during the fracture reduction and implant positioning. The fragment was pulled laterally by the strong force of the traction devices and then fixed with monocortical, self-drilling, self-tapping screws.

b In the course of the healing process, the implant has loosened on the shaft after 6 months (one sees that the implant has again resumed its regular form. Here the monocortical screws were pulled out of the bone axially).

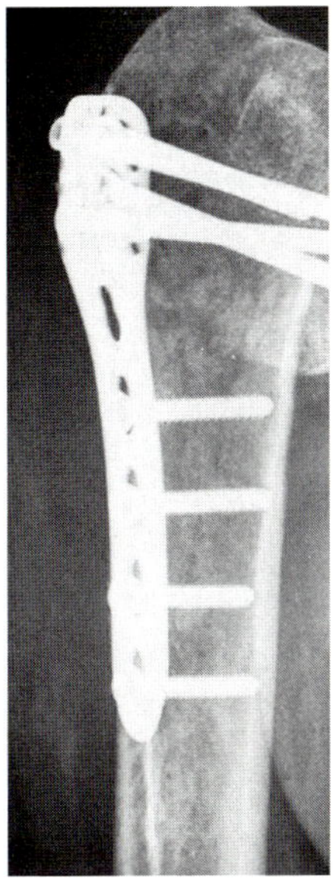

Fig 4-10 Loosening of LHS despite the use of a torque-limiting screwdriver.

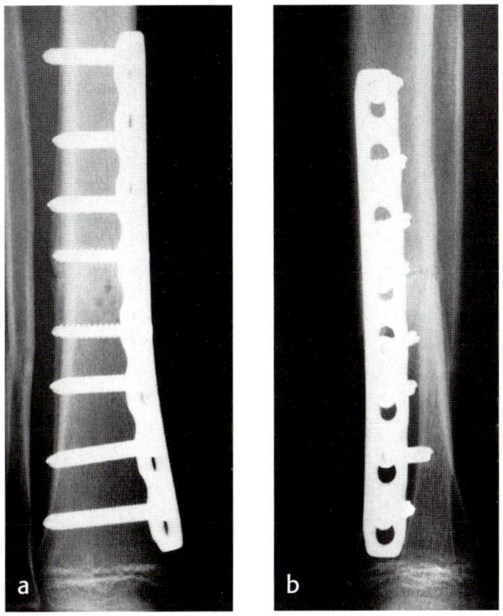

Fig 4-11a–b Misplacement of the most proximal LHS.

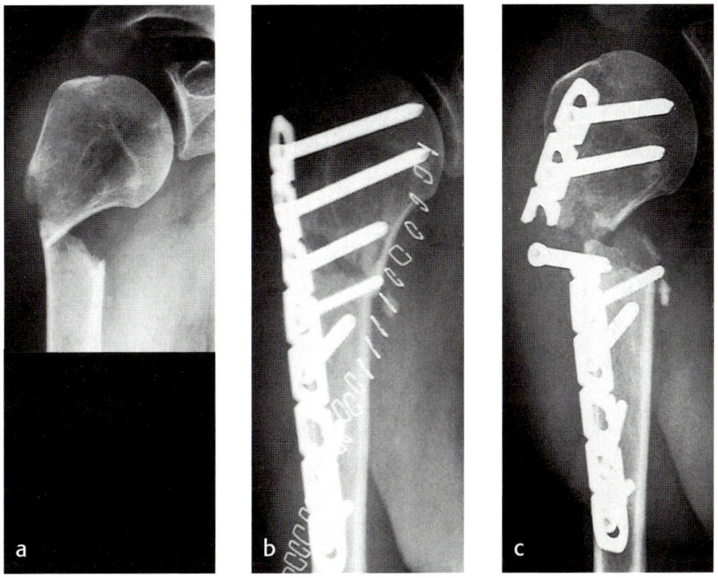

4-12a–c 44-year-old woman with subcapital proximal humeral shaft fracture.

- a Injury x-ray.
- b Postoperative x-ray shows the third proximal screw crosses the unreduced fracture line. The second technical error is the use of a reconstruction plate for a humeral shaft fracture.
- c Implant failure after 3 weeks.

LHS crossing an unreduced fracture line, leading to delayed fracture union. LHS were designed to optimize the fixation of a plate to the bone. In contrast to lag screws, locking head screws are not designed to produce compression. A locking head screw crossing an unreduced fracture line works as a position screw while maintaining the distance of the two fragments relative to each other. A fracture gap locked with an LHS is therefore unable to produce callus due to micromotion (Fig 4-12).

Solution: LHS should never cross a fracture line.
Exception: In articular fractures after precise reduction and compression with a reduction tool. Therefore the required reduction must be achieved before placement of the locking head screw. This will avoid loss of reduction and delayed union or nonunion.

LHS are never lag screws. They can only serve as fixation screws or position screws. When interfragmentary compression has been obtained using a reduction forceps or a lag screw, the positioning of the bone fragments that has been achieved can be maintained using LHS.

Incorrect positioning of the plate. This can cause the plate to impinge on the soft tissues, and it may lead to the LHS missing the bone (Fig 4-13).
Solution: Check plate position with image intensifier or by palpation if required.

Pullout of the pulling device for the LISS ("whirlybird"). In osteoporotic bone or when the reduction pathway is too large, it is possible for the pulling device ("whirlybird") to pull out.
Solution: Reduce the distance between the plate and the bone, eg, with a collinear reduction clamp.

2.2 Insufficient reduction and demanding MIPO

Difficult indirect closed reduction. MIPO with locked internal fixators requires closed indirect reduction. Incorrect reduction can lead to malalignment.
Solution: The procedure has to be learned and is a difficult one. Reduction has to be checked during the operation both clinically and radiographically.

Minimally invasive plate osteosynthesis (MIPO). With the small access routes that are used (small incisions, stab incisions), the procedure is difficult and injury to vessels or nerves can occur (Fig 4-14). Minimal invasive fixation of a 13-hole LISS-PLT: The superficial peroneal nerves and vessels are at risk when seating the monocortical LHS through stab incisions at the distal end of the plate.
Solution: Do not overuse the minimal invasive approach. MIPO should only be done by surgeons with a lot of experience. Otherwise use a less invasive approach.

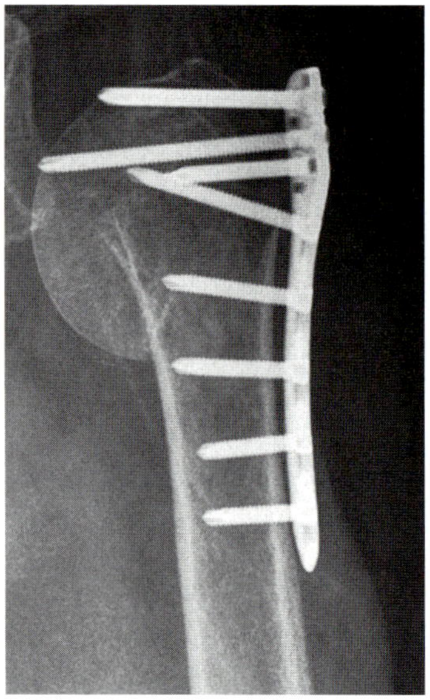

Fig 4-13 Inadequate reduction and position of the locking proximal humeral plate (LPHP) leads to a subacromial impingement.

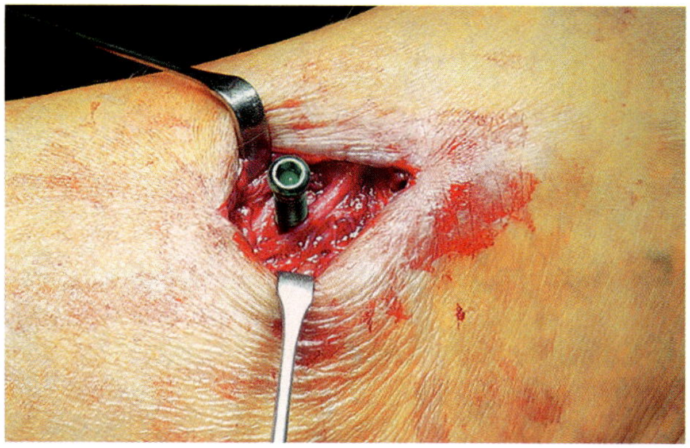

Fig 4-14 The superficial peroneal nerves and vessels are at risk seating the monocortical LHS through stab incisions at the end of the plate on the distal tibia.

2.3 Incorrect principle and method of fracture fixation

- As a result of lack of planning.
- May also result from an attempt to combine two methods of fracture fixation in a single fracture.

Solution: see Tab 1-10

2.4 Incorrect choice of plate

Examples include:

- Wrong choice of plate (eg, reconstruction plate for humeral shaft fractures (Fig 4-12)
- Too short plate (Fig 4-8)

Solution: Choice of proper implants. Please see Tab 3-6 and Tab 3-9.

3 Pitfalls and complications during rehabilitation

3.1 Secondary plastic deformation of the LCP/locked internal fixator

Bridge osteosynthesis with locked internal fixators (using the splinting method based on the principle of relative stability in fracture fixation) provides very little primary stability. As the fragments are not precisely reduced, the bone does not contribute to primary stability. This type of osteosynthesis, with reduced and relative stability, allows reversible elastic deformation of the locked internal fixator implant in the area of the fracture zone. This effect is desirable and stimulates indirect bone healing.

If unacceptable early loading or overloading of the fracture area occurs, irreversible secondary plastic bending of the fixator can occur (Fig 4-15). Assessing the degree of stability achieved can be carried out clinically or using a radiographic stress examination. After completion of the bridging osteosynthesis for a multifragmentary fracture using an internal fixator, it is necessary to check the stability of the fixation intraoperatively using an image intensifier. This allows assessment of the degree of remaining elasticity (ie, reversible deformation) of the osteosynthesis. In lower leg fractures, additional plating of the fibula or placement of an additional temporary external fixator on the opposite side of the locked internal fixator may be necessary.

The fracture care follow-up treatment needs to be adjusted to the individual fracture situation and the cooperation of the patient. In the case of internal extramedullary splint fixation (ie, locked internal fixator), rehabilitation and physical therapy has to be slightly altered. Since this is an elastic method of fixation and the bone does not contribute to the primary stability, the implant initially has to bear initially the entire load.

Callus formation must occur before weight bearing can be initiated and gradually increased.

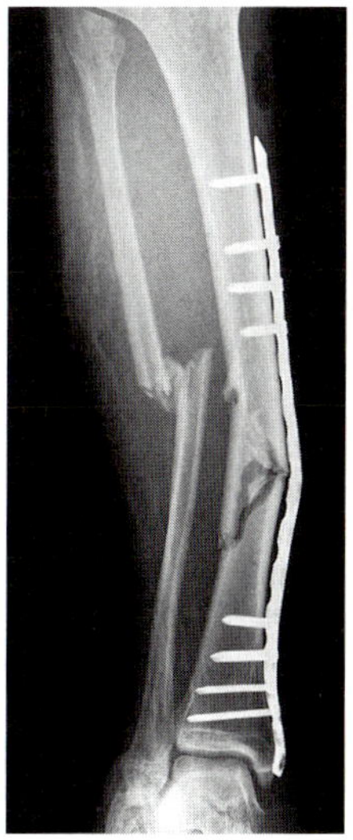

Fig 4-15 Single overload situation which leads to a plastic deformation of the implant. On the first postoperative night, the patient mobilized with full weight bearing.

3.2 Difficult implant removal: LHS are difficult or impossible to remove

Difficulty in removing LHS can occur for the following reasons:

- **Damaged recess of the screw head.** Causes might be:
  - A worn screwdriver tip.
  - Only partially introduction of the screwdriver tip into the deep recess of the screw head.
  - Tipping or gyration of the screwdriver when screwing in the screws manually.
- **LHS which are too tight locked.** This can occur if the torque-limiting device was not used and the screw was introduced using a power tool drive.
- **Screw heads jammed in the plate hole.** Causes might be:
  - A wrong direction of LHS—not perpendicular to the axis of the threaded part of the combination hole.
  - The positioning of the LHS in the wrong part of the LCP combination hole.
- **Too long self-drilling, self-tapping LHS.**

When the tip of a self-drilling, self-tapping LHS ends in the opposite cortex, screw removal can be difficult due to bony ingrowth into the drill flutes.

- **Bone on growth to LHS**

As locking head screws are locked to the plate, micromovement in the bone, especially for slide loosening, not exists. This mechanical advantage can lead to a strong integration of the screw into the bone. The increased torque needed to remove such a screw can exceed the applicable torque to the screw drive.

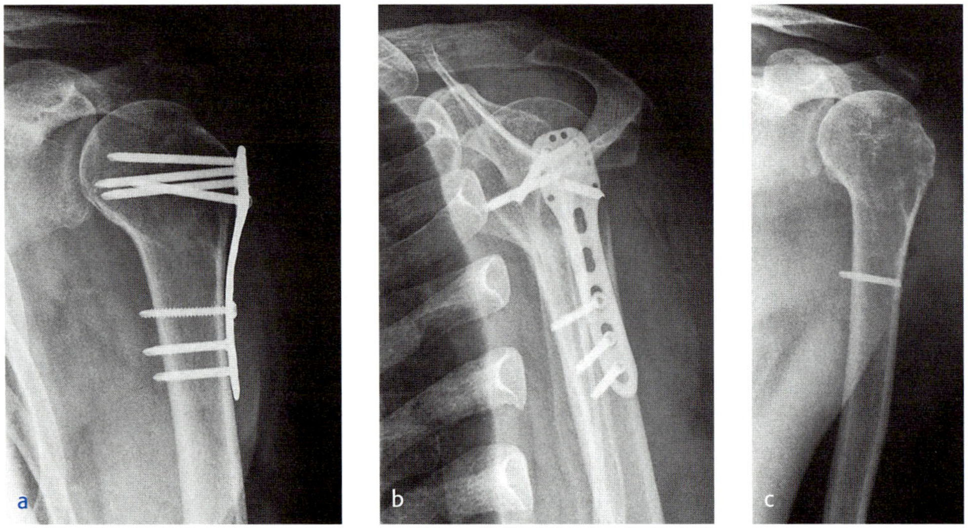

Fig 4-16a–c

- a AP view.
- b Axillary view. Shows a bony healing 8 months after surgical treatment of a proximal humeral fracture—1-B1. One of the LHS in the shaft (ie, second screw from distal) is in the wrong part of the combination hole of the LPHP. This leads to screw jamming and problem by implant removal.
- c Screw head turned of by the implant removal.

Removal of LHS (with a destroyed drive)

- For screws with an empty destroyed drive recess without broken instrument the following steps are required: 1, 3, 5, 6, 7, 8. Check for appropriate drill bit.
- For screw with broken instrument in the screw recess the following steps are required: 2, 3, 4, 5, 6, 7, 8.

Step 1

a Before using the drill bit, try to remove the screw with the conical extraction screw. Insert the extraction screw under axial load and by left-wise rotation (anticlockwise) (Fig 4-17a). Do not use excessive force to avoid breaking the extraction screw. If this fails, a second approach may be attempted.

b If the conical extraction screw does not get purchased it is advisable to take the appropriate drill bit to prepare the recess (Fig 4-17b).

Try step 1a again.

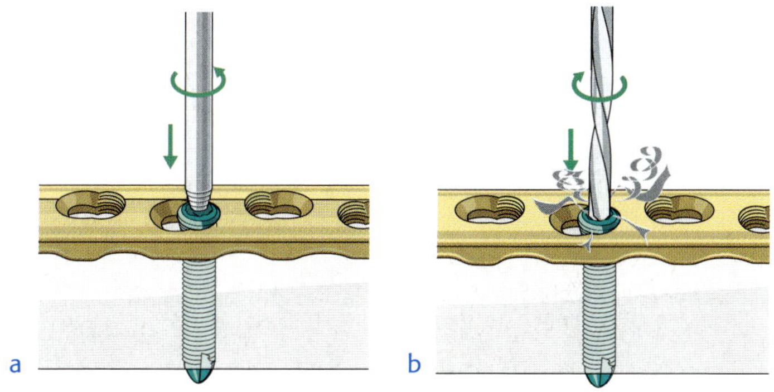

Fig 4-17a–b

Step 2

Attempt to remove the broken part of the instrument using a sharp hook and/or forceps. If this is unsuccessful, proceed to the next step (Fig 4-18).

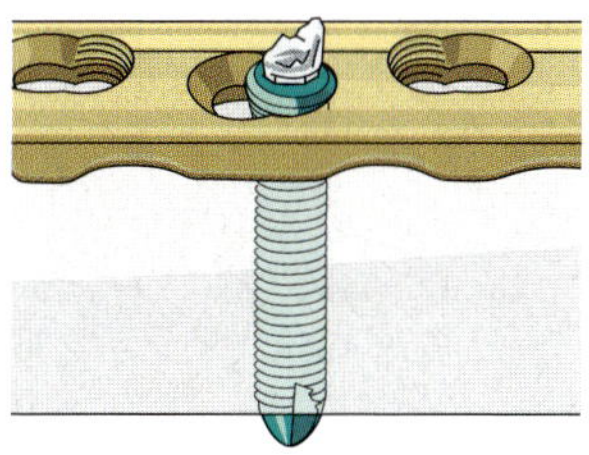

Fig 4-18

Step 3

Prepare the instruments checking Tab 4-1. It is recommended to cover the area around the screw removal site with sterile adhesive film to protect the surrounding soft tissue. Prepare the suction device and the irrigation system.

Screw/recess type	Instruments
Small fragment screws (recess: Stardrive T15 or Hex 2.5)	■ Appropriate drill bit ■ Irrigation system (syringe and water) and suction device ■ Extraction screw, conical, for screws Ø 2.7, 3.5 and 4.0 mm ■ Extraction bolt for 3.5/4.0 mm screws ■ Spare reamer tube ■ Pliers for screw removal ■ Adhesive film (optional)
Large fragment screws (recess: Stardrive T25 or Hex 3.5)	■ Appropriate drill bit ■ Irrigation system (syringe and water) and suction device ■ Extraction screw, conical, for screws Ø 4.5 and 6.5 mm ■ Extraction bolt, for screws Ø 4.5 and 5.0 mm; or extraction bolt, for screws Ø 6.0, 6.5 and 7.0 mm ■ Spare reamer tube ■ Pliers for screw removal ■ Adhesive film (optional)

Tab 4-1 Instruments required for complete screw removal.

Step 4

Drill bits made out of carbides are very brittle and sensitive to strokes. To avoid damages of carbidge drill bits, start the drill prior of touching the screw head with the drill bit. Keep the drill running until the drill bit is removed from the screw head. Start drilling with revolving carbide drill bit with the irrigation system and suction device in operation. The direction of drilling should be perpendicular to the fractured surface of the instrument. Smooth the rough surface. The suction device should be placed close to the tip of the drill bit (Fig 4-19).

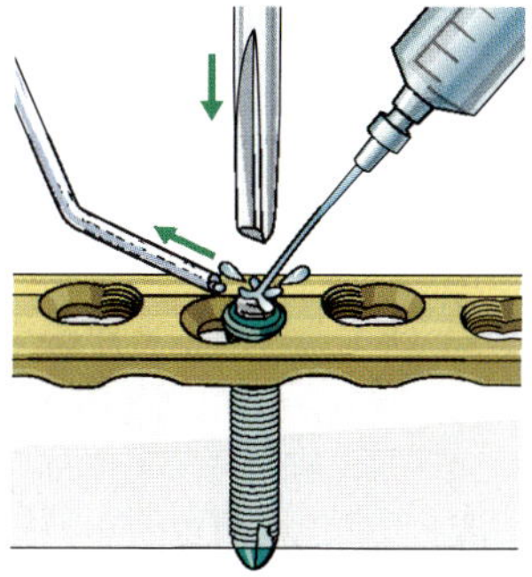

Fig 4-19

Step 5

Drill continuously without stopping. Axial force is required for efficient drilling. It is recommended to align the axis of the drill bit with the axis of the screw.

Note: If axial alignment cannot be achieved, a larger diameter drill bit may be required to separate the plate completely from the screw.

The 6.0 mm carbide drill bit can only be used after predrilling with the 4.0 mm carbide drill bit.

Step 6

Drill into the head of the screw until there is no longer a physical connection between the screw and the plate. Then remove the plate (Fig 4-20).

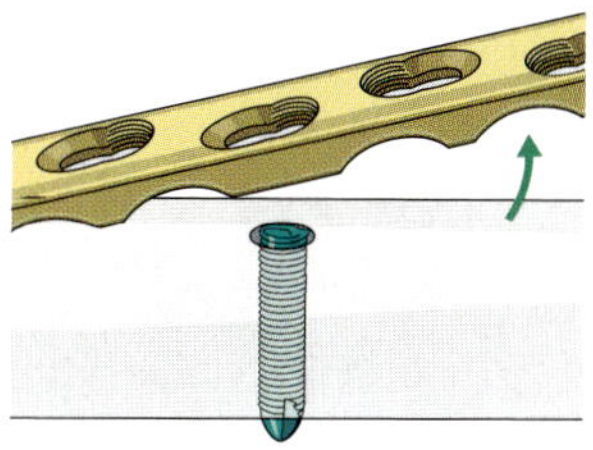

Fig 4-20

Step 7

Remove the screw shaft (Fig 4-21):

a If the screw protrudes from the bone, use the pliers for screw removal. Grip the screw and turn counter-clockwise. Do not pull.

b If the screw does not protrude from the bone, use the spare reamer tube and the extraction bolt. Align the axis of the spare reamer tube with the axis of the screw. Ream to a depth of 5 mm.

c Place the extraction bolt over the screw. While pushing, turn the screw counterclockwise. This will create a tight connection between the conical shape of the thread of the extraction bolt and the screw shaft.

d Turn counterclockwise until the screw shaft is completely removed.

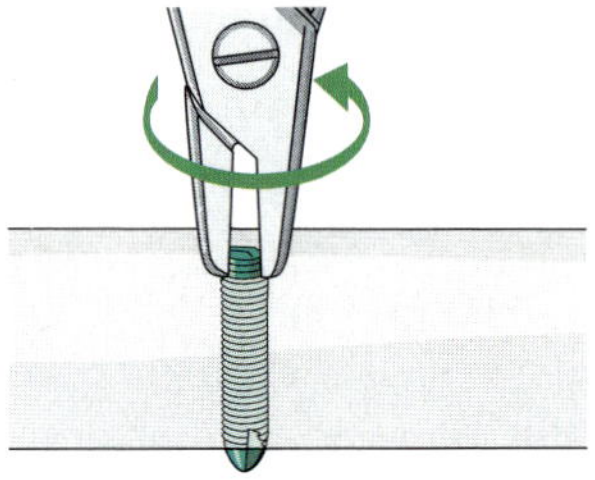

Fig 4-21a

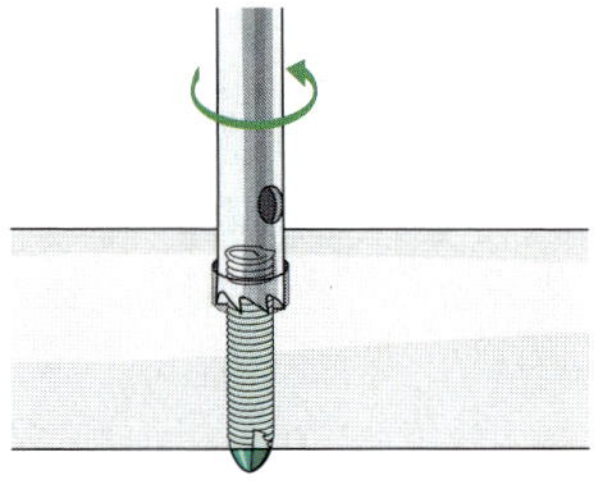

Fig 4-21b

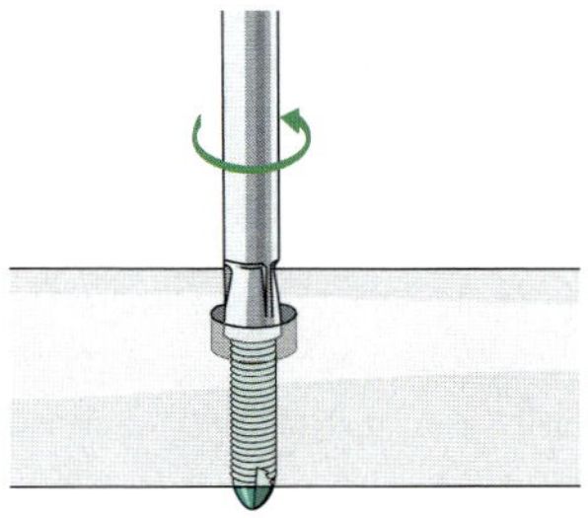

Fig 4-21c

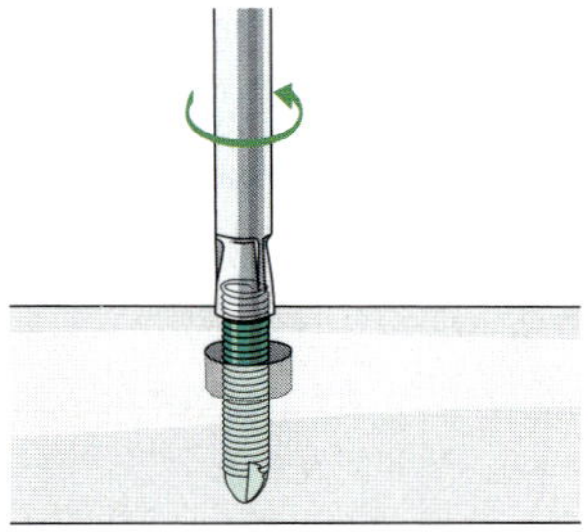

Fig 4-21d

Step 8

It is recommended to perform a final x-ray control examination to ensure no undesired material has been left in the body.

Difficult implant removal because of bony ingrowth into plates and screws

Reasons for difficult removal of plates with angular stability due to bony ingrowth may include (Fig 4-22):

- The callus may grow into the plate holes.
- Titanium implants in particular are associated with marked bone ingrowth.
- Delay in removing implants in children.

3.3 Delayed union, nonunion

Indirect bone healing is expected in a fixation by splinting method such as bridging the fracture zone with a locked internal fixator, resulting in timely callus formation in the fracture site and gradual maturation. If there is excessive elasticity, bridging of the callus may be delayed, necessitating some modification of the postoperative treatment or a second operation to add more stability (additional strategic screws, external fixator).

Fractures with severe soft-tissue trauma and subsequent disturbance of the periostal blood supply require a longer time for bone consolidation.

Locked splinting of simple fractures with internal fixators sometimes shows delayed healing.

In most cases treated with biological fracture fixation—bridging with LIF, primary bone grafting is not required, but a secondary bone grafting should be considered if no clear healing signs are given within 6 months (mostly in open fractures with bone loss.)

3.4 Refracture after implant removal

Recurring fractures following implant removal in fractures with indirect bone healing and callus formation are rare. The incidence of refracture after removal of implants is considered lower in the splinting method than in conventional compression plating, but no evidence has been obtained to support this. The use of monocortical screws and a reduced number of screws appear to be beneficial.

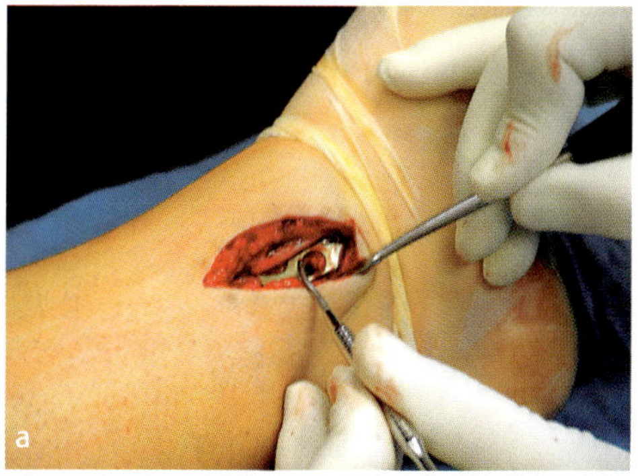

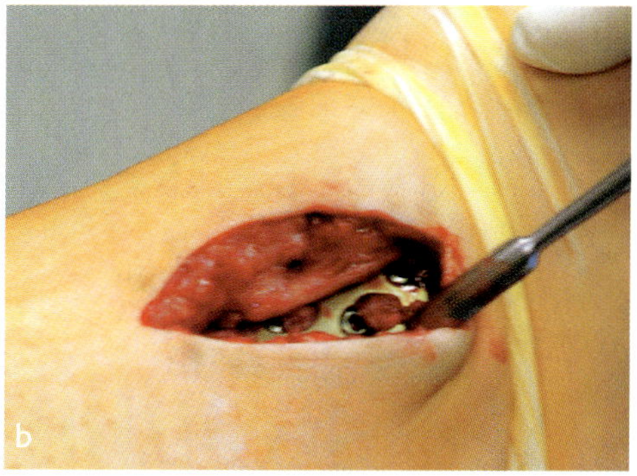

Fig 4-22a–b Callus growth into the plate holes.

3.5 Infection

Infections rarely occur following fracture fixation with locked internal fixator. The progression of such infections is also less severe than those seen with compression plates, as the periosteal blood supply is not additionally damaged by the plate. If an infection near the implant used in MIPO is suspected, its removal should be considered. However, the implant should be removed only after bone union has been obtained, unless it shows signs of loosening, implying no stability of fragments (Fig 4-23).

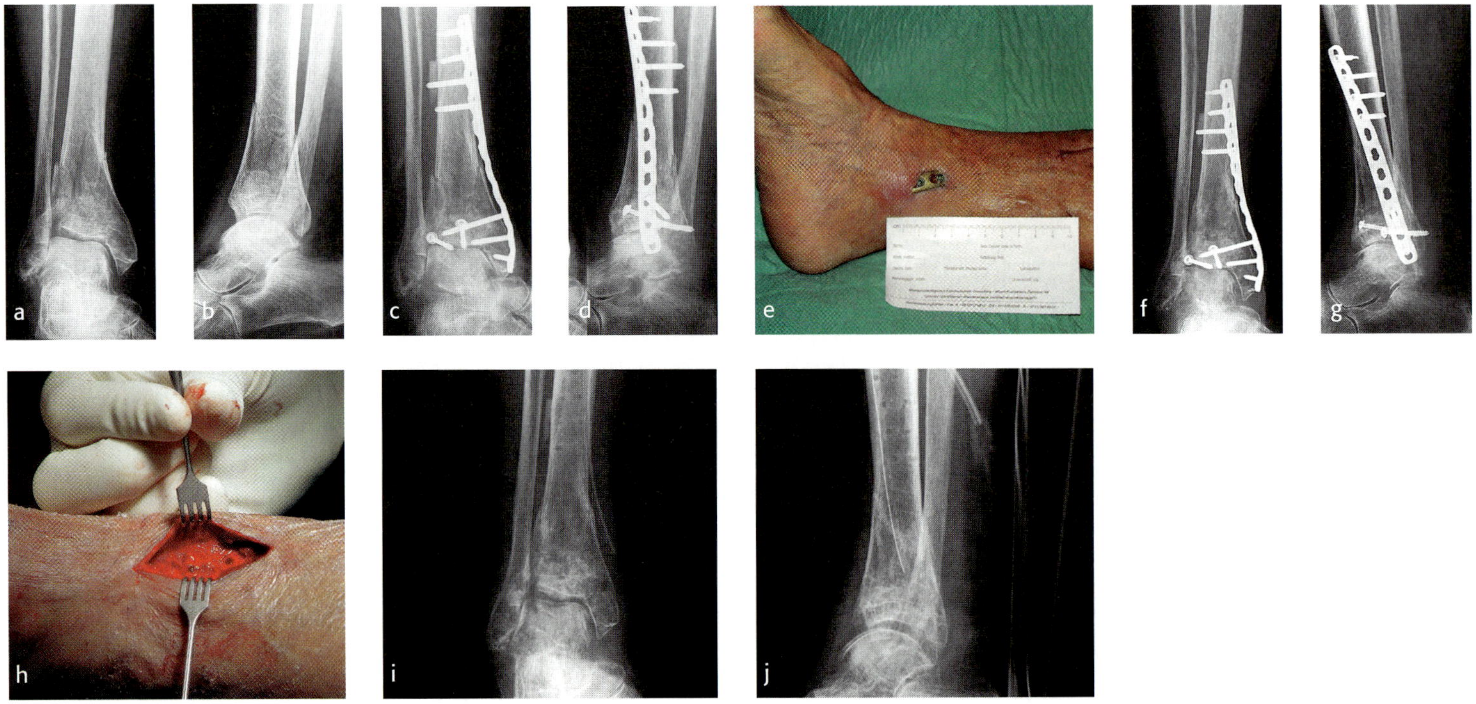

Fig 4-23a–j Infection.

a–b Fracture of the right distal tibia 43-C2; nicotine abuse.

c–d Postoperative x-rays: MIPO with percutaneous lag screws for the articular fracture and bridging of the metaphyseal fracture with LCP and LHS. The anterolateral tibial key fragment is not reduced.

e After a few days infection of the wound and skin lesion over the distal part of the plate. Wound therapy with the vacuum method.

f–g Bony consolidation after 5 weeks and implant removal.

h After implant removal good granulative soft tissue under the plate and good blood supply.

i–j X-rays after implant removal.

4 Suggestions for further reading

Boldin C, Fankhauser F, Hofer HP, et al (2006) Three-year Results of Proximal Tibia Fractures Treated with the LISS. *Clin Orthop Relat Res*; Publish Ahead of Print

Cole PA, Zlowodzki M, Kregor PJ et al (2003) Less Invasive Stabilization System (LISS) for fractures of the proximal tibia: indications, surgical technique and preliminary results of the UMC Clinical Trial. *Injury*; 34 Suppl1:A16–29.

Gautier E, Sommer C (2003) Guidelines for the clinical application of the LCP. *Injury*; 34 Suppl2:B63–76.

Gautier E, Sommer Ch (2003) [Biological internal fixation—guidelines for the rehabilitation]. *Ther Umsch*; 60(12):729–735. German.

Kääb MJ, Stockle U, Schütz M, et al (2005) Stabilisation of periprosthetic fractures with angular stable internal fixation: a report of 13 cases. *Arch Orthop Trauma Surg*; 23:1–6.

Korner J, Lill H, Müller LP, et al (2003) The LCP-concept in the operative treatment of distal humerus fractures—biological, biomechanical and surgical aspects. *Injury*; 34 Suppl2:B20–30. Review.

Messmer P, Regazzoni P, Gross T (2003) [New stabilization techniques for fixation of proximal tibial fractures (LISS/LCP)]. *Ther Umsch*; 60(12):762–767. German.

Ricci WM, Rudzki JR, Borrelli J Jr (2004) Treatment of complex proximal tibia fractures with the less invasive skeletal stabilization system. *J Orthop Trauma*; 18(8):521–527.

Rikli DA, Babst R (2003) [New principles in the surgical treatment of distal radius fractures—locking implants]. *Ther Umsch*; 60(12):745–750. German.

Ryf C, Götsch U, Perren T, et al (2003) [New surgical treatment procedures in fractures of the distal tibia (LCP, MIPO)]. *Ther Umsch*; 60(12):768–775. German.

Schandelmaier P, Partenheimer A, Koenemann B, et al (2001) Distal femoral fractures and LISS stabilization. *Injury*; 32 Suppl3:SC55–63. Review.

Schütz M, Kolbeck S, Spranger A, et al (2003) [Palmar plating with the locking compression plate for dorsally displaced fractures of the distal radius—first clinical experiences] *Zentralbl Chir*; 128(12):997–1002. German.

Schütz M, Müller M, Kääb M, et al (2003) Less invasive stabilization system (LISS) in the treatment of distal femoral fractures. *Acta Chir Orthop Traumatol Cech*; 70(2):74–82.

Schütz M, Müller M, Krettek C, et al (2001) Minimally invasive fracture stabilization of distal femoral fractures with the LISS: a prospective multicenter study. Results of a clinical study with special emphasis on difficult cases. *Injury*; 32 Suppl3:SC48–54.

Schütz M, Müller M, Regazzoni P, et al (2005) Use of the less invasive stabilization system (LISS) in patients with distal femoral (AO33) fractures: a prospective multicenter study. *Arch Orthop Trauma Surg*; 125(2):102–108.

Sommer C, Babst R, Müller M, et al (2004) Locking compression plate loosening and plate breakage: a report of four cases. *J Orthop Trauma*; 18(8):571–577.

Sommer C, Gautier E, Müller M, et al (2003) First clinical results of the Locking Compression Plate (LCP). *Injury*; 34 Suppl2:B43–54.

Sommer Ch, Gautier E (2003) [Relevance and advantages of new angular stable screw-plate systems for diaphyseal fractures (locking compression plate versus intramedullary nail]. *Ther Umsch*; 60(12):751–756. German.

Weight M, Collinge C (2004) Early results of the less invasive stabilization system for mechanically unstable fractures of the distal femur (AO/OTA types A2, A3, C2, and C3). *J Orthop Trauma*; 18(8):503–508.

Wick M, Müller EJ, Kutscha-Lissberg F, et al (2004) [Periprosthetic supracondylar femoral fractures: LISS or retrograde intramedullary nailing? Problems with the use of minimally invasive technique]. *Unfallchirurg*; 107(3):181–188. German.

Cases

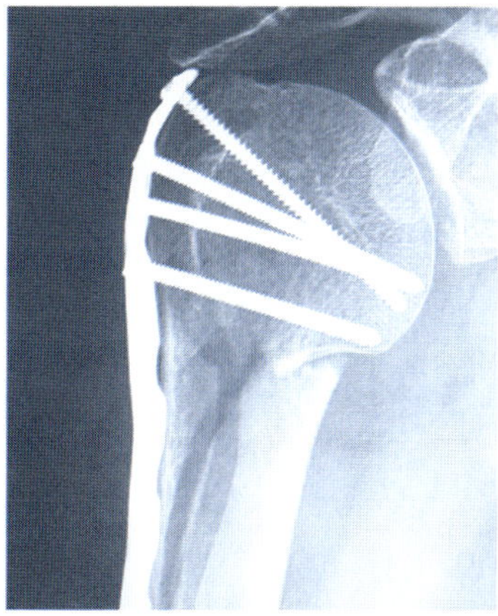
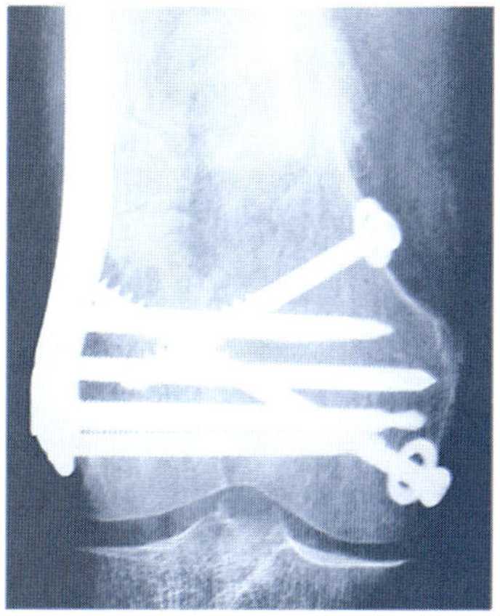
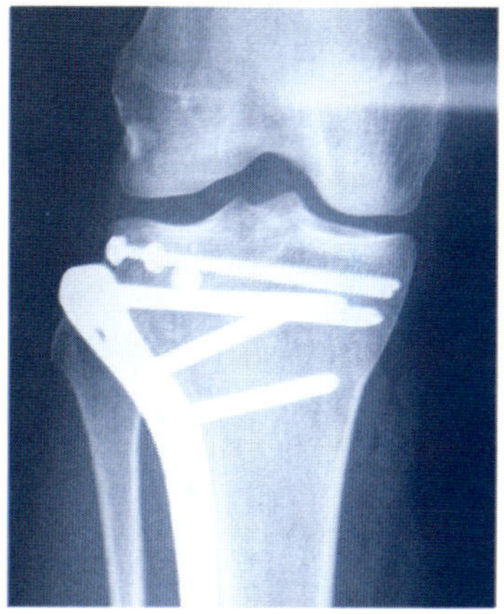

Cases

5 Shoulder girdle

Cases

5 Shoulder girdle

Author Christoph Sommer

5.1 Clavicle

1 Incidence of fractures

Fractures of the clavicle are very common and are mostly caused by a simple fall on the shoulder with direct impact over the lateral part of the clavicle. It is a typical sport injury (bicycle, ski, and ball sports), and therefore most often seen in young and healthy people. The clavicle is often broken in polytraumatized patients involved in a high-energy trauma (road traffic accident), often as part of a complex chest injury with serial rib fractures and pulmonary contusion. In these high-energy injuries, associated neurovascular injuries are common and careful attention must be paid to these.

2 Classification

Midshaft fractures (OTA 06) are classified according to the classification of the diaphyseal parts of the long bone in A, B, and C types (simple, wedge, and complex). The fractures of the medial or lateral part of the clavicle can be divided into extraarticular or intraarticular and nondisplaced or displaced fractures [1].

3 Treatment methods

Most fractures of the clavicle are successfully treated conservatively with a figure-of-eight strapping which relieves pain and allows early motion [2]. The nonunion rate varies widely in the literature and ranges at about 1–10%.

Displaced and unstable fractures of the lateral (and very rarely the medial) end are indications for surgery, usually stabilized by open reduction and internal fixation (ORIF) using various small traditional or specialized plates (eg, clavicular hook

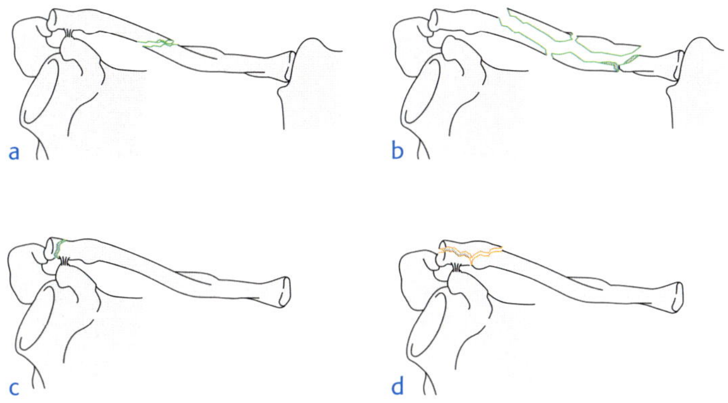

Fig 5.1-1a–d OTA clavicle classification.
a 06-A1 Diaphysis, simple spiral
b 06-C1 Diaphysis, complex spiral
c 07-A1 Lateral end, extraarticular metaphysis, impacted.
d 07-B2 Lateral end, intraarticular wedge fracture with dislocation

plate for the lateral part), tension band wiring, or position screws between the clavicle and the coracoid process.

Absolute indications for operative stabilization of midshaft fractures are open fractures (or impending perforation of the skin by a sharp irreducible fragment) and fractures with associated vascular injury requiring surgical repair. Another indication for primary stabilization of the clavicle includes the displaced floating shoulder injury. Painful nonunions are an indication for operative treatment and many other situations are described as relative indications for a stabilization of the clavicle: in combination with ipsilateral serial rib fractures and flail chest (low-standing shoulder girdle), in cases of a polytraumatized patient requiring crutches, bilateral fractures, and fractures with major displacement, especially a shortening of more than 2 cm [3, 4].

The gold standard in the stabilization of midshaft fractures or nonunions of the clavicle is the open anatomical reduction and plate fixation in a traditional compression method using either a standard straight plate 3.5 (LC-DCP or LCP in an anterior plate position) or a reconstruction plate 3.5 (superior plate position) [5–7]. The open approach is either in the sagittal plane ("coup de sabre") or more horizontal and parallel to the bone, recommended in more complex fracture patterns requiring longer (bridging) plates.

Due to the quite high rate of nonunions and refractures after implant removal (up to 10–20%), which might be partially caused by the open approach with iatrogenic damage of the blood supply of intermediate fragments, a less invasive approach may reduce this risk. Intramedullary stabilization using a titanium elastic nail (TEN) is a promising method for simple fractures (type A) requiring operative treatment [8, 9]. In more complex fractures (types B and C) or in combination with chest instability or scapular neck fracture a more stable implant is required. The minimally invasive plate osteosynthesis (MIPO) technique using a straight anteriorly placed LCP 3.5 is a less invasive but demanding way to stabilize these fractures, in cases where a closed reduction is successful [10].

4 Implant overview

a

b

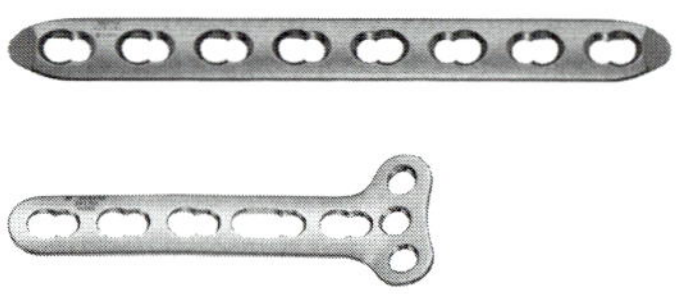

Fig 5.1-2a–b
a LCP 3.5
b LCP T-plate 3.5

5 Bibliography

1. **Orthopedic Trauma Association** (1996) Fracture and Dislocation Compendium. *J Orthop Trauma;* 10 (Suppl 1).
2. **Nordqvist A, Petersson CJ, Redlund-Johnell I** (1998) Mid-clavicle fractures in adults: end result study after conservative treatment. *J Orthop Trauma;* 12(8):572–576.
3. **Robinson CM, Court-Brown CM, McQueen MM, et al** (2004) Estimating the risk of nonunion following nonoperative treatment of a clavicular fracture. *J Bone Joint Surg Am;* 86–A(7):1359–1365.
4. **Wick M, Muller EJ, Kollig E, et al** (2001) Midshaft fractures of the clavicle with a shortening of more than 2 cm predispose to nonunion. *Arch Orthop Trauma Surg;* 121(4):207–211.
5. **Geel CW** (2000) 4.1 Scapula and clavicle. *Rüedi TP, Murphy WM (eds), AO Principles of Fracture Management.* Stuttgart New York: Thieme-Verlag, 255–268.
6. **Shen WJ, Liu TJ, Shen YS** (1999) Plate fixation of fresh displaced midshaft clavicle fractures. *Injury;* 30(7):497–500.
7. **Wu CC, Shih CH, Chen WJ, et al** (1998) Treatment of clavicular aseptic nonunion: comparison of plating and intramedullary nailing techniques. *J Trauma;* 45(3):512–516.
8. **Jubel A, Andermahr J, Faymonville C, et al** (2002) [Reconstruction of shoulder-girdle symmetry after midclavicular fractures. Stable, elastic intramedullary pinning versus rucksack bandage]. *Chirurg;* 73(10):978–981. German.
9. **Jubel A, Andermahr J, Schiffer G, et al** (2003) Elastic stable intramedullary nailing of midclavicular fractures with a titanium nail. *Clin Orthop Relat Res;* (408):279–285.
10. **Reckord U, Walliser M, Sommer C** [Percutaneous LCP osteosynthesis (MIPO) of the clavicle treating the floating shoulder]. *Swiss Surg;* 9 (Suppl 1):34. German.

Author Christopher G Finkemeier

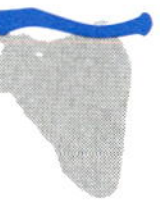

5.1.1 Nonunion after nonoperative treatment of a displaced transverse clavicular midshaft fracture—OTA 06-A1

1 Case description

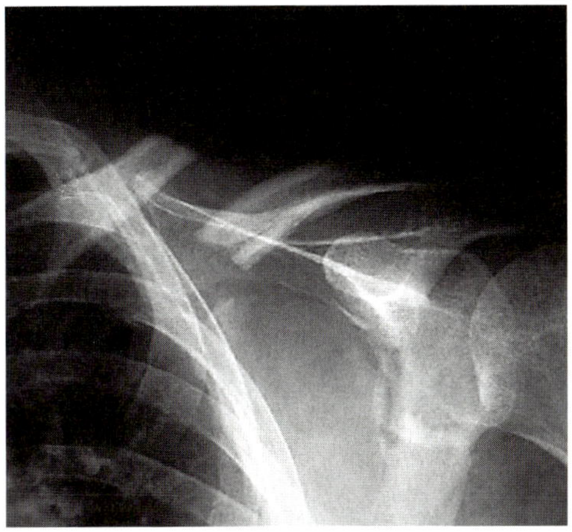

41-year-old man injured in a motor vehicle collision showing fracture of the left clavicle.
Type of injury: high-energy, monotrauma.
Closed fracture.

Fig 5.1.1-1
Nonunion. AP view.

Indication

Nonunion is a good indication for operative treatment. This case shows a midshaft clavicle fracture 6 months after an injury presenting with wide displacement and no evidence of healing. The patient complains of pain and associated loss of power in active use of left shoulder. He also complains of pain when sleeping on the left side. A clavicular fracture with no evidence of bone healing after 6 months of nonoperative treatment in a patient with significant pain and reduced function of the involved extremity is an indication for operative treatment.

Preoperative planning

Equipment

- LCP 3.5, 9 holes
- 4.0 mm self-tapping locking head screws (LHS)
- 3.5 mm cortex screw
- 1.6 mm K-wire
- Bone graft

(Size of system, instruments, and implants can vary according to anatomy.)

Place an x-ray plate under the patient prior to draping. This ensures that the film is in the correct position.

Patient preparation and positioning

Antibiotics: single dose 1st generation cephalosporin

Fig 5.1.1-2 Beach chair position. Prepare the entire upper extremity, the upper chest wall, and be sure to include the sternum and manubrium. If taking a bone graft, prepare the ipsilateral iliac crest as well.

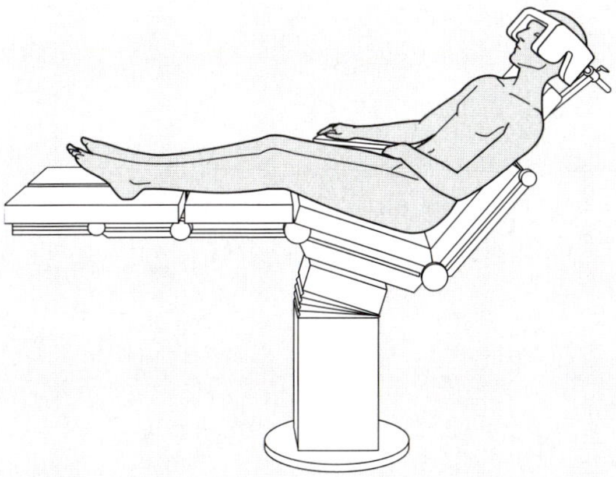

2 Surgical approach

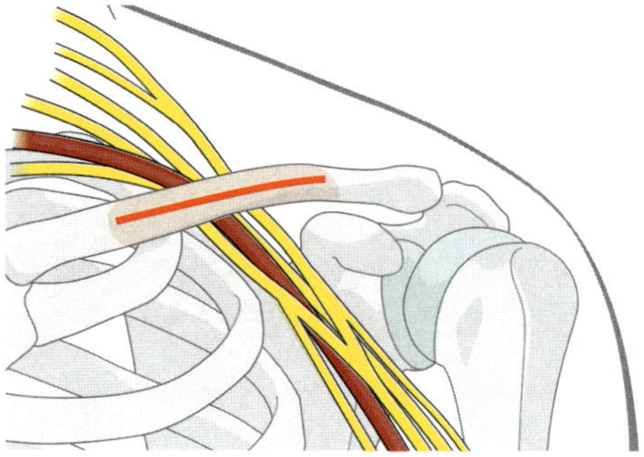

Fig 5.1.1-3 A straight incision is made over the clavicle and is centered over the fracture. Sharply divide the thin fibers of the platysma overlying the clavicle being careful to avoid transecting the supraclavicular nerves.

If possible, identify and tag the supraclavicular nerves with small vessel loops. Many of these nerves are thin and very friable. Only the larger nerves are likely to be protected and preserved.

Avoid elevating the periostium and the subclavious muscle attachments to preserve as much blood supply as possible.
Clear out the fibrous tissue from within the nonunion site.

Open the medullary canal of each fracture fragment and resect any nonviable bone at the ends of the fracture fragments. Look for punctual bleeding as evidence of viability. Try to keep soft-tissue attachments to wedged fragments as they should be preserved to help maintain the length of the clavicle.

3 Reduction

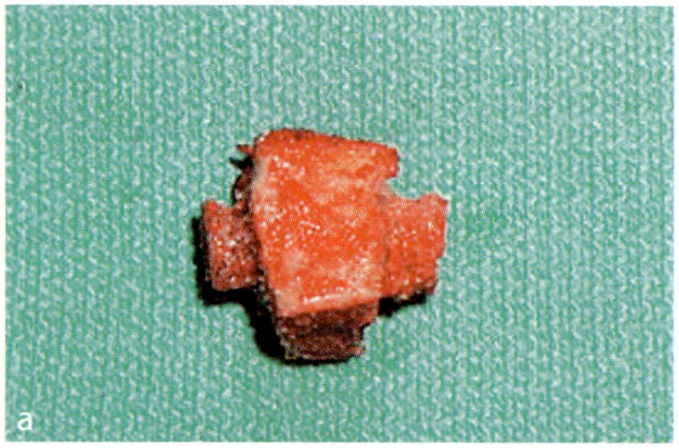

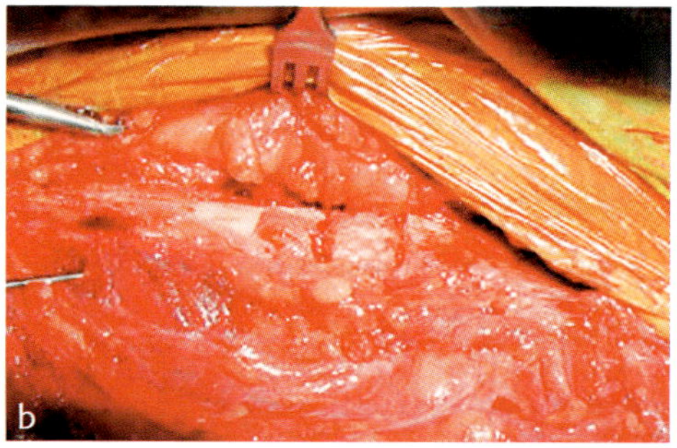

Fig 5.1.1-4a–b Fixation using bone graft.

a The tricortical graft should be harvested almost twice the size necessary to fill the gap.

b Small dowels are fashioned from each end of the graft so they can be inlaid into the intramedullary canal of each end of the fragment.

If the bone ends are angled or oblique, reduction with a pointed reduction forceps is recommended.

If the bone ends are straight (90°) then fix a plate to one part and reduce the other fragment to the plated fragment. This is best done with a pointed reduction forceps, but a serrated jaw clamp can occasionally be of use.

If there is a segmental defect greater than 1 cm, a tricortical graft should be placed to maintain length and function. If the gap is less than a centimeter, bringing the bone ends together should not shorten the clavicle too much and should result in normal function.

If necessary, a 1.6 mm K-wire can be used to hold the tricortical bone graft in place.

4 Fixation

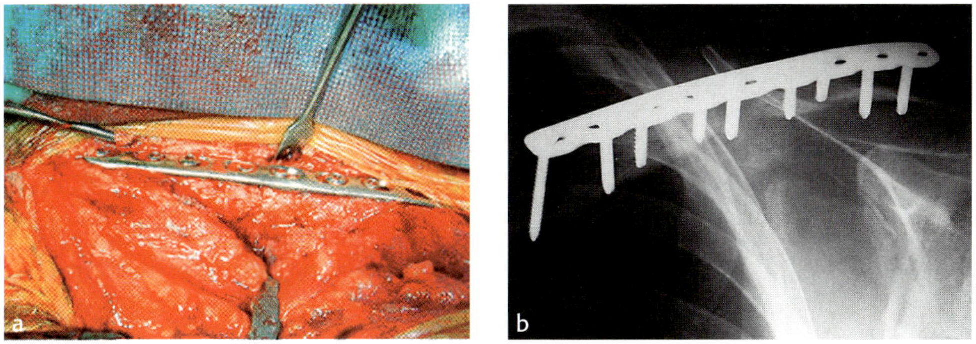

Fig 5.1.1-5a–b

a Once the graft is placed with the dowels in the intramedullary canal of each bone end it should then be compressed between the two ends of the fractured clavicle using the dynamic compression feature of the plate.

b After the graft is compressed and the plate is in the appropriate position at least two additional 4.0 mm locking head screws can be placed on each side of the intercalary bone graft.

5 Rehabilitation

Additional immobilization: a sling is recommended only for comfort.
Mobilization: passive and active mobilization after one day postoperative.
Physiotherapy: started postoperatively on day one.
Pharmaceutical treatment: mild narcotics such as hydrocodone or codeine are usually adequate for pain control. Nonsteroid antiinflammatory agents should not be used after bone grafting. Local analgesics such as lidocaine or bupivicaine injected immediately postoperative are helpful in decreasing postoperative narcotic use.

Implant removal
After 12 months.
Implant removal is recommended for patients with prominent hardware which causes pain.

---

6 Pitfalls –

Equipment
Using weak implants that are likely to fail such as one-third semi-tubular plates.

Approach
Severing the supraclavicular nerves.
Stripping too much soft tissue off the bone during exposure.

Reduction and fixation
Over-shortening the clavicle.

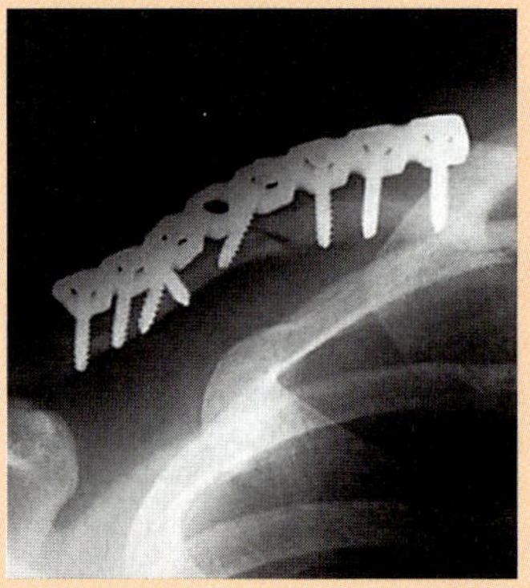

Fig 5.1.1-6 A reconstruction plate can be contoured to better fit the clavicle if so desired. A straight LCP may lie slightly off the bone due to the curved nature of the clavicle.

Rehabilitation
Immobilizing the patient.

7 Pearls +

Equipment
The LCP 3.5 provides sufficient fixation to allow immediate weight bearing on the ipsilateral upper extremity.

Approach
Once the outer fibers of the platysma are incised with the scalpel, spread the last few fibers with scissors to identify and preserve the supraclavicular nerves.

Reduction and fixation
Fashion a tricortical iliac crest intercalary graft with dowels to maintain length of the clavicle and allow for compression of the bone fragments.

The major benefit of the LCP over the reconstruction plate is better resistance to bending forces.

Rehabilitation
Allow immediate range of motion of the shoulder to prevent stiffness and atrophy.

Author Michael Wagner

5.1.2 Lateral extraarticular metaphyseal impacted clavicular fracture—OTA 07-A1

1 Case description

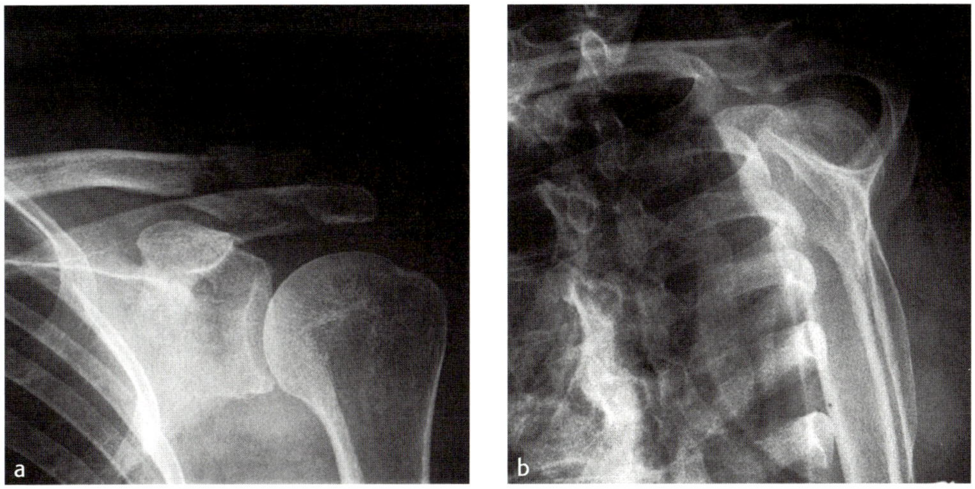

64-year-old woman fell when she was skiing and fractured the left lateral clavicle.

Fig 5.1.2-1a–b
a AP view.
b Oblique view.

Indication

Lateral clavicular fracture with avulsion of the coracoclavicular ligament, closed fracture, monotrauma, open technique. Internal fixator method, bridging the fracture with an LCP T-plate.

Preoperative planning

Equipment

- LCP T-plate 3.5, 6 holes
- 3.5 mm self-tapping locking head screws (LHS)

(Size of system, instruments, and implants can vary according to anatomy.)

The 4 holes in the crossbar of the T-plate facilitate stable fixation of the small lateral fragment. The alternative implants would be the narrow LCP 3.5 and/or the reconstruction plate. However, in this case these plates would be disadvantageous because it would only be possible to insert a maximum of one or two screws into the small lateral fragment.

Patient preparation and positioning

Antibiotics: none
Thrombosis prophylaxis: none

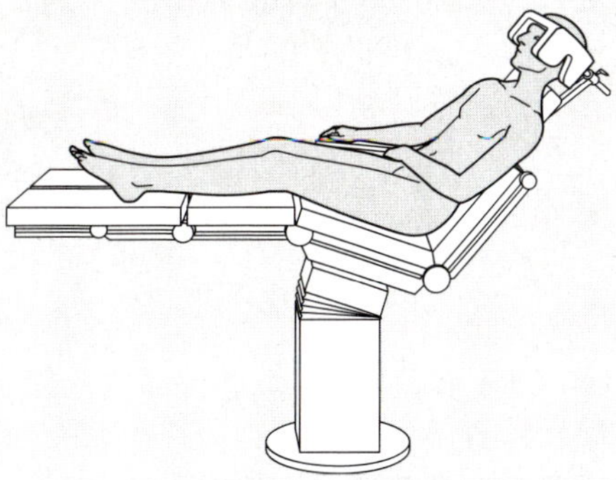

Fig 5.1.2-2 Beach chair position. Prepare the entire upper extremity, the upper chest wall, and be sure to include the sternum and manubrium. The arm is draped but not immobilized.

2 Surgical approach

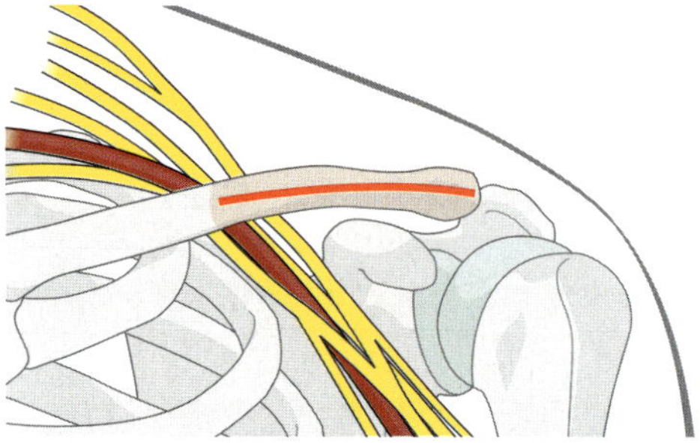

Fig 5.1.2-3 Straight incision over the lateral clavicle.

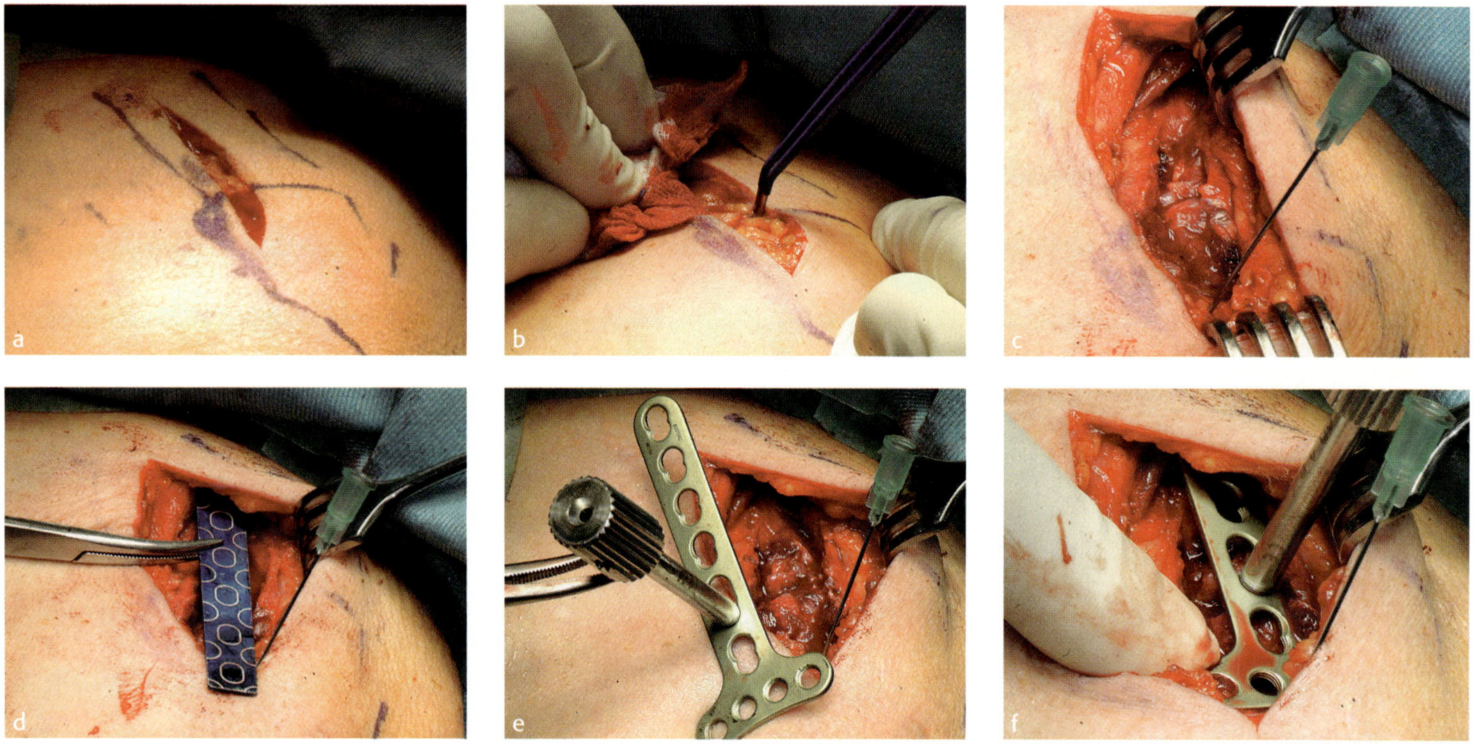

Fig 5.1.2-4a–f

a–c After sterile washing and free draping for intraoperative mobility of the upper extremity, a straight incision over the lateral end of the clavicle/acromioclavicular joint is made. After division of the subcutis, injury to the muscle attachments of the clavicular part of the deltoid muscle is identified. The acromioclavicular joint is marked with a needle.

d–f The size and shape of the plate is determined using a template. The threaded drill sleeve serves as a gripping and manipulation handle for the insertion of the LCP T-plate 3.5 that is applied to the cranial surface of the clavicle.

3 Reduction and fixation

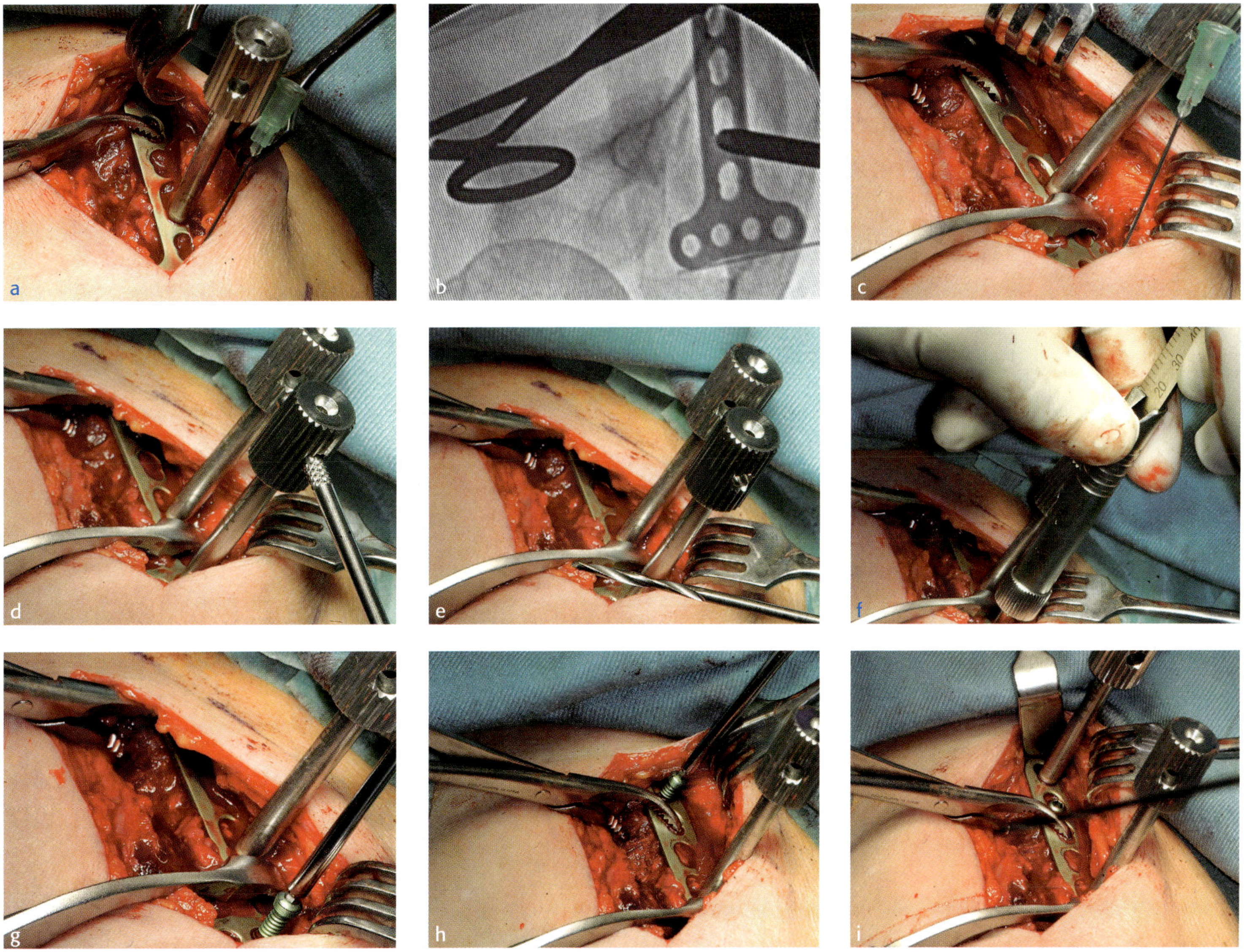

Fig 5.1.2-5a–i Reduction of the fracture by manipulating the freely mobile draped upper extremity and temporary fixation of the plate to the fragments with the reduction forceps. The plate position is assessed with the image intensifier.
For the fixation of the plate an additional threaded drill sleeve is screwed into the T-bar and tightened with a pin wrench. This is followed by drilling, length measurement, and insertion of a locking head screw (LHS). The next step is to stabilize the plate by anchoring the screws in the central clavicular fragment. The drill sleeves guarantee a perpendicular orientation for drilling and screw insertion.

3 Reduction and fixation (cont)

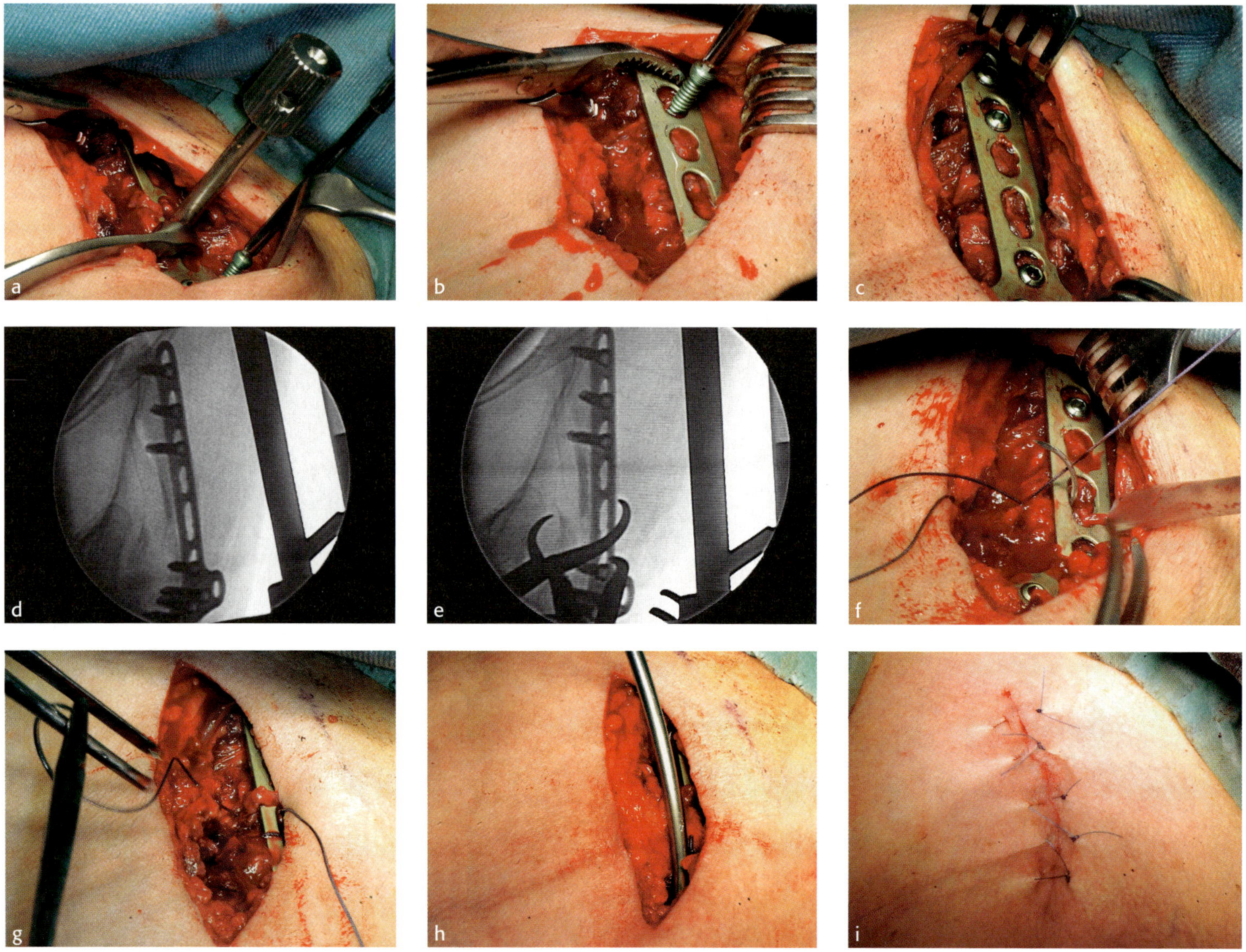

Fig 5.1.2-6a–i After length measurement the LHS are inserted. Then, additional LHS are anchored in the distal peripheral fragment and thus complete the bridging osteosynthesis according to the internal fixator method—three LHS in the central fragment, four LHS in the small peripheral fragment. Suture fixation of the avulsion fragment of the coracoclavicular ligament. Wound closure, reinsertion of the partially detached muscles, insertion of the redon drains, layered wound closure.

4 Rehabilitation

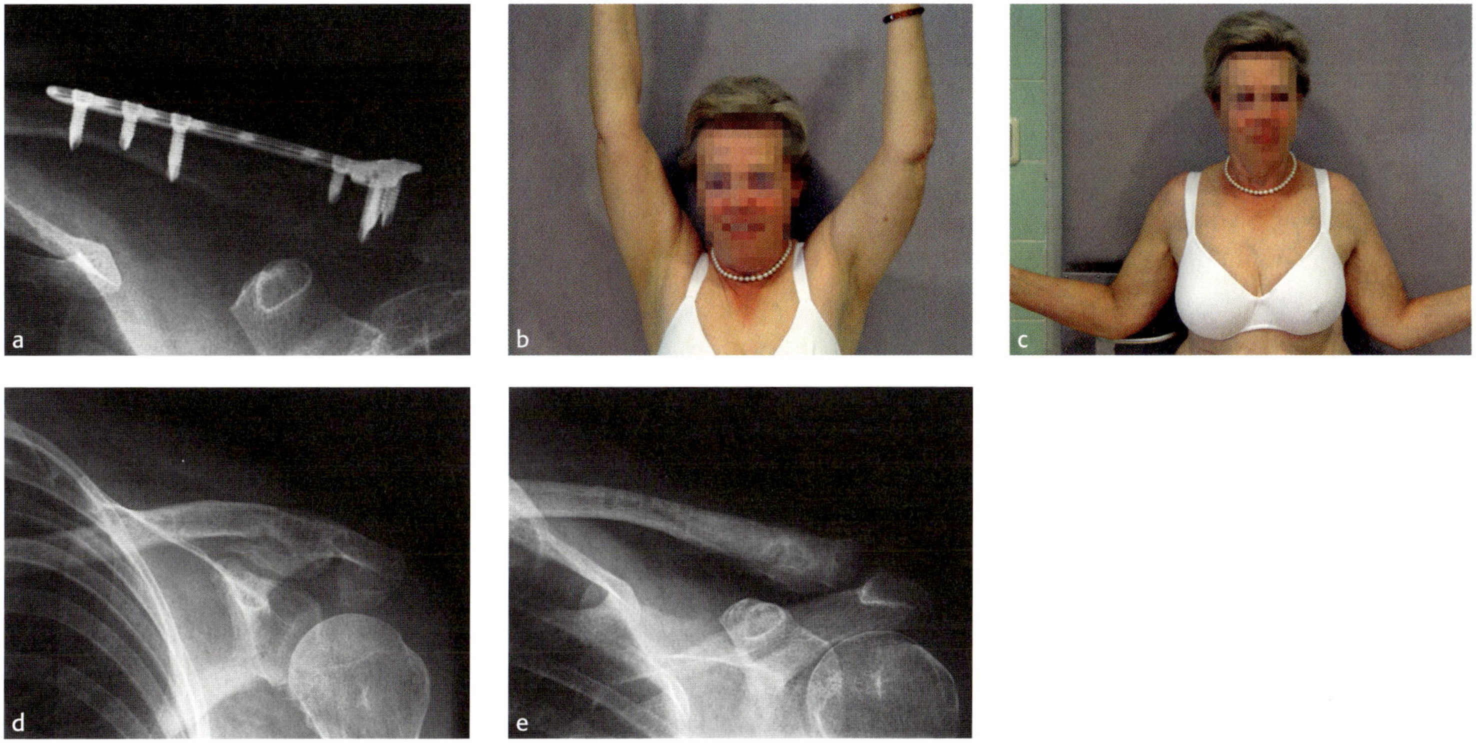

Fig 5.1.2-7a–e
a Postoperative x-ray after 6 months. AP view.
b–c Functional outcome after 5 months.
d X-ray after implant removal. AP view.
e X-ray after implant removal. Oblique view.

Gilchrist bandage for 2 weeks, removal of the redon drains on the first postoperative day.

Removal of the sutures 12 days after the operation. Start of passive exercises for the shoulder from third postoperative day.

5 Pitfalls –

Reduction and fixation

Fig 5.1.2-8a–d The avulsed coracoclavicular ligament remains displaced. The next step is to try and reduce this fragment with the help of the reduction forceps. Any attempt to stabilize this fragment with the aid of a lag screw will fail. The lag screw will not find sufficient anchorage in the small fragment. Therefore, suture fixation of the coracoclavicular ligament is preferred. Bone healing with a slight displacement of the avulsion fragment.

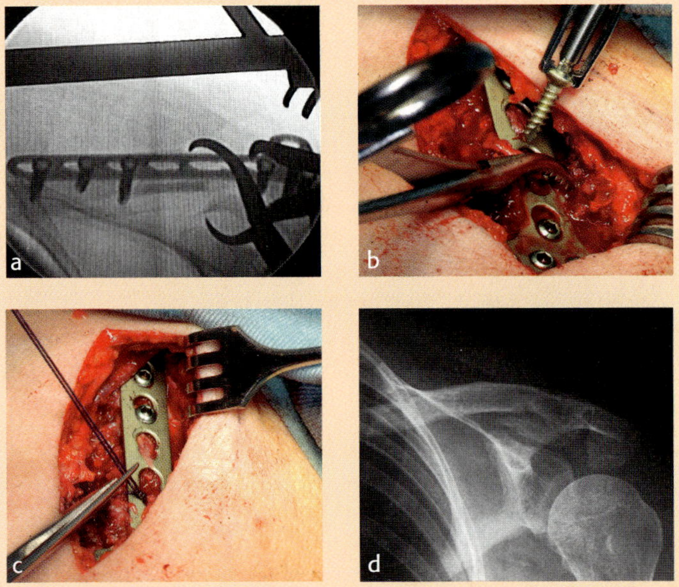

6 Pearls +

Reduction and fixation

Reduction onto the plate with small reduction forceps.

The 4 holes in the crossbar of the LCP T-plate 3.5 facilitate stabile fixation of the small lateral fragment.

Suture fixation of the osseous avulsion.

Author Michael Wagner

5.1.3 Displaced clavicular fracture with loss of length—OTA 06-C1

1 Case description

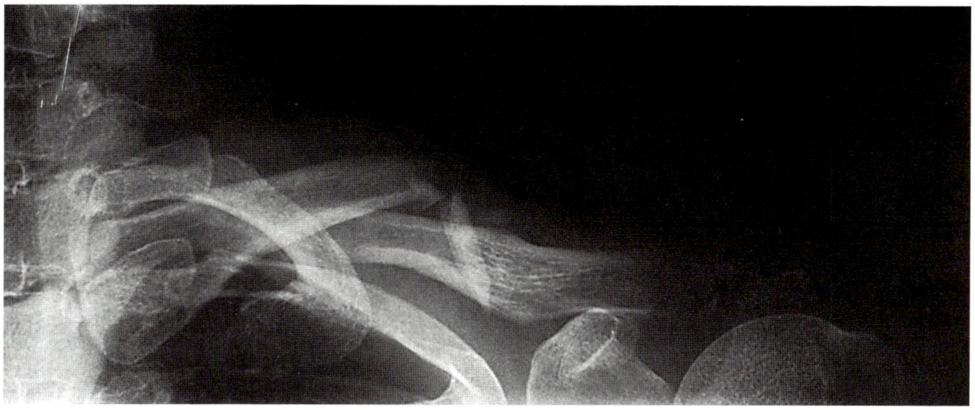

38-year-old woman fell from a horse 4 weeks before treatment, injuring the left clavicle.
Low-energy trauma; monotrauma.
Closed fracture.

Fig 5.1.3-1 AP view.

Indication

Fracture of the clavicle with a displacement of more than one shaft width. Loss of approximately 2 cm of length, accompanied by neurological deficit and sensory disorder affecting all fingers. The indication for operative treatment is based on the diagnosis of shortening of the clavicle and the neurological deficits.

Preoperative planning

Equipment

- LCP 3.5, 8 holes
- 3.5 mm locking head screws (LHS)
- 2.7 mm cortex screws
- Reduction forceps

(Size of system, instruments, and implants can vary according to anatomy.)

Patient preparation and positioning

Antibiotics: none
Thrombosis prophylaxis: none

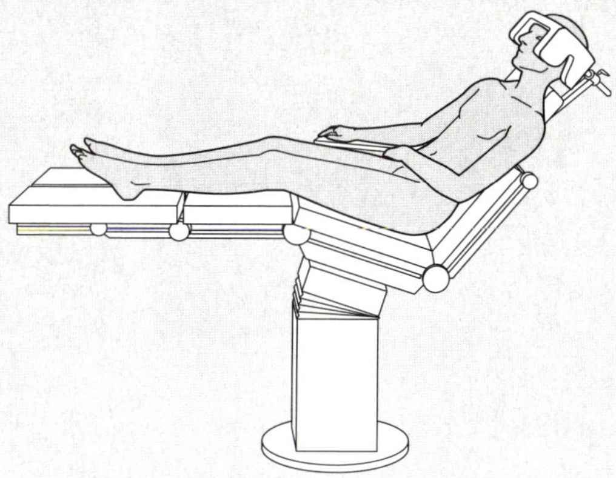

Fig 5.1.3-2 Beach chair position. Prepare the entire upper extremity, the upper chest wall, and be sure to include the sternum and manubrium of sternum. The arm is draped but not immobilized.

2 Surgical approach

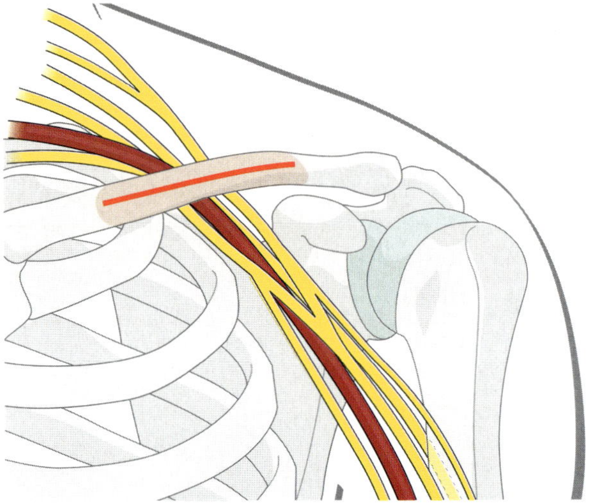

Fig 5.1.3-3 A straight incision, centered over the fracture, is made over the clavicle.

3 Reduction

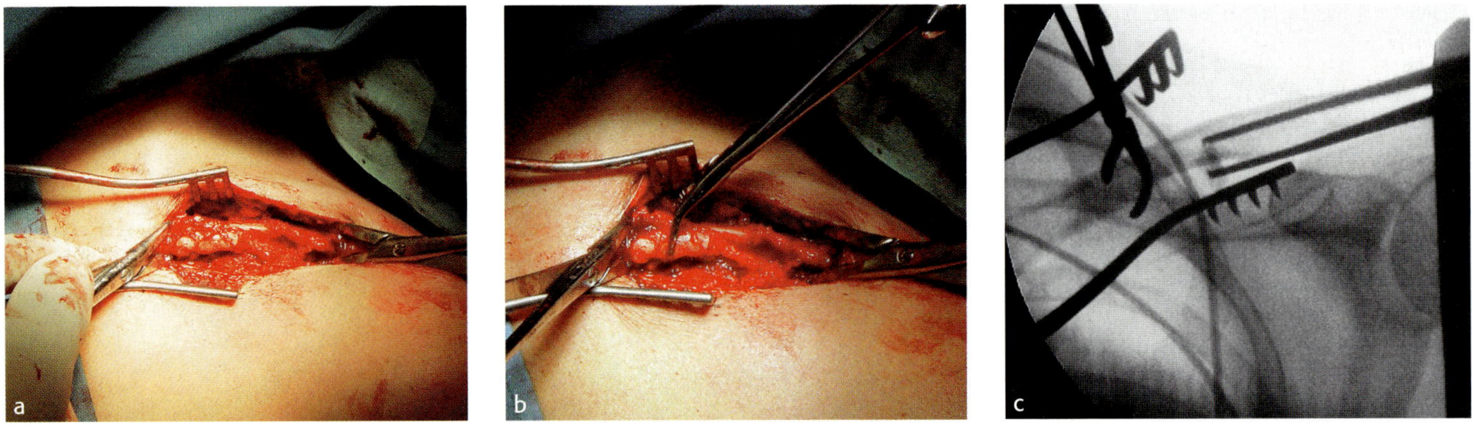

Fig 5.1.3-4a–c

a After exposing the fracture and freeing the main fragments from recently formed callus, the two main fragments are distracted and the length of the clavicle is restored.
The two main fragments are held with serrated reduction forceps.

b–c As soon as the exact length has been restored, the reduction is secured with a third reduction forceps.

3 Reduction (cont)

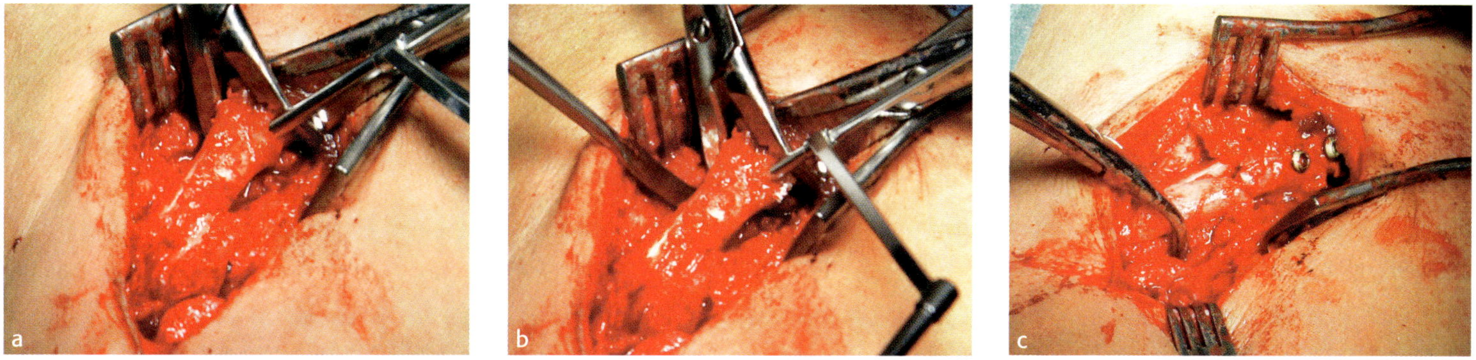

Fig 5.1.3-5a–c

a A 2.7 mm lag screw is inserted. The gliding hole for another lag screw is drilled with the 2.7 mm drill bit.

b The appropriate drill bit is inserted into the drill sleeve and the hole is tapped. A bone rasp protects the soft tissue on the opposite side.

c The reduced fracture is fixed with two 2.7 mm lag screws. The additional intermediary fragment is stabilized with a third lag screw.

4 Fixation

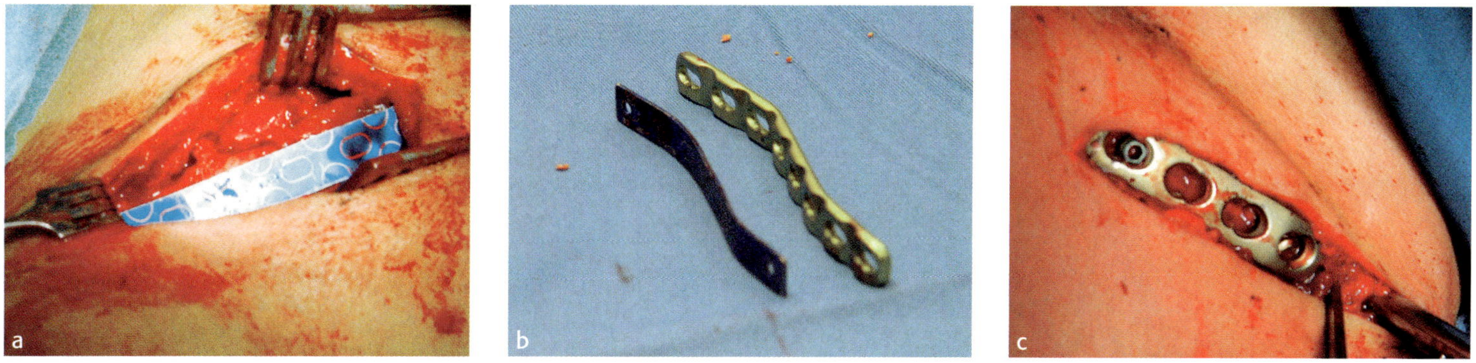

Fig 5.1.3-6a–c

a The shape of the bone is determined with the help of a template in preparation for the application of a protection plate to the anterior side of the clavicle.

b An LCP 3.5, 8 holes, is precontoured based on the bending template. The plate needs not be bent to an absolutely anatomical shape if locking head screws are used.

c Application of the protection plate to bridge the independent lag screws. The screw heads lie beneath the plate. In the medial and lateral part, the plate is slide-inserted beneath the muscle attachments and the locking head screws are inserted via small incisions through the muscle fibers.

4 Fixation (cont)

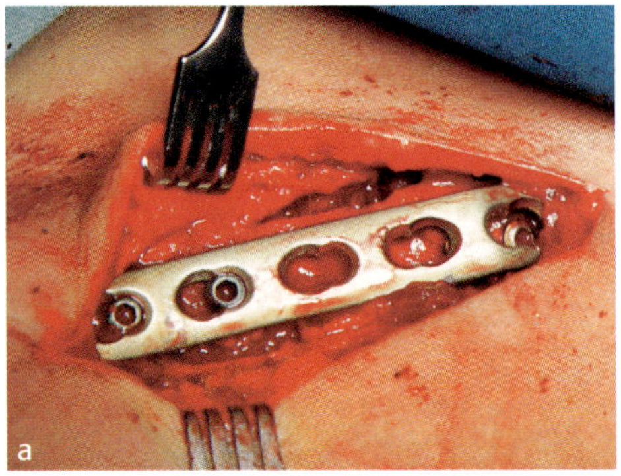

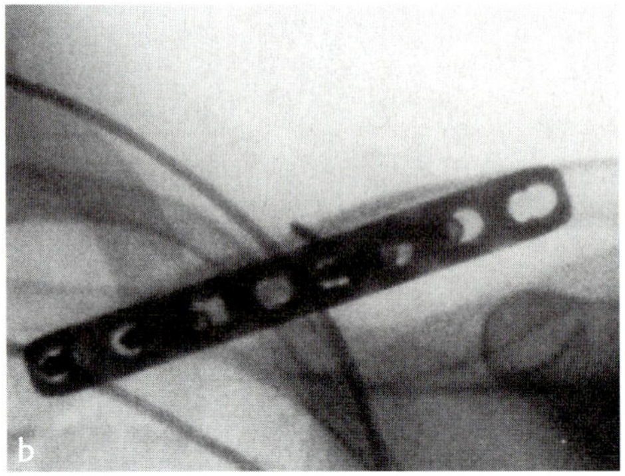

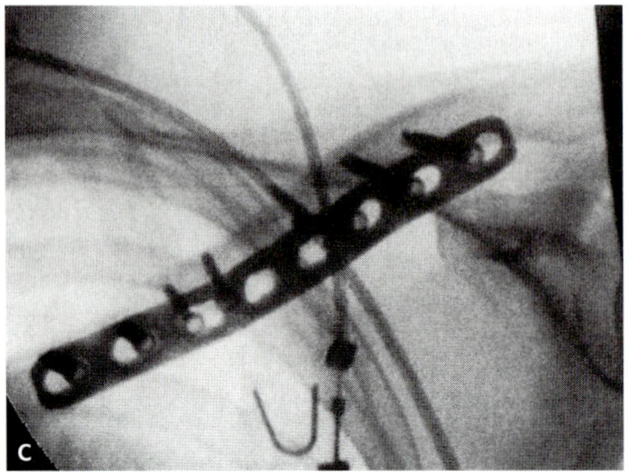

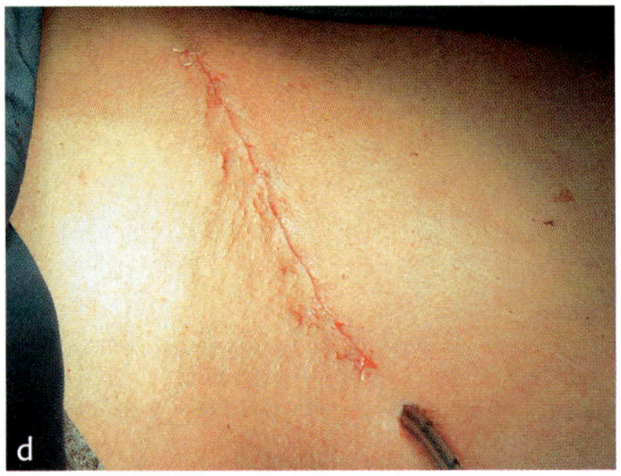

Fig 5.1.3-7a–d

a Intraoperative image showing the middle section of the protection plate that has been stabilized with locking head screws. In the lateral corner of the incision one of the independently used lag screws is seen through the plate hole.

b AP view, intraoperative x-ray.

c Oblique view. The fracture is well reduced in both planes and has been stabilized with three 2.7 mm lag screws and an additional LCP as a protection plate stabilized with five locking head screws. These were inserted as bicortical screws because of the small diameter of the clavicle.

d Skin closure.

5 Rehabilitation

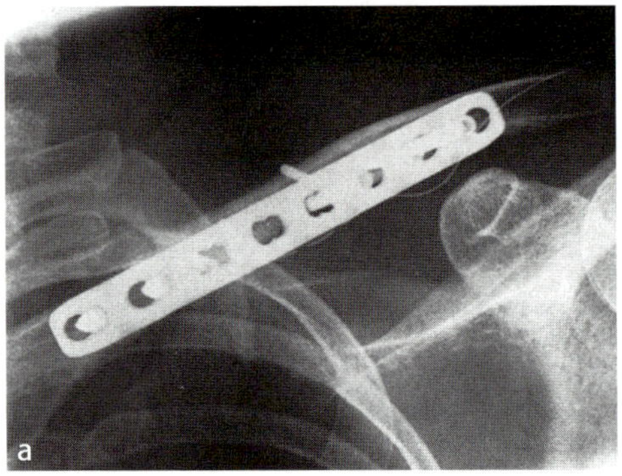

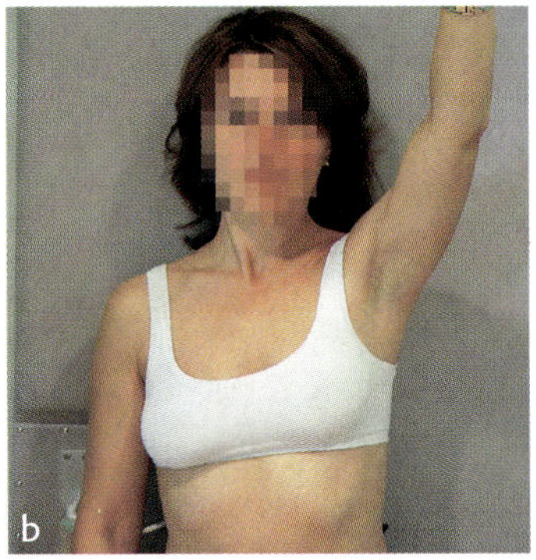

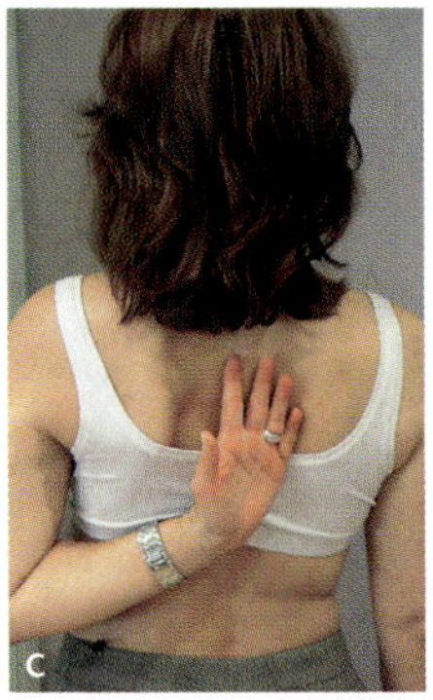

Immediate postoperative functional treatment without immobilization started with passive mobilization after 2 days.

Fig 5.1.3-8a–c

a Postoperative x-ray.

b–c Functional outcome after 2 weeks.

5 Rehabilitation (cont)

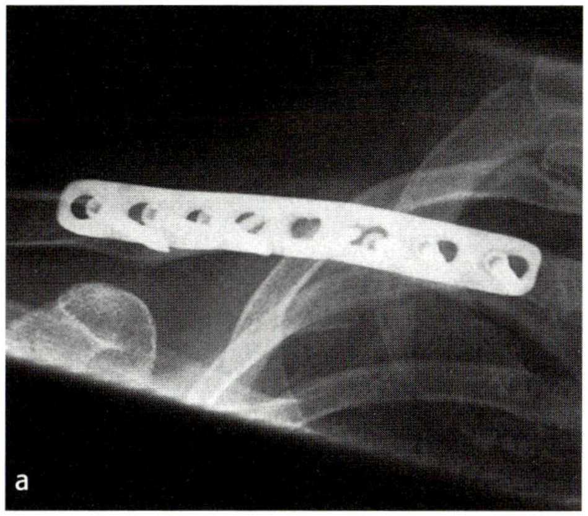

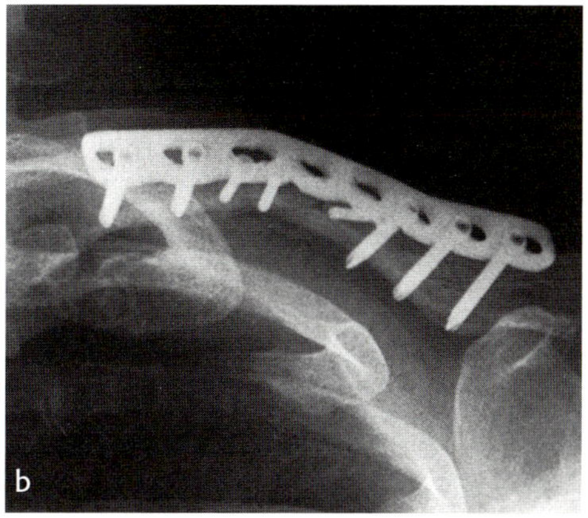

Fig 5.1.3-9a–b Postoperative x-rays after 6 weeks.
a AP view.
b Oblique view.

6 Pitfalls –

Equipment

Approach
Injury to the neurovascular structures.

Reduction and fixation
ORIF needs an open technique.

7 Pearls +

Equipment
The LCP with LHS needs not be contoured absolutely to the anatomical shape.

Approach
Better overview during reduction and less damage to the soft tissues.

Reduction and fixation
Anterior application of the plate so that an LCP 3.5 can be used. This is far more stable than the reconstruction plate 3.5 that would have to be used for cranial plate application.

Bending of the LCP 3.5 is easier to fit the anterior aspect of the clavicle. This plate is stronger than the reconstruction plate.

Interfragmentary compression with lag screws. Plate-independent lag screws are not restricted in direction and angulation.

6 Pitfalls – (cont)

7 Pearls + (cont)

Reduction and fixation (cont)

Fixation of the protection plate with LHS: This noncontact plate allows a positioning above the screw heads from the lag screws.

Rehabilitation

With a good and stable osteosynthesis, early functional rehabilitation is possible

Author Christoph Sommer

5.1.4 Clavicular midshaft fracture and serial rib fractures—OTA 06-B1

1 Case description

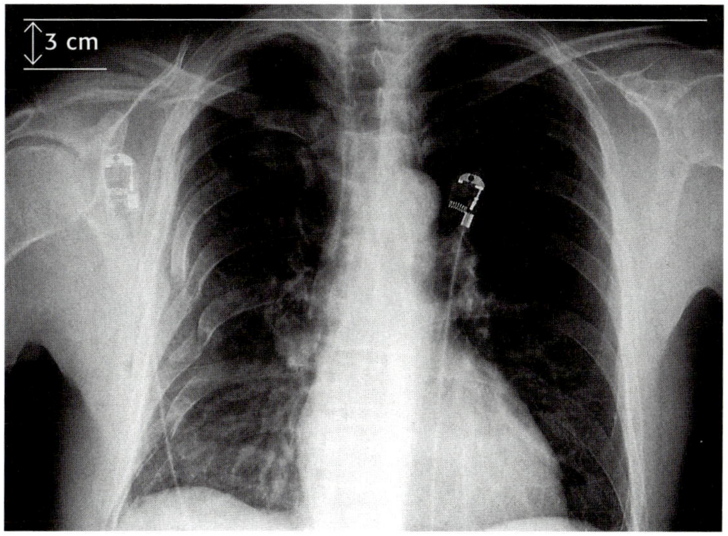

50-year-old man collided with another skier and sustained a lateral thorax trauma. He fractured ribs 2–8 on his right side, suffered pneumothorax and fracture of the right clavicle in the middle part. Initially, a chest drain was applied.

Fig 5.1.4-1 The x-ray in upright position after the first few days showed a displacement of the clavicle and an unstable thorax. The right shoulder was 3 cm lower than the left shoulder.

Indication

The combination of serial rib fractures and an ipsilateral clavicular fracture is a relative indication for operative intervention. If, as in this case, the shoulder drops several centimeters, osteosynthesis of the clavicle can improve the position of the shoulder considerably.

In this combined injury, stable plate osteosynthesis is preferred. An elastic intramedullary nail is not likely to improve the shoulder height. The expected forces on the clavicle, due to the unstable thorax, favor ventral positioning of the plate. A minimally invasive approach helps support the blood supply to the fragments but requires closed reduction.

Preoperative planning

Equipment

- LCP 3.5, 10 holes
- 3.5 mm locking head screws (LHS)
- 1.6 mm K-wires

(Size of system, instruments, and implants can vary according to anatomy.)

Patient preparation and positioning

Antibiotics: single dose 2nd generation cephalosporin

Thrombosis prophylaxis: low-molecular heparin

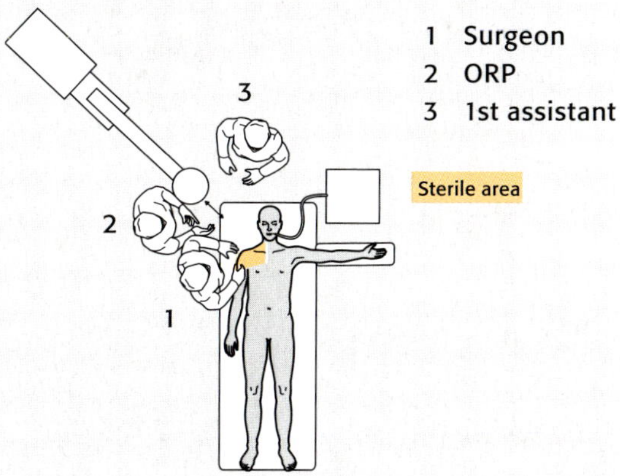

Fig 5.1.4-2 The image intensifier must be positioned to allow projection of the entire clavicula. From ventrocaudal to posterocranial and also across from ventrocranial to posterocaudal.

2 Surgical approach

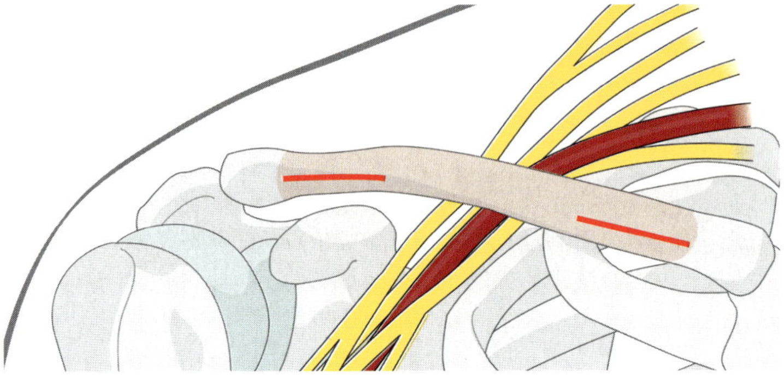

Fig 5.1.4-3 Two incisions are made one at each end of the plate on the medial and lateral sides of the fracture and parallel to the clavicle extending for about 2–3 cm of the clavicula caudal. Skin and fascia of the muscle are cut; dissection to the clavicle with a bone rasp. The fracture zone is not exposed.

3 Reduction and fixation

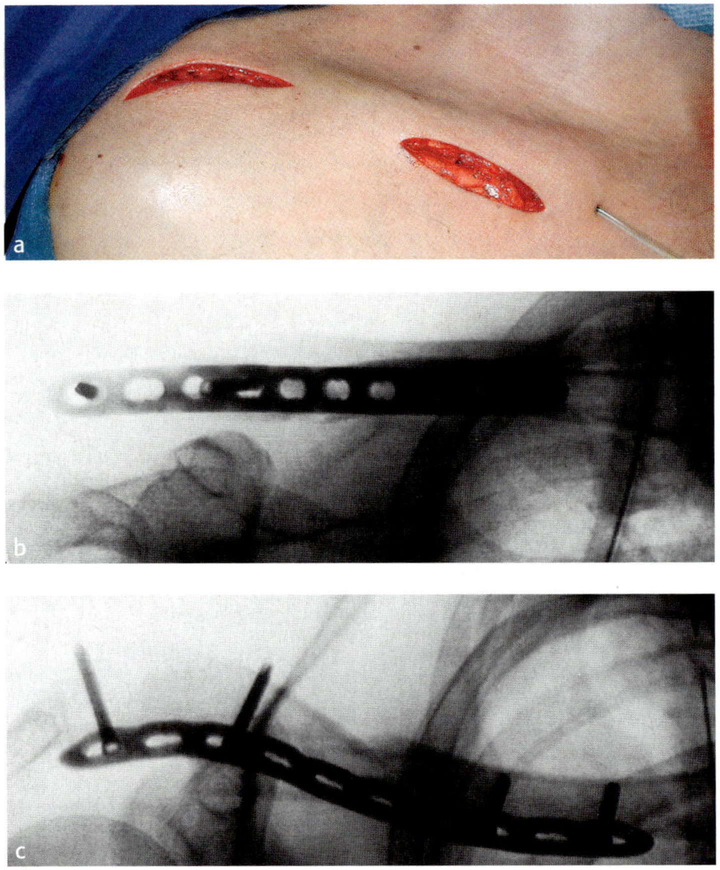

Fig 5.1.4-4a–c
The chosen 10-hole LCP 3.5 is adapted to the shape of the ventral contour of the left clavicle. The plate needs not be bent to an absolutely anatomical form if locking head screws are used.
The plate bed on the ventral side of the clavicle is tunneled.
If a drill sleeve is inserted into the lateral hole and used as a handle, the plate can easily be inserted from the lateral to the medial side.
The plate position has to be checked by image intensifier to ensure that it does not interfere with the acromioclavicular joint.
Temporary fixation with K-wire through the lateral drill sleeve and trocar.
A drill sleeve is now inserted into the medial hole and the fracture is reduced manually and indirectly by manipulation of the plate.
A second K-wire is inserted into the medial hole through a trocar. The plate position and the reduction must now be checked with the image intensifier.
The K-wires are replaced by locking head screws. The fracture can now only be corrected in the frontal plane.
A second locking head screw can be inserted on both sides; ideally one hole is left unoccupied.

3 Reduction and fixation (cont)

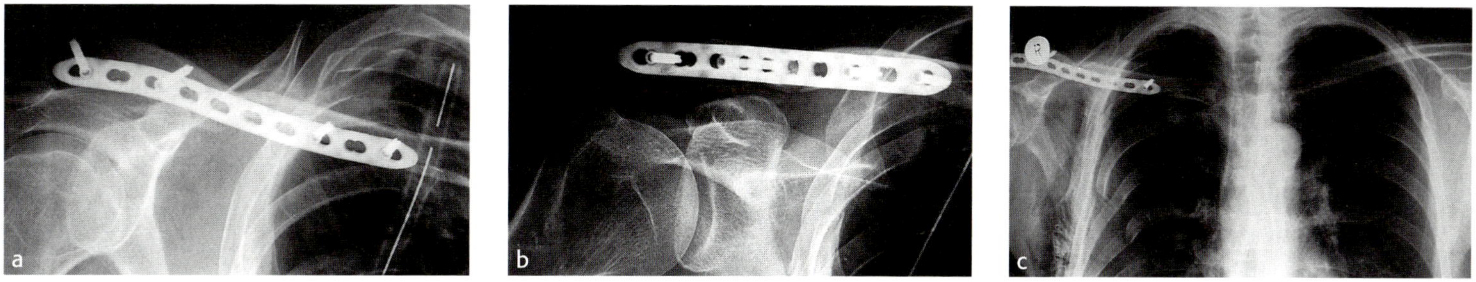

Fig 5.1.4-5a–c The x-ray taken immediately postoperatively confirms correct central plate and screw placement on the clavicle.

4 Rehabilitation

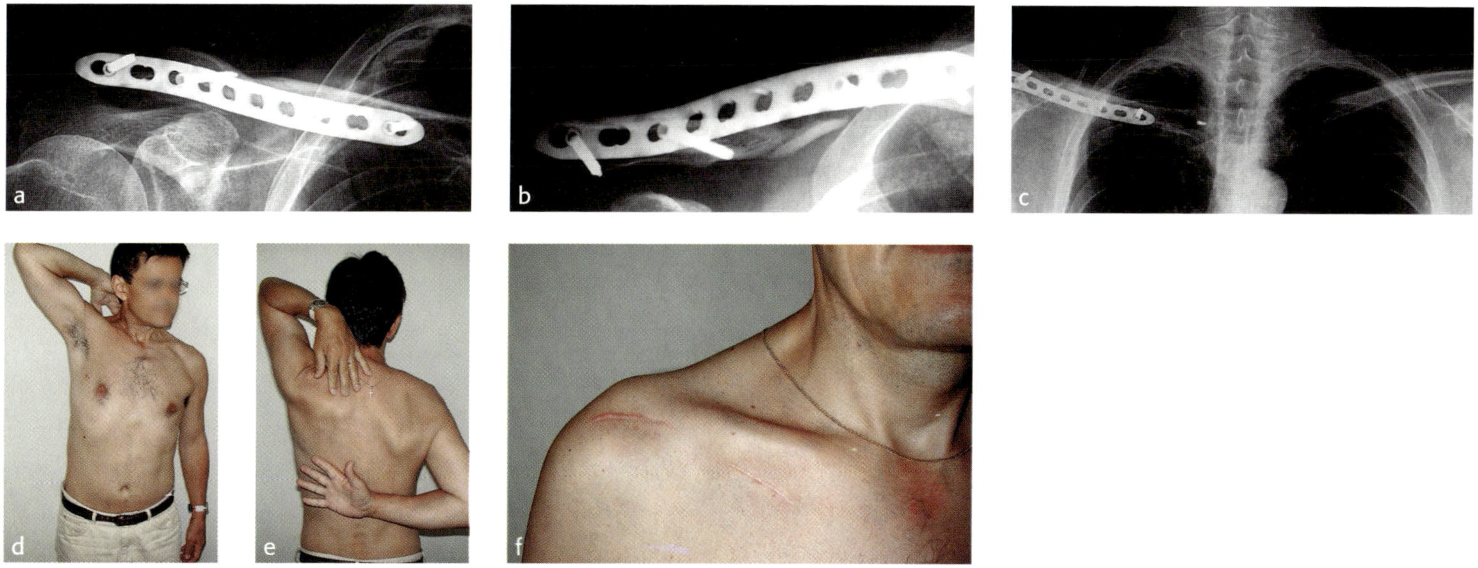

Fig 5.1.4-6a–f

a–c Functional rehabilitation followed. In addition to breathing therapy, guided movement of the shoulder was performed. The clinical and radiological check-up after 3 months confirmed consolidation of the fracture and a painfree patient. Shoulder height on both sides was the same.

d–f Clinically, shoulder function on both sides was the same. The scar had a satisfactory appearance and the plate was causing no disturbance to the patient but remains visible.

5 Pitfalls –

Equipment

Approach
Reduction by means of this minimally invasive procedure is difficult.

Reduction and fixation
Tangential screws in this ventral position could provoke loosening of the screws and plate.

Rehabilitation

6 Pearls +

Equipment
The LCP instruments facilitate minimally invasive techniques. The plate needs not be contoured absolutely to the anatomical shape. The drill sleeves are ideal for holding the plate so that it can be temporarily stabilized with K-wires.

Approach
A minimally invasive procedure can be an advantage if there is soft-tissue injury.

Reduction and fixation
The ventrocaudal position allows insertion of a straight plate whereas a weaker reconstruction plate is more appropriate in the cranial position.

Rehabilitation
Early functional rehabilitation is possible with a good and stable osteosynthesis. Implant removal is also possible by a minimally invasive approach.

Author Christoph Sommer

5.1.5 Displaced oblique clavicular midshaft fracture—OTA 06-A1 and scapular neck fracture—OTA 09-B3 (floating shoulder)

1 Case description

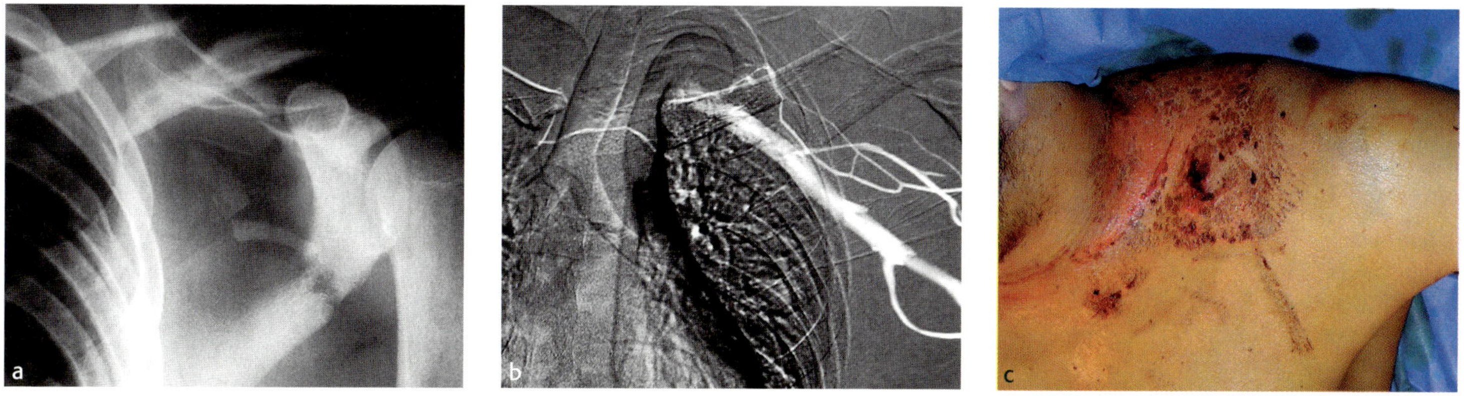

23-year-old man was struck on the left shoulder by a falling tree. He suffered direct trauma with a resulting floating shoulder (clavicular midshaft fracture and displaced scapular fracture). The patient had extensive closed soft-tissue damage across the left shoulder and concomitant paresis of the plexus. In addition, he had a dislocation and fracture of the C5/6 vertebra without neurological deficit. Venography of the massively swollen left arm showed normal arterial circulation and drainage over the subclavian vein. The soft tissue showed great improvement 7 days after initial emergency treatment of the C5/6 vertebra fracture and local treatment of the skin lesion.

Fig 5.1.5-1a–c
a Midclavicle fracture and displaced scapula fracture.
b Venography.
c Skin lesion.

Indication

A combination of a clavicular fracture and a scapular fracture (floating shoulder) may be an indication for operative stabilization. With a clear displacement, as in this case, stable plate osteosynthesis of the clavicle is sufficient for the stabilization of the shoulder girdle. Standard procedure would be an open anatomical reduction and internal fixation. Unfortunately, the patient had a skin lesion at the site of the planned incision. A minimally invasive approach in this case would be ideal. Intramedullary fixation with an elastic nail is generally not the preferred procedure for this type of combination fracture. Stabilization with a small external fixator would be another alternative.

Preoperative planning

Equipment

- LCP 3.5, 12 holes
- 3.5 mm locking head screws (LHS)
- K-wires

(Size of system, instruments, and implants can vary according to anatomy.)

Patient preparation and positioning

Antibiotics: single dose 2nd generation cephalosporin
Thrombosis prophylaxis: low-molecular heparin

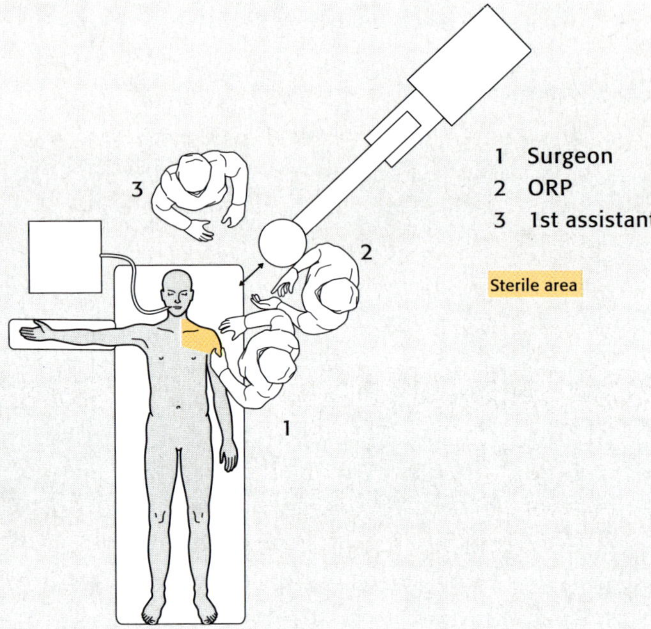

Fig 5.1.5-2 The image intensifier must be positioned to allow projection of the entire clavicle. From ventrocaudal to posterocranial and also across from ventrocranial to posterocaudal.

2 Surgical approach

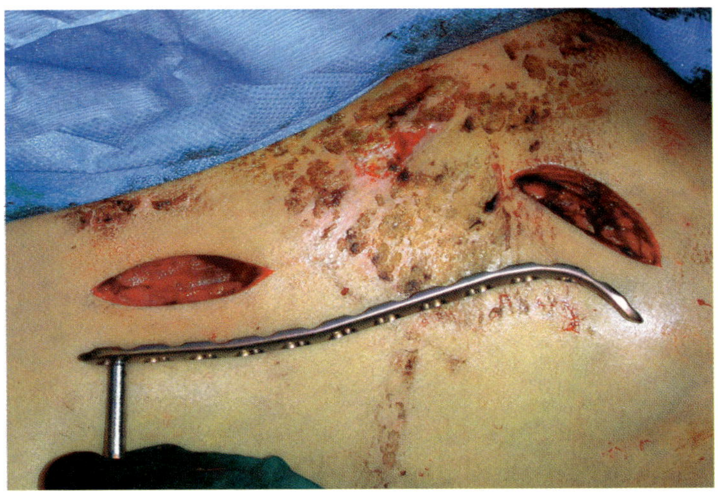

Fig 5.1.5-3 The length of the LCP 3.5 is chosen according to the length of the fracture on the ventrocaudal aspect. Two incisions are made horizontally 2 cm caudal to the clavicle over the planned positions of the plate ends. In this case, the traumatic skin lesion could be avoided. Incision of the subcutaneous fascia is made and the inserting muscles are slightly detached from the anterior border of the clavicle medial and lateral of the fracture.

3 Reduction and fixation

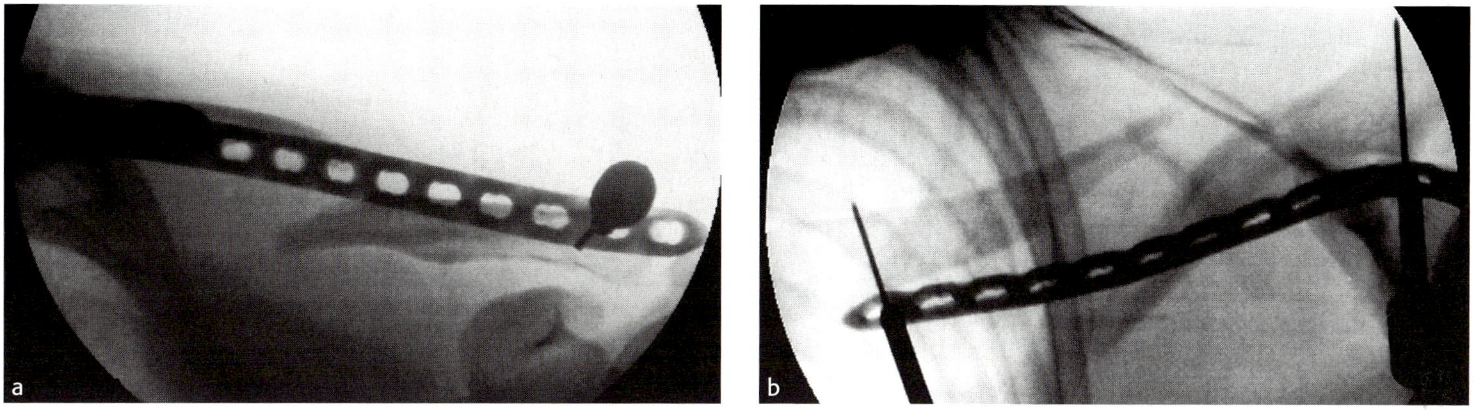

Fig 5.1.5-4a–d

a A subcutaneous tunnel is made with the help of a blunt instrument (elevator, bone rasp) ventrocaudally at the anterior surface of the clavicle. With the help of a drill sleeve inserted into the lateral hole, the precontoured plate can be inserted from lateral to medial. Aided by the image intensifier, the plate is positioned with the most lateral hole slightly medial to the acromioclavicular joint. The plate is then fixed temporarily to the clavicle with a K-wire inserted through the drill sleeve and K-wire trocar. The fracture can now be reduced indirectly.

b Next, temporary fixation of the plate is performed medially by insertion of a K-wire. Image intensification shows good plate positioning at each end, but still angulation of the fracture.

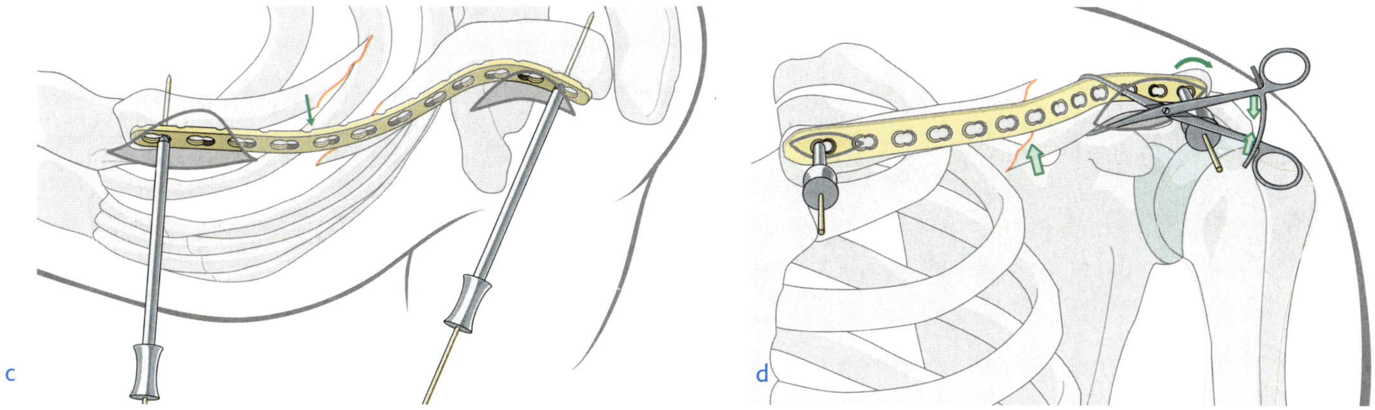

c–d The fracture can now be finally reduced towards the plate using a reduction forceps inserted through the small medial and lateral incisions. After correct reduction has been achieved, the locking head screws can be inserted. The plate has to be centered to the clavicle (AP direction) to avoid tangential insertion of the screws. Two LHS on each side are sufficient in good bone quality. In osteoporotic bone or tangential screw position, three LHS on each side are recommended.

3 Reduction and fixation (cont)

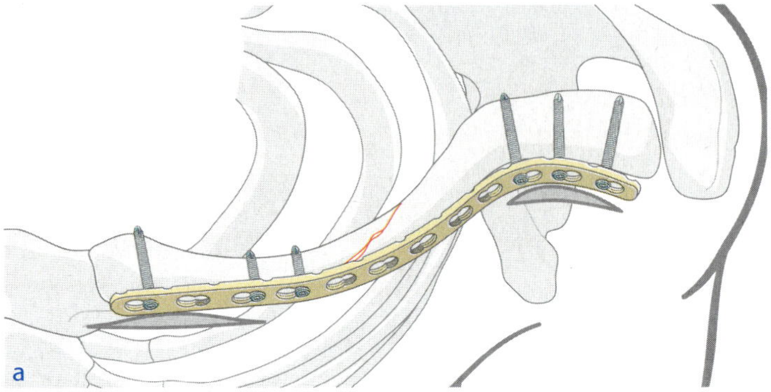

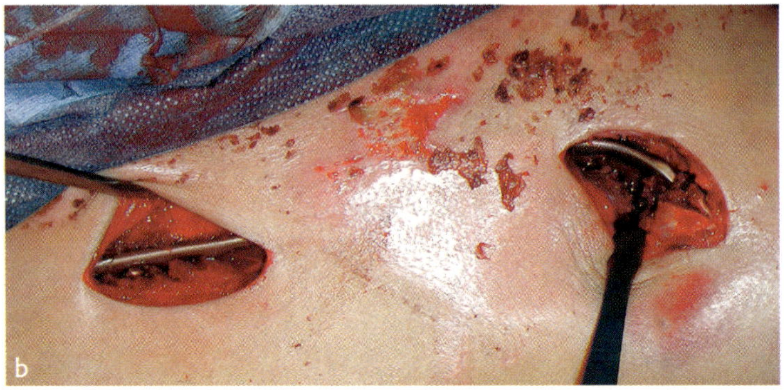

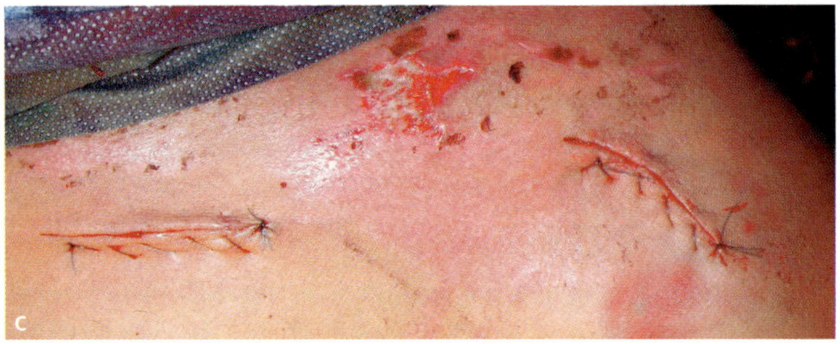

Fig 5.1.5-5a–c
- a–b Fixed fracture prior to wound closure.
- c The approaches required to avoid soft-tissue damage can be seen here. A standard approach would have interfered with the injury.

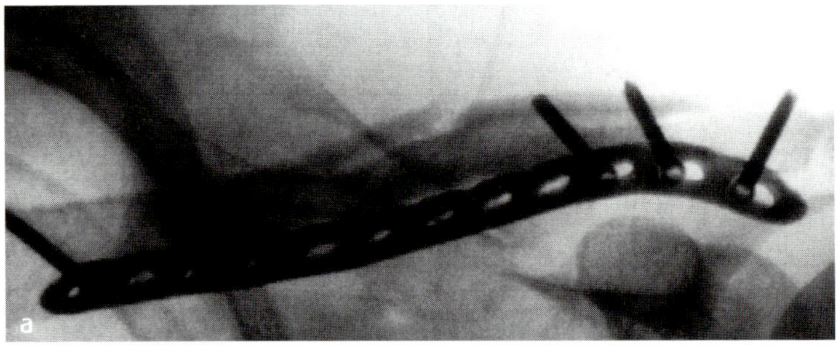

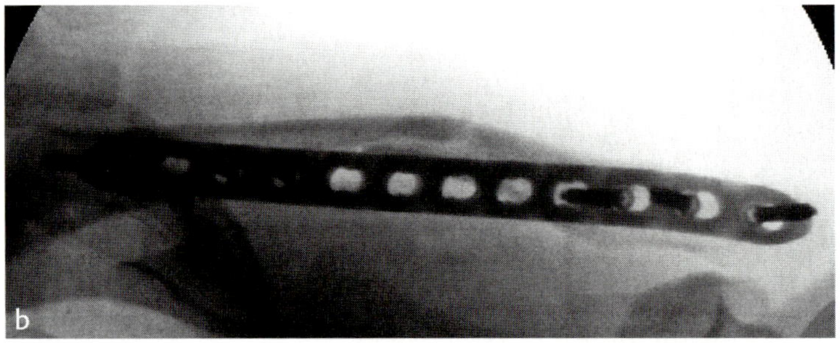

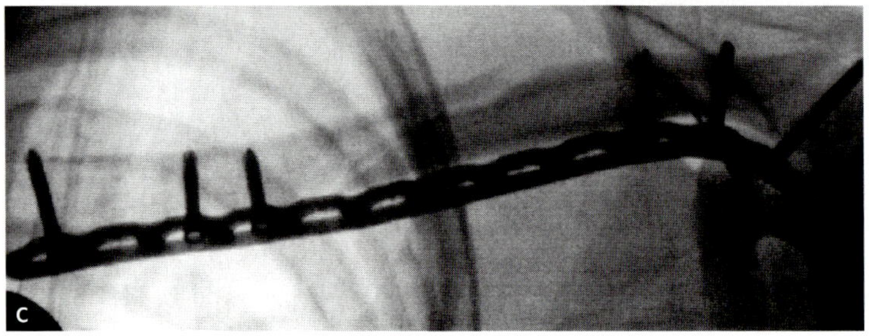

Fig 5.1.5-6a–c The final x-rays show correct reduction of the fracture with clavicle lengthening by 2 mm.
- a AP view.
- b 30° AP cranial tilt view.
- c Craniocaudal view.

4 Rehabilitation

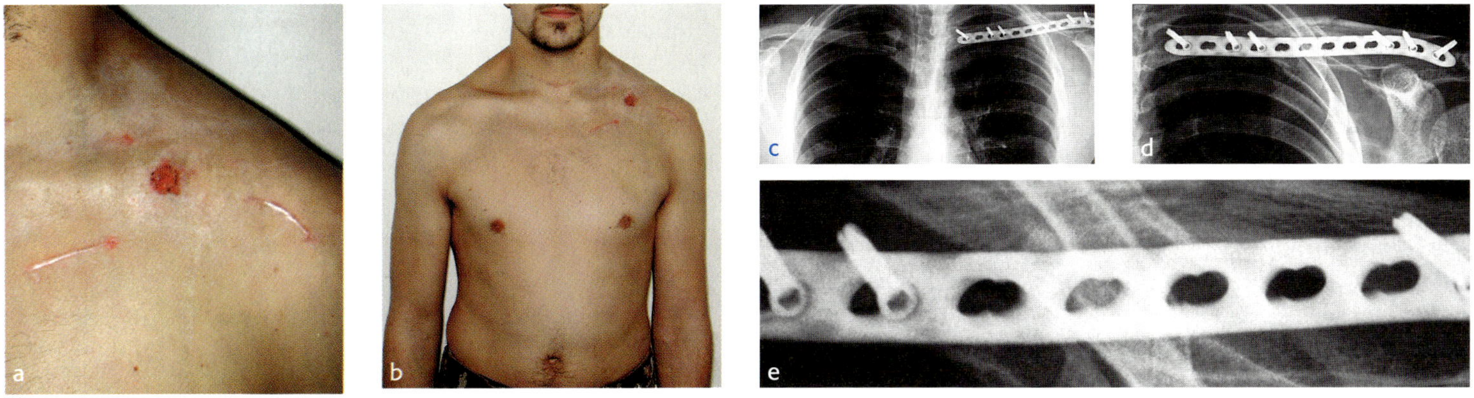

Fig 5.1.5-7a–e

a–b Functional rehabilitation follows the operation. Extensive physiotherapy and ergotherapy for the preexisting plexus paresis is performed. No major loading is recommended for 6 weeks. The paresis of the plexus recovered completely during the course of treatment.

c–d The fracture of the clavicle and the scapula showed good healing with symmetrical shoulder height.

e The clavicle fracture healed endosteally with minimal periosteal callus.

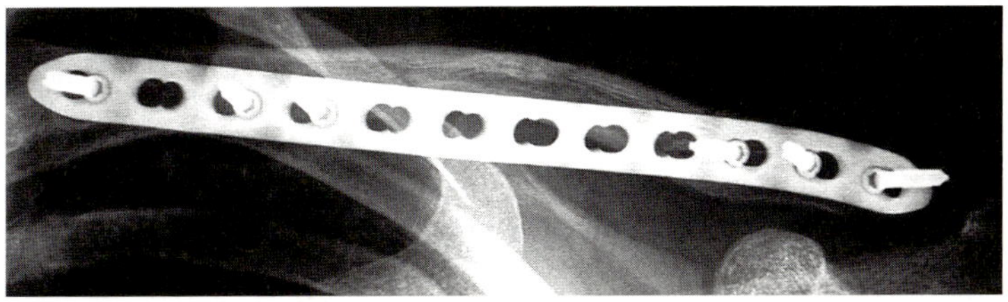

Fig 5.1.5-8 After 3 months the fracture had consolidated.

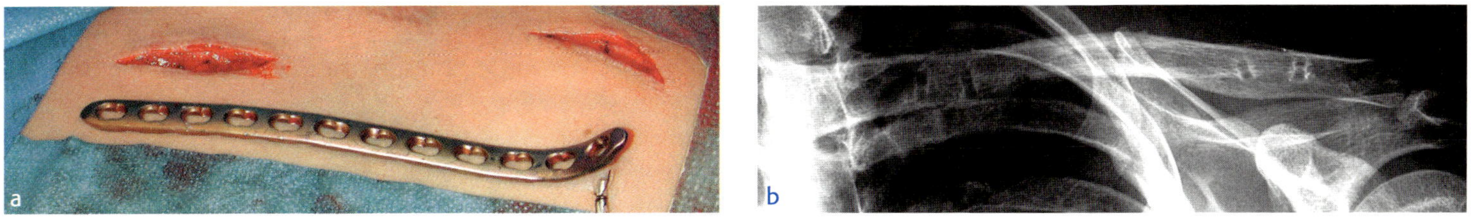

Fig 5.1.5-9a–b

a After 18 months and achieving full function without pain, the patient wished to have the implant removed. The removal procedure was performed percutaneously through the existing incisions.

b The control x-ray shows the consolidated fracture.

5 Pitfalls –

Equipment

Approach
A minimally invasive approach is only possible if the fracture can be reduced easily. In a normal fracture without soft-tissue injury, a standard approach is preferred.

Reduction and fixation
Reduction by a minimally invasive approach is quite difficult. The plate should be bent anatomically (contralateral side as reference). The position of the LCP 3.5 must be strictly anterocaudal to avoid tangential orientation of the screws (the locking head screws can only be inserted at a right angle).

Rehabilitation

6 Pearls +

Equipment
The LCP instruments facilitate minimally invasive techniques. The plate needs not be contoured absolutely to the anatomical shape. The drill sleeves are ideal for holding the plate so that it can be temporarily stabilized with K-wires.

Approach
A minimally invasive procedure can be an advantage if there is soft-tissue injury.

Reduction and fixation
The ventrocaudal position allows insertion of a straight plate whereas a weaker reconstruction plate is more appropriate in the cranial position.

Rehabilitation
Early functional rehabilitation is possible with a good and stable osteosynthesis. Implant removal is also possible by minimally invasive approach.

Author Christoph Sommer

5.2 Scapula

1 Incidence of fractures

Fractures of the scapula occur quite often and are usually caused by a high-energy direct impact over the scapular region. Most of these patients have associated injuries such as thoracic rib fractures and other fractures of the shoulder girdle [1].

2 Classification

In the OTA classification the fractures are divided into extraarticular (type A) and intraarticular (type B). A1-type concerns fractures of the processes (acrominon and coracoid), A2-type stays for body fractures and A3-type represents complex extraarticular fractures. B type fractures are subgrouped as simple impacted (B1), not impacted (B2), or as complex (B3) glenoid fractures [2]. The combination of a scapular neck fracture with a clavicular fracture is also called floating shoulder.

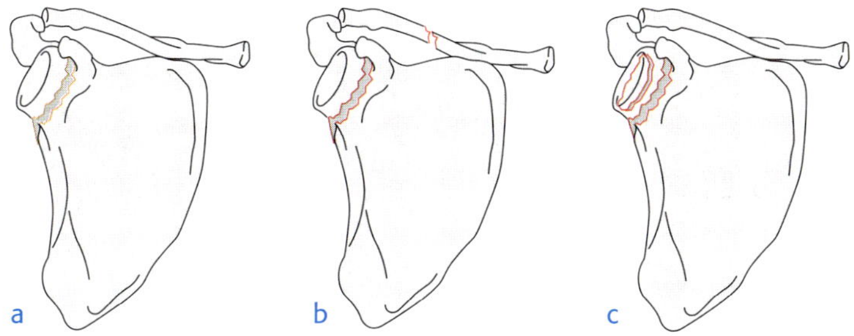

Fig 5.2-1a–c OTA classification.
a 09-A2.3 Body fracture
b 09-A3.2 Complex extraarticular fracture
c 09-B2.3 intraarticular glenoid, nonimpacted

3 Treatment method

Most scapular fractures can be treated conservatively with short immobilization time and early motion. Indications for surgery are established in cases of displaced intraarticular (glenoid) fracture with large fragments and shoulder instability, displaced floating shoulder injuries, and the rare situation of an open fracture [3].

Glenoid fractures are articular fractures and require an anatomical reduction and stable fixation, usually with one or two lag screws depending on the size of the displaced fragment(s). These fractures are usually located anterior-inferiorly and occur in combination with a shoulder dislocation in the same direction. They therefore require an anterior standard approach with open reduction and stable screw fixation. Alternatively, if closed reduction is successful, a percutaneous approach and stabilization with cannulated screws can be performed. In rare situations, the glenoid fracture is part of a complex fracture of the scapula, involving other parts of this bone (neck and body). In case of major intraarticular displacement, an operative treatment with open reduction and stable internal fixation using screws and/or plates is required. The only possible approach for these rare fractures is posterior through the interface between infraspinatus and teres minor muscle. Great care must be taken to preserve the neurovascular structures (axillary and suprascapular nerve, humeral circumflex artery) [4]. Plate fixation on the inferior or superior border of the scapular body may be difficult due to the thin bony structure. In these regions, the locking head screws of the LCP system offer a great advantage and can improve the achieved stability (see case 5.2.1).

Displaced floating shoulder injuries (fracture of the scapular neck associated with a fracture of the midshaft of the ipsilateral clavicle) are usually very unstable and show a tendency for caudal rotational displacement with low standing shoulder girdle. These injuries can often be treated successfully by stable plate fixation of the clavicle alone [5–7]. Conservative treatment for less displaced fractures may also be successful [8].

4 Implant overview

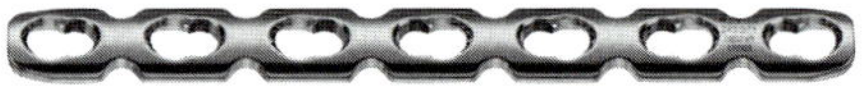

Fig 5.2-2 LCP reconstruction plate 3.5

5 Bibliography

1. **Geel CW** (2000) 4.1 Scapula and clavicle. *Rüedi TP, Murphy WM (eds), AO Principles of Fracture Management.* Stuttgart New York: Thieme-Verlag, 255–268.
2. **Orthopedic Trauma Association** (1986) Fracture and Dislocation Compendium. *J Orthop Trauma;* 10(Suppl 1).
3. **Hardegger FH, Simpson LA, Weber BG** (1984) The operative treatment of scapular fractures. *J Bone Joint Surg Br;* 66(5):725–731.
4. **Ebraheim NA, Mekhail AO, Padanilum TG, et al** (1997) Anatomic considerations for a modified posterior approach to the scapula. *Clin Orthop Relat Res;* (334):136–143.
5. **Egol KA, Connor PM, Karunakar MA, et al** (2001) The floating shoulder: clinical and functional results. *J Bone Joint Surg Am;* 83-A(8):1188–1194.
6. **Herscovici D, Fiennes AG, Allgower M, et al** (1992) The floating shoulder: ipsilateral clavicle and scapular neck fractures. *J Bone Joint Surg Br;* 74(3):362–364.
7. **Labler L, Platz A, Weishaupt D, et al** (2004) Clinical and functional results after floating shoulder injuries. *J Trauma;* 57(3):595–602.
8. **Ramos L, Mencia R, Alonso A, et al** (1997) Conservative treatment of ipsilateral fractures of the scapula and clavicle. *J Trauma;* 42(2):239–242.

Author Christoph Sommer

5.2.1 Intraarticular multifragmentary scapular fracture—OTA 09-B3

1 Case description

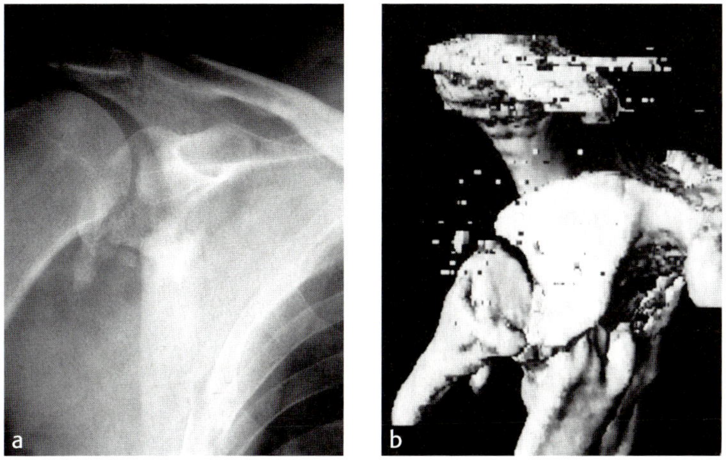

53-year-old motorcyclist fell and suffered a direct trauma to his right shoulder girdle. He had serial fractures of ribs 1–5 on his right side with a hematopneumothorax and was treated with a chest tube. He suffered a multifragmentary intraarticular scapular fracture with a clear step in the joint surface, diagnosed as a OTA 09-B3.2 injury (multifragmentary with glenoid neck and body). There were no neurovascular injuries.

Fig 5.2.1-1a–b
a AP view.
b The CT scan showed a fracture of the glenoid with three fragments and a large posterocaudal, severely displaced glenoid part.

Indication

This severely displaced fracture is a clear indication for open reduction and internal fixation. When there is a fracture line through the scapular body and neck, a posterior approach and a plate osteosynthesis is ideal. A plate system with locking head screws is of great advantage at the small scapular rim.

Preoperative planning

Equipment

- LCP reconstruction plate 3.5, 5 holes
- LCP reconstruction plate 3.5, 6 holes
- 3.5 mm locking head screws (LHS)
- 3.5 mm cortex screws
- K-wires
- Weber reduction forceps

(Size of system, instruments, and implants can vary according to anatomy.)

Patient preparation and positioning

Antibiotics: single dose 2nd generation cephalosporin
Thrombosis prophylaxis: low-molecular heparin

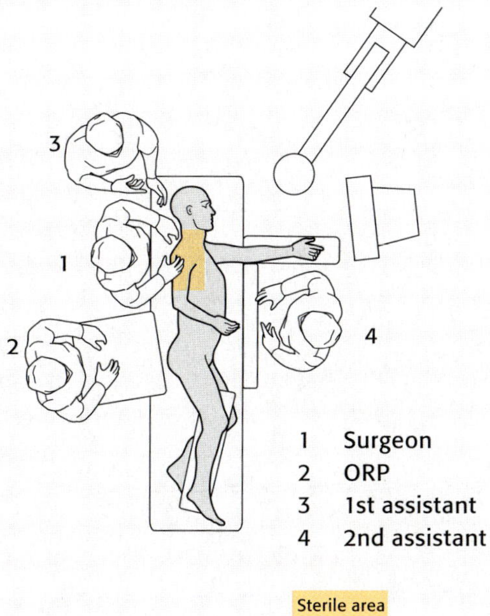

Fig 5.2.1-2 Lateral position. Entire right arm freely moveable including shoulder girdle.

2 Surgical approach

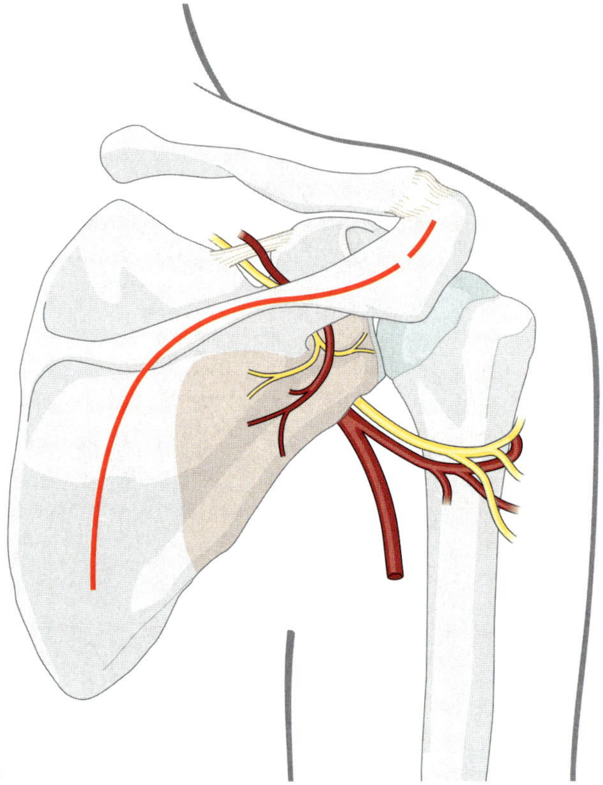

a

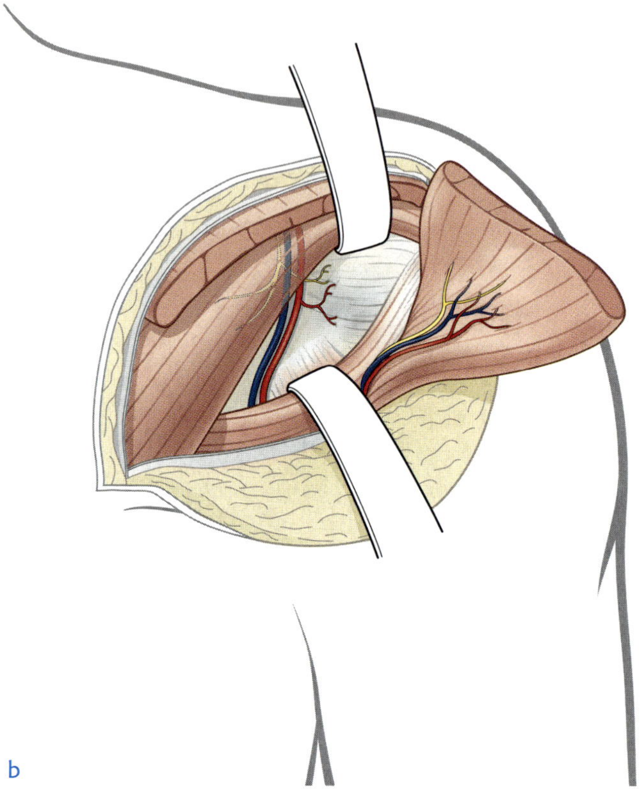

b

Fig 5.2.1-3a–b A curved incision at the inferior rim of the spine of scapula is performed from lateral to medial. The medial curve runs along the medial scapula rim and extends to the inferior scapula edge. The deltoid muscle is detached sharply from the spine of scapula and the basis of the acromion leaving a small residue on the bone for refixation. The deltoid muscle with the neurovascular bundle is held laterally. The approach is continued by entering the gap between the infraspinatus and the teres minor muscles. The suprascapular nerve is traced on its way from lateralcaudal to the entrance to the infraspinatus muscle. Capsulotomy should be performed in the region of the dorsal labrum if it has not already been torn apart. The shoulder joint is now freely visible and the humeral head can be subluxated in a ventral direction or the subluxation can be supported with a Hohmann retractor for a better overview.

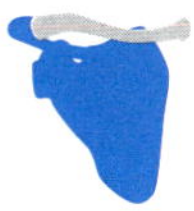

3 Reduction and fixation

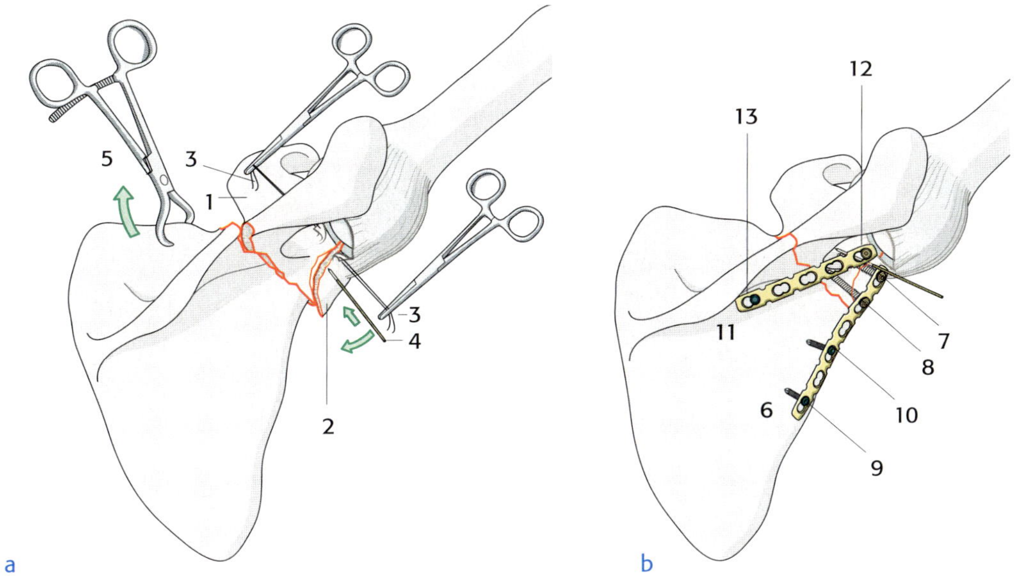

1 Glenoid fragment
2 Inferior glenoid fragment
3 Threads for holding the lateral capsule
4 K-wire used as a joystick
5 Small Weber reduction foreceps to reduce the glenoid fragments
6 Preshaped LCP reconstruction plate 3.5, 6 holes
7 Cortex lag screw 3.5 mm
8 Cortex lag screw 3.5 mm
9 Self-tapping LHS
10 Self-tapping LHS
11 Preshaped LCP reconstruction plate 3.5, 5 holes
12 Cortex screw 3.5 mm
13 Self-tapping LHS

Fig 5.2.1-4a–b
The joint surface is reduced anatomically under vision.
A K-wire is drilled into the inferior glenoid fragment and used as a joystick. If the K-wire has been inserted in a correct position, it can be used to fix the caudal fragment temporarily onto the second glenoid fragment.
The lateral capsule can be held aside with threads.
After reduction the glenoid fragments are reduced onto the scapula with the help of the Weber reduction forceps.
The definitive stabilization begins caudally with a bent LCP reconstruction plate 3.5 that is fixed with two cortex screws onto the glenoid. These cortex screws provide interfragmentary compression and stabilization of the glenoid. Locking head screws are ideal for the thin scapula. Conventional cortex or cancellous bone screws would normally not find sufficient anchorage.
A second LCP reconstruction plate 3.5 is needed at the craniodorsal aspect to complete the definitive stabilization of the glenoid and scapula. Locking head screws are also used to ensure firm connections between screw, plate, and bone.

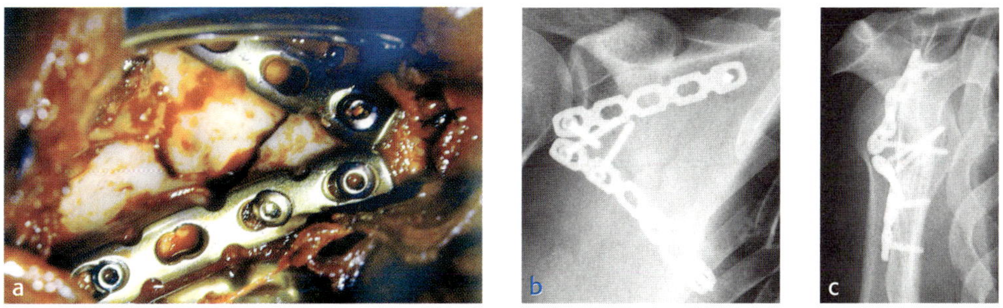

Fig 5.2.1-5a–c
a The intraoperative picture shows the two dorsal reconstruction LCP 3.5.
b–c The postoperative x-rays (AP and tangential view) confirm the anatomical reconstruction of the glenoid and the stable bridging to the scapula body.

4 Rehabilitation

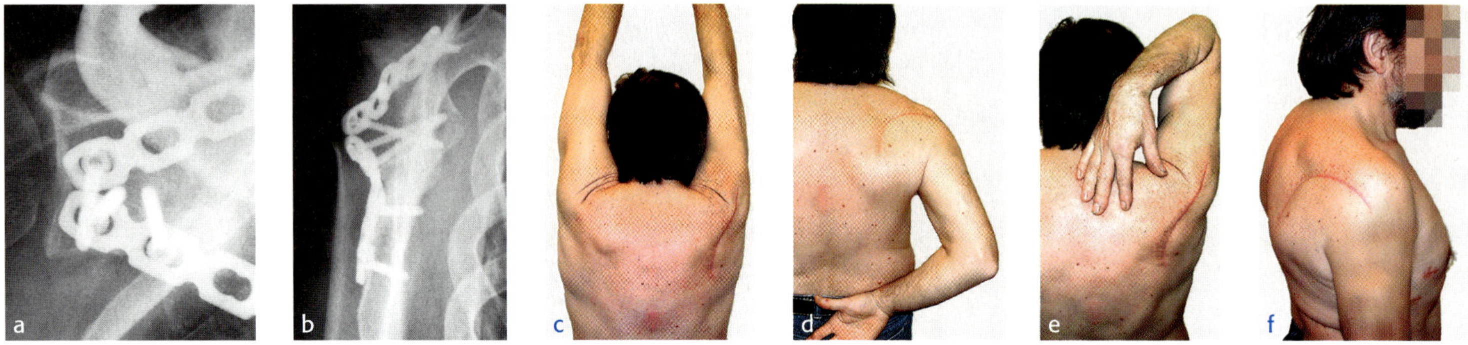

Fig 5.2.1-6a–f In a stable shoulder girdle without dislocation tendency, functional treatment begins on the first postoperative day. Active assisted exercise is done as far as tolerated. Load bearing can be started 6 weeks after trauma. The x-rays after 3 months show complete consolidation. A very good clinical result is achieved after 3 months with early functional treatment.

5 Pitfalls –

Equipment

Approach

The suprascapular nerve supplying the infraspinatus muscle is at risk.

Reduction and fixation

A nonanatomic reconstruction can lead to osteoarthrosis of the glenohumeral joint.

Rehabilitation

Early loading or poor compliance of the patient can lead to instability and nonunion.

6 Pearls +

Equipment

Locking head screws and LCP system allow good anchorage in the thin scapular body and also offer the possibility of plate depending lag screws (combination of different screws).

Approach

A displaced intraarticular glenoid fracture requires open reduction. A dorsal approach for the scapula neck or scapula body is recommended.

Reduction and fixation

The LCP with LHS allows good anchorage in the thin scapular body.

Rehabilitation

Stable fixation of the scapula with plate and locking head screws allows early functional treatment and good shoulder function is obtained.

Author Christopher G Finkemeier

5.2.2 Intraarticular displaced glenoid fossa fracture and scapular neck fracture—OTA 09-B3

1 Case description

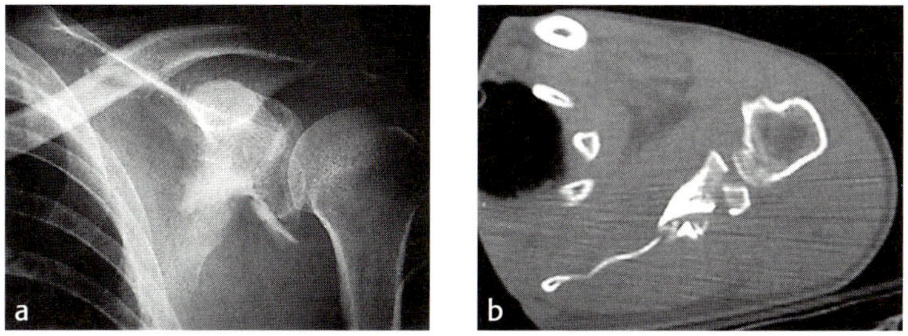

45-year-old male, fracture of left glenoid.
Type of injury: low-energy, monotrauma. Closed fracture.

Fig 5.2.2-1a–b
a AP view of left shoulder.
b CT scan (axial cut).

Indication

This case shows a displaced intraarticular glenoid fossa fracture and a scapular neck fracture. The articular fracture is significantly displaced and rotated. This is not acceptable for an intraarticular fracture and could lead to nonunion or painful posttraumatic arthritis. The displaced articular fracture with the additional scapular neck fracture makes this an injury that has a high probability of doing poorly without anatomic reduction and stable fixation.

Preoperative planning

Equipment

- LCP reconstruction plate 3.5, 6 holes
- 3.5 mm self-tapping locking head screws (LHS)
- 3.5 mm cortex screws
- K-wires
- Small and large pointed reduction forceps
- Tag sutures for the infraspinatus tendon and the edges of the joint capsule

(Size of system, instruments, and implants can vary according to anatomy.)

Patient preparation and positioning

Antibiotics: single dose 2nd generation cephalosporin

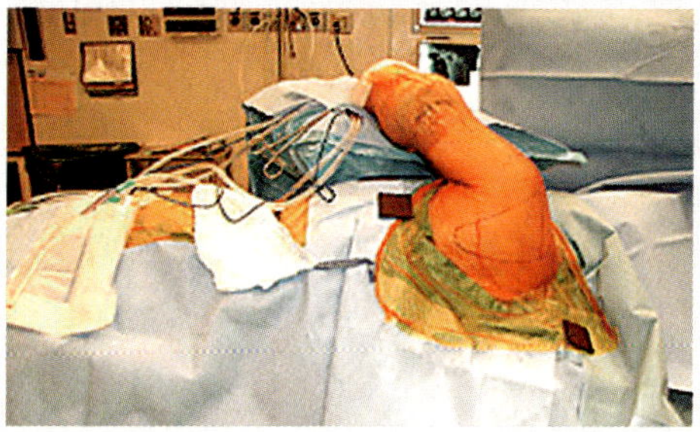

Fig 5.2.2-2 The majority of glenoid fractures are best treated posteriorly. Patients can be placed in a lateral or prone position for the best exposure of the glenoid. The lateral position is preferable as it allows the involved upper extremity to be moved into different positions during surgery, if needed.

2 Surgical approach

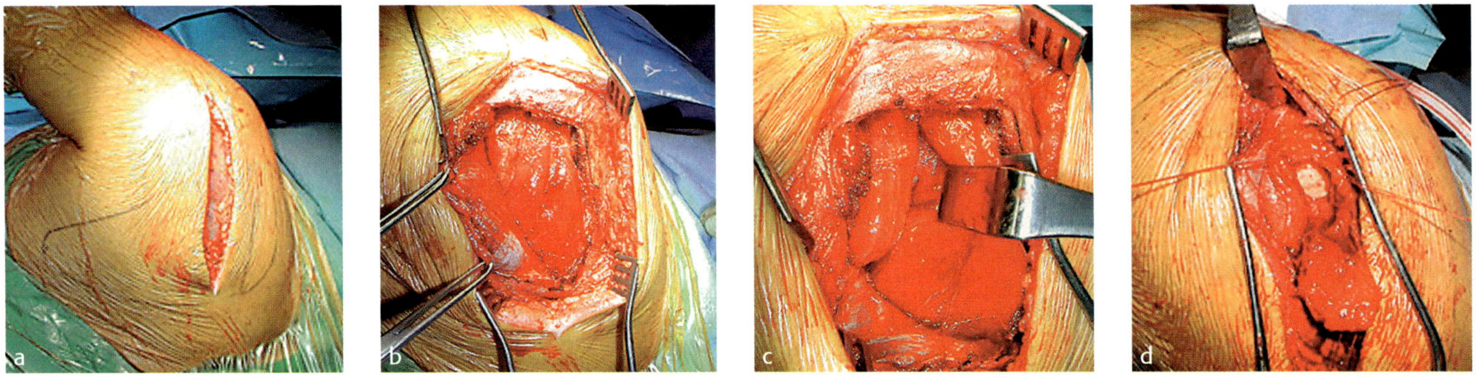

Fig 5.2.2-3a–d

a The incision is made along the inferior border of the scapular spine. It can be extended down over the lateral aspect of the deltoid if more exposure is needed such as when performing a glenohumeral arthrotomy.

b The posterior and lateral heads of the deltoid are then sharply detached from the scapular spine. The deltoid is encased by a superficial and deep fascial layer. Be careful to identify both fascial layers so that the entire muscle can be retracted to expose the external rotators of the shoulder. Avoid the muscle fibres of the deltoid which make it difficult to distinctly identify the external rotator muscles below. Once the surgeon is out of the correct plane of dissection, it is difficult to find the correct plane. Other problems can also occur such as increased bleeding and poor visualization as well as wide areas of muscle damage.

c With the deltoid retracted inferiorly, bluntly develop the interval between teres minor and infraspinatus muscles along their scapular body origins up to the humeral head insertions. This interval will take the surgeon directly to the scapular body and the joint capsule. At this stage look for the suprascapular nerve and accompanying blood vessels coursing through the spinoglenoid notch and entering the infraspinatus muscle belly.

d Incise and dissect off the tedonous portion of the infraspinatus insertion on the humeral head, keeping the underlying capsule intact. Once the tendon is elevated and tagged with a suture, perform a T-capsulotomy of the glenohumeral capsule to expose the glenoid articular surface. A shoulder retractor is helpful to retract the humeral head sufficiently to see the entire glenoid fossa. At this stage, the glenoid fossa should be exposed as well as the proximal lateral border of the scapular body and the glenoid neck.

3 Reduction and fixation

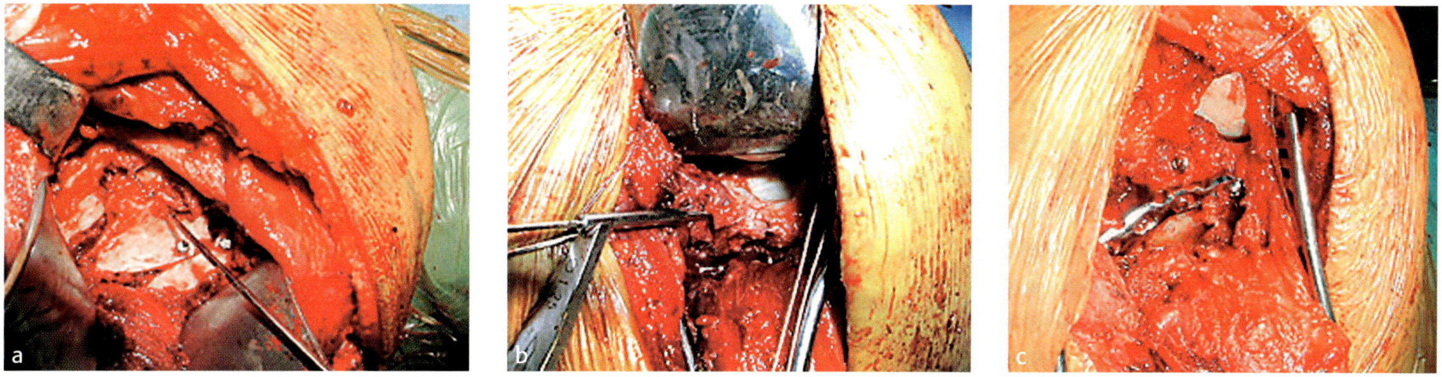

Fig 5.2.2-4a–c

a Reduction begins with cleaning of the fracture surfaces and identifying the key fragments that need reduction.
As with all periarticular fractures the articular surface is reduced first. K-wires may need to be inserted into the fragments to control their rotation and angulation.
Reduction screws or drill holes may need to be placed into the fragments to provide holding points for pointed reduction forceps.

b Once the articular fragments are reduced, K-wires can be placed to provisionally maintain the reduction prior to interfragmentary lag screws. The surgeon may decide to forego the placement of provisional K-wires and proceed directly to lag screw placement.
If there are multiple articular fragments, the surgeon should reconstruct the joint beginning with deepest fragments and building outward. Bioabsorbable pins are useful to fix the interior articular fragments in order to prevent burying hardware in locations that will not be accessible after the outer portions of the joint are reduced and instrumented. If bioabsorbable implants are not available, then the surgeon should use K-wires to hold the intercalary pieces. The K-wires need to be cut fl ush with the bone surface so that the next articular piece will fit anatomically into place.
Articular fragments should be fixed with implants appropriate for their size. 3.5 mm screws are most commonly used, but 2.7 mm and 2.0 mm screws can also be used for smaller pieces. As with most articular fractures, the surgeon should try to compress the fragments, which can be accomplished with overdrilling the near cortex or using shaft screws.

c Once the glenoid fossa has been reconstructed, the next step is to reduce and fix it to the rest of the scapula.
There are four main areas of the scapula where adequate fixation can be accomplished: the lateral border of the scapula, the coracoid process, the glenoid neck or process, and the base of the scapular spine.
The typical fixation method consists of a small fragment reconstruction plate that runs along the lateral border of the scapula and up onto the back of the scapular neck. Locking head screws are helpful in these cases as comminution may result in monocortical fixation in several locations.
One-third semi-tubular locking plates are adequate to fix fractures of the thin scapula body if needed.

4 Rehabilitation

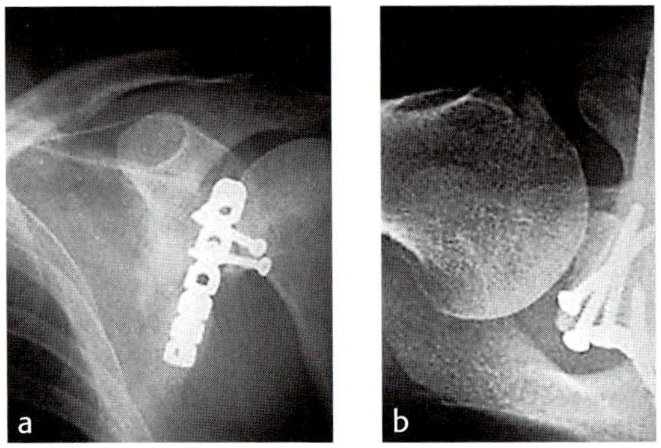

Fig 5.2.2-5a–b Postoperative x-rays after 6 weeks.

Additional immobilization: a sling or shoulder immobilizer can be used to support the involved shoulder for 1–2 weeks or until the patient's pain subsides.
Mobilization: passive mobilization after 1 day. Active mobilization after 21 to 42 days depending on the adequacy of the repair of the infraspinatus and the deltoid muscles.
Physiotherapy: begin first postoperative day for passive and active-assisted exercises.
Pharmaceutical treatment: hydrocone and acetaminophen.

Implant removal

Implant removal is not usually necessary and should be avoided due to the added soft-tissue trauma and the risk of injuring the suprascapular nerve.

5 Pitfalls –

Approach
Working outside of the correct tissue plane.

Reduction and fixation
Attempting to obtain adequate fixation in the thin portion of the scapular body.

Rehabilitation
Immobilizing the shoulder or delaying physiotherapy beyond 2–3 weeks.

Implant removal
Removing implants for reasons other than infection or mechanical impingement.

6 Pearls +

Approach

Reduction and fixation
Remember the four areas of the scapula where adequate fixation can be obtained: the lateral border of the scapula, the glenoid neck, the coracoid process, and the base of the scapular spine.

Rehabilitation
Start physiotherapy immediately.

Implant removal
Do not remove implants unless absolutely necessary.

6.1 Humerus, proximal

Cases

Case		Classification	Method	Implant used	Implant function	Page
6.1.1	Extraarticular unstable subcapital humeral fracture with diaphyseal involvement	11-A3	compression and locked splinting	LCP metaphyseal plate 3.5/4.5/5.0	locked internal fixator and reduction screw	231
6.1.2	Extraarticular bifocal proximal humeral fracture with rotatory displacement of the epiphysis	11-B2	compression	LPHP	protection plate and reduction screw [1]	235
6.1.3	Extraarticular bifocal proximal humeral fracture without metaphyseal impaction	11-B2	compression	PHILOS	blade plate [1]	243
6.1.4	Extraarticular bifocal proximal humeral fracture with proximal diaphyseal extension	11-B2	compression	PHILOS	compression plate and lag screw [1]	249
6.1.5	Extraarticular bifocal proximal humeral fracture with glenohumeral dislocation	11-B3	locked splinting	PHILOS	locked internal fixator [1]	253
6.1.6	Intraarticular proximal humeral fracture with slight displacement	11-C1	locked splinting	LPHP	locked internal fixator and reduction screw [1]	259
6.1.7	Intraarticular proximal humeral fracture with valgus malalignment	11-C2	locked splinting	LPHP	locked internal fixator and reduction screw [1]	265
6.1.8	Intraarticular impacted proximal humeral fracture with displacement	11-C2	locked splinting	LPHP	locked internal fixator and reduction screw [1]	271
6.1.9	4-part proximal humeral fracture	11-C2	locked splinting	PHILOS	locked internal fixator and reduction screw [1]	279

[1] Additional tension band with sutures for the head fragment.

6 Humerus

Author Michael Plecko

6.1 Humerus, proximal

1 Incidence of fractures

Fractures of the proximal humerus are common injuries, accounting for about 4–5% of all fractures and 45% of fractures of the humerus [1]. Depending on the fracture types included, incidence rates vary from 73/100,000 [2] to 105/100,000 [1]. The incidence of proximal humeral fractures is age dependent, with a marked increase beyond the fifth decade of life [3] and a female preponderance of 1.5–3:1 [1, 2]. Detailed age and sex distribution according to the type of fracture is provided in a recent study [4]. According to the Müller AO Classification the majority of proximal humeral fractures can be assigned to type A (66%) and B (27%) fractures with a tendency towards more complex fractures with age [4].

While in the younger patient high-energy trauma predominates, low-energy trauma is the most common injury in the older patient. The rise in fracture incidence with age, especially with only moderate trauma, and the higher incidence among women are characteristic epidemiologic features of fractures associated with osteoporosis.

In younger patients with high-energy trauma, accompanying injuries of the axillary nerve or brachial plexus, as well as soft-tissue damage are frequently observed. This is rare in elderly patients with low-energy trauma.

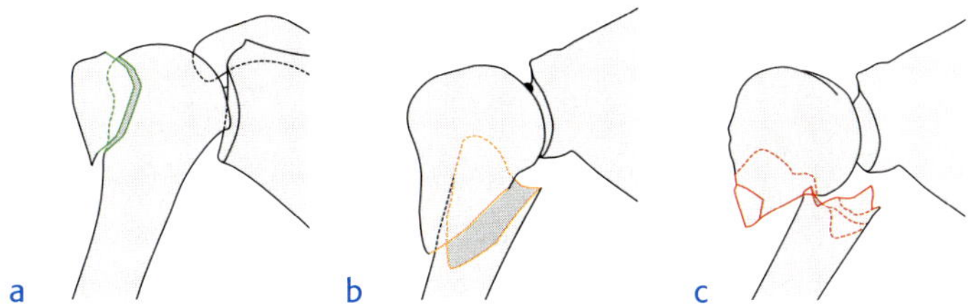

Fig 6.1-1a–c 11-A Extraarticular unifocal fracture.
a 11-A1 tuberosity
b 11-A2 impacted metaphyseal
c 11-A3 nonimpacted metaphyseal

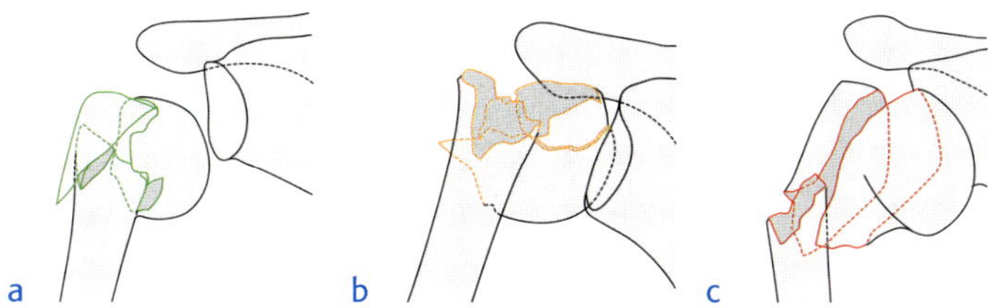

Fig 6.1-2a–c 11-B Extraarticular bifocal fracture.
a 11-B1 with metaphyseal impaction
b 11-B2 without metaphyseal impaction
c 11-B3 with glenohumeral dislocation

2 Classification

Proximal humeral fractures are classified according to the Müller AO classification system and Neer´s Classification [5, 6], though both classification systems have limited reproducibility [7]. Classification is useful for comparison of study populations and allows guidelines to be set for treatment and rehabilitation.

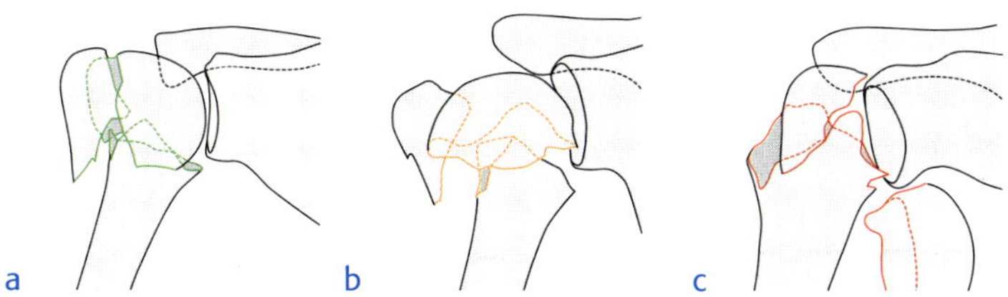

Fig 6.1-3a–c 11-C Articular fracture.
a 11-C1 with slight displacement
b 11-C2 impacted with marked displacement
c 11-C3 dislocated

The Müller AO Classification categorizes proximal humeral fractures according to fracture localization and fracture pattern: type A represents extraarticular unifocal fractures, type B concerns extraarticular bifocal fractures and type C classifies articular fractures.

3 Treatment methods and indications

Nondisplaced or minimally displaced proximal humeral fractures according to types 11-A1.1, 11-A2.1, 11-A2.2, 11-A2.3, 11-A3.1, 11-B1.1, 11-B1.2, 11-B1.3, 11-C1.1, 11-C1.2, and 11-C1.3 are usually treated conservatively by early functional treatment or immobilization. More complex and/or unstable fracture types usually require operative treatment. Decision making should include:

- fracture type,
- patient age,
- individual functional demands, and
- expected compliance with rehabilitation.

Additional injuries and biological criteria, such as bone density, circulation, preexisting arthrosis of the shoulder, integrity of the rotator cuff, and comorbidity have to be considered.

For open fractures as well as for fractures with accompanying vascular or nerve lesions, immediate operative treatment is recommended. In severely displaced fractures, early reduction and osteosynthesis should be achieved.

Operative techniques for proximal humeral fractures include minimally invasive techniques like percutaneous pinning [8] and/or percutaneous screw fixation [9–11]. To avoid migration of the pins, a humerus block—as described by Resch [12]—may be used. In some cases with a limited open approach for reduction, screw fixation with additional tension band osteosynthesis may enable increased stability [13, 14]. Minimally invasive techniques has the advantage of lesser soft-tissue damage, but demand optimal percutaneous reduction of the fracture fragments and often additional sling immobilization for 3–4 weeks.

Although minimally invasive techniques have widely been promoted over the past decade, some fracture types seem to be more suitable for these minimally invasive techniques than others. Good indications for percutaneous techniques are: type 11-A1 fractures with more than 3 mm displacement of the greater tuberosity, 11-A3.1 and 11-A3.2 fractures if good closed reduction can be achieved, and 11-B1 fractures with more than 3 mm displacement of the greater or lesser tuberosity. Valgus impacted 4-part fractures type 11-C2.1 with minor lateral displacement between the articular segment and the shaft can successfully be reduced percutaneously due to intact periosteum and soft-tissue support. In contrast, 11-B2, 11-B3, some 11-C2 and most 11-C3 fractures may need open reduction techniques.

Intramedullary fixation has primarily been applied in humeral shaft fractures and has later on been extended to subcapital 11-A2 and 11-A3 fractures. Standard intramedullary nail designs as well as elastic intramedullary pins have been used [15, 16]. In the last few years special intramedullary implants for proximal humeral fractures have been developed. The newly designed proximal humeral nail with a spiral blade (PHN) provides improved rotational stability compared with nails using locking screws only [17] and combines the advantage of a stable implant with a limited open access. 11-A3 fractures are most suitable for operative treatment with the PHN, although the inevitable approach through the rotator cuff has to be considered in younger patients. Indications for intramedullary implants may be extended towards more complex fractures like 11-B2 with additional fixation of the tuberosities by secure sutures or by screws.

The classic open reduction technique and conventional plate fixation, mainly using the T-plate, has been performed for many years. Exact preparation of the fracture fragments led to additional damage of the blood supply with a high rate of avascular necrosis of the humeral head [18–20]. This problem

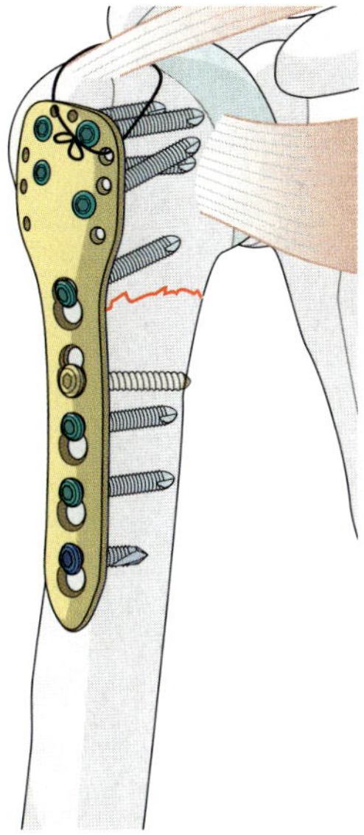

Fig 6.1-4 Proximal humeral fracture with restored medial buttress in the metaphyseal area.

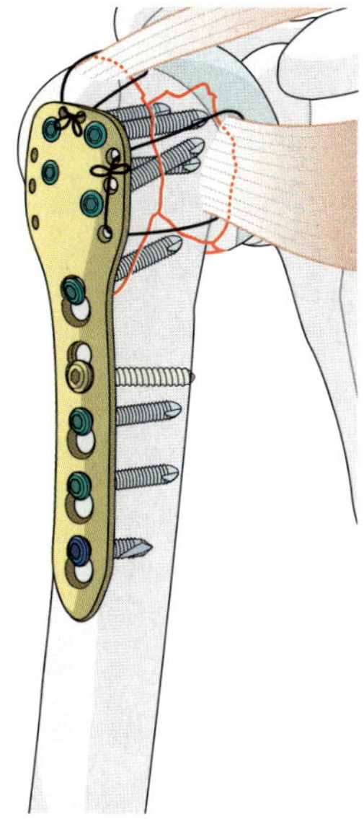

Fig 6.1-5 Proximal humeral fracture with restored medial buttress by impacting the shaft into the humeral head.

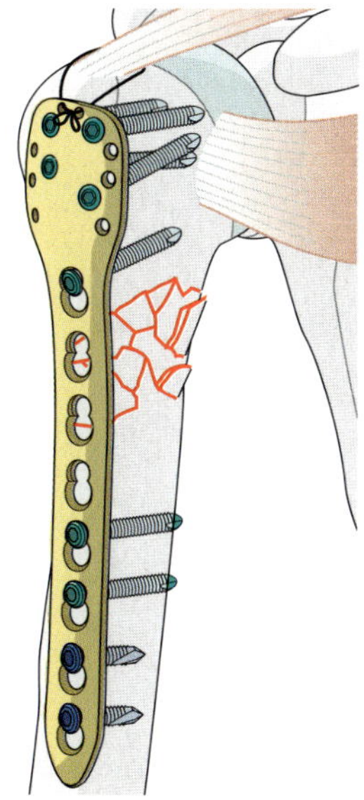

Fig 6.1-6 Proximal humeral fracture with deficient medial buttress due to metaphyseal comminution. An 8-hole LPHP is used as a locked bridging plate splinting the fracture zone.

Video 6.1-1

has been overcome by using indirect reduction techniques and careful soft-tissue dissection. Using the same implants this modified technique reduced the rate of avascular necrosis to 0–4% [21, 22]. In addition, especially in osteoporosis, conventional screws may disengage, leading to secondary displacement.

In the last few years the development of angular stable implants for fractures of the proximal humerus, according to the locking compression plate (LCP) concept, has initiated a new era in the operative treatment of these fractures. Anatomically preshaped implants like the locking proximal humeral plate (LPHP), proximal humerus internal locking system (PHILOS), or modified conventional implants like the cloverleaf plate with locking head screws can be used for this new concept. Sometimes fixation with two small LCPs may be useful. The combination of locking head screws with the three dimensional positioning of the screws within the humeral head leads to improved stability. Application of these new angular stable implants is mainly considered when open reduction is necessary. Therefore fractures 11-A3, 11-B2, 11-B3, 11-C2, and reconstructable 11-C3 fractures are the most frequent indications for these new techniques.

Fixation of proximal humeral fractures with angular stable plate osteosynthesis can be performed either through a deltopectoral or a delta splitting approach. Special attention to the axillary nerve and careful preservation of the periosteal blood supply by indirect reduction maneuvers are essential (no-touch technique).

Reconstruction of the medial buttress in the metaphyseal area of the humerus is a key point in fracture fixation with locking proximal humeral plates. If the medial buttress can be restored by indirect reduction, this leads to a very stable construct and allows early functional rehabilitation (Fig 6.1-4). If there is medial comminution or bone defect, the medial buttress may be restored by impacting the shaft into the head and fixing it in this position with the LPHP or PHILOS which, in most cases, is stable enough for active-assisted mobilization (Fig 6.1-5). If the comminution is too extensive to allow restoration of the medial buttress, the locking compression plate may be used as a locked internal fixator bridging the fracture zone with empty plate holes over the fracture (Fig 6.1-6).

In these cases the rehabilitation protocol has to be adapted and only passive exercises should be performed. Otherwise stress concentration will lead to implant failure.

When dealing with angular stable implants in the treatment of proximal humeral fractures, a few guidelines have to be considered [25]. Thorough analysis of the fracture type with respect to residual blood supply of the articular head segment, in order to avoid extensive preparation of the fracture lines to preserve the periosteal blood supply, and for careful reduction of the humeral fracture, preferably by indirect technique.

Adequate reduction techniques are manual longitudinal traction, rotation, lateralization of the shaft, and gentle manipulation of the tuberosities and the humeral head segment, using suture loops through the rotator cuff tendons close to their bony insertion, gentle reduction of the medialized shaft to the plate, using a conventional screw as reduction screw.

Later on, correct positioning of the implant to avoid subacromial impingement, correct length of the locking head screws within the humeral head, nonperforation of the articular surface, use of self-tapping (not self-drilling, self-tapping) screws within the humeral head, use of additional strong nonabsorbable sutures through the rotator cuff tendons and the plate as tension banding are highly recommended as well as application of at least two bicortical locking head screws within the humeral shaft (in osteoporotic bone three locking head screws are recommended).

Although long-term experience with angular stable proximal humeral implants in a larger patient cohort is pending, biomechanical studies as well as first clinical data are promising [17, 23–25].

4 Implant overwiew

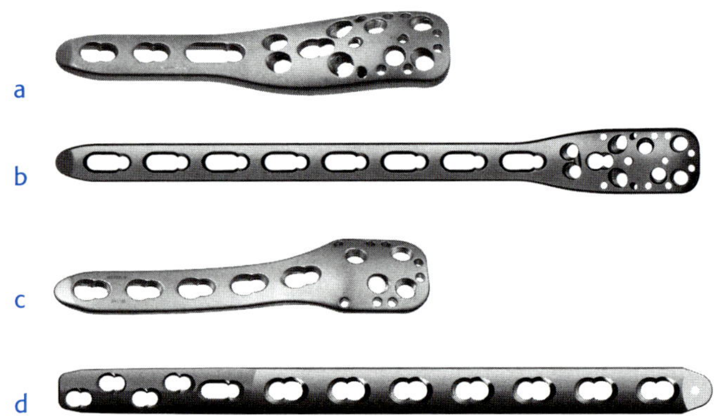

Fig 6.1-7a–d
a PHILOS—proximal humeral plate 3.5
b PHILOS long—proximal humeral plate 3.5
c LPHP—locking proximal humeral plate 3.5
d LCP metaphyseal plate 3.5/4.5/5.0

5 Bibliography

1. **Rose SH, Melton LJ 3rd, Morrey BF, et al** (1982) Epidemiologic features of humeral fractures. *Clin Orthop;* 168:24–30.
2. **Lind T, Krøner K, Jensen J** (1989) The epidemiology of fractures of the proximal humerus. *Arch Orthop Trauma Surg;* 108(5):285–287.
3. **Kristiansen B, Barford G, Bredesen J, et al** (1987) Epidemiology of proximal humeral fractures. *Acta Orthop Scand;* 58(1):75–77.
4. C**ourt-Brown CM, Garg A, Mc Queen MM** (2001) The epidemiology of proximal humeral fractures. *Acta Orthop Scand;* 72(4):365–371.
5. **Mueller ME, Nazarian S, Koch P, et al** (1990) *The comprehensive classification of fractures of long bones.* Berlin Heidelberg New York: Springer-Verlag.
6. **Neer CS 2nd** (1970) Displaced proximal humeral fractures. I. Classification and evaluation. *J Bone Joint Surg Am;* 52(6):1077–1089.
7. **Siebenrock KA, Gerber Ch** (1993) The reproducibility of classification of fractures of the proximal end of the humerus. *J Bone Joint Surg Am;* 75:1751–1755.
8. **Jaberg H, Warner JJ, Jakob RP** (1992) Percutaneous stabilization of unstable fractures of the humerus. *J Bone Joint Surg;* 74(4):508–515.
9. **Resch H, Povacz P, Froehlich R, et al** (1997) Percutaneous fixation of three-and four- part fractures of the proximal humerus. *J Bone Joint Surg Br;* 79(2):295–300.
10. **Szyszkowitz R, Schippinger G** (1999) [Fractures of the proximal humerus.] *Unfallchirurg;* 102(6):422–428.
11. **Fankhauser F, Schippinger G, Weber K, et al** (2003) Cadaveric-biomechanical evaluation of bone-implant construct of proximal humerus fractures (Neer type 3). *J Trauma;* 55(2):345–349.
12. **Resch H** (2003) [Fractures of the humeral head.] *Unfallchirurg;* 106(8):602–617.
13. **Rüedi TP** (1989) The treatment of displaced metaphyseal fractures with screws and wiring systems. *Orthopedics;* 12(1):55–59.
14. **Ochsner PE, Ilchmann T** (1991) [Tension band osteosynthesis with absorbable cords in proximal comminuted fractures of the humerus.] *Unfallchirurg;* 94(10):508–510.
15. **Zifko B, Poigenfürst J, Pezzei C** (1992) [Intramedullary nailing of unstable proximal humeral fractures.] *Orthopäde;* 21(2):115–120.
16. **Blum J, Rommens PM, Janzing H** (1998) [Retrograde nailing of humerus shaft fractures with the unreamed humerus nail. An international multicenter study.] *Unfallchirurg;* 101(5):342–352.
17. **Hessmann MH, Rommens PM** (2003) [*The biomechanical behavior of angular stable implants at the proximal.*] 1st ed. Bern Göttingen Toronto Seattle: Hans Huber Verlag. German
18. **Kuner EH, Siebler G** (1987) [Dislocation fractures of the proximal humerus—results following surgical treatment. A follow-up study of 167 cases.] *Unfallchirurg;* 13(2):64–71.
19. **Speck M, Lang FJH, Regazzoni P** (1996) [Multifragmentary proximal humeral fractures—Failures after T-plate fixation.] *Swiss Surg;* 2:51–56. German
20. **Lill H, Lange K, Prasse-Badde J, et al** (1997) [T-plate osteosynthesis in dislocated proximal humerus fractures] *Unfallchirurg;* 23(5):183–190.
21. **Hessmann M, Baumgaertel F, Gehling H, et al** (1999) Plate fixation of proximal humeral fractures with indirect reduction: surgical technique and results utilizing three shoulder scores. *Injury;* 30(7):453–462.
22. **Esser RD** (1994) Treatment of three-and four-part fractures of the proximal humerus with a modified cloverleaf plate. *J Orthop Trauma;* 8(1):15–22.
23. **Plecko M, Kraus A** (2004) Internal fixation of proximal humerus fractures using the locking proximal humeral plate. *Oper Orthop Traumatol;* 17:25–50.

24. **Lill H, Hepp P, Korner J, et al** (2003) Proximal humeral fractures: how stiff should an implant be? A comparative mechanical study with new implants in human specimens. *Arch Orthop Trauma Surg;* 123:74–81.
25. **Lill H, Hepp P, Rose T, et al** (2004) [The angle stable locking-proximal-humerus-plate (LPHP) for proximal humeral fractures using a small anterior-lateral-deltoid-splitting-approach - technique and first results] *Zentralbl Chir;* 129(1):43–48.

Author Christoph Sommer

6.1.1 Extraarticular unstable subcapital humeral fracture with diaphyseal involvement—11-A3

1 Case description

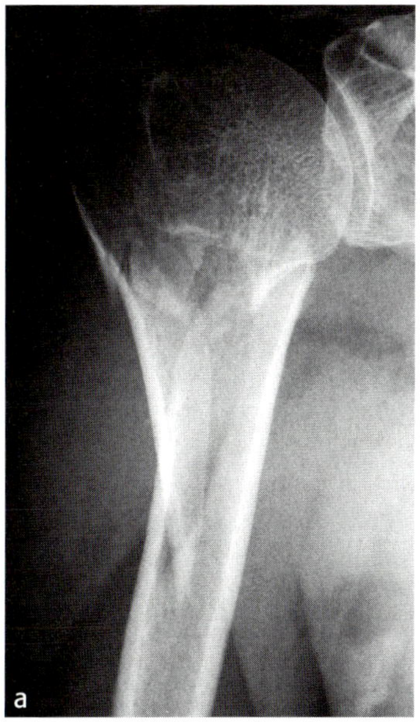

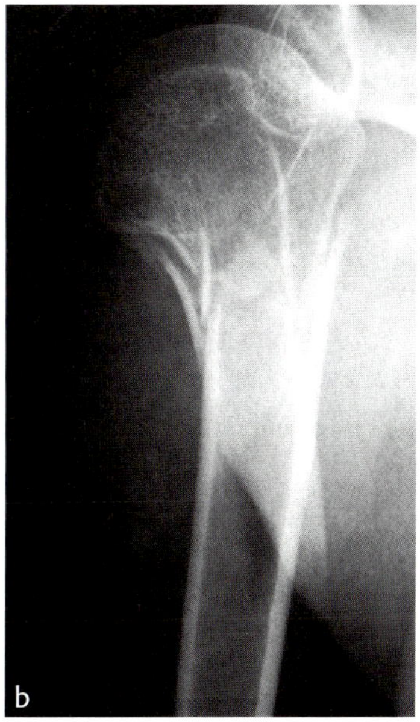

63-year-old active business woman (self-employed), skiing injury to the right dominant arm.

Fig 6.1.1-1a–b
a AP view.
b Axillary view.

Indication

Proximal extraarticular humeral fracture with comminution and diaphyseal extension (11-A3.3), very unstable and painful.
Operative treatment reduces pain, instability is overcome, and patient's request to use the right dominant arm as soon as possible is met.
Nonoperative treatment is a valid option, since there are few displacements and no neurovascular injuries. However, fixation with a Velpeau bandage for 4–6 weeks is required, and subsequent impairment of shoulder movement is to be expected.

Preoperative planning

Equipment

- LCP metaphyseal plate 3.5/4.5/5.0, 5+8 holes
- 3.5 mm locking head screws (LHS)
- 3.5 mm cortex screw
- 2.0 mm K-wires

(Size of system, instruments, and implants can vary according to anatomy.)

Patient preparation and positioning

Antibiotics: single dose 2nd generation cephalosporin
Thrombosis prophylaxis: low-molecular heparin

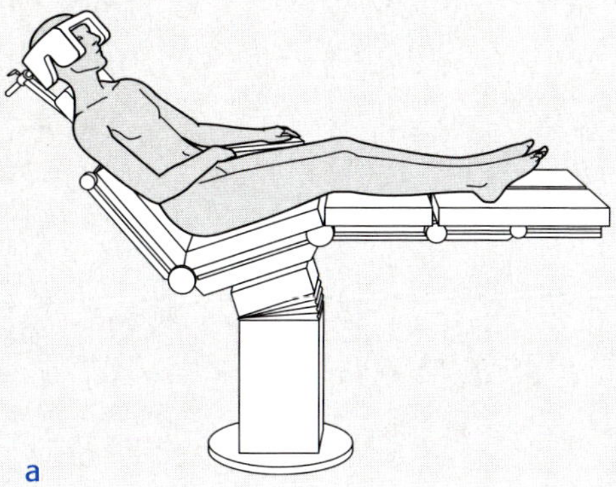

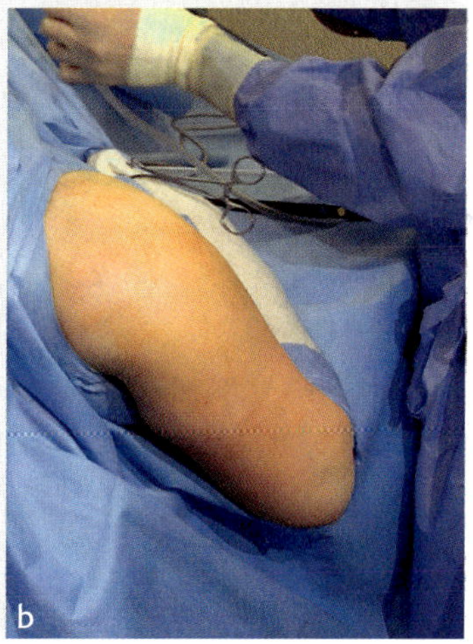

Fig 6.1.1-2a–b
Beach chair position.
Arm freely moveable.

2 Surgical approach

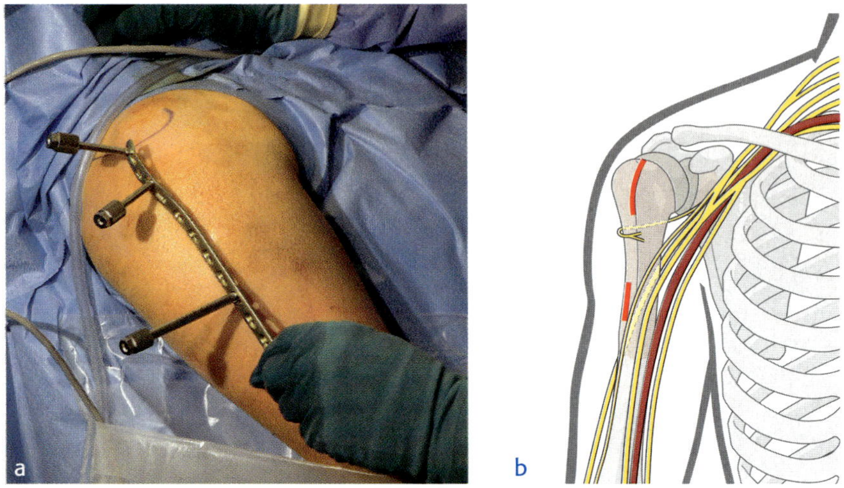

a b

Fig 6.1.1-3a–b

a A straight LCP metaphyseal plate 3.5/4.5/5.0 is slightly contoured to approximately fit the shape of the humeral head.

b A minimally invasive approach (anterolateral deltoid split) with two small incisions (2–3 cm long) is sufficient. This preserves vascularity, but does not allow full view of the fracture site. Care must be taken not to injure the axillary nerve. It should be noted that only approximate alignment of axis and rotation is possible.

Alternatively, an open approach offers a direct view of the fracture, but it is not preferable because of additional damage to vascularity.

3 Reduction and fixation

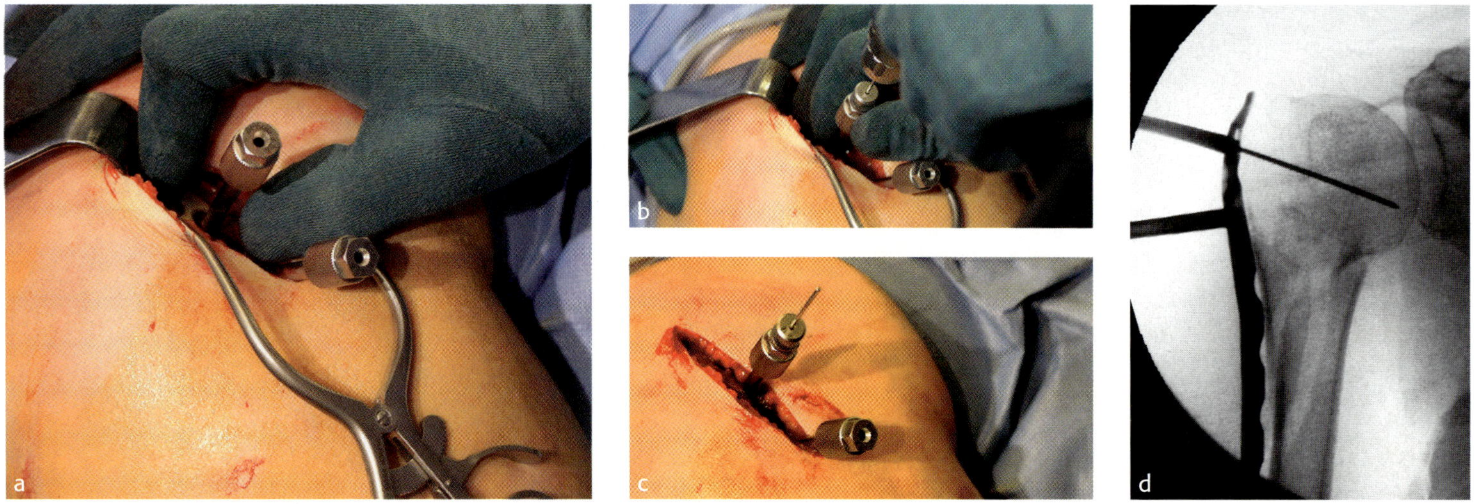

a b c d

Fig 6.1.1-4a–j

a After epiperiosteal tunneling with an elevator, the plate is gently inserted along the anterolateral aspect of the humeral shaft. The two drill sleeves, firmly anchored in the proximal part of the plate act as handles.

b–d Preliminary fixation of the plate with a K-wire placed into the humeral head. Image intensifier shows the position of the plate relative to the humeral head and shaft and the closed reduction obtained.

3 Reduction and fixation (cont)

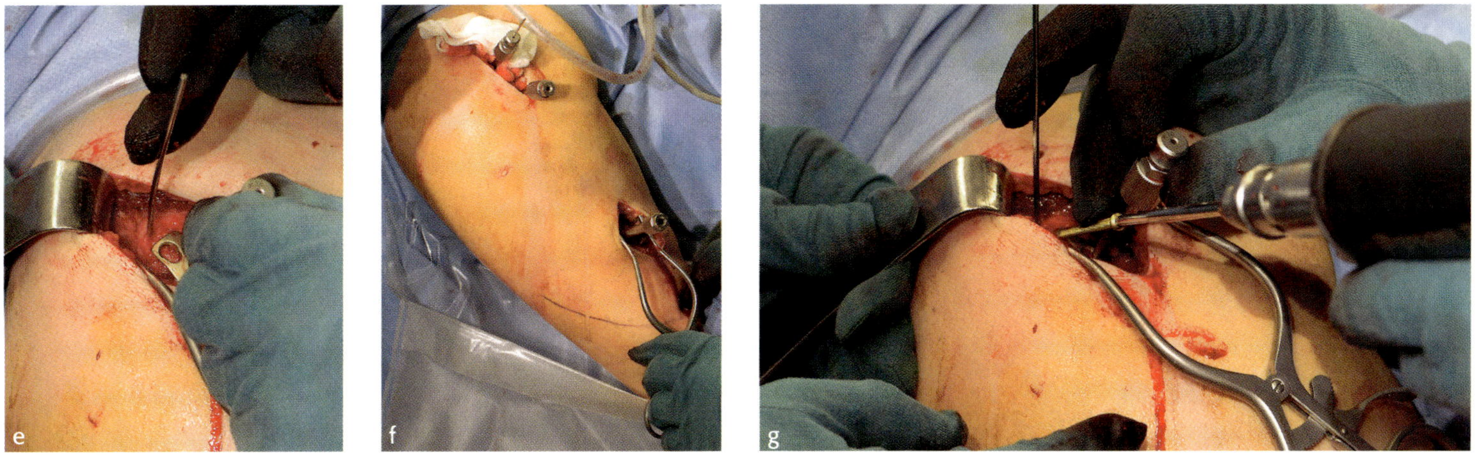

Fig 6.1.1-4a–j (cont)

e Reduction can be adjusted by means of the 2.0 mm K-wire used as joystick.

f A drill sleeve is placed in the most distal hole of the plate. A 2.0 mm K-wire is inserted and positioning of the plate is controlled.

g Fixation of the humeral head with one 3.5 mm cortex screw and a 3.5 mm self-tapping locking head screw.
Before fixing the bridging plate to the humerus distally the fracture reduction and axial alignment should be checked by image intensification once more.

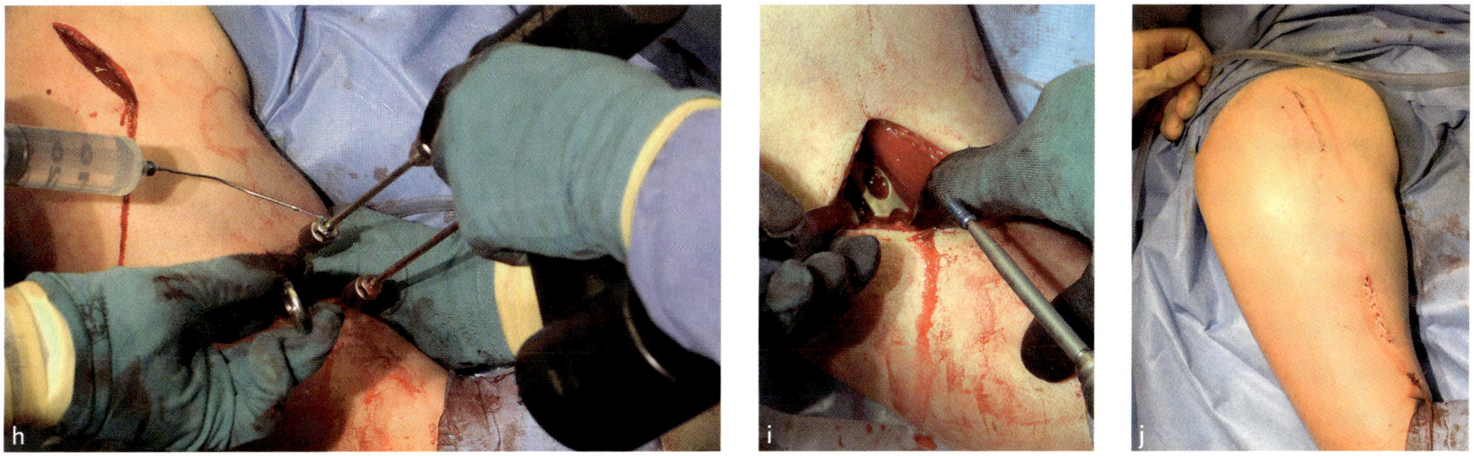

h The most distal hole is drilled, the drill bit remaining in place to secure the correct length, while axial alignment is still possible. A further check with the image intensifier is advisable before the two self-tapping LHS are inserted bicortically.

i The fixation is completed by inserting a third LHS distally and two LHS proximally.

j Free arm motion and abduction must be checked prior to skin closure.

4 Rehabilitation

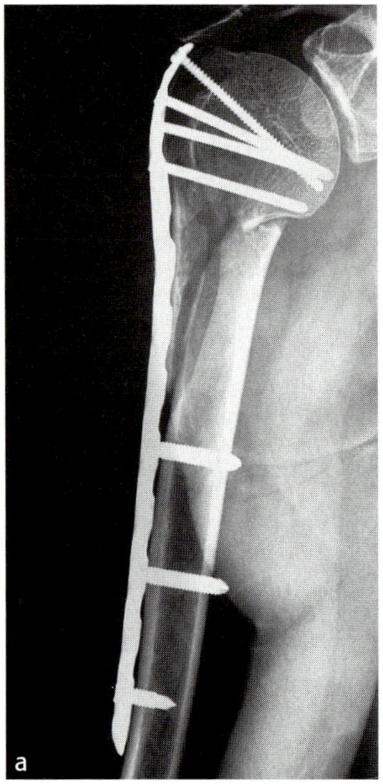

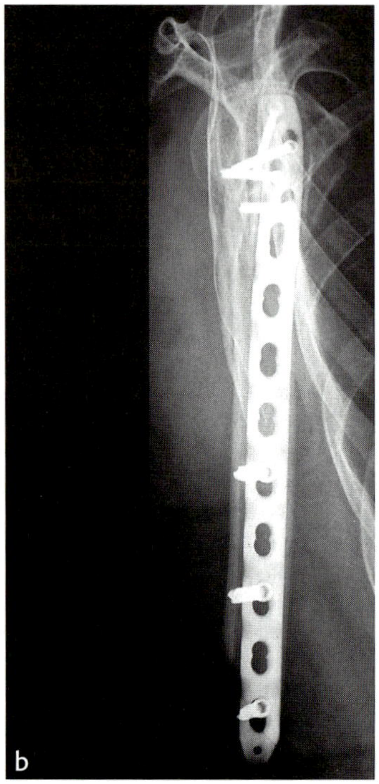

No additional immobilization.
Weight bearing: partial after 6 weeks; full after 8 weeks.
Physiotherapy: functional postoperative treatment with active-assisted movement with a physiotherapist as of the first postoperative day.
Pharmaceutical treatment: analgesics if required.
Implant removal: only if patient suffers from the implant.

Fig 6.1.1-5a–b Postoperative x-rays (bridging the fracture zone with the internal fixator method).

5 Pitfalls -

Approach
Open approach with additional damage to vascularity.
Damage to the anterior branch of the axillary nerve.

Reduction and fixation

6 Pearls +

Approach
A minimally invasive technique does not require exposure of the fracture focus and preserves vascularity.

Reduction and fixation
Note that except for the most distal LHS, all screws are bicortical, which appears mandatory in the humerus due to the wide range of motion, especially rotation of the arm.

Author Wilson Li

6.1.2 Extraarticular bifocal proximal humeral fracture with rotatory displacement of the epiphysis—11-B2

1 Case description

49-year-old man slipped and fell on his shoulder. Type of injury: low-energy, monotrauma. Closed fracture.

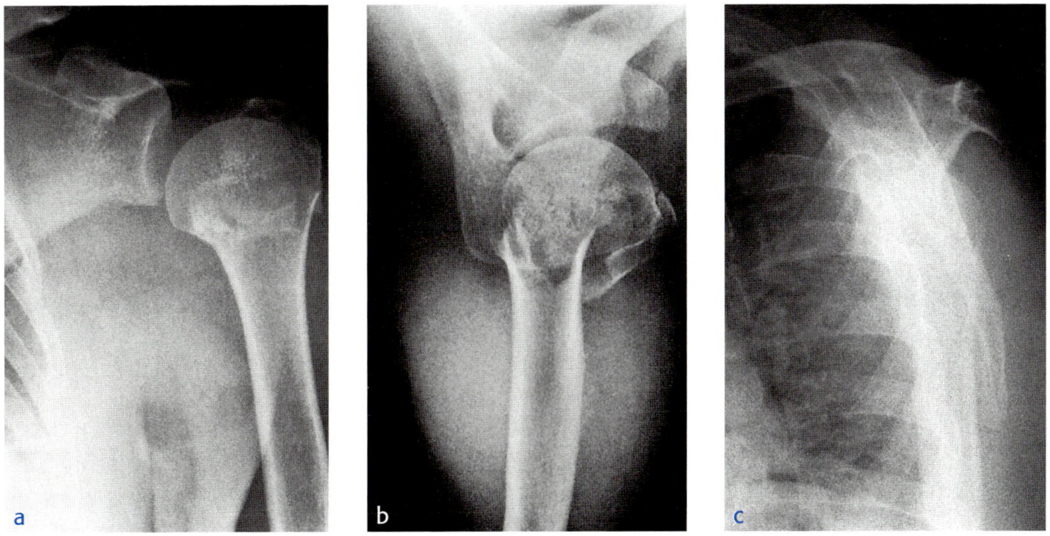

Fig 6.1.2-1a–c
a AP view.
b Axillary view.
c Lateral view.

Indication

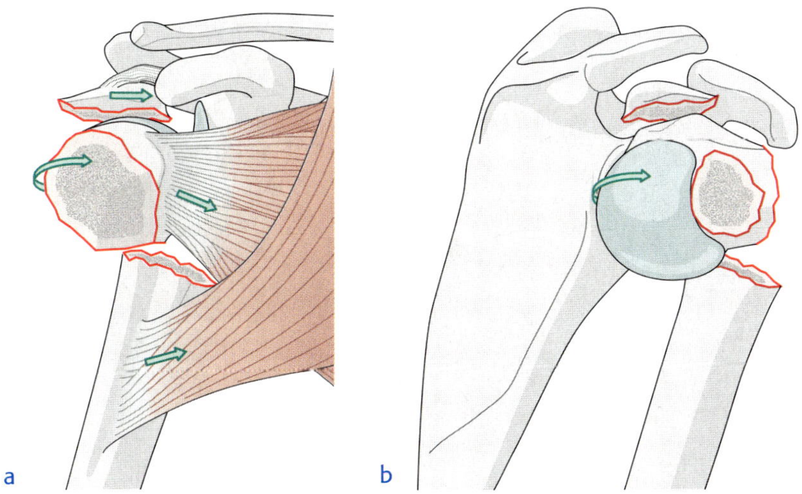

Bifocal fracture of the surgical neck of the humerus is very painful and disabling as the segments are pulled by respective muscle attachments into typical displacement patterns. Nonoperative treatment often results in painful nonunion or malunion with restricted range of motion. Percutaneous pinning may result in loss of initial reduction, while plating with traditional implants may not be stable in osteoporotic bone.

Fig 6.1.2-2a–b
Deforming forces acting on the fragments the supraspinatus pulls the greater tuberosity into abduction, the subscapularis pulls the lesser tuberosity into medial rotation, and the pectoralis major pulls the shaft into medialization.

Indication (cont)

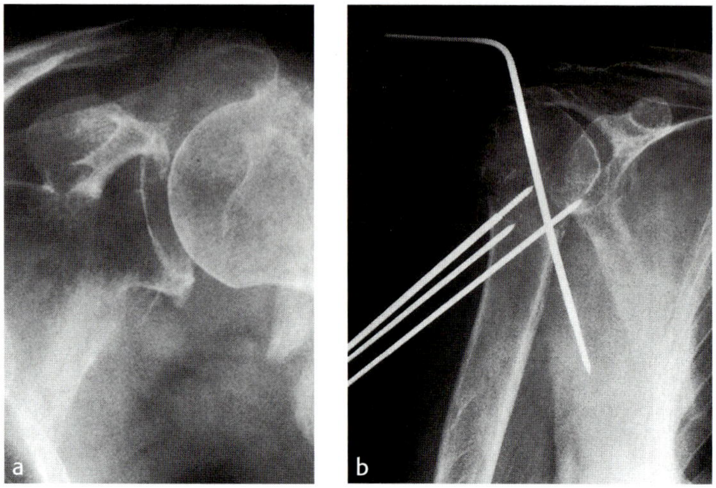
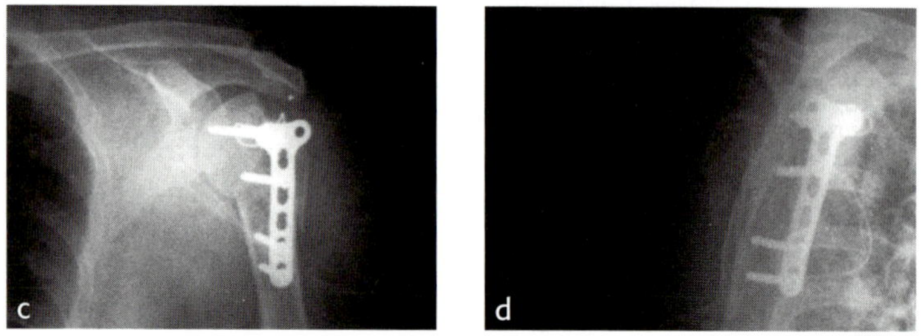

Fig 6.1.2-3a–d Examples of failed osteosynthesis.
a Nonunion after nonoperative treatment.
b Loosening and migration of pins with loss of reduction.
c–d Secondary loss of reduction with conventional plate due to inadequate stability.

Preoperative planning

Equipment

- Locking proximal humeral plate (LPHP) 3.5, 5 holes
- 3.5 mm self-tapping locking head screws (LHS)
- 3.5 mm cortex screws
- 2.0 mm K-wires
- Nonabsorbable sutures

(Size of system, instruments, and implants can vary according to anatomy.)

Patient preparation and positioning

Antibiotics: single dose 2nd generation cephalosporin
Thrombosis prophylaxis: none

Image intensifier on same side as operating team, able to swing 90° without moving the arm.

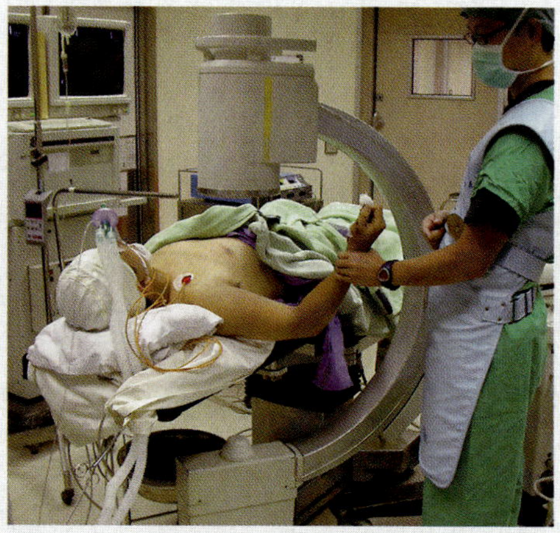

Fig 6.1.2-4 Semi beach chair position with arm freely moveable.

2 Surgical approach

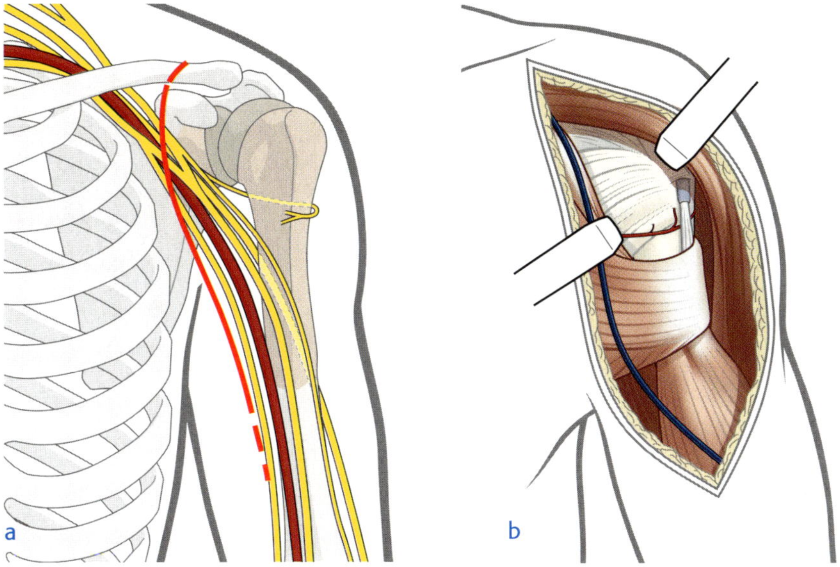

Fig 6.1.2-5a–b

- a Deltopectoral approach, cephalic vein protected medially. The bicipital groove and tendon are useful landmarks.
- b No violation of the rotator cuff. There is a small risk of injuring the axillary artery and axillary nerve.

3 Reduction

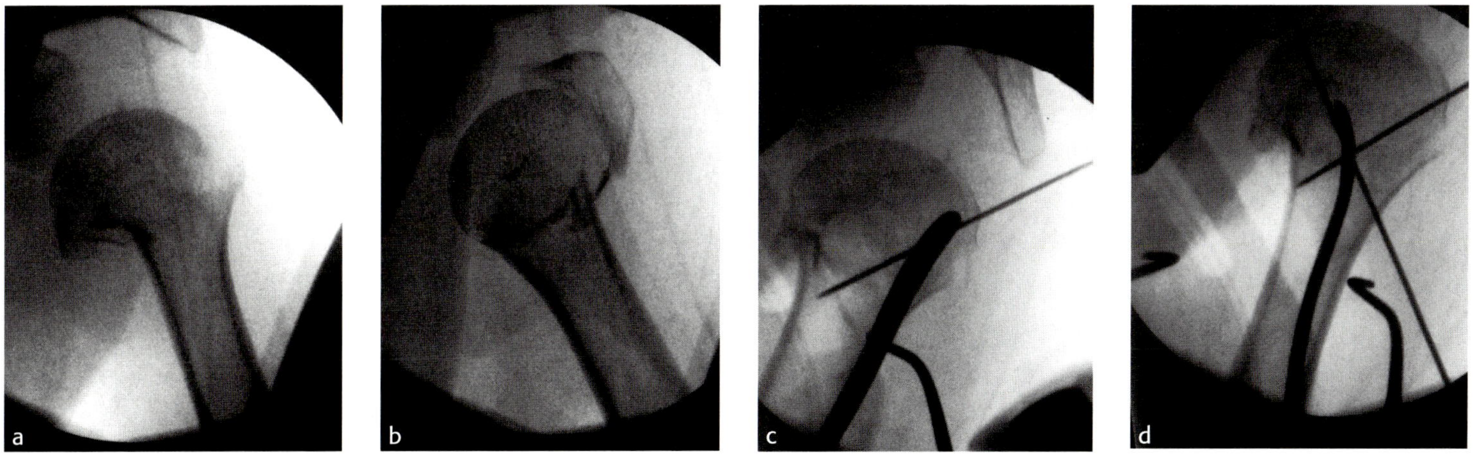

Fig 6.1.2-6a–d

- a–b Gentle reduction with the aid of bone spikes to derotate the tuberosity segment and to align the cervicotubercular cortex, especially the medial calcar.
- c–d Hold the reduction temporarily with at least two K-wires in two different planes. Check with the image intensifier to confirm reduction, axial and rotational alignment.

3 Reduction (cont)

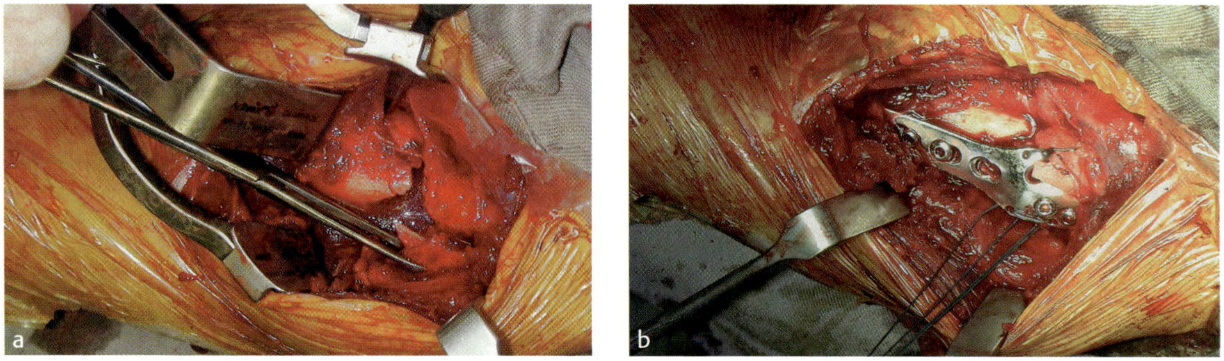

Fig 6.1.2-7a–b

a Metaphyseal comminution may be brought together by forceps and intraosseous sutures.

b Sutures tied to tubercles and brought through suture holes on the plate neutralize muscle tension and help to maintain reduction. A displaced fracture can be reduced using the plate as a reduction tool.

4 Fixation

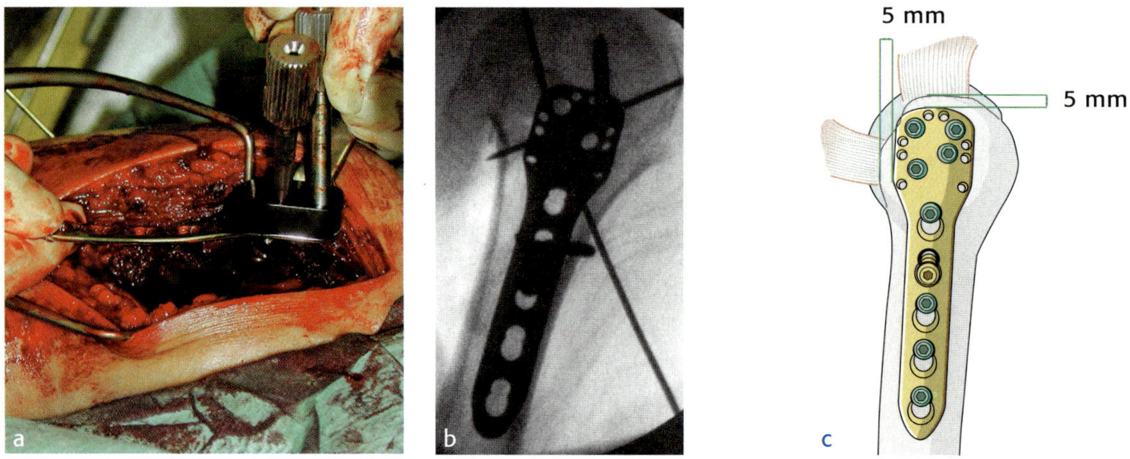

Fig 6.1.2-8a–c

a Apply the locking proximal humeral plate (LPHP) 3.5 with 5 holes to the anterolateral cortex 5 mm caudal to the proximal end of the greater tubercle and about 5 mm dorsal to the lateral edge of the bicipital groove, with drill sleeves attached to the plate as handles through the guiding block.

b–c Fix the plate onto the cortex of the shaft with one 3.5 mm cortex screw at the second most proximal combination hole. Check with the image intensifier to confirm position and to exclude overhang on the sides.

4 Fixation (cont)

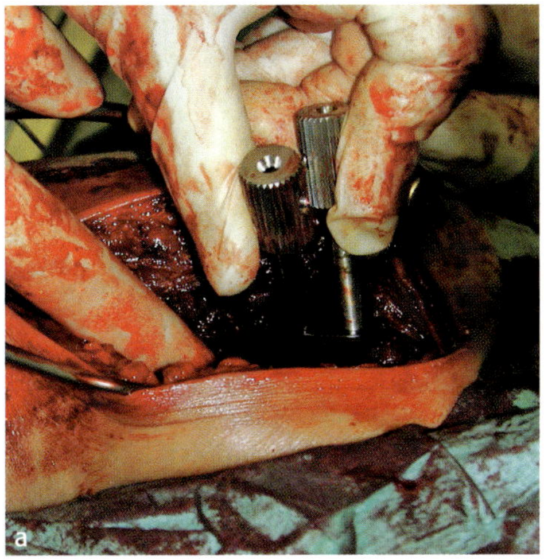

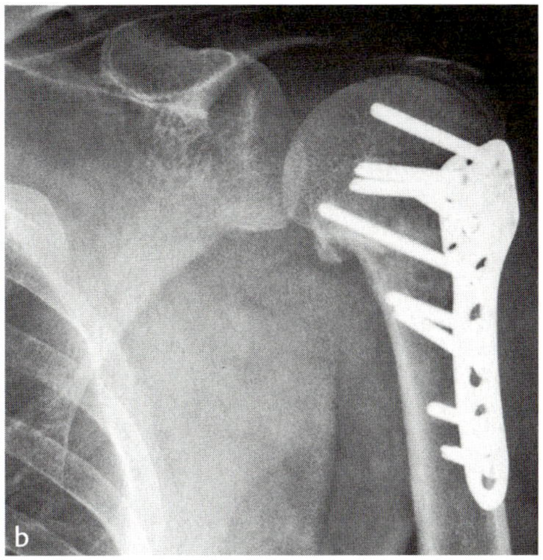

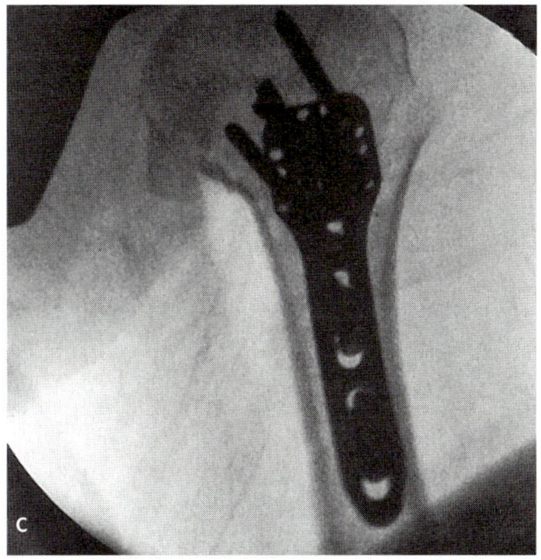

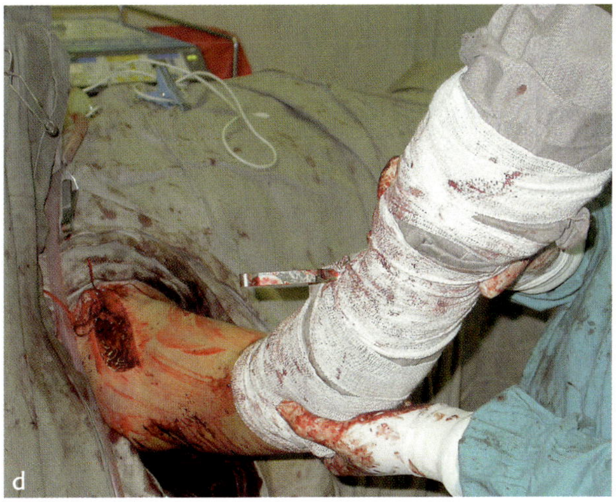

Fig 6.1.2-9a–d

- a Fix the proximal (head and neck) segment with four 3.5 mm self-tapping locking head screws in angular fashion with the aid of the guiding block.
- b Depending on the degree of metaphyseal comminution and bone quality, the most proximal combination hole can be filled with a cortex screw or a locking head screw in a cranial direction as a triangulation screw, or it can be left empty. Remove all K-wires. Fill the three distal holes with cortex screws or locking head screws.
- c Check with the image intensifier for alignment of the whole construct.
- d Ensure free arm motion before skin closure.

5 Rehabilitation

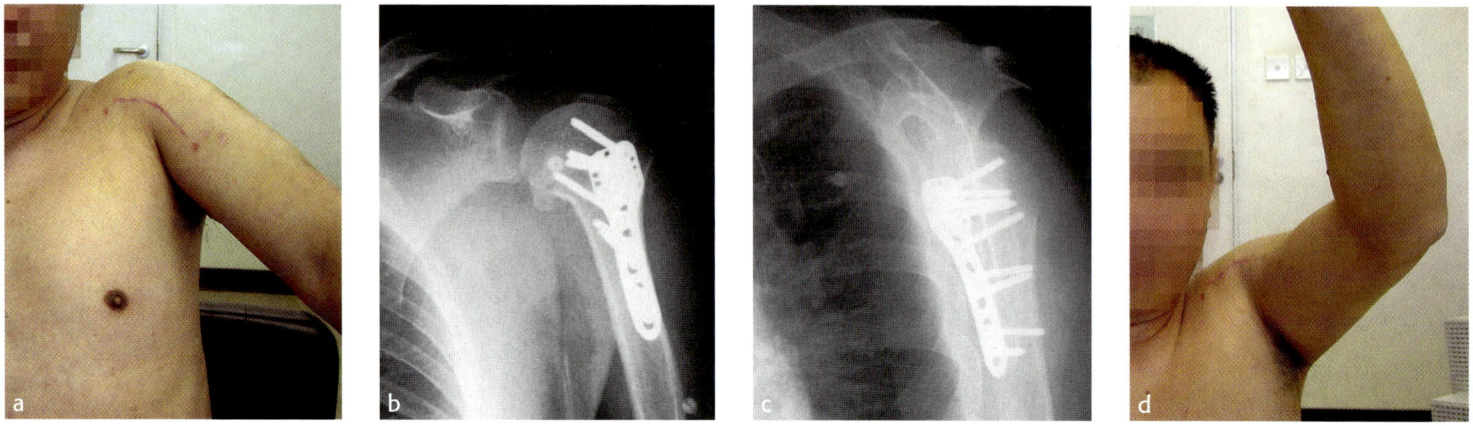

Fig 6.1.2-10a–d
a Clinical picture after 6 weeks.
b–c Postoperative x-ray after 2 weeks.
d Clinical picture after 18 weeks.

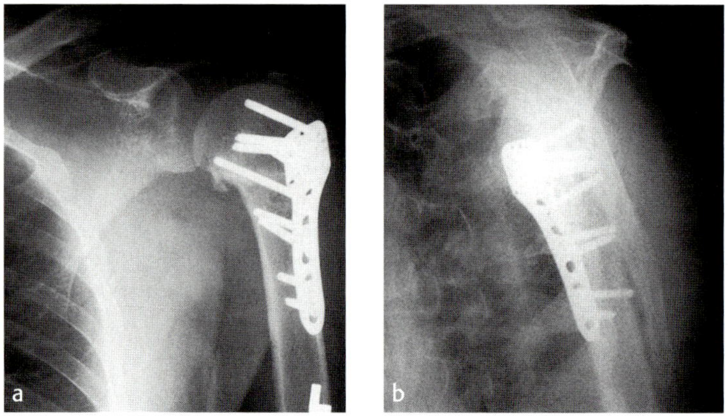

Fig 6.1.2-11a–b Postoperative x-rays after 8 months.
a AP view.
b Axial view.

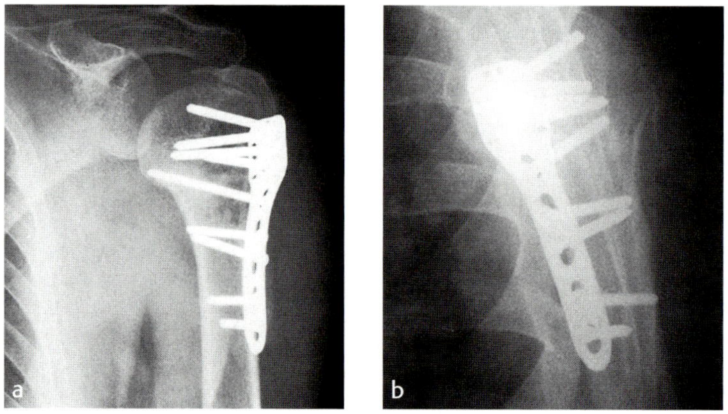

Fig 6.1.2-12a–b Postoperative x-rays after 1 year.
a AP view.
b Axial view.

Additional immobilization: arm sling for comfort.
Physiotherapy: pendulum exercises from first postoperative day. Gentle passive and active-assisted mobilization exercises under supervision of a physiotherapist by the first week.
Pharmaceutical treatment: analgesics if required.

6 Pitfalls –

Equipment
Insecure temporary fixation may push the proximal segment into varus, especially in osteoporotic bone.

Approach
Open approach may add damage to vascularity in this fracture.

Reduction and fixation
Axillary nerve and artery may be in danger. Metaphyseal comminution is difficult to control.

7 Pearls +

Equipment
The plate can be used to reduce the fracture. Plate precontoured to anatomy. Preset screw placement orientation provides angular stability. LHS are good for osteoporotic bone.

Approach
Direct assessment of vascularity through an open approach, proceed to hemiarthroplasty in elderly patients if complete disruption.

Reduction and fixation
Fig 6.1.2-13a–b Additional fragments may be fixed by intraosseous sutures brought through suture holes in the plate.

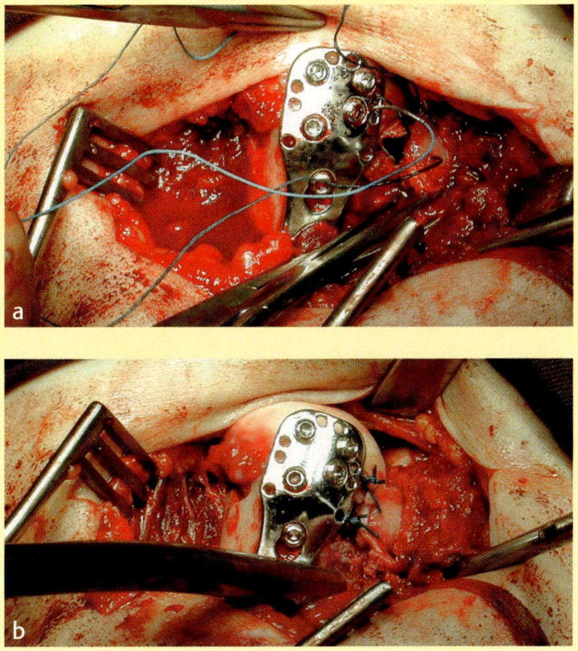

6 Pitfalls (cont) –

Rehabilitation

Too early overzealous exercise in type C fractures may result in loss of reduction.

7 Pearls (cont) +

Rehabilitation

The only implant that enables immediate mobilization with the potential to restore best possible mobility.

Author Reto Babst

6.1.3 Extraarticular bifocal proximal humeral fracture without metaphyseal impaction—11-B2

1 Case description

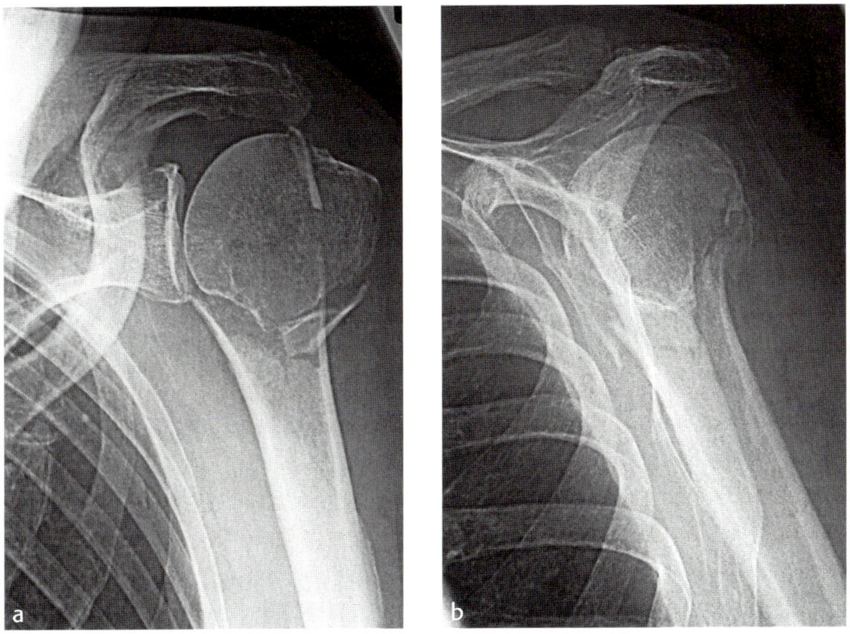

69-year-old man was caught in a machine and experienced rapid torsion of the upper extremity causing an open degloving wound around the elbow and a rupture of the brachioradial nerve.

The proximal humerus sustained a 3-part fracture, initially slightly displaced and was first treated conservatively.

The x-ray revealed a secondary displaced head fragment with minimal displacement of the greater tubercle, an impression between the greater tubercle and the bicipital groove, and an extension of the fracture through the lesser tubercle, with an additional metaphyseal fragment below the lesser tubercle.

Fig 6.1.3-1a–b
a AP view.
b Axial view.

Indication

Relevant dislocation with the danger of vascular compromise of the humeral head due to the displacement. Consider 2-D or 3-D CT scan for proper preoperative planning.

Preoperative planning

Equipment
- PHILOS proximal humeral plate 3.5, 3 holes
- 3.5 mm self-tapping locking head screws (LHS)
- 3.5 mm cortex screws
- 2.0 mm K-wires
- Bone punch
- Strong nonabsorbable sutures
- Equipment for bone graft harvesting
- Optional: calcium triphosphate bone substitute in block form

(Size of system, instruments,
and implants can vary according to anatomy.)

Patient preparation and positioning
Antibiotics: single dose 2nd generation cephalosporin
Thrombosis prophylaxis: low-molecular heparin

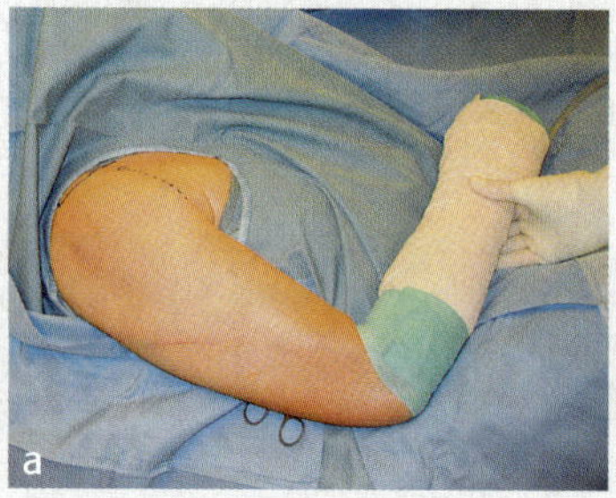
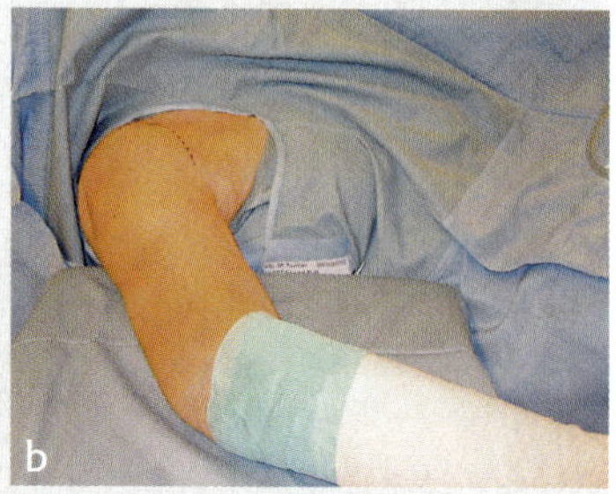

Fig 6.1.3-2a–b The beach chair position with an additional table allows the arm to be positioned in abduction. The deltoid muscle is therefore not under tension which also eases the approach to the posterior parts of the greater tubercle.
a Beach chair position.
b Beach chair position with an additional table.

2 Surgical approach

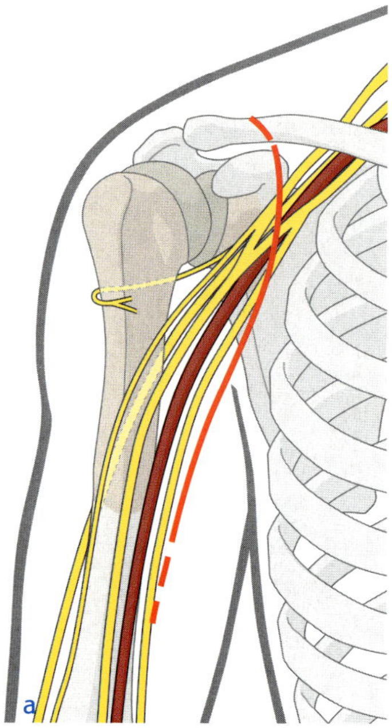
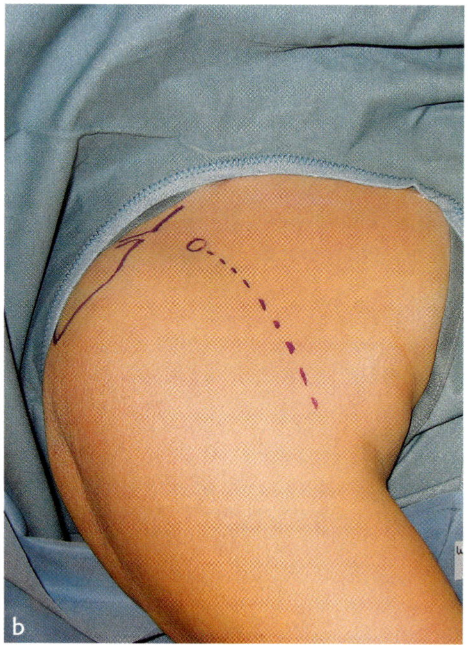

Fig 6.1.3-3a–b A slightly curved incision, starting below the coracoid process, of 6–8 cm is usually sufficient. Care should be taken to spare the cephalic vein, which is left on the lateral side. The clavipectoral fascia is incised lateral to the conjoint tendon.

3 Reduction and fixation

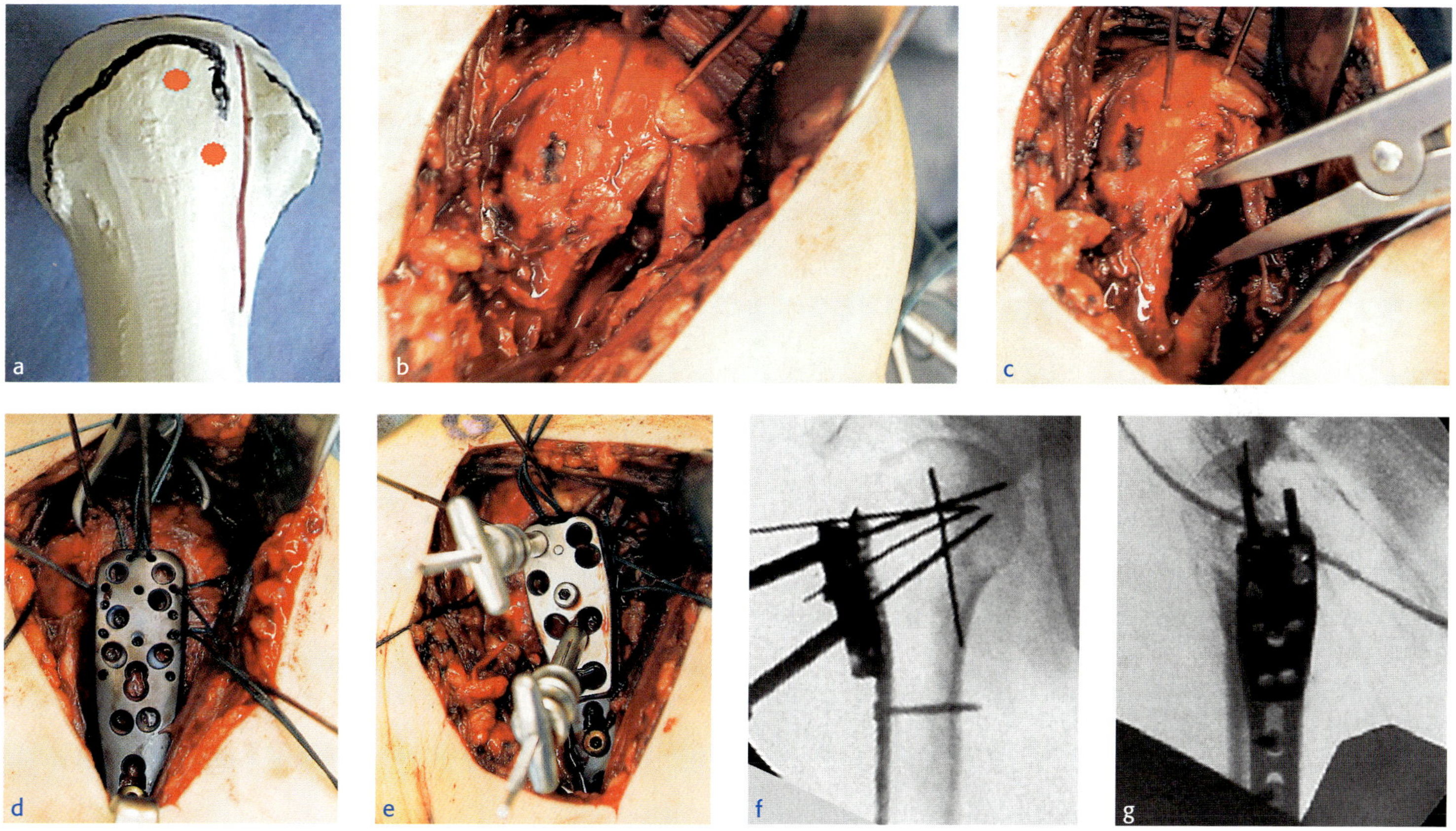

Video 6.1-1

Fig 6.1.3-4a–g

a–b The tubercles are fitted with 6.0 mm sutures as tension bands to help reduction. They can be used at the end of the fixation to tension band the tubercles against the plate. Two K-wires are placed as an orientation aid 5 mm below the top of the greater tubercle and 2–5 mm lateral to the bicipital groove.

c The fracture is then approximately reduced through the fracture gap with the help of a bone spreader and/or traction on the arm.

d The PHILOS plate is now brought onto the shaft by inserting the tension band sutures through the prepared holes in the plate. The plate is then fixed with a cortex screw through the gliding hole against the shaft. When tightening the screw, the head fragment is held with the tension band sutures (or with a pointed reduction forceps against the plate). Reduction is then achieved with the plate

e The aiming device (threaded drill sleeve) is then attached to the plate and the reduction is maintained with blocked 2.5 mm K-wires.

f–g Reduction is controlled with the image intensifier in AP/axial view.

When anatomical alignment is achieved, the locking head screws are inserted according to the needs of the fracture pattern. The screws in the shaft can either be locking head screws or cortex screws. If we use the latter in osteopenic bone they should be directed slightly obliquely, to get more threads engaged in the thin osteopenic cortex.

4 Rehabilitation

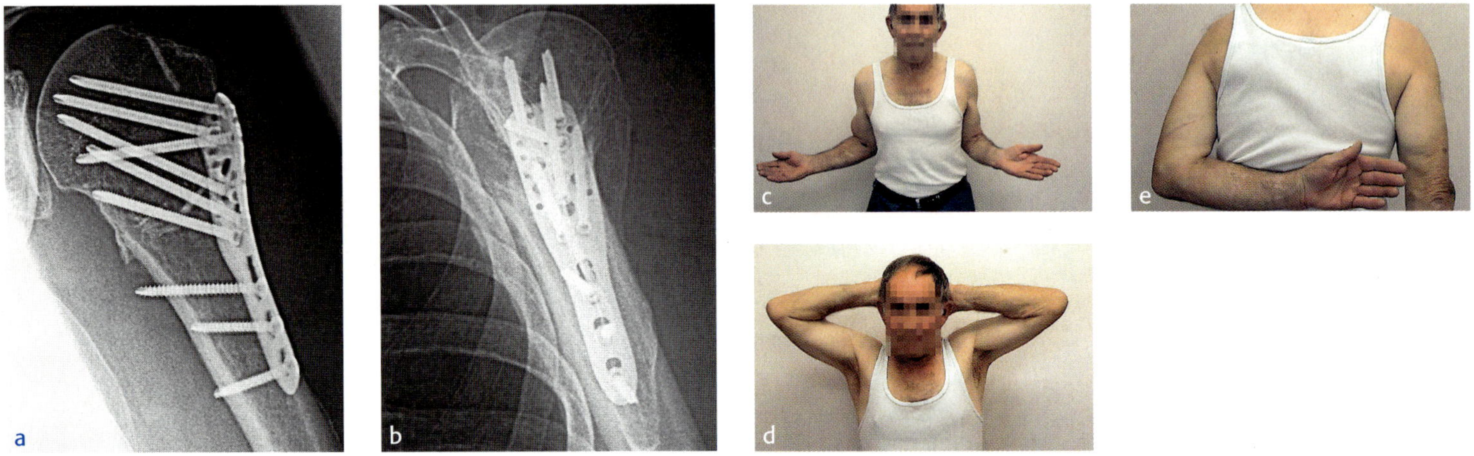

Postoperative immobilization with a Gilchrist bandage during the night; during the day a simple sling for 6 weeks is recommended.

Physiotherapy: functional rehabilitation with active-assisted movements with a physiotherapist as of the first postoperative day.

Weight bearing after 6 weeks and active and resistive training.

Pharmaceutical treatment: analgesics depending on the postoperative pain.

Fig 6.1.3-5a–e

a–b Postoperative x-rays 1 year after operation. The first screw through the gliding hole is too long since it was used to reduce the fracture with the plate. No signs of osteonecrosis.

c–e The patient has regained an almost full range of motion.

Implant removal

After 8–12 months if symptomatic.

5 Pitfalls –

Patient preparation and positioning

6 Pearls +

Patient preparation and positioning

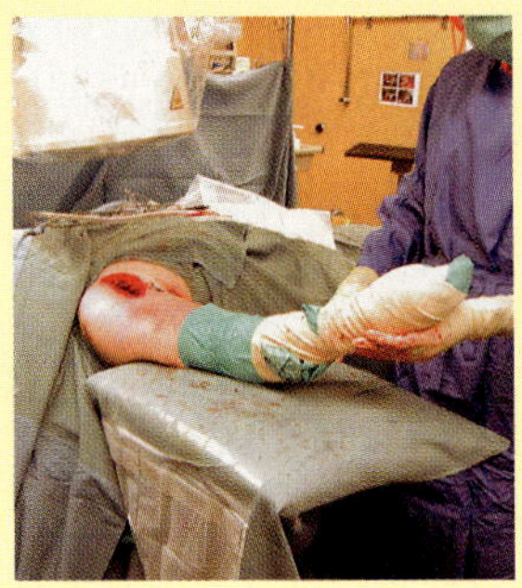

Fig 6.1.3-6 For elderly patients the beach chair position may be hazardous for cerebral perfusion, therefore a supine position on a radiolucent table using a side table allows exactly the same access for ORIF of the proximal humerus as the beach chair position.

5 Pitfalls – (cont)

Reduction and fixation

Placing the PHILOS plate too high will cause an impingement.

Reduction of the head fragment without maintaining its position against the plate will easily result in a varus position.

If there is comminution on the medial side of the neck, the head fragment tends to fall into varus.

Vigorous reduction maneuvers with reduction forceps have the potential to devascularize the head fragment.

6 Pearls + (cont)

Reduction and fixation

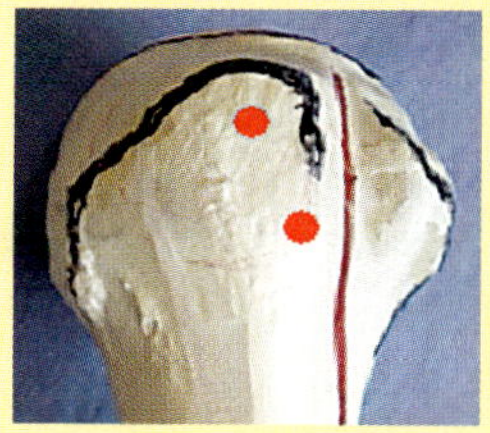

Fig 6.1.3-7 Put K-wires in the planned position of the plate. The red spots mark the proximal and anterior borderline of the plate.

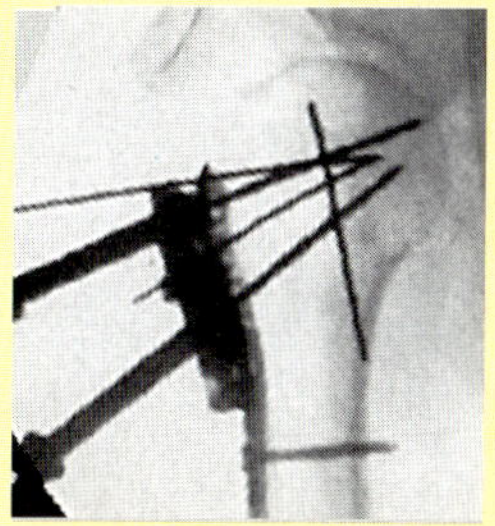

Fig 6.1.3-8 Maintain the head position with K-wires. This can also be achieved by 2.5 mm threaded K-wires locked with clamps from mini external fixator set.

Video 6.1-1

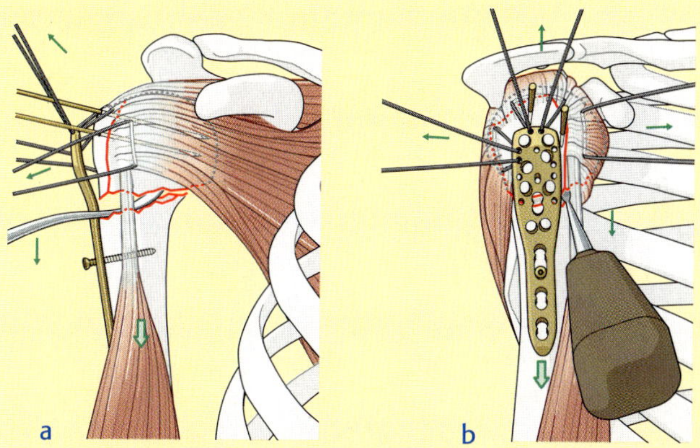

Fig 6.1.3-9a–b Use direct reduction techniques through the fracture gap, fix the head fragments temporarily and then use the plate to obtain reduction, especially in 3- and 4-part fractures.
A K-wire medially directed to support the head fragment until the proximal LHS are positioned can help to maintain the correct position.
Also, tension band sutures secure the fragments against the plate and help to hold the tubercle and the head in position.

Author Michael J Gardner, Dean G Lorich, David L Helfet

6.1.4 Extraarticular bifocal proximal humeral fracture with proximal diaphyseal extension—11-B2

1 Case description

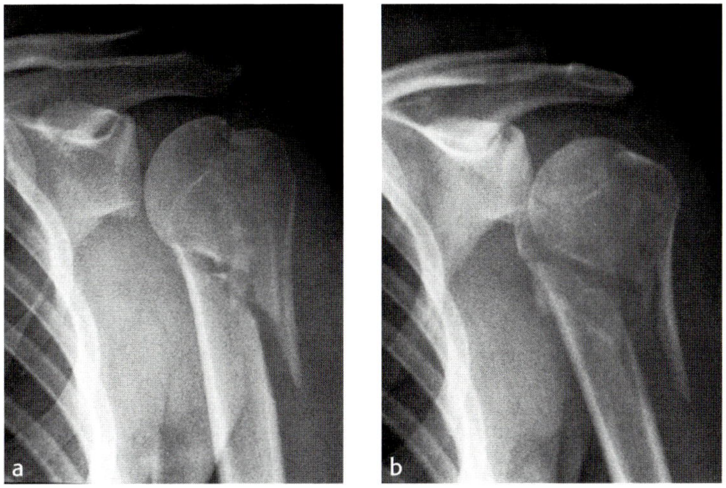

21-year-old active female fell from a height and landed on her left side. She sustained a spiral proximal humeral fracture and a greater tuberosity fracture. She also sustained several lumbar vertebral fractures.

Fig 6.1.4-1a–b
a AP view.
b Axial view.

Indication

Extraarticular proximal humeral neck fracture with a displaced proximal diaphyseal fragment and posteromedial butterfly fragment. The displacement, as well as the fracture obliquity, make this fracture very unstable and mandates reduction and fixation.

Preoperative planning

Equipment

- PHILOS proximal humeral plate 3.5, 5 holes
- Reconstruction plate 3.5, 5 holes
- 3.5 mm locking head screws (LHS)
- 3.5 mm cortex screws
- 2.0 mm K-wires with threaded tip
- Nonabsorbable sutures

(Size of system, instruments, and implants can vary according to anatomy.)

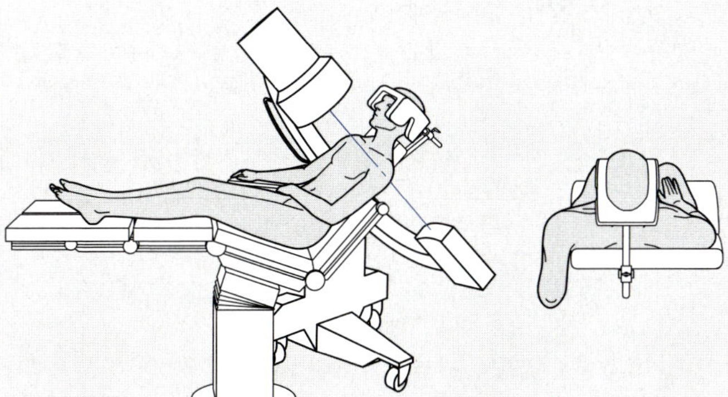

a b

Fig 6.1.4-2a–b The patient is placed in the beach chair position, with the back elevated 30° from the horizontal, and with the injured arm free from the edge of the table. The left shoulder and arm prepped and free draped for intraoperative mobility.

Patient preparation and positioning

Antibiotics: 2nd generation cephalosporin
Thrombosis prophylaxis: none

2 Surgical approach

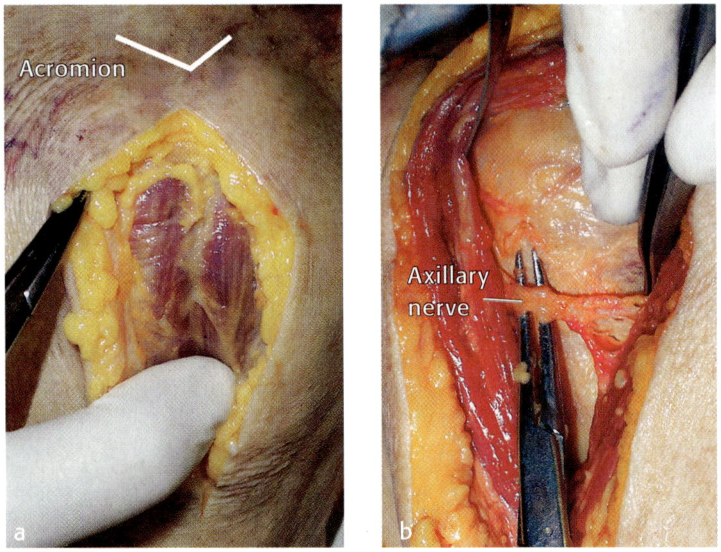

8 cm incision from the anterolateral corner of the acromion. Identify the anterior deltoid raphe. Sharply divide the raphe, beginning proximally.

Identify the axillary nerve motor branch and posterior humeral circumflex artery, which cross the humerus approximately 6.5 cm from the undersurface of the acromion and 3.5 cm from the lateral prominence of the greater tuberosity. Protect the neurovascular bundle with a vessel loop. Extend raphe incision distally down the humeral shaft as necessary.

Fig 6.1.4-3a–b Extended anterolateral acromial approach.

a Dissection in a cadaver using the extended anterolateral acromial approach demonstrates the appearance of the anterior deltoid raphe.

b Splitting the raphe in a cadaver reveals the axillary nerve, with no branches other than the main anterior motor branch crossing at this level.

3 Reduction and fixation

- Use threaded 2.0 mm K-wires as joysticks in the head fragment to reduce the fracture. Pay close attention to length, rotation, and alignment.
- Attach the aiming device to the plate and slide it distally along the head and shaft underneath the axillary nerve and vessel.
- Loop nonabsorbable sutures through the small holes in the proximal part of the plate.
- Insert cortex screws into the distal shaft fragment to stabilize the plate on the bone distally.
- Use K-wires to reduce the fracture and for temporary fixation.
- Attach threaded guides to the proximal part of the plate, and insert K-wires into the humeral head provisionally.
- Recheck reduction with the image intensifier.
- Insert locking head screws through the plate into the humeral head.
- In the case of an oblique or spiral fracture with extension to the proximal diaphysis, place a reconstruction plate anteriorly at the apex of the spike to buttress the reduction.
- Use threaded K-wires to reduce and stabilize the greater tuberosity, and place the proximal end of the plate to buttress the fragment. Using a free needle, pass the sutures through the rotator cuff tendons to supplement fixation. These act as tension bands to indirectly reduce and stabilize the tuberosity and head fragments to the shaft.

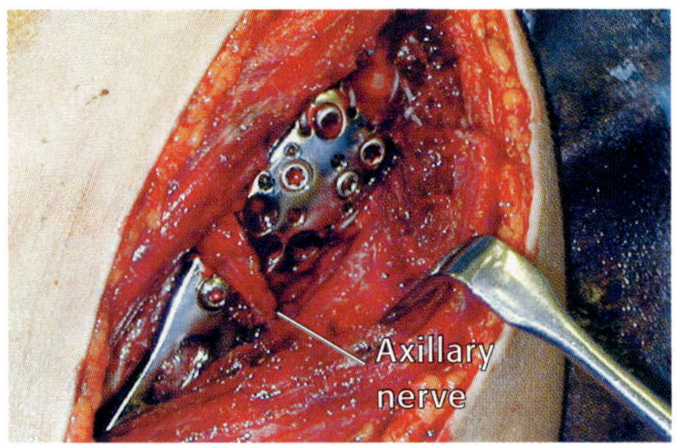

Fig 6.1.4-4 Intraoperatively, the plate was slid underneath the protected axillary nerve. The holes in the plate are used for sutures to tension band the rotator cuff tendons to enhance stability.

4 Rehabilitation

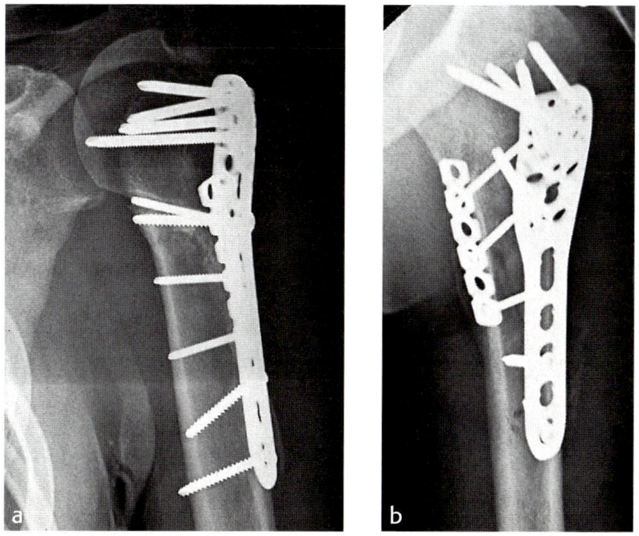

Apply sterile dressings and place the extremity in sling immobilization.

Administer prophylactic postoperative antibiotics for 24 hours.

Physiotherapy: begin gentle active and passive range of motion immediately on postoperative day one. A continuous passive motion machine is often helpful to prevent stiffness.

Fig 6.1.4-5a–b 5 months postoperatively. Significant healing of the fracture and maintenance of implant position is seen.

Implant removal

If the fracture is healed and the implant becomes symptomatic, it may be removed through a similar approach at a minimum of 12 months.

5 Pitfalls –

Approach

The main risk with this approach is damage to the anterior motor branch of the axillary nerve at the level of the deltoid raphe.

Reduction and fixation

The axillary nerve and vessel may be injured during hardware and fracture manipulation.

Rehabilitation

Prolonging physiotherapy may lead to shoulder dysfunction and aggressive therapy may lead to fixation failure.

6 Pearls +

Approach

This surgical approach is a more direct and less-invasive approach to proximal humeral fractures and is particularly useful for greater tuberosity fractures. It allows direct access to the lateral metaphysis while requiring less soft-tissue stripping. The neurovascular bundle must be sought, based on anatomical landmarks, through careful dissection. Although the posterior humeral circumflex artery contributes to only a small portion of the humeral head blood supply, this should be protected as well.

Reduction and fixation

The neurovascular bundle must be visualized and handled carefully during manipulation.

Rehabilitation

A careful balance between early physiotherapy to prevent shoulder stiffness, and gentle mobilization to avoid stressing the implant must be found.

Author James P Stannard

6.1.5 Extraarticular bifocal proximal humeral fracture with glenohumeral dislocation—11-B3

1 Case description

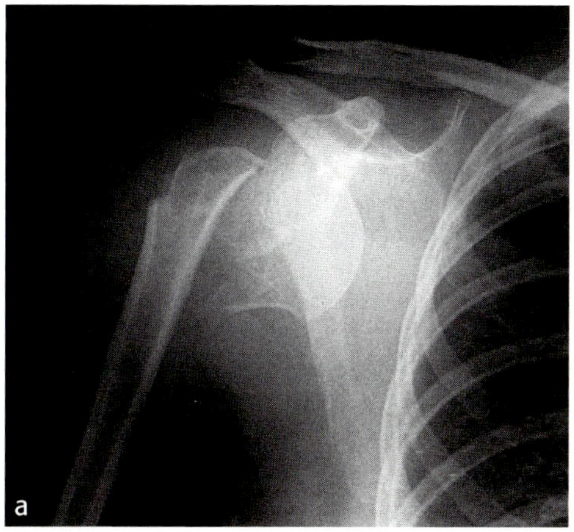

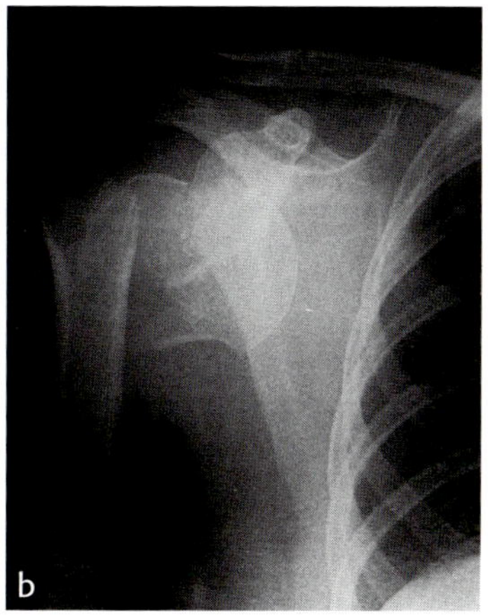

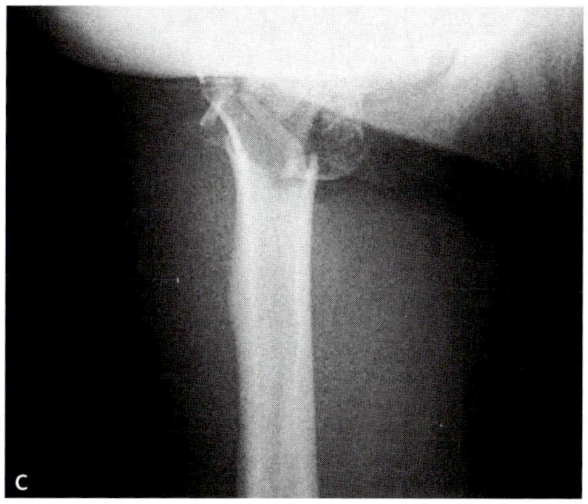

Fig 6.1.5-1a–c
a AP view.
b True AP view.
c Axillary lateral view.

36-year-old woman fell on her right dominant shoulder in a motorcycle accident.
Type of injury: high-energy. Multiple trauma: liver laceration.
Closed head injury, shoulder dislocation, closed fracture.

Indication

Most proximal humeral fractures are low energy injuries with minimal displacement and are suitable for nonoperative treatment. The advantages of nonoperative treatment include a lower complication rate and acceptable functional outcome as long as the fracture has adequate stability to allow early motion of the shoulder. Disadvantages of the nonoperative approach include frequent loss of some motion, primarily forward flexion and abduction above shoulder height.

Indications for surgical treatment include:

- displaced 2-, 3-, or 4-part fractures that cannot be reduced to a stable position using closed reduction,
- medial comminution and instability,
- irreducible fracture dislocations,
- head splitting fractures, and
- open proximal humeral fractures.

Relative indications include:

- multiple trauma patients who need partial use of their upper extremity for weight bearing,
- bilateral proximal humeral fractures,
- fracture dislocations, and
- dominant arm in younger, active patients.

Advantages of surgical treatment of unstable fractures include improved restoration of the anatomy of the proximal humerus and improved stability to allow early motion of the shoulder. Disadvantages include an increased incidence of complications such as: infection, nonunion, hardware complications, heterotopic ossification, and osteonecrosis of the humeral head.

Preoperative planning

Equipment
- PHILOS proximal humeral plate 3.5, 3 holes
- 3.5 mm locking head screws (LHS)
- K-wires
- Sutures

(Size of system, instruments, and implants can vary according to anatomy.)

Patient preparation and positioning
Antibiotics: cephalosporin
Thrombosis prophylaxis: low-molecular heparin

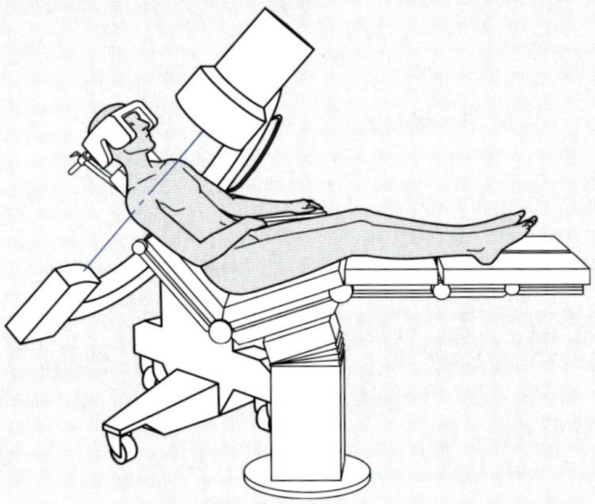

Fig 6.1.5-2 The most useful position for the patient is to be either supine or in the beach chair position with a roll under the affected shoulder elevating that side approximately 30°. A radiolucent table should be used to allow x-ray views to be obtained. The entire arm receives a sterile preparation and is draped free so that it is freely mobile. This position allows the surgeon and assistants to have full access to the proximal humerus while significantly improving the ability to obtain appropriate x-rays using the image intensifier.

2 Surgical approach

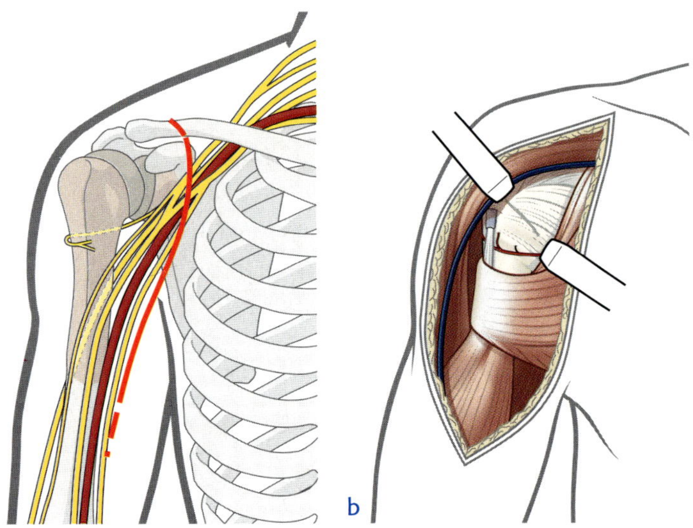

Fig 6.1.5-3a–b
- a Deltopectoral approach. The incision is made in a straight 10–15 cm line from just above the coracoid process in the line of the deltopectoral groove.
- b The internervous plane is between the deltoid muscle (axillary nerve) and the pectoralis major muscle (medial and lateral pectoral nerve).
  The deep anatomy is frequently distorted due to the trauma. The short head of the biceps and the coracobrachialis muscle are both retracted medially, allowing access to the anterior part of the shoulder. Beneath these muscles are the transversely oriented fibers of the subscapularis muscle, which forms the only remaining anterior covering of the joint capsule. If this muscle has not already been torn from its insertion, it will have to be released and tagged with stay sutures for repair at the end of the case.

2 Surgical approach (cont)

The cephalic vein is identified and generally retracted laterally along with the deltoid muscle. The pectoralis major is retracted medially.
It is frequently helpful to gently place a blunt retractor superiorly and posteriorly to help reduce the greater tuberosity back to the remainder of the humeral head.

Dangers of this approach include the musculocutaneous nerve, and the axillary nerve at the inferior border of the subscapularis tendon.

3 Reduction

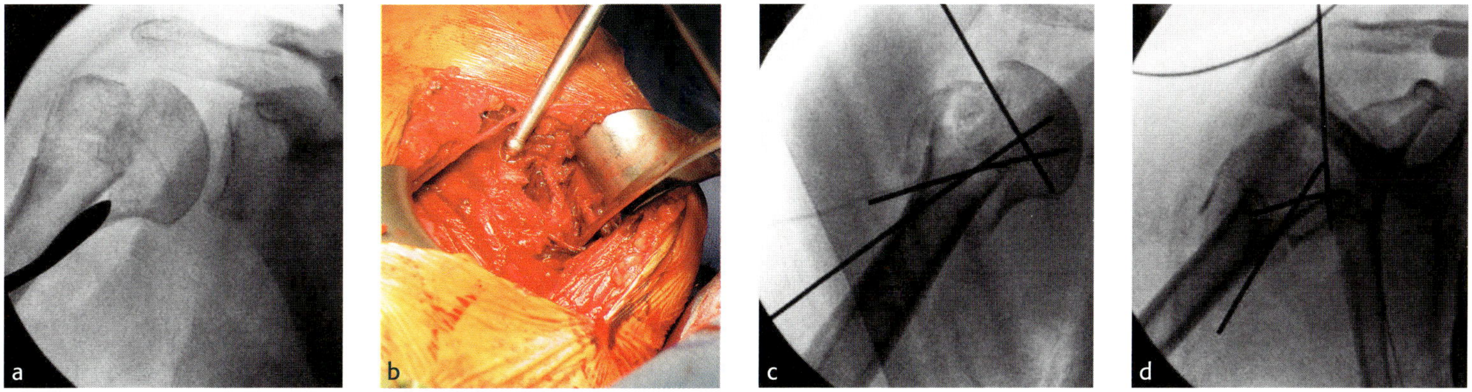

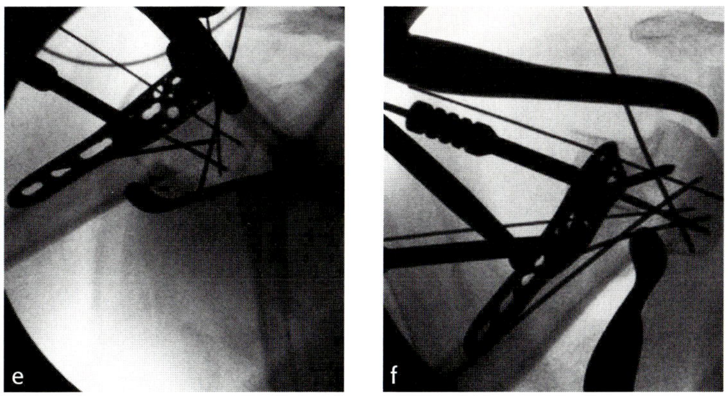

Fig 6.1.5-4a-f
- a Gentle reduction of the humeral head from subcoracoid dislocation using longitudinal traction combined with manipulation from either the surgeon's finger or a blunt instrument, such as a blunt Hohmann retractor, around the head of the humerus.
- b Carefully place the blunt Hohmann retractor around the greater tuberosity to assist in reduction of the tuberosity and improve visualization.
  Reduce the shaft to the humeral head using traction with assistance from the ball spike if necessary.
- c–d Hold the reduction of the fracture by placing temporary K-wires to stabilize the shaft and greater tuberosity to the humeral head.
- e–f Pin plate in place with K-wires after checking the reduction and making adjustments as necessary.

4 Fixation

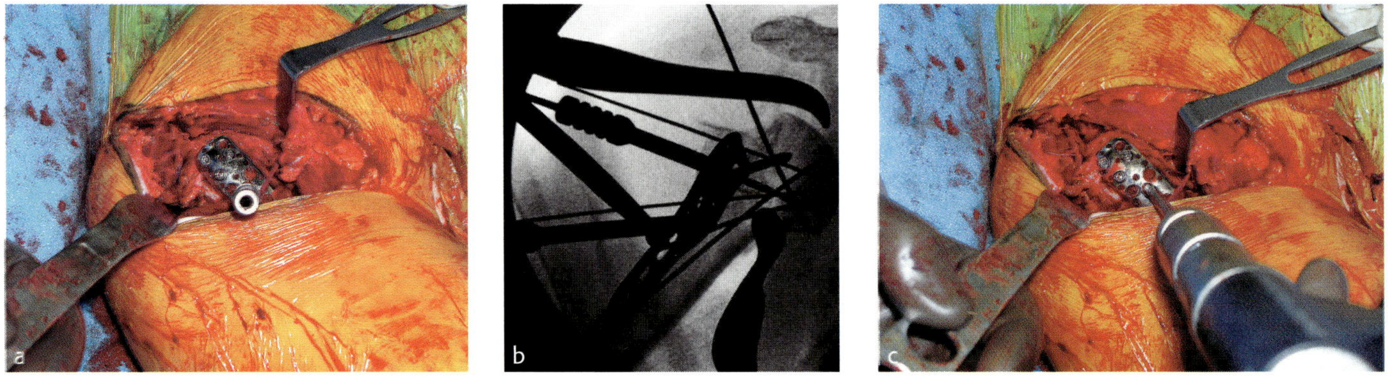

Fig 6.1.5-5a–j

a–b Thread the 2.8 mm drill guide into the PHILOS plate, and drill with a 2.8 mm drill bit to the subchondral bone. This step should be done using image intensification in both the AP and lateral planes by rotating the image intensifier. After completing the drilling, remove the drill guide and measure the screw length using a standard small fragment depth gauge.

c Apply a locking head screw (LHS) using power with the torquelimiting attachment to the screwdriver. The final tightening must be done by hand using the torque-limiting screwdriver.

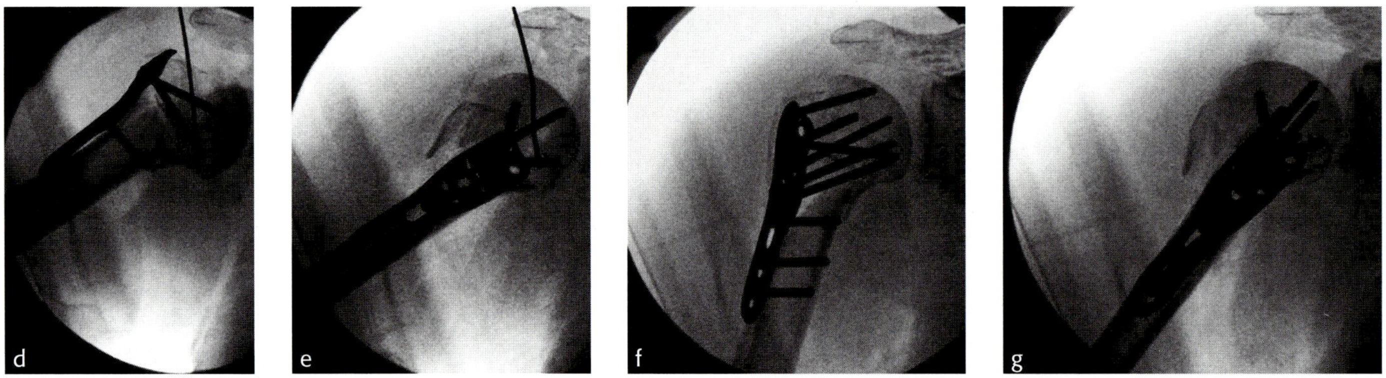

d–e The process is then repeated placing multiple screws at divergent angles.

f–g The diaphyseal screws are placed through the combination holes that can be either locking head screws or cortex screws, depending upon the fracture pattern, the bone quality, and surgeon's preference.

4 Fixation (cont)

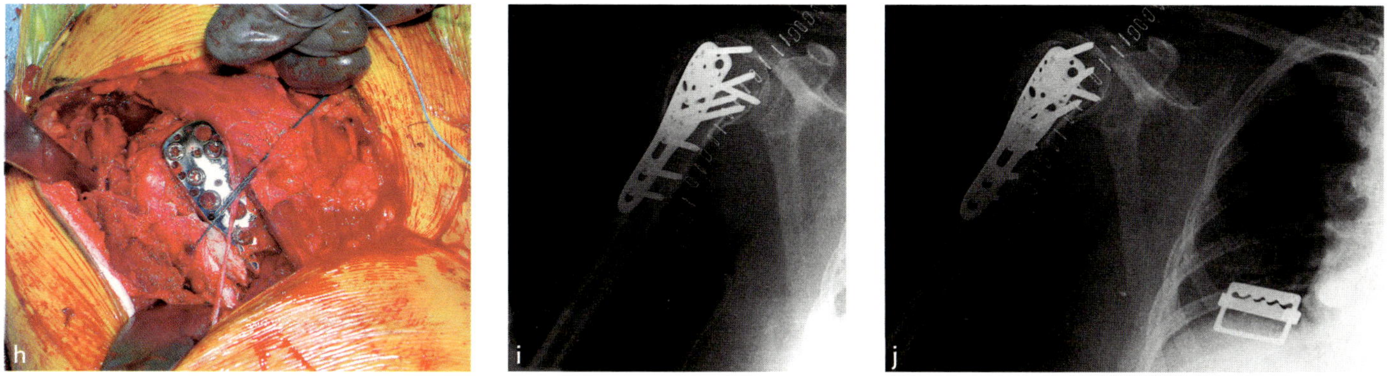

Fig 6.1.5-5a-j (cont)

h–j Holes have been manufactured into the proximal plate to allow placement of sutures to reduce and stabilize large fragments not captured by the locking plate and screws. Suture stabilization was very helpful with one large fragment in this case.

Irrigate the surgical site and close the wound.

5 Rehabilitation

Additional immobilization: sling or shoulder immobilizer for comfort only.
Mobilization: passive mobilization after one day. Active mobilization after 4 weeks.
Physiotherapy: beginning on first postoperative day.

6 Pitfalls –

Equipment

Reduction can be difficult to achieve with 3- and 4-part fractures.

Reduction and fixation

Be aware of medial column comminution. The fracture will tend to fall into a varus mal- or nonunion if locking head screws that approach the subchondral bone are not used.

Alternatively, attach the aiming device to the proximal end of the plate and use the triple trocar system to place a wire and measure the screw length. It is preferred to use the technique described above in this case rather than the technique here, because the aiming device is bulky and requires more extensive exposure and consequent soft-tissue stripping.

Rehabilitation

7 Pearls +

Equipment

A ball spike can aid in obtaining the reduction. Also, use temporary K-wires and a blunt Hohmann retractor over the greater tuberosity to obtain an adequate reduction.

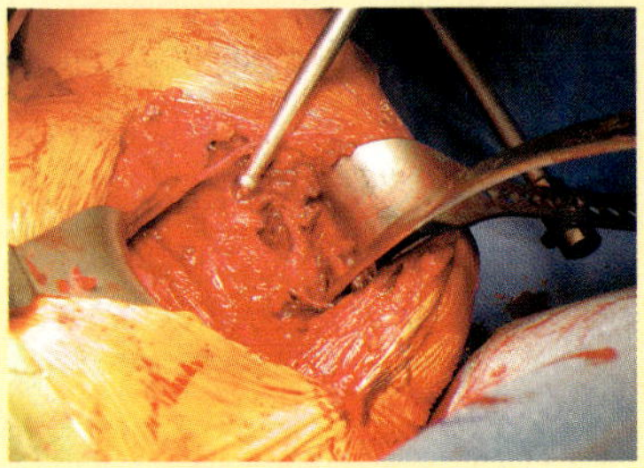

Fig 6.1.5-6 Hohmann retractor over the tuberosity.

Reduction and fixation

The first hole coming down the shaft is oblong and allows the plate to be moved a short distance either proximally or distally as needed to improve the fit.

Use a suture through the plate holes and at the insertion of the supraspinatus to stabilize the greater tuberosity or other major fragments if they are not stabilized adequately by the plate and screws.

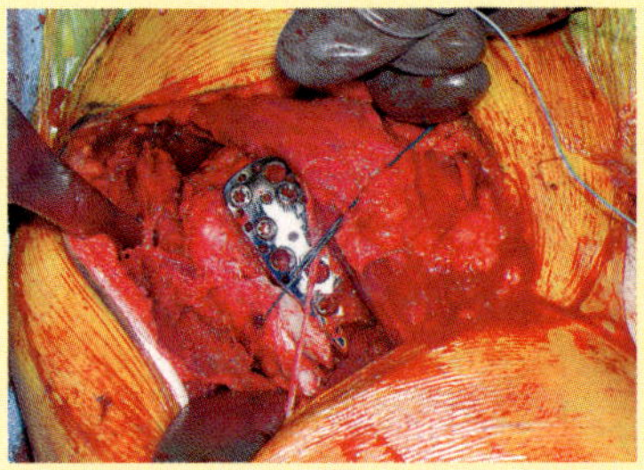

Fig 6.1.5-7 Suture fixation.

Rehabilitation

Early motion beginning on postoperative day number one is critical to the final result. Adequate stability must be achieved to allow early motion.

Author Norbert Südkamp

6.1.6 Intraarticular proximal humeral fracture with slight displacement—11-C1

1 Case description

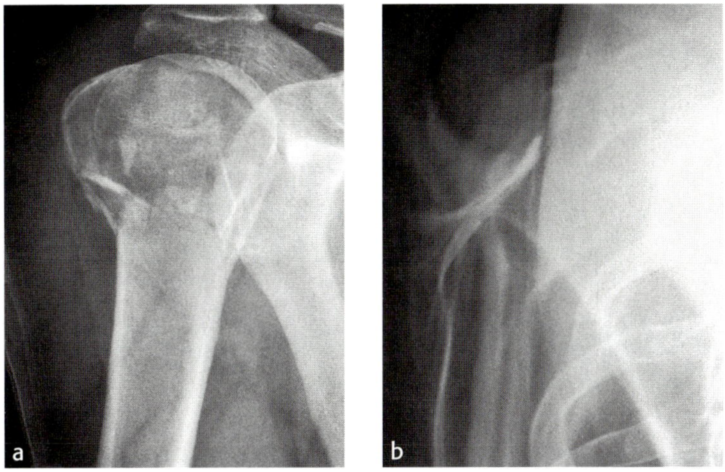

55-year-old man had a fall during skiing resulting in low energy monotrauma and closed fracture.

Fig 6.1.6-1a–b
a AP view.
b Lateral view.

Indication

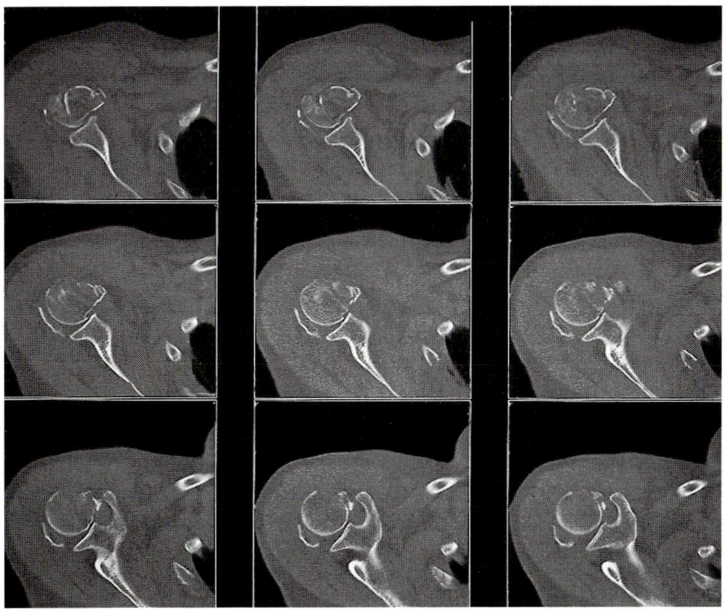

This valgus impacted 3-part fracture is an indication for surgery in this age group (even in elderly patients)—if there is a functional demand. Restoration of the anatomy of the proximal humerus is a prerequisite for correct function of the rotator cuff and the shoulder joint.
To fully analyze the extent of the injury, it is usually necessary to conduct a CT scan from the injury region.
Nevertheless, a conservative treatment could be discussed in such a case. Advantages, disadvantages, and probable outcomes of the different treatment options have to be discussed with the patients to enable them to make this personal choice.

Fig 6.1.6-2 CT scans of the valgus impacted 3-part fracture.

Preoperative planning

Equipment

- Locking proximal humeral plate (LPHP), 5 holes
- 3.5 mm self-tapping locking head screws (LHS)
- 3.5 mm cortex screws
- 1.8 mm K-wires
- Reduction forceps

(Size of system, instruments, and implants can vary according to anatomy.)

Patient preparation and positioning

Antibiotics: single dose 2nd generation cephalosporin

Thrombosis prophylaxis: low-molecular heparin

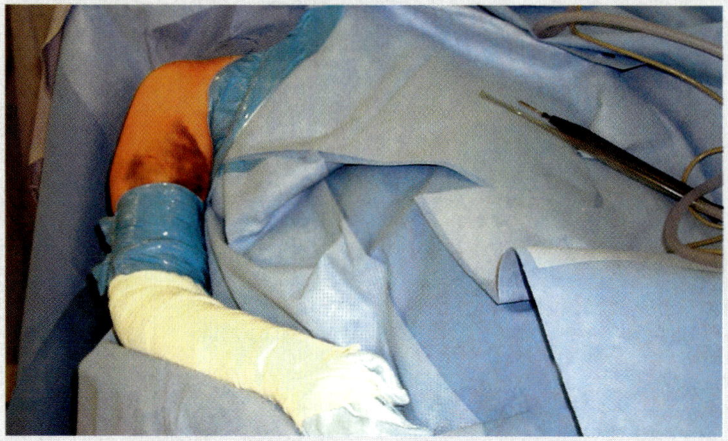

Fig 6.1.6-3 Supine position of the patient with separate arm rest.

2 Surgical approach

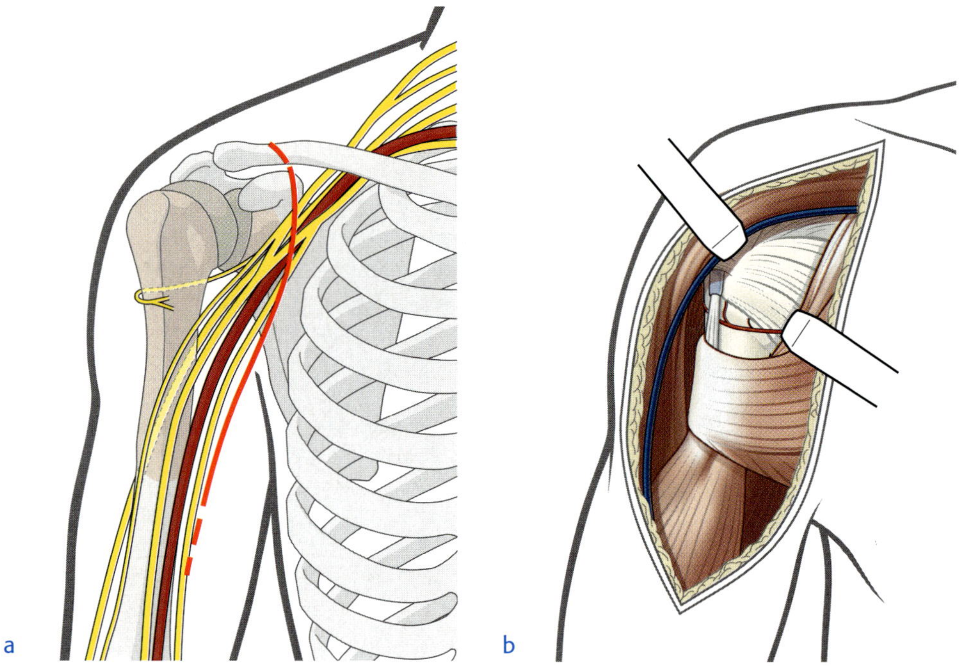

Fig 6.1.6-4a–b Deltopectoral approach. The anterior approach in the deltopectoral groove is used. Starting at the coracoid process, a skin incision of approximately 10 cm is performed along the deltopectoral groove.

The subcutaneous tissue is split. The muscle fascia is incised and the cephalic vein is prepared. The vein will be kept to the lateral side with the deltoid muscle since it is the draining vein for the deltoid. The muscles are split and the proximal humerus exposed. The fragments are carefully treated so as not to violate the vascular supply of the attached soft tissues.

3 Reduction

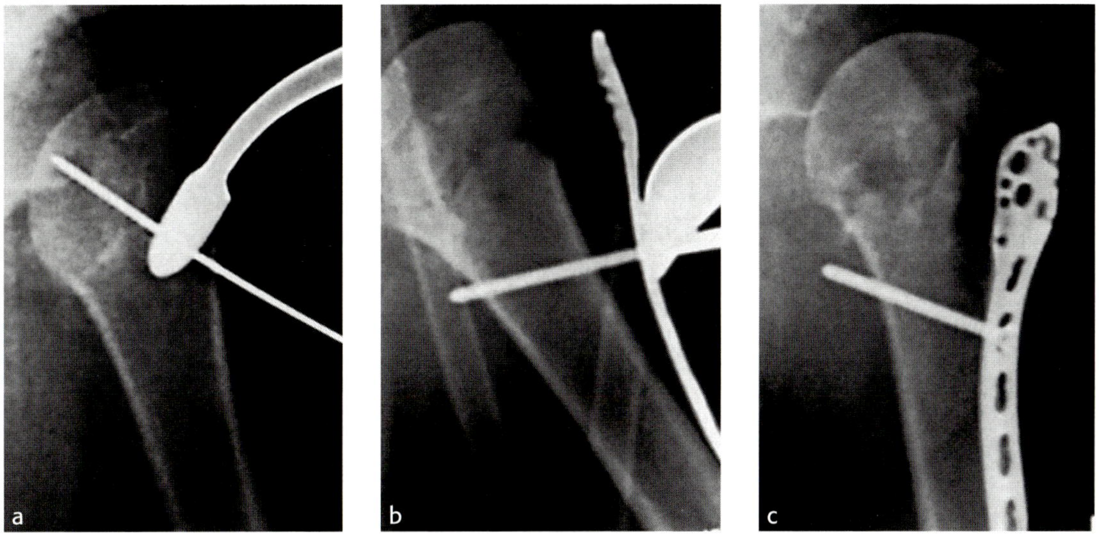

Fig 6.1.6-5a–c Reduction with an elevator through the fracture and indirect reduction with the help of the locking proximal humeral plate and a 3.5 mm cortex screw.

To ease reduction, long-term absorbable sutures are placed in all three tendons of the rotator cuff. Next to the sutures an elevator can be inserted through the fracture, with which the fragment is manipulated into the correct position. In some cases, the plate that is positioned lateral to the bicipital groove can also be used for indirect reduction to reduce the head fragment from its valgus position into an anatomical one.

Reduction can then be maintained temporarily with K-wires or a pointed reduction forceps. The locking proximal humeral plate can be fixed to the head fragment with K-wires through the suture holes in the proximal plate section.
The image intensifier is used to verify correct reduction in two planes. If the reduction is not satisfactory, these steps are repeated until the reduction is acceptable.

4 Fixation

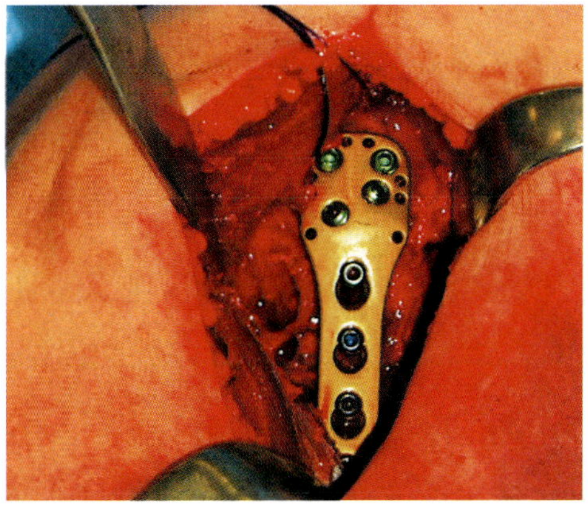

Fixation is then performed with locking head screws in the proximal part of the fracture, using the appropriate drill guide. Care must be taken not to perforate the head or rather the cartilage with the drill bit and to have the correct lengths of the screws so as not to injure the joint during early functional treatment with too long screws. The shaft portion can be fixed with 3.5 mm cortex screws or locking head screws. In elderly patients with some osteoporosis, locking head screws are preferred while for younger patients with good bone quality 3.5 mm cortex screws are used.

Fig 6.1.6-6 Finished fixation using locking head screws. Suture fixation is not yet finished at this stage.

4 Fixation (cont)

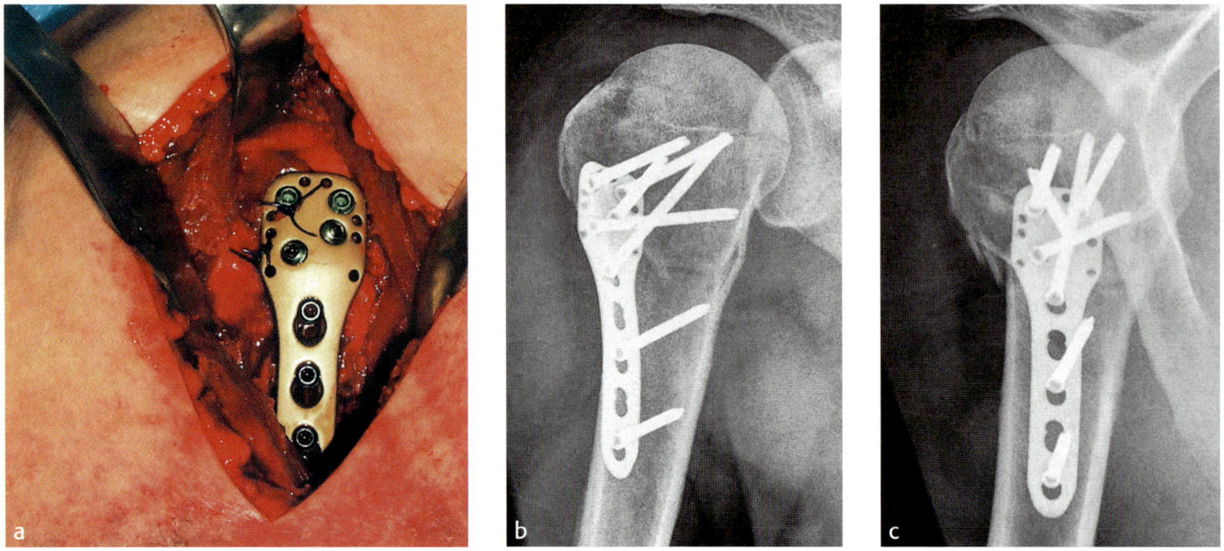

The fixation is controlled with the image intensifier and finally the prepositioned sutures are fixed to the plate. This increases the intrinsic stability of the construct and enhances stability of the fixation for early functional postoperative treatment.

Fig 6.1.6-7a–c
a Final result with LPHP and attached sutures.
b Postoperative x-ray control, AP view.
c Postoperative x-ray control, lateral view.

5 Rehabilitation

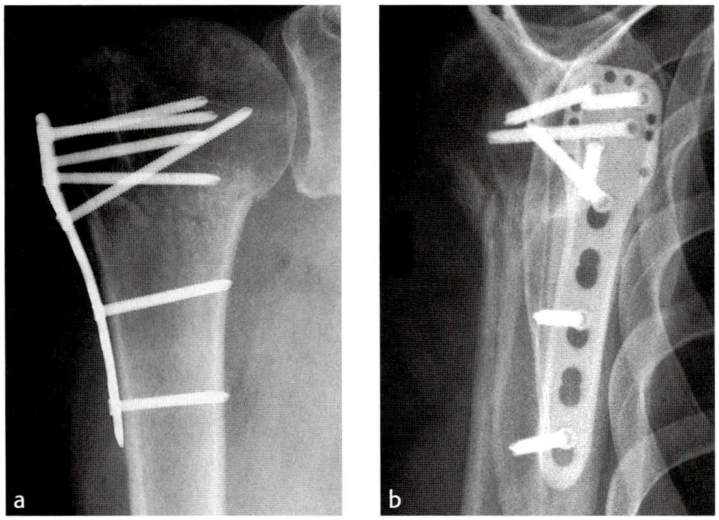

Postoperatively, the arm was put in an arm sling for 2 days and early functional postoperative treatment was started on day three with pendulum exercises. Active-assisted and passive motion exercises. Additionally, a continuous passive motion machine is advantageous.
Thrombosis prophylaxis is terminated after 5 days.

Fig 6.1.6-8a–b Follow up x-rays after 9 weeks.
a AP view.
b Lateral view.

5 Rehabilitation (cont)

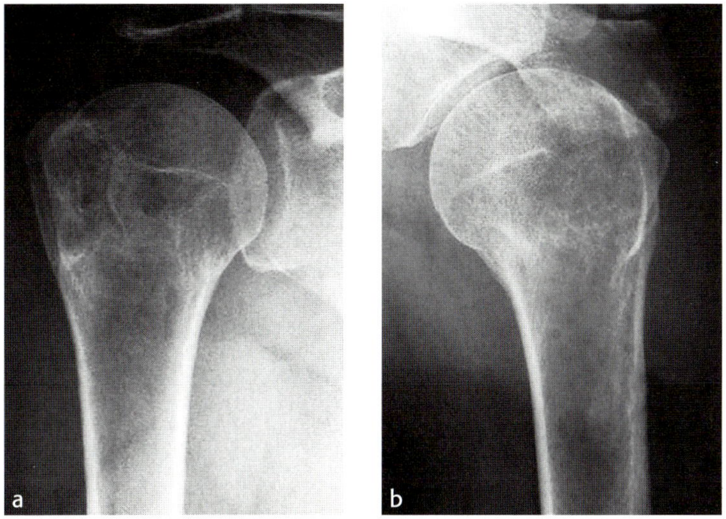

Implant removal

Implant removal is not mandatory. If necessary or desired by the patient, it is usually performed after 3–6 months.

Fig 6.1.6-9a–b Follow up x-rays after 1 year.
a AP view.
b Lateral view.

6 Pitfalls –

Equipment

Inadequate preoperative imaging may result in poor understanding of the fracture pattern and position of the fragment. Intraoperative denuding of fragments for better visualization is necessary and may result in avascular necrosis.

Reduction

Incorrect reduction and failure to maintain reduction is mostly due to inadequate intraoperative imaging. Usually in the beach chair position, the second plane can only be obtained with movement of the arm—this may result in loss of reduction.

Fixation

Incorrect intraoperative imaging may also result in improper screw lengths, which then perforate the head. This is only detected at postoperative x-ray control.
Violation of subchondral bone in the head area with the drill bit can later result in secondary screw perforation through the head.

7 Pearls +

Equipment

With increasing experience only standard shoulder instruments and the instrumentation for the LPHP/ PHILOS are necessary to successfully complete the case. For improved intraoperative visualization, the supine position usually allows better access with the image intensifier. A lateral approach with two incisions (sparing the axillary nerve) can also be considered.

Reduction

Prior to reducing the fracture it is advisable to insert sutures into the three tendons of the rotator cuff. Pulling on these sutures improves reduction maneuvers and helps to maintain reduction.

Fixation

The use of the aiming block improves the precision of screw direction.

Author Frankie Leung

6.1.7 Intraarticular proximal humeral fracture with valgus malalignment—11-C2

1 Case description

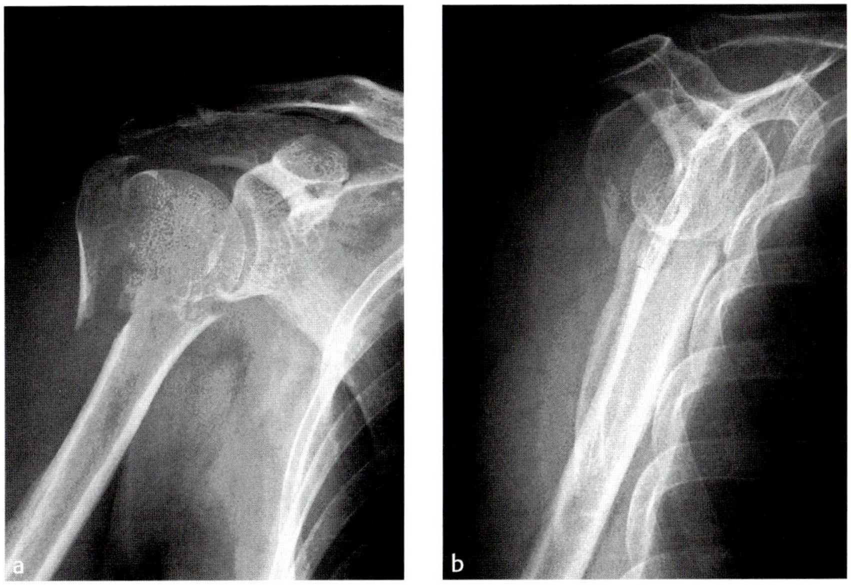

69-year-old woman fell on level ground.
Type of injury: low-energy, monotrauma.
Closed fracture.

Fig 6.1.7-1a–b
a AP view.
b Lateral view.

Indication

The articular fracture of the proximal humerus with valgus malalignment is unstable and painful. If left unreduced, the fracture will heal with malunion causing shoulder stiffness and prolonged pain.
Operative fixation reduces the acute pain, achieves a better reduction of the fracture, and allows for early mobilization of the shoulder joint. However, if the fracture is not stably fixed there may be a complication of nonunion after surgical fixation, particularly in the anatomical neck region.

A locking proximal humeral plate (LPHP) will be the implant of choice as there is a need for stable fixation of both the humeral head and the diaphysis.
An alternative fixation method is by wiring in a figure-of-eight manner. The surgical dissection is the same but the stability achieved will be less.
Nonoperative treatment is used only in patients unsuitable for surgery. A collar and cuff bandage can be given for 4–6 weeks and subsequent shoulder stiffness is expected.

Preoperative planning

Equipment

- Locking proximal humeral plate (LPHP) 3.5, 5 holes
- 3.5 mm self-tapping locking head screws (LHS)
- 3.5 mm cortex screws
- 2.0 mm K-wires
- Bone punch
- Strong nonabsorbable sutures
- Equipment for bone graft harvesting
- Optional: calcium triphosphate bone substitute in block form

(Size of system, instruments, and implants can vary according to anatomy.)

Patient preparation and positioning

Antibiotics: single dose 2nd generation cephalosporin

Thrombosis prophylaxis: none

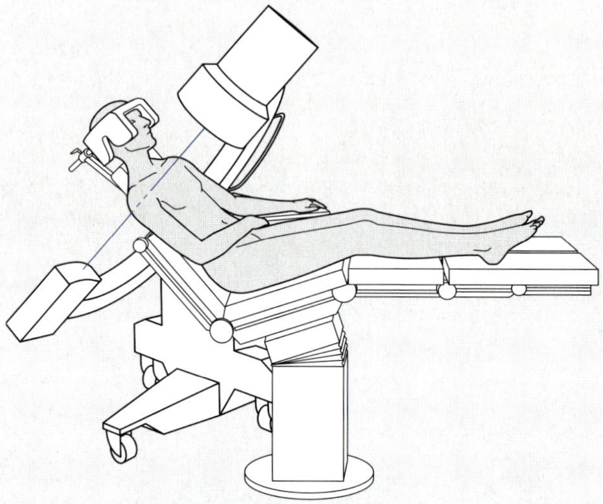

Fig 6.1.7-2 Beach chair position.

2 Surgical approach

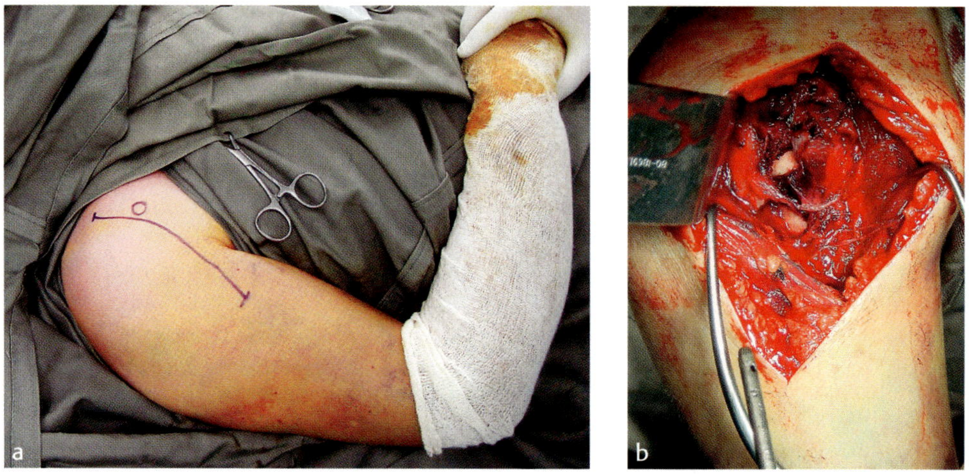

Fig 6.1.7-3a–b

a The coracoid process is palpated and marked. A standard deltopectoral approach with a 10–12 cm incision is used.

b Care must be taken to preserve the cephalic vein in order to decrease postoperative edema of the affected limb. The interval between the deltoid and pectoralis major muscle is developed. Retraction of the deltoid muscle laterally will expose the fracture.

3 Reduction

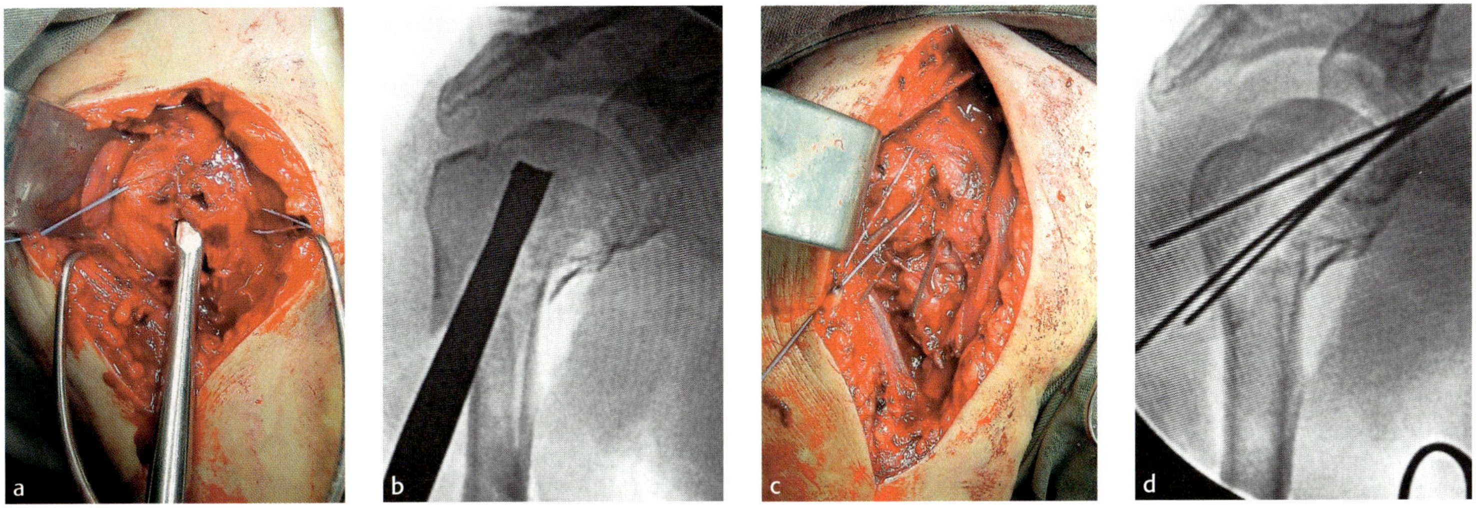

Fig 6.1.7-4a–d

a Place nonabsorbable sutures above the greater tuberosity into the tendon. The humeral head is reduced with the aid of a bone punch.

b Image intensifier shows the reduction of the humeral head fragment. Make sure that the head fragment is supported by pulling down the displaced greater tuberosity.

c Fix the reduced fracture with three K-wires.

d Check the reduction with the image intensifier. In osteoporotic bone the K-wire can be driven into the glenoid temporarily.

4 Fixation

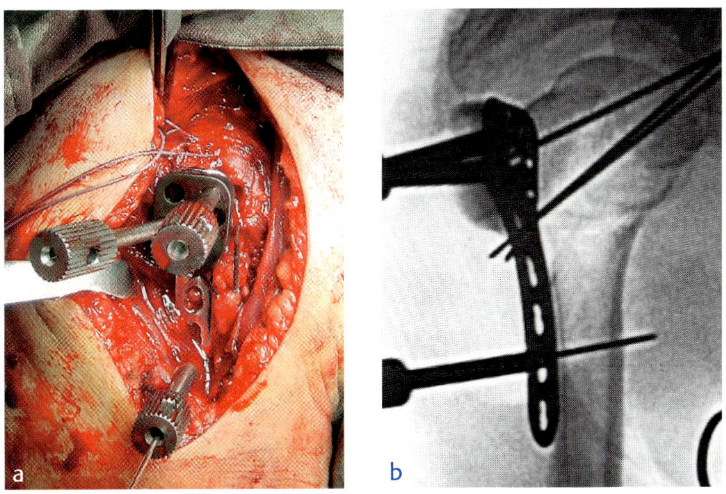

Fig 6.1.7-5a–i

a Place the LPHP over the anterolateral aspect of the proximal humerus and fix it temporarily with a K-wire placed into the diaphysis. The suture holding the greater tuberosity is passed through one of the small holes on the plate.

b The position of the plate is checked with the image intensifier. Avoid placing the plate too superiorly which will cause shoulder impingement.

4 Fixation (cont)

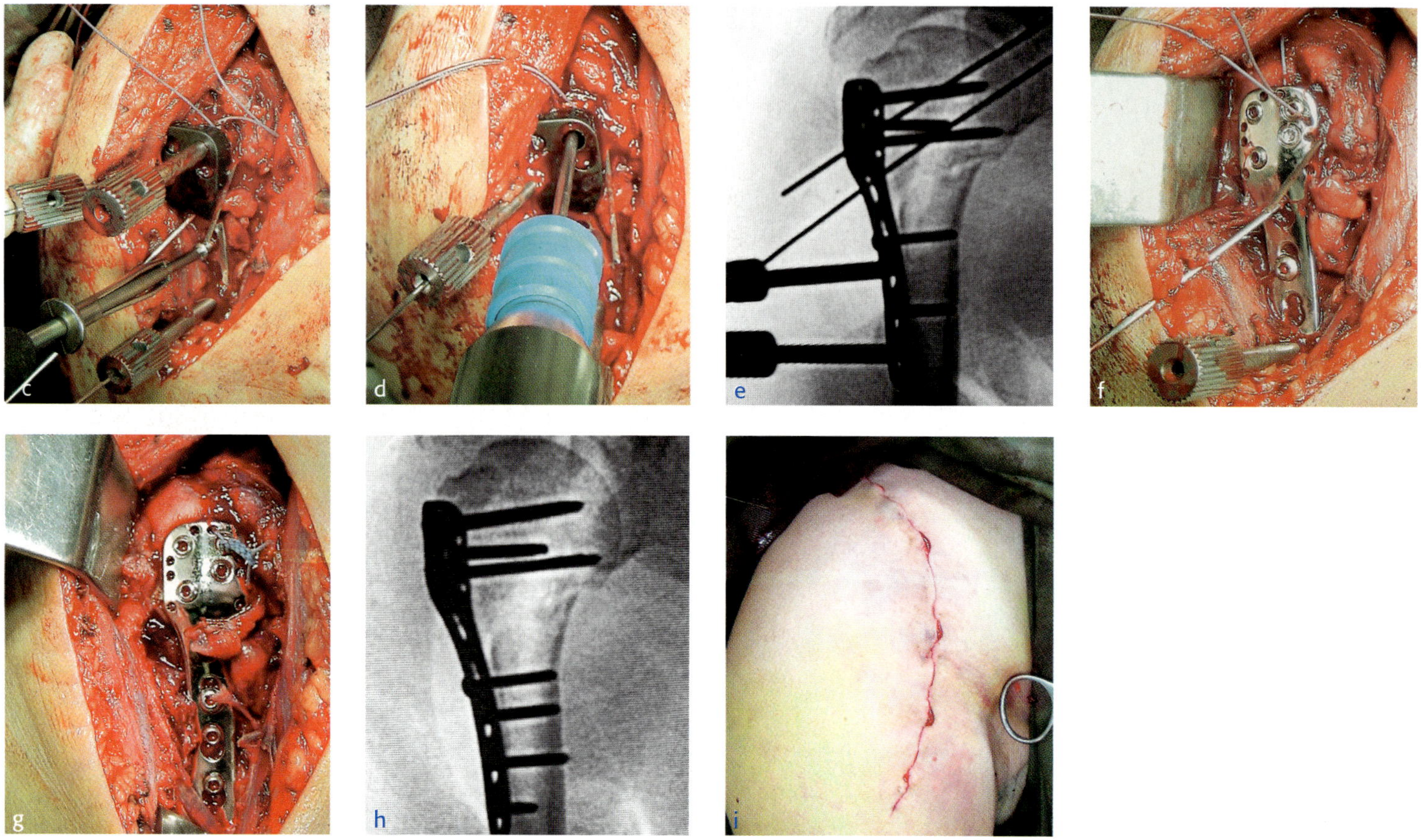

Fig 6.1.7-5a–i (cont)

c Insert a 3.5 mm cortex screw into the hole below the anatomical neck fracture. This will greatly facilitate insertion of the remaining screws.

d Fix the humeral head with a self-tapping 3.5 mm LHS. Make sure the drilling is done with the guiding block so that proper locking of the screw head is ensured. There is no need to perforate the articular surface. Deduct 5 mm from the measured length to avoid inadvertent screw perforation of the articular surface.

e Insert the remaining LHS into the humeral head fragment. Check the screw length by image intensification.

f Insert LHS into the diaphyseal portion. Bicortical screws are used, except for the most distal one.

g Tie the nonabsorbable suture to secure the position of the greater tuberosity.

h Check the position of the screws and the reduction with the image intensifier.

i Skin closure.

5 Rehabilitation

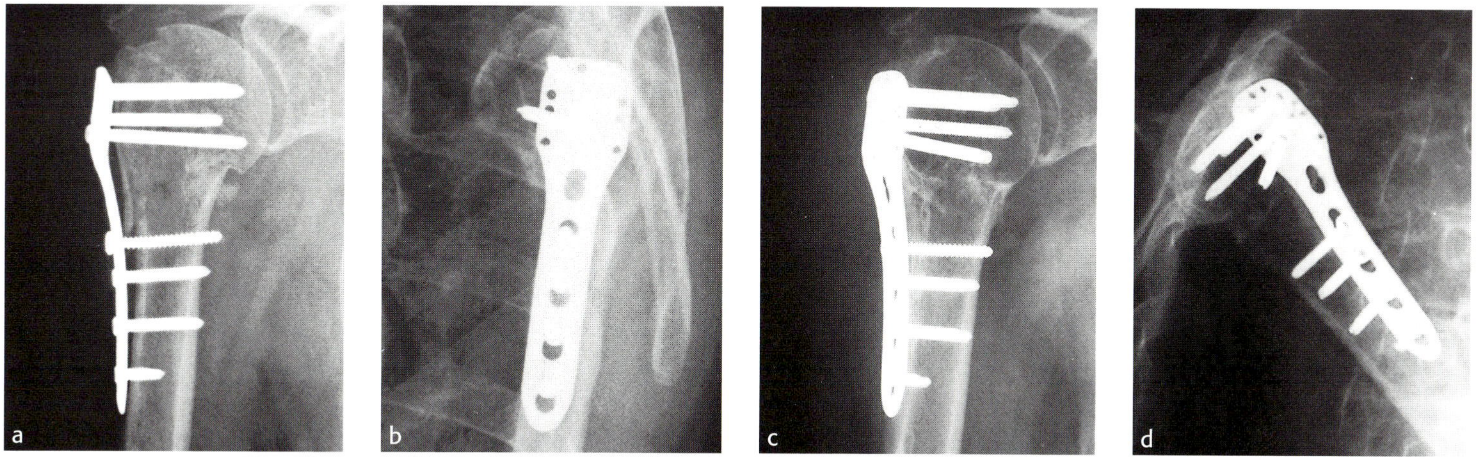

Additional immobilization: arm sling.
Physiotherapy: active-assisted exercise with the physiotherapist as of the first post operative day.

Fig 6.1.7-6a–d
- a Postoperative x-ray after 6 weeks. AP view.
- b Postoperative x-ray after 6 weeks. Lateral view.
- c Follow-up x-ray after 15 months. AP view.
- d Follow-up x-ray after 15 months. Axial view.

6 Pitfalls –

Reduction and fixation

It may be difficult to pass sutures through small holes once the screws are inserted.

Often, after the humeral head is reduced, there is a bone defect.

Loss of fixation of the humeral head fragment can occur if the screws are too short.

7 Pearls +

Reduction and fixation

It is easier if sutures are passed around the small holes before any screw fixation.

Careful depth gauge measurement and confirmation with the image intensifier is recommended.

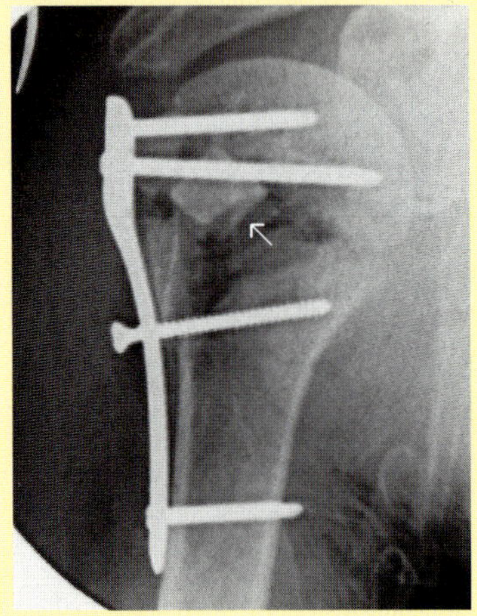

Fig 6.1.7-7 The use of autogenous corticocancellous bone graft from the iliac crest or the insertion of a block of calcium triphosphate (white arrow) will increase the stability of the fixation and enhance bone healing.

Author Michael Plecko

6.1.8 Intraarticular impacted proximal humeral fracture with displacement—11-C2

1 Case description

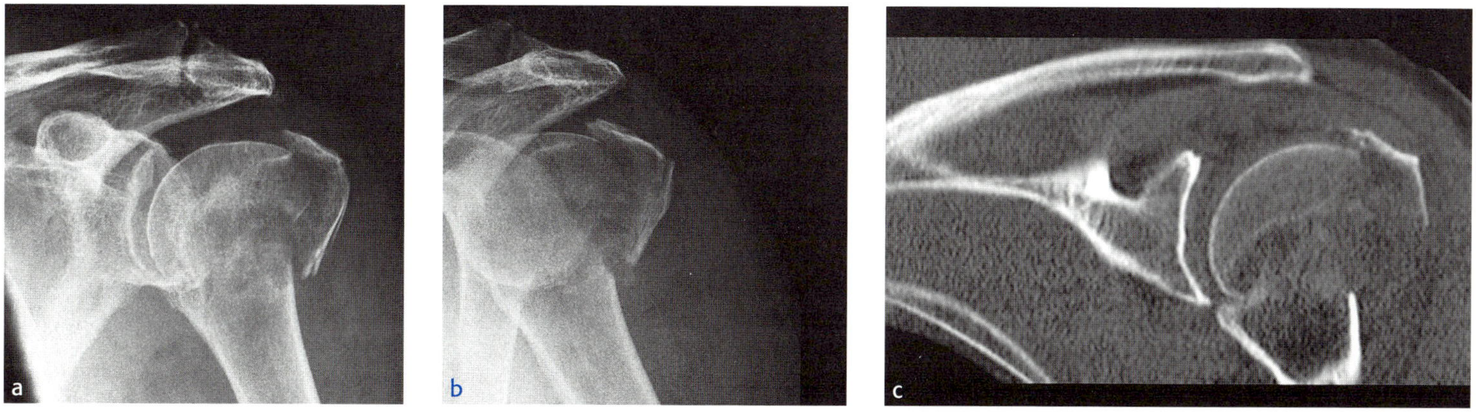

75-year-old very active woman, fell on the stairs in her house. Lived alone before the accident, did all housework and gardening by herself. Unstable painful fracture of her left proximal humerus, nondominant arm.
11–C2.1 fracture with valgus impaction of the articular segment, posterior—superior dislocation of the greater tuberosity, an additional fracture of the lesser tuberosity with multiple fragments, and a medial displacement of the humeral shaft. Marked osteoporosis.

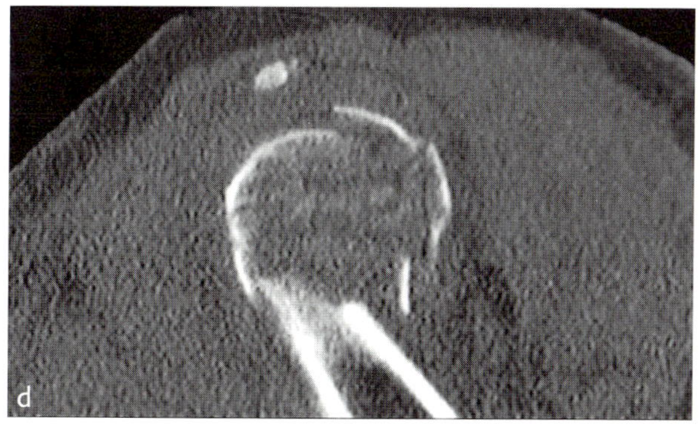

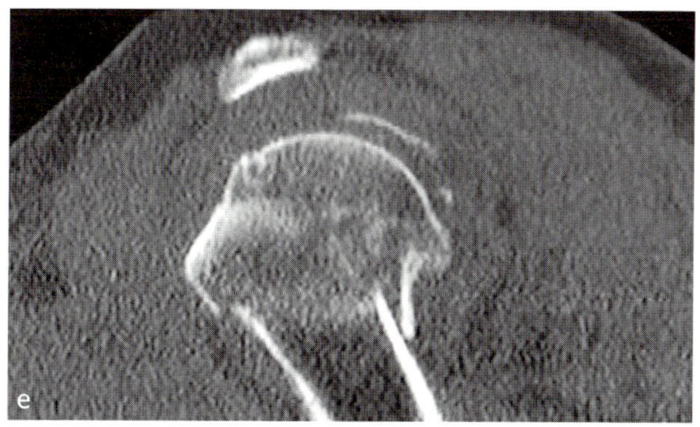

Fig 6.1.8-1a–e
- a AP view.
- b Axial view.
- c CT scan in frontal plane.
- d–e CT scan in sagittal plane showing comminution and dislocation of the greater tuberosity.

Indication

Unstable intraarticular proximal humeral fracture with valgus impaction of the articular segment, posterior and superior displacement of the multiple fractured greater tuberosity, medial displacement of the shaft, marked osteoporosis, severe pain, no additional nerve lesion or vascular damage.
Conservative treatment is not a good option in this case due to marked displacement. It would only be considered if operative treatment would appear too risky due to comorbidity in a low demand patient.
Closed reduction and percutaneous pinning with additional screw fixation is possible but, due to the multiply fractured greater tuberosity and additional osteoporosis, percutaneous screw fixation may provide insufficient stability and could lead to secondary displacement. Due to displacement of the shaft, closed and percutaneous pinning reduction may be difficult. An additional immobilization for 3–4 weeks as well as a second operation for pin removal would be necessary.
Considering this and the patients request for early independence, careful open reduction under visual control and internal fixation with locking proximal humeral plate and additional tension banding is chosen. This offers the advantage of open reduction and preservation of the periosteal bridges to the fracture fragments and a stable fixation with early functional rehabilitation. Quick pain relief is achieved.

Preoperative planning

Equipment

- Locking proximal humeral plate (LPHP), 5 holes (alternatively: 8 holes)
- 3.5 mm self-tapping locking head screws (LHS)
- 3.5 mm cortex screw
- 1.8 mm K-wires
- Nonabsorbable sutures

(Size of system, instruments, and implants can vary according to anatomy.)

Patient preparation and positioning

General anesthesia is recommended, alternatively a scalene block can be used.

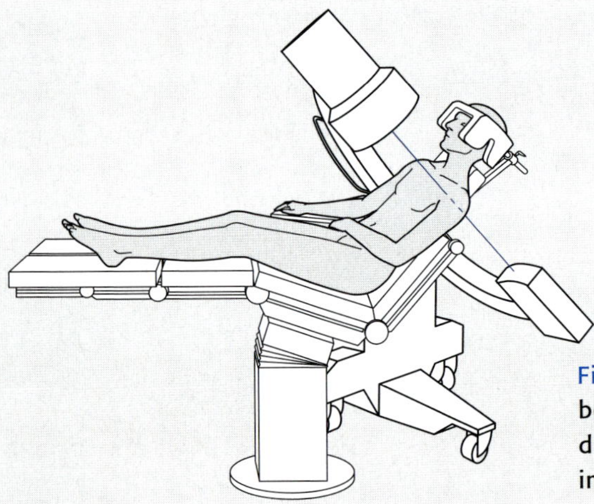

Fig 6.1.8-2 Patient is placed in beach chair position. The arm is free-draped for intraoperative mobility. An image intensifier is helpful.

2 Surgical approach

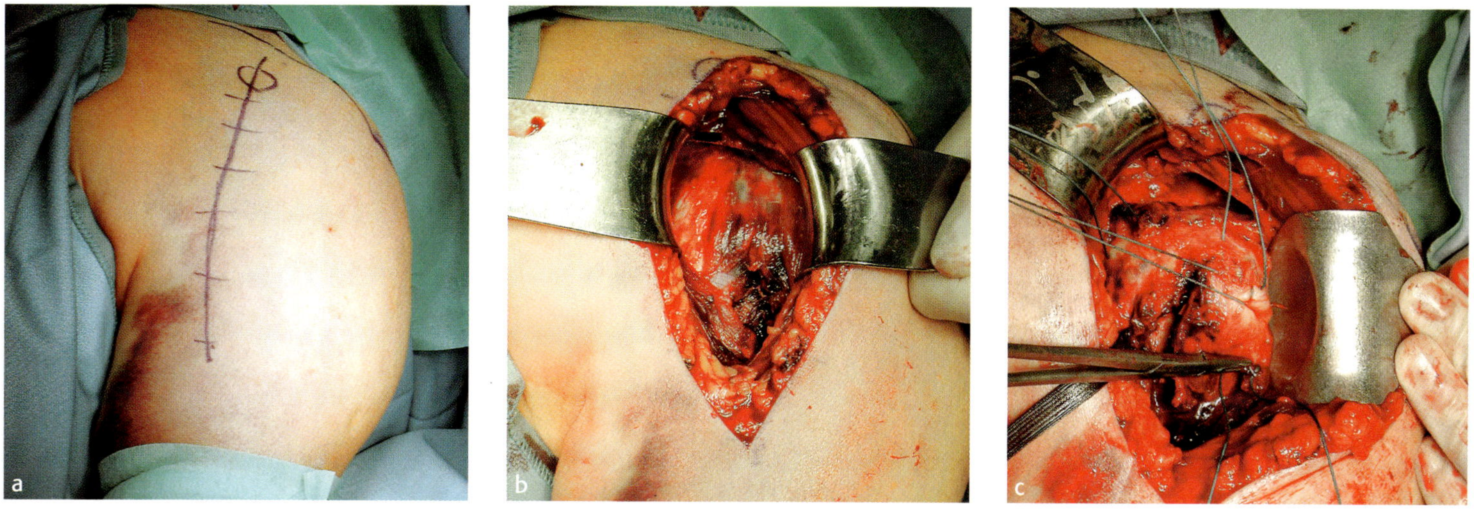

Fig 6.1.8-3a–c

a–b Deltopectoral approach. Perform a 12 cm incision from the coracoid process to the deltoid insertion, split the deltoid and the pectoralis major. Use the cephalic vein as a landmark and leave the cephalic vein with the deltoid to the lateral side. Cautious blunt preparation of the subdeltoid space with the fingers.

c Identify the tendon of the long head of the biceps brachii muscles and anchor strong nonabsorbable sutures through the supraspinatus, infraspinatus, and subscapularis tendon at the tendon-bone interface. These sutures allow gentle manipulation of the humeral head fragments. Fracture lines should be identified but not completely exposed.

3 Reduction

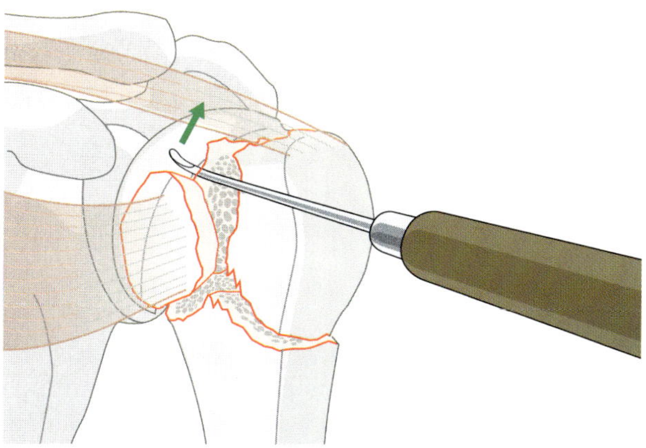

Fig 6.1.8-4 Reduce the humeral head fragments by gently pulling the sutures anchored in the supraspinatus, infraspinatus, and subscapularis tendon. Reduce the articular segment by using a small elevator. In unstable situations temporary pinning may be advisable.

3 Reduction (cont)

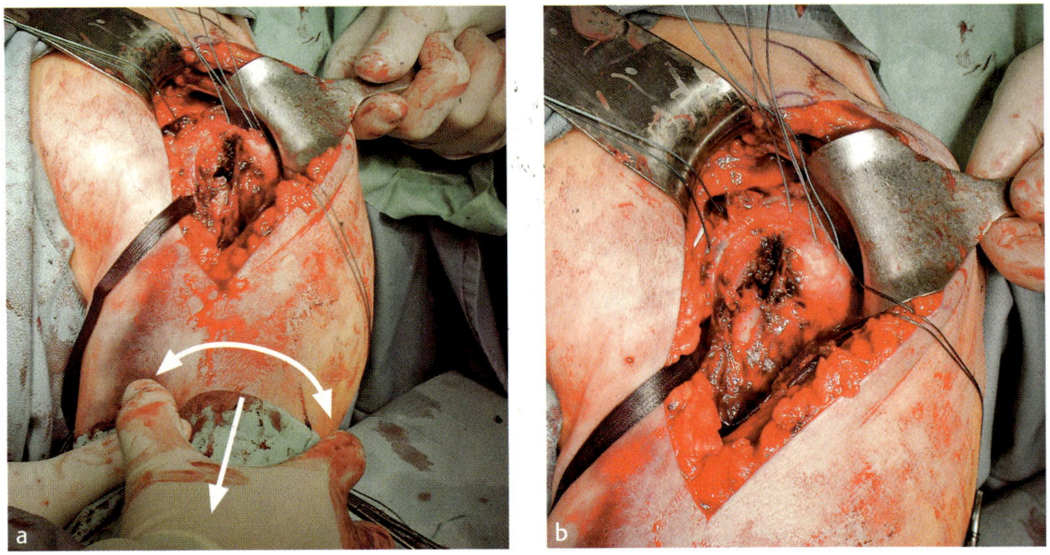

Fig 6.1.8-5a–b Reduce the shaft approximately by an indirect reduction maneuver.

a Pull and rotate the distal part of the humerus.
b Control of the reduced fragments.

4 Fixation

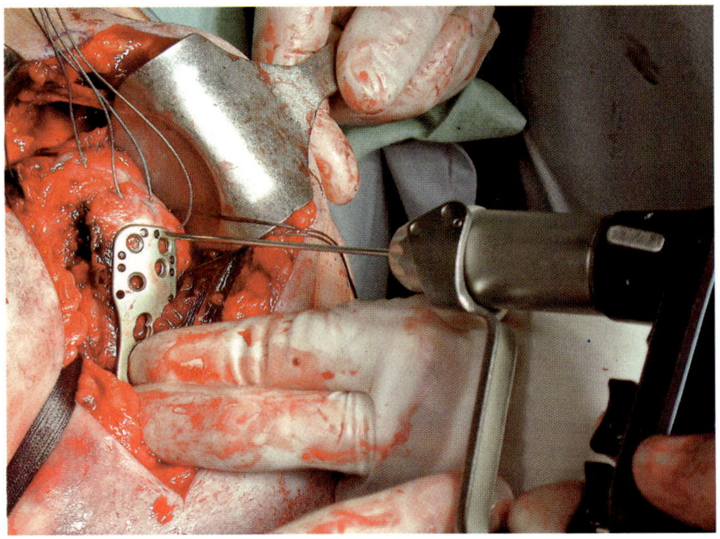

Fig 6.1.8-6 Adapt the 5-hole locking proximal humeral plate (LPHP) to the proximal part of the humerus and fix it temporarily with 1.8 mm K-wires through the suture holes. Place the upper end of the plate 5–7 mm below the tip of the greater tuberosity and about 5 mm posterior to the bicipital groove. Checking the correct position of the implants with the image intensifier is advisable.

4 Fixation (cont)

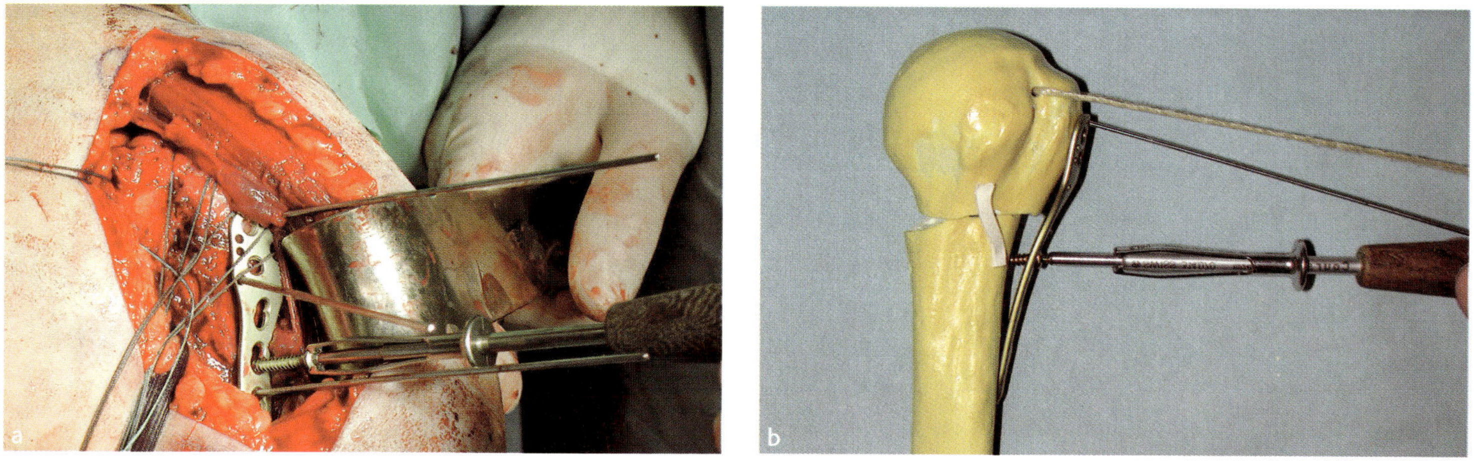

Fig 6.1.8-7a–b Insert a 3.5 mm cortex screw through the first hole below the subcapital fracture line. By tightening the screw the humeral shaft will be gently reduced towards the plate, against the medializing muscle forces of the pectoralis major muscles.

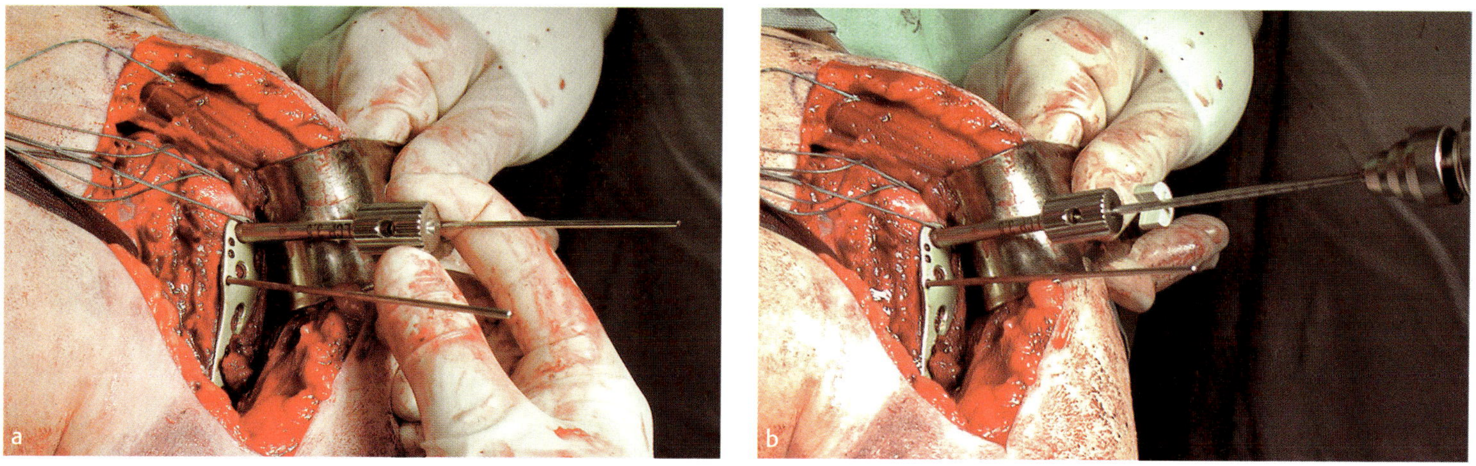

Fig 6.1.8-8a–b Insert the threaded drill guide into the two proximal parallel locking holes and use the 2.8 mm drill bit for the preparation of the holes. Do not perforate the articular surface. Lasermarks and a plastic ring on the drill bit facilitate direct reading of the drilled depth.

4 Fixation (cont)

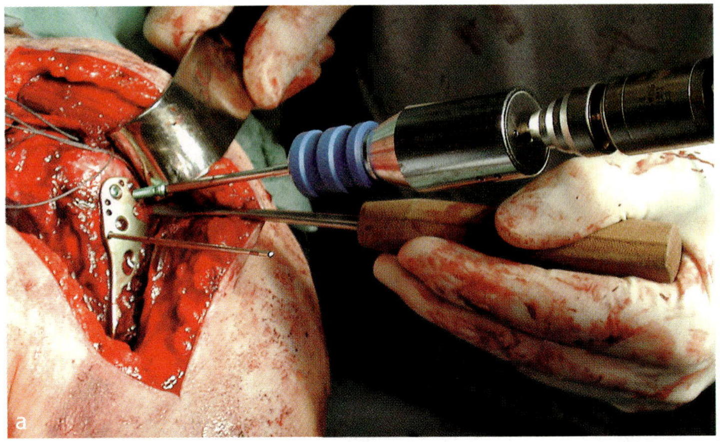

Fig 6.1.8-9a–c

a Insert two 3.5 mm self-tapping locking head screws (LHS) into the upper holes using the torque-limiting attachment to the screwdriver. Check ideal length of these locking head screws by image intensifier in order not to penetrate the articular surface (leave about 3 mm between the tip of the screw and the articular surface).

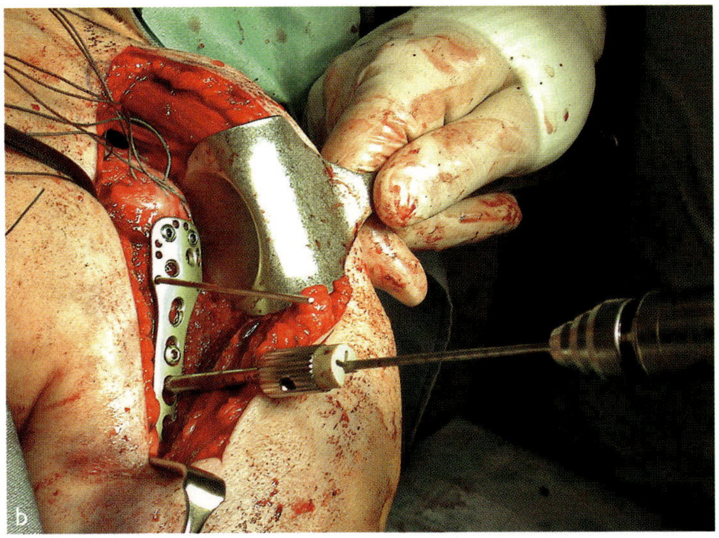

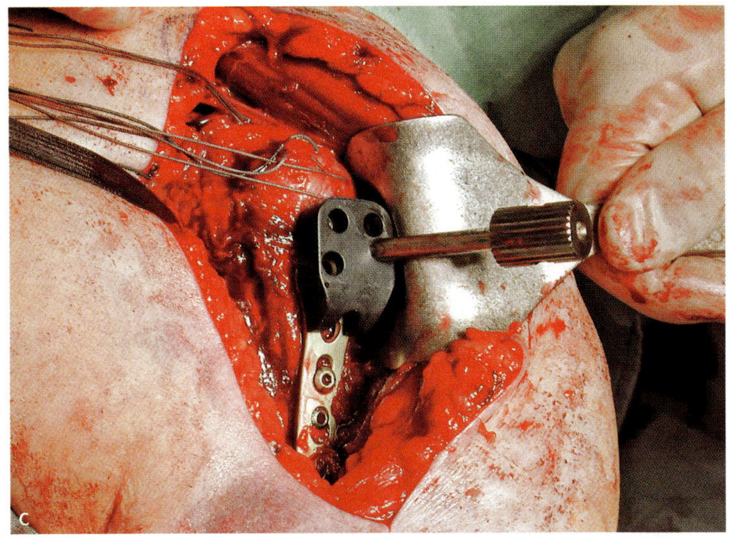

b Insert the threaded LCP drill guide into the holes at the humeral shaft. Use a 2.8 mm drill bit and, after measurement of the length, insert a bicortical 3.5 mm self-tapping LHS into each hole using the torque-limiting attachment on the screwdriver. Notice that a minimum of two bicortical 3.5 mm self-tapping LHS should be placed in the shaft fragment. The hole at the end of the plate may be equipped with a monocortical 3.5 mm, self-drilling, self-tapping LHS.

c Insert the threaded LCP drill guide into the remaining three divergent drill holes in the proximal part of the plate using the guiding block. After drilling, insert 3.5 mm self-tapping LHS using the torque-limiting attachment on the screwdriver in each of these holes. Check all screw lengths carefully with the image intensifier.

4 Fixation (cont)

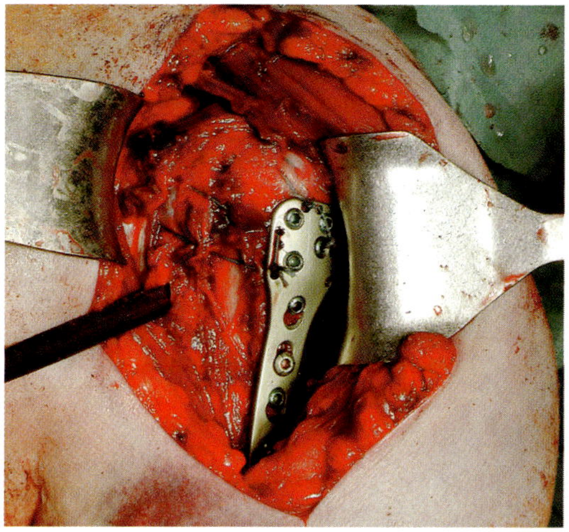

Fig 6.1.8-10 Fix the anchored sutures through the suture holes in the plate and tie them tightly to neutralize the muscle forces of the rotator cuff.

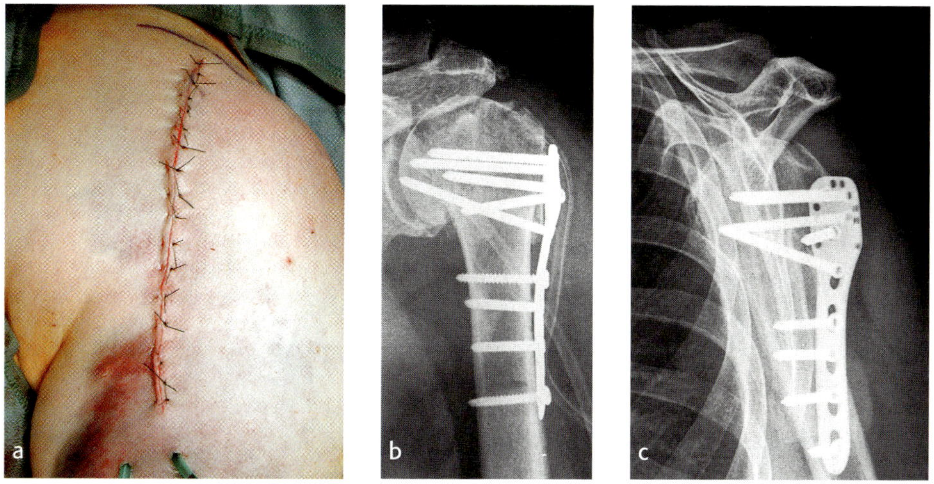

Fig 6.1.8-11a–c

a Check shoulder mobility and fracture stability by passive motion. Perform wound closure after irrigation and drainage.

b–c Postoperative x-rays show good reduction and positioning of the implant.

5 Rehabilitation

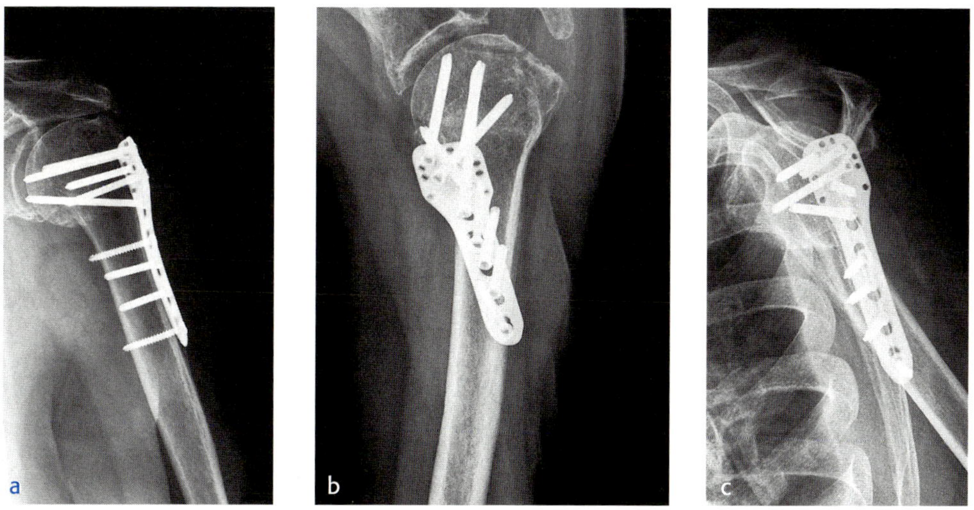

Additional immobilization: bandage for 2–3 weeks.

Physiotherapy: passive and active-assisted mobilization as of the second postoperative day.

Unrestricted active mobilization after 3–4 weeks.

Pharmaceutical treatment: painkillers in the early postoperative period, thereafter when needed.

Fig 6.1.8-12a–c X-rays at one year follow-up show complete healing of the fracture without signs of avascular necrosis. One screw seems to penetrate the articular surface without causing any clinical symptoms.

5 Rehabilitation (cont)

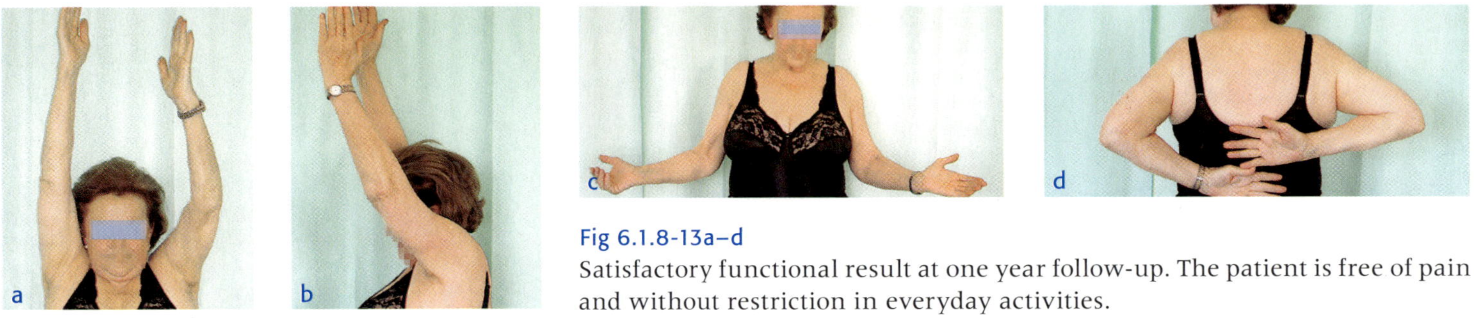

Fig 6.1.8-13a–d
Satisfactory functional result at one year follow-up. The patient is free of pain and without restriction in everyday activities.

6 Pitfalls –

Approach
Too extensive exposure of the fracture fragments may damage vascularity and lead to a high rate of avascular necrosis.

Reduction
Brisk reduction maneuvers with reduction forceps may damage blood supply and any residual intact periostieum on the fragments.
Incorrect positioning of the plate may lead to subacromial impingement and restricted range of motion.

Fixation
Incorrect length of the LHS leads to perforation of the articular surface of the humeral head.
3.5 mm cortex screws may lead to reduced stability in osteoporotic bone and premature loosening.
Lack of sufficient medial buttress without adjustment of the rehabilitation protocol may lead to implant failure.

7 Pearls +

Approach
Open procedure without extensive exposure of the fracture lines may help to preserve the blood supply of the segments. Alternative: small anterolateral splitting of the deltoid muscle.

Reduction
Indirect reduction maneuvers help to preserve blood supply and residual periostieum in this open procedure.
Optimal positioning of the anatomically preshaped plate, controlled by image intensification, prevents hardware impingement and enables unrestricted range of motion.

Fixation
Optimal length, especially of the LHS, avoids perforation of the articular surface.
LHS, in combination with 3-D orientation, lead to improved stability even in osteoporotic bone, but exact locking remains essential.
Reconstruction of the medial buttress leads to sufficient stability for early functional rehabilitation.

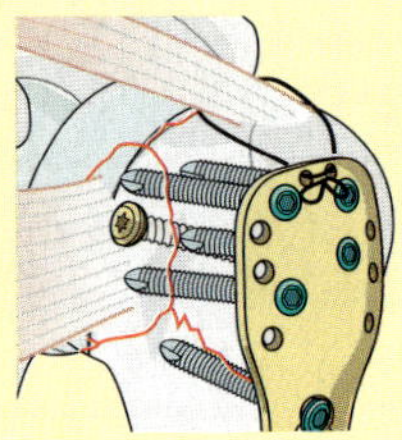

Fig 6.1.8-14 In the case of a homogeneous fragment of the lesser tuberosity, the suture through the subscapularis tendon may be replaced by a 3.5 mm cortex screw from the lesser tuberosity to the humeral shaft.

Author Christian Ryf

6.1.9 4-part proximal humeral fracture—11-C2

1 Case description

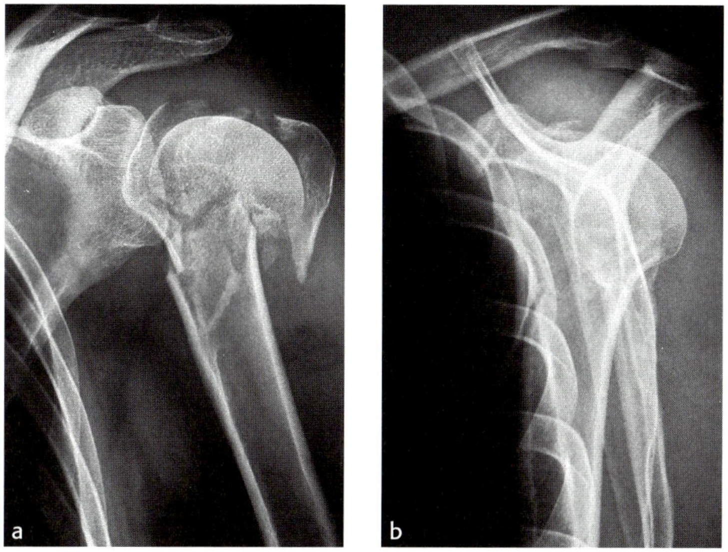

23-year-old man fell while skiing and suffered a 4-part proximal humeral fracture on the left side. He had no further injuries. A CT scan was carried out for fracture study.

Fig 6.1.9-1a–b
a AP view.
b Lateral view.

Indication

The decision for an osteosynthesis in this rather young patient was taken. The risk of aseptic necrosis in this fracture with subluxation of the humerus head is considerable.

Preoperative planning

Equipment

- PHILOS proximal humeral plate 3.5, 3 holes
- 3.5 mm cortex screws
- 3.5 mm locking head screws (LHS)
- 2.5 mm K-wire
- Partially threaded K-wires 2.0 mm
- Osteosutures

(Size of system, instruments, and implants can vary according to anatomy.)

Patient preparation and positioning

Antibiotics: single dose 2nd generation cephalosporin
Thrombosis prophylaxis: low-molecular heparin
A conventional x-ray and a CT scan were carried out for operation planning. The valgization, subluxation, and the four main fragments are shown.

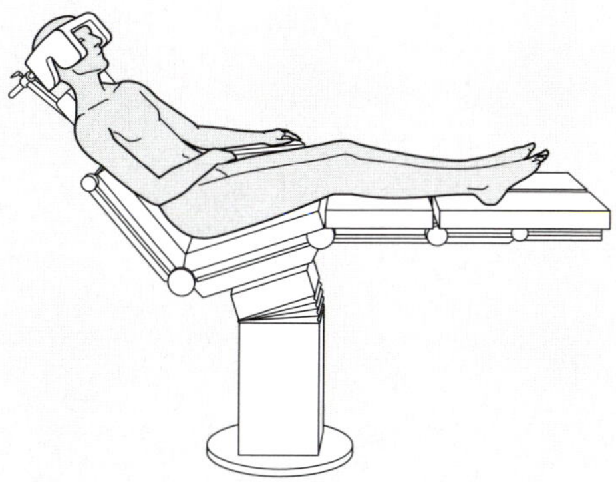

Fig 6.1.9-2 The patient is placed in the beach chair position. Left arm freely moveable.

2 Surgical approach

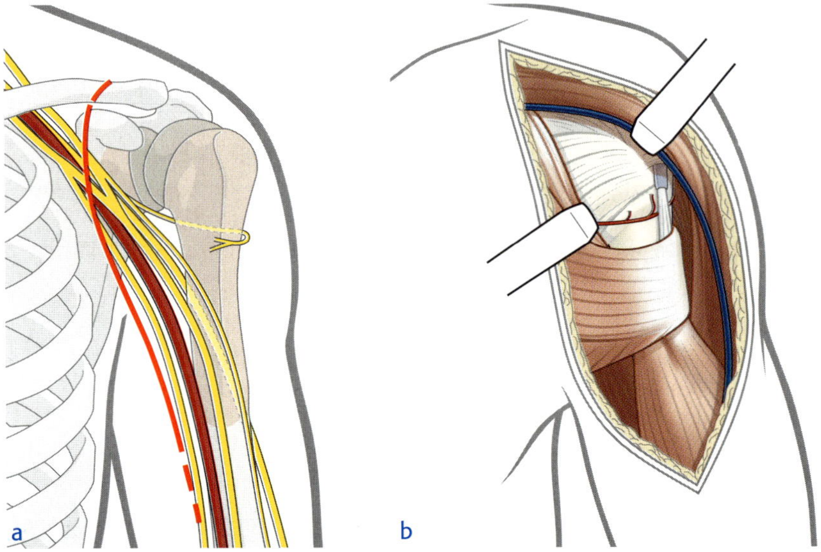

Fig 6.1.9-3a–b A deltopectoral approach is performed, sparing the cephalic vein. The deltoid is partially detached from the clavicle at the anterior aspect.

There is multifragmentary fracture of the greater and lesser tubercles, a longitudinal split, and cranial displacement as had been expected from the preoperative x-rays.

Some small fragments are removed and reimplanted later.

3 Reduction and fixation

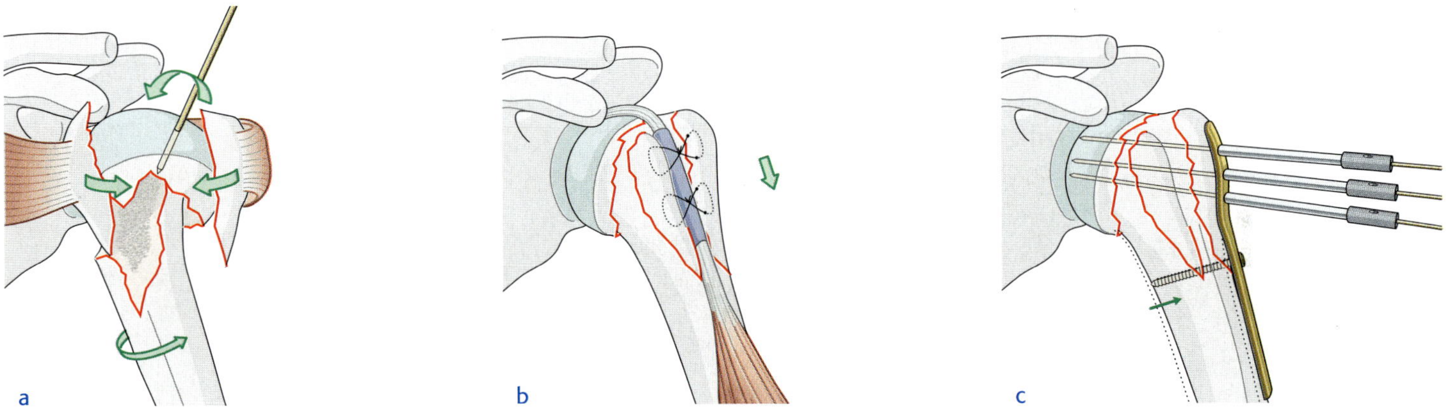

Fig 6.1.9-4a–g

a A 2.5 mm K-wire is drilled into the massively valgizated humeral head fragment in the sense of a joystick support. With axial traction and rotation of the arm and the joystick, head reduction can be accomplished.

b Now the tubercules are pulled into position and provisionally fixed with a fiber-wire osteosuture.

c The 3-hole PHILOS plate is applied laterally and provisionally fixed with a conventional cortex screw onto the shaft. Definitive reduction under image intensification control and fine tuning of the plate follows.

3 Reduction and fixation (cont)

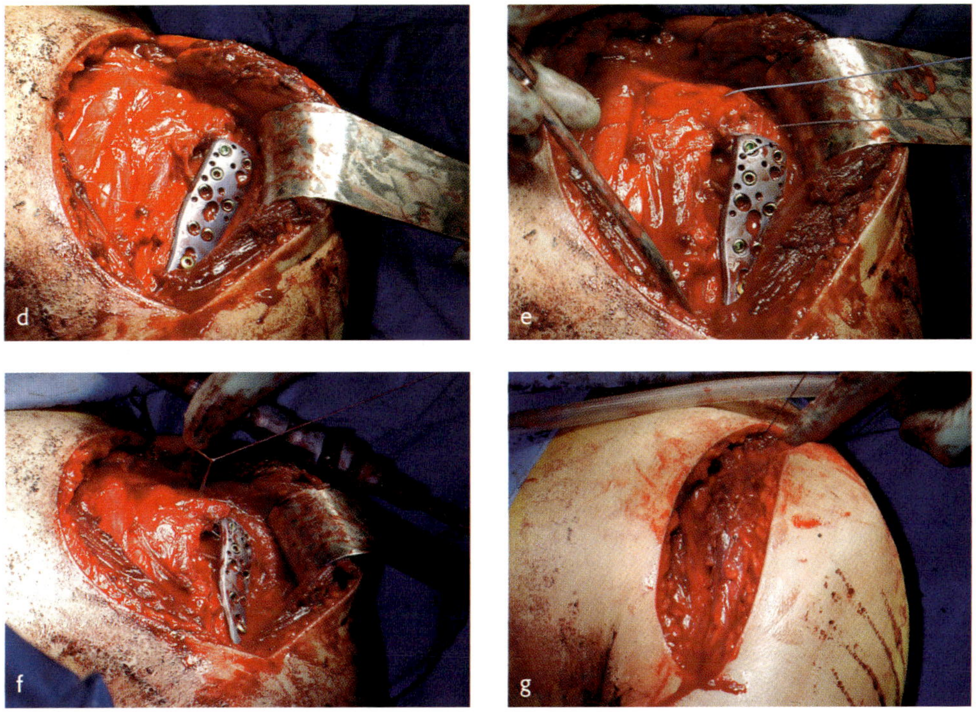

Fig 6.1.9-4a–g (cont)

d To increase the bone-to-bone contact, the shaft is impacted into the humeral head. Now all other plate holes are occupied with locking head screws.

e–f Osteosuture of the smaller tubercular fragments, mainly from the greater tubercle, with fiber-wire, completing the stable osteosynthesis.

g The partially removed deltoid muscle is readapted and the fascia sutured.

4 Rehabilitation

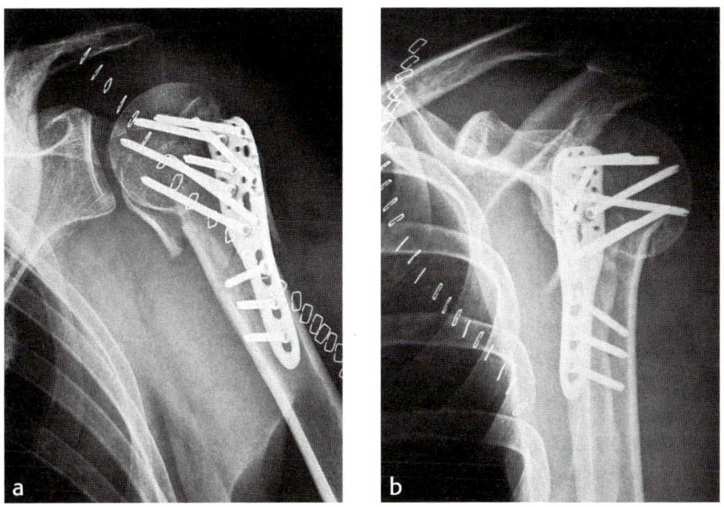

Gentle active-assisted physiotherapy begins on the second postoperative day for at least 3–4 weeks. A desault gilet is used for fixation.

Active motion should begin after 4 weeks if supported by the x-ray findings.

Fig 6.1.9-5a–b Postoperative x-rays after 4 weeks.

a AP view.

b Lateral view.

6.2 Humerus, shaft

Cases

Case		Classification	Method	Implant used	Implant function	Page
6.2.1	Spiral wedge humeral shaft fracture with humeral head involvement	12-B1	locked splinting	LCP metaphyseal plate 3.5/4.5/5.0	locked internal fixator	289
6.2.2	Fragmented humeral shaft wedge fracture	12-B3	locked splinting	LCP metaphyseal plate 3.5/4.5/5.0	locked internal fixator	293
6.2.3	Gunshot fracture of the humeral shaft	12-C1	locked splinting	LCP 4.5	locked internal fixator	299
6.2.4	Complex segmental proximal humeral shaft fracture	12-C2	locked splinting	LCP metaphyseal plate 3.5/4.5/5.0	locked internal fixator and reduction screw	305
6.2.5	Complex segmental humeral shaft fracture	12-C2	locked splinting	LCP metaphyseal plate 3.5/4.5/5.0	locked internal fixator	311
6.2.6	Simple transverse humeral shaft fracture and partial intraarticular sagittal lateral humeral condyle fracture	12-A3 13-B1	locked splinting	LCP metaphyseal plate 3.5/4.5/5.0	locked internal fixator	317
6.2.7	Pathological humeral shaft fracture		locked splinting	LCP 4.5/5.0, narrow	locked internal fixator	321
6.2.8	Intercalary reconstruction of the humerus following oncological resection			LPHP; LCP reconstruction plate 3.5; LCP metaphyseal plate 3.5/4.5/5.0	locked internal fixator	325

6 Humerus

Author Christoph Sommer

6.2 Humerus, shaft

1 Incidence

Fractures of the humeral shaft are quite rare in an average population and occur in about 1–2% of all fractures. In men, bimodal age distribution with a peak in the third decade is the result of moderate to severe injury. For women, a larger peak can be expected in the seventh decade after a simple fall [1]. Most fractures occur in the midthird third of the diaphysis with about 30% in the proximal and about 10% in the distal thirds.

2 Classification

Fractures are categorized according to the Müller AO Classification as A-, B- and C-type fractures [2]. Low-energy mechanisms (simple fall, arm wrestling) usually lead to closed fractures with more simple fracture patterns (A1, B1), whereby high-energy traumas result in a high rate of open fractures with either transverse (A3, B3) or complex fractures (C1–3), often associated with neurovascular injuries.

3 Treatment methods

Conservative treatment is still the gold standard for many humeral shaft fractures. Different methods have been described; the most accepted is functional bracing, resulting in a high rate of union (94–98%) and in good to excellent function in most cases [3]. However, there are clinical situations where operative stabilization is more appropriate. Absolute indications for operative treatment are higher degree open fractures II–III (Tscherne classification), fractures with vascular injury requiring vascular repair, and pathological fractures. The list of relative indications is long and includes special fracture types (transverse, long spiral), multiple trauma, floating elbow, bilateral fractures, radial nerve palsy, poor patient compliance

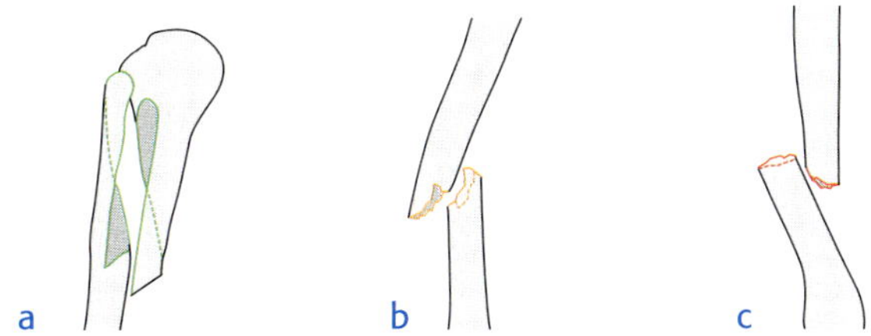

Fig 6.2-1a–c 12-A Simple fracture.
a 12-A1 spiral
b 12-A2 oblique (≥ 30°)
c 12-A3 transverse (< 30°)

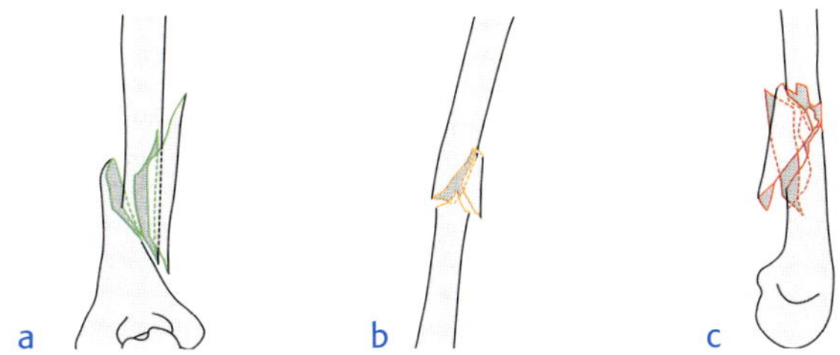

Fig 6.2-2a–c 12-B Wedge fracture.
a 12-B1 spiral wedge
b 12-B2 bending wedge
c 12-B3 fragmented wedge

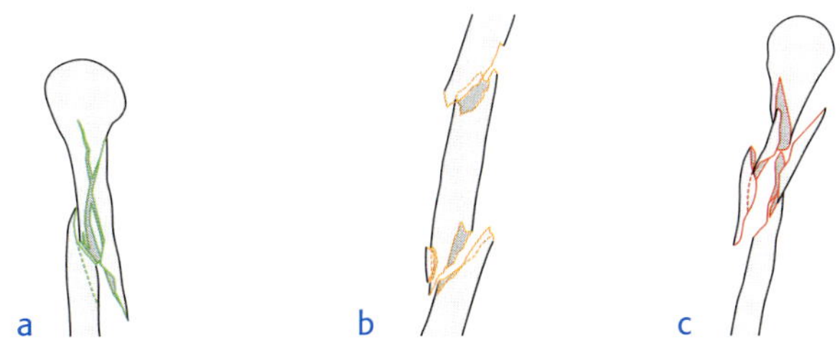

Fig 6.2-3a–c 12-C Complex fracture.
a 12-C1 spiral
b 12-C2 segmental
c 12-C3 irregular

and obesity, which may complicate an alternative conservative treatment. In all these situations, individual decisions for conservative or operative treatment have to be chosen according to different factors such as patient's expectation, surgical experience, available infrastructure and others.

Primary radial nerve palsy usually recovers spontaneously in cases with closed and not largely displaced fractures (low-energy mechanism) and therefore operative exploration seems to be unnecessary [4]. On the other hand, in high-energy traumas that often result in open fractures, primary nerve palsy is not infrequently caused by a nerve tear, which requires surgical repair. In these cases, operative treatment with radial nerve exploration seems to be justified [4, 5].

Different implants are available for the operative stabilization of humeral shaft fractures. It is still controversial whether plate fixation or intramedullary nailing is more appropriate. There are many pros and cons for each treatment option. In general, similar union rates can be expected for either plating or nailing [6–9]. Shoulder function seems to be more impaired after antegrade nailing compared to plate fixation [6, 8, 10] or retrograde nailing [11], whereby elbow function on the other hand may be more impaired after plate fixation. This is especially true for fractures of the distal third of the humerus compared to antegrade nailing [6]. In summary, the choice of implant depends on many different factors, but is mainly influenced by the preference and experience of the surgeon.

The development of the angular stable screw-plate system (LCP) offers further advantages in the plating of humeral shaft fractures or nonunions, especially in cases of osteoporotic bone and in fractures extending to the metaphysis or the joint [12]. The first clinical experience with the LCP in this region however showed several complications that were mainly caused by wrong applications due to the unknown new system. General guidelines for the use of the LCP, especially in the humerus, have been provided. Possibly the most important piece of advice is to insert the locking head screws bicortically in the diaphysis in the case of poor bone quality.

The standard approach for plate fixation in the proximal half of the shaft is the anterolateral and for the distal half the dorsal approach. In situations with vascular injury, a medial approach is mandatory. Recently, minimally invasive plating techniques even in the humerus have been described. An antero-anterolateral approach at each end of the inserted plate can give safe access to the humerus, provided the surgeon knows the anatomy precisely. Together with the applied bridging technique (using a DCP) good results have been reported in a small group of patients.

4 Implant overview

a

b

c

d

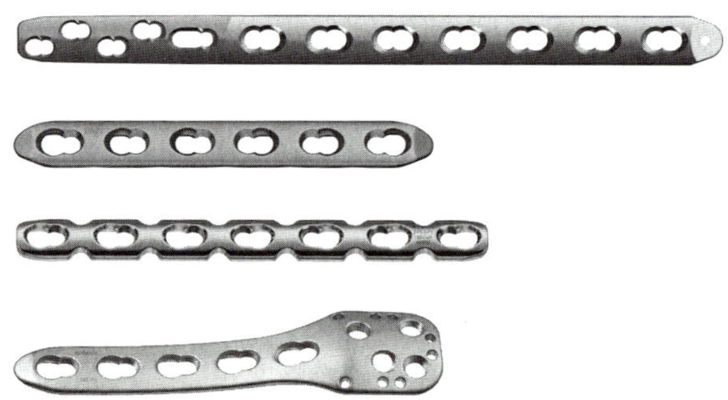

Fig 6.2-4a–d

a LCP metaphyseal plate 3.5/4.5/5.0
b LCP 4.5/5.0
c LCP reconstruction plate 3.5
d LPHP—Locking proximal humeral plate 3.5

5 Bibliography

1. **Tytherleigh-Strong G, Walls N, McQueen MM** (1998) The epidemiology of humeral shaft fractures. *J Bone Joint Surg Br;* 80(2):249–253.
2. **Müller ME, Nazarian S, Koch P, et al** (1990) The comprehensive classification of fractures of long bones. Berlin Heidelberg New York: Springer-Verlag.
3. **Sarmiento A, Zagorski JB, Zych GA, et al** (2000) Functional bracing for the treatment of fractures of the humeral diaphysis. *J Bone Joint Surg Am;* 82(4):478–486.
4. **Alnot J, Osman N, Masmejean E, et al** (2000) [Lesions of the radial nerve in fractures of the humeral diaphysis. Apropos of 62 cases]. *Rev Chir Orthop Reparatrice Appar Mot;* 86(2):143–150.
5. **Ring D, Chin K, Jupiter JB** (2004) Radial nerve palsy associated with high-energy humeral shaft fractures. *J Hand Surg [Am];* 29(1):144–147.
6. **Chapman JR, Henley MB, Agel J, et al** (2000) Randomized prospective study of humeral shaft fracture fixation: intramedullary nails versus plates. *J Orthop Trauma;* 14(3):162–166.
7. **Lin J** (1998) Treatment of humeral shaft fractures with humeral locked nail and comparison with plate fixation. *J Trauma;* 44(5):859–864.
8. **McCormack RG, Brien D, Buckley RE, et al** (2000) Fixation of fractures of the shaft of the humerus by dynamic compression plate or intramedullary nail. A prospective, randomised trial. *J Bone Joint Surg Br;* 82(3):336–339.
9. **Rommens PM, Blum J, Runkel M** (1998) Retrograde nailing of humeral shaft fractures. *Clin Orthop;* (350):26–39.
10. **Ajmal M, O'Sullivan M, McCabe J, et al** (2001) Antegrade locked intramedullary nailing in humeral shaft fractures. *Injury;* 32(9):692–694.
11. **Blum J, Janzing H, Gahr R, et al** (2001) Clinical performance of a new medullary humeral nail: antegrade versus retrograde insertion. *J Orthop Trauma;* 15(5):342–349.
12. **Ring D, Kloen P, Kadzielski J, et al** (2004) Locking compression plates for osteoporotic nonunions of the diaphyseal humerus. *Clin Orthop;* (425):50–54.

Author Michael Wagner

6.2.1 Spiral wedge humeral shaft fracture with humeral head involvement—12-B1

1 Case description

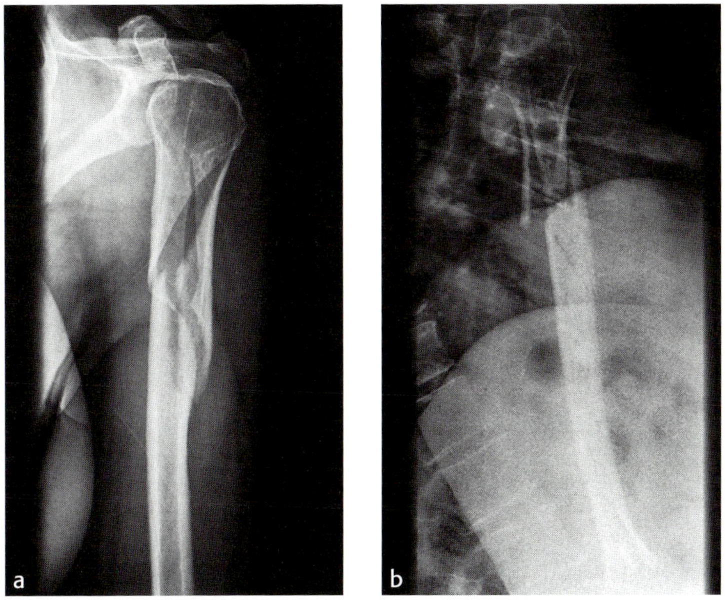

55-year-old woman fell down the stairs and suffered a monotrauma to her left arm.

Fig 6.2.1-1a–b
a AP view.
b Lateral view.

Indication

Painful and unstable fracture of the humeral shaft is an indication for operative treatment. Antegrade intramedullary nailing is possible but not a good option because of the small proximal head fragment. Conservative treatment is possible but requires a long immobilization period.

Preoperative planning

Equipment

- LCP metaphyseal plate 3.5/4.5/5.0, 4 + 12 holes
- 3.5 mm locking head screws (LHS)
- 4.5 mm LHS
- 1.25 mm K-wires
- 2.0 mm K-wires

(Size of system, instruments, and implants can vary according to anatomy.)

Patient preparation and positioning

Antibiotics: none
Thrombosis prophylaxis: low-molecular heparin

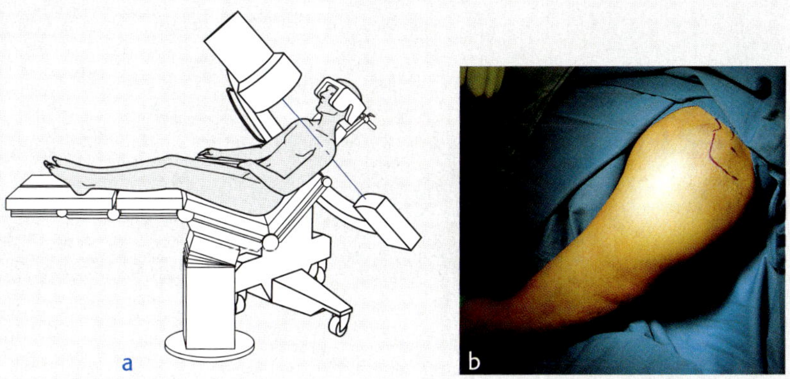

Fig 6.2.1-2a–b
Beach chair position.

2 Surgical approach

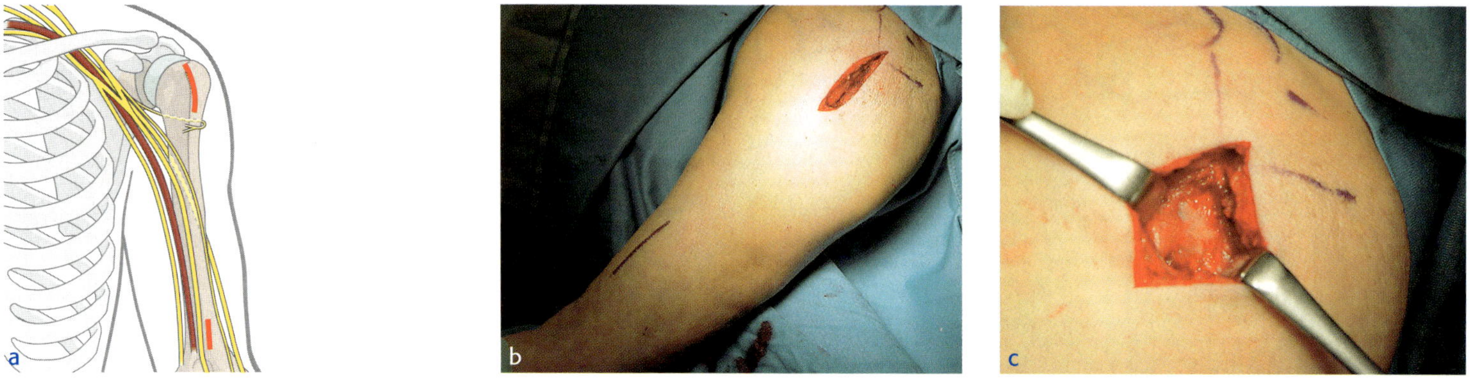

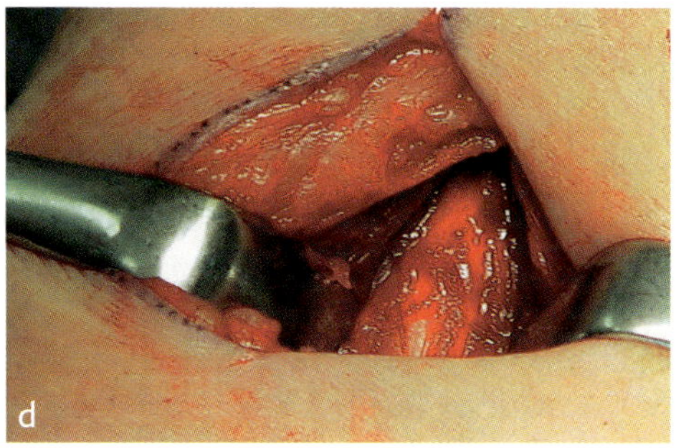

Fig 6.2.1-3a–d

a In order to perform minimally invasive plate osteosynthesis, a deltoid splitting approach proximally, and an anterolateral approach to the distal shaft was chosen.

b Splitting of the deltoid starting from the anterolateral side of the acromion.

c Splitting of the deltoid at the level of the raphe. In a deltoid splitting approach it is necessary to preserve the axillary nerve.

d Anterolateral approach to the humeral shaft.

3 Reduction and fixation

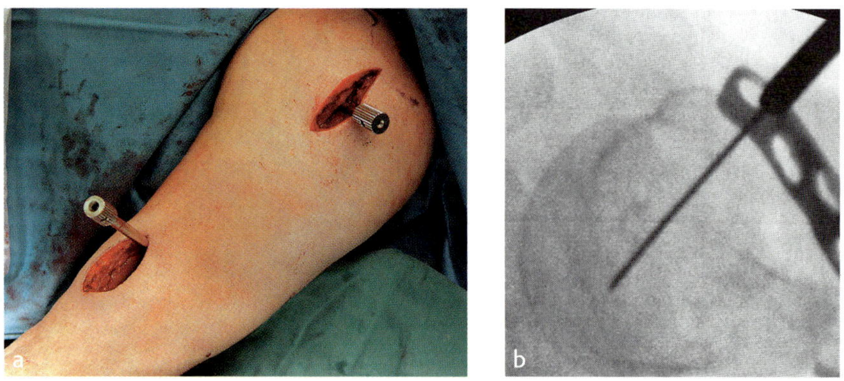

Fracture reduction with manual traction, control using image intensifier.

Twisting of a 3.5/4.5/5.0 metaphyseal LCP for the distal tibia like a helical plate.

Epiperiosteal tunneling with a blunt raspatory and submuscular plate insertion in a proximal to distal direction.

Fig 6.2.1-4a–b

a Positioning of the plate opposite the bone with the aid of threaded drill sleeves.

b Temporary plate fixation proximally and distally with a 1.25 mm K-wire.

3 Reduction and fixation (cont)

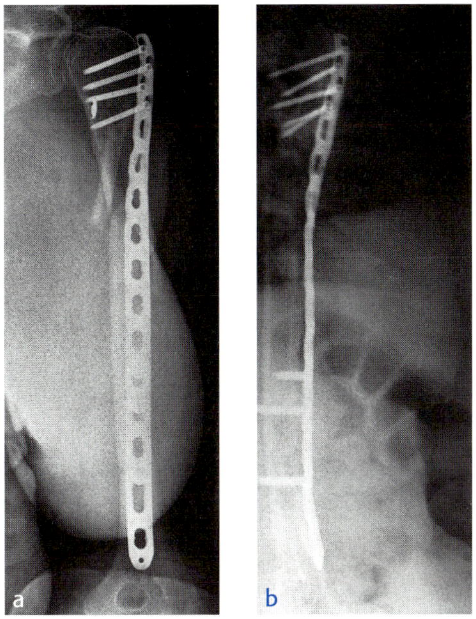

Fixation of the metaphyseal LCP proximally with four 3.5 mm LHS, distally with three 4.5 mm LHS, two of these bicortical. A drill bit broke while drilling, but was left in place. Due to the torque of the plate, the proximal, metaphysis-oriented part of the plate lies against the lateral side of the humeral head. The distal part is situated anterior to the shaft.

Fig 6.2.1-5a–b Postoperative x-rays.
a AP view.
b Lateral view.

4 Rehabilitation

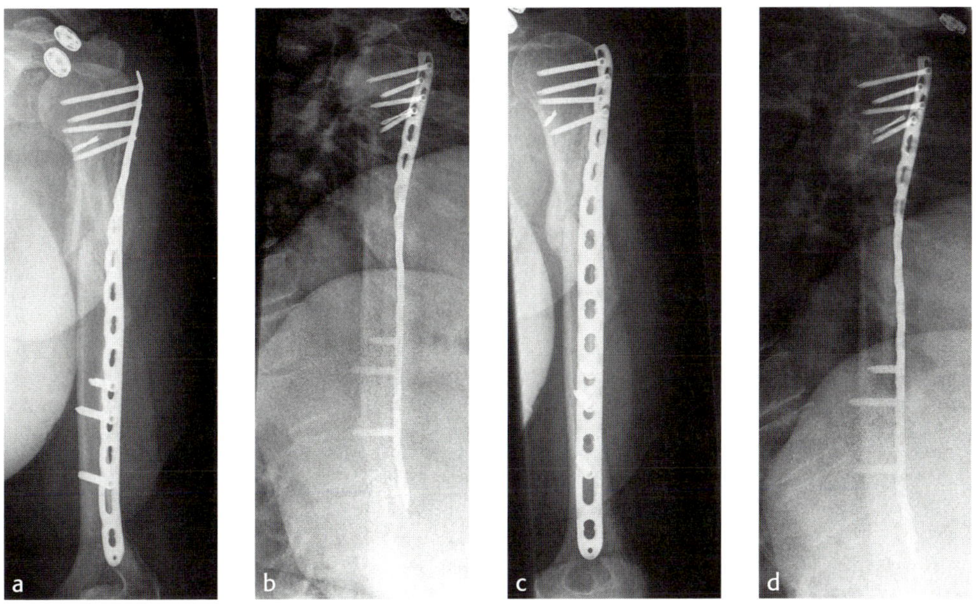

Immobilization in a Gilchrist bandage for 3 weeks. Passive exercise from day 2 postoperatively. Elbow, wrist, and finger exercises allowed from day 1 postoperatively. Exercises following removal of the Gilchrist bandage.

Fig 6.2.1-6a–d
a–b Follow-up x-rays after 2 months. Incipient callus bridging of the fracture.
c–d X-rays after 4 months. Bone healing of the fracture.

4 Rehabilitation (cont)

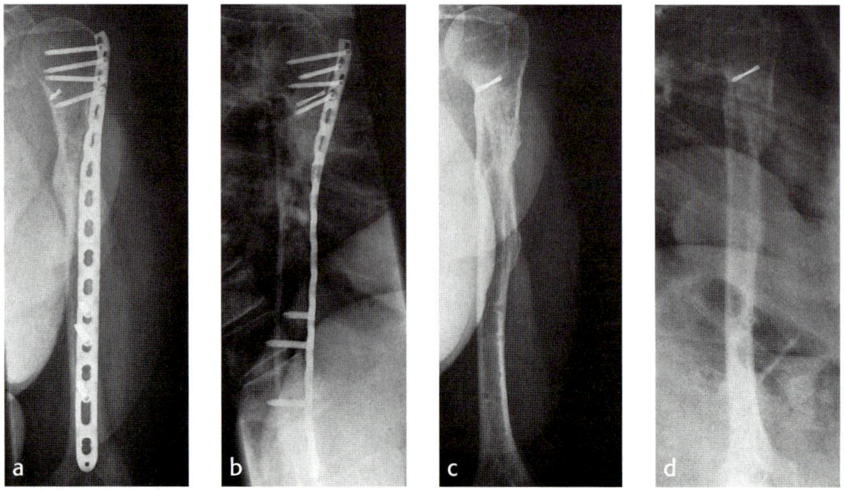

Fig 6.2.1-7a–b Postoperative x-rays after 7 months.

Implant removal

Fig 6.2.1-7c–d Implant removal after 9 months to reduce pain caused by proximal soft-tissue impingement.

5 Pitfalls –

Approach

Deltoid splitting approach: danger of axillary lesion, strictly epiperiosteal preparation and plate insertion is necessary.

Anterior incision to the humeral shaft: preservation of the brachioradialis and radial nerve is necessary. After pushing the belly of the biceps to the medial side, the brachialis muscle is split anteriorly above the bone in the direction of its fibers. The muscle structure pushed to the lateral side protects the radialis nerve like a cushion. Use of a Hohmann retractor should be avoided, so as not to inflict any tensive/compressive forces.

Reduction and fixation

Closed reduction and MIPO are demanding.

Implant removal

Due to a slight protrusion of the plate proximally, impingement occurred with some pain. This required removal of the implant.

6 Pearls +

Equipment

The metaphyseal LCP, which was prebent similar to a "helical plate", fits to the anatomical conditions of the proximal humerus.
LHS allow stable fixation and early functional postoperative care.

Reduction and fixation

The splinting method with an internal fixator combined with MIPO techniques offers a good solution for multifragmentary fractures in the shaft and metaphysis region.

Author Christoph Sommer

6.2.2 Fragmented humeral shaft wedge fracture—12-B3

1 Case description

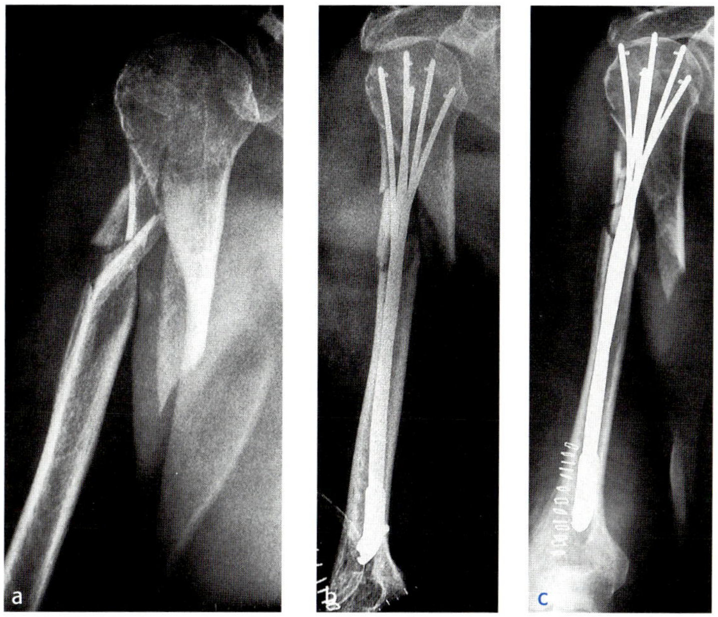

72-year-old woman had a fall while traveling abroad and injured her right arm. She suffered a torsional fracture of the proximal humeral shaft with an avulsed intermediate wedge.

Four days later she was treated by osteosynthesis in the form of retrograde insertion of a flexnail. Just a few days later there was slight collapse of the fracture with penetration of the nail tip into the humeral head. In addition, the patient was now complaining of a sensory disorder in the region served by the ulnar nerve and of loss of strength in the forearm muscles innervated by the median nerve. The patient, who had now returned home, presented at our hospital. Her condition at that time is demonstrated in Fig 6.2.2-1c.

Fig 6.2.2-1a–c

a Preoperative x-ray, AP view.

b Postoperative x-ray after insertion of a flexnail.

c Postoperative x-ray 1 week after insertion of the flexnail.

Indication

The fracture was clearly in incorrect alignment with the insufficient intramedullary nail in situ. This was combined with moderate symptoms of neurological deficit, possibly caused by the persisting dislocation of the fracture, and represented a clear indication for revision osteosynthesis. One possible procedure would be the antegrade insertion of an intramedullary nail with locking options in the region of the humeral head, but the patient vehemently rejected this proposal. An alternative procedure would be plate osteosynthesis performed either in open technique via an anterolateral standard approach or in MIPO technique.

Preoperative planning

Equipment

- LCP metaphyseal plate 3.5/4.5/5.0, 5 + 8 holes
- 3.5 mm locking head screws (LHS)
- 5.0 mm LHS
- 3.5 mm cortex screws
- K-wire

(Size of system, instruments, and implants can vary according to anatomy.)

Patient preparation and positioning

Antibiotics: single dose 2nd generation cephalosporin

Thrombosis prophylaxis: low-molecular heparin

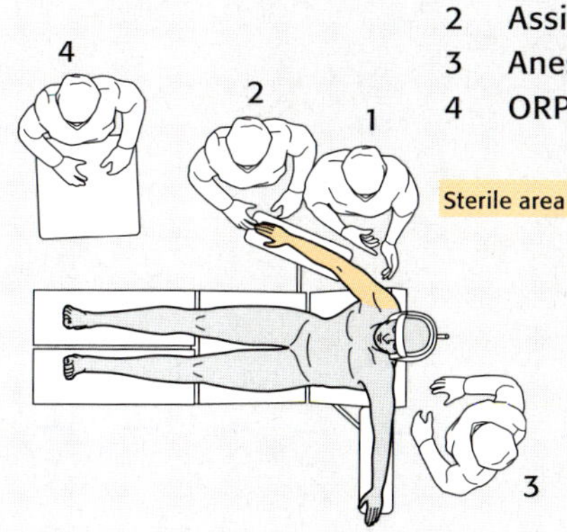

1 Surgeon
2 Assistant
3 Anesthetist
4 ORP

Fig 6.2.2-2 Beach chair position.

2 Surgical approach

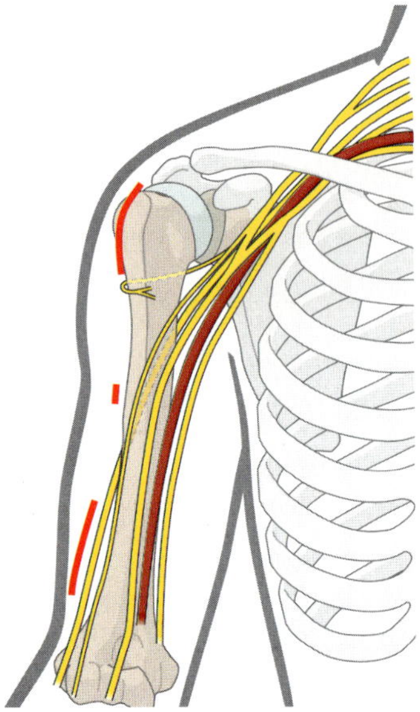

Fig 6.2.2-3 The proximal location of the fracture requires fixation of the plate in the region of the humeral head, which can best be achieved by means of an anterolateral deltoid split approach. The incision is made from the lower margin of the acromion and runs approximately 6 cm in a distal direction. Division of the deltoid muscle in the direction of its fibers, approach and dissection of the subacromial bursa. Exposure of the most superior branch of the axillary nerve that is clearly visible at the lower margin of the incision.
Taking care to preserve this nerve, the plate bed is created by epiperiosteal tunneling with the distal plate end with blunt penetration of the insertion of the deltoid muscle close to the bone. Since the plate is only inserted as far as the junction of the mid to the distal thirds of the shaft and comes to rest in an anterolateral position, the radial nerve need not be identified in the distal region. The approach is made anterolaterally next to the biceps muscle and runs through the upper regions of the brachialis muscle to the distal humeral shaft.

3 Reduction and fixation

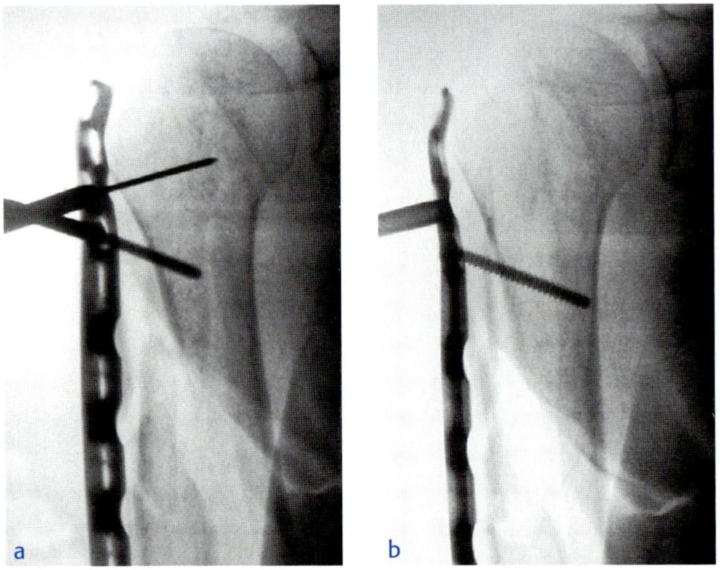

Fig 6.2.2-4a–b

a The plate is bent slightly at its proximal end (to correspond to the contours of the greater tubercle), slide-inserted and initially fixed at the upper end in the humeral head with a K-wire that is introduced through a threaded drill guide. A K-wire is also introduced through the distal incision, likewise through a threaded drill guide, into the distal shaft once length and rotation have been adjusted to be as correct as possible (indirectly by the weight and position of the forearm).

b The gaping and angularly displaced fracture can now be indirectly reduced to the plate by inserting a 3.5 mm cortex screw into the proximal part as a first step so that the proximal fragment is approximated to the plate.

3 Reduction and fixation (cont)

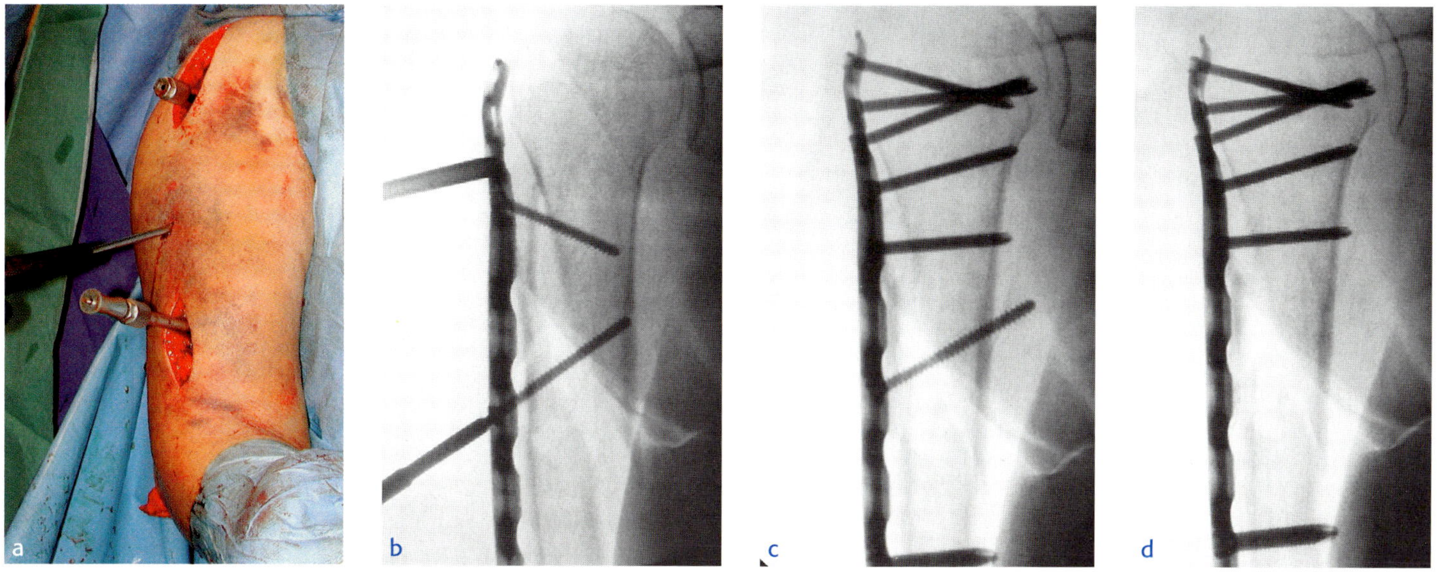

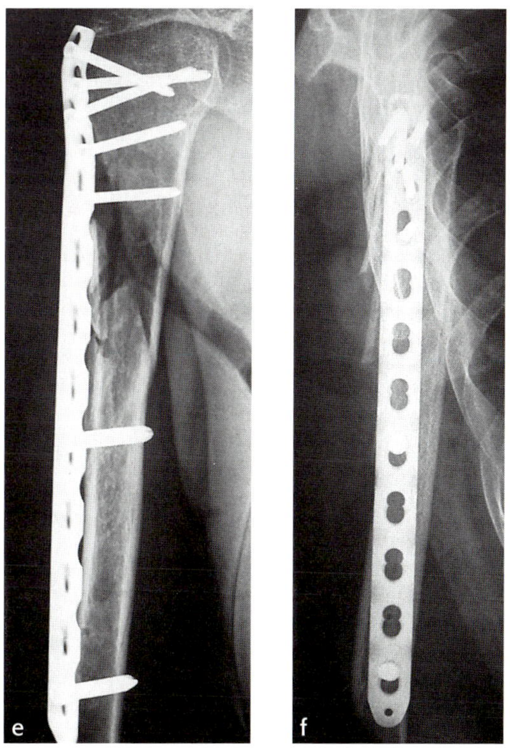

Fig 6.2.2-5a–f

a–c Since the fracture gap is still open, an identical 3.5 mm cortex screw is inserted as the next step via a separate stab incision and tightened to act as a reduction screw. In this way the displaced fracture can be pulled together and reduced in a more or less anatomically correct position. Alternatively, this procedure could be performed with collinear reduction forceps inserted percutaneously, which would require a slightly larger incision.

d After evaluating axial alignment in the lateral view, definitive fixation is performed by insertion of five 3.5 mm bicortical or sub-bicortical locking head screws proximally in the humeral head section and by two 5.0 mm bicortical locking head screws distally. The interfragmentary lag screw inserted earlier as a reduction screw is now too long and is removed.

e–f At completion, correct axial alignment was apparent in both planes as well as an almost anatomically reduced main fracture zone with a slightly dehiscent anterior intermediary fragment.

4 Rehabilitation

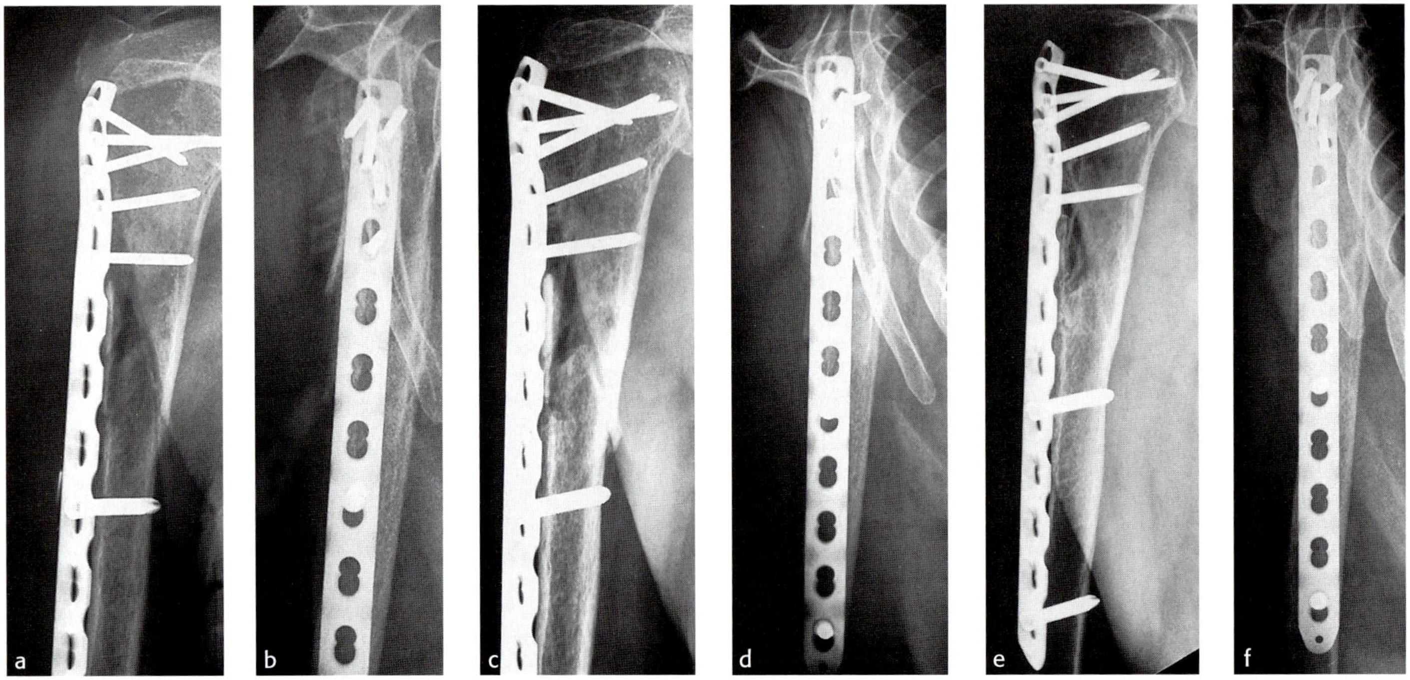

Early functional rehabilitation without immobilization with active-assisted exercises to stimulate shoulder and elbow mobility.

Fig 6.2.2-6a–f
- a–b After 6 weeks the neurological deficit had completely disappeared. There were radiological signs of initial consolidation in the medial segments with slow formation of callus.
- c–d Increasing consolidation was visible even endosteally after 3 months with unchanged stable seating of the locking head screws.
- e–f After 14 months completely consolidated fracture zone in the advanced stages of remodeling and completely normal shoulder and elbow function.

5 Pitfalls –

Equipment

Approach
Deltoid splitting approach: danger of axillary lesion. Risk of lesion of the radial nerve due to:
- an approach too lateral or too distal, or
- incorrect exposure of the nerve.

Reduction and fixation
A minimally invasive approach makes it more difficult to align the fracture in terms of axes, length, and rotation. Tangential screw insertion is to be avoided since this may lead to plate pull-out.

Rehabilitation

6 Pearls +

Equipment
Plate systems with locking head screws facilitate a minimally invasive procedure. There is less risk of infection compared to conventional plates because there is less need to cause additional damage to the vascularity of the periosteum and the fracture zone. An internal osteosynthesis procedure has advantages over an external fixator because a very long time to healing must be expected and, therefore, there will be a correspondingly long period with the fixator in situ.

Approach
The minimally invasive approach reduces the risk of additional iatrogenic damage to the biologically severely injured fracture zone.

Reduction and fixation
A cortex screw can be used as a reduction screw:
- to reduce the bone fragment onto the plate
- to reduce the fracture gap

The insertion of locking head screws increases the primary and secondary stability of the osteosynthesis.

Rehabilitation
An internal fixation procedure offers greatly improved patient comfort compared to stabilization with an external fixator.

Author Christoph Sommer

6.2.3 Gunshot fracture of the humeral shaft—12-C1

1 Case description

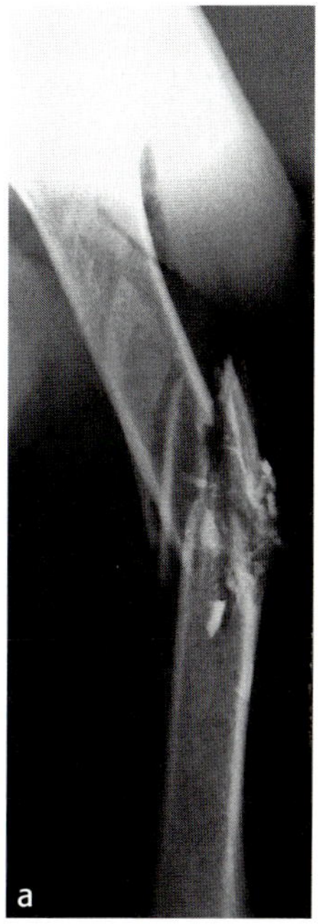

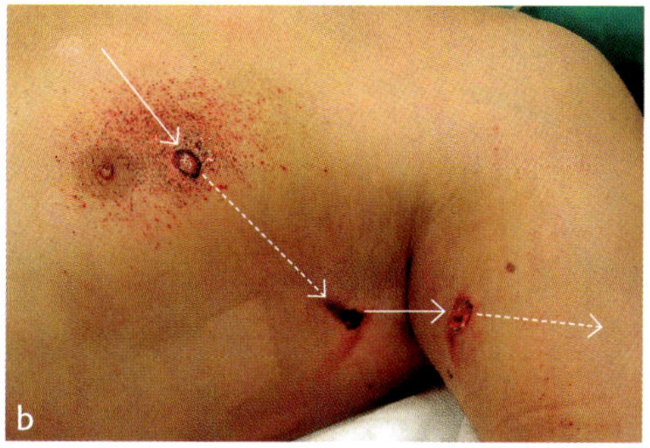

42-year-old man attempting suicide shot a bullet diagonally through the left hemithorax and into the left upper arm. The thoracic injury (right through the lung) was treated by thorax drainage and healed. The shot through the upper arm caused a shaft fracture in the midthird (12-C1). There were no concomitant neurovascular injuries.

Fig 6.2.3-1a–b
a AP view.
b Clinical picture.

Indication

Gunshot fracture of the humerus is a clear indication for operative treatment. Soft tissue debridement and stabilization of the fracture is essential. One possibility would be standard osteosynthesis with an external fixator. Intramedullary nailing or plate osteosynthesis procedures can also be recommended. In an open procedure, which would be indicated in any case with concomitant neurovascular injuries, plate osteosynthesis with primary and secondary cancellous bone grafting would be preferred. In the case presented here, it was decided to perform minimally invasive insertion of an internal fixator after surgical debridement of the entry and exit sites and irrigation of the gunshot channel.

Preoperative planning

Equipment
- LCP 4.5, 13 holes
- 5.0 mm locking head screws (LHS)

(Size of system, instruments, and implants can vary according to anatomy.)

Patient preparation and positioning
Antibiotics: single shot 2nd generation cephalosporin
Thrombosis prophylaxis: low-molecular heparin

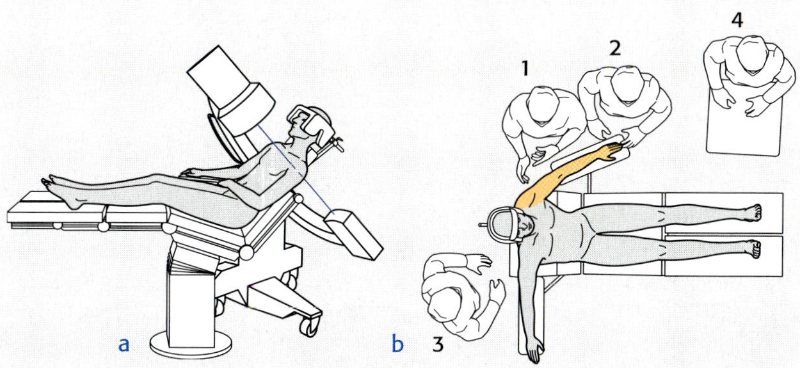

1 Surgeon
2 Assistant
3 Anesthetist
4 ORP

Sterile area

Fig 6.2.3-2a–b Beach chair position.

2 Surgical approach

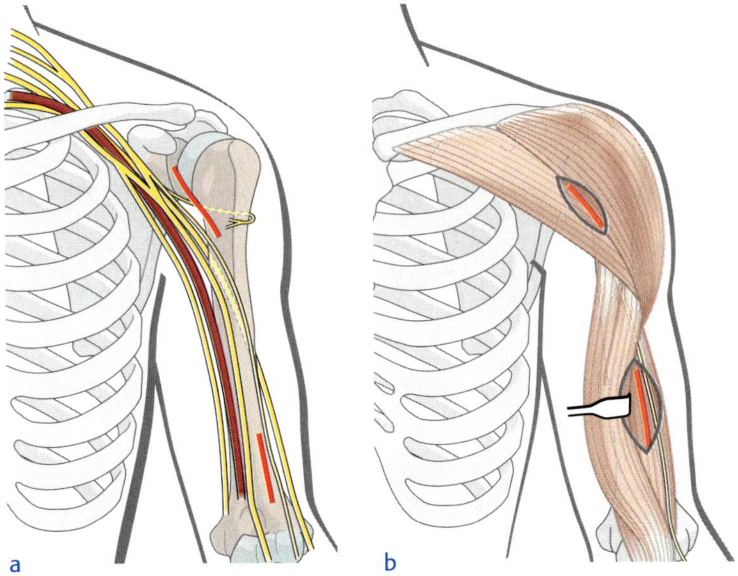

Incisions were made at the proximal and distal humerus without exposing the actual fracture zone.

Fig 6.2.3-3a–b Proximally, a short standard incision is made in the line of the deltopectoral groove, taking care to avoid injury of the cephalic vein. The approach passes under the deltoid muscle which is reflected laterally. Distally, a standard anterolateral approach to the lateral humerus is performed. Identification of the groove between the brachialis and brachioradialis muscles in which the radial nerve lies. After visualization and preservation of the radial nerve, the brachialis muscle is divided at the junction of the lateral and mid thirds in the direction of its fibers, thus facilitating direct access to the humeral shaft.

3 Reduction and fixation

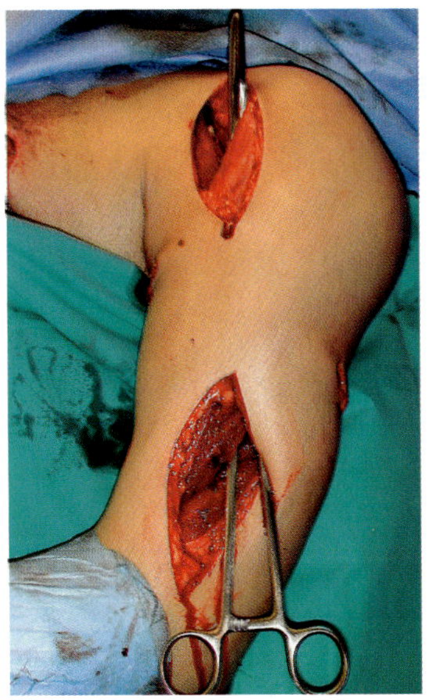

Fig 6.2.3-4 A tunnel is now created across the unexposed fracture zone close to the bone starting proximally or distally. This maneuver can be performed either with the plate itself or with a large pair of tweezers.
Blunt penetration of the distal insertion of the deltoid muscle is necessary.

3 Reduction and fixation (cont)

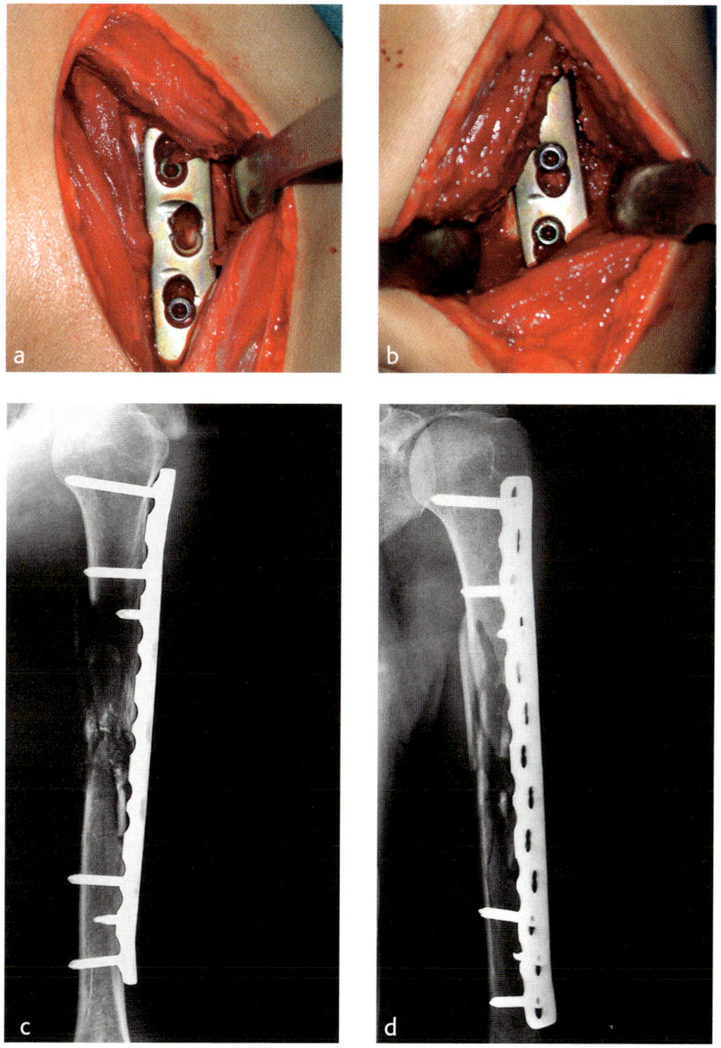

Fig 6.2.3-5a–d

a–b The beach chair position with the arm dangling automatically leads to a fairly good indirect reduction in terms of length and axes. If the forearm is held in the neutral position, the rotational alignment will more or less correct itself. The LCP, bent slightly outwards at its proximal and distal ends, can now be inserted into the prepared plate bed. Primary fixation is achieved by insertion of a long, bicortical locking head screw into the most proximal hole. After fine-tuning the reduction of length and rotation, a 5.0 mm bicortical locking head screw is inserted into the most distal plate hole. With the arm hanging loosely and the patient relaxed, care should be taken not to stabilize the fracture zone in over-distraction. Fine-tuning of axial alignment can be undertaken in the lateral view by applying manual pressure and counter-pressure at the level of the fracture zone and/or at the elbow to realign any residual angular deformity. Further stabilization is achieved by insertion of additional locking head screws proximally and distally. It is recommended that 4–5 cortices should be fixed. Bicortical screws increase rotational stability, which is strongly recommended if bone quality is poor.

c–d The postoperative x-rays confirm that the comminuted zone has been bridged in correct alignment as the result of osteosynthesis with a locked internal fixator.

4 Rehabilitation

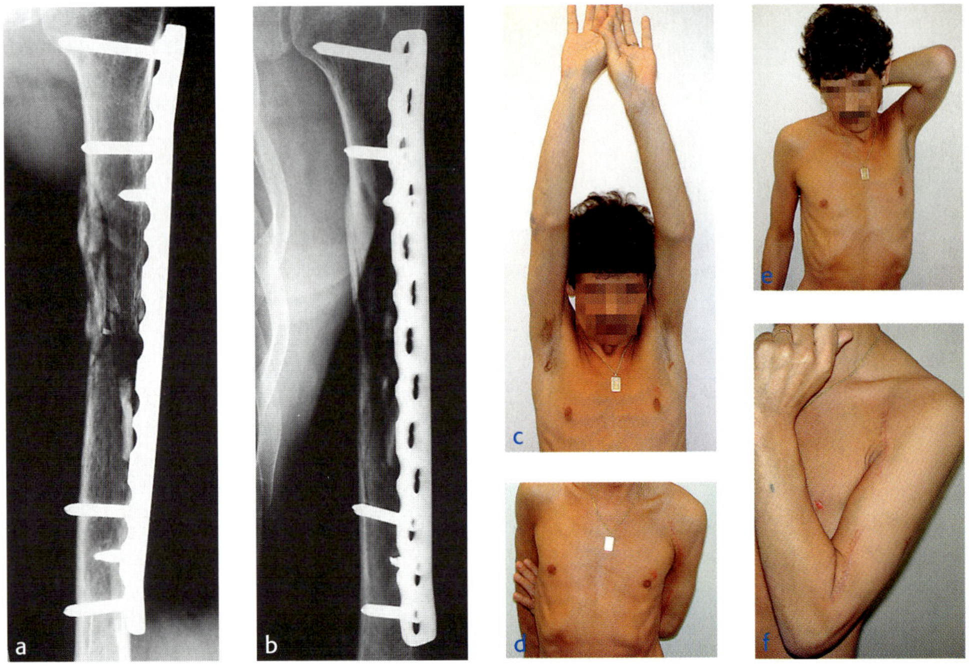

Open wound treatment of the gunshot entry and exit sites was continued and led to uneventful wound closure within a few days. Early functional rehabilitation without immobilization of the left upper arm.

Fig 6.2.3-6a–f
a–b After 7 weeks clear signs of early callus formation in the comminuted zone with unchanged stable seating of the plate and screws.
c–f At this time the patient demonstrated normal function of the shoulder and elbow joints. From this point on loading was gradually increased until full loading was achieved at 3 months.

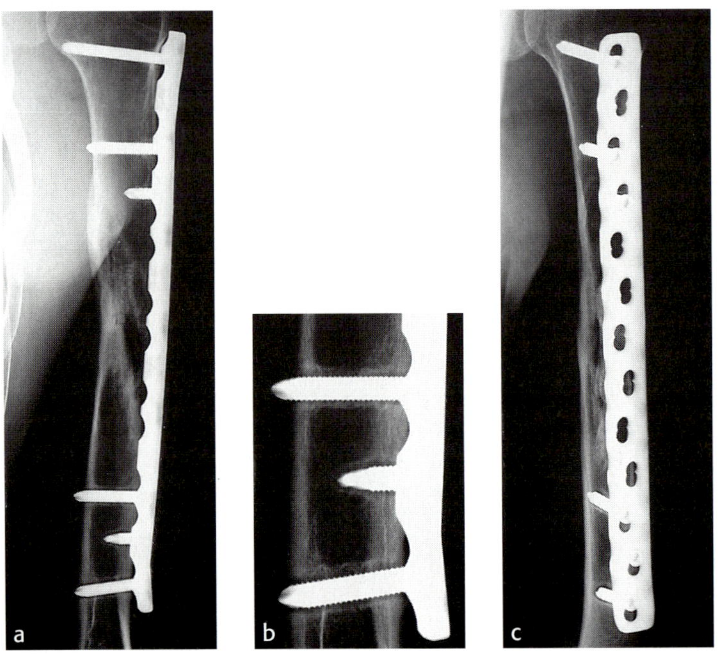

Fig 6.2.3-7a–c After one year the fracture zone had been partially bridged. Resorption lucencies around the screws were clearly visible on the detailed images, especially around the distal screws, whereby there are also signs of reossification of these areas as an indication that complete stability of the former fracture zone has been regained.

4 Rehabilitation (cont)

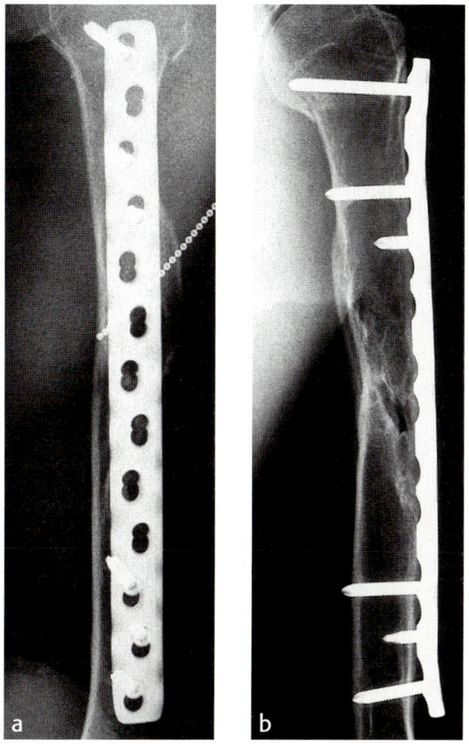

Fig 6.2.3-8a–b A subsequent examination after 4 1/2 years showed predominantly endosteal consolidation of the fracture zone with almost complete remodeling. The resorption lucencies around the distal locking head screws were now completely reossified. The implants will not be removed if the patient remains free of symptoms.

5 Pitfalls –

Equipment

6 Pearls +

Equipment

Plate systems with locking head screws facilitate a minimally invasive procedure. There is less risk of infection compared to conventional plates because there is less need to cause additional damage to the vascularity of the periosteum and the fracture zone. An internal osteosynthesis procedure has advantages over an external fixator because a very long time to healing must be expected and, therefore, there will be a correspondingly long period with the fixator in situ.

5 Pitfalls – (cont)

Approach
Lesion of the radial nerve due to incorrect exposure of the nerve.

Reduction and fixation
A minimally invasive approach makes it more difficult to align the fracture in terms of axes, length, and rotation. Tangential screw insertion is to be avoided since this may lead to plate pull-out.

Rehabilitation
Due to a slight protrusion of the plate, proximal impingement occurred with some pain, which required removal of the implant.

6 Pearls + (cont)

Approach
The minimally invasive approach reduces the risk of additional iatrogenic damage to the biologically severely injured fracture zone.

Reduction and fixation
The insertion of locking head screws increases the primary and secondary stability of the osteosynthesis.

Rehabilitation
An internal fixation procedure offers greatly improved patient comfort compared to stabilization with an external fixator.

Author Christoph Sommer

6.2.4 Complex segmental proximal humeral shaft fracture—12-C2

1 Case description

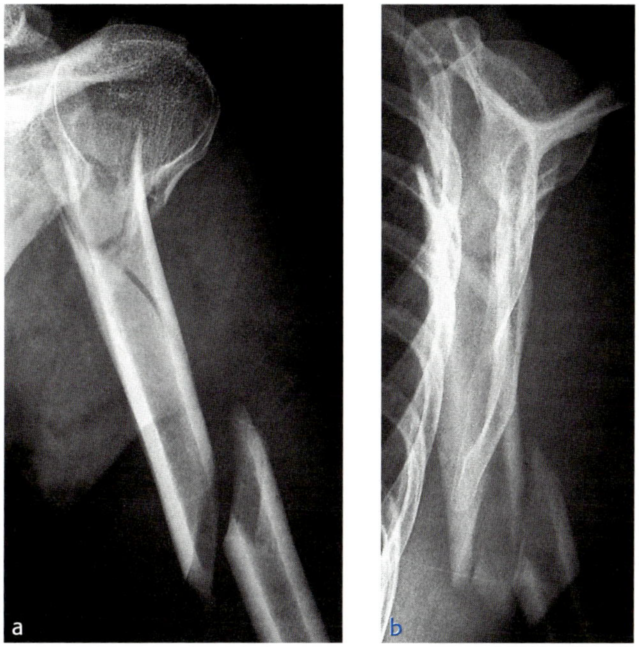

45-year-old man fell while skiing and suffered a bifocal fracture of the left proximal humerus. The injury was a subcapital oblique fracture combined with a proximal shaft fracture, whereby the intermediary fragment was split longitudinally (12-C2.2). No concomitant neurovascular injuries.

Fig 6.2.4-1
a AP view.
b Lateral view.

Indication

This very unstable fracture is not well suited to nonoperative treatment, in particular, because the proximal fracture showed evidence of substantial lateral displacement. Surgical alternatives would include the antegrade insertion of an intramedullary nail with proximal locking option in the area of the humeral head or plate osteosynthesis. Minimally invasive plate osteosynthesis is an elegant way to minimize the surgical trauma of an extensive anterolateral approach.

Preoperative planning

Equipment

- LCP metaphyseal plate, 3.5/4.5/5.0, 5 + 11 holes
- 3.5 mm locking head screws (LHS)
- 3.5 mm cortex screws

(Size of system, instruments, and implants can vary according to anatomy.)

Patient preparation and positioning

Antibiotics: single dose 2nd generation cephalosporin
Thrombosis prophylaxis: low-molecular heparin

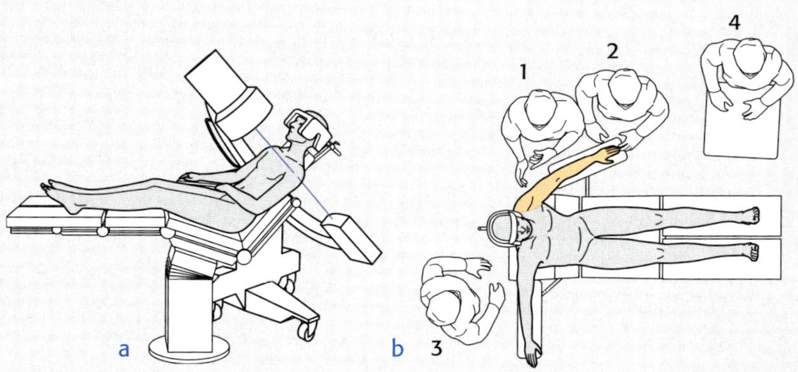

Fig 6.2.4-2a–b Beach chair position.

2 Surgical approach

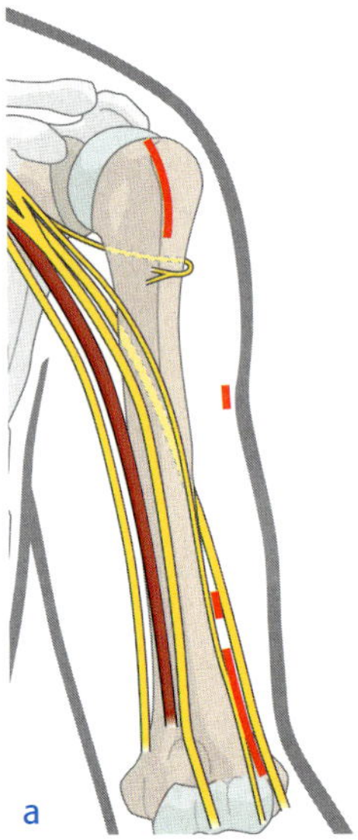

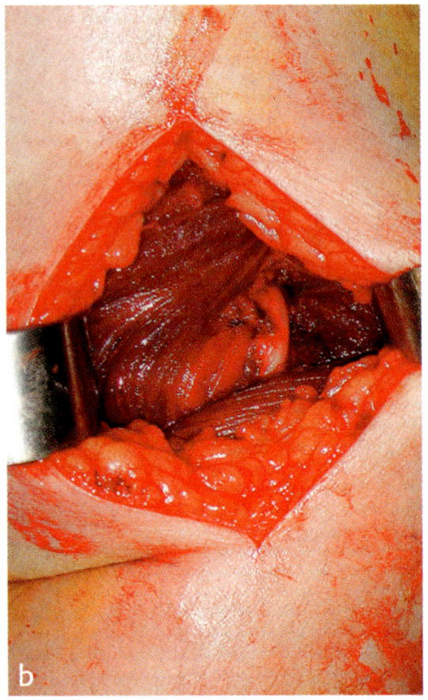

Fig 6.2.4-3a–b

a Since the proximal fracture runs beneath the humeral head, adequate fixation in that region is essential. Therefore, an anterolateral deltoid split approach is the optimal procedure. The approach starts at the lower margin of the acromion and extends approximately 6 cm in a distal direction as far as the subcapital zone. Division of the deltoid in the direction of its fibers, whereby the most superior branch of the axillary nerve and its accompanying vessels can be identified at the lower margin of the incision.
Incision of the subacromial bursa and epiperiosteal tunneling in a distal direction with a blunt instrument or the distal plate end with reflection and preservation of the branch of the axillary nerve. Since a long plate is necessary to reach the distal section of the humeral shaft, an open distal approach should be chosen, with identification of the groove between the brachialis and brachioradialis muscles and exposure of the radial nerve.

b Anterior to the visible radial nerve, transmuscular incision through the brachialis muscle at the junction of the lateral and mid thirds by muscle division in the direction of its fibers. Direct approach to the distal humeral shaft, which can be exposed by application of two small Hohmann retractors. The plate can be slid into the prepared plate bed from proximal to distal.

3 Reduction and fixation

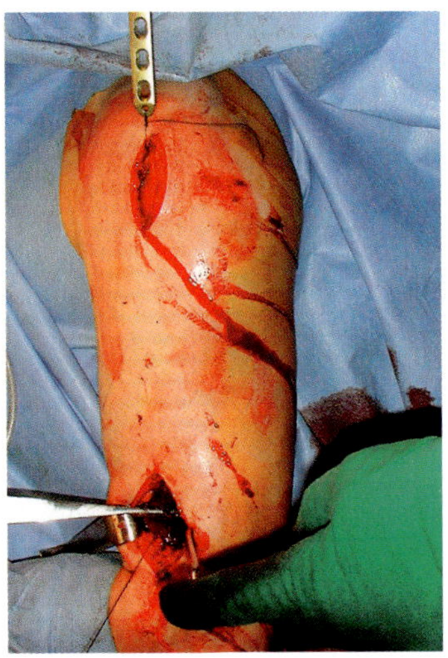

Fig 6.2.4-4 Another possibility is to insert a long, strong thread first by means of a tunneling device and to attach the plate to it. The plate can now be pulled in a distal direction with the help of this thread.

3 Reduction and fixation (cont)

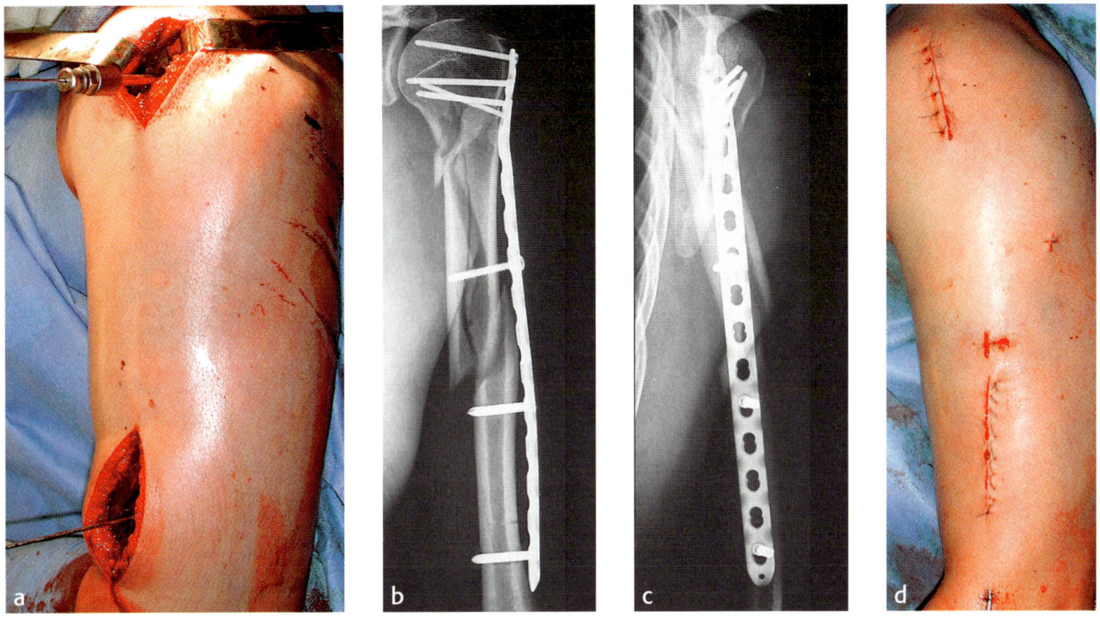

Fig 6.2.4-5a–d

a The proximal plate end has to be bent slightly outwards prior to insertion to achieve optimal adaptation to the greater tubercle. Once the plate has been inserted, it is first secured proximally in the correct position with one screw. In this case, a conventional 3.5 mm cortex screw that pressed the plate optimally towards the greater tubercle and avoided irritation of the soft tissues was chosen. Reduction of the main fracture zone is achieved indirectly by the weight of the forearm as the arm hangs down, whereby axial, length and rotational alignment of the proximal fragment in relation to the distal fragment are adequately restored in the usual way. After evaluation of fracture alignment, a 4.3 mm drill bit is inserted through the 5.0 mm threaded drill guide in the most distal plate hole, whereby the drill bit penetrates both cortices. Before inserting any further screws, axial deviation can be assessed in the lateral view and can be corrected indirectly via the plate by manual pressure and counterpressure. After placing additional screws in the region of the humeral head (if possible, locking head screws depending on the situation and screw orientation), a bicortical screw is introduced adjacent to the fracture in the distal main fragment. Only then is the drill bit in the most distal plate hole replaced by a bicortical locking head screw. Since the intermediate fragment was in marked anteromedial dislocation, it was pulled into position by insertion of a conventional 4.5 mm cortex screw through a stab incision which then functioned as a reduction screw.

b–c The final x-rays confirmed bridging of the fracture zone in correct axial alignment with the plate well positioned close to the bone.

d Wound closure.

4 Rehabilitation

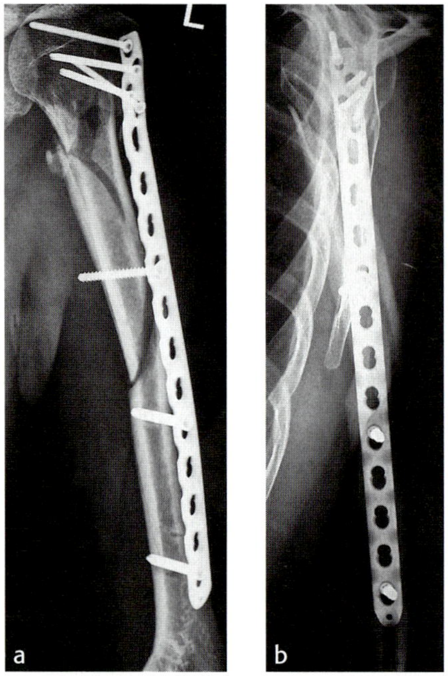

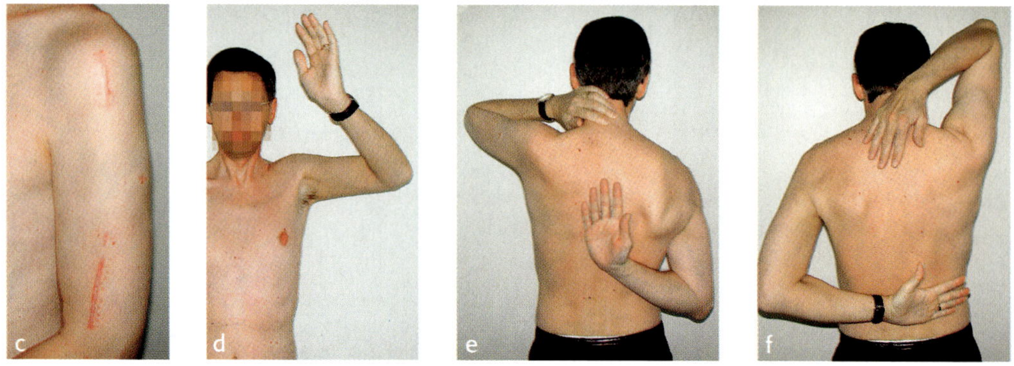

Early functional rehabilitation without immobilization. No loading for the first 6 weeks, whereby shoulder and elbow motion was strengthened in guided active exercises.

Fig 6.2.4-6a–f

a–b After 6 weeks, initial callus formation was visible at the proximal fracture location; the distal location showed signs of resorption of the fracture margins, indicating the start of consolidation.

c–f The patient demonstrates very good function of the left shoulder with active flexion and abduction to 100° as well as almost normal inner and outer rotation.

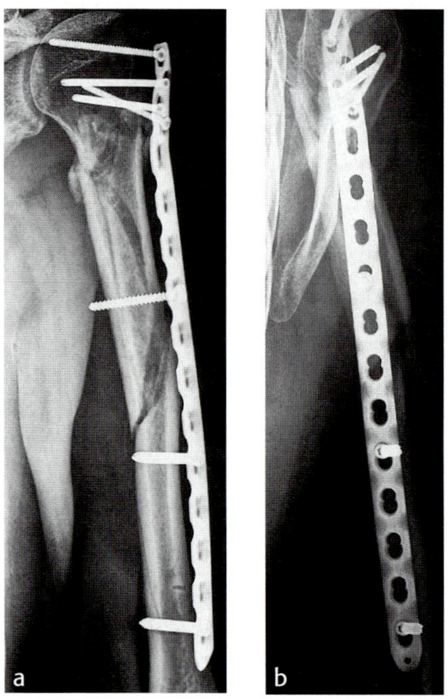

Fig 6.2.4-7a–b

After 3 months, increasing periosteal and endosteal consolidation of the proximal fracture site. Likewise, increasing endosteal consolidation at the distal fracture site.

4 Rehabilitation (cont)

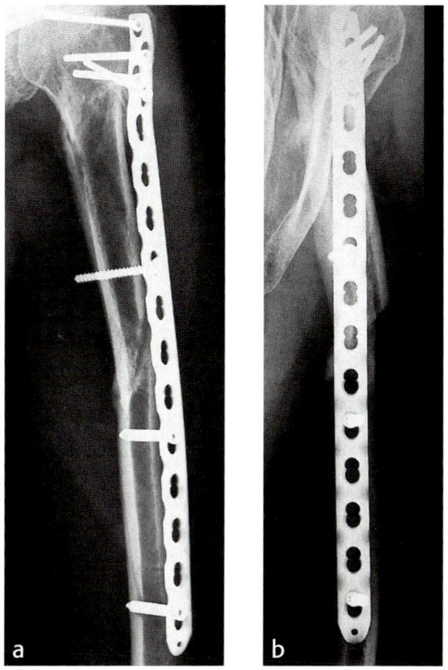

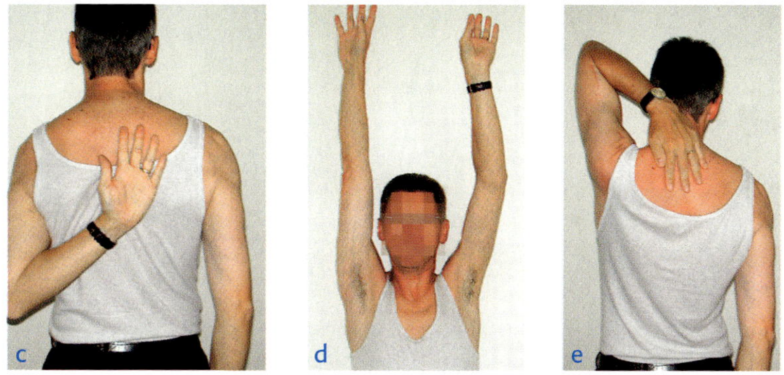

Fig 6.2.4-8a–e

a–b After 7 months, complete fracture consolidation was documented, whereby remodeling was still in progress.

c–e At this time, unrestricted shoulder and elbow function with the affected and contralateral limbs showing almost equal performance.

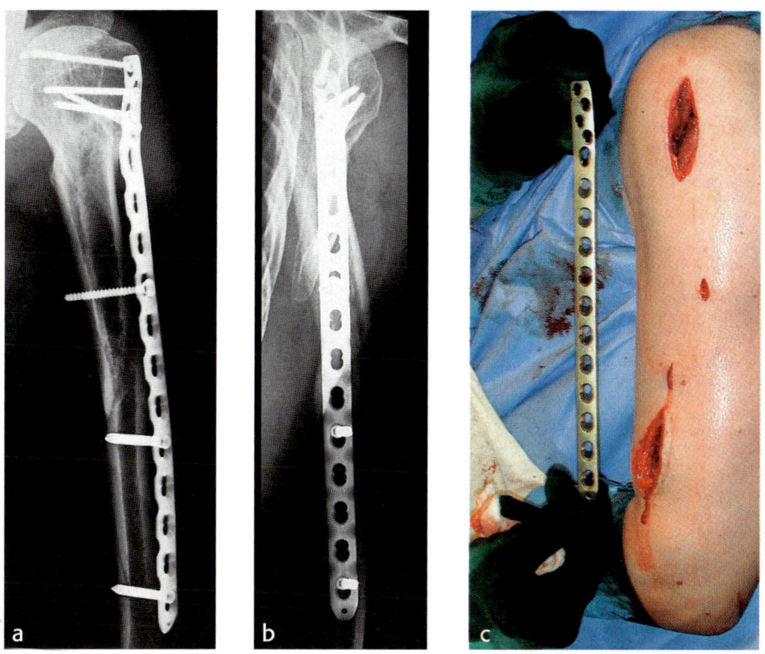

Implant removal

Fig 6.2.4-9a–c After 16 months the patient requested implant removal although there were not really any symptoms. The fracture completely remodeled.

Implant removal was performed through the same incisions as the osteosynthesis, making sure that the radial nerve in the distal region was carefully identified, exposed, and retracted.

5 Pitfalls –

Equipment

Approach
Lesion of the radial nerve due to incorrect exposure of the nerve.

Reduction and fixation
A minimally invasive approach makes it more difficult to align the fracture in terms of axes, length, and rotation. Tangential screw insertion is to be avoided since this may lead to plate pull-out.

Rehabilitation

6 Pearls +

Equipment
Plate systems with locking head screws facilitate a minimally invasive procedure. There is less risk of infection compared to conventional plates because there is less need to cause additional damage to the vascularity of the periosteum and the fracture zone. An internal osteosynthesis procedure has advantages over an external fixator because a very long time to healing must be expected and, therefore, there will be a correspondingly long period with the fixator in situ.

Approach
The minimally invasive approach reduces the risk of additional iatrogenic damage of the biologically severely injured fracture zone.

Reduction and fixation
The insertion of locking head screws increases the primary and secondary stability of the osteosynthesis.

Rehabilitation
An internal fixation procedure offers greatly improved patient comfort compared to stabilization with an external fixator.

Author Christoph Sommer

6.2.5 Complex segmental humeral shaft fracture—12-C2

1 Case description

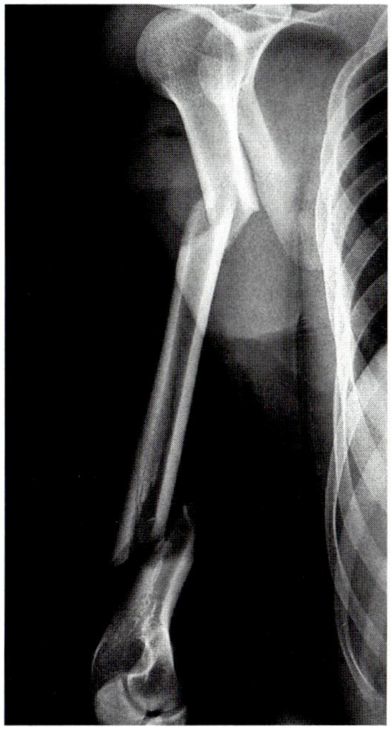

21-year-old snowboarder collided with a marker post and injured his right arm. During the fall he sustained a closed bifocal fracture of the right humeral shaft (12-C2.1). No concomitant neurovascular injuries.

Fig 6.2.5-1 AP view.

Indication

This bifocal fracture is not well suited to nonoperative treatment, in particular because these were more or less transverse fractures situated relatively far proximally and distally. The distal fracture component is not suited to intramedullary nail fixation. Other options would include external fixator or plate osteosynthesis. The open procedure for conventional plate osteosynthesis requires an extensive approach along the entire length of the humerus. Minimally invasive slide-insertion technique reduces the length of the approach considerably.

Preoperative planning

Equipment

- LCP metaphyseal plate 3.5/4.5/5.0, 5 + 11 holes
- 3.5 mm locking head screws (LHS)

(Size of system, instruments, and implants can vary according to anatomy.)

Patient preparation and positioning

Antibiotics: single dose 2nd generation cephalosporin

Thrombosis prophylaxis: low-molecular heparin

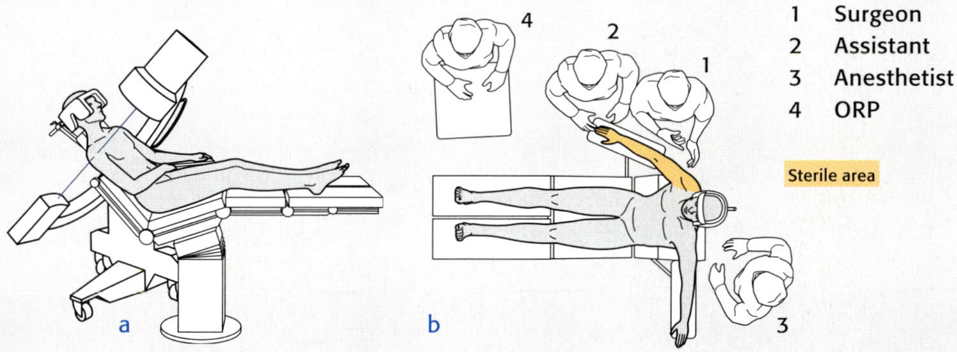

Fig 6.2.5-2a–b Beach chair position.

2 Surgical approach

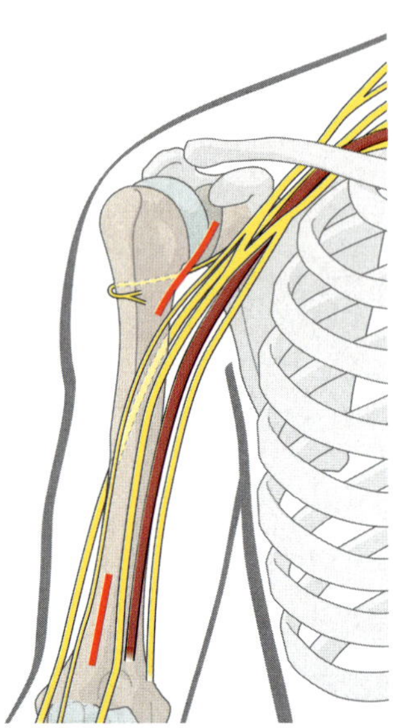

a

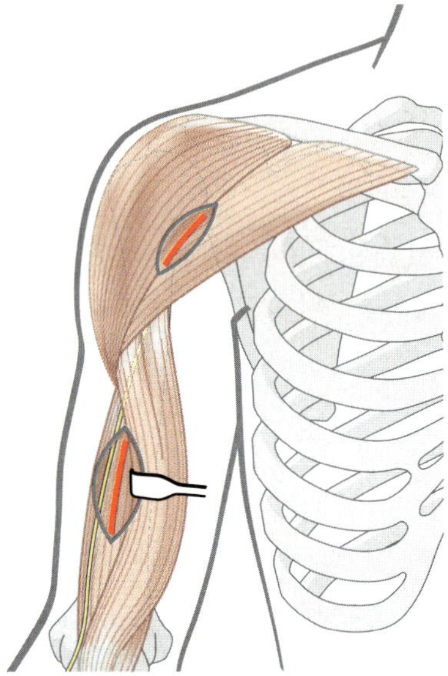

b

Fig 6.2.5-3a–b Incisions were made at the proximal and distal humerus without exposing the actual fracture zone. Proximally, a short standard incision is made in the line of the deltopectoral groove, taking care to avoid the cephalic vein. The approach passes under the deltoid muscle which is reflected laterally. Distally, a standard anterolateral approach for the lateral humerus is performed. Identification of the groove between the brachialis and brachioradialis muscles in which the radial nerve lies. After visualization and preservation of the radial nerve, the brachialis muscle is divided at the junction of the lateral part and the midthird in the direction of its fibers, thus facilitating direct access to the humeral shaft.

3 Reduction and fixation

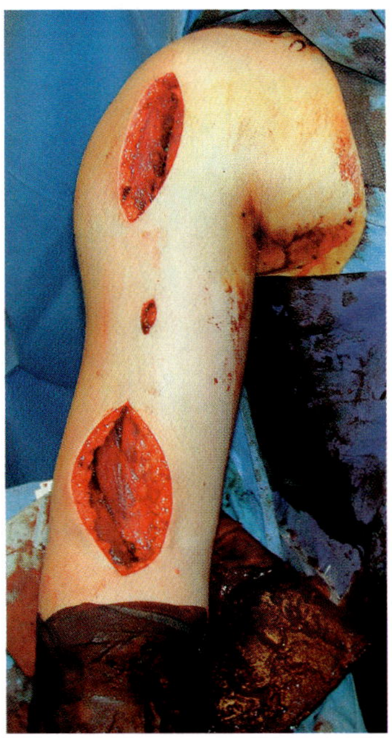

Fig 6.2.5-4 A tunnel is now created across the unexposed fracture zone close to the bone starting proximally or distally. This maneuver can be performed either with the plate itself or with a large pair of tweezers. Blunt penetration of the distal insertion of the deltoid muscle is necessary.

3 Reduction and fixation (cont)

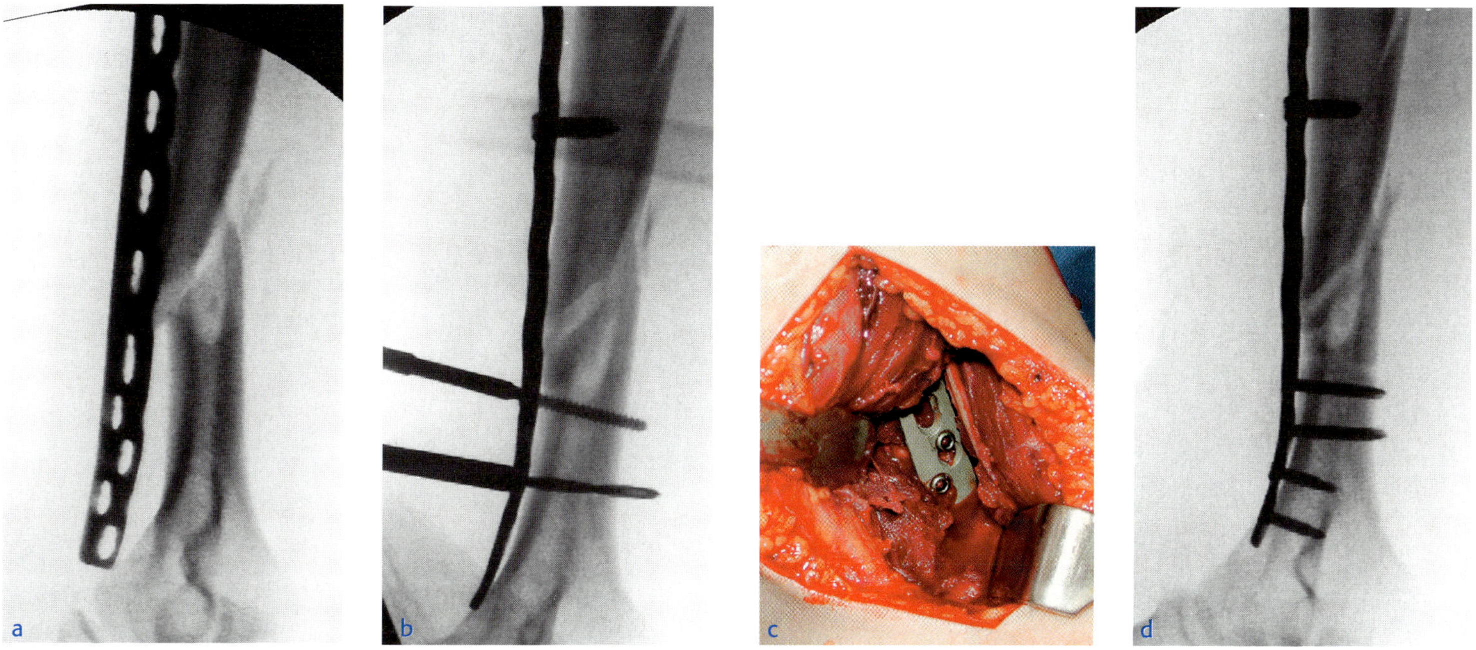

Fig 6.2.5-5a–d

a The proximal deltopectoral approach permits tunneling in a distal direction and, likewise, the distal incision permits tunneling in a proximal direction under the distal portion of the fracture zone. The LCP metaphyseal plate, appropriately bent at its distal and proximal ends, can be slid from the proximal aspect in a distal direction into the prepared plate bed. Fracture reduction is achieved by means of the plate, whereby this is first anchored proximally by insertion of a bicortical locking head screw in the subcapital region.

b The middle segment does not have to be anatomically adapted but should be reduced in correct axial and length alignment, if possible. This can be achieved by manual counterpressure exerted on the medial aspect of the humerus or by application of percutaneously inserted collinear reduction forceps. The middle segment is secured with two screws, whereby two monocortical screws are sufficient. If bone quality is poor, bicortical screw insertion should be chosen. To complete the procedure, the distal main fragment is reduced by means of the plate. This can be achieved either by use of the collinear reduction forceps, the insertion of conventional reduction screws or by means of the distraction instruments.

c Subsequent distal fixation was achieved in this case by insertion of four 3.5 mm LHS, whereby bicortical screws are inserted for proximal fixation and monocortical screws for distal fixation.

d The last two screws are inserted into one cortex only to avoid irritation of the olecranon in the region of the olecranon fossa.

3 Reduction and fixation (cont)

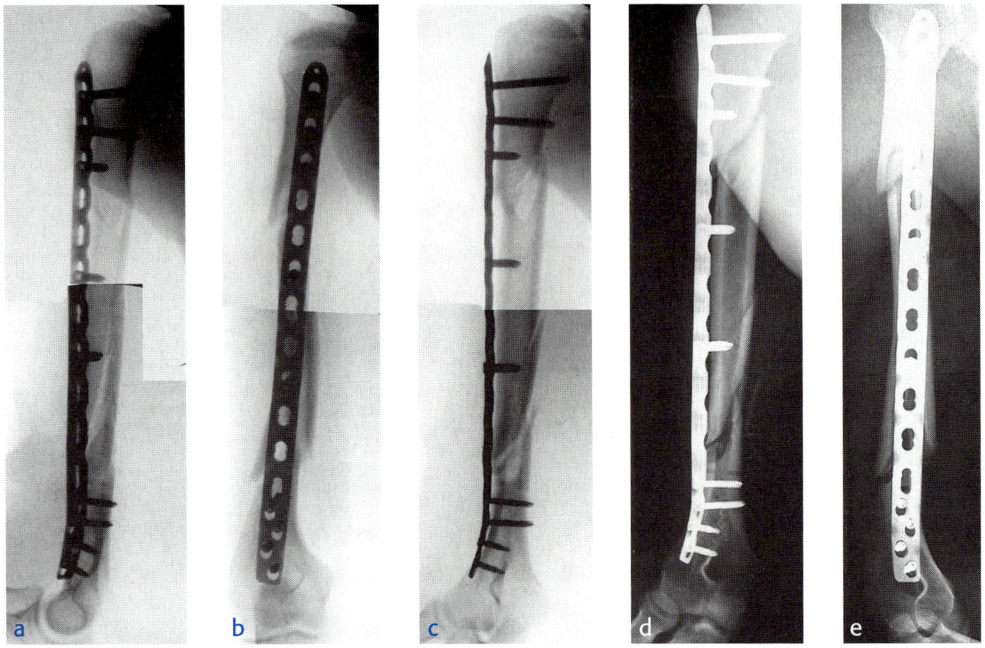

Fig 6.2.5-6a–e
a–c Intraoperative imaging in three planes confirms correct axial bridging of the bifocal fracture, whereby the lateral view shows evidence of a slight axial deviation at the level of the upper fracture focus.
d–e The postoperative situation is documented.

4 Rehabilitation

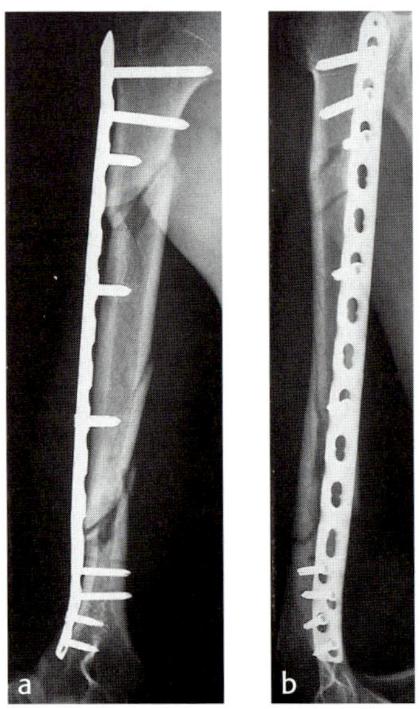

Early functional rehabilitation without any form of immobilization. No loading for the first 6 weeks. Guided active exercises for the shoulder and elbow up to the pain threshold.

Fig 6.2.5-7a–b X-rays at 6 weeks show the start of callus formation at the level of the proximal fractured area. Distally, there are only signs of a certain blurring of the fracture margins as a sign of initial consolidation. The screws are all in stable anchorage without resorption zones.

4 Rehabilitation (cont)

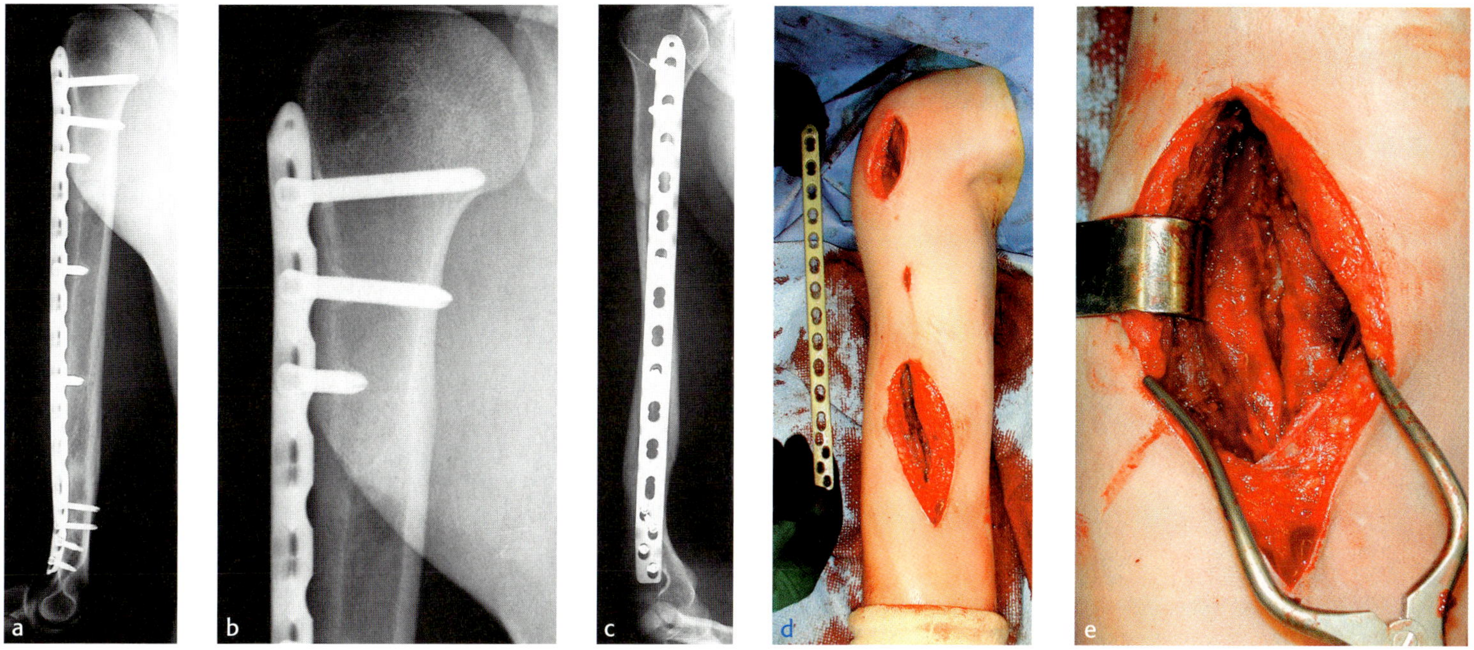

Implant removal

Fig 6.2.5-8a–e

a–c After 6 weeks, increased loading with transition to unrestricted full loading after 3 months. After 16 months final examination of the symptom-free patient shows evidence of total consolidation, whereby the remodeling process has been completed. The fracture zones are no longer visible.

d–e The implants were removed at the request of the patient. This was performed through the same approaches, whereby the distal approach was slightly extended to ensure a clear view and preservation of the radial nerve.

5 Pitfalls –

Equipment

Approach
Lesion of the radial nerve due to incorrect exposure of the nerve.

Reduction and fixation
A minimally invasive approach makes it more difficult to align the fracture in terms of axes, length, and rotation. Tangential screw insertion is to be avoided since this may lead to plate pull-out.

Rehabilitation

6 Pearls +

Equipment
Plate systems with locking head screws facilitate a minimally invasive procedure. There is less risk of infection compared to conventional plates because there is less need to cause additional damage to the vascularity of the periosteum and the fracture zone. An internal osteosynthesis procedure has advantages over an external fixator because a very long time to healing must be expected and, therefore, there will be a correspondingly long period with the fixator in situ.

Approach
The minimally invasive approach reduces the risk of additional iatrogenic damage of the biologically severely injured fracture zone.

Reduction and fixation
The insertion of locking head screws increases the primary and secondary stability of the osteosynthesis.

Rehabilitation
An internal fixation procedure offers greatly improved patient comfort compared to stabilization with an external fixator.

Author Christoph Sommer

6.2.6 Simple transverse humeral shaft fracture—12-A3 and partial intraarticular sagittal lateral humeral condyle fracture—13-B1

1 Case description

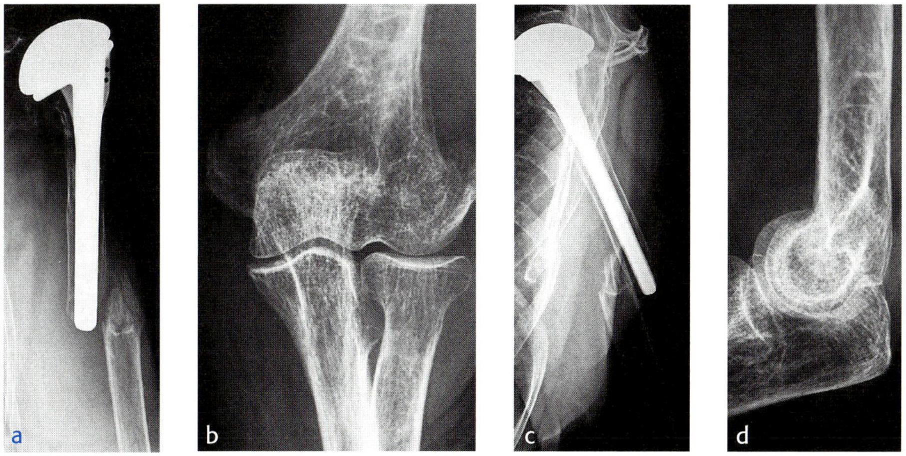

87-year-old woman, mentally still reasonably active, fell on her left arm and sustained a periprosthetic fracture of the humeral diaphysis (12-A3) and a distal, moderately displaced intraarticular fracture of the humeral condyle (13-B1.1). Status after implantation of a humeral head prosthesis three years ago with poor shoulder function and rotator cuff insufficiency. Osteoporosis with a very thin diaphyseal cortex.

Fig 6.2.6-1a–d
a–b AP view.
c–d Lateral view.

Indication

Nonoperative treatment of this laterally displaced periprosthetic oblique fracture is not expected to lead to a successful outcome. Alternative procedures would be a replacement prosthesis with implantation of a long stem prosthesis although the in situ cemented prosthesis should not be removed from this very thin, poor quality bone. Therefore, a decision was taken to perform plate osteosynthesis, whereby a plate system with locking head screws would seem highly appropriate in view of the severely osteoporotic bone. The distal intraarticular fracture can be stabilized at the same time to facilitate early functional rehabilitation.

Preoperative planning

Equipment

- LCP 4.5/5.0, narrow, 10 holes
- LCP T-plate 3.5, 4 holes
- Locking head screws (LHS)

(Size of system, instruments, and implants can vary according to anatomy.)

Patient preparation and positioning

Antibiotics: single dose 2nd generation cephalosporin
Thrombosis prophylaxis: low-molecular heparin

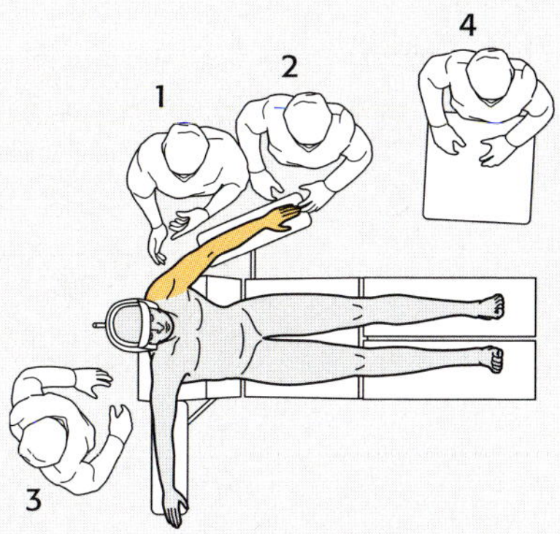

1 Surgeon
2 Assistant
3 Anesthetist
4 ORP

Sterile area

Fig 6.2.6-2 Beach chair position.

2 Surgical approach

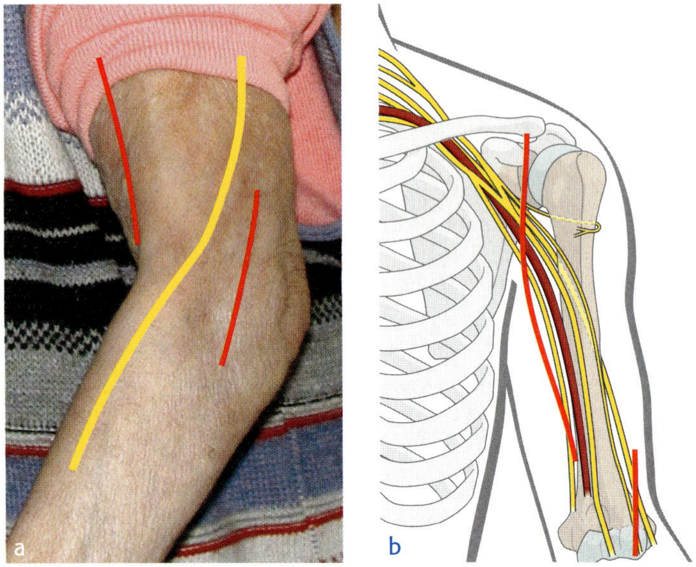

Fig 6.2.6-3a–b In this situation, a standard anterior open approach is preferred for the diaphyseal fracture, proximally through the deltopectoral groove preserving the cephalic vein. Lateral to the biceps tendon/muscle, the approach is continued distally to the distal third of the diaphysis, splitting the brachial muscle between the medial and middle thirds. The radial nerve remains more lateral, and is not visualized.
The distal articular fracture is approached through a strict lateral radial incision between the triceps and brachioradial muscles. The radial nerve runs more anteriorly and therefore does not need to be exposed.

3 Reduction and fixation

In a first step, the proximal periprosthetic fracture is treated. Open approach and reduction by means of the plate, which is slightly bent at its distal end, permitting divergent insertion of the two most distal locking head screws. This increases the stability and reduces the risk of en bloc plate pull-out. Proximal anchorage is difficult in view of the very thin bone. A short monocortical, locking head screw is inserted into the most proximal plate hole. It is not possible to anchor screws into any of the other proximal plate holes, not even cortex screws inserted diagonally. For this reason, the plate is anchored in the proximal main fragment almost exclusively by fixation with two cerclage wires and two additional titanium rings. Distal fixation is achieved by insertion of four bicortical locking head screws, which provide very good stability.
Direct reduction of the dislocated radial condyle is performed by way of the second approach as described above. An LCP T-plate 3.5 is applied as the fixation device. It is appropriately precontoured and anchored in the manner of an internal fixator, ie, exclusively with locking head screws. Intraoperative evaluation confirmed that stable conditions had been achieved at both fracture sites.

4 Rehabilitation

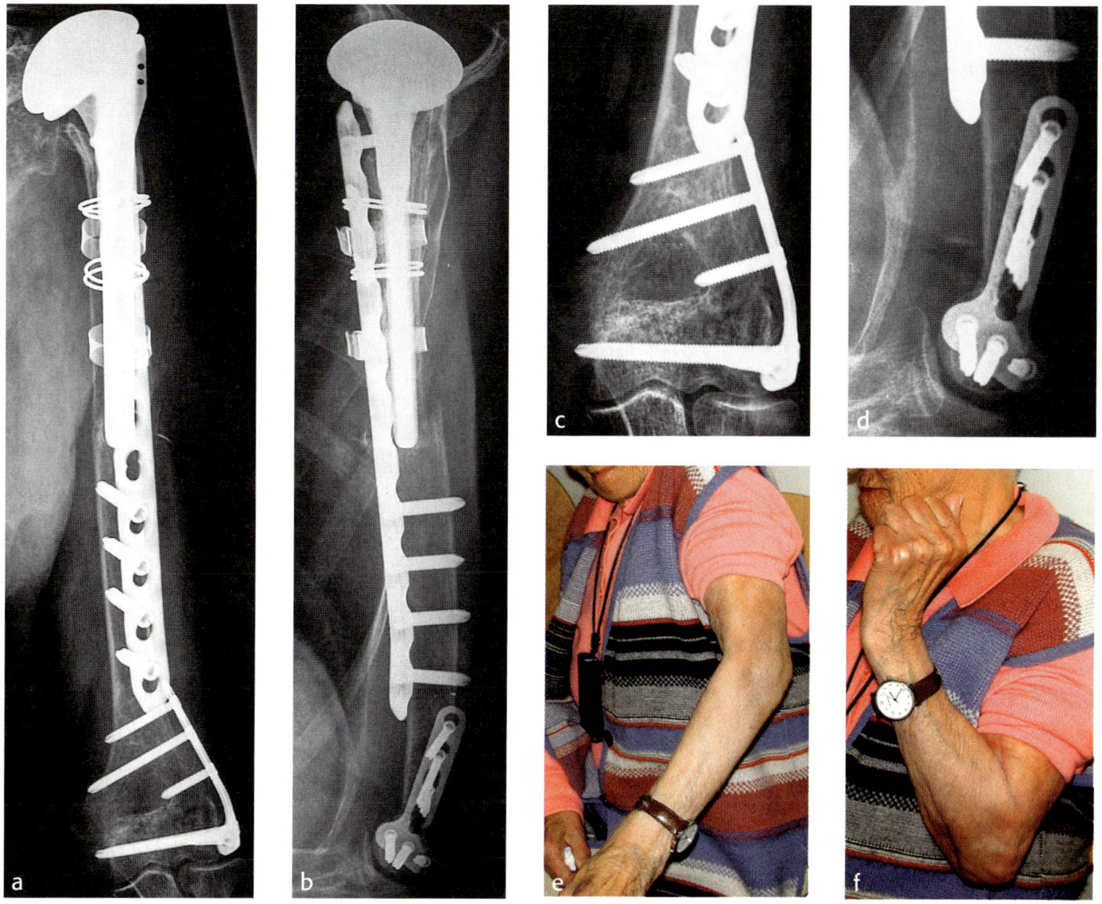

Fig 6.2.6-4a–f

a–d Early functional rehabilitation was started cautiously, whereby the limb was immobilized during the night as a precaution. X-ray assessment after 2 months revealed increasing consolidation of both fractures, unchanged, stable seating of the implants without resorption lucencies around the screws.

e–f The patient was more or less free of symptoms and demonstrated a moderate extension restriction at the elbow with a deficit of approximately 30°. The range of motion at the shoulder was clearly restricted both actively and passively (preoperative status).

Further clinical and x-ray examinations will not be undertaken provided the patient remains free of symptoms.

5 Pitfalls –

Approach
Correct intramuscular layers have to be identified to preserve the radial nerve.

Reduction and fixation
Stabilization in the proximal part may fail.

Rehabilitation
Stability is critical, and therefore too aggressive rehabilitation may cause a failure of fixation.

6 Pearls +

Approach
Double approach (proximal anterior; distal lateral) preserves the radial nerve.

Reduction and fixation
The locking screw-plate system is very helpful for periprosthetic and osteoporotic fractures.

Rehabilitation
Early functional rehabilitation is essential to preserve the already diminished preoperative shoulder mobility.

Author Michael Wagner

6.2.7 Pathological humeral shaft fracture

1 Case description

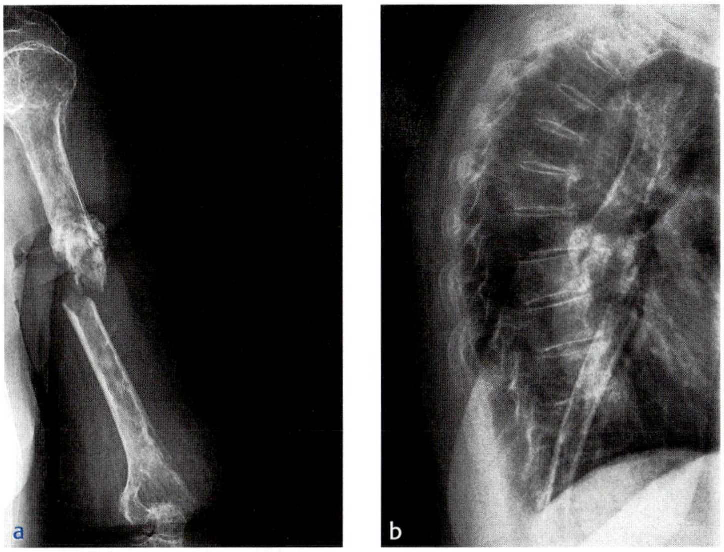

75-year-old woman with pathological fracture of the left humeral shaft and multiple myeloma.

Fig 6.2.7-1a–b
a AP view.
b Lateral view.

Indication

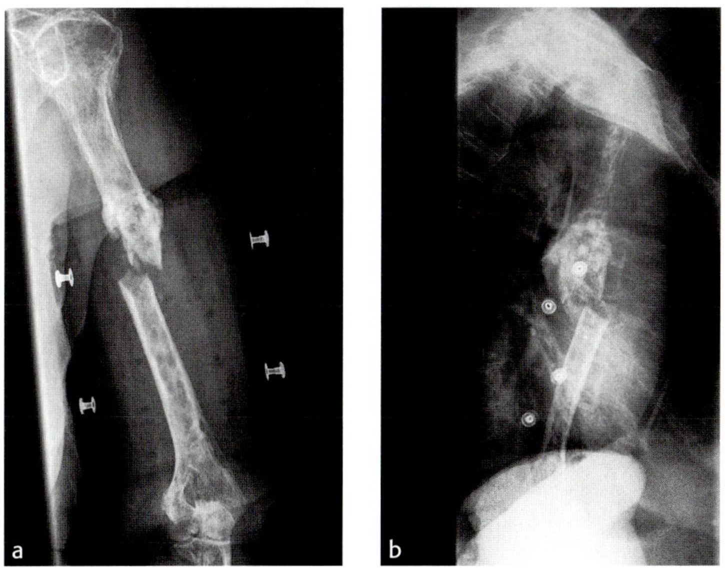

Pathological fracture of the humeral shaft in the presence of multiple myeloma. Osseous healing after nonoperative treatment, namely, immobilization in a brace. Refracture immediately adjacent and distal to the previously healed fracture. The unstable, displaced fracture without signs of neurological deficit was again treated nonoperatively, however, after 8 weeks follow-up assessment revealed nonunion.

Fig 6.2.7-2a–b
a AP view.
b Lateral view.

Preoperative planning

Equipment
- Metaphyseal LCP 3.5/4.5/5.0, 4 + 10 holes
- 3.5 mm locking head screws (LHS)
- 5.0 mm LHS
- 3.5 mm cortex screw
- 2.0 mm K-wires

(Size of system, instruments, and implants can vary according to anatomy.)

Patient preparation and positioning
Antibiotics: 3rd generation cephalosporin
Thrombosis prophylaxis: low-molecular heparin

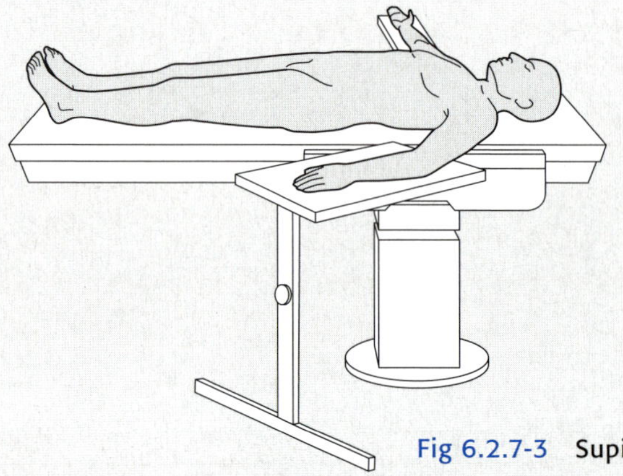

Fig 6.2.7-3 Supine position with hand table.

2 Surgical approach

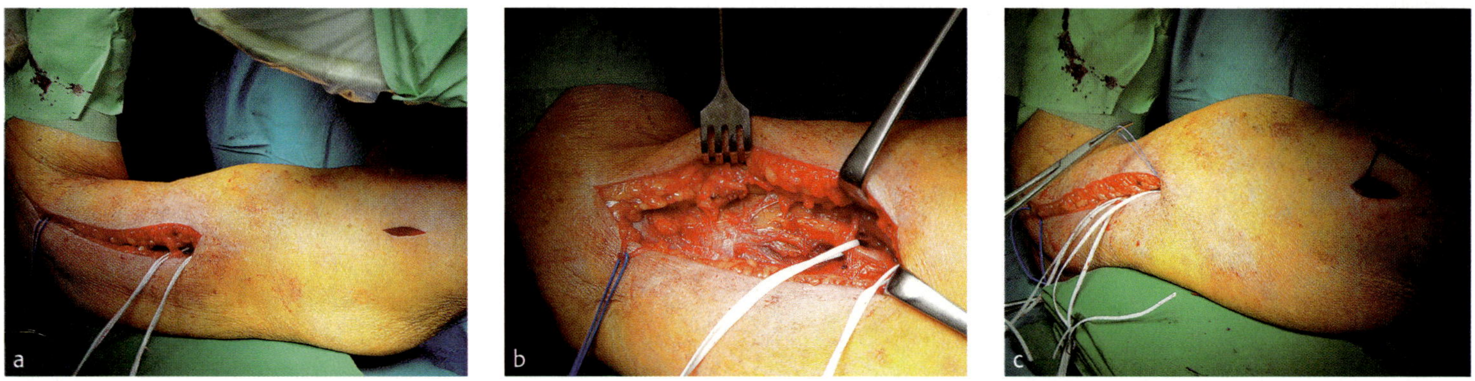

Fig 6.2.7-4a–c
- a Lateral approach to the distal part of the humerus and anterolateral incision at the proximal shaft.
- b Careful preparation of the radial nerve which is retracted with the vessel loop (white).
- c Submuscular tunneling in preparation for subsequent slide-insertion of the plate and insertion of a guide thread.

3 Reduction and fixation

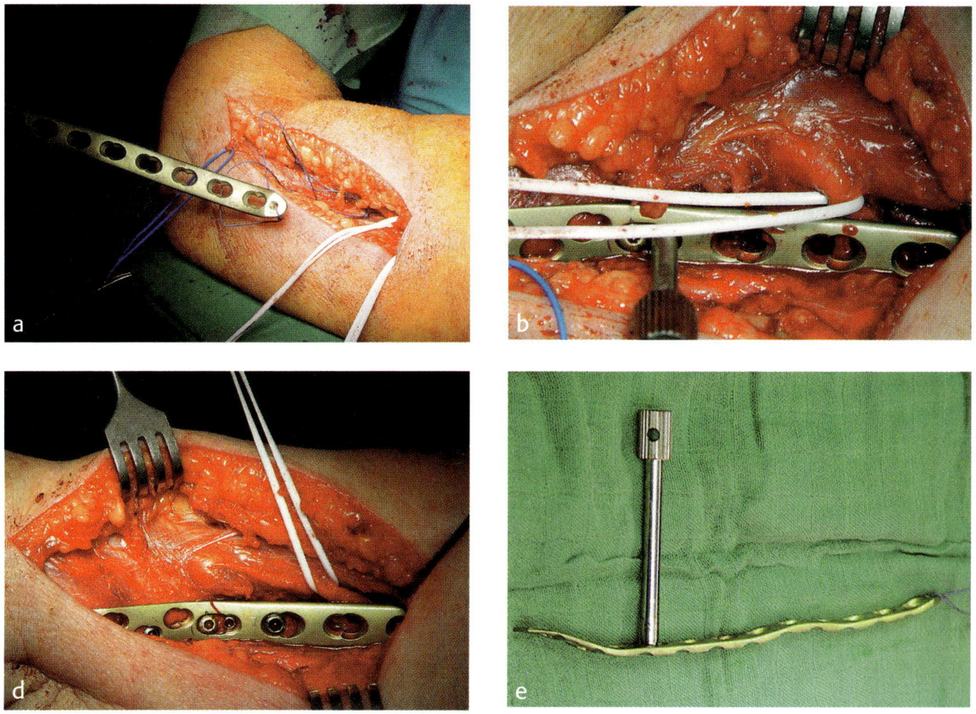

Fig 6.2.7-5a–e Fracture reduction by manual traction; control using image intensifier.

- a Insertion of the narrow 3.5/4.5/5.0 metaphyseal LCP from the distal aspect in a proximal direction with the help of the guide thread that has been passed through the hole at the proximal end of the plate.
- b Since the plate will be stabilized as a noncontact internal fixator with locking head screws, ie, distant from the bone, the radial nerve is left beneath the fixator.
- c Temporary fixation of the distal fragment is performed by means of the attachable centering sleeve and drill bit at the distal end of the plate first and then at the proximal end.
- d Fixation of the metaphyseal plate with LHS at the distal humeral fragment. A 3.5 mm cortex screw is inserted into the long oval hole and acts as a reduction screw and is left in situ. The radial nerve (white vessel loop) runs beneath the laterally positioned plate. The radial nerve was not mobilized because it had become immobilized in its sulcus by callus formation related to the previous fracture.
- e To accommodate this, the plate was contoured to a wave shape.

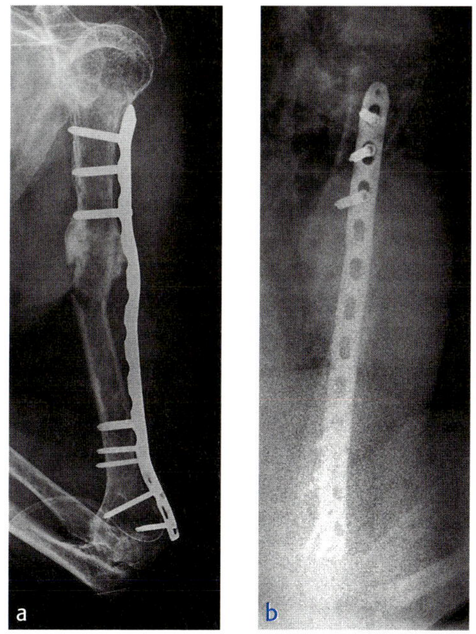

Fig 6.2.7-6a–b Postoperative x-rays.

- a AP view. The gap between the bone and the plate is clearly visible. The radial nerve is situated in this gap.
- b Lateral view.

Elastic fixation of the nonunion with locked internal fixator. The nonunion was not exposed surgically.

4 Rehabilitation

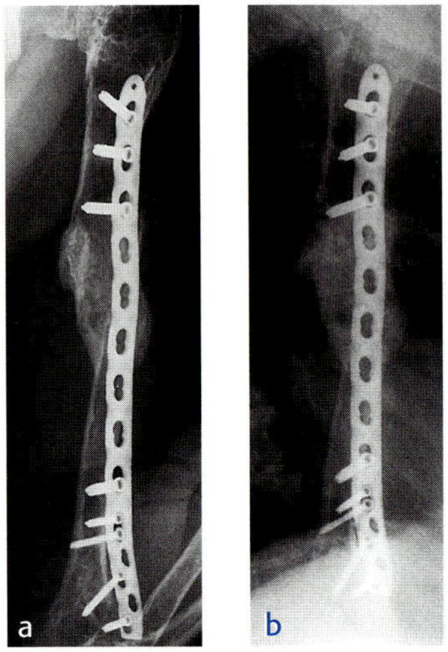

Full active and passive therapy was commenced from the first postoperative day.

Fig 6.2.7-7a–b X-rays after 2 1/2 years show callus bridging of the fracture, no loosening of the implants despite osteoporosis and partial pathological osteolysis.
a AP view.
b Lateral view.

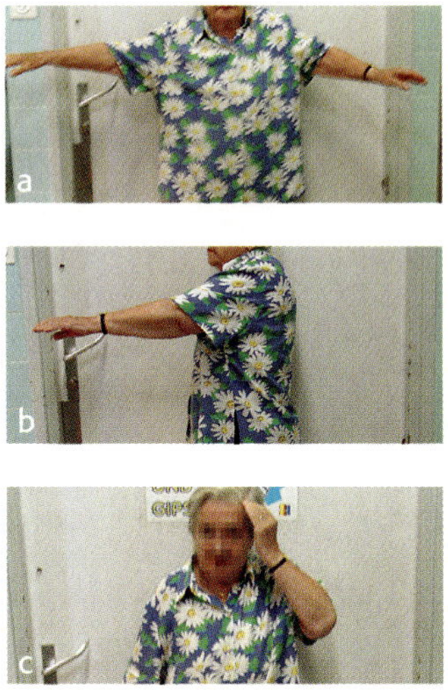

Fig 6.2.7-8a–c Functional pictures after 2 1/2 years. Painfree, partially restricted function at the shoulder joint. No neurological deficit.

5 Pitfalls –

Approach
Any lateral approach to the humerus requires retraction and preservation of the radial nerve.

Reduction and fixation

6 Pearls +

Equipment
Noncontact plates can be stabilized at a fixed distance from the bone, consequently, the radial nerve can be permitted to pass beneath the plate.

Reduction and fixation
Less invasive plate osteosynthesis of a nonunion with elastic fixation leads to rapid, indirect bone healing due to the preservation of optimal biological conditions.

Authors Klaus-D Schaser, Norbert P Haas, Ingo Melcher

6.2.8 Intercalary reconstruction of the humerus following oncological resection

1 Case description

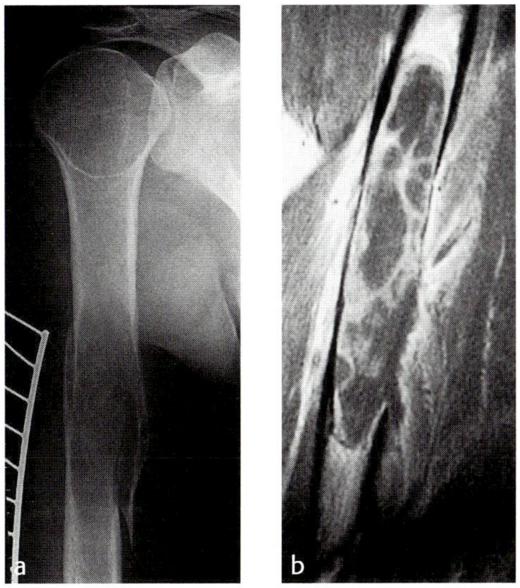

32-year-old man sustained a spontaneous, pathological fracture of the humeral shaft due to first manifestation of a Ewing sarcoma of the humeral diaphysis. The AP x-ray and MRI show a diaphyseal osteolysis without sclerosis and a tumor matrix and surrounding edema.

Fig 6.2.8-1a–b
a–b AP x-ray and MRI scan showing the diaphyseal osteolysis and intraosseous tumor matrix (Ewing Sarcoma) with surrounding edema and pathological fracture of the humeral diaphysis.

Indication

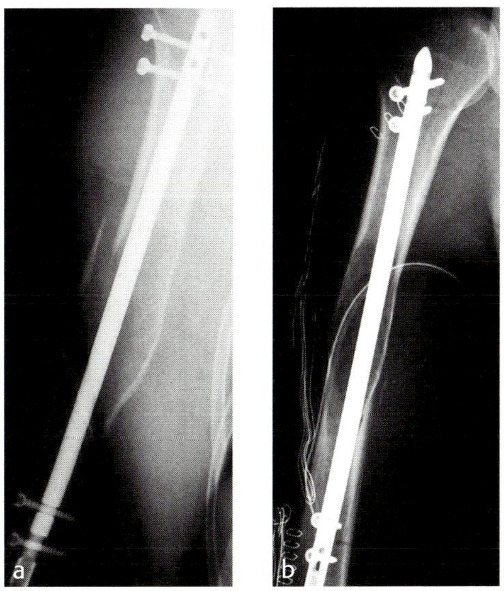

The pathological fracture was erroneously thought to be caused by a juvenile solid (unicameral) bone cyst and subsequently treated by closed reduction and retrograde intramedullary nailing using a solid nail (other hospital, not a tumor center). After prolonged immobilization of the shoulder and arm the fracture showed no healing response, however, a progressively growing paraosteal soft-tissue tumor mass caused painful swelling. Secondary incisional biopsy revealed the final histopathological diagnosis of Ewing sarcoma. Subsequently, the patient (no metastatic disease) was included in established oncological treatment protocols (EURO-Ewing) and a preoperative neoadjuvant polychemotherapy was performed.

Fig 6.2.8-2a–b
Immediate postoperative x-rays after closed reduction and retrograde nailing, performed under suspicion of a unicameral solid (juvenile) bone cyst (external hospital, not a tumor center).

Indication (cont)

Overall onco-surgical treatment protocol:

1. Neoadjuvant (preoperative) polychemotherapy
2. Surgical resection: wide resection of the tumor and tumor-cell dissemination tissue areas (entire diaphysis with nail)
3. Skeletal reconstruction (free vascularized autologous fibula transfer and osteosynthesis to the residual proximal and distal humerus using LCP 3.5)
4. Soft-tissue coverage and muscle transfers to restore function.
5. Adjuvant (postoperative) polychemotherapy

Preoperative planning

Equipment

- Locking proximal humerus plate (LPHP), 8 holes
- LCP metaphyseal plate 3.5/4.5/5.0, 13 holes
- LCP reconstruction plates 3.5, 6 holes
- LCP 3.5, 9 holes
- LCP reconstruction plates 3.5, 10 holes
- LCP metaphyseal plate 3.5/4.5/5.0, 5 + 13 holes
- Locking head screws (LHS)

(Size of system, instruments, and implants can vary according to anatomy.)

Patient preparation and positioning

Antibiotics: cephalosporin

Thrombosis prophylaxis: low-molecular heparin

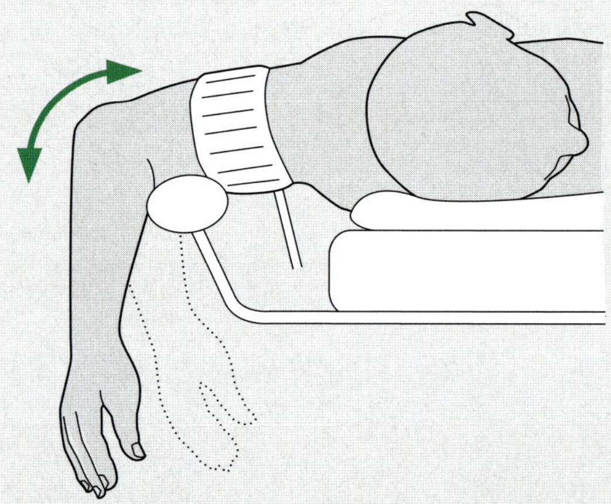

Fig 6.2.8-3 Patient in prone position with arm on arm table with 90° abduction in the shoulder joint and the elbow in 90° flexion (hanging L position).

2 Tumor resection

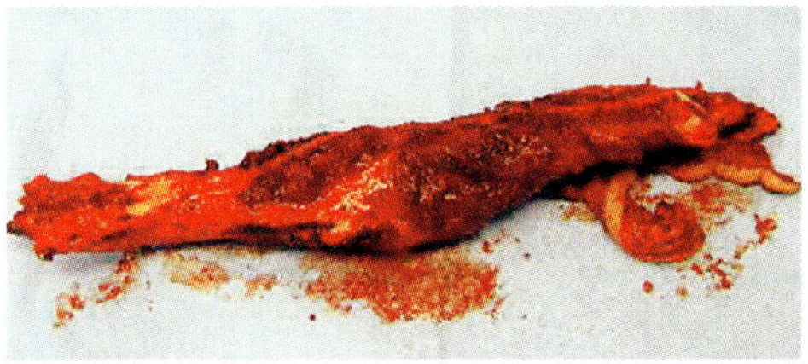

Fig 6.2.8-4 For resection the dorsal approach to the humerus was used, leaving the biopsy tract untouched and en-bloc to the specimen. To perform a wide and safe oncological resection the entire extraarticular humeral diaphysis was resected leaving the intramedullary nail in situ and without contact to the biopsy tract. The radial nerve (not involved in the tumor) was preserved. The intraoperative clinical image shows the surgical specimen with tumor-free resection margins (R0) as verified by intraoperative histopathological analysis of both the bone marrow and soft-tissue margins.

3 Skeletal reconstruction

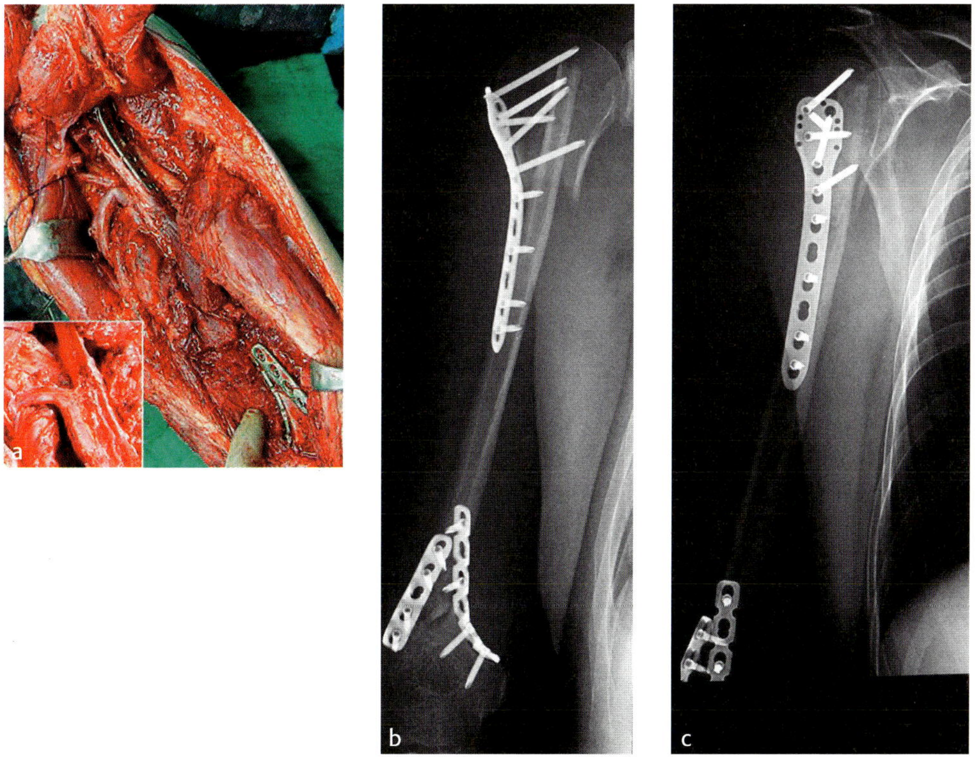

Fig 6.2.8-5a–c

- a Biological reconstruction of the intercalary defect was performed by free vascularized autologous fibula transfer. After the fibula, including the nutrient vessels (fibular artery and vein), had been harvested (preserved periosteum and soft-tissue envelope) microvascular anastomosis was performed end-to-side to the brachial artery and vein. Proximal stabilization of the fibular graft after reperfusion was achieved by using a locking proximal humerus plate (LPHP, 8-hole), while distal fixation was performed with a LCP reconstruction plate 3.5 and a LCP 3.5.
- b–c AP and lateral x-rays 10 days after surgery.

4 Motor reconstruction and soft-tissue coverage

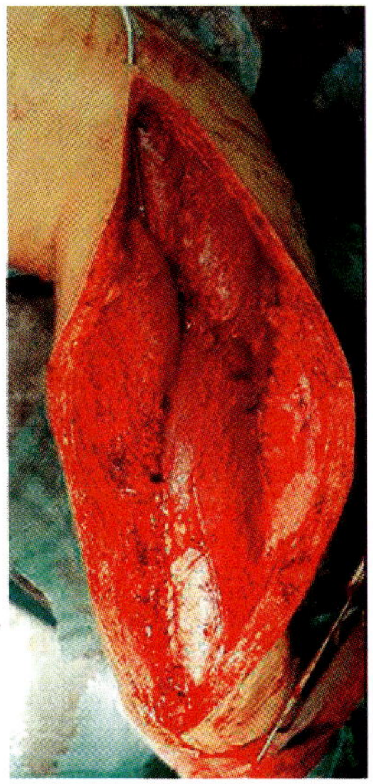

Fig 6.2.8-6 To provide forward flexion of the shoulder the pectoralis muscle was secured to the periosteum of the proximal fibular graft. Shoulder extension and arm elevation occurs through the transfer of the deltoid, trapezius, latissimus dorsi to the proximal part of the fibular graft. Extension of the elbow is ensured by refixation of the triceps muscle to the distal dorsal aspect of the fibular graft. The biceps and brachioradialis were left untouched. The radial nerve was transpositioned to the anterior aspect of the graft.

5 Revision surgery and follow-up

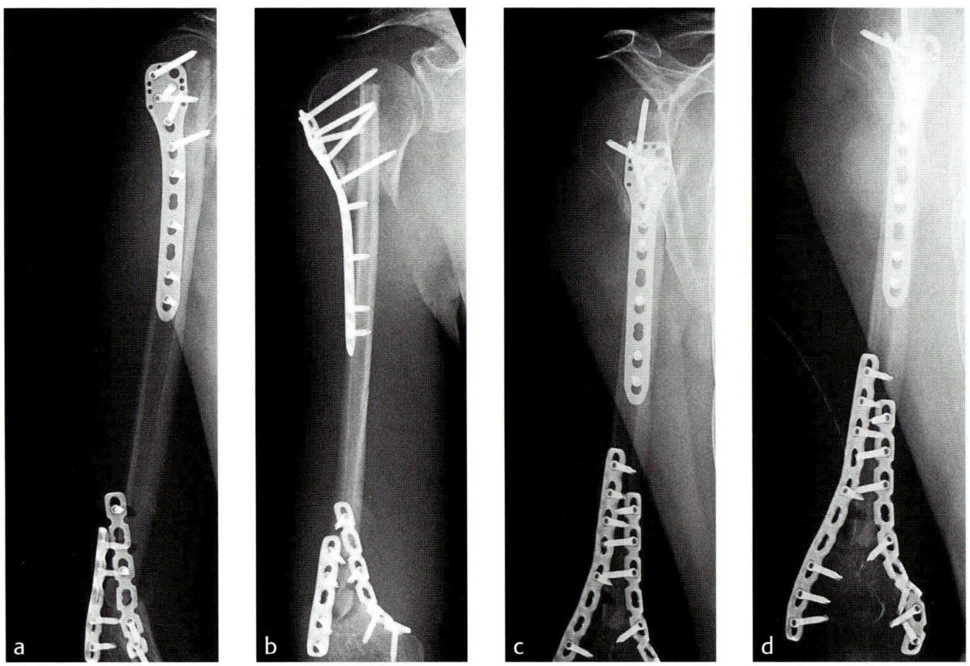

Fig 6.2.8-7a–c

a–b 4 months after surgery the proximal aspect of the graft showed an excellent healing to the humeral head. At the distal part both plates showed loosening and pull-out of the screws. Doppler ultrasound analysis at this time revealed regular flow of the arterial and venous microvessels.

c–d Consequently, implant removal and reosteosynthesis was performed using two longer LCP 3.5 that provided stability and extended more proximally on the graft.

5 Revision surgery and follow-up (cont)

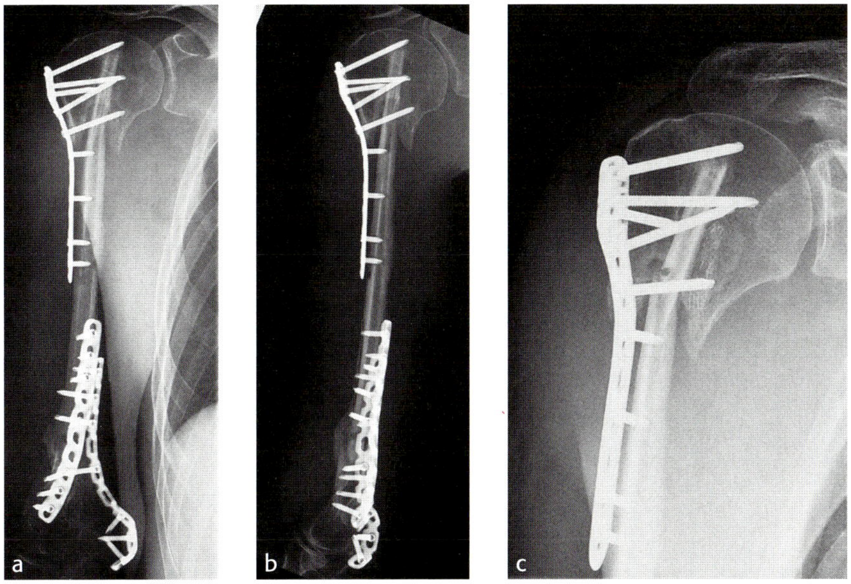

Fig 6.2.8-8a–c At 8 months after surgery a fracture of the proximal part of the fibular graft occurred while its end showed bony consolidation within the humeral head. The distal aspect of the graft displayed completed consolidation. Again, re-osteosynthesis was performed by removal of the locking proximal humerus plate (LPHP) and bridging the entire fibular graft by a long, prebent, and torqued 4.5 metaphyseal LCP. In addition, cancellous bone grafting of the subcapital fracture region was performed.

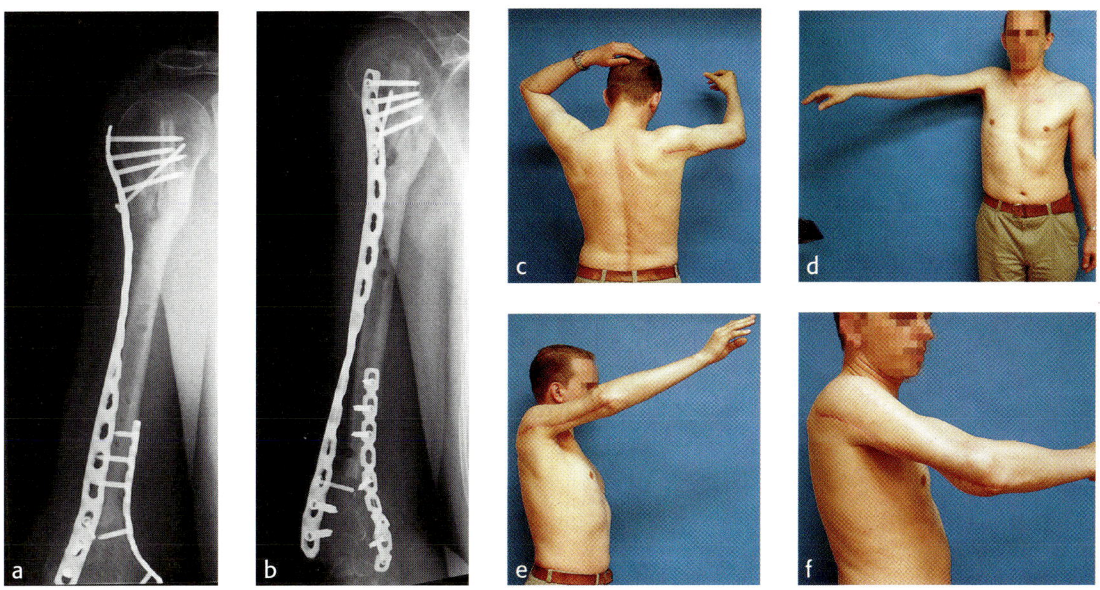

Fig 6.2.8-9a–f Clinical images and x-rays at one year follow-up demonstrate completed proximal and distal bone consolidation and acceptable motor function. At present the patient is free from local or systemic tumor recurrence.

6 Pitfalls –

Diagnosis
Incorrect diagnosis and interpretation of radiographic findings.

Failure to perform an incisional biopsy in questionable lesions.

Preoperative planning and subsequent surgery based on the incorrect diagnosis leads to serious consequences which compromise and possibly prevent limb sparing surgery as well as impair the patient's overall prognosis.

Approach
Humerus: radial nerve injury due to circumferential preparation of the diaphysis.

Fibula: morbidity with the risk of peroneal nerve injury during harvesting of the vascularized graft.

Resection
Intraoperative tumor-cell dissemination due to preparation-induced manipulation at the tumor site and tumor-derived blood loss.

Reconstruction
Insufficient performance of microvascular surgery may lead to stenosis of the anastomosis and thrombosis of the nutrient vessels.

Badly bent plates may interfere with the radial or ulnar nerve.

Intraoperative fracture of the fibular graft due to multiple perforation of the graft (reaming) and insertion of too many screws.

7 Pearls +

Diagnosis
On suspicion of malignant bone tumor refer the patient to a musculoskeletal tumor center prior to incisional biopsy.

Approach
The dorsal approach allows complete resection of diaphyseal and distal bone tumors of the humerus without interfering with neurovascular structures and other compartments.

Resection
If possible an external fixator may be used to maintain length and rotation after resection.
Intraoperative histopathological analysis is mandatory to ensure tumor-cell free surgical margins.

Reconstruction
The LCP appears to be an ideal implant for primary and revision surgical treatment of segmental intercalary skeletal defects.
If oncologically justifiable, preserve the rotator cuff insertion at the proximal humerus for improved motor function.

6.3 Humerus, distal

Cases

Case		Classification	Method	Implant used	Implant function	Page
6.3.1	Supracondylar distal humeral fracture with extension into the shaft and proximal ulnar fracture	13-A2; 11-B1; 21-B1	compression	LCP 3.5; LCP distal medial humerus (DHM); LCP olecranon plate	lag screw, cerclage protection plates	339
6.3.2	Open displaced complete articular distal humeral fracture	13-C1	compression	LCP reconstruction plate 3.5	lag screws and compression plates	345
6.3.3	Open complete intraarticular distal humeral fracture	13-C2	compression	LCP reconstruction plate 3.5	lag screws and compression plates	349
6.3.4	Displaced intraarticular distal humeral fracture	13-C3	compression	DHP distal humeral plate 2.7/3.5	lag screws and compression plates	353
6.3.5	Displaced intraarticular distal humeral fracture	13-C3	compression	LCP reconstruction plate 3.5	lag screws and compression plates	357
6.3.6	Pathology of the elbow		locked splinting	LCP 3.5	locked internal fixator	361

6 Humerus

Author Reto Babst

6.3 Humerus, distal

1 Incidence rate

Distal humeral fractures are rare injuries in adults, comprising 2% of all fractures [1] but approximately 1/3 of all humeral fractures [2]. A recent epidemiologic report showed an incidence for distal humeral fractures of 5.7%, [3] with an even distribution among the sexes. Distal humeral fractures show a bimodal distribution regarding age and gender with the highest incidence for males below the age of 20 and females above the age of 80. Detailed sex and age distribution according to the fracture types is reported in the cited study. The majority of distal humeral fractures comprise extraarticular fractures (38.7%). Partial articular fractures have an incidence of 24.1% and intraarticular fractures (37.2%) have a slightly lower incidence than extraarticular fractures [3].

2/3 of the distal humeral fractures are caused by simple falls (predominantly in females), whereas 1/3 concerns high-velocity injuries (fall from a height, road traffic accidents, sport accidents, mainly in males) [3].

Depending on the mechanism of injury, complementary lesions are not unusual such as additional fractures around the elbow combined with ligamentous injuries, which are often not evident due to osseous instability at the initial assessment. Vascular lesions in combination with isolated distal humeral fractures are very rare and mostly associated with high-velocity mechanisms. Ulnar nerve palsies are mostly seen in medial epicondylar fractures (13-A1.2) in young adults, due to a simple fall or a sports injury [3]. Open distal humeral fractures are predominant in type C fractures and their incidence varies from 20–50% in different series [3, 4].

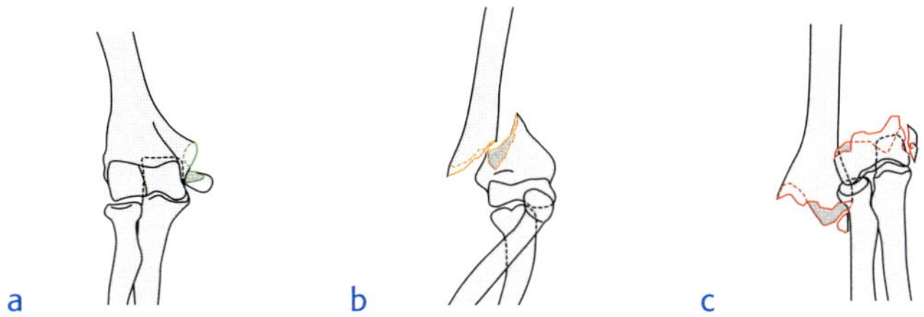

Fig 6.3-1a–c 13-A Extraarticular fracture.
a 13-A1 apophyseal avulsion
b 13-A2 metaphyseal simple
c 13-A3 metaphyseal multifragmentary

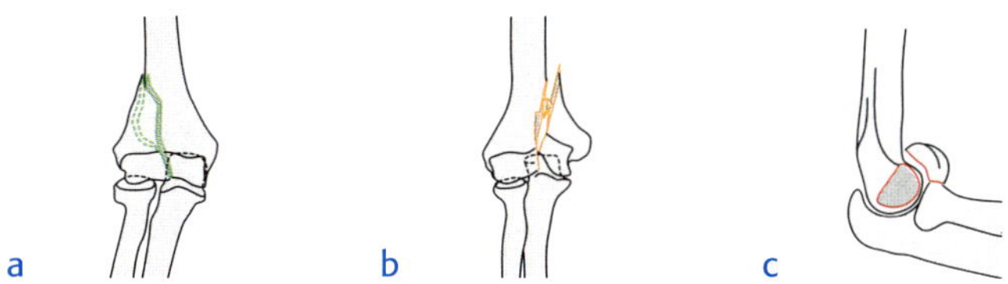

Fig 6.3-2a–c 13-B Partial articular fracture.
a 13-B1 sagittal lateral condyle
b 13-B2 sagittal medial condyle
c 13-B3 frontal

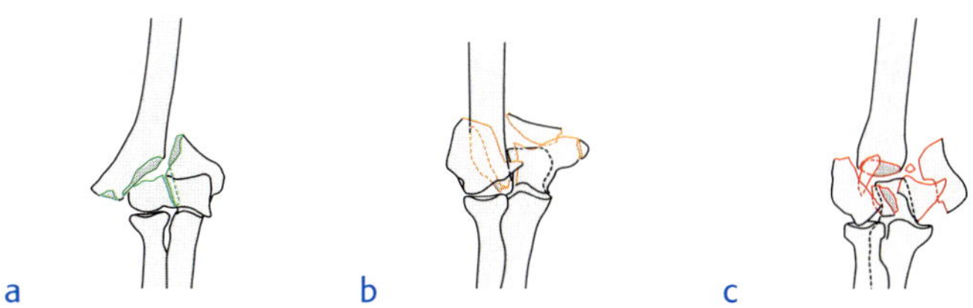

Fig 6.2-3a–c 13-C Complete articular fracture.
a 13-C1 articular simple, metaphyseal simple
b 13-C2 articular simple, metaphyseal multifragmentary
c 13-C3 articular multifragmentary

2 Classification

Several classification systems are used for the description of distal humeral fractures. The Müller AO Classification [5] and the Jupiter-Mehne classification [6] are descriptive classifying systems that include most fracture patterns of the distal humerus. The latter is more distinctive concerning the mechanism of extraarticular and partial articular fractures and differs between high and low fracture patterns in respect of the olecranon fossa. Since low fracture configurations are associated with a higher risk of union complications [3], this classification has a more detailed prognostic value than the Müller AO Classification.

However, the reliability of the Müller AO Classification is high with a value of 0.94 when using the preoperative x-rays and the summary of intraoperative findings [3]. In contrast to the Jupiter-Mehne classification with a value of 0.295, the Müller AO Classification results in a substantial agreement (0.52 and 0.66) using just the preoperative x-rays [7]. Despite its limitations, today the Müller AO Classification seems to be the most valuable descriptive classification system for distal humeral fractures, especially in combination with the intraoperative findings.

Video 6.3-1

3 Treatment methods

Regarding assessment and procedural setting, the complex anatomy of the distal humerus presents a diagnostic and therapeutic challenge, in particular, due to small osseous fragments, sparse subchondral bone, a great amount of joint cartilage and the frequent presence of relevant osteoporosis.

Standard x-rays (AP/lateral view) of the elbow are often sufficient to appreciate the main fracture pattern. An additional oblique view is recommended to view other fracture planes. The value of 2-D and 3-D imaging is not yet clear, but has the potential to add important information regarding fracture lines involving the articular portion in the sagittal and coronal planes. A preoperative extension view under anesthesia using an image intensifier may add additional information to the preoperative assessment, thus optimizing the surgical procedure.

The approach is adapted to the fracture pattern: Partial articular fractures may be treated using a direct lateral or medial approach, whereas a dorsal incision offers the best approach conditions to extraarticular and intraarticular fractures. Displaced extraarticular fractures may be exposed by choosing a triceps splitting procedure as well as following the medial or lateral margin of the muscle. When treating intraarticular fractures, different forms of triceps reflecting approaches like the olecranon osteotomy [12], the triceps anconeus pedicle (TRAP) [8] or the triceps sparing approach [9] are recommended. The majority of intraarticular fractures is approached using an olecranon osteotomy as recommended by the AO. In elderly patients with multifragmentary fractures, olecranon preserving approaches are preferable [9, 8]. The latter are also a good option for the fixation of simple intraarticular fractures. The semilunar notch serves as a template for the reconstruction of the trochlea.

Although ORIF of distal humeral fractures is challenging and has complications [3, 4, 10, 11, 15] such as implant failure, malunion, nonunion, elbow stiffness, infection, heterotopic bone formation, and ulnar neuropathy, it is generally accepted to be the better choice of treatment for displaced extraarticular, partial articular, and intraarticular fractures than a conservative procedure.

Conservative treatment may be an option for nondisplaced extraarticular (13-A) and partial articular fractures (13-B). For intraarticular fractures (13-C), it should be restricted to inoperable patients [3, 16]. However, 4–6 weeks immo-bilization is marked by a high risk of secondary displacement, elbow stiffness, nonunion, and malunion leading to instability and posttraumatic arthritis.

Minimally invasive approaches using percutaneous K-wire fixation may be considered in some extraarticular and partial articular fractures (13-A1, 13-B1-3) as well as in high-risk patients with osteoporosis and displaced extraarticular fractures of the type 13-A2.3, 13-A3.1-2. These might profit from a percutaneous fixation by K-wires combined with tension band fixation including 4–6 weeks immobilization in a 90° cylinder cast. The limited functional demand of this patient group outweighs the possible drawbacks of elbow stiffness, nonunion, and malunion.

Only ORIF with stable fragment fixation by screws and plates using the appropriate technique allows early active postoperative motion. This concerns all fractures of the distal humerus and is a prerequisite for an optimal functional result; the success rate is 75–85% [3, 4, 10, 11, 15]. Due to the complex anatomy of the distal humerus, reconstruction plates 3.5, and easily contoured or preshaped plates are recommended [11, 12]. One-third tubular plates, although easier to adapt, are not strong enough and will fail [11]. Plate fixation of both, the medial and the lateral column is necessary to achieve adequate stability of the distal humerus. Two posterior plates are biomechanically less stable than two sidewise parallel plates or bilateral perpendicular plates as recommended by the AO [4, 11–15]. Coronal shearing fragments are best fixed either by Herbert screws or by subcartilaginous countersunk 1.5–2.0 mm mini fragment screws.

The problem of fixation of small and osteoporotic fragments using conventional reconstruction plates can be solved by perpendicular screw placement through well adapted plates which "cradle" the medial epicondyle and the dorsal aspect of the lateral epicondyle [16]. The new LCP concept with angular stable locking head screws in converging directions within LCP reconstruction plates 3.5 has the potential to increase screw anchorage in those fragments. First clinical trials with form plates using locking head screws with smaller diameters in the articular area have shown promising results.

Regarding any fixation system, the stabilizing technique should aim for anatomical joint reconstruction with preliminary K-wire fixation of the articular block. Interfragmentary compression is achieved in well reconstructed articular segments with a short threaded cancellous bone screw, whereas a positioning screw maintains the correct position of the trochlea if further bone fragments are missing. The latter are replaced by bone grafts. The joint block is then fixed by well adapted plates, screw insertion starting in the distal plate holes and using eccentric proximal screws to achieve interfragmentary compression between the articular block and the meta-/diaphyseal area. Whenever possible, a compression screw is placed between the articular and the metaphyseal block to increase stability.

A transposition of the ulnar nerve is not routinely performed. If interference or scarring by a plate is expected, a subcutaneous transposition is recommended [17].

An olecranon osteotomy is usually fixed by two K-wires and a tension band or by a cancellous bone screw using a washer, combined with a tension band.

To check the intraarticular screw position, an intraoperative x-ray or an image intensifier control should be examined carefully. Intraoperative range of motion and stability should be checked for immediate postoperative treatment setting.

Postoperative immobilization in a splint to deal with pain and swelling is recommended for the first 3–4 days. Immediate active-assisted mobilization takes place depending on swelling and pain for 6 weeks. The role of continuous passive motion is not yet defined [11, 16]. Resistive training starts after radiological control and confirmation of healing progression at 8–12 weeks.

In elderly patients with poor bone stock due to age, rheumatoid arthritis or long-term steroid medication, the treatment of multifragmentary intraarticular fracture types 13-C2 and

C3 by a primary elbow arthroplasty may be considered. Despite lack of strong evidence favoring this approach, small data series including elderly patients show comparable results to ORIF [18–20].

6 Implant overview

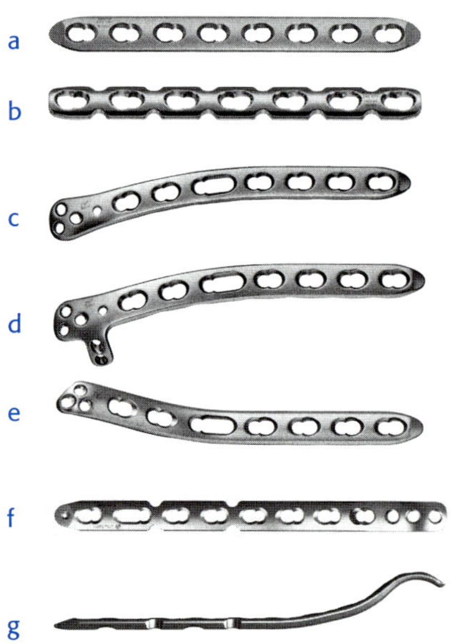

Fig 6.3-4a–g
a LCP 3.5
b LCP reconstruction plate 3.5
c DHP—distal humeral plate dorsolateral 2.7/3.5
d DHP—distal humeral plate dorsolateral 2.7/3.5 with lateral support
e DHP—distal humeral plate medial 2.7/3.5
f–g LCP metaphyseal plate 3.5, for distal medial humerus

6 Bibliography

1. **Jupiter JB, Morrey BF** (1993) Fractures of the distal humerus in the adult. *Morrey BF, (ed), The Ellbow and its disorders.* 2nd edition Philadelphia, PA: WB Saunders, 328–366.
2. **Rose SH, Melton LJ, Morrey BF, et al** (1982) Epidemiologic features of humeral fractures. *Clin Orthop*; 168:24–30.
3. **Robinson CM, Hill RM, Jacobs N, et al** (2003) Adult distal humeral metaphyseal fractures: epidemiology and results of treatment. *J Orthop Trauma*; 17 (1):38–47.
4. **Jupiter JB, Neff U, Holzach P, et al** (1985) Intercondylar fractures of the humerus. *J Bone Joint Surg Am*; 67(2):226–239.
5. **Müller ME, Nazarian S, Koch P, et al** (1990) The comprehensive classification of fractures of long bones. Berlin Heidelberg New York: Springer.
6. **Jupiter JB, Mehne DK** (1992) Fractures of the distal humerus. *Orthopedics*; 15(7):825–833.
7. **Wainwright AM, Williams JR, Carr AJ** (2000) Interobserver and intraobserver variation in classification systems for fractures of the distal humerus; *J Bone Joint Surg Br*; 82(5):636–642.
8. **O'Driscoll SW** (2000)The triceps-reflecting anconeus pedicle (TRAP) approach for distal humeral fractures and nonunions. *Orthop Clin North Am*; 31(1):91–101.
9. **Bryan RS, Morrey BF** (1982) Extensive posterior exposure of the elbow: A triceps-sparing approach; *Clin Orthop Relat Res*;166:188–192.
10. **John H, Rosso R, Neff U, et al** (1994) Operative treatment of distal humerus fractures in the elderly; *J Bone Joint Surg Br*; 76(5):93–96.
11. **O' Driscoll SW, Sanchez-Sotelo J, Torchia ME** (2002) Management of the smashed distal humerus; *Orthop Clin North Am*; 33(1):19–33.
12. **Holdsworth BJ** (2000); Humerus: Distal. In AO principles of fracture management: Rüedi TP, Murphy WM, ed. Stuttgart New York, Thieme.
13. **Schemitsch EH, Tencer AF, Henley MB** (1994) Biomechanical evaluation of methods of internal fixation of the distal humerus; *J Orthop Trauma*; 8(6):468–475.

14. **Helfet DL, Hotchkiss RN** (1990) Internal fixation of the distal humerus: a biomechanical comparison of methods; *J Orthop Trauma*; 4(3):260–264.
15. **Waddell JP, Hatch J, Richards R** (1988) Supracondylar fractures of the humerus: Results of surgical treatment; *J Trauma*; 28(12):1615–1621.
16. **Mehne DK, Jupiter JB** (1992) Skeletal Trauma. Part II Fractures of the distal humerus. *Browner BD, Jupiter JB, Levine AM, Trafton PG (eds), Skeletal Trauma*. Philadelphia London Toronto Montreal Sydney Tokyo; WB Saunders.
17. **Ring D, Jupiter JB** (1999) Complex fractures of the distal humerus and their complications; *J Shoulder Elbow Surgery*; 8(1):85–97.
18. **Frankle MA, Herscovici D Jr, DiPasquale TG, et al** (2003) A comparison of open reduction and internal fixation and primary total elbow arthroplasty in the treatment of intraarticular distal humerus fractures in women older than age 65; *J Orthop Trauma*; 17(7):473–480.
19. **Obremskey WT, Bhandari M, Dirschl DR, et al** (2003) Internal fixation versus arthroplasty of comminuted fractures of the distal humerus; *J Orthop Trauma*; 17(6):463–465.
20. **Gambirasio R, Riand N, Stern R, et al** (2001) Total elbow replacement for complex fractures of the distal humerus. An option for the elderly patient; *J Bone Joint surgery Br*; 83(7):974–978.

Author **Michael Plecko**

6.3.1 Supracondylar distal humeral fracture—13-A2 with extension into the shaft—11-B1 and proximal ulnar fracture—21-B1

1 Case description

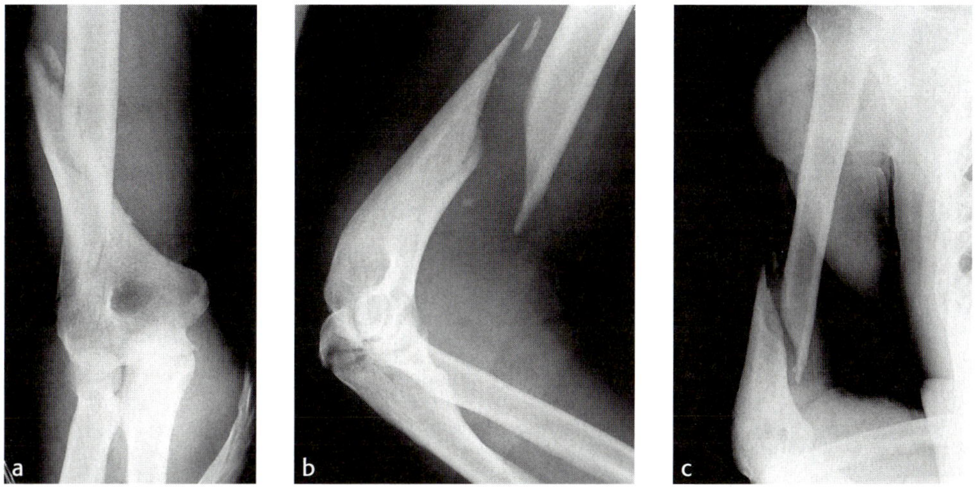

41-year-old, mentally disabled man injured his right dominant arm in a car accident. Displaced fracture of the humeral shaft (11-B1), extraarticular supracondylar fracture of the humerus (13-A2) and fracture of the proximal ulna with comminution (21-B1). Immediate radial nerve palsy after the accident.

Fig 6.3.1-1a–e
a AP view.
b Lateral view.
c Oblique view.
d CT scan distal humerus, frontal plane.
e CT scan shaft fracture, sagittal plane.

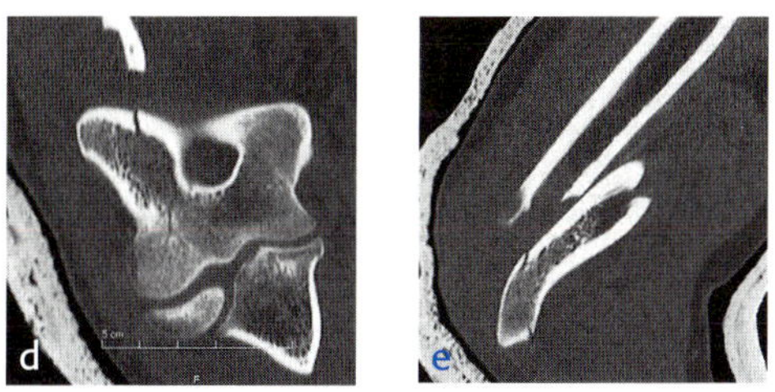

The patient received first aid in a small hospital. Reduction maneuvers were performed but were ineffective and the arm was stabilized in a plaster cast for transportation purposes only.

Note: In displaced oblique fractures of the distal third of the humerus, there is a high risk that the radial nerve may be caught between the fracture fragments and become damaged.

Indication

Unstable displaced fracture at the middle to distal third. Some minimally displaced fracture lines in the supracondylar region extending into the lateral condyle. Fracture of the proximal ulna with comminution zone. Primary radial nerve palsy immediately after the accident. No vascular damage. Closed soft-tissue trauma grade I according to Tscherne and Oestern.

Nonoperative management was not an option because of the likelihood that soft tissue and the radial nerve might be situated in the fracture gap. In addition, fracture of the olecranon with a comminution zone is an unstable fracture pattern. Stable fixation of all fractures seemed to be the best option because of the low compliance of the patient due to his mental disability. Minimally invasive stabilization was not considered because of the required revision of the radial nerve. Additionally, the distal humeral fragment was too short to offer sufficient anchorage for an intramedullary device. The decision was made to perform an open procedure, revision and decompression of the radial nerve, reduction and stable fixation of the humeral fracture with cerclage wires and interfragmentary cortex lag screws (interfragmentary compression). A double plate osteosynthesis with two LCP 3.5 secured with locking head screws had to be performed to increase stability.

At the proximal ulna open reduction and angular stable plate osteosynthesis was performed to stabilize the olecranon fracture.

Preoperative planning

Equipment
- LCP 3.5, 12 holes
- LCP metaphyseal plate 3.5, for distal medial humerus, 13 holes
- LCP olecranon plate 3.5 (right), 8 holes (cut to 5 holes)
- 3.5 mm self-tapping locking head screws (LHS)
- 3.5 mm cortex screws
- Cerclage wires

(Size of system, instruments, and implants can vary according to anatomy.)

Patient preparation and positioning
Antibiotics: cephalosporin
Thrombosis prophylaxis: none

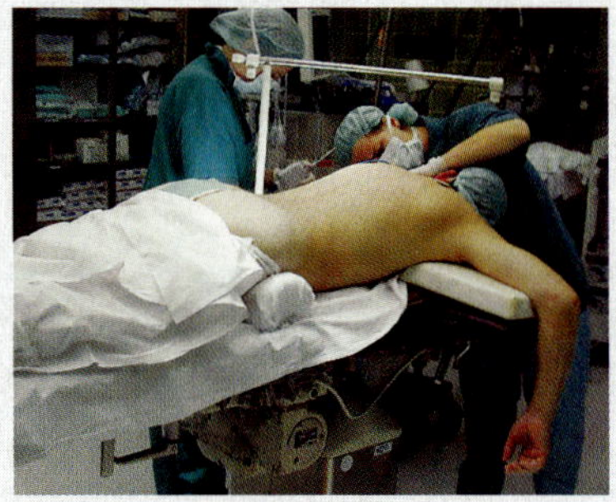

Fig 6.3.1-2 The patient is in the prone position. The arm is freely draped and positioned on a radiolucent arm table. No tourniquet is used in this fracture situation although it would be helpful in a more distal humeral fracture.

2 Surgical approach

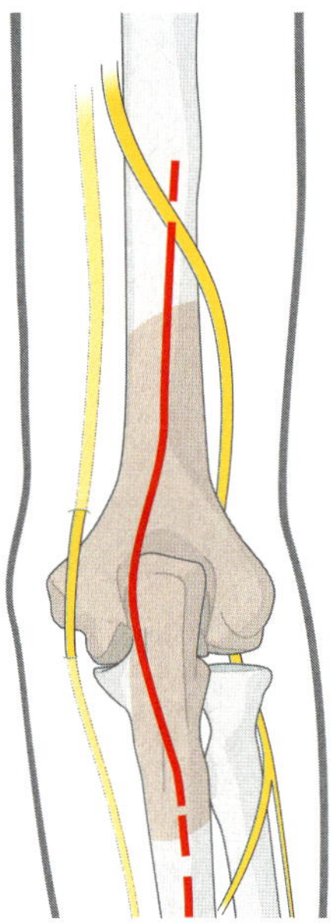

a

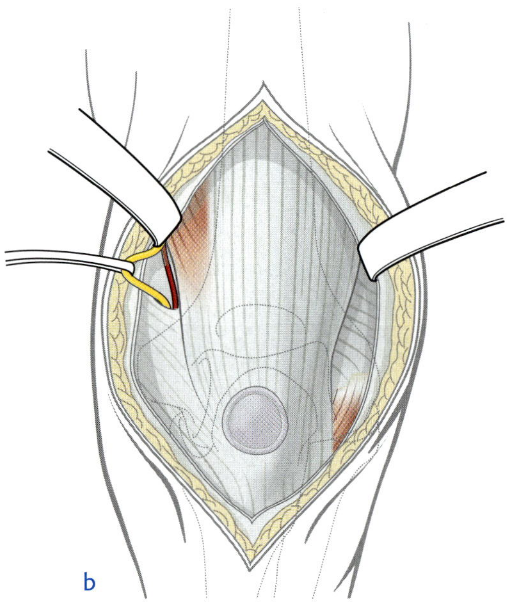

b

Fig 6.3.1-3a–d
- a A straight posterior incision is made from the midthird of the humerus, medial to the tip of the olecranon, down to the forearm. Alternatively, the incision may be curved around the tip of the olecranon on the radial side. The hematoma in the olecranon bursa is evacuated and in this case the bursa was resected.
- b The ulnar nerve is identified, released to the first motor branch and protected. The triceps muscle is mobilized. In complex olecranon fracture situations, the muscle is reflected to proximal with one or more olecranon fragments in continuity with the tendon.

2 Surgical approach (cont)

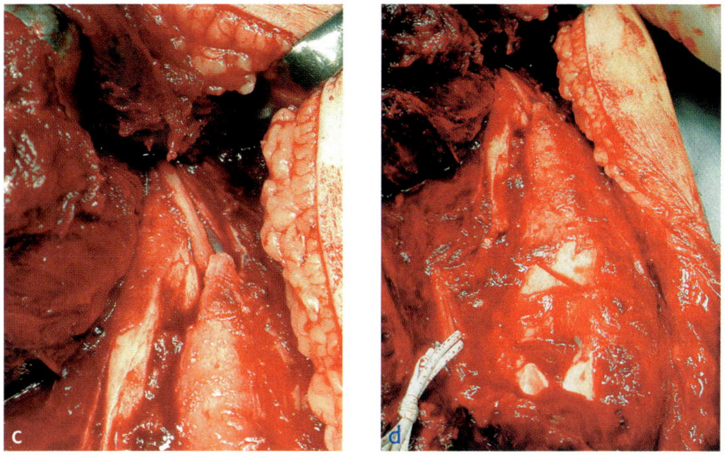

Fig 6.3.1-3a–d (cont)
c–d The radial nerve is identified and, as expected, the nerve has suffered damage between the two main humeral shaft fragments. All fracture lines are identified, but are not completely exposed in an effort to keep the periosteal blood supply intact.

3 Reduction and fixation

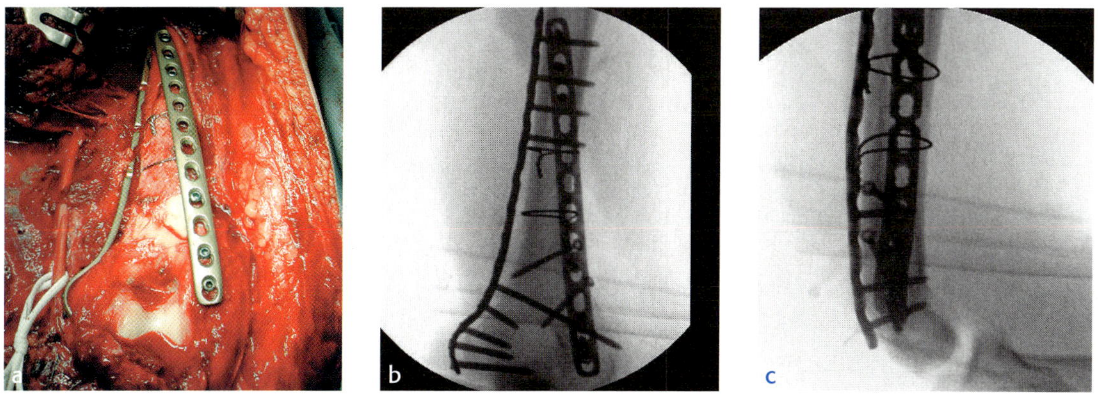

Reduce the fracture fragments with pointed reduction forceps without additional damage to the periosteal blood supply to the bone. When reduction is optimal, cerclage wires and interfragmentary cortex lag screws are inserted to stabilize the fracture. This leads to interfragmentary compression and good bone healing.

Fig 6.3.1-4a–d To improve stability two protection plates are used. First an LCP 3.5 is prepared for the dorsal side of the shaft and the radial column. The plate is slightly precontoured and fixed proximally with three 3.5 mm locking head screws and distally with two. Afterwards, an LCP metaphyseal plate 3.5 for distal medial humerus is chosen. The plate is fixed with locking head screws to the lateral side of the medial column as a protection plate. This noncontact plate is not pressed to the bone so that the periosteal blood supply is preserved. Image intensification shows a gap of a few millimeters between the plate and the medial cortex. The ulnar nerve is retracted with a white vessel loop.

3 Reduction and fixation (cont)

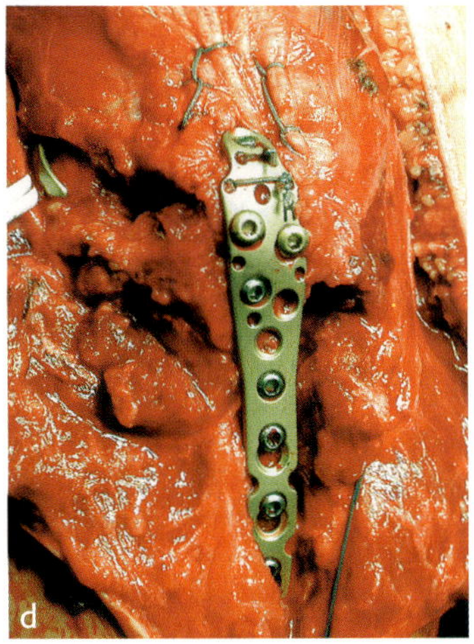

Fig 6.3.1-4a–d (cont) After irrigation the final procedure is reduction of the fragments of the olecranon without any step-off at the articular surface. Temporary K-wire fixation may be helpful. For definitive fracture stabilization of this multifragmented fracture plate fixation with an angular stable LCP olecranon plate is preferred. If the fragments at the tip of the olecranon are small, additional heavy, nonabsorbable sutures that fix the triceps tendon to the plate may help to improve stability.
The ulnar nerve is either transposed to the anterior side of the epicondyle or repositioned in its bed in the bicipital groove.
After irrigation and drainage careful wound closure has to be performed and a soft bandage is applied.

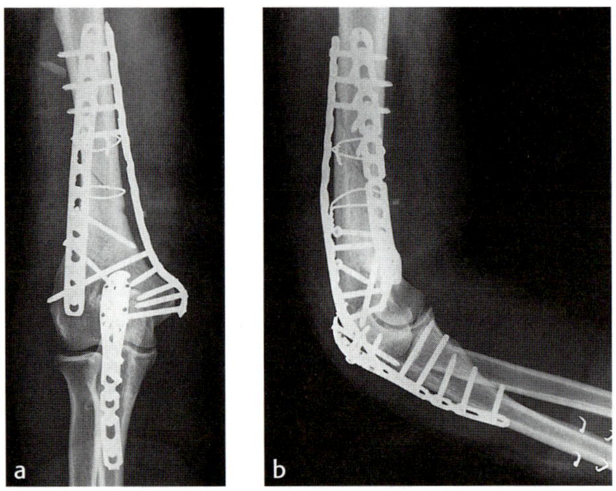

Fig 6.3.1-5a–b Postoperative x-rays show a good reduction of the fracture of the humerus and the ulna and good positioning of the implants.
a AP view.
b Lateral view.

4 Rehabilitation

No additional external fixation is used. After removal of the drains, the patient starts with active motion. He uses the arm up to his comfort threshold for activities of daily living. A special splint extending his wrist and fingers is used because of radial nerve palsy. No special rehabilitation protocol is prescribed because of the reduced compliance of the patient due to his mental disability.
Pharmaceutical treatment: painkillers in the early postoperative period, thereafter, as required.

4 Rehabilitation (cont)

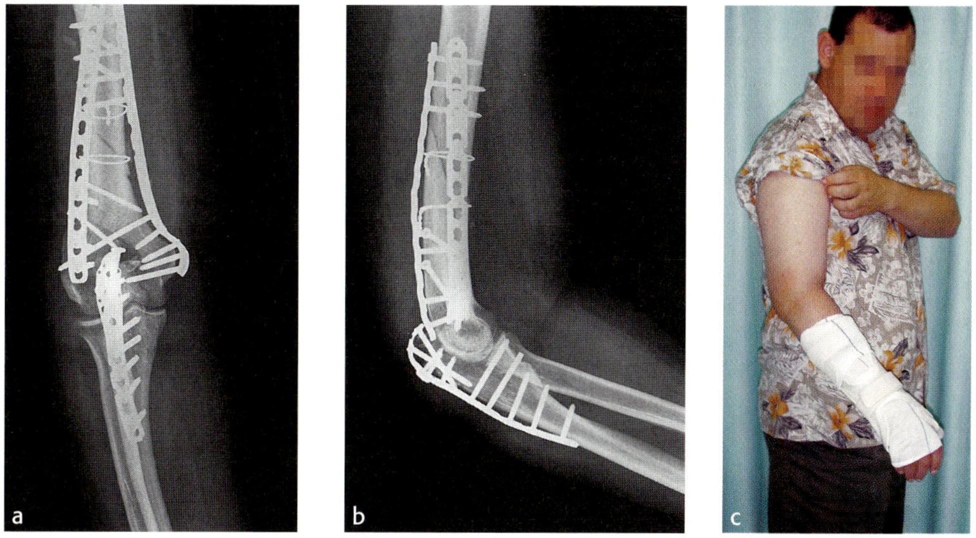

Fig 6.3.1-6a–c 8 weeks follow-up.
a AP view.
b Lateral view.
c Functional result with flexion up to 110° and an extension deficit of 30°.

The fractures remained stable and the x-rays after 8 weeks showed no loosening of the implants and good healing. The forearm splint was still needed and no regeneration of the radial nerve could be achieved. The patient did not complain of pain and had a satisfactory range of motion with flexion up to 110° and an extension deficit of 30°. Usually, active-assisted and active physiotherapy is performed to improve the range of motion of the elbow joint and passive exercises help to mobilize the wrist joint and the finger joints. A neurological examination, nerve conduction velocity and an EMG (electromyography) is planned at 3 months after the injury to assess recovery of nerve function.

5 Pitfalls –

Approach
Extensive exposure of the fracture, leading to additional damage to the periosteal blood supply to the humerus.
Ulnar and radial nerve are in danger.
There is a lot of scarring after such an extensive approach, leading to some restriction in range of motion.

6 Pearls +

Approach
Although this is an extensile approach, careful preservation of the periosteum will help to avoid additional damage to the blood supply to the bone. An open approach to this humeral fracture, identification and careful preservation of the ulnar and radial nerve will help to avoid aggravation of the nerve lesion.

In the case of a dislocated, multifragmentary fracture of the olecranon, the proximal fragments are still attached to the tendon insertion and can be retracted proximally as a single structure, thus exposing the humeral fracture.

5 Pitfalls – (cont)

Reduction

Insufficient reduction and residual diastasis between the fracture fragments will lead to malunion or nonunion in a high percentage of cases, especially in fractures of the humerus.

In oblique or spiral fractures of the distal third of the humeral shaft, closed reduction maneuvers may damage the radial nerve because, in a high percentage of cases, the nerve will be situated between the fractured surfaces.

Fixation

Although the standard implant for humeral shaft fractures is a broad LCP, the use of this type of plate as a single posterior implant will not sufficiently stabilize a fracture that extends into the condylar region of the distal humerus.

K-wire fixation and tension band osteosynthesis will not be suitable for a proximal ulnar fracture with a multifragmentary zone.

6 Pearls + (cont)

Reduction

Precise reduction of the fractured surfaces is important in open osteosynthesis of humeral fractures, especially in the supracondylar region. Reduction maneuvers have to be performed with respect to the periosteal blood supply by traction, rotation, and the use of pointed reduction forceps to apply interfragmentary compression.

Fixation

Fractures of the distal third of the humeral shaft and the supracondylar region should be fixed by the principles of absolute stability. Interfragmentary compression is necessary and is implemented by interfragmentary cortex lag screws or cerclage wires. To improve stability two protection plates are advantageous. The use of locking compression plates like the LCP metaphyseal plate 3.5, for distal medial humerus, fixed with locking head screws, make precise precontouring of the plates unnecessary. There is no risk of primary loss of reduction.

Using the LCP as a noncontact plate a small gap is left between the plate and the bone for better preservation of the periosteal blood supply.

Angular stable plating of the proximal ulna leads to greater stability even in multifragmentary fracture situations. This permits an early active rehabilitation program to be followed.

Authors Michael J Gardner, Dean Lorich, David L Helfet

6.3.2 Open displaced complete articular distal humeral fracture–13-C1

1 Case description

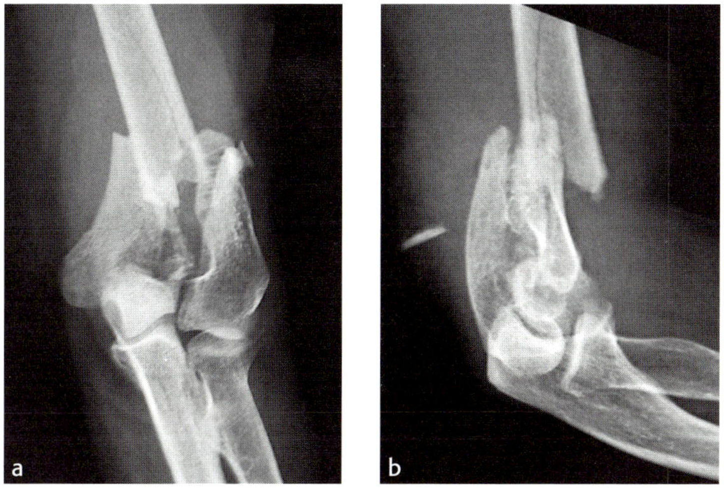

Fig 6.3.2-1a–b 74-year-old woman slipped and fell on her right flexed elbow and sustained a Gustilo type IIIA open distal humeral fracture. There were no associated neurovascular injuries or gross wound contamination.

Indication

Bicolumnar fracture of the distal humerus with intraarticular displacement. The intraarticular nature of this fracture and significant displacement of the fracture fragments are the main indications for operative intervention.

Preoperative planning

Equipment

- LCP reconstruction plate 3.5, 7 holes
- LCP reconstruction plate 3.5, 8 holes
- 3.5 mm locking head screws (LHS)
- 3.5 mm cortex screws
- 2.7 mm cortex screw
- Threaded 2.0 mm K-wires

(Size of system, instruments, and implants can vary according to anatomy.)

Patient preparation and positioning

Antibiotics: 1st or 2nd generation cephalosporin. The injured arm is placed over a padded bolster. The elbow is flexed 90°. The arm is prepped and draped free to the axilla. A sterile tourniquet is placed on the proximal arm.

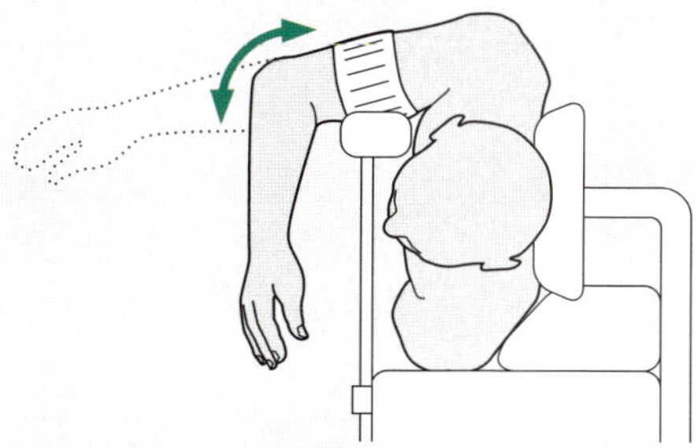

Fig 6.3.2-2 Place the patient in the left lateral decubitus position with the operative side up; a beanbag is used for stabilization of the body.

2 Surgical approach

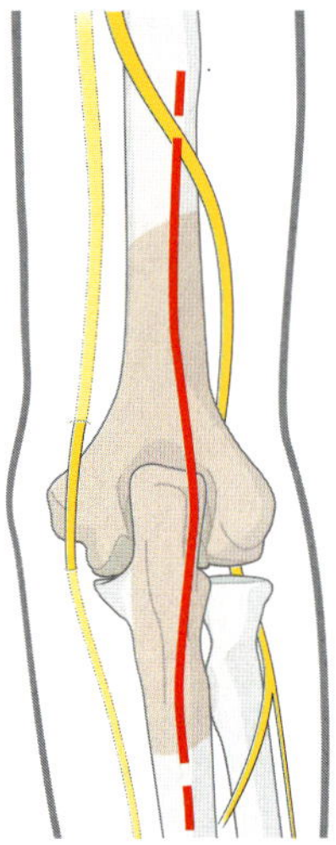

Fig 6.3.2-3 Irrigate and debride the open wound.
Make a midline incision over the posterior arm incorporating the traumatic wound, approximately 15 cm proximal to the olecranon. Curve laterally around the tip of the olecranon and continue in the midline 5 cm distally.

Raise full-thickness flaps medially and laterally.

Identify the ulnar nerve behind the medial epicondyle and protect it with a vessel loop.
Dissect the medial border of the triceps muscle free from the joint capsule. Develop this plane distally, and sharply release the triceps muscle insertion on the ulna, reflecting the entire muscle-tendon unit laterally, while taking care not to disrupt continuity of the extensor mechanism. Alternatively, an olecranon osteotomy or triceps split may be performed.

3 Reduction and fixation

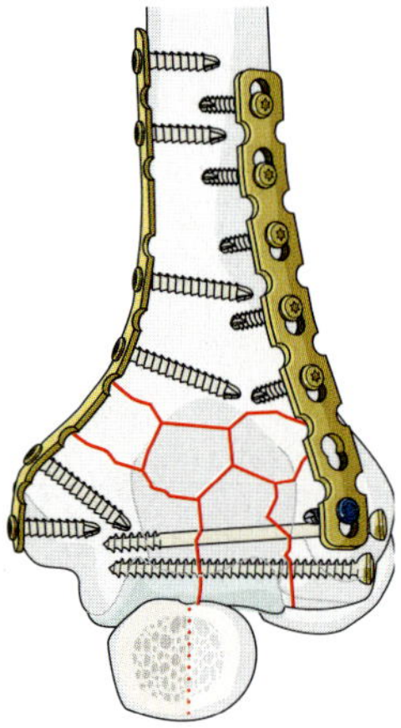

Fig 6.3.2-4 Use threaded K-wires as a joystick to reduce the vertical intraarticular split with the aid of a pointed reduction forceps. A pointed reduction forceps may be helpful to control fracture fragments. As with all intraarticular fractures, anatomical reduction of articular fragments is critical.
Place an interfragmentary 2.7 mm or 2.4 mm fully-threaded cortex screw to stabilize the trochlea. When minimal comminution is present the fragments may be compressed, taking care not to overcompress. The olecranon may serve as a useful template for the trochlear width when comminution is present.
With the trochlea stabilized, reduce this distal block to the medial and lateral columns. Precisely contour the reconstruction LCP 3.5 to fit appropriately. Reduce and stabilize the lateral column provisionally using K-wires and reduction forceps. The medial plate should then be placed on the medial edge of the humerus, and may hook distally over the nonarticular medial epicondyle.
Definitively stabilize the lateral column with another reconstruction LCP 3.5 applied to its posterior surface, allowing the plates to be placed perpendicular to each other. The lateral plate should extend as distally as possible to ensure rigid fixation. When the proximal limbs of the "T" have an oblique component, interfragmentary screws may be placed additionally. Insert monocortical or bicortical 3.5 mm locking head screws to complete the construction.
Repair the triceps tendon to the ulna with interrupted nonabsorbable sutures through transverse drill holes in the olecranon distally.
The ulnar nerve may be transposed to the subcutaneous tissues anteriorly to minimize hardware irritation and scar encasement.
Passively flex and extend the elbow and rotate the forearm to assess range of motion and stability prior to wound closure.

4 Rehabilitation

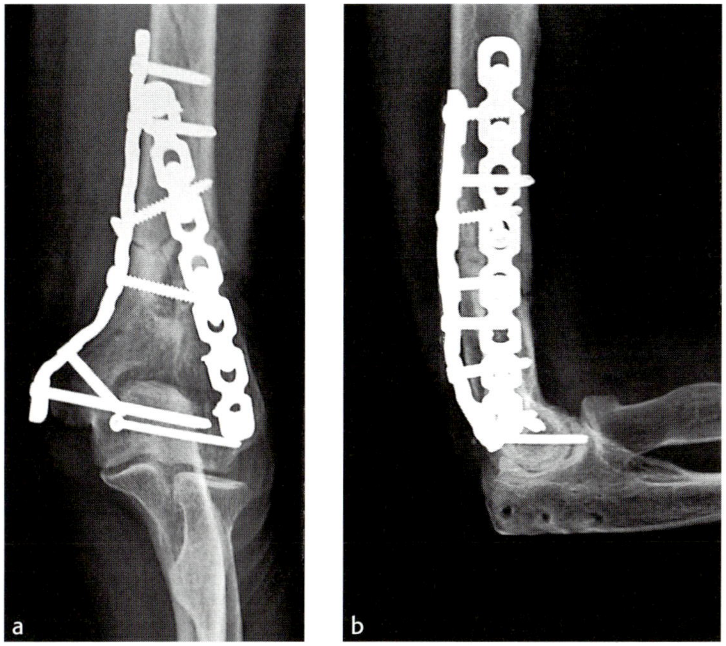

Continue antibiotic therapy with cephalosporin for 48–72 hours and monitor the wound closely for signs of infection.

Prescribe indomethacin for heterotopic ossification prophylaxis, along with a gastrointestinal protective agent.

From the first postoperative day the splint should be removed and a hinged elbow brace should be applied.

Aggressive active and passive range of motion exercises should be initiated, as well as an elbow continuous passive motion machine.

Fig 6.3.4-5a–b At 6 months postoperatively, the fracture is well aligned with evidence of healing.

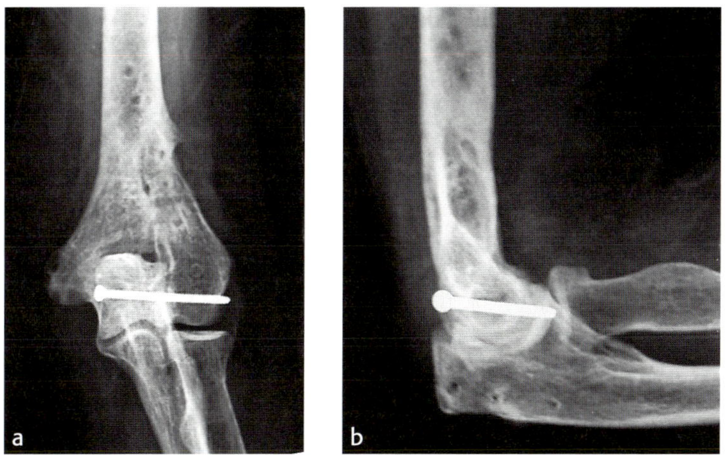

Implant removal

Fig 6.3.4-6a–b Following implant removal 10 months postoperatively, the patient had good elbow function and a healed fracture.

If the hardware becomes symptomatic and the fracture is shown to have healed both in x-ray and clinically, the implant may be removed, followed by protection of the distal humerus and limited weight bearing for 6–12 weeks.

5 Pitfalls –

Approach
The radial nerve may be injured proximally if the triceps muscle is split, or while exposing the lateral humeral shaft.

The ulnar nerve may be injured by direct injury or traction.

This approach may lead to subluxation of the triceps mechanism.

Reduction and fixation
When significant intraarticular comminution is present reconstructing the trochlea anatomically may be very difficult.

Bending the plates through the screw holes will not allow the use of locking head screws.

Hardware irritation may cause ulnar neuritis.
Screws in the olecranon or coronoid fossa may limit elbow motion.

Rehabilitation
Elbow stiffness and heterotopic ossification are not infrequent following intraarticular distal humeral fractures.

6 Pearls +

Approach
If a triceps muscle split is used, the triceps muscle should not be split more than 10 cm proximal to its insertion to avoid radial nerve injury. Though radial nerve exposure is not necessary, be aware of its position during lateral dissection.

Initial dissection and protection of the ulnar nerve with a Penrose drain, and freeing the nerve 6–8 cm proximal to the medial epicondyle will minimize damage.

It is critical to reapproximate the triceps tendon anatomically and securely reattach it to the olecranon with nonabsorbable sutures.

Reduction and fixation
When significant fragmentation of the articular fracture is present, use the dimensions and contour of the olecranon to reconstruct the trochlea anatomically.

When the preoperative plan dictates the use of a locking head screw in a certain hole, take care to bend the plate through the notch and not the screw hole.

Ulnar neuritis may be prevented by anterior transposition of the nerve during the primary procedure. The ulnar nerve is transposed as subsequent hardware removal and soft tissue release does not require dissecting the nerve out of scar tissue.

Special anatomically formed plates—distal humeral plate—make the fixation easier. No bending is required.

Rehabilitation
Early physical therapy and indomethacin prophylaxis can maximize postoperative restoration of elbow motion.
A stable fixation is necessary.

Author Reto Babst

6.3.3 Open complete intraarticular distal humeral fracture—13-C2

1 Case description

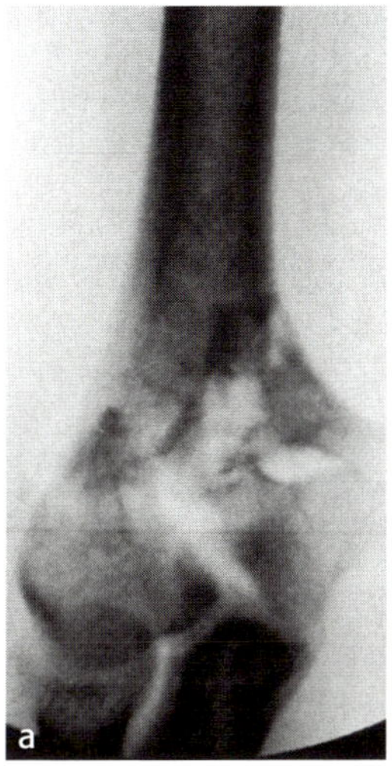

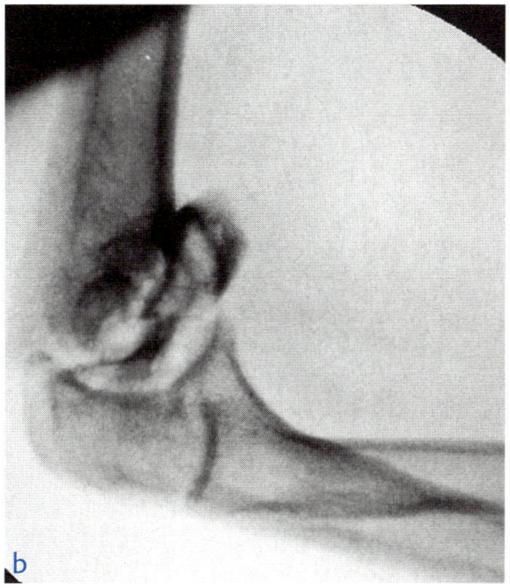

51-year-old man sustained a displaced distal humeral fracture of his dominant arm when falling down stairs.

Fig 6.3.3-1a–b
a AP view.
b Lateral view.

Indication

Displaced intraarticular fracture with a simple articular fracture pattern and some comminution in the epimetaphyseal part. If additional information is needed, either a traction view intraoperatively or a CT scan is recommended for proper preoperative planning.

Preoperative planning

Equipment

- LCP reconstruction plate 3.5, 6 holes on the radial column and LCP reconstruction plate 3.5, 8 holes on the ulnar column
- 3.5 mm self-tapping locking head screws (LHS)
- 3.5 mm cortex screws
- 4.0 mm cancellous bone screw
- 1.6 mm K-wires
- 1.6 mm nonabsorbable sutures

(Size of system, instruments, and implants can vary according to anatomy.)

Patient preparation and positioning

Antibiotics: single dose 2nd generation cephalosporin
Thrombosis prophylaxis: low-molecular heparin

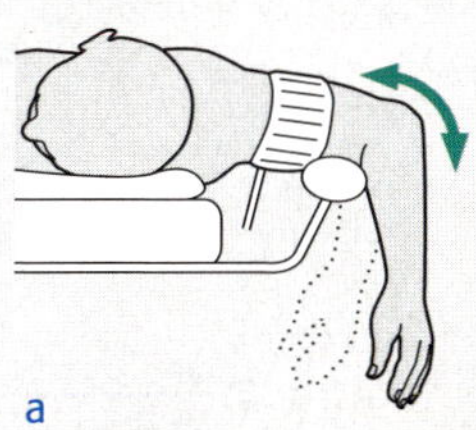

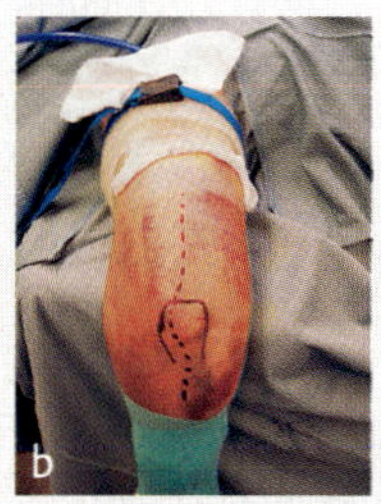

Fig 6.3.3-2a–b The patient is in a prone position with his arm on a short arm table. Arm freely movable with the possibility to flex more than 90°

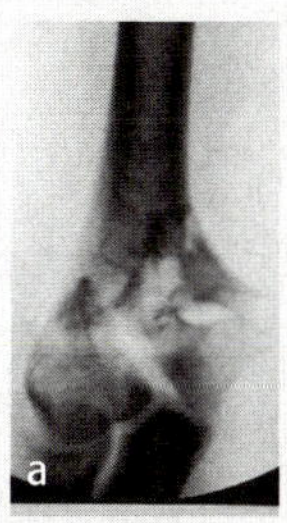

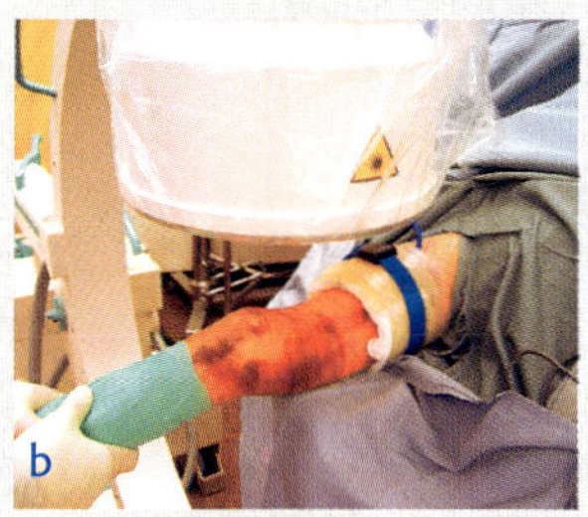

Fig 6.3.3-3a–b Preoperative extension view with the patient under anesthesia using the image intensifier is recommended to obtain additional information if the preoperative x-rays are not conclusive. Consider also CT scans for preoperative planning.

2 Surgical approach

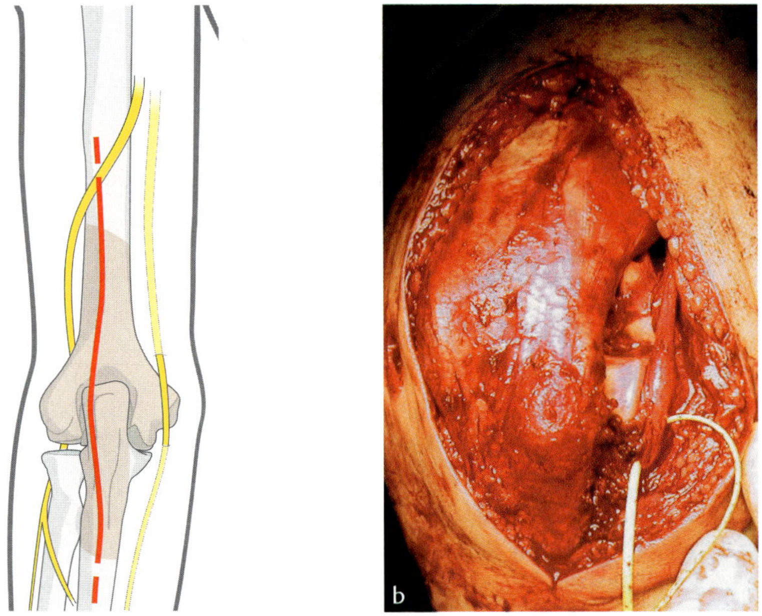

a b

Fig 6.3.3-4a–b Slightly curved incision radial to the olecranon tip. Isolation of the ulnar nerve and opening the joint on the ulnar side. Osteotomy of the tip of the olecranon leaving the extensor apparatus intact. The intact olecranon provides a template for joint reconstruction. This approach is only advisable when dealing with a simple articular fracture.

3 Reduction and fixation

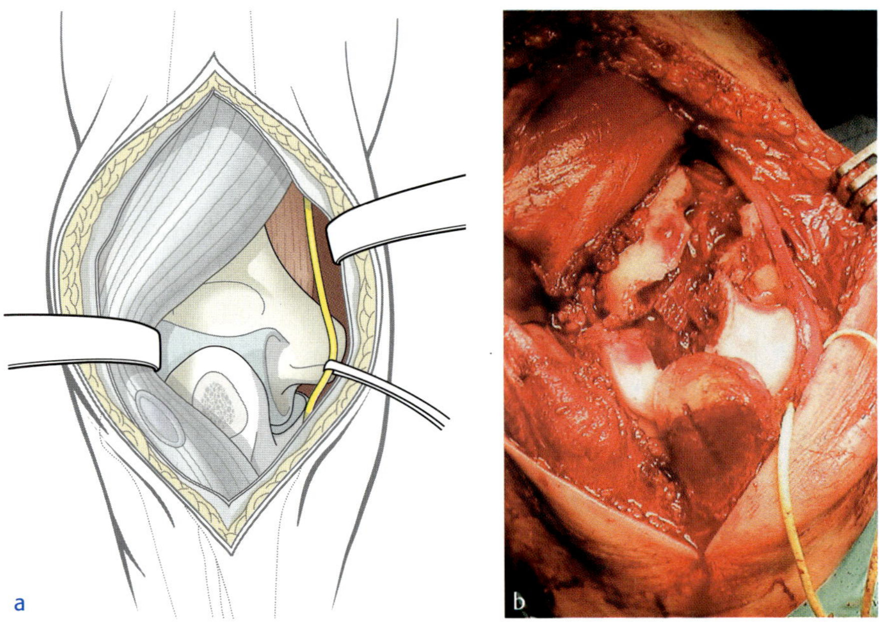

a b

Fig 6.3.3-5a–d

a–b The triceps muscle, together with its tendinous attachments are displaced radially and the articulation becomes visible. Note the olecranon joint remains intact. This is a modification of the Bryan-Morrey approach which is used for total elbow arthroplasty, and to release not only Sharpey's fibers but the attached cortical bone of the olecranon as well.

3 Reduction and fixation (cont)

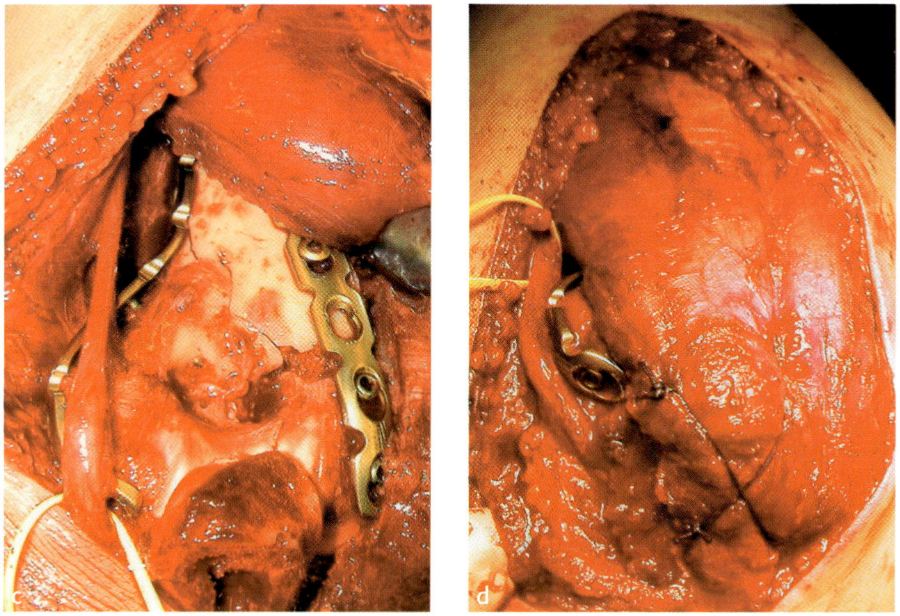

Fig 6.3.3-5a–d (cont)

c As a first step the articular block was reduced and fixed with a 4.0 mm cancellous bone screw. Then the articular block was temporarily fixed with K-wires and the radial column was stabilized, first using a LHS distally and then three cortex screws proximally. The first screw proximal to the fracture was placed in an eccentric mode. Thereafter the ulnar plate was adapted and proximally fixed with cortex screws and distally with three LHS.

d The olecranon tip osteotomy is then flipped back and tension banded in a figure-of-eight with a nonabsorbable suture.

4 Rehabilitation

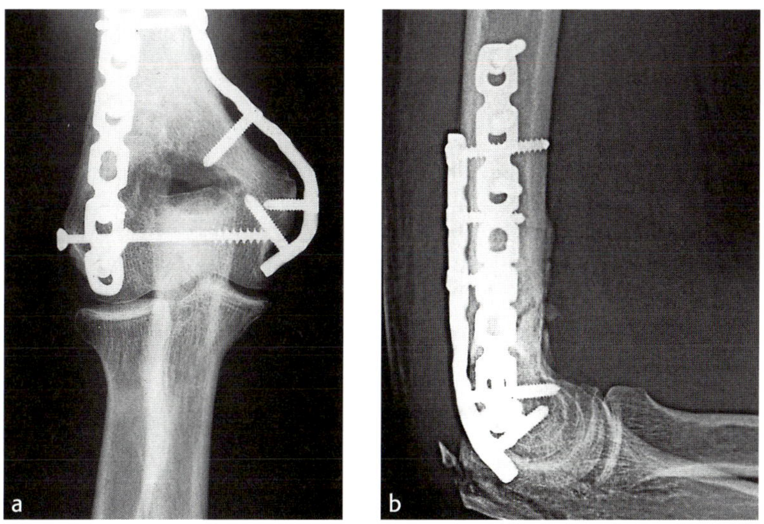

Fig 6.3.3-6a–b Postoperative x-rays, AP- and lateral view 12 weeks postoperative. The flip osteotomy is clinically healed, even though the osteotomy line is still visible.

Additional immobilization: splint for 3–4 days.
Weight bearing: depending on the x-ray, starting after 6–10 weeks.
Physiotherapy: functional aftercare with active assisted movement with a physiotherapist as of postoperative day 1.
Pharmaceutical treatment: pain medication on demand during the first postoperative days.

Implant removal
Only due to mechanical irritation.

5 Pitfalls –

Approach

The modified Bryan-Morrey approach allows a good visualization of the distal humerus when dealing with simple fracture patterns. It is important that the triceps muscle is released together with the forearm fascia and the ulnar periosteum incontinuity so that the extensor apparatus remains intact. This can be achieved either by dissection of Sharpey's fibers (Bryan-Morrey approach) or with a minimal flip osteotomy of the olecranon tip.

Reduction and fixation

The ulnar nerve should not lie directly on the plate. Either the plate is covered by soft tissue or the nerve should be transposed out of groove for ulnar nerve. Its position should be noted in the operative report.

Rehabilitation

In polytraumatized patients with head injuries, prophylaxis against periarticular bone formation has to be considered.

6 Pearls +

Approach

A simple extraarticular fracture pattern might be stabilized with a bilateral approach from each side of the triceps without osteotomy of the olecranon.

Reduction and fixation

Complex articular fractures with a simple fracture pattern of one column are often easier to fix when the simple column fracture is reduced and fixed first to the shaft fragment. Subsequently, reconstruction and fixation of the articular block against the correctly reduced and fixed column fragment.

Author Reto Babst

6.3.4 Displaced intraarticular distal humeral fracture—13-C3

1 Case description

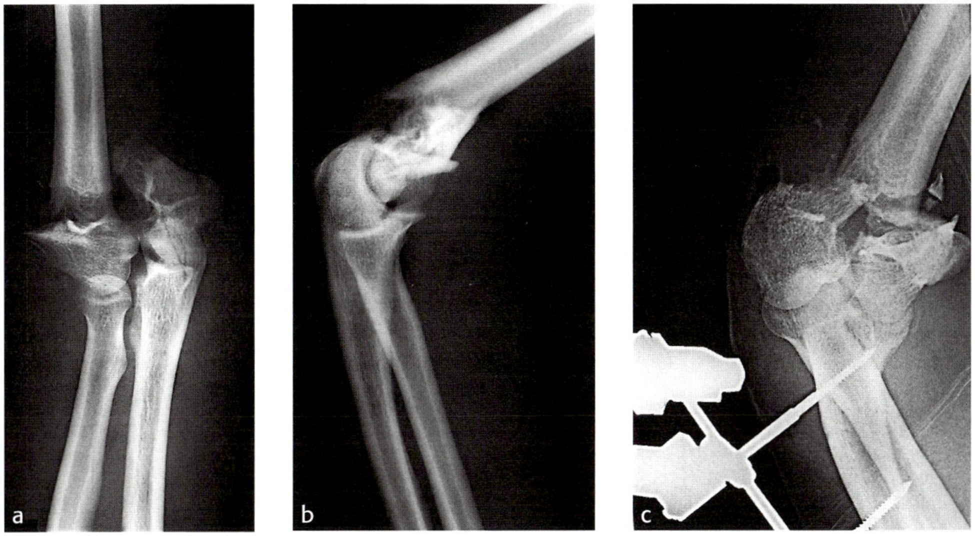

23-year-old man polytraumatized, with an open displaced right distal humeral fracture of the dominant arm, with fracture of the right acetabulum, the right femur, and rib fractures with lung contusion of the right hemithorax.

Fig 6.3.4-1a–c
a AP view.
b Lateral view.
c Temporary joint-spanning external fixator.

Indication

Displaced distal intraarticular humeral fracture without comminution but an intermediate fragment of the radial column was left on the scene. There is also an undisplaced fracture of the tip of the proximal ulna. If additional information is necessary, a CT scan will provide further information for adequate preoperative planning.

Due to displacement there is a danger of compromising the ulnar nerve and there is a need to mobilize the elbow as soon as possible after stable fixation. Nonoperative treatment is not an option for this open fracture as it is the dominant arm of a young laborer.

Due to general conditions, the fracture was first immobilized with a temporary joint-spanning external fixator (Fig 6.3.4-1c) after debridement and pulse irrigation during the first operation for fixation of the femoral fracture. The final fixation of the distal humerus took place 7 days after the accident.

Preoperative planning

Equipment

- DHP—distal humeral plate 2.7/3.5, 7 holes on the radial column, 6 holes on the ulnar column
- 3.5 mm and 2.7 mm self-tapping locking head screws (LHS)
- 3.5 mm cortex screw
- 1.6 mm K-wires

(Size of system, instruments, and implants can vary according to anatomy.)

Patient preparation and positioning

Antibiotics: single dose 2nd generation cephalosporin

Thrombosis prophylaxis: low-molecular heparin

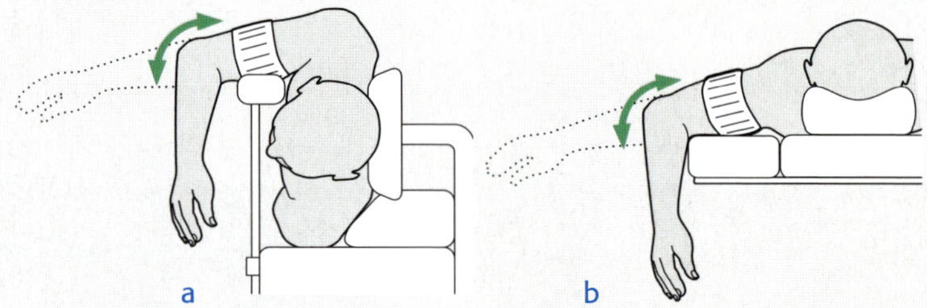

Fig 6.3.4-2a–b
a Lateral decubitus.
b Prone position.

2 Surgical approach

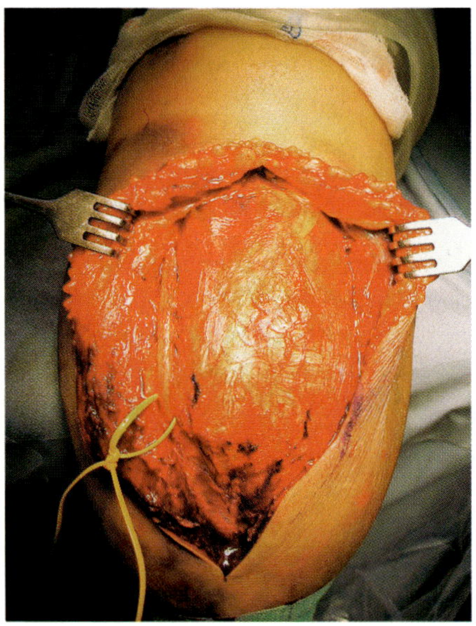

Fig 6.3.4-3 Straight incision along the axis of the humeral shaft curving on the radial side of the olecranon straight along the axis of the ulna. Preparation of the triceps muscle and isolation of the ulnar nerve.

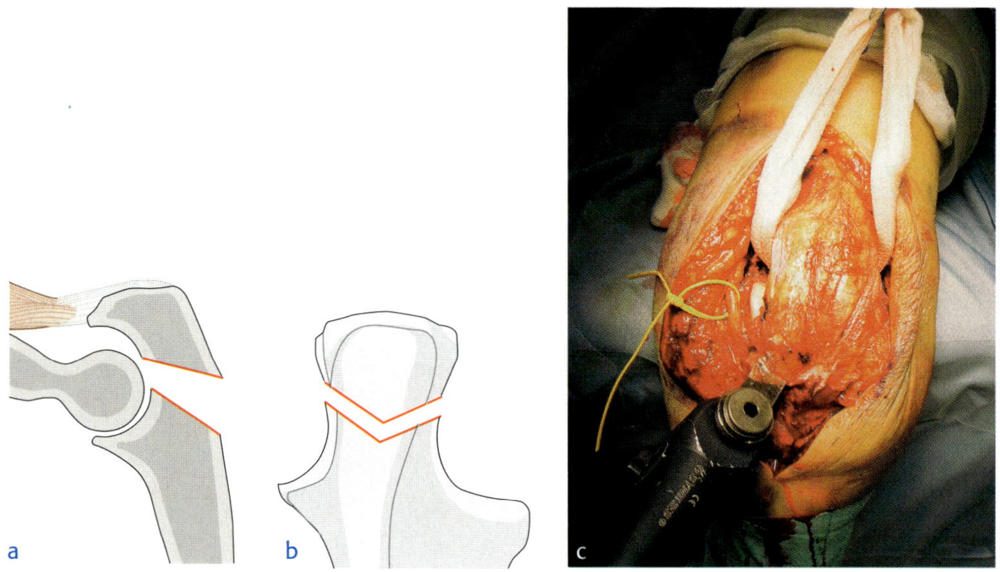

Fig 6.3.4-4a–c The Chevron type osteotomy is planned at the level of the deepest concavitiy of the ulnar joint. In situations with a simple intraarticular fracture, an olecranon tip osteotomy might also be sufficient to achieve a good view for an anatomical joint reconstruction.

3 Reduction and fixation

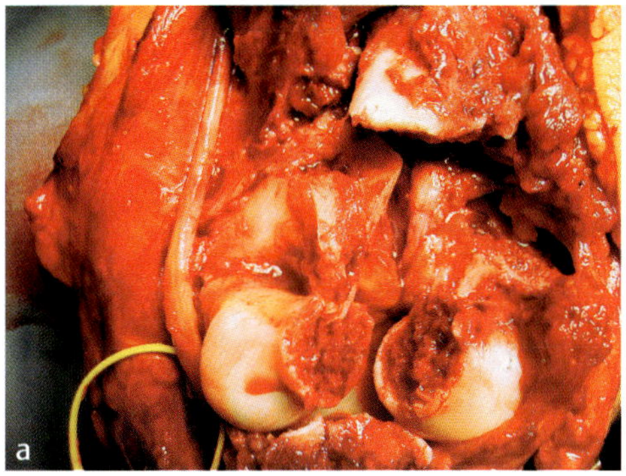
a

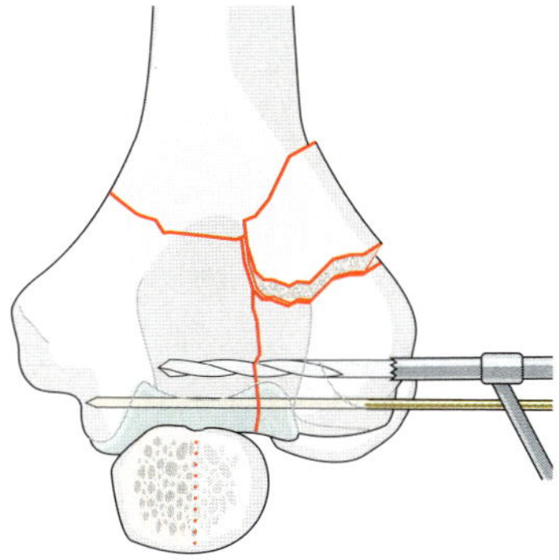
b

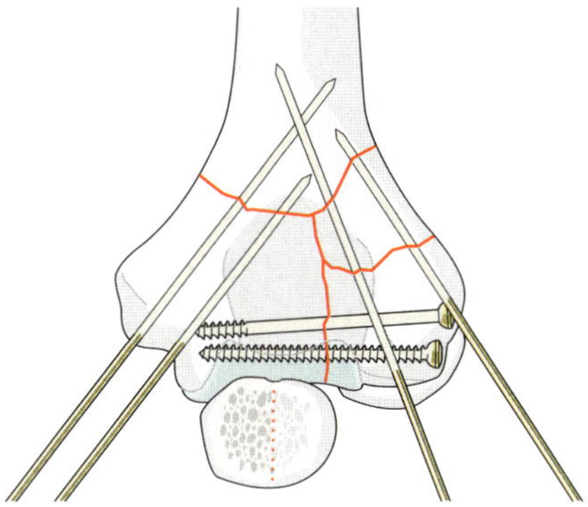
c

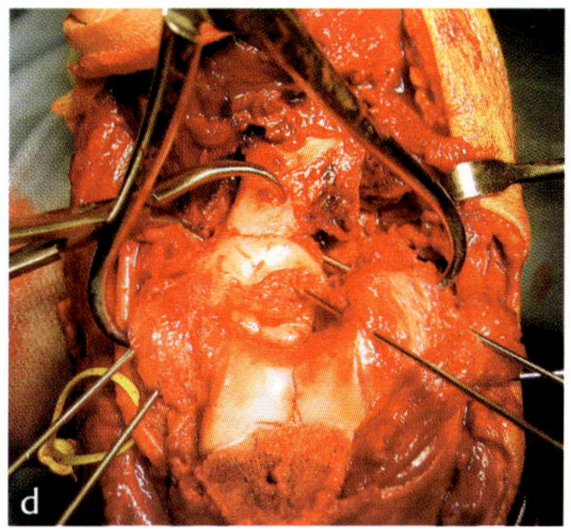
d

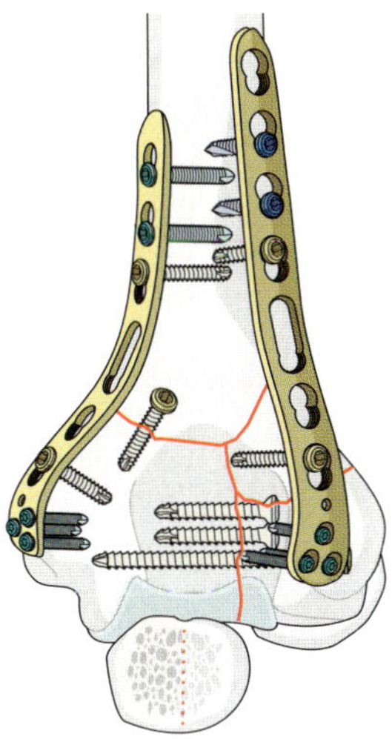
e

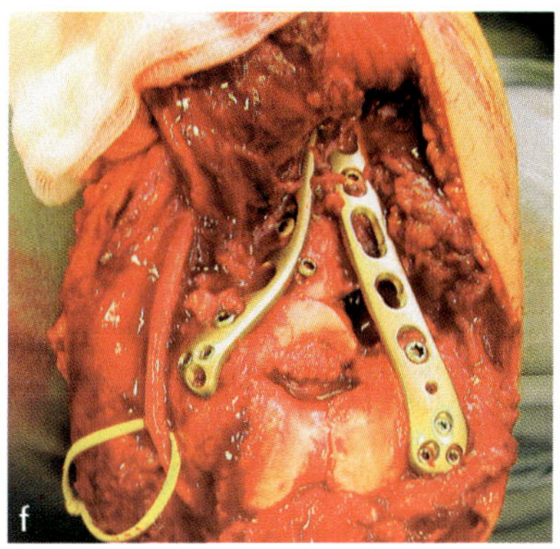
f

Fig 6.3.4-5a–f

- a The tip of the olecranon is then reflected with the triceps muscle.
- b With this simple trochlea fracture pattern the joint block is reduced first and temporarily fixed with a K-wire and then with a cortex screw.
- c–d The joint block is then temporarily fixed against the shaft using pointed reduction forceps and then K-wires.
- e–f After placing a cortex screw between the shaft and the ulnar fragment, the distal humeral plate (6-hole DHP) is first fixed with cortex screws on the shaft on the ulnar side and then with LHS distally. The defect on the radial side is then bridged with the radial distal humeral plate (7-hole DHP). The plate is then fixed with cortex screws on the shaft and with LHS in the distal fragment. Note the defect on the radial side due to the fragment left on the scene.

4 Rehabilitation

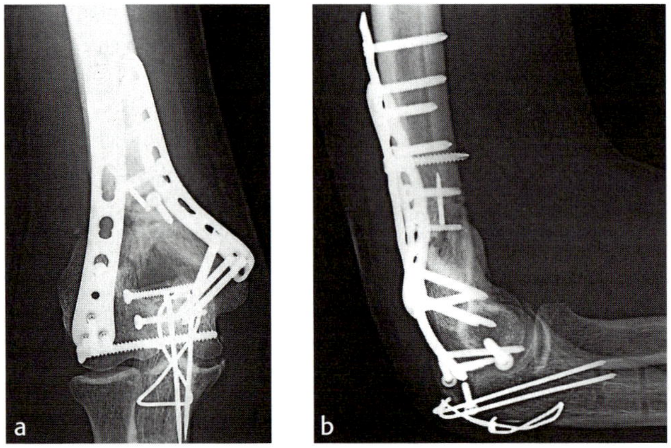

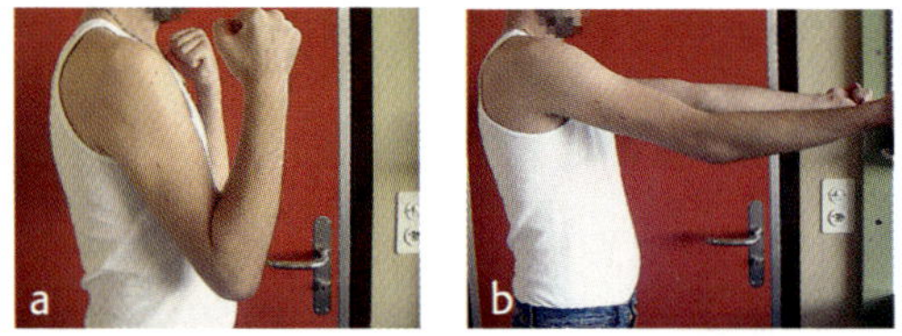

Fig 6.3.4-7a–b Function after 3 months was extension/flexion 0/20/130.

Fig 6.3.4-6a–b X-ray 12 weeks postoperative. Note the defect on the radial side. Since this was a second degree open fracture and the radial column fragments had contact to the posterior cortex, no cancellous bone graft was primarily added. The articular fracture was fixed with a 3.5 mm lag screw. The tip of the olecranon was stabilized with two 2.7 mm cortex lag screws. The osteotomy was closed with K-wires and a tension band fixation.

Additional immobilization: splint 3–4 days.
Pharmaceutical treatment: painkillers on demand during the first postoperative days.
Physiotherapy: functional aftercare with active assisted movement with a pyhsiotherapist as of postoperative day 1.
Weight bearing: depending on the x-ray, starting after 6–10 weeks.

5 Pitfalls –

Approach
The osteotomy of the olecranon with a chisel or a saw should be performed within the bone and not include the cartilage.

Reduction and fixation
The ulnar nerve should not lie directly on the plate. Either the plate is covered by soft tissue or the nerve should be transposed out of the groove for ulnar nerve. Its position should be noted in the operative report.

Rehabilitation
In polytraumatized patients with head injuries prophylaxis against periarticular bone formation has to be considered.

6 Pearls +

Approach
Simple articular fracture pattern might be stabilized with a bilateral approach from each side of the triceps muscle without osteotomy of the olecranon.

Reduction and fixation
Complex articular fractures with a simple fracture pattern of one column are often easier to fix when the column with its articular attachment is fixed first before the articular part of the other column is reduced against the now stabilized articular fragment.

Author Michael Schütz

6.3.5 Displaced intraarticular distal humeral fracture—13-C3

1 Case description

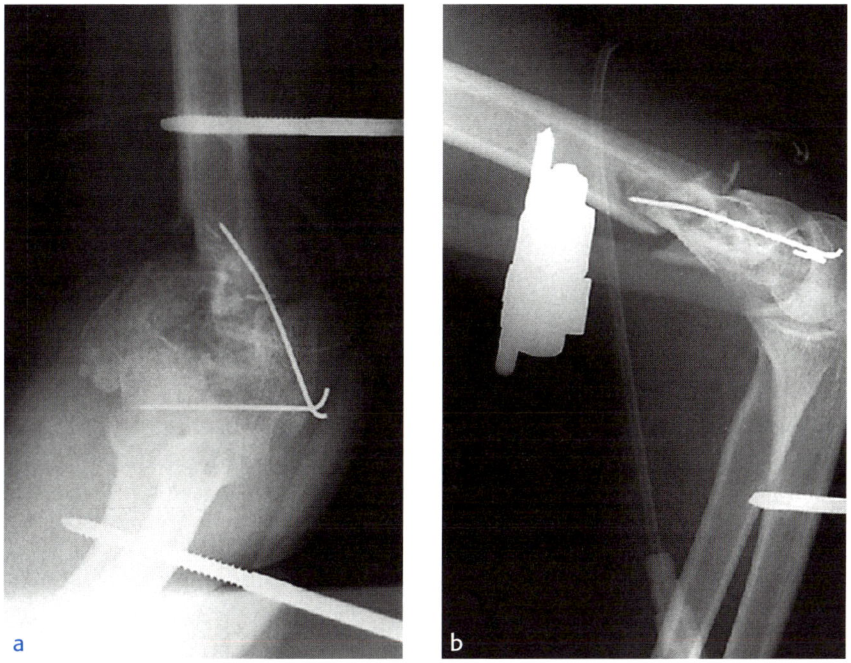

A 19-year-old woman fell out of a window and was polytraumatized. The injuries she sustained were complex with fracture of the pelvis, thoracic injuries, and a third degree open distal humeral fracture with bone defect. In the initial hospital, her elbow was treated with two K-wires and elbow transfixation.
After stabilization of her general condition, she received a definitive osteosynthesis of the distal humeral fracture on the fourth day after the accident.

Fig 6.3.5-1a–b
a AP view.
b Lateral view.

Indication

A dislocated intraarticular distal humeral fracture is a clear indication for operation in young patients.

Preoperative planning

Equipment
- LCP reconstruction plate 3.5, 8 holes
- Reconstruction plate 3.5, 6 holes
- 3.5 mm self-tapping locking head screws (LHS)
- 3.5 mm cortex screw
- 1.6 mm K-wires

(Size of system, instruments, and implants can vary according to anatomy.)

Patient preparation and positioning
Antibiotics: single dose 2nd generation cephalosporin
Thrombosis prophylaxis: low-molecular heparin

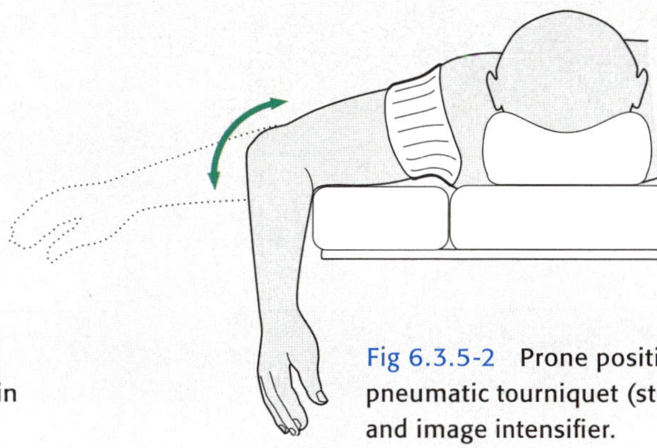

Fig 6.3.5-2 Prone position, arm on an arm table, pneumatic tourniquet (sterile or unsterile), x-ray and image intensifier.

2 Surgical approach

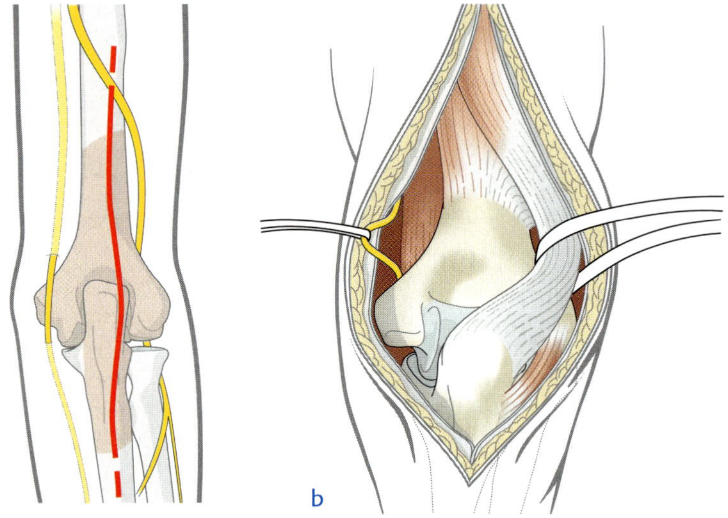

a b

Fig 6.3.5-3a–b Posterior approach with integration of the wound. The ulnar nerve is exposed and retracted.
An olecranon osteotomy may be required in more complex intraarticular fractures.

3 Reduction and fixation

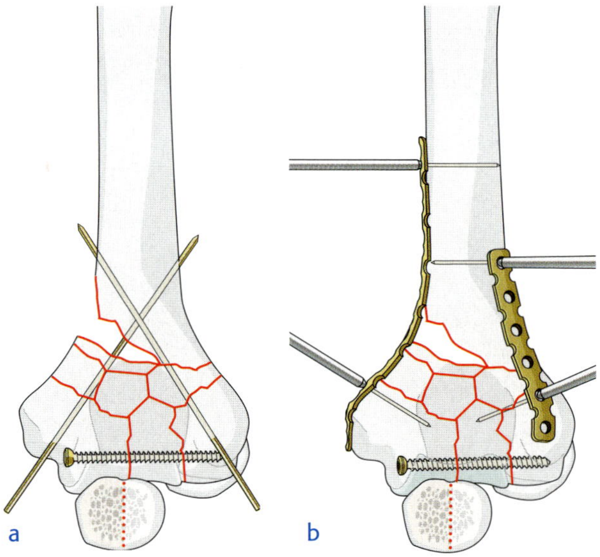

a b

Fig 6.3.5-4a–f

a The external fixator is removed before sterile draping of the patient. Debridement of the wound follows. The joint fragments are cleaned. The articular fracture is reduced with the pointed reduction forceps. The reduction is maintained with two 1.6 mm K-wires. An isolated 3.5 mm interfragmentary cortex screw is inserted as a lag screw to maintain the reconstruction of the trochlea. Reduction of the trochlea over the radial supracondylar column to the meta-/diaphysis should be performed first because of bone loss on the ulnar side. To achieve correct axial alignment, the two ulnar fragments must be held apart.

b The fragments are initially fixed with two 1.6 mm K-wires inserted through the joint block into the shaft.
The LCP reconstruction plates 3.5 are contoured using the bending template so that they fit the lateral supracondylar column (5-hole plate) and the medial supracondylar column (8-hole plate).
First one reconstruction plate is fixed to the posterior aspect of the radial column with one locking head screw proximally and one distally. This allows the joint block to rotate slightly around the distal screw and facilitates the exact alignment of the medial supracondylar column (complication due to the bone defect).

3 Reduction and fixation (cont)

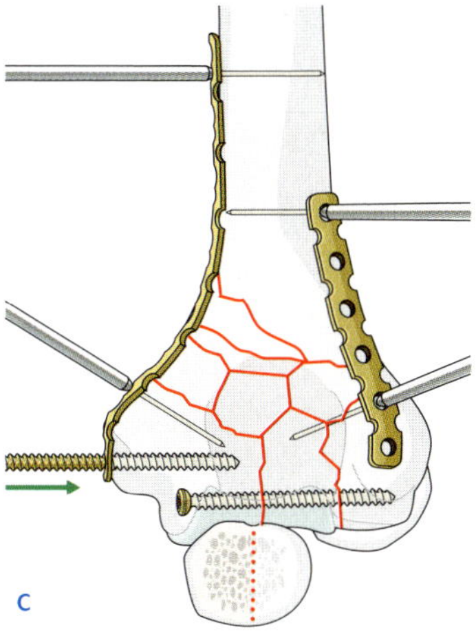

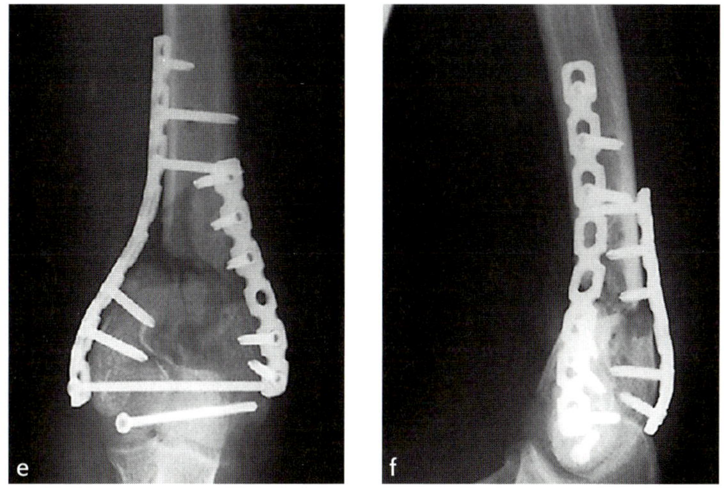

Fig 6.3.5-4a–f (cont)

c The ulnar reconstruction plate is bent into its final shape and fixed to the shaft by inserting a K-wire through the trocar.

d An additional interfragmentary lag screw is inserted through the distal hole in the ulnar plate. Whereas only monocortical screws are inserted to stabilize the radial plate, two bicortical screws are used to secure the other plate to the ulnar diaphysis in order to neutralize the prevailing rotational forces. Primary bone grafting of the defect was not carried out.

e–f Intraoperative, clinical assessment of the range of motion (passive movement in all planes) and final radiological control of plate position prior to wound closure.

4 Rehabilitation

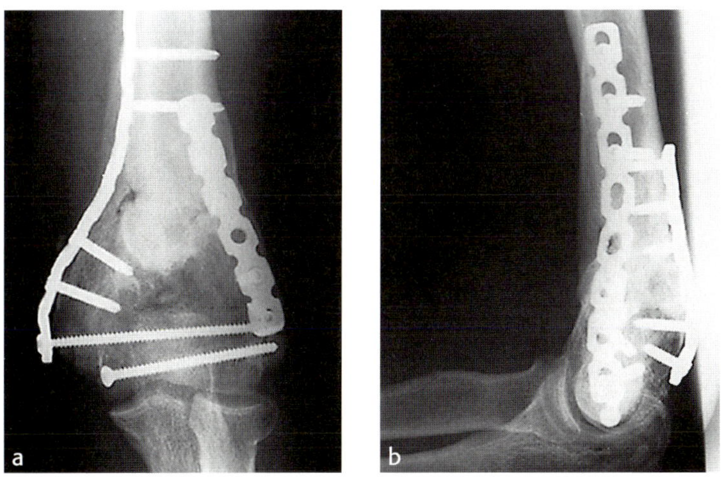

Sterile wound dressing. A dorsal splint is applied until definitive wound healing. On the second day active and passive physiotherapy was commenced with the splint in situ. Continued antibiotic treatment to ensure wound healing of the open fracture.

Fig 6.3.5-5a–b Good consolidation of the fracture after 9 months without the need for further surgery (eg, cancellous bone grafting).

a AP view.

b Lateral view.

4 Rehabilitation (cont)

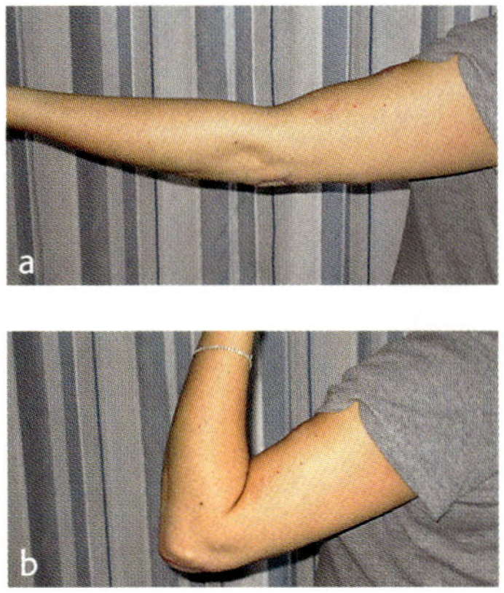

Fig 6.3.5-6a–b At the end of the treatment, the patient had an unlimited elbow function with a range of motion of 0/10/120 and unrestricted rotation.

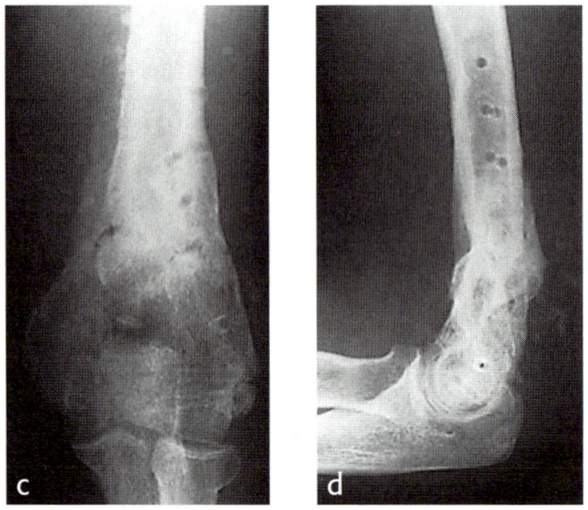

Implant removal

Fig 6.3.5-6c–d In the further course of consolidation, a heterotopic ossification, mainly at the posterior aspect, was excised at implant removal.

5 Pitfalls –

Approach

The ulnar nerve may be injured by direct injury or traction.
This approach may lead to subluxation of the triceps mechanism.

Reduction and fixation

When significant intraarticular comminution is present, reconstructing the trochlea anatomically may be very difficult.
Bending the plates through the screw holes will not allow the use of locking head screws.
Hardware irritation may cause ulnar neuritis.
Screws in the olecranon or coronoid fossa may limit elbow motion.

Rehabilitation

Elbow stiffness and heterotopic ossification are not infrequent following intraarticular distal humeral fractures.

6 Pearls +

Approach

Initial dissection and protection of the ulnar nerve with a Penrose drain, and freeing the nerve 6–8 cm proximal to the medial epicondyle will minimize damage.
It is critical to reapproximate the triceps tendon anatomically and securely reattach it to the olecranon with nonabsorbable sutures.

Reduction and fixation

When significant fragmentation of the articular fracture is present, use the dimensions and contour of the olecranon to reconstruct the trochlea anatomically.
When the preoperative plan dictates the use of a locking head screw in a certain hole, take care to bend the plate through the notch and not through the screw hole.
Ulnar neuritis may be prevented by anterior transposition of the nerve during the primary procedure.

Rehabilitation

Early physiotherapy and indomethacin prophylaxis can maximize postoperative restoration of elbow motion.

Authors Thomas Hockertz, Andreas Gruner, Gabriele Streicher, Heinrich Reilmann

6.3.6 Pathology of the elbow

1 Case description

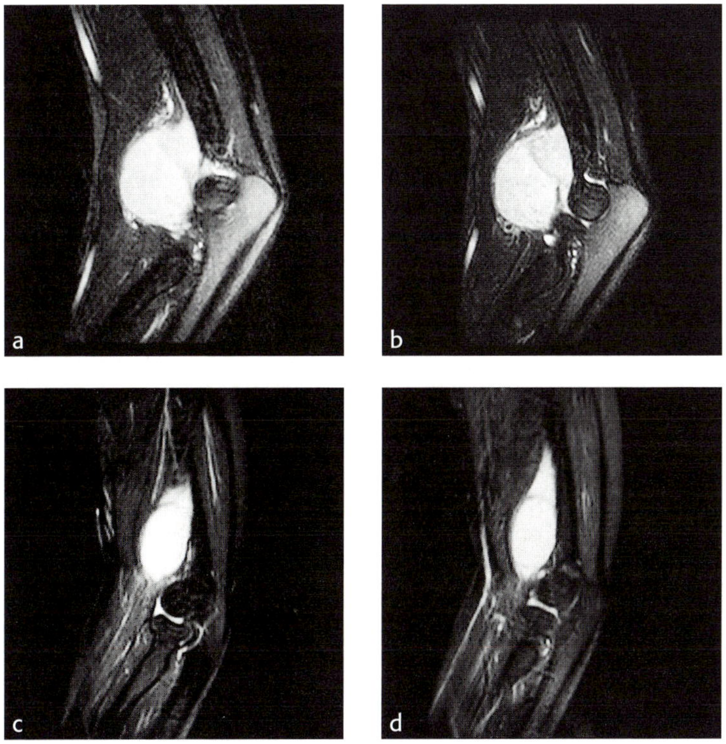

16-year-old female patient with pathology of the left elbow.

Fig 6.3.6-1a–d Nuclear magnetic resonance spectroscopy (NMR).

a NMR of primary tumor—sarcoma.
b NMR of primary tumor—sarcoma.
c NMR of recurrent sarcoma.
d NMR of recurrent sarcoma.

Indication

Young female patient with recurrent sarcoma of the left arm requiring stable fixation after compartment resection and iliac crest bone grafting. Since the proximal bone segment was very short, locking head stabilization.

Preoperative planning

Equipment

- LCP 3.5, 8-holes
- 3.5 mm locking head screws (LHS)
- 3.5 mm cortex screws

(Size of system, instruments, and implants can vary according to anatomy.)

Patient preparation and positioning

Antibiotics: 2nd generation cephalosphorin
Thrombosis prophylaxis: low-molecular heparin

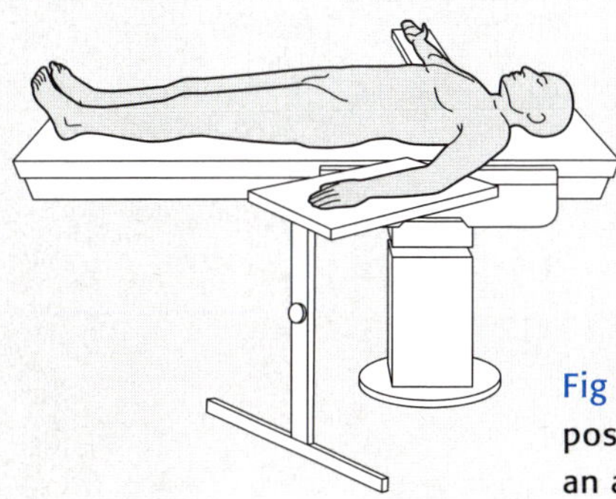

Fig 6.3.6-2 Patient in supine position with the arm resting on an arm table.

2 Surgical approach

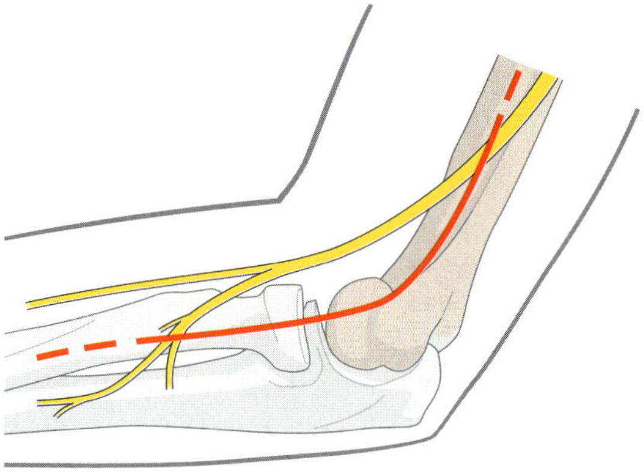

Fig 6.3.6-3 Extended radial approach to the left elbow.

3 Reduction and fixation

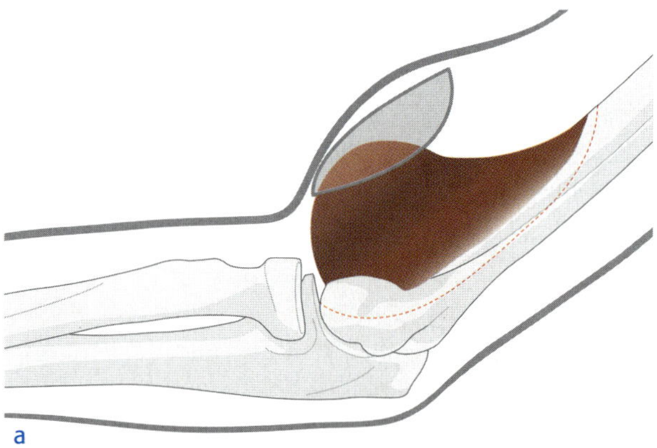

Fig 6.3.6-4a–f

a Location of the tumor on the distal humerus.

b–c Excision of the tumor including the underlying bone without disturbing the continuity of the humerus and tourniquet of the radial nerve.

d Prebending and adaptation of an LCP to fit the specific bone shape of the lateral distal humerus—stabilization of the LCP in the region of the distal joint by insertion of a cortex screw and a locking head screw.

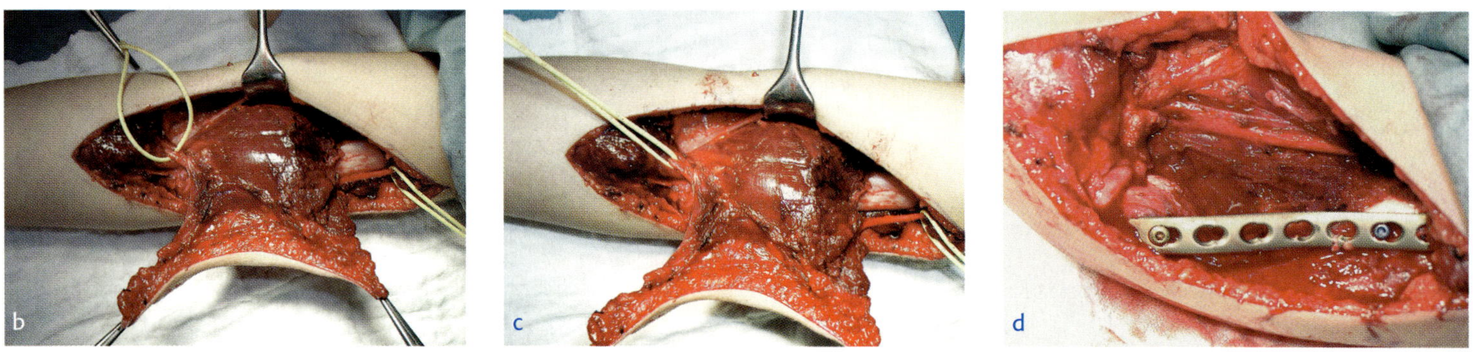

3 Reduction and fixation (cont)

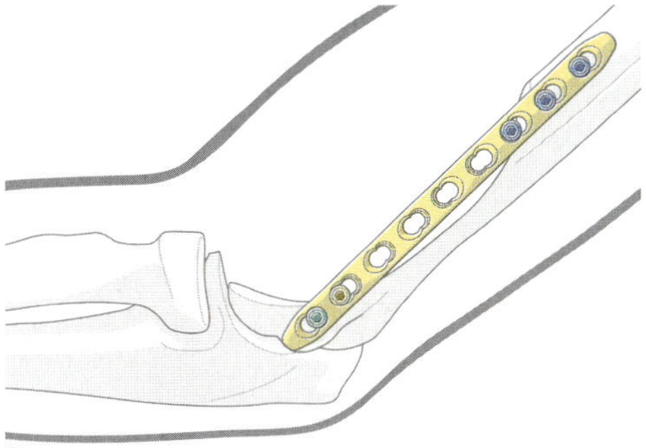

e

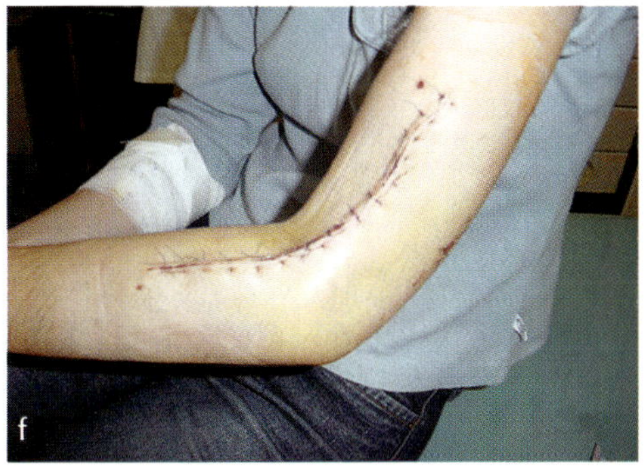

Fig 6.3.6-4a–f (cont)

e Proximal fixation in the area of the resected bone by insertion of two locking head screws—bridging of the bone defect to maintain mobility and weight bearing capabilities.

f Clinical view postoperatively.

4 Rehabilitation

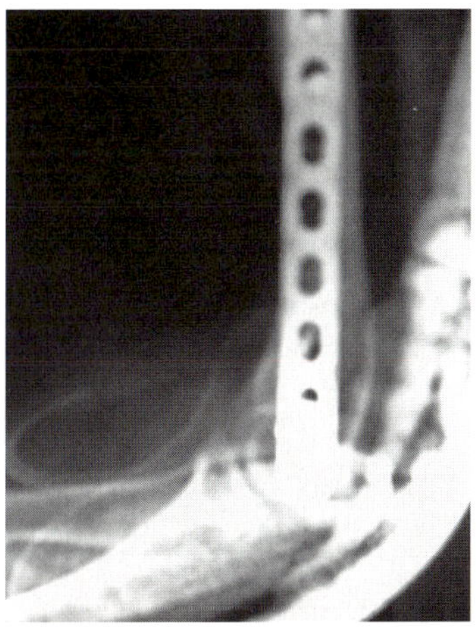

Additional immobilization: Upper arm plaster cast until soft-tissue healing.

Mobilization:
- Immobilization for 2 weeks
- Passive mobilization after 4 days
- Active mobilization after 14 days

Physiotherapy: from the 14th postoperative day.
Pharmaceutical treatment: Nonsteroid antiinflammatory drugs.

Fig 6.3.6-5 Postoperative x-ray lateral view.

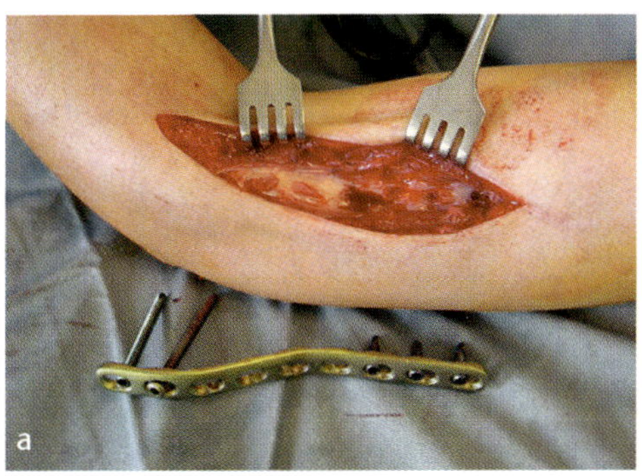

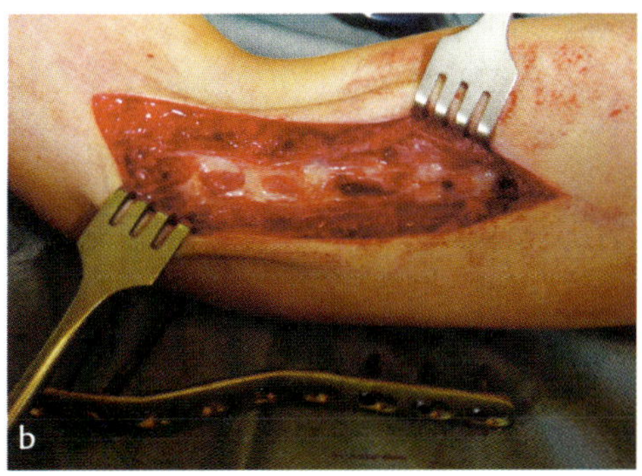

Implant removal
Implant removal after 6 months because of definitive bone healing.
Technique for implant removal: Same approach as for insertion of the implant.

Fig 6.3.6-6a–b Intraoperative situation at implant removal.

5 Pitfalls –

Rehabilitation

Implant removal

6 Pearls +

Rehabilitation

Early functional treatment may be possible even under difficult circumstances.

Implant removal

Fig 6.3.6-7 Good healing of the bone graft.

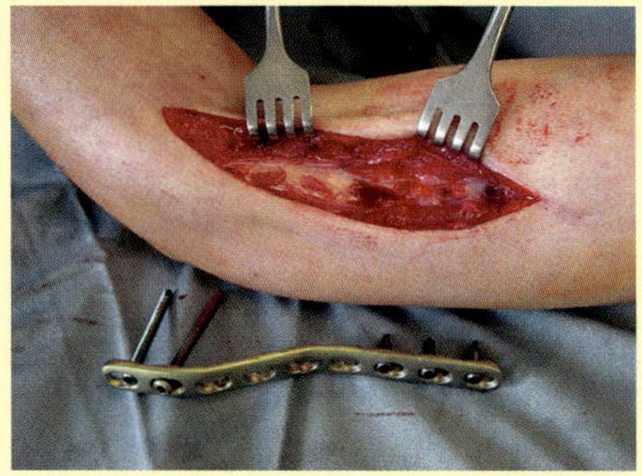

7.1 Radius and ulna, proximal

Cases

Case		Classification	Method	Implant used	Implant function	Page
7.1.1	Articular olecranon fracture	21-B1	compression	LCP metaphyseal plate 3.5	lag screws and protection plate	371
7.1.2	Olecranon fracture	21-B1	compression	LCP metaphyseal plate 3.5	tension band plate	375
7.1.3	Open proximal ulnar fracture; simple ulnar shaft fracture; anterior dislocation of the radial head	21-B1; 22-A1	compression and locked splinting	LCP olecranon plate 3.5	lag screws and protection plate and locked internal fixator	381
7.1.4	Complex radial head fracture and extraarticular olecranon fracture	21-B3	compression	LCP 3.5	lag screws and protection plate	385
7.1.5	3-part radial head and transverse radial neck fracture; intraarticular proximal ulnar fracture	21-B3	compression	Mini condylar plate; LCP 3.5	lag screws and protection plate	389
7.1.6	Extraarticular proximal ulnar fracture with pseudarthrosis	21-A1	compression	LCP 3.5	compression plate	395

7 Radius and ulna

Author Christopher W Geel

7.1 Radius and ulna, proximal

1 Incidence

Treatment of proximal forearm fractures carries unique problems, as the involvement of elbow joint structures needs to be considered. Instability, malunion, nonunion, and impingement may result in severe posttraumatic dysfunction. The anatomical and functional complexity of the elbow joint has to be restored with utmost care and precision. Therefore, fracture reduction and fixation remain as crucial as restoration of additional avulsions and lacerations of ligamentous and capsular lesions.

The complexity of the elbow function is based on a three-component buildup and structure of the joint entity, including the ulnatrochlear joint, the radiocapitellar joint and the radioulnar joint. Conservative closed treatment is followed by 92% unsatisfactory results [1]. Lack of early motion leads to functional deficiencies, particularly concerning pronation and supination. Only strict observance of biological and biomechanical principles of stability reproduces 90% excellent functional results [2].

Osteochondral fragments or loose bodies are not uncommon with radial head injuries. Capitellar abrasions are frequently observed. High-energy fractures may be associated with distal injuries such as additional fractures, interosseous membrane injuries and distal radioulnar joint disruptions [3].

In consequence, restoration of the interosseous membrane as well as of associated ligamentous and capsular injuries around the radial head and proximal ulna are mandatory.

Primary objectives are the restoration of the radial bow to boost pro- and supination and the stable fixation allowing early mobilization regarding pro- and supination and adjacent joints such as elbow and wrist.

2 Classification

The prime characteristics of fracture types are defined by the Müller AO Classification:

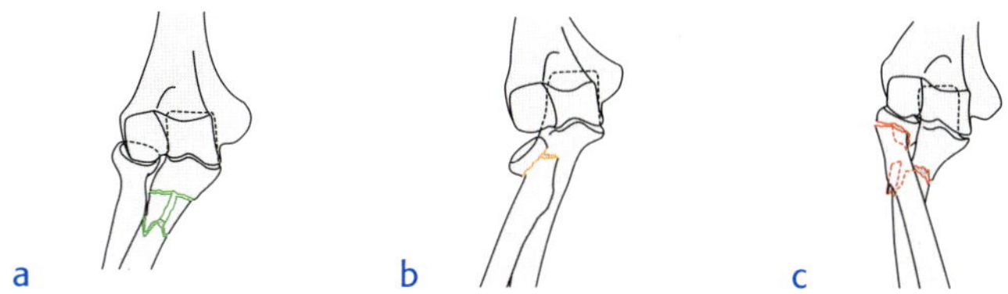

Fig 7.1-1a–c 21-A extraarticular fracture.
a 21-A1 ulna, radius intact
b 21-A2 radius, ulna intact
c 21-A3 both bones

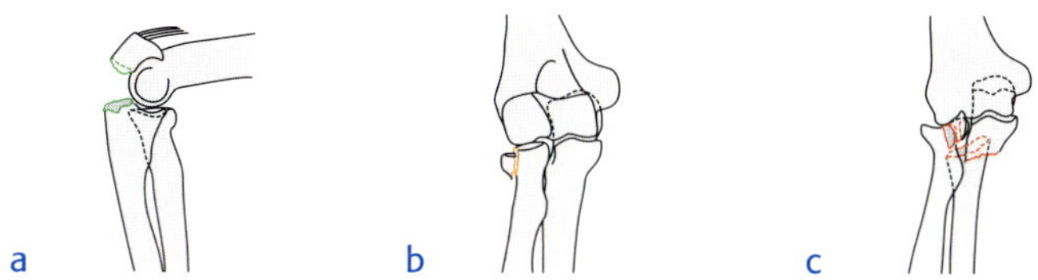

Fig 7.1-2a–c 21-B articular fracture.
a 21-B1 ulna, radius intact
b 21-B2 radius, ulna intact
c 21-B3 one bone, other extraarticular

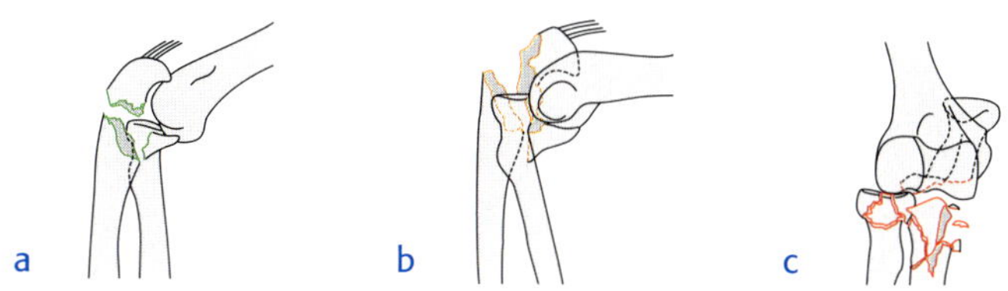

Fig 7.1-3a–c 21-C articular fracture of both bones.
a 21-C1 simple
b 21-C2 one articular simple other articular multifragmentary
c 21-C3 multifragmentary

3 Treatment methods

The radioulnar joint is always to be checked for subluxation proximally (Monteggia fracture) and distally (Galeazzi fracture). Proximal ulna fractures result in loss of tension mechanism at the triceps tendon insertion. Direct high-energy forces create a comminution and fragmentation with possible intraarticular comminution and cartilage damage. Involvement of the coronoid process or proximal ulna are presently associated with high-energy trauma and multifragmentary fractures. Radial head fractures from wedge fractures to subcapital fractures and multifragmentary fractures can be associated with or without dislocation.

High-energy trauma to the elbow often results in bruises of the skin with delayed surgery as a consequence. Diagnostic elbow x-rays as well as wrist x-rays are mandatory. To clarify radial head fractures, a 45-degree radial head oblique view magnifies the radial head and separates the results from the ulna to achieve a better overview [4].

Restoration of dorsoradial bow and anatomic length of radius and ulna with adequate tensioning of the interosseous membrane are of basic consideration. Priority is to be given to stable fixation for early mobilization, in particular regarding pro- and supination. However, differential procedures have to be respected case wise; anatomical reduction is to be limited to length, axis and rotation, while "chasing all fragments" is to be considered useless.

Regarding surgical procedures, different techniques may be discussed:

As only rotational stable internal fixation lets await good functional results, intramedullar radial bow restoration is currently not satisfactory. Due to danger of radial nerve injury, percutaneous plating is suitable more likely for ulna shaft fractures than for proximal radial fractures. Multifragmentary fractures require bridge plating, short oblique fractures with or without wedge fragment need interfragmentary compression support.

Interfragmentary compression is to be achieved by lag screw technique, screw external articulated tension device and use of push-pull compression plate technique. In radial head fractures the use of mini fragment instrumentation is desirable [5].

Preference is given to arm board supine position. The lateral decubitus is especially suitable for regional anesthesia. The prone position is not advisable, especially in obese patients and multiple traumas (chest wall and ventilation problems). The use of a tourniquet is advantageous.

In radial fractures, a modified Boyd approach with osteotomy of the lateral humeral condyle to improve visualization of the radial head and to reduce the risk of superficial radial nerve damage is recommended. The radial head fracture reduction uses thin wires as a sling for temporary reduction maneuver as well as pointed reduction forceps. The restoration of the depressed radial head central zone is important to regain normal anatomy and to improve functional outcome.

In ulnar fractures, the skin incision and the subcutaneous approach are corresponding with the interspace between flexor and extensor carpi ulnaris muscle. However, the skin incision should not directly correlate with the future implant position. Moreover, a wide skin bridge is needed if an additional, radial incision is used. Comminuted fractures require a LC-DCP 3.5 or LCP 3.5 and a one-third tubular plate only engaged as tension band function. Finally, plate bending is to be foreseen outside the plate holes to prevent distortion of the locking holes.

4 Implant overview

a

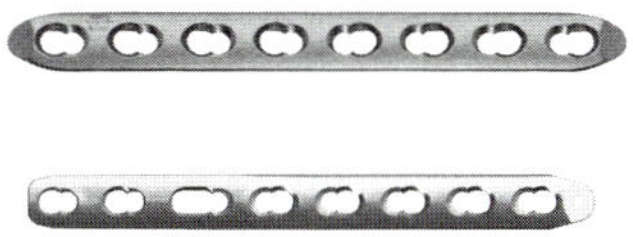

b

Fig 7.1-4a–b
a LCP 3.5
b LCP metaphyseal plate 3.5

5 Bibliography

1. **Hughston JC** (1957) Fractures of the distal radial shaft; mistakes in management. *J Bone Joint Surg Am*; 39-A(2):249–264.
2. **Tile M, Petrie D** (1969) Fractures of radius and ulna. *J Bone J Joint Surg*; 51-B:193–199.
3. **Heim U** (1998) [Combined fractures of the radius and the ulna at the elbow level in adults. Analysis of 120 cases after more than 1 year]. *Rev Chir Orthop Reparatrice Appar Mot*; 84(2):142–153.
4. **Moed BR, Kellam JF , Foster RJ, et al** (1986) Immediate internal fixation of open fractures of the diaphysis of the forearm. *J Bone Joint Surg Am*; 68(7):1008–1017.
5. **Geel CW, Palmer AK** (1992) Radial head fractures and their effect on the distal radioulnar joint A rational for treatment. *Clin Orthop Relat Res*; 275:79–84.

Author Michael Schütz

7.1.1 Articular olecranon fracture—21-B1

1 Case description

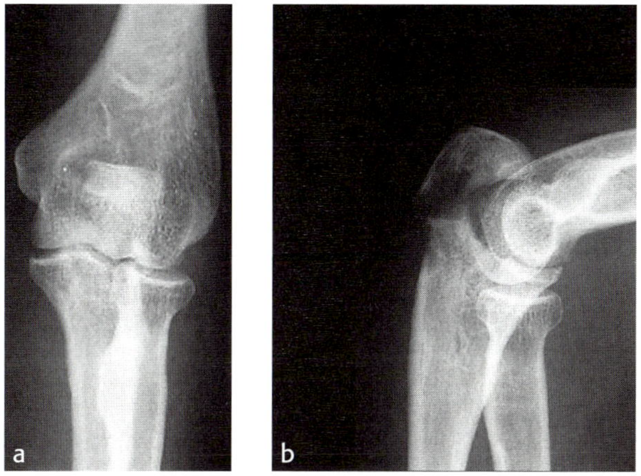

46-year-old patient fell and sustained an olecranon fracture. There were no other injuries.

Fig 7.1.1-1a–b
a AP view.
b Lateral view.

Indication

According to the principles of articular fracture management, a stable osteosynthesis permitting early functional treatment with or without a splint should be achieved. Due to an intermediate intraarticular fragment, plate osteosynthesis was performed instead of K-wire or cerclage fixation.

Preoperative planning

Equipment

- LCP metaphyseal plate 3.5, 6 holes
- 3.5 mm locking head screws (LHS)
- 3.5 mm cortex screws
- 1.25 and 1.6 mm K-wires

(Size of system, instruments, and implants can vary according to anatomy.)

Patient preparation and positioning

Antibiotics: single dose 2nd generation cephalosporin
Trombosis prophylaxis: low-molecular heparin

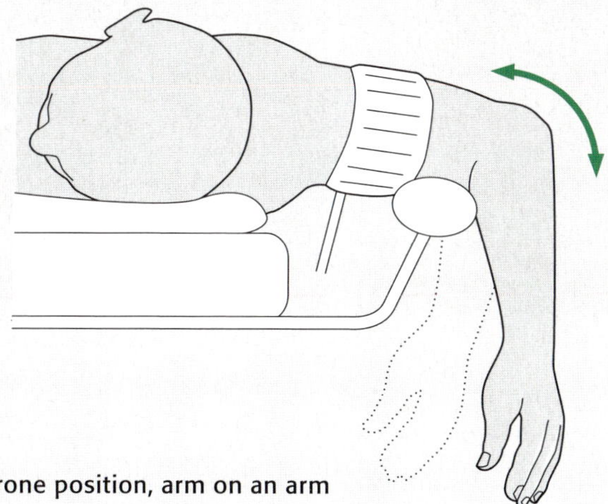

Fig 7.1.1-2 Prone position, arm on an arm table, pneumatic tourniquet (sterile or unsterile), radiography and image intensification.

2 Surgical approach

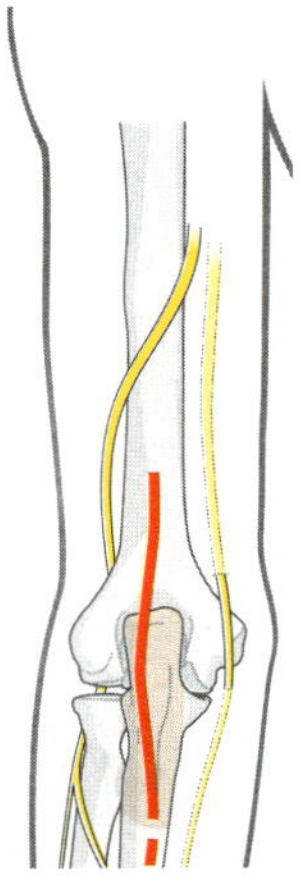

Fig 7.1.1-3 Posterior incision to the olecranon.

3 Reduction and fixation

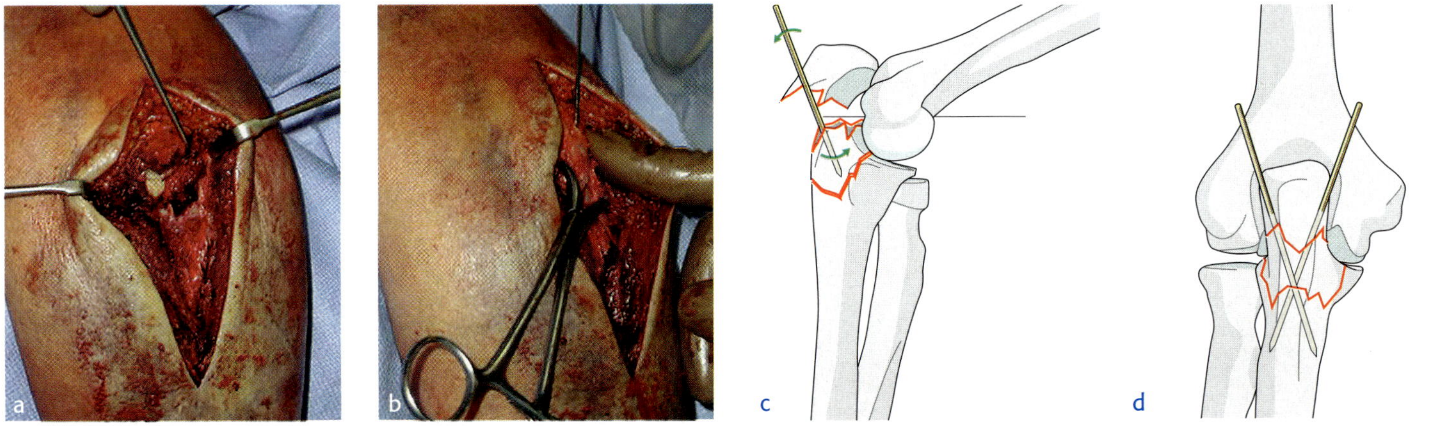

Fig 7.1.1-4a–i

a The articular fracture zone is exposed.

b–d The intermediate fracture fragment is reduced, under vision, in correct alignment to the distal joint fragment, and temporarily fixed with two K-wires. The K-wires must be inserted so that they will not interfere with the planned position of the plate.

The proximal main fragment is then reduced anatomically onto the distal fragment with the help of the pointed reduction forceps. The complete reduction is stabilized with 1.6 mm K-wires.

3 Reduction and fixation (cont)

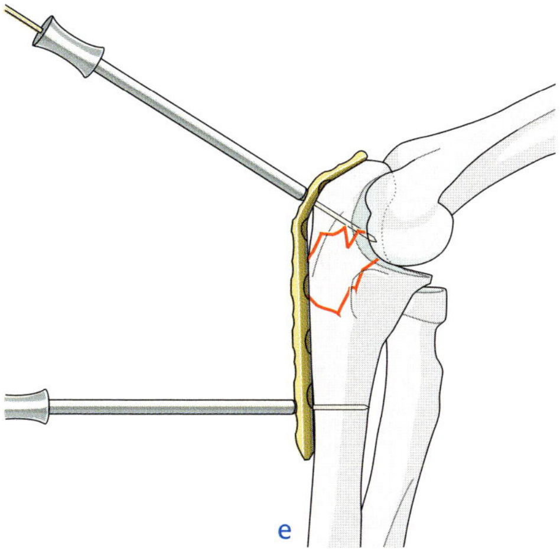

e

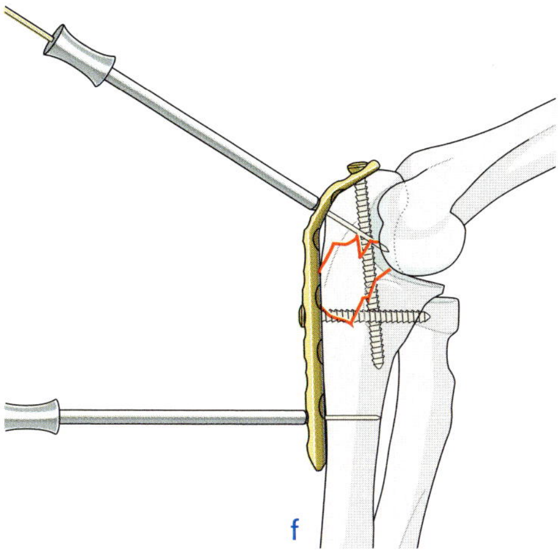

f

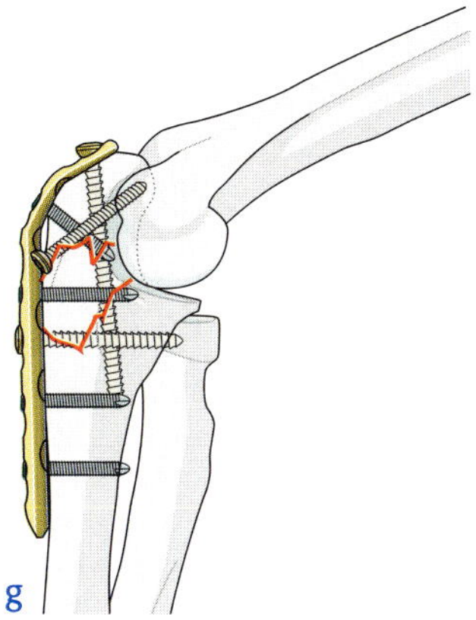

g

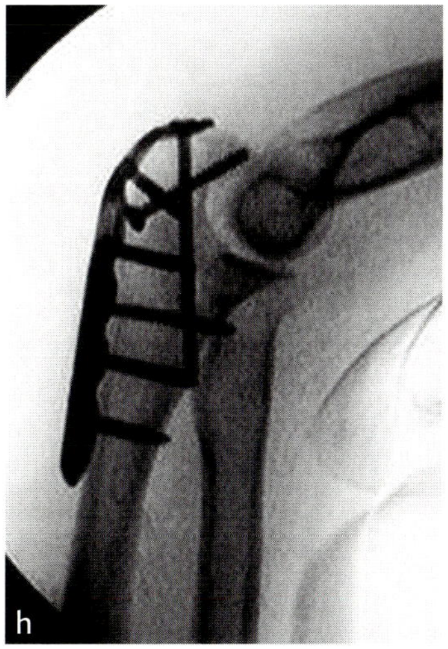

h

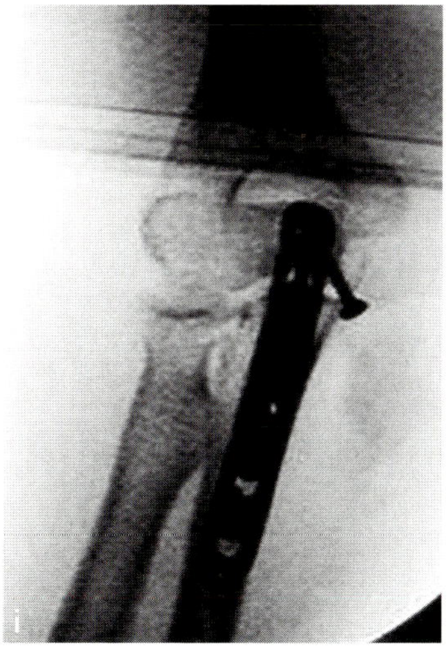

i

Fig 7.1.1-4a–i (cont)

e The 6-hole metaphyseal LCP is bent anatomically at its proximal end to encompass the olecranon. To achieve close bone plate contact, the triceps attachment is split and the plate is positioned. The plate is fixed with two K-wires inserted through the two trocars.

f The first screw is a 3.5 mm cortex lag screw positioned subchondrally as proximally as possible. This step is monitored by image intensification. Another 3.5 mm cortex screw is inserted into the shaft. The intermediate metaphyseal fragment is fixed with a 3.5 mm cortex lag screw oriented towards the olecranon.

g Four locking head screws are inserted for final fixation.

h–i Clinical testing of the range of motion and radiological control ends the operation.

4 Rehabilitation

A posterior upper arm splint is applied until wound healing has occurred.

Physiotherapy begins on postoperative day two, initially with passive movement and later with active movement.

Implant removal

Implant removal may be necessary due to the very thin soft-tissue coverage and the probability of irritation.

5 Pitfalls –

Reduction and fixation
If cortex screws and locking head screws are both being inserted into the same plate, there is a risk that the fixation techniques will interfere with each other, which may lead to implant loosening.

Rehabilitation
Prolonging physiotherapy may lead to elbow stiffness, and aggressive therapy may lead to fixation failure (radial head).

6 Pearls +

Reduction and fixation
It is highly recommended to insert all cortex (conventional) screws before inserting the locking head screws.

Rehabilitation
A careful balance between early physiotherapy to prevent elbow stiffness (especially pronation and supination), and gentle mobilization must be found.

Author Christian Ryf

7.1.2 Olecranon fracture—21-B1

1 Case description

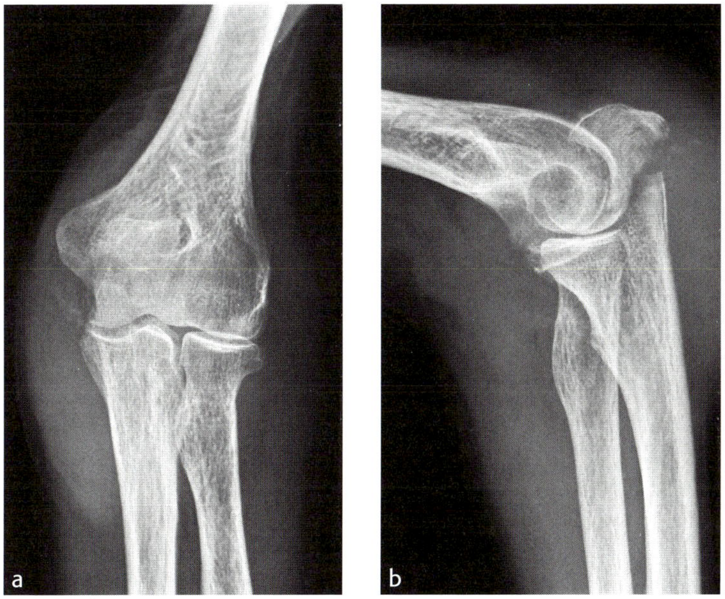

88-year-old woman fell on the street and suffered a closed olecranon fracture of her left arm.

Fig 7.1.2-1a–b
a AP view.
b Lateral view.

Indication

Tension band fixation is required due to severe osteoporosis. Tension band plating was indicated.

Preoperative planning

Equipment

- LCP metaphyseal plate 3.5, 8 holes
- 3.5 mm self-tapping locking head screws (LHS)
- 3.5 mm cortex screws
- 1.6 mm K-wires

(Size of system, instruments, and implants can vary according to anatomy.)

Patient preparation and positioning

Antibiotics: single dose 2nd generation cephalosporin
Thrombosis prophylaxis: low-molecular heparin

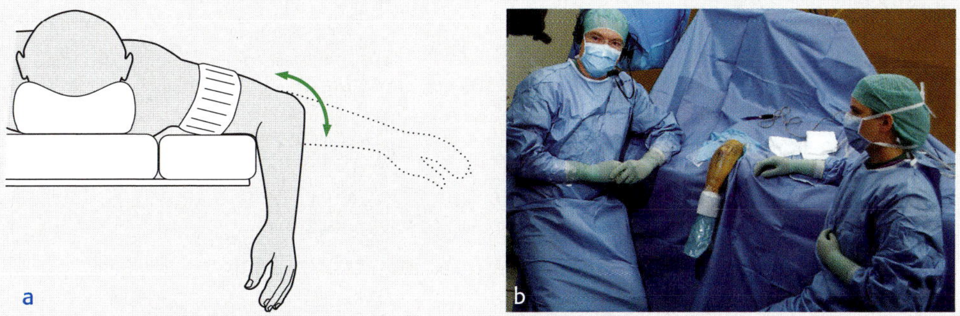

Fig 7.1.2-2a–b Prone position, arm on an arm table, pneumatique tourniquet.

2 Surgical approach

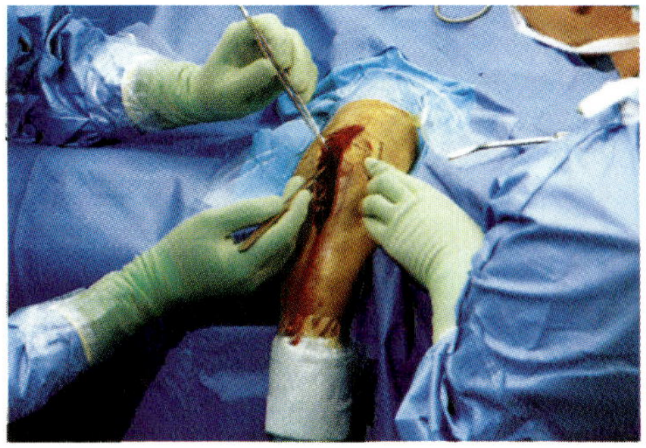

Fig 7.1.2-3 Sligthly curved posteroradial approach.

3 Reduction and fixation

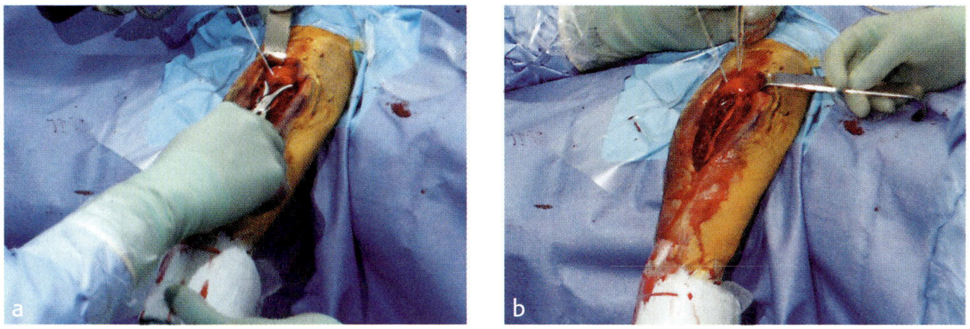

Fig 7.1.2-4a–b Open reduction with small pointed reduction forceps and preliminary fixation of the olecranon main fragment with two 1.6 mm K-wires.

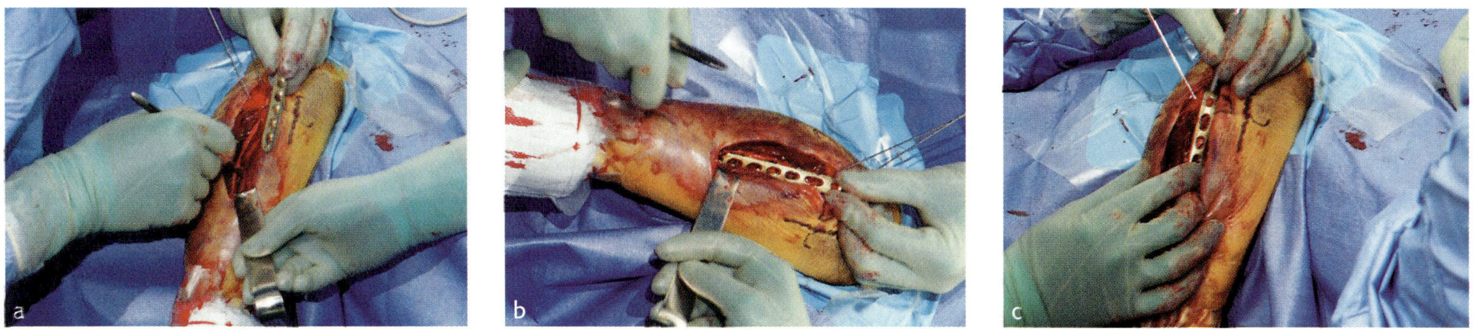

Fig 7.1.2-5a–c Shaping of the plate.
The thinner part of the LCP metaphyseal plate with converting screw holes is bent towards the proximal main fragments.

3 Reduction and fixation (cont)

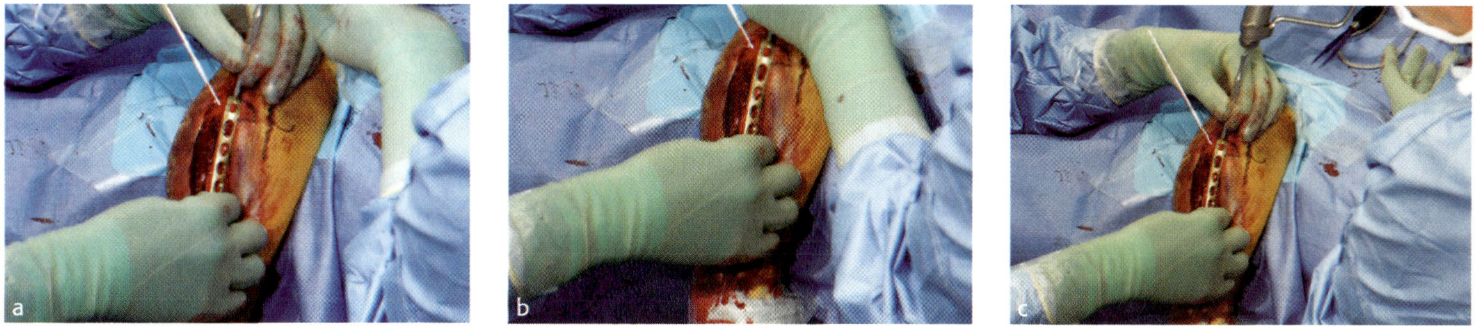

Fig 7.1.2-6a–c Preliminary fixation of the plate with K-wires and corresponding drill sleeves.

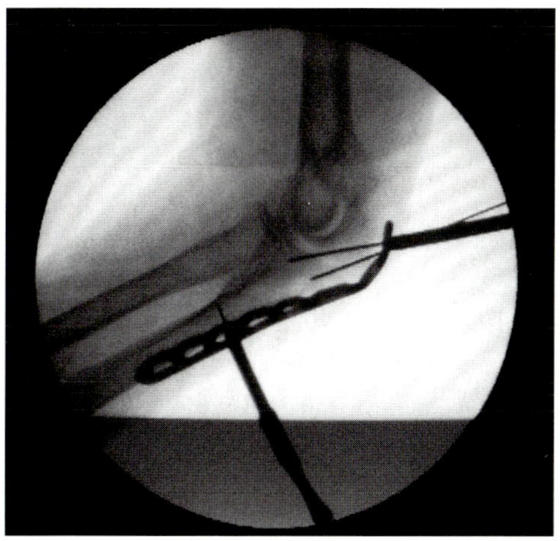

Fig 7.1.2-7 Check reduction and plate position with image intensifier.

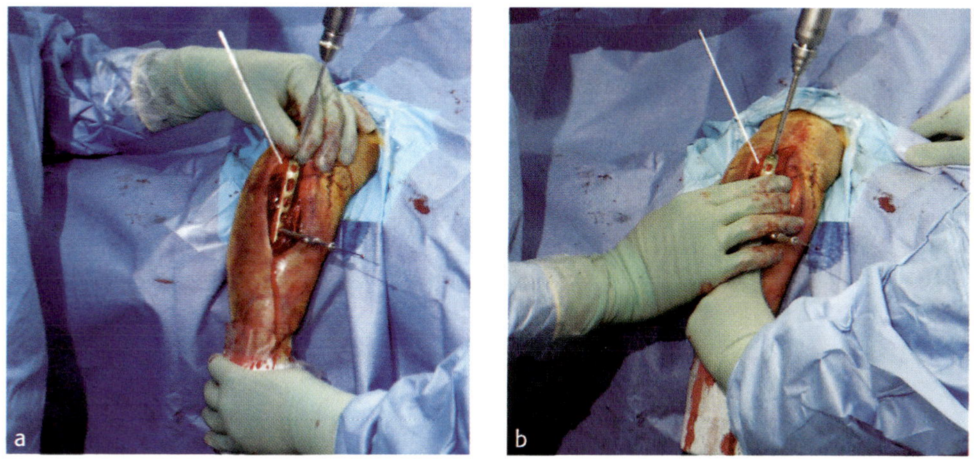

Fig 7.1.2-8a–l Definitive fixation of the plate.
Order of screw insertion: First a 3.5 mm self-tapping LHS is inserted (in a perpendicular direction to the plate) in the most proximal plate hole to hold the proximal main fragment.

3 Reduction and fixation (cont)

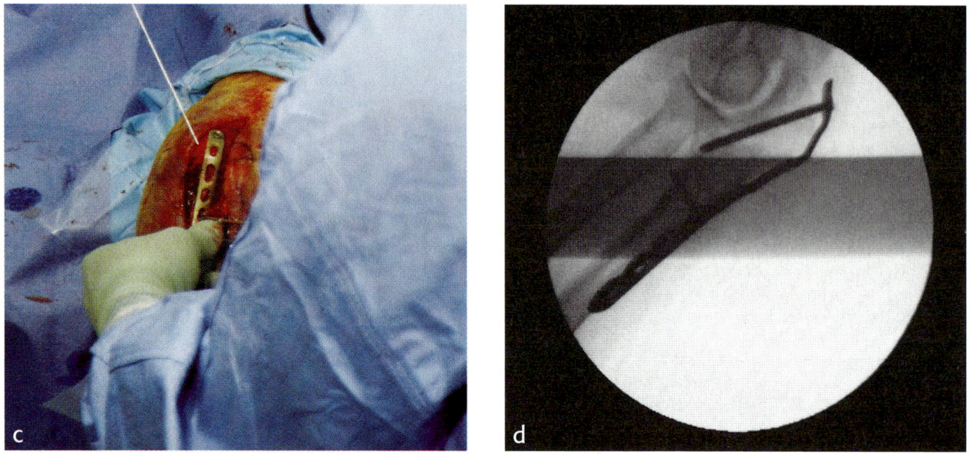

Fig 7.1.2-8a–l (cont) A 3.5 mm cortex screw is eccentrically drilled in order to apply the tension band principle.

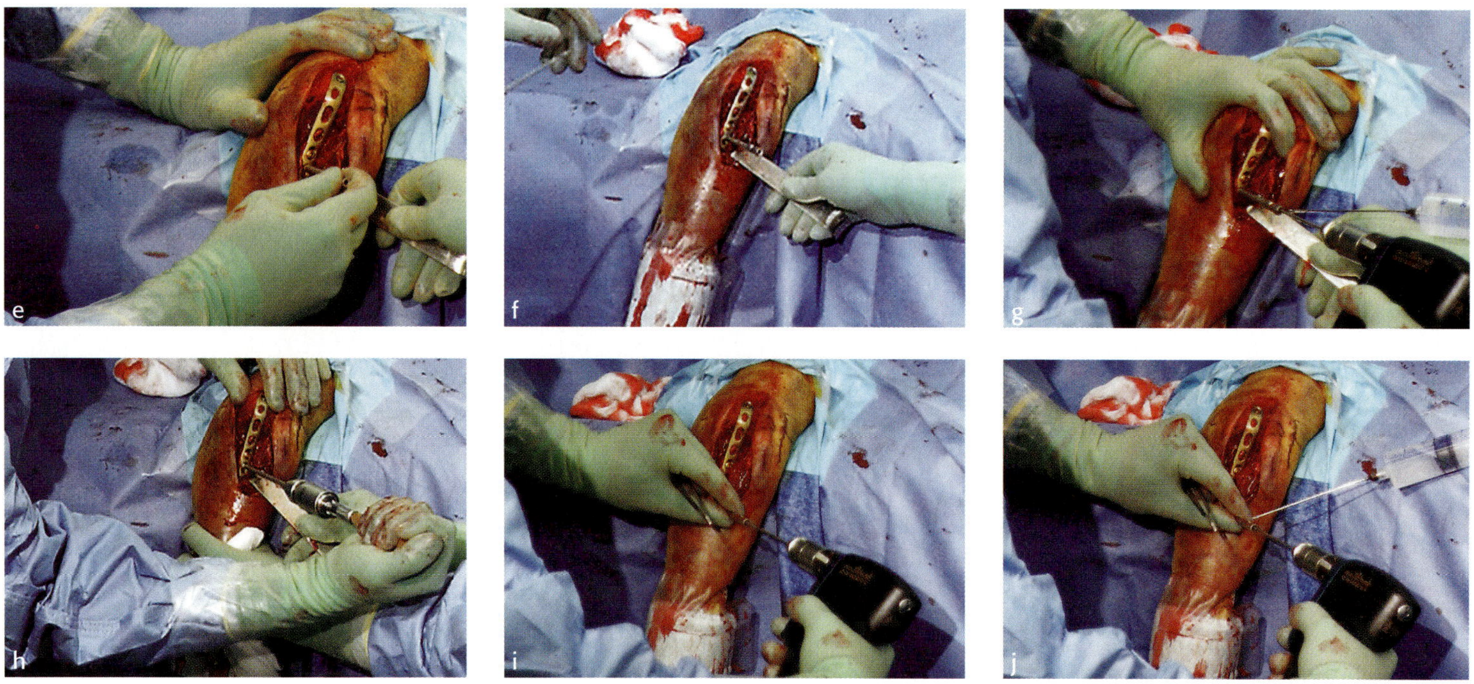

3 Reduction and fixation (cont)

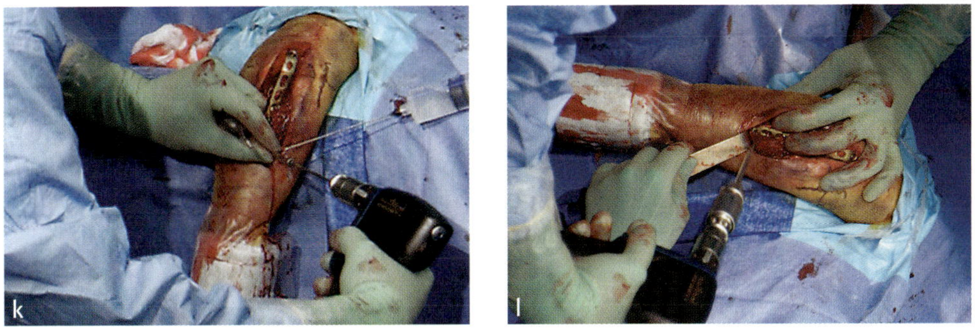

Fig 7.1.2-8a–l (cont) Fixation is completed with two additional bicortical self-tapping 3.5 mm LHS in both main fragments.

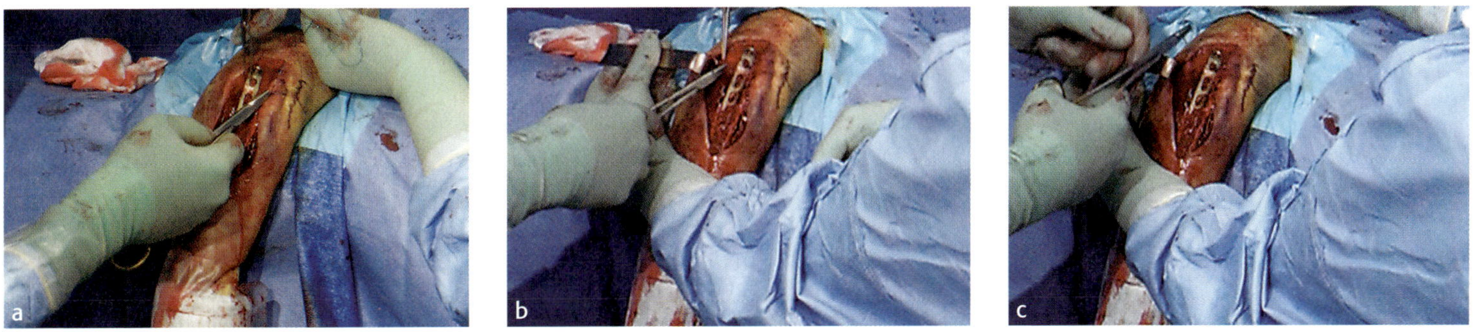

Fig 7.1.2-9a–c Very small articular fragments attached to the soft tissue are fixed with resorbable osteosutures.

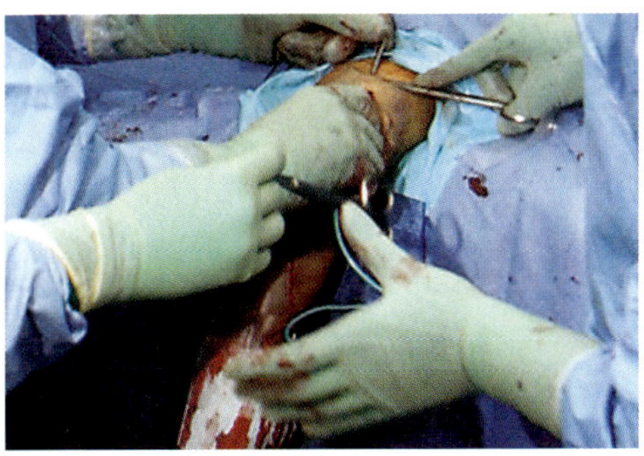

Fig 7.1.2-10 Vacuum drain and wound closure.

4 Rehabilitation

Functional postoperative care for unlimited range of motion, pain limited weight bearing for 6 weeks, full weight bearing after x-ray examination and documented undisturbed bone healing.

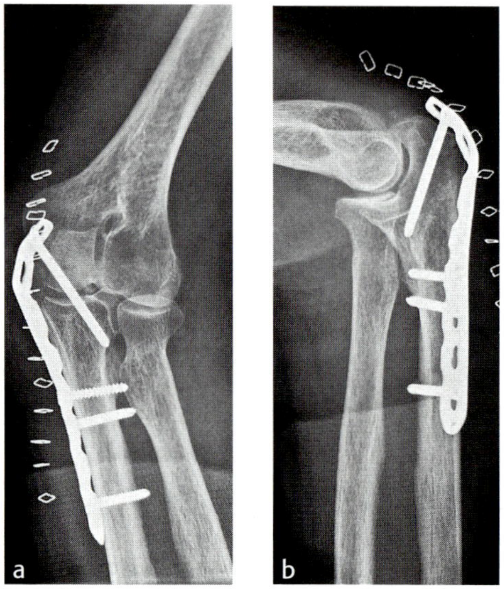

Fig 7.1.2-11a–b Postoperative x-rays after 1 week.
a AP view
b Lateral view.

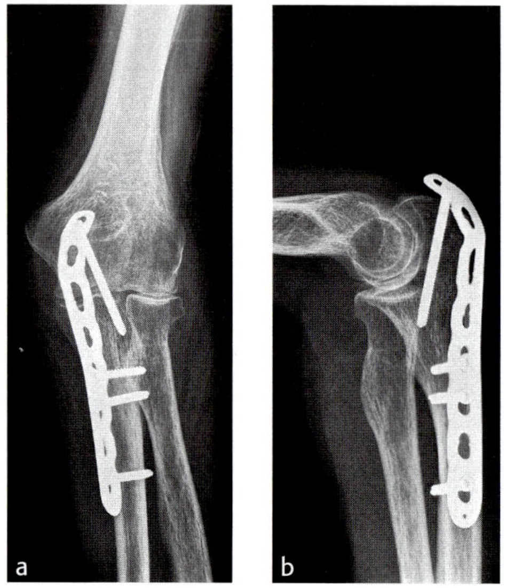

Fig 7.1.2-12a–b Postoperative x-rays after 5 weeks.
a AP view
b Lateral view.

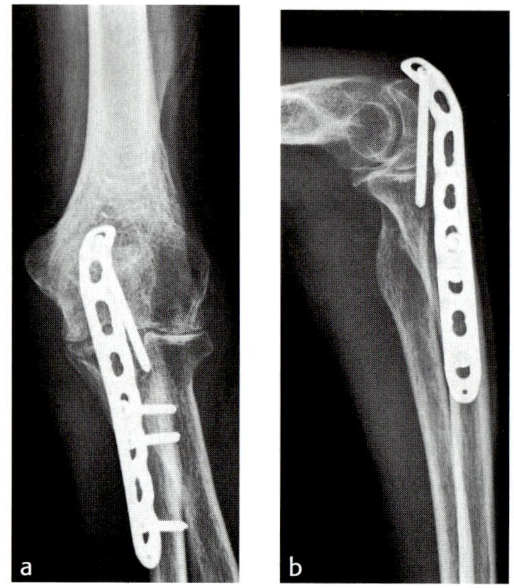

Fig 7.1.2-13a–b Postoperative x-rays after 10 weeks.
a AP view
b Lateral view.

5 Pitfalls –

Equipment
Severe bending of the plate may lead to deformation of the threaded part of the combination hole, making the hole incapable of holding LHS.

Approach
Damage of the ulnar nerve.

6 Pearls +

Equipment
Anatomically preshaped plates may be useful.
The LCP is an ideal implant fort he treatment of forearm fractures especially in osteoporotic bone.

Approach
Adequate posteroradial approach and careful preparation.

Author Michael Plecko

7.1.3 Open proximal ulnar fracture—21-B1; simple ulnar shaft fracture—22-A1; anterior dislocation of the radial head

1 Case description

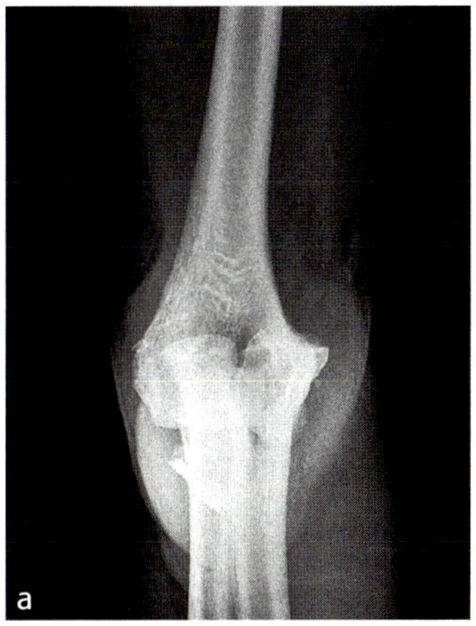

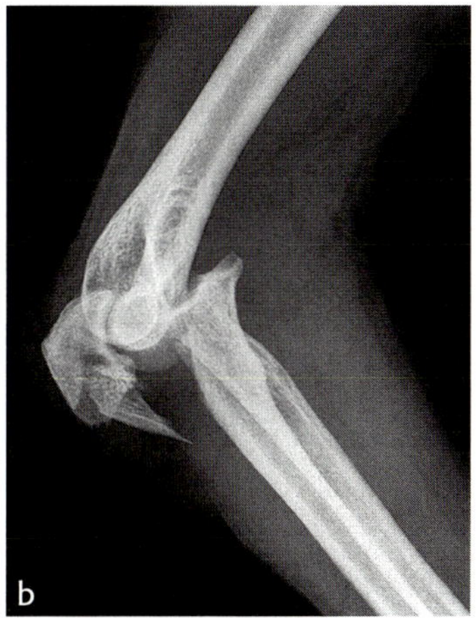

79-year-old man fell from a ladder, suffered a Gustilo type I open, multifragmentary fracture of the proximal ulna (21-B1) with anterior dislocation of the radial head and an undisplaced simple fracture of the ulnar shaft (22-A1). His right dominant arm was affected. Additionally, he had a severe thorax trauma with multiple rib fractures and a hematopneumothorax.

Fig 7.1.3-1a–b
a AP view of the right elbow.
b Lateral view.

After stabilizing his general condition, open reduction and internal fixation with additional reduction of the radial head had to be performed within the first 48 hours.

Indication

Segmental fracture of the ulna 21-B1, multifragmentary Gustilo type I open fracture of the proximal ulna, anterior dislocation of the radial head, and additional simple undisplaced 22-A1 fracture at the shaft of the ulna.

Preoperative planning

Equipment
- LCP olecranon plate 3.5, 8 holes
- 3.5 mm self-tapping locking head screws (LHS)
- 3.5 mm cortex screws
- 2.4 mm cortex screw

(Size of system, instruments, and implants can vary according to anatomy.)

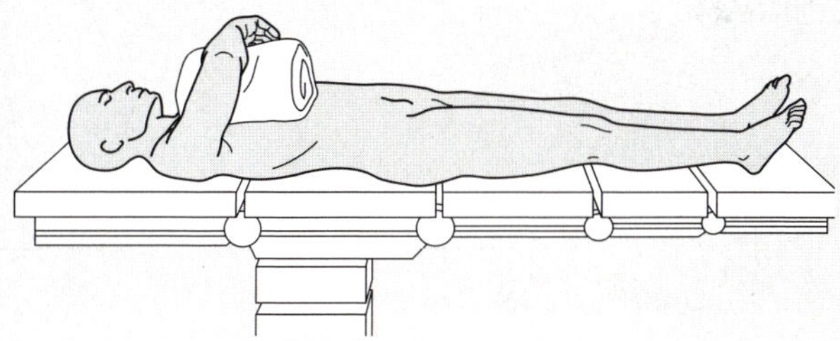

Fig 7.1.3-2 Supine position with towel roll at the level of the rib cage with the injured arm placed on it. Sterile tourniquet.

Patient preparation and positioning
Antibiotics: none
Thrombosis prophylaxis: none

2 Surgical approach

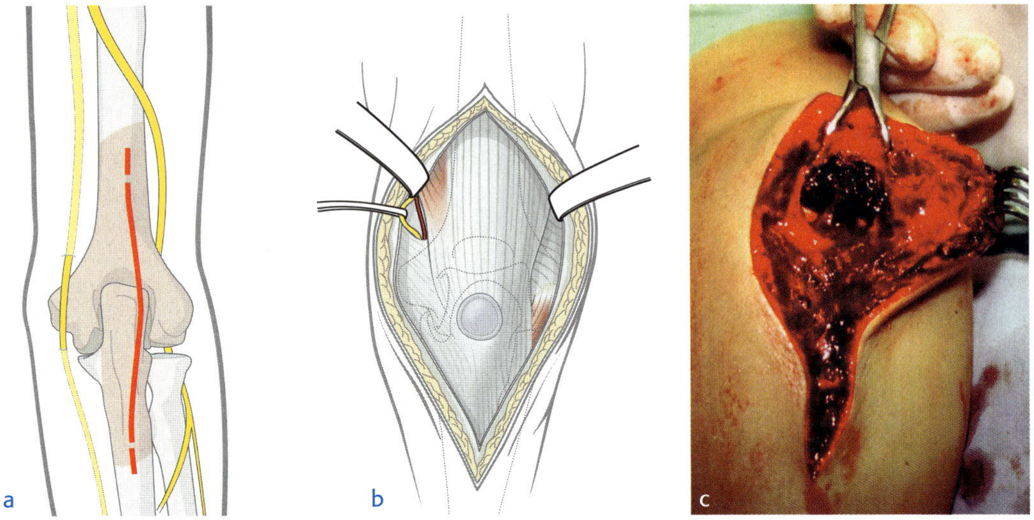

Fig 7.1.3-3a–c Posterior approach to the ulna. Excision of blood clot and of the olecranon bursa. Preparation of the ulnar nerve with a vessel loop.

3 Reduction and fixation

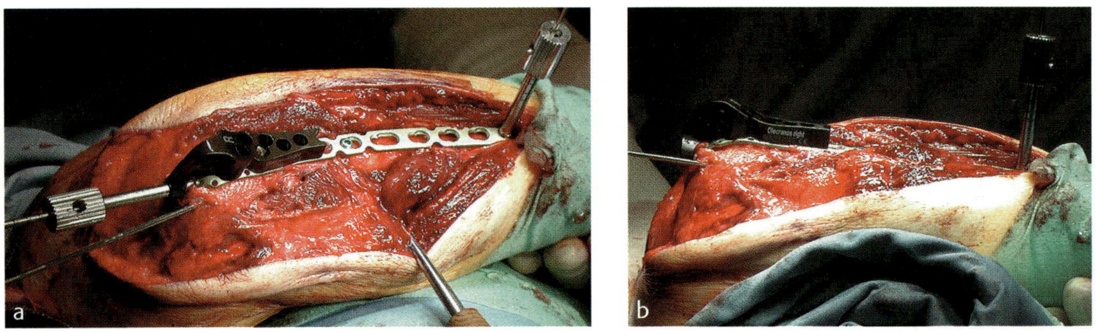

Fig 7.1.3-4a–c

a–b Anatomical reduction of the olecranon fracture with a pointed reduction forceps and temporary fixation with a K-wire from proximal to distal. Positioning of an 8-hole LCP olecranon plate and temporary fixation of the proximal end of the plate by insertion of a K-wire through the threaded drill sleeve. The drill sleeve is correctly positioned with the help of the aiming block.
The first screw to be introduced through the plate is a cortex screw to fix the coronoid process. The second screw, a 3.5 mm LHS, is inserted into the shaft fragment. The cortical fragment on the radial side is fixed with a plate-independent 2.4 mm cortex screw using the compression method.

3 Reduction and fixation (cont)

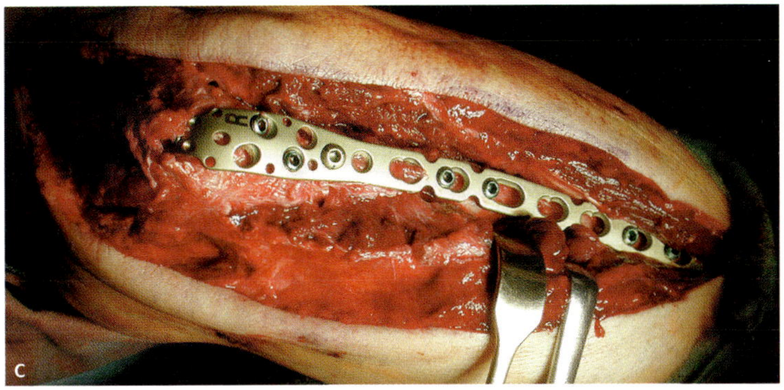

Fig 7.1.3-4a–c (cont)
c The fixation of the plate is finalized with four LHS in the proximal fragment, two in the intermediate shaft fragment, and three in the distal shaft fragment.

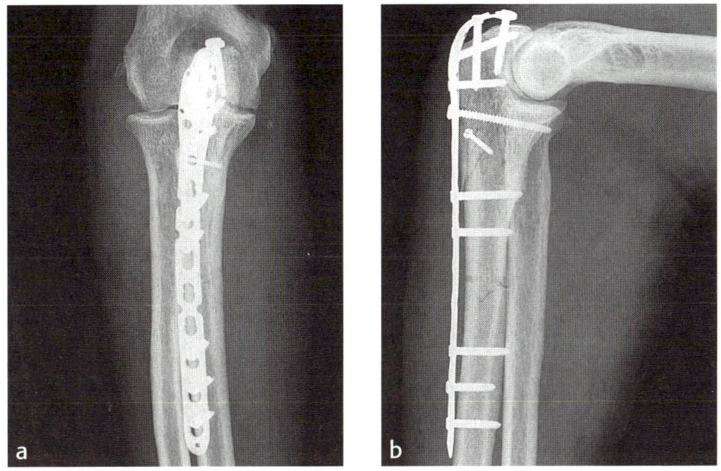

Fig 7.1.3-5a–b The lateral postoperative x-rays show an additional undisplaced shaft fracture of the ulna. The radial head is reduced.
a AP view.
b Lateral view.

4 Rehabilitation

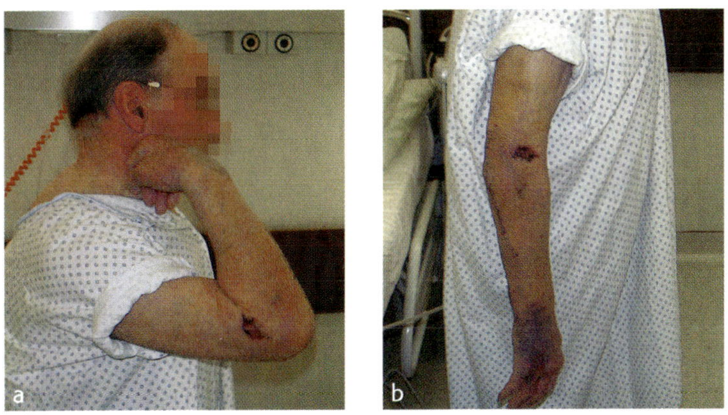

Functional treatment started on postoperative day one with active and passive movement of the elbow joint and the forearm.

Fig 7.1.3-6a–b Range of motion 12 days after the operation.

4 Rehabilitation (cont)

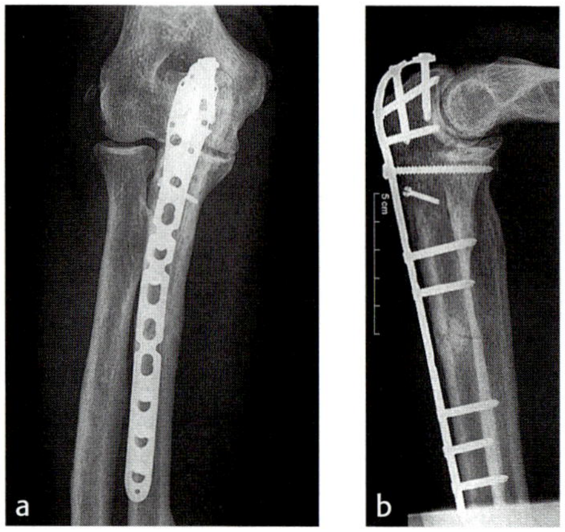

Fig 7.1.3-7a–b Postoperative x-rays after 6 months show bone consolidation of both fractures with the radial head in correct alignment.

a AP view.

b Lateral view.

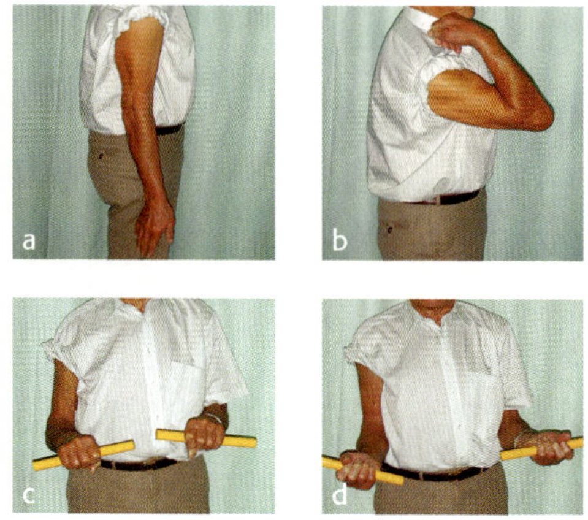

Fig 7.1.3-8a–d 6 months after the operation the patient was painfree, had only slightly functional restrictions, and equal strength on both sides.

a–b Range of motion: flexion/extension 0°/5°/140°.

c–d Range of motion: pronation/supination 70°/0°/70°.

5 Pitfalls –

Equipment

Reduction and fixation

In this case, the undisplaced additional shaft fracture was not clearly seen on the preoperative x-rays.

The correct reduction and fixation of this multifragmentary olecranon fracture is the precondition for the reduction of the displaced radial head.

6 Pearls +

Equipment

Anatomical preshaped plates are helpful in complex fracture situations.

Reduction and fixation

The special, anatomically preshaped LCP olecranon plate 3.5 with the combination hole allowed stable fixation of this segmental fracture by two different methods: the compression method for the olecranon fracture and splinting methode for the undisplaced shaft fracture. Angular stable plating of the proximal ulna leads to higher stability also in multifragmentary fracture situations. This permits an early active rehabilitation program.

Author Michael Schütz, Norbert P Haas

7.1.4 Complex radial head fracture and extraarticular olecranon fracture—21-B3

1 Case description

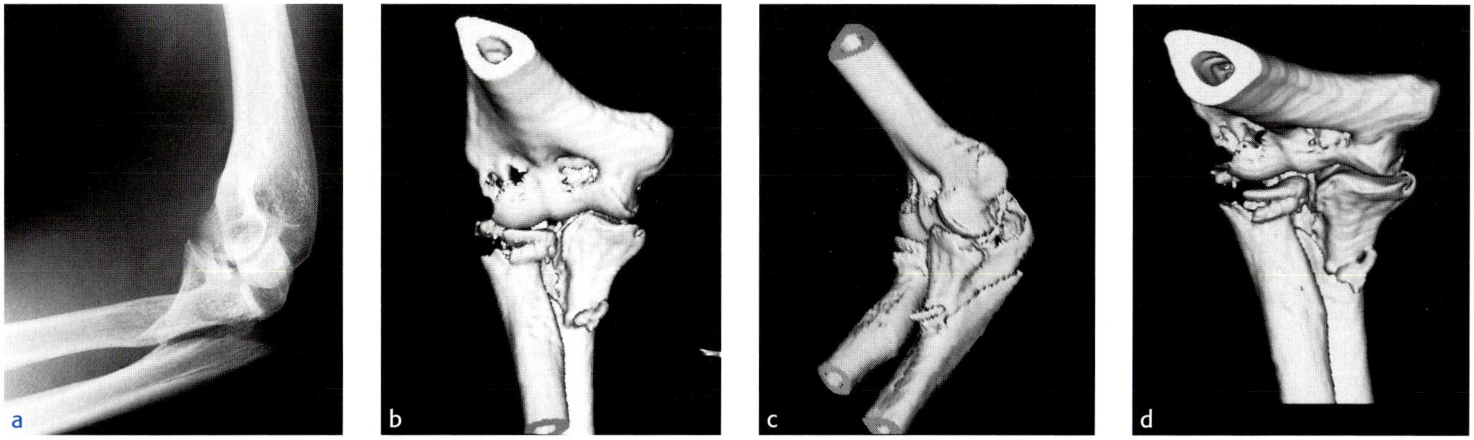

53-year-old man fell while riding his bicycle and sustained an elbow fracture. There were no other injuries. After a CT scan, the patient was operated on the same day.

Fig 7.1.4-1a–d
a Preoperative x-ray, lateral view.
b–d CT scans.

Indication

According to the principles of intraarticular fracture management, a stable osteosynthesis and, depending on the ligamentous lesions, early functional treatment with or without a splint should be achieved.

Preoperative planning

Equipment

- LCP 3.5, 8 holes
- 2.0 mm cortex screws
- 3.5 mm cortex screws
- 3.5 mm locking head screws (LHS)
- 1.25 mm K-wires
- 1.6 mm K-wires

(Size of system, instruments, and implants can vary according to anatomy.)

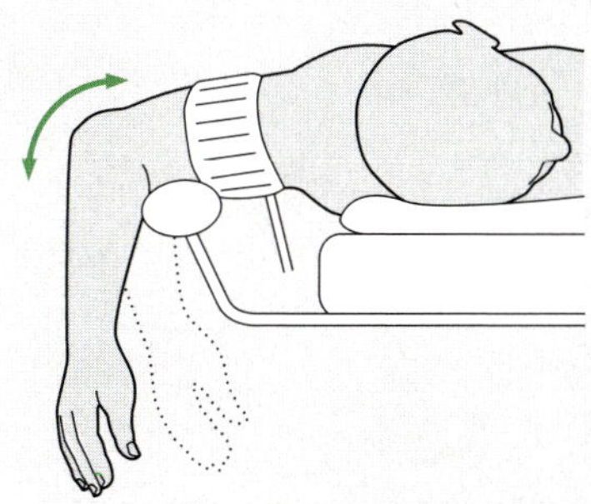

Fig 7.1.4-2 Prone position, arm on an arm table, pneumatic tourniquet, radiography and image intensifier.

Patient preparation and positioning

Antibiotics: single dose 2nd generation cephalosporin
Trombosis prophylaxis: low-molecular heparin

2 Surgical approach

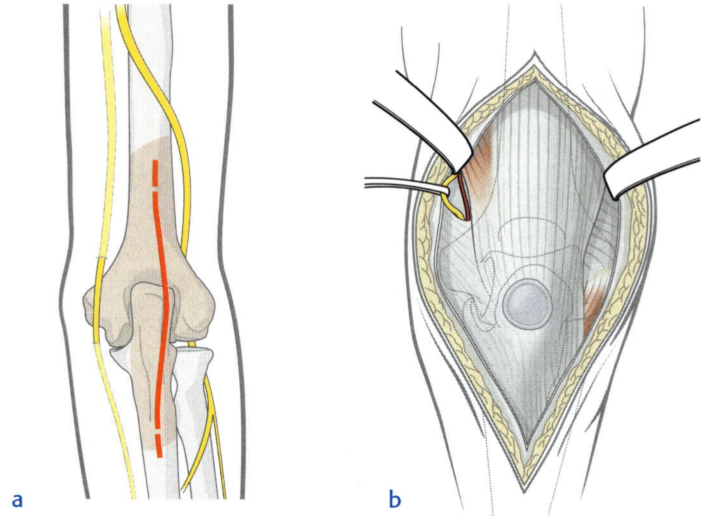

Fig 7.1.4-3a–b Posterior incision. The radial fracture can be exposed through the olecranon fracture.

3 Reduction and fixation

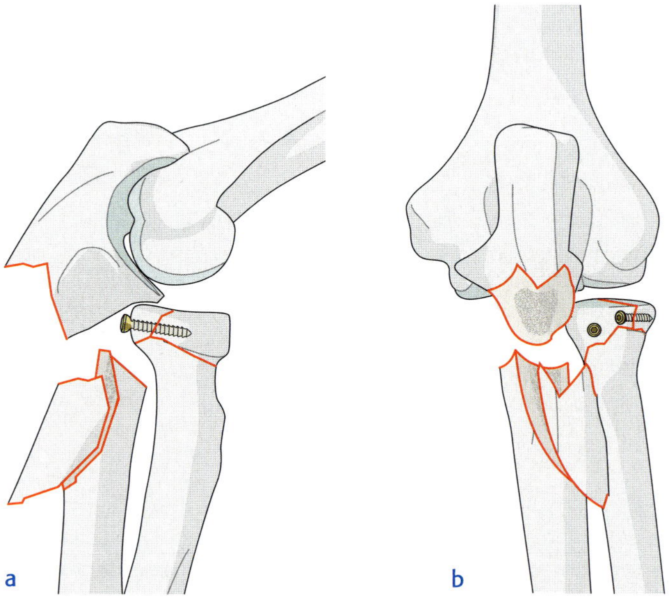

Fig 7.1.4-4a–h

a–b The impacted radial joint fragment is elevated and initially fixed with 1.25 mm K-wires. Two 2.0 mm lag screws are inserted to stabilize the main radial fracture fragments. One of the screws must have contact with the intact radial neck zone.

3 Reduction and fixation (cont)

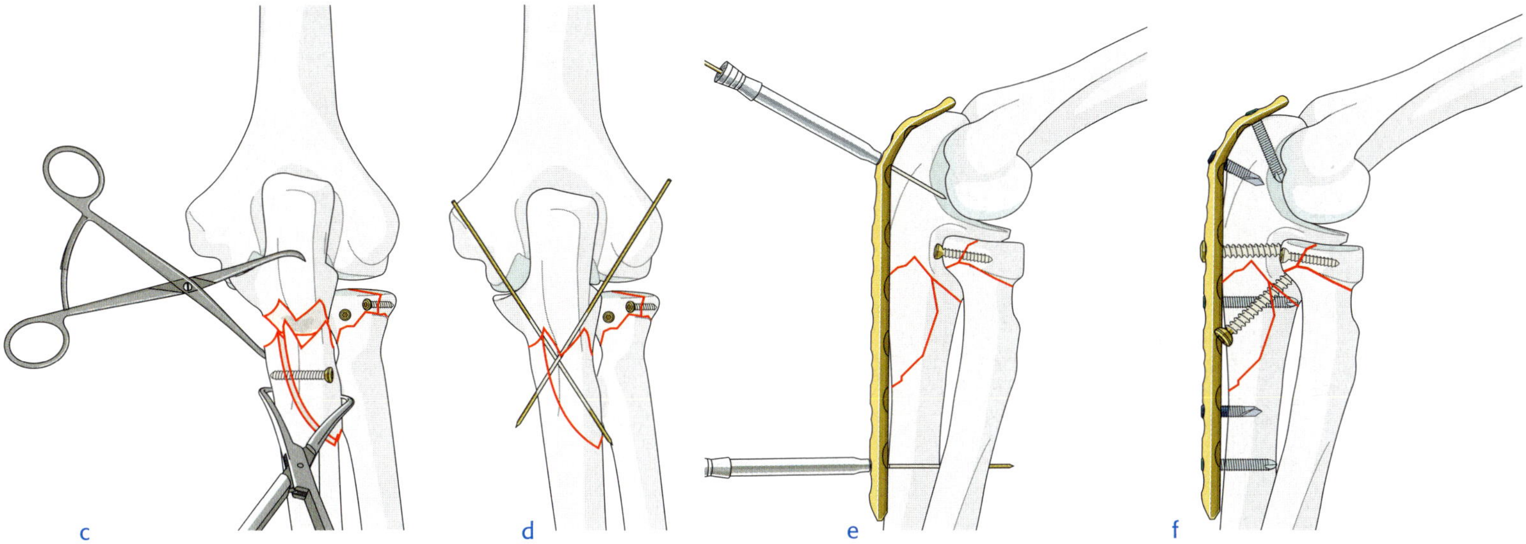

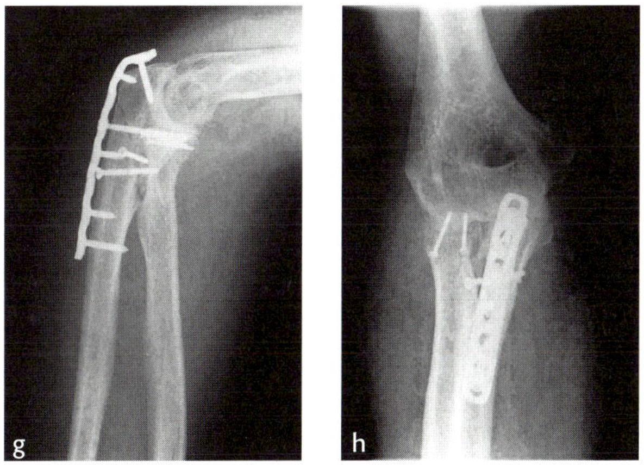

Fig 7.1.4-4a–h (cont)

c–d Reduction of the extraarticular fracture and the additional metaphyseal fragment. Two small pointed reduction forceps are used to hold the main fragments. The reduction and the additional fragment are initially fixed with three K-wires. While positioning the K-wires, the planned plate position must be taken into account. The 8-hole LCP is bent to encompass the tip of the olecranon. To achieve tight bone-plate contact, the triceps muscle attachment is split and the plate positioned. At the end of the operation, the muscle must be sutured.

e The plate is aligned and drill sleeves are inserted proximally and distally. The plate is now secured with two 1.6 mm K-wires.

f A 3.5 mm cortex screw is inserted through the fifth hole and directed toward the coronoid process. Drilling is performed under image intensification control in lateral projection to ensure the exact placement of this essential screw.
The intermediate fragment is secured with an additional isolated lag screw inserted in a radioulnar direction.
Two locking head screws proximally and three locking head screws distally stabilize the fracture in internal fixator technique.

g–h Clinical assessment of the range of motion in pronation and supination (radial head) and a radiological control ends the operation.

4 Rehabilitation

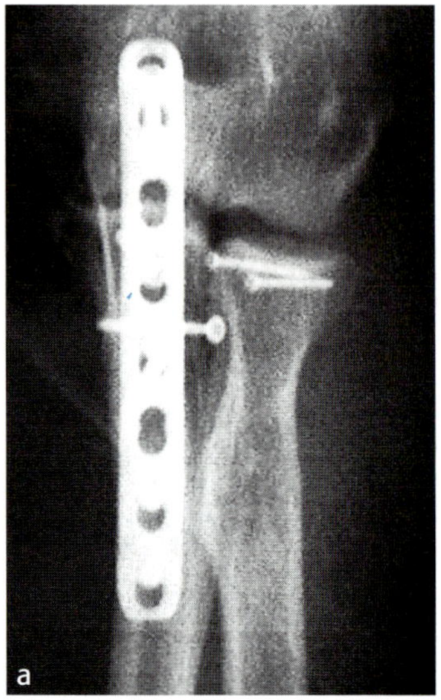

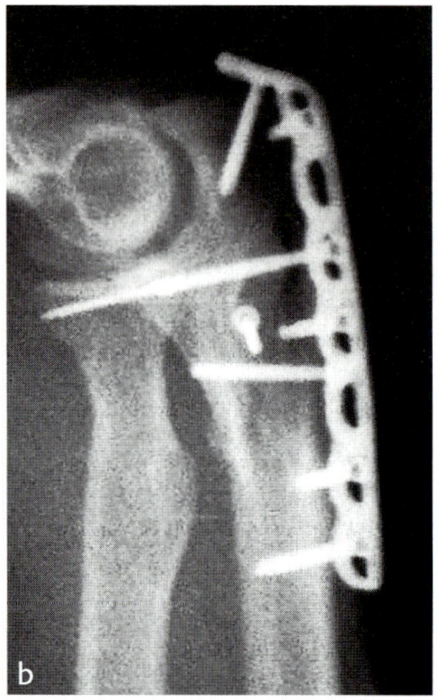

A posterior upper arm splint is applied until definitive wound healing has occurred.
Physiotherapy begins on postoperative day two initially with passive movement, followed later with active movement.

Fig 7.1.4-5a–b Postoperative x-rays after 9 months.

Implant removal
Implant removal may be necessary because of the very thin soft-tissue coverage and the probability of irritation.

5 Pitfalls –

Reduction and fixation
If cortex screws and locking head screws are both being inserted into the same plate, there is a risk that the fixation techniques will interfere with each other, and this may lead to implant loosening.

Rehabilitation
Delayed physiotherapy may lead to elbow stiffness, and aggressive therapy may lead to fixation failure (radial head).

6 Pearls +

Reduction and fixation
It is highly recommended to insert all cortex (conventional) screws before inserting the locking head screws.

Rehabilitation
A careful balance between early physiotherapy to prevent elbow stiffness (especially pronation and supination), and gentle mobilization must be found.

Author Christopher W Geel

7.1.5 3-part radial head and transverse radial neck fracture; intraarticular proximal ulnar fracture—21-B3

1 Case description

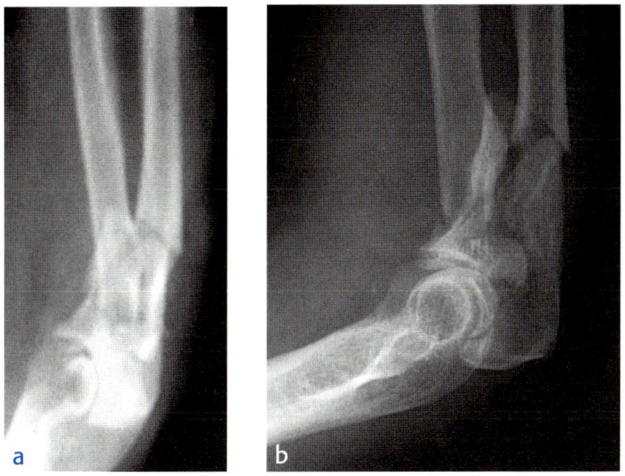

56-year-old man fell from a tree stand during hunting season. Type of injury: high-energy trauma, multiple trauma with chest contusion with pneumothorax left, closed fracture.

Fig 7.1.5-1a–b
a AP view.
b Lateral view.

Indication

3-part radial head fracture and transverse radial neck fracture associated with multifragmentary, intraarticular proximal ulnar fracture, with fracture of coronoid process. This combination fracture renders the elbow joint unstable and, because of intraarticular involvement, is best treated by ORIF.

Preoperative planning

Equipment

Radius:
- Mini condylar plate 2.0, 7 holes
- 2.0 mm and 2.7 mm cortex screw
- 3.5 mm screw with spiked washer

Ulna:
- LCP 3.5, 9 holes
- Locking head screws (LHS)
- 3.5 mm cortex screw

(Size of system, instruments, and implants can vary according to anatomy.)

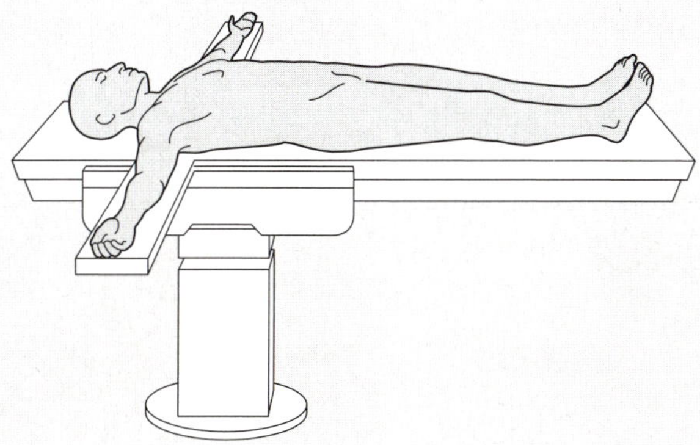

Fig 7.1.5-2 Supine position on operating table with radiolucent arm board.

Patient preparation and positioning

Antibiotics: 2nd generation cephalosporin
Thrombosis prophylaxis: low-molecular heparin

2 Surgical approach

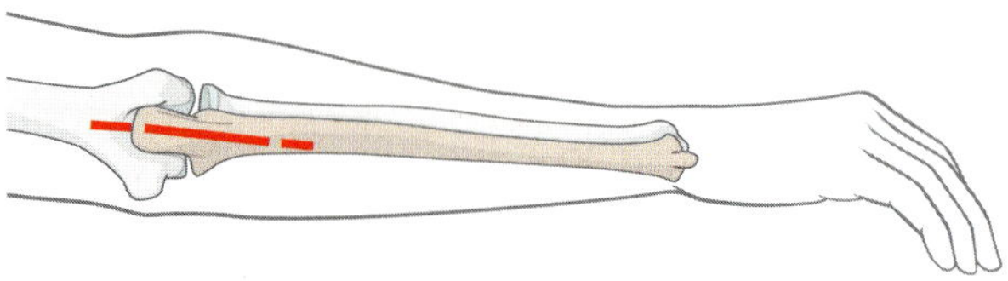

Fig 7.1.5-3 Ulna:
ORIF as first step to secure proper length of forearm and to facilitate the ORIF of the multifragmentary radial head fracture.
Incision posteriorly over subcutaneous border of ulna.
Identification of ulnar border without violating periosteal coverage.
Irrigation of elbow joint and securing ulnar nerve with vessel loop.

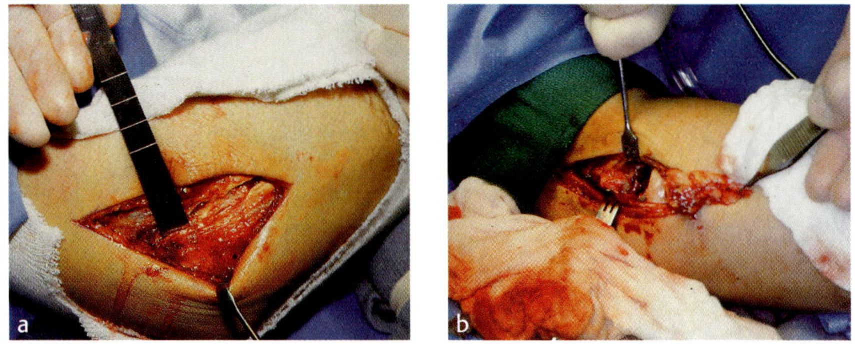

Fig 7.1.5-4a–b Radius:
Wide skin bridge between the two incisions. Radial head approach used modified Gordon-Boyd's approach with osteotomy radial collateral ligament after predrilling of the future anchoring hole.

3 Reduction

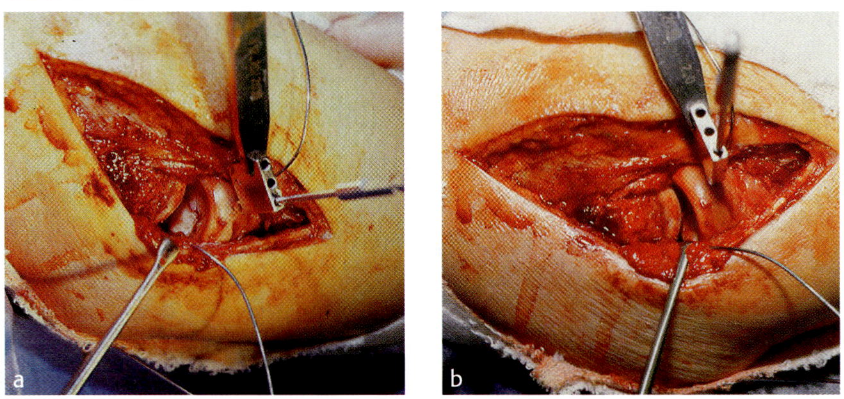

Fig 7.1.5-5a–b Radius: Temporary cerclage around radial head after inspection of joint surface and irrigation of elbow joint.
Drilling with parallel soft-tissue protector to ensure proper placement of lag screws parallel to radial head joint surface.

Ulna: indirect reduction of ulnar fracture with plate in situ using push-pull technique.

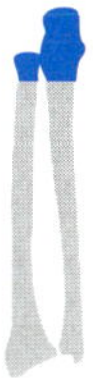

4 Fixation

First step—fixation of ulna:
Anchoring and fixation of plate proximally with combination of screw to prevent plate spinning, followed by LHS.
Lag screw fixation of cornoid process fragment.
Interfragmentary additional compression through the plate.
Insertion of distal LHS in monocortical fashion.

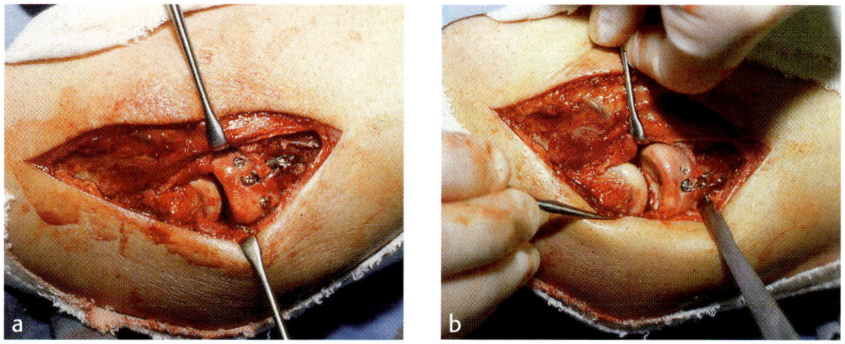

Fig 7.1.5-6a–b Second step—fixation of radius:
a Insertion of 2.7 mm and 2.0 mm cortex lag screws.
b Reduction of the now stable radial head fixation to the radial shaft with a mini, condylar plate 2.0, extraarticular proximally without interference with joint congruencey.

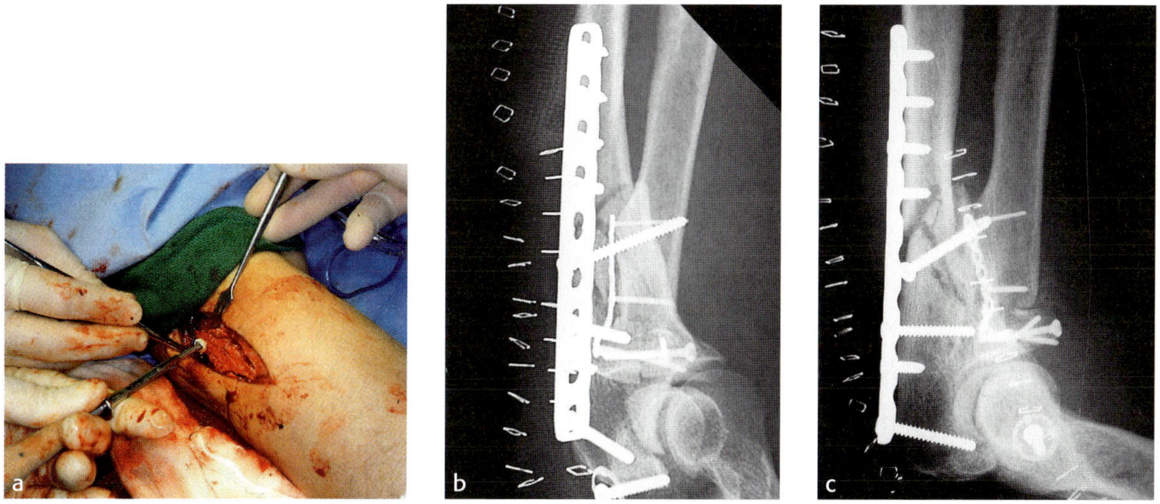

Fig 7.1.5-7a–c Second step—fixation of radius:
Refixation of osteotomized radial collateral ligament insertion with spiked washer and 3.5 mm cortex screw.

5 Rehabilitation

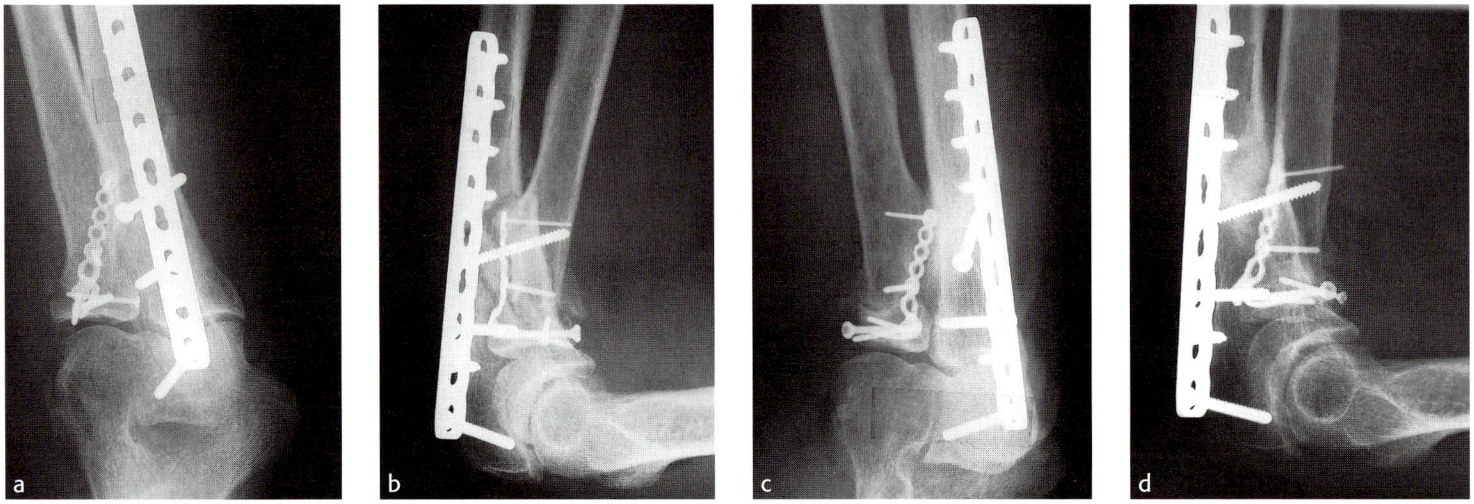

Active mobilization after 1 day.
Bone healing after 12 weeks.

Fig 7.1.5-8a–d Postoperative x-rays.
a AP view after 6 weeks.
b Lateral view after 6 weeks.
c AP view after 6 months.
d Lateral view after 6 months.

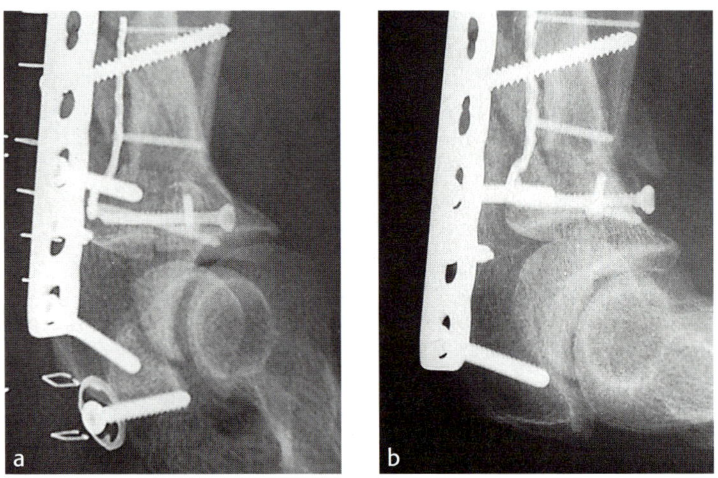

Implant removal

Partial implant removal after 1 month.
Technique for implant removal: stab incision under local anaesthetic.

Fig 7.1.5-9a–b
a Reason for implant removal: screw with spiked washer is protruding under skin.
b Lateral x-ray after partial implant removal.

6 Pitfalls –

Approach

Rehabilitation

7 Pearls +

Approach

Osteotomy of the radial collateral ligament allows excellent view of articular surface.

Rehabilitation

Early active rather than passive motion allows for a controlled recovery.

Author Christoph Sommer

7.1.6 Extraarticular proximal ulnar fracture with pseudarthrosis—21-A1

1 Case description

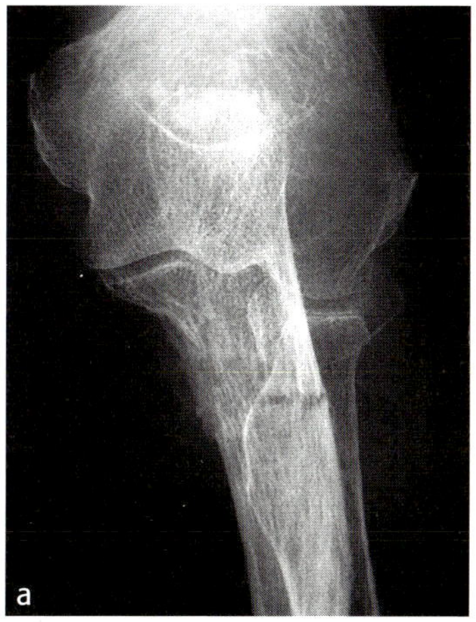

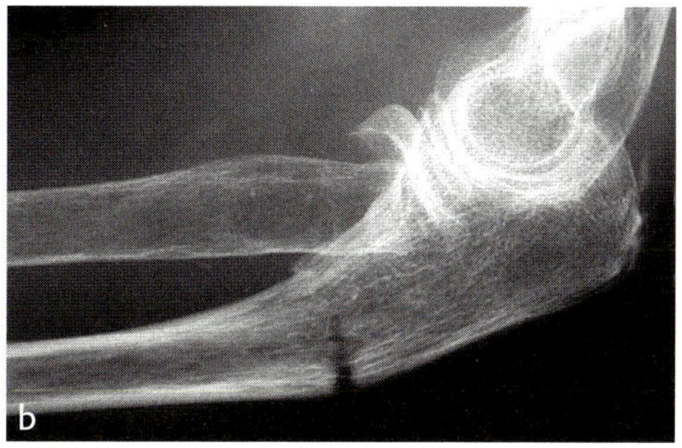

Fig 7.1.6-1a–b
a AP view.
b Lateral view.

80-year-old woman fell at home and landed on her left elbow. She sustained an extraarticular, closed, slightly angulated diaphyseal fracture of the left proximal ulna (21-A1.2). The patient has had an asymptomatic pseudarthrosis beneath the head of the radius since childhood.

Indication

This is only a relative indication for surgery because nonoperative fracture treatment would also be possible. Given the pseudarthrosis at the head of the radius, a surgical procedure is preferred so that there can be early functional rehabilitation. Since there is obvious osteoporosis, a plate system with locking head screws such as the LCP is especially suitable. The treatment goal for this simple fracture pattern (oblique fracture) is anatomical reduction and compression plate osteosynthesis to achieve absolute stability.

Preoperative planning

Equipment

- LCP 3.5, 7 holes
- 3.5 mm locking head screws (LHS)
- 3.5 mm cortex screws

(Size of system, instruments, and implants can vary according to anatomy.)

Patient preparation and positioning

Antibiotics: 2nd generation cephalosporin
Thrombosis prophylaxis: low-molecular heparin

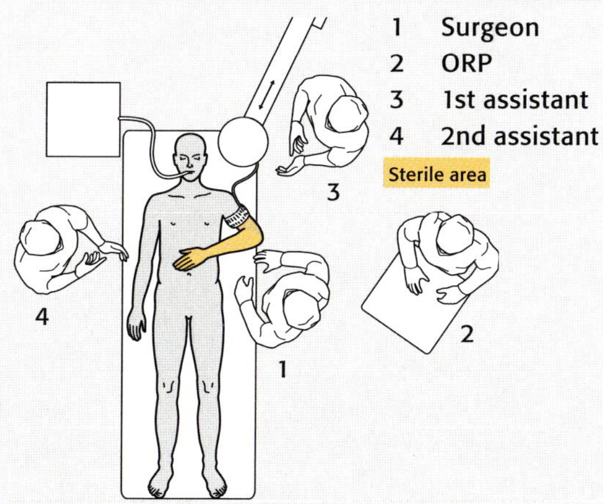

Fig 7.1.6-2 Supine position, left upper extremity is sterile draped and intraoperatively mobile. Nonsterile tourniquet on the upper arm (insufflated only if required). The freely mobile arm is positioned on the patient's stomach; this requires a second assistant.

2 Surgical approach

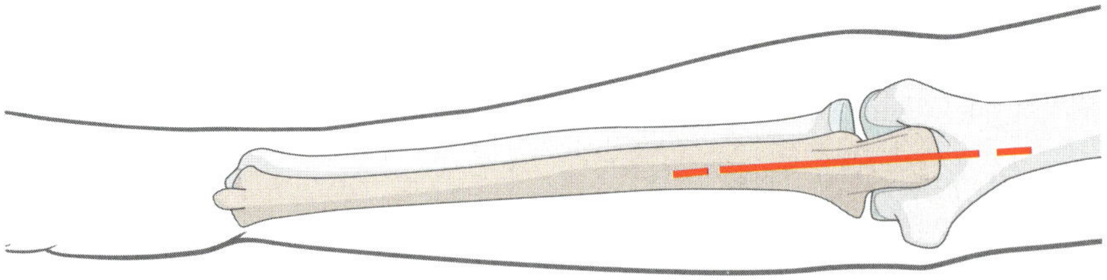

Fig 7.1.6-3 Standard proximal posterior approach to the ulna from the tip of the olecranon to the junction of the proximal and mid thirds. Incision of the muscle fasciae at the posterior ulnar aspect, with careful exposure of the ulnar crest.

3 Reduction and fixation

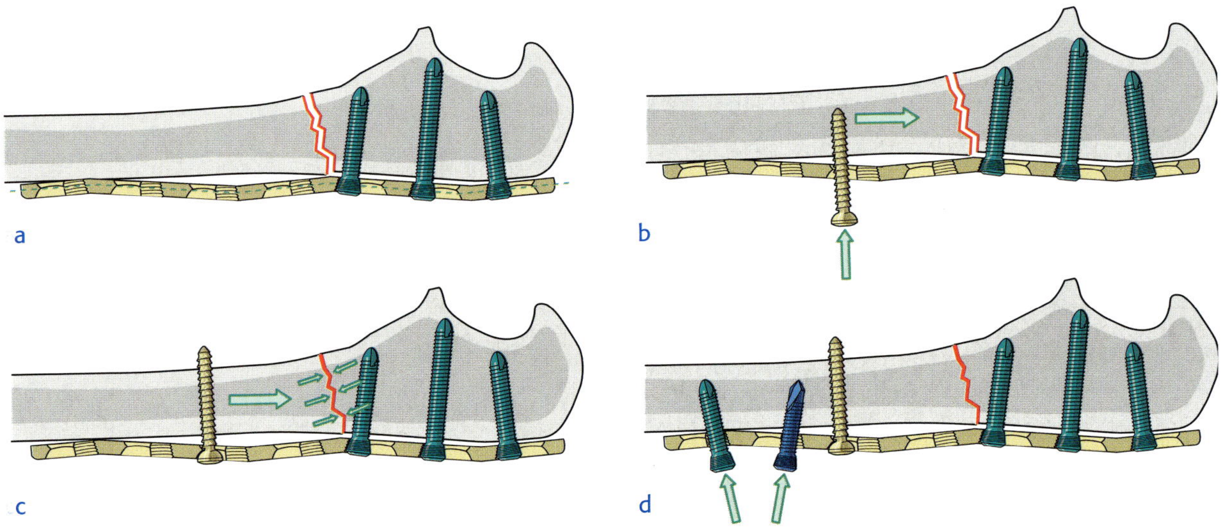

Fig 7.1.6-4a–d

a In the presence of severe osteoporosis, the so-called "wave plate" technique is a suitable treatment, whereby the plate is slightly bent between the individual plate holes so that a flat, wave-shaped plate is created. This permits the insertion of locking head screws in different, nonparallel directions, thus increasing the pull-out force of the implant. In a first step, the precontoured plate is secured to the proximal main fragment of the ulna with three locking head screws as long as possible.

b–c In the next step, eccentric insertion of a 3.5 mm cortex screw in the proximal diaphysis to create interfragmentary compression.

d The anatomically reduced and compressed fracture is now definitively stabilized by insertion of two locking head screws into the shaft at the distal end of the plate. These are oriented divergently and thus increase the primary stability.

3 Reduction and fixation (cont)

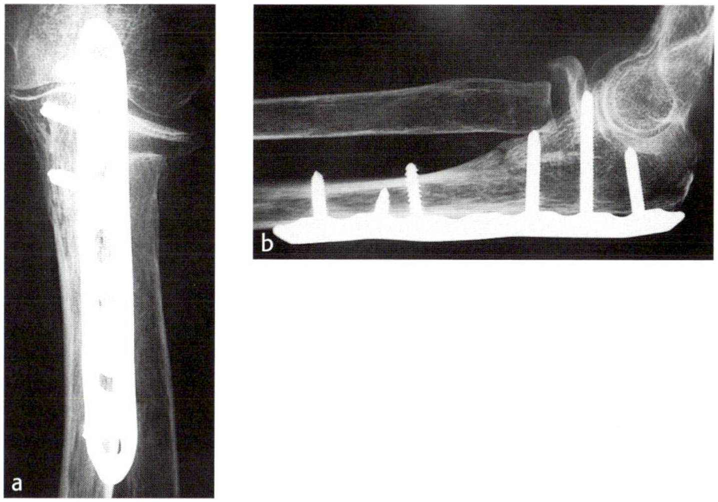

Fig 7.1.6-5a–b The postoperative x-rays confirm the anatomical reduction and interfragmentary compression of the fracture.

4 Rehabilitation

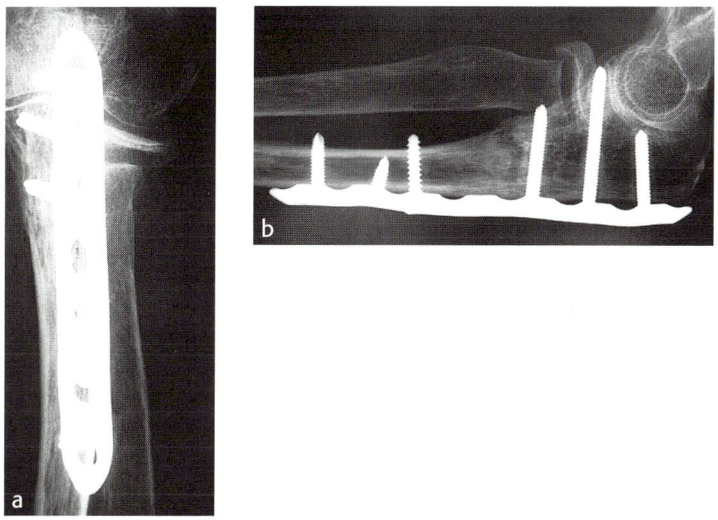

Fig 7.1.6-6a–b Early functional rehabilitation without any form of immobilization. After 6 weeks the x-rays show clear consolidation of the fracture with some blurring of the former fracture gap and signs of periosteal callus formation indicating slight micromotion related to this bridging osteosynthesis.

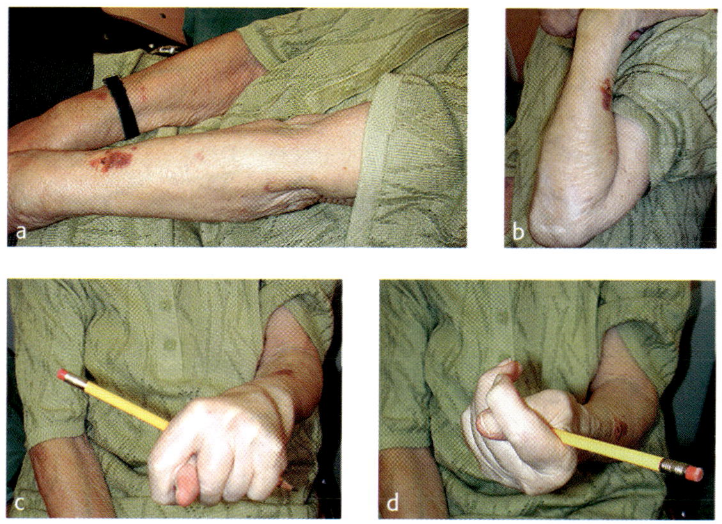

Fig 7.1.6-7a–d Elbow function is almost normal at this time and identical to the level of function before the accident. Further clinical and radiological examinations will not be undertaken provided the patient remains free of symptoms. The implants are not removed.

5 Pitfalls –

Equipment

During preshaping of the LCP 3.5 the holes may become bent and the locking head screws will not hold properly. Therefore, the plate should always be bent and twisted between the holes.

Approach

This standard approach to the proximal ulna is not usually problematic.

Reduction and fixation

The reduction is easy and can be performed using the principle of reduction onto the plate. In severe osteoporotic bone, it may not be possible to achieve axial compression by eccentric insertion of cortex screw because there is a risk of the screw pulling out of the bone. The proximal locking head screw should be as long as possible but should not penetrate the opposite cortex since it is undesirable to have the screw tips in an intra-articular position.

Rehabilitation

6 Pearls +

Equipment

The LCP is an ideal implant for the treatment of forearm fractures especially in osteoporotic bone.

Approach

Reduction and fixation

The so-called ″wave plate“ technique allows the insertion of locking head screws in different, nonparallel directions, which increases the primary stability of the whole construct. There is higher resistance to tensioning forces.

Rehabilitation

The LCP applied as described in this case provides optimal stabilization allowing for early functional aftertreatment.

7.2 Radius and ulna, shaft

Cases

Case		Classification	Method	Implant used	Implant function	Page
7.2.1	Displaced radial shaft fracture	22-A2	compression	LCP 3.5	lag screw protection plate	403
7.2.2	Wedge radial and ulnar shaft fracture	22-B3	compression	LCP 3.5	compression plate	407
7.2.3	Open radial and ulnar shaft fractures and complex articular distal radial fracture	22-B3; 23-C	compression	LCP 3.5; LCP T-plate 3.5	compression plate	411
7.2.4	Complex radial and ulnar shaft fracture	22-C3	locked splinting	LCP 3.5	locked internal fixator and reduction screw	415

7 Radius and ulna

Author Thomas P Rüedi

7.2 Radius and ulna, shaft

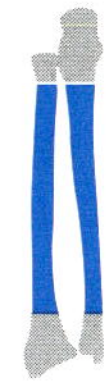

1 Incidence

In the adult, fractures of the forearm comprise about 10–15% of all fractures treated surgically. This is due to the fact that the anatomical relationship of the radius and ulna and of the adjacent joints requires a precise reconstruction and alignment and absolutely stable fixation of both bones in order to allow for early motion and restitution of function. The indications for nonoperative treatment in a functional brace are therefore limited to nondisplaced fractures of the midshaft, preferably of one bone only.

2 Classification

According to the Müller AO Classification, radial and ulnar shaft fractures are classified in A, B, and C types.

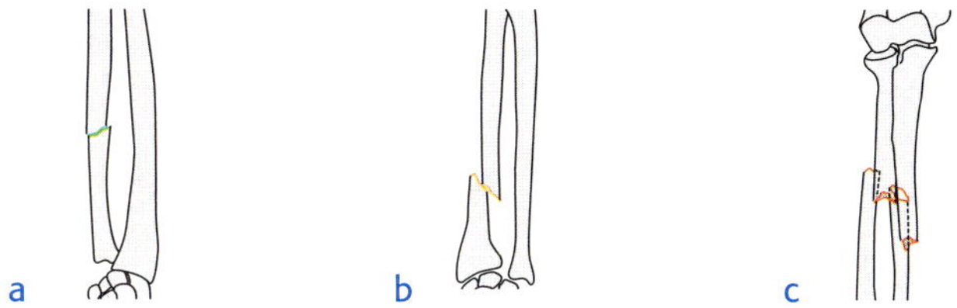

Fig 7.2-1a–c 22-A simple fractures.
a 22-A1 ulna, radius intact
b 22-A2 radius, ulna intact
c 22-A3 both bones

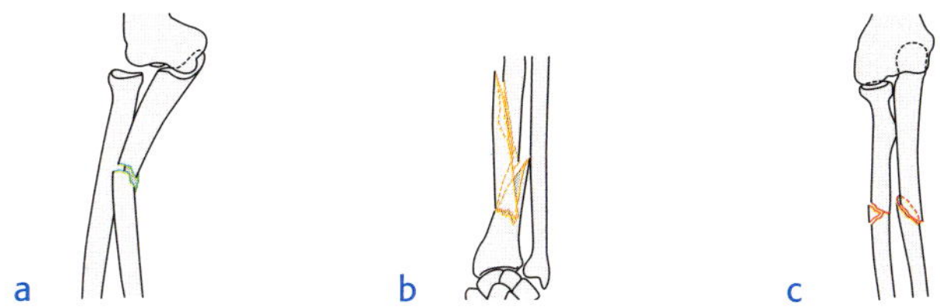

Fig 7.2-2a–c 22-B wedge fractures.
a 22-B1 ulna, radius intact
b 22-B2 radius, ulna intact
c 22-B3 one bone wedge, other simple or wedge

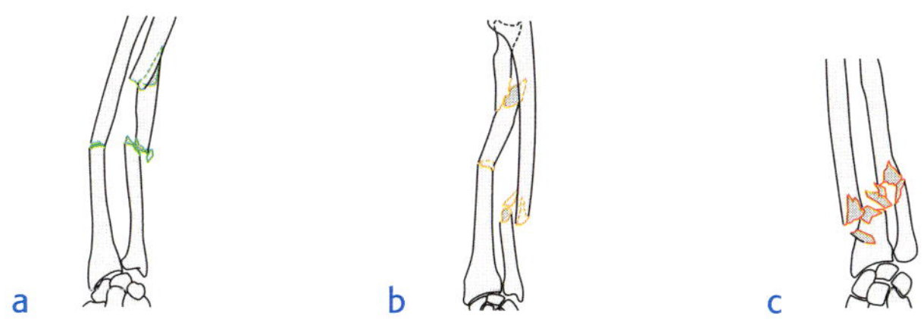

Fig 7.2-3a–c 22-C complex fractures.
a 22-C1 ulna complex, radius simple
b 22-C2 radius complex, ulna simple
c 22-C3 both bones complex

3 Treatment methods

As already mentioned, the forearm as such should be regarded as an articulation with several facets that contribute to pro- and supination as well as flexion and extension in the wrist and elbow. This demands rigid fixation which is currently best achieved with plates and screws. Intramedullary devices with interlocking are under development but have not yet reached the reliability of plating.

The well established and successful techniques with the 3.5 DCP and LC-DCP have recently been challenged by the internal fixator principle. The PC-Fix was originally introduced in different clinical studies for the forearm bones. It proved its innovative qualities in over 1,000 applications with a very high success rate. Nevertheless, the further development of the LCP 3.5 with its combination holes has now replaced the PC-Fix, as it offers the same biological advantages as the latter, but with higher versatility and a broader spectrum of indications.

In simple type A fractures it is recommended that the LCP 3.5 be applied in conventional technique with 3.5 mm cortex screws and interfragmentary compression. For more complex type C fractures, the LCP can be applied purely as an internal

Video 7.2-1

fixator bridging the multifragmentary fracture zone and at the same time securing the correct axial alignment and rotation. While the radius usually requires an open exposure, the ulna can be approached by minimally invasive techniques, sliding the plate along the easily palpable bone. Thanks to the locking head screws precise contouring of the LCP is not necessary; however the use of bicortical self-tapping locking head screws is recommended.

4 Implant overview

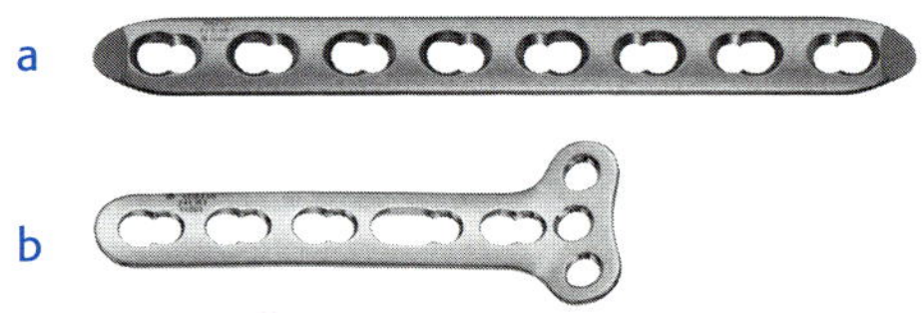

Fig 7.2-4a–b
a LCP 3.5
b LCP T-plate 3.5

5 Suggestions for further reading

Chapman MW, Gordon JE, Zissimos AG (1989) Compression-plate fixation of acute fractures of the diaphyses of the radius and ulna. *J Bone Joint Surg Am*; 71(2):159–169.

De Pedro JA, Garcia-Navarrete F, Garcia De Lucas F, et al (1992) Internal fixation of ulnar fractures by locking nail. *Clin Orthop*; 283:81–85.

Duncan R, Geissler W, Freeland AE, et al (1992) Immediate internal fixation of open fractures of the diaphysis of the forearm. *J Orthop Trauma*; 6(1):25–31.

Heim U, Zehnder R (1989) Analysis of failures after osteosynthesis of diaphyseal fractures of the forearm. *Hefte Unfallheilkd*; 201:243–258.

Hertel R, Pisan M, Lambert S, et al (1996) Plate osteosynthesis of diaphyseal fractures of the radius and ulna. *Injury*; 27(8):545–548.

Oestern HJ, Tscherne H (1983) [Results of a collective AO follow-up of forearm shaft fractures]. *Unfallheilkunde*; 86(3):136–142.

Author Michael Wagner

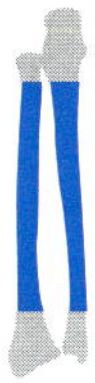

7.2.1 Displaced radial shaft fracture—22-A2

1 Case description

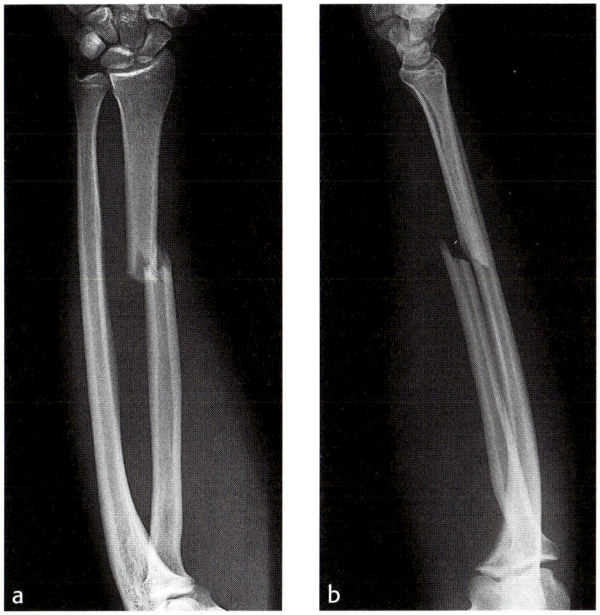

25-year-old man fell and suffered a monotrauma to his right arm.

Fig 7.2.1-1a–b
a AP view.
b Lateral view.

Indication

This displaced radial shaft fracture is an indication for operative intervention. Shaft fractures of the forearm require accurate reduction so ORIF is indicated. Plate osteosynthesis offers the opportunity to restore the anatomical shape of the bone, accurately which is a prerequisite to regaining full forearm pronation and supination. Intramedullary nailing would be an alternative procedure in this for radial shaft fracture but would not permit immediate functional postoperative care.

Preoperative planning

Equipment

- LCP 3.5, narrow, 8 holes
- 2.7 mm cortex screw
- 3.5 mm locking head screws (LHS)
- 1.25 mm K-wires
- Pointed reduction forceps

(Size of system, instruments, and implants can vary according to anatomy.)

Patient preparation and positioning

Antibiotics: none
Thrombosis prophylaxis: none

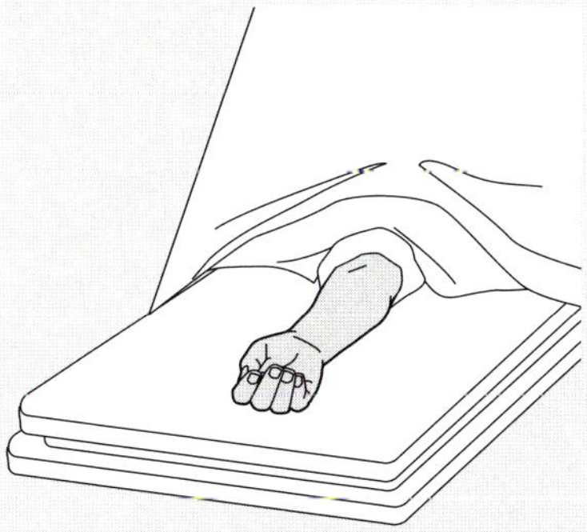

Fig 7.2.1-2 Supine position, arm table, blood tourniquet, arm in abduction.

2 Surgical approach

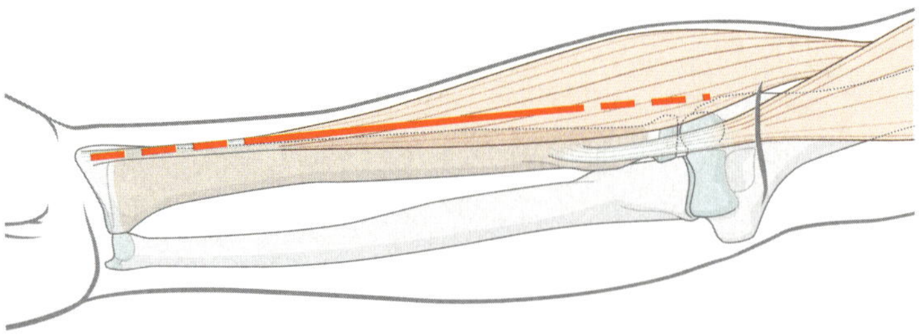

a

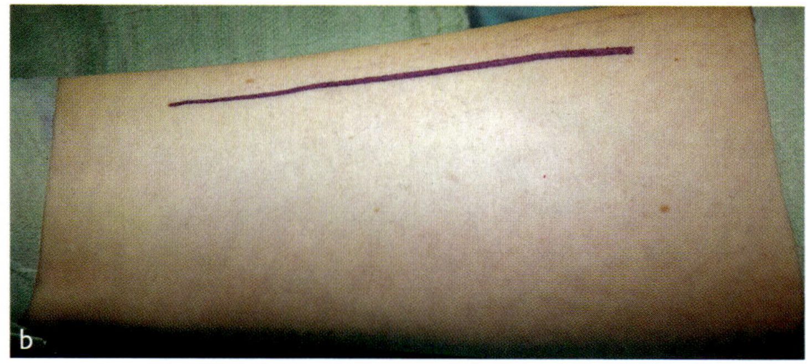

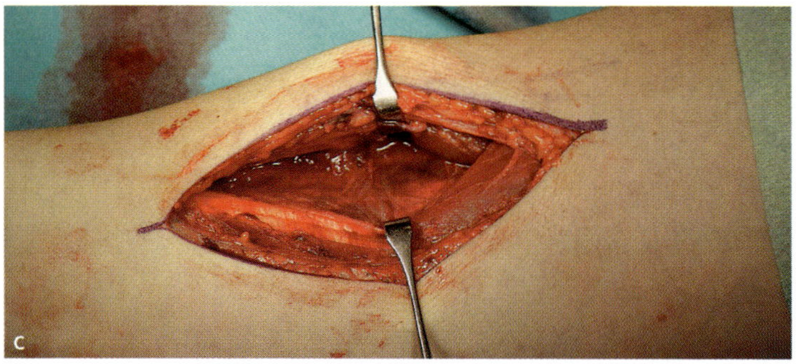

Fig 7.2.1-3a–c
a Palmar approach according to Henry.
b An incision for a palmar approach is marked on the skin preoperatively.
c Splitting of the fascia and procedure at the edge of the brachioradialis muscle.

3 Reduction and fixation

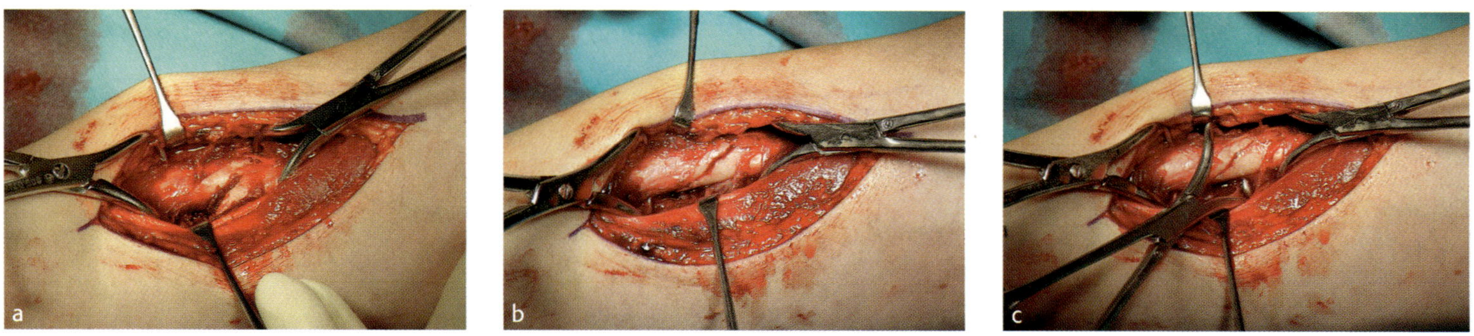

Fig 7.2.1-4a–l
a–c After exposure of the shaft fracture both the proximal and distal fragments are held with a pointed reduction forceps and the reduction is performed under longitudinal traction and direct vision. The reduction result is held in place with a third pair of pointed reduction forceps.

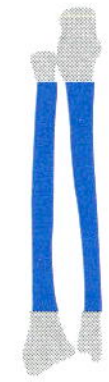

3 Reduction and fixation (cont)

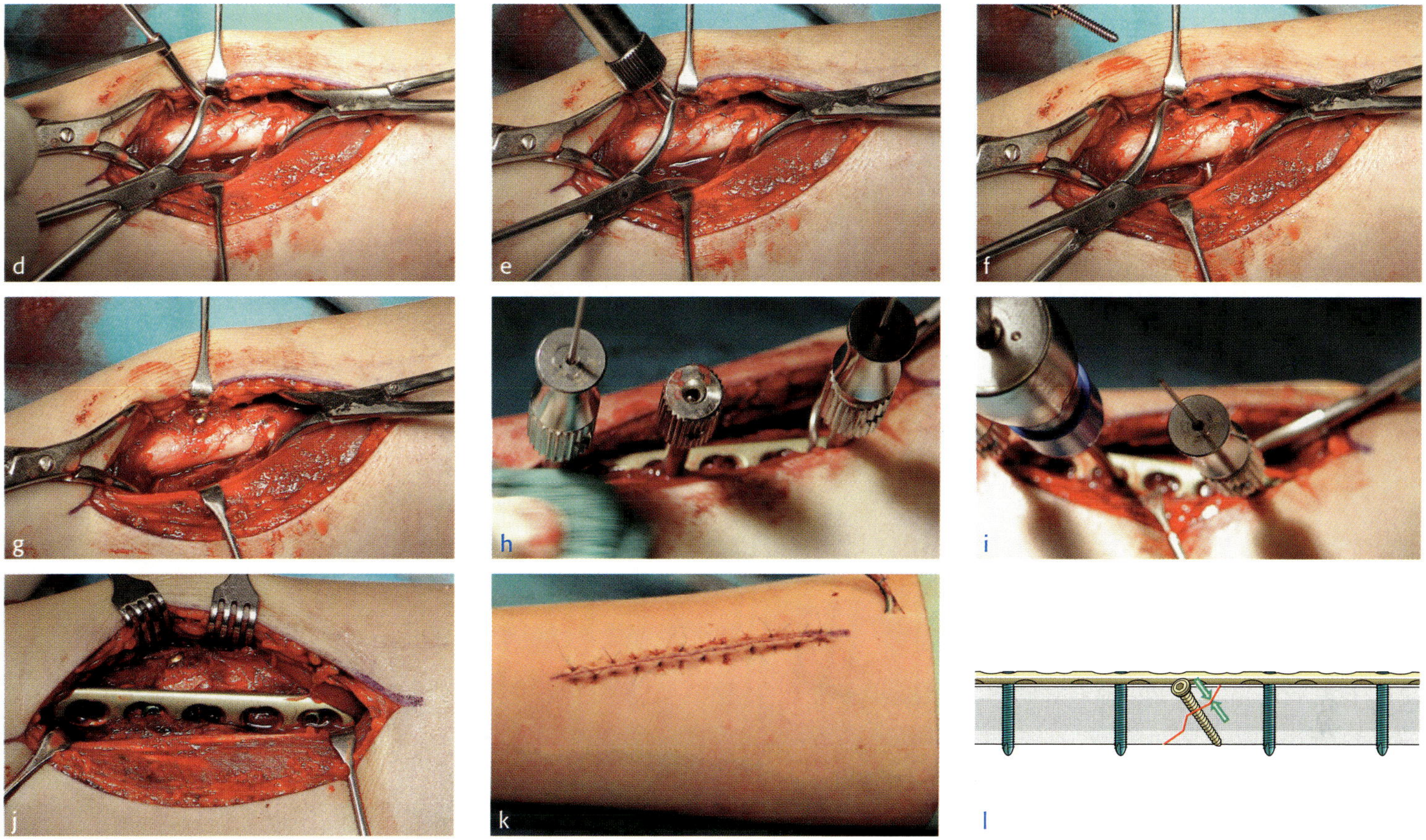

Fig 7.2.1-4a–l (cont)

- d Predrilling of the holes for the 2.7 mm cortex screw with various drill bits for the gliding and threaded holes.
- e Length measurement.
- f Insertion of the lag screw (2.7 mm cortex screw).
- g Fracture stabilization with an independent lag screw for interfragmentary compression.
- h Insertion of the LCP 3.5, 8 holes and temporary fixation with K-wires in the proximal and distal fragment. After x-ray control of plate position, definitive fixation with the protection plate following using four LHS, two per fragment.
- i Drilling through a threaded drill sleeve and locking of the LHS with the torque-limiting screwdriver.
- j Osteosynthesis after completion.
- k Redon drainage and suture.
- l This simple radial shaft fracture was stabilized by an open, precise reduction and compression method using a 2.7 mm lag screw. An angular stable noncontact plate fixed with LHS was inserted to act as a protection plate.

4 Rehabilitation

No additional immobilization. Active mobilization starts on day one postoperatively, including active-assisted physiotherapy of the elbow and wrist.

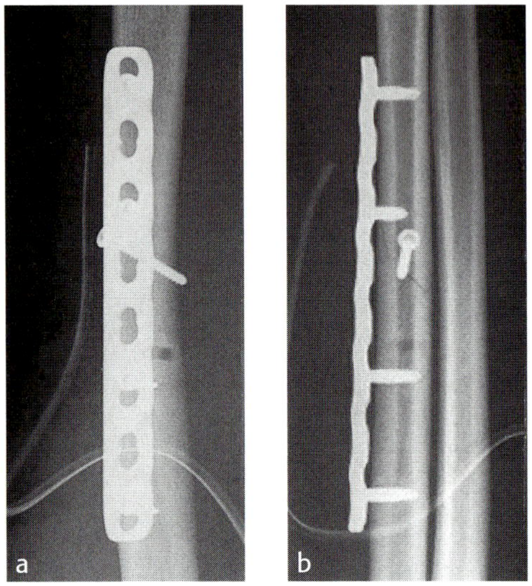

Fig 7.2.1-5a–b Postoperative x-rays after 1 day.
- a AP view.
- b Lateral view. The gap between the non-contact plate and the bone is visible.

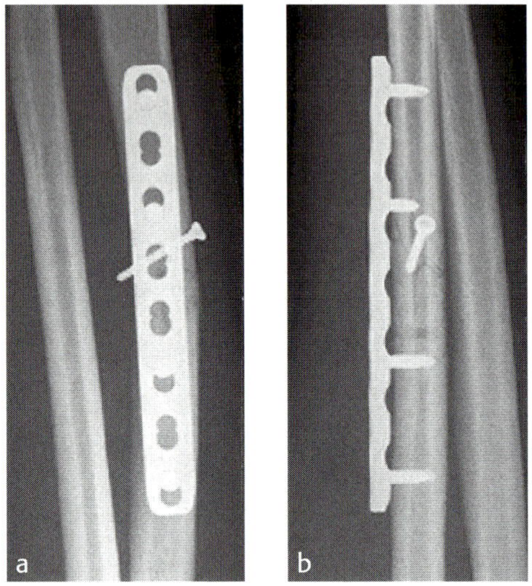

Fig 7.2.1-6a–b Postoperative x-rays after 6 weeks.
- a AP view.
- b Lateral view.

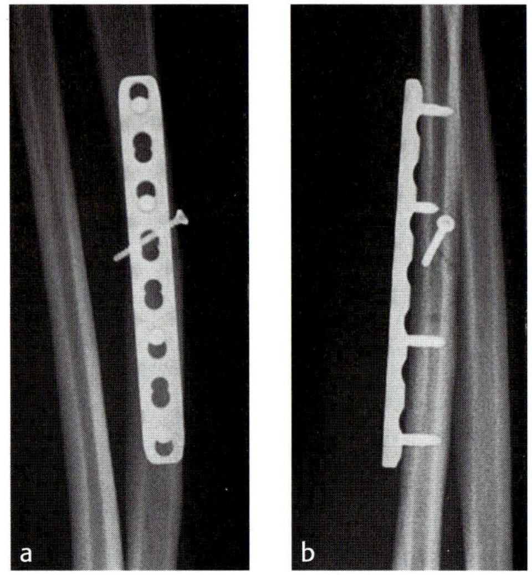

Fig 7.2.1-7a–b Postoperative x-rays after 5 months. Direct bone healing.
- a AP view.
- b Lateral view.

5 Pitfalls –

Approach

Lesion of the radial nerve.
Circulatory damage caused by open reduction and compression osteosynthesis in conventional plate technique.

Reduction and fixation

Fixation of a conventional plate with cortex screws requires precise prebending of the plate. Otherwise there is a risk of primary loss of reduction.

6 Pearls +

Reduction and fixation

A plate-independent lag screw is technically simpler than a lag screw through a plate hole. A protection plate secured with LHS has the following advantages:
- Precise prebending of the plate on to the bone surface is not necessary as the plate is secured as a noncontact plate.
- No primary loss of reduction.
- Minimal periosteal circulatory damage.
- Reduced risk of refracture on potential implant removal.

Authors Emanuel Gautier, Georges Kohut

7.2.2 Wedge radial and ulnar shaft fracture—22-B3

1 Case description

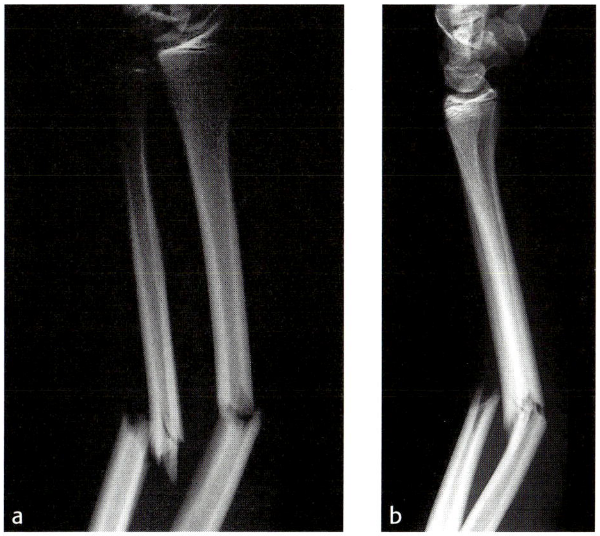

15-year-old man fell while playing soccer and suffered a monotrauma to his left arm.

Fig 7.2.2-1a–b
a AP view showing transverse fractures of both forearm bones. The radius has a simple fracture, the ulna an additional small bending wedge.
b Lateral view.

Indication

This displaced forearm fracture (22-B3.1) is in this age group an absolute indication for open reduction and internal fixation using plates. Intramedullary nailing would be difficult because of the narrow medullary cavity. Plate osteosynthesis offers the opportunity to restore accurately the anatomical shape of both forearm bones, which is a prerequisite to regaining full forearm pronation and supination.

Preoperative planning

Equipment

- LCP 3.5, 7 holes
- 3.5 mm locking head screws (LHS)
- 3.5 mm cortex screws

(Size of system, instruments, and implants can vary according to anatomy.)

Patient preparation and positioning

Antibiotics: 2nd generation cephalosporin for 48 hours
Thrombosis prophylaxis: none

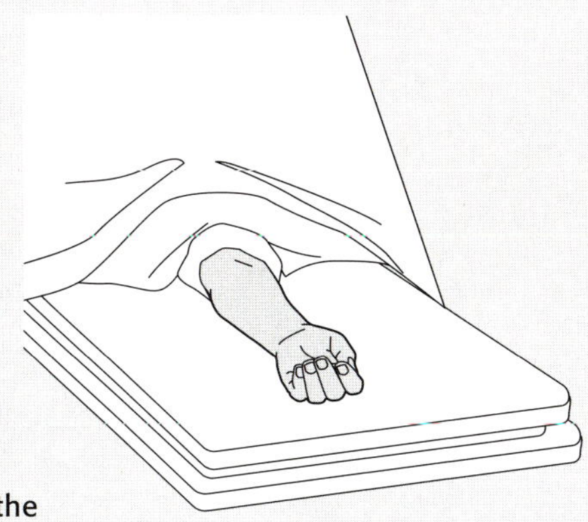

Fig 7.2.2-2 Position the patient supine on the table, with the upper extremity abducted and supported on a hand table.
A tourniquet is placed on the upper arm.
Approach to the ulna is performed with the elbow in flexion and the forearm pronated.
Approach to the radius with extension of the elbow and the forearm supinated.

2 Surgical approach

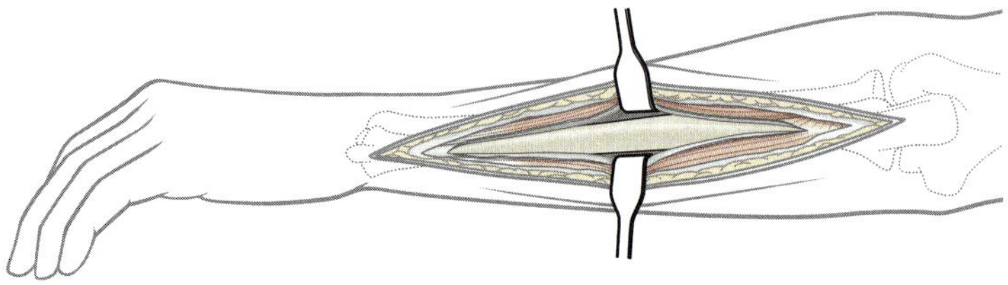

a

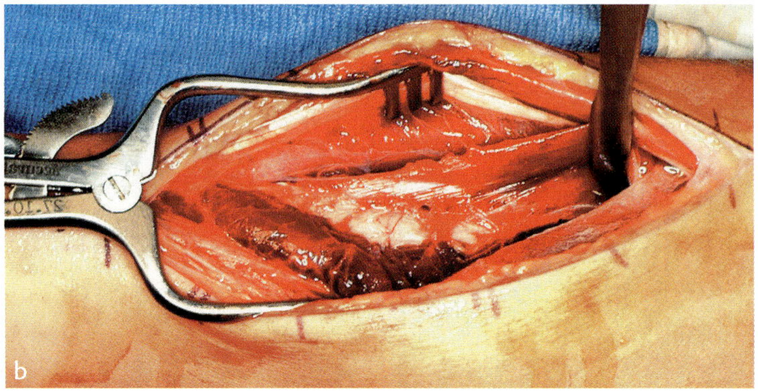

b

Fig 7.2.2-3a–b
a Standard approach to the ulna.

b Approach to the radial shaft according to Henry.

3 Reduction and fixation—ulna

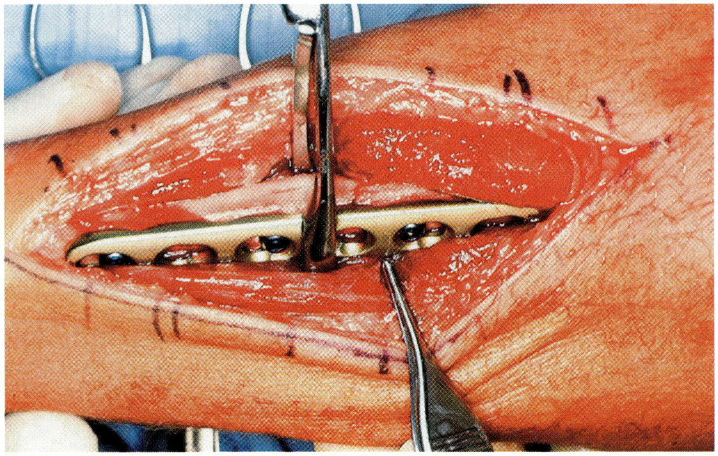

After epiperiosteal exposure of the ulnar shaft the plate is anchored on the distal fragment with two LHS prior to reduction. The reduction is performed by manual traction and the proximal fragment is held in position using a small Verbrugge clamp. Interfragmentary compression of the fracture is generated using a conventional cortex screw inserted eccentrically at the proximal end of the plate. Fixation is completed with a LHS inserted close to the fracture.

Fig 7.2.2-4 Intraoperative view of the ulna showing the plate in position fixed to the distal fragment with two LHS, and the proximal fragment held in position with the Verbrugge clamp. Extensive traumatic periosteal stripping mainly of the proximal fragment is visible.

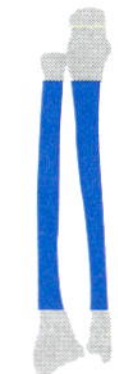

4 Reduction and fixation—radius

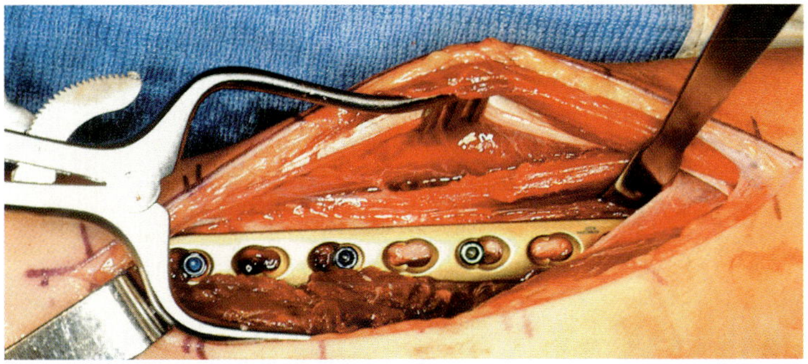

Identical procedure for reduction and fixation of the radial shaft as described for the ulna.

Fig 7.2.2-5 Intraoperative view showing the completed fixation using a 7-hole LCP 3.5.

5 Rehabilitation

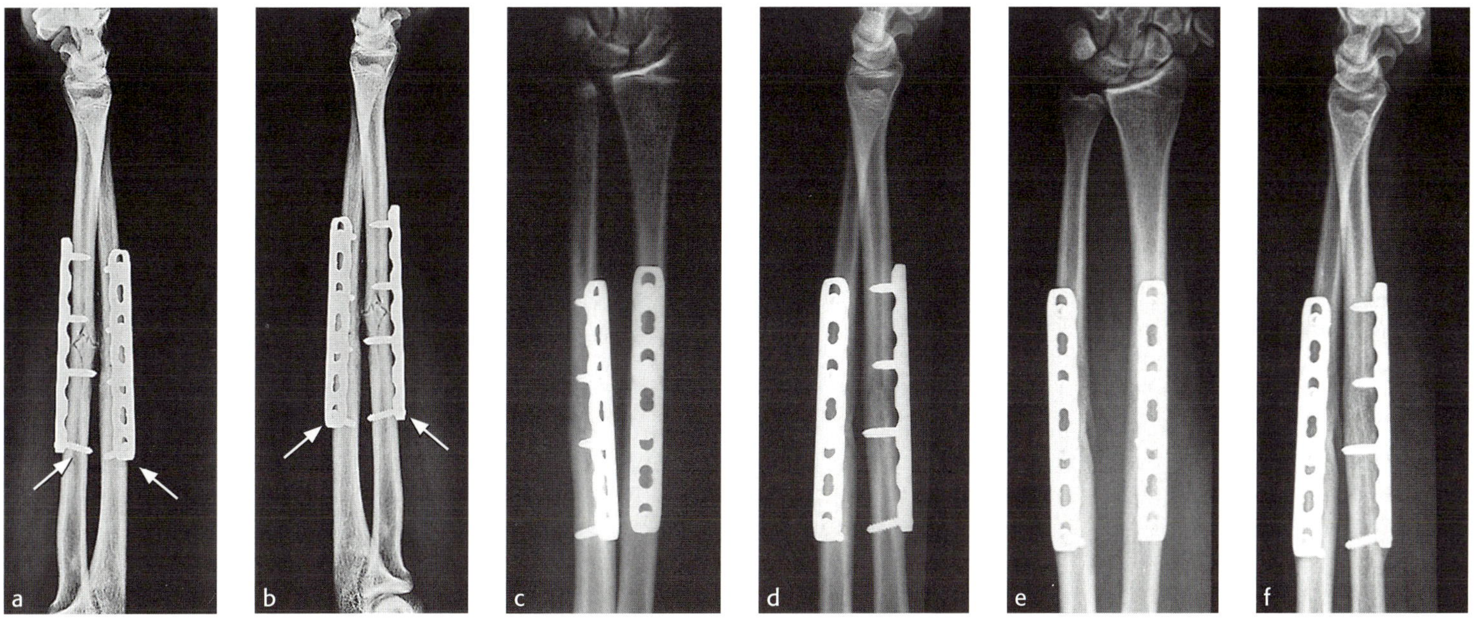

Postoperatively no additional immobilization is needed, the forearm is elevated. Active mobilization starts on the second day including pronation and supination of the forearm and flexion and extension of the elbow and wrist joints.

Fig 7.2.2-6a–f
- a–b Postoperative x-rays: AP view, lateral view. Note the weccentric cortex screws in the proximal combination hole of each plate (arrow).
- c–d X-rays after 19 weeks: AP view, lateral view.
- e–f X-rays after 15 months: AP view, lateral view.

5 Rehabilitation (cont)

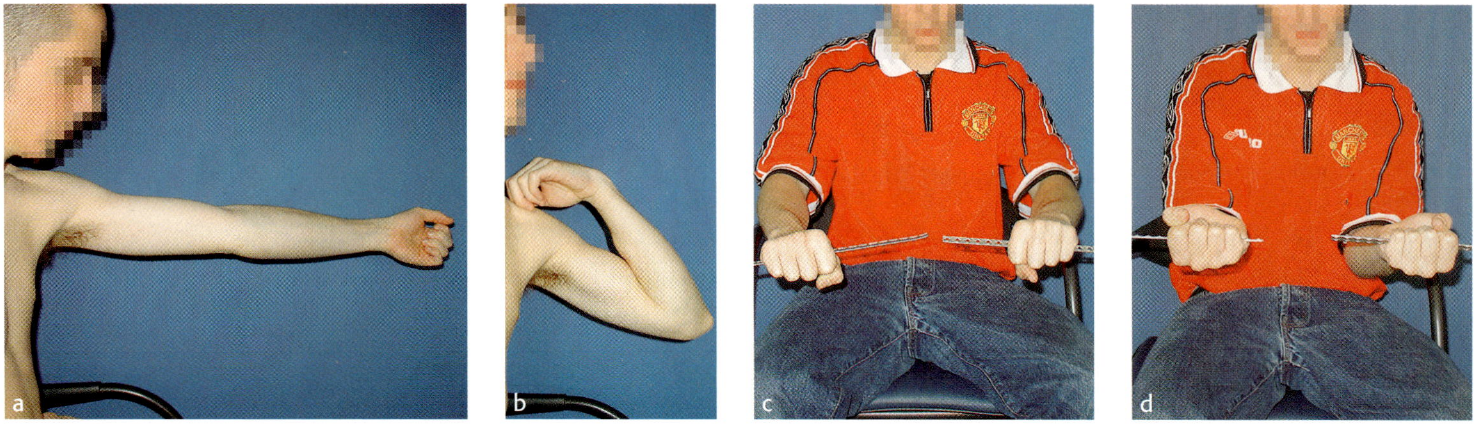

Fig 7.2.2-7a–d Functional results after four years.
a–b Showing full extension and flexion of the elbow.
c–d Showing full pronation and supination of the forearm.

Implant removal
No implant removal because the plates do not hinder or bother the patient.

6 Pitfalls –

Reduction and fixation
Extensile exposure with damage to the blood supply of the cortex to achieve anatomical reduction.

A 7-hole plate is the minimal length of plate for stabilization of a transverse forearm fracture. Comminuted fractures need a much longer plate, at least a 10–12-hole plate.

Two screws per main fragment is the absolute minimum for plate fixation from the mechanical point of view. This is sufficient only in good bone quality. For safety reasons at least three screws (mono- or bicortical) are recommended.

7 Pearls +

Reduction and fixation
Anatomical reduction of both bones of the forearm in the case of a relatively simple fracture configuration to allow complete pronation and supination of the forearm to be regained.

Use of interfragmentary compression as a tool for load sharing between implant and bone, thus, unloading the implant.

The combination hole permits the use of eccentric standard screws to achieve interfragmentary compression and also stable plate fixation to the bone with a minimum of LHS.

Early unrestricted mobilization of all adjacent joints.

Author Michael Wagner

7.2.3 Open radial and ulnar shaft fractures—22-B3 and complex articular distal radial fracture—23-C

1 Case description

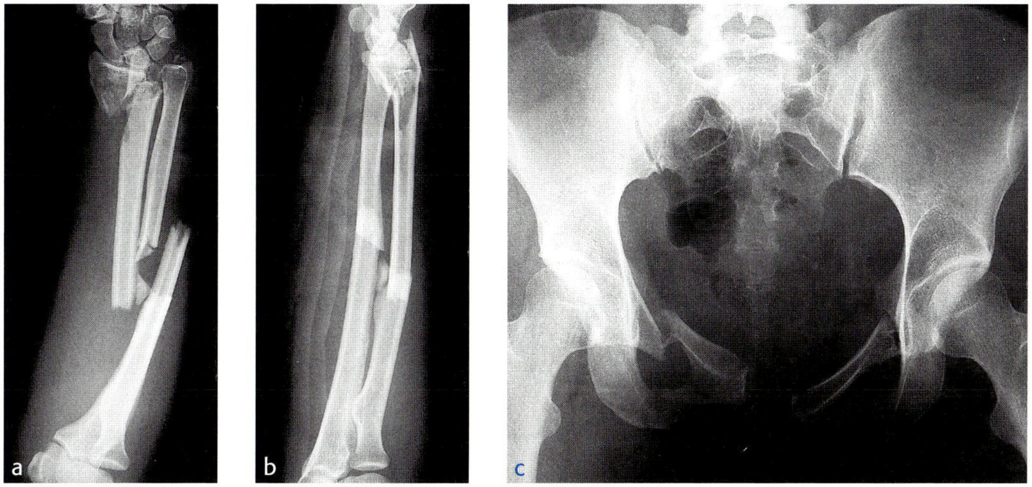

25-year-old woman fell off her motorcycle and suffered multiple injuries.

Fig 7.2.3-1a–c
a–b Open diaphyseal fractures of the radius and ulna. AP view and lateral view.
c Open pelvic ring fracture (61-C) with avulsion of the symphysis and lesion of the sacroiliac joint including injury to the vagina. Not described in this case.

Indication

Open unstable shaft fractures of the forearm bones (Gustilo type I), with additional fracture of the distal radius and joint involvement, provide the indication for surgery on this multiply injured female patient. Treatment for shock and stabilization of the unstable pelvic ring fracture with treatment of the vaginal injury with subsequent intensive care in the intensive care unit. Treatment of the open diaphyseal fractures of the forearm bones was carried out as an emergency procedure on the first day once the patient's condition was stable.

Primary traumatic paralysis of the radial nerve.

Preoperative planning

Equipment

- LCP 3.5, narrow, 10 holes
- LCP 3.5, narrow, 9 holes
- LCP T-plate 3.5, 5 holes
- 3.5 mm locking head screws (LHS)
- 3.5 mm cortex screws
- 1.8 mm K-wires

(Size of system, instruments, and implants can vary according to anatomy.)

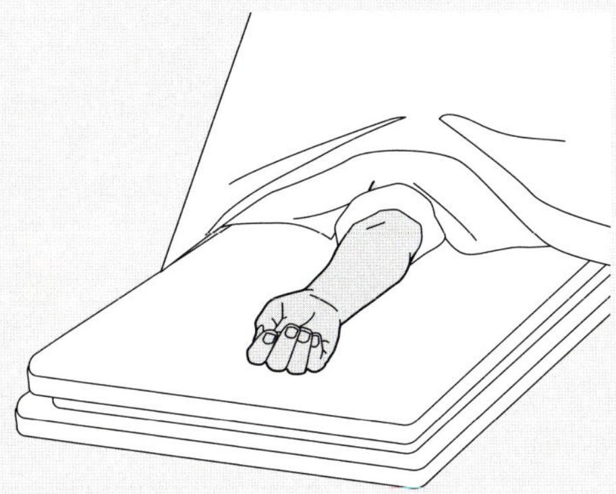

Patient preparation and positioning

Antibiotics: 3rd generation cephalosporin

Thrombosis prophylaxis: low-molecular heparin

Fig 7.2.3-2 Supine position, arm table, blood tourniquet, arm in abduction.

2 Surgical approach

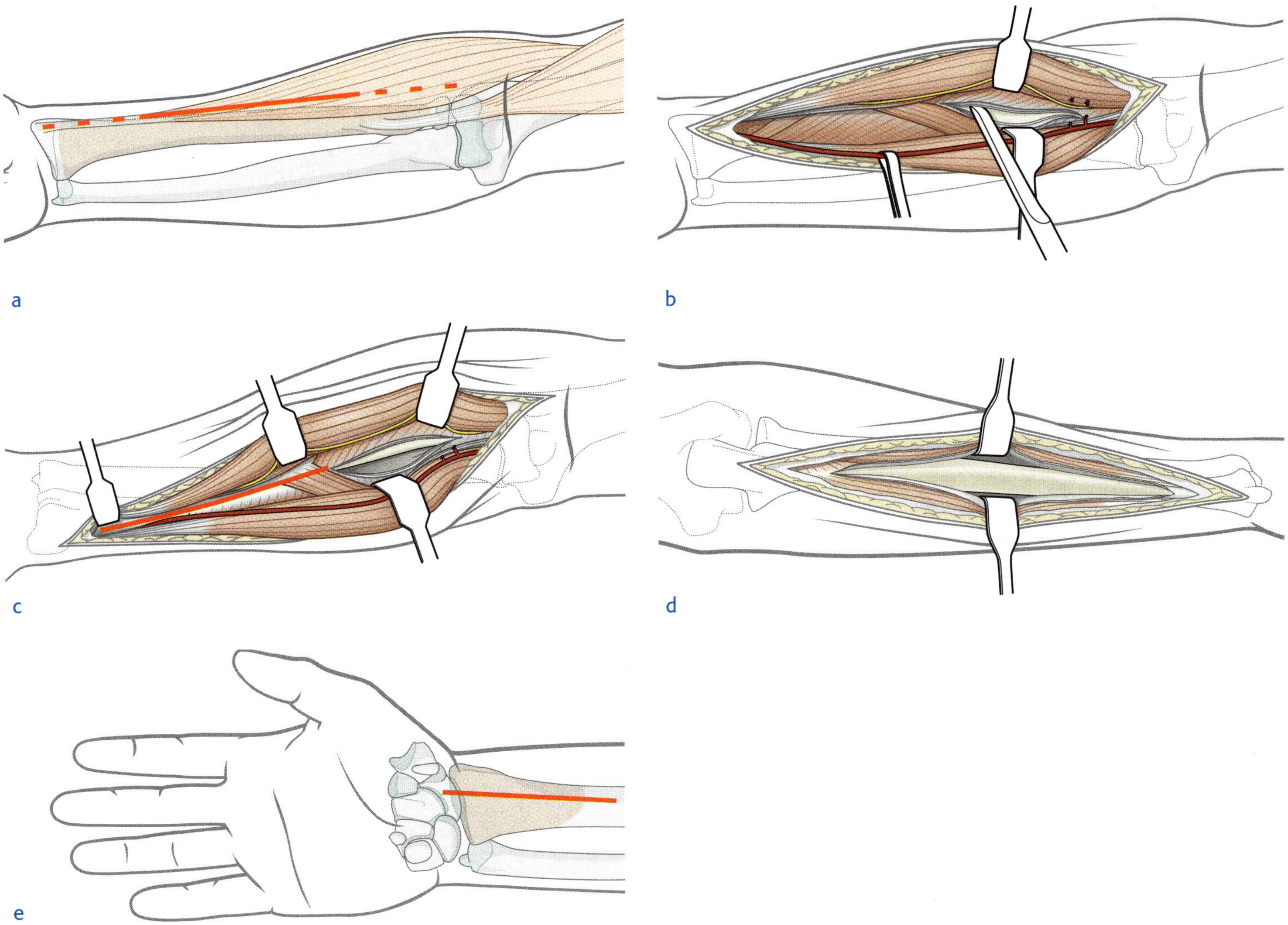

Fig 7.2.3-3a–e

a–c Treatment of the diaphyseal fracture of the radius. Palmar approach according to Henry.

d Treatment of the diaphyseal fracture of the ulna. Posterior approach to the ulna shaft.

e Treatment of the distal radius fracture. Palmar approach to the distal radius.

3 Reduction and fixation

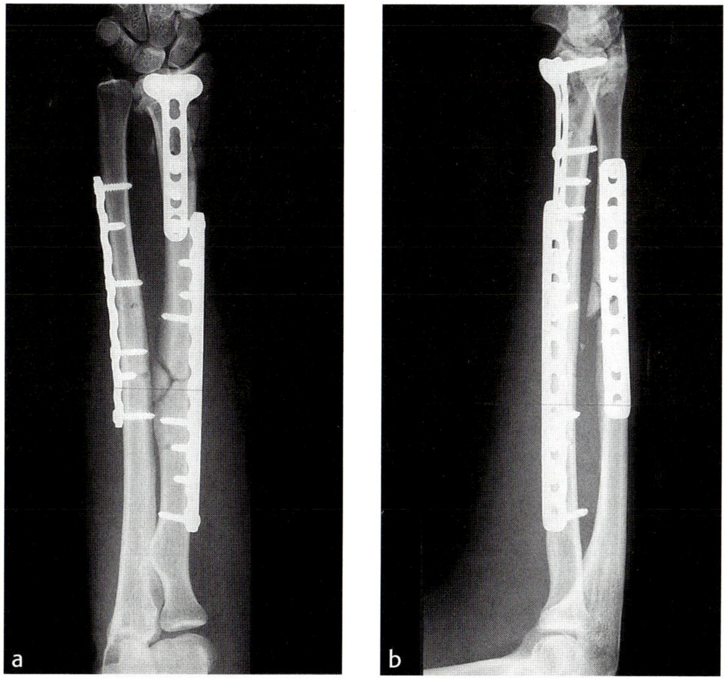

Fig 7.2.3-4a–b
a AP view.
b Lateral view.

Treatment of the radial shaft fracture.
Open reduction. The wedge fragment still attached to the periosteum is realigned. The two main fragments were then compressed and stabilized by application of a 10-hole LCP 3.5 as a compression plate. Eccentrically positioned cortex screws are inserted into both the proximal and distal main fragments. Definitive stabilization of the plate is achieved by insertion of two monocortical LHS each in the proximal and distal main fragments.
Treatment of the diaphyseal fracture of the ulna.
Open reduction. Stabilization with a 9-hole LCP. Utilization of the compression method by eccentric positioning of the cortex screws and additional fixation of the plate with monocortical LHS.
Treatment of the distal radial fracture.
Open reduction of the distal ulnar fracture and stabilization by application of a LCP 3.5. Indirect reduction and temporary fixation with K-wires. To complete the procedure, the plate is precontoured and then definitively stabilized by insertion of LHS distally and then proximally.
Wound closure, redon drainage.

4 Rehabilitation

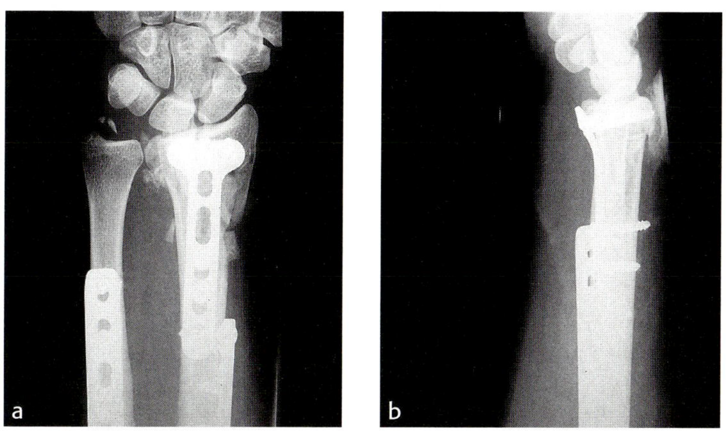

Immobilization for 3 weeks followed by physiotherapy. Spontaneous remission of the radial nerve paralysis after 6 weeks.

Fig 7.2.3-5a–b Postoperative x-rays of the distal radial fracture.
a AP view.
b Lateral x-ray showing avulsion of a posterior bone fragment that was realigned by posterior open reduction in a revision operation 1 week later and secured by insertion of a 3.0 mm cannulated screw.

4 Rehabilitation (cont)

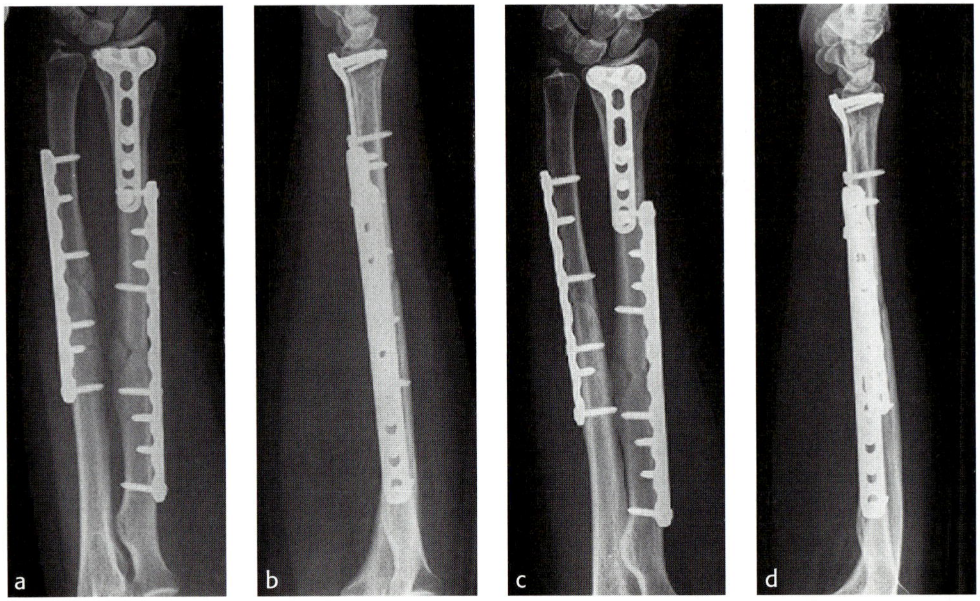

Fig 7.2.3-6a–d
a X-ray after 4 months, AP view.
b X-ray after 4 months, lateral view.
c X-ray after 18 months, AP view.
d X-ray after 18 months, lateral view.

5 Pitfalls –

Approach

It is especially important at the proximal shaft to be careful not to damage the radial nerve.

Reduction and fixation

Fig 7.2.3-7 Reduction maneuvers should be as indirect and tissue-friendly as possible even in open reduction and be performed exclusively with the pointed reduction forceps and not with clamps with serrated jaws.

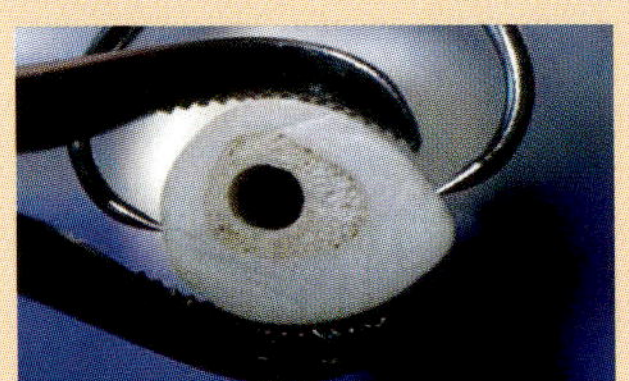

6 Pearls +

Approach

Reduction and fixation

Thanks to its combination holes, the LCP can be applied as a compression plate by the insertion of eccentrically placed cortex screws. The additional fixation of the plate with LHS provides greater stability and enhances the following technical and biological benefits:

- Precise prebending of the plate onto the bone surface is not necessary, as the plate is secured as a noncontact plate.
- No primary loss of reduction.
- Minimal periosteal circulatory damage.
- Reduced risk of refracture on potential implant removal.

Authors Michael J Gardner, Dean L Lorich David L Helfet

7.2.4 Complex radial and ulnar shaft fracture—22-C3

1 Case description

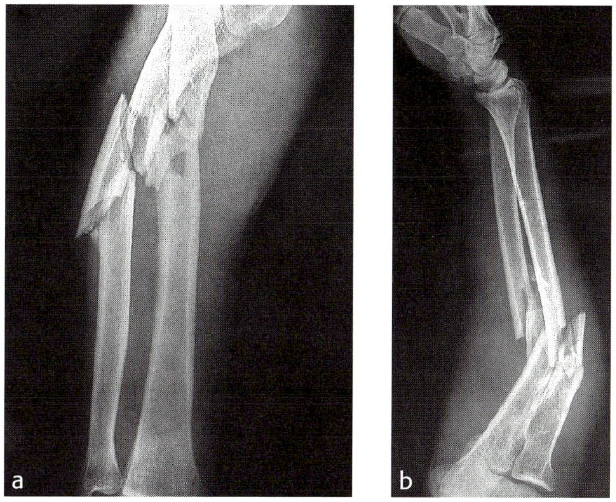

58-year-old male pedestrian was struck by a car and knocked into a brick wall. He was brought to the emergency department with evident left forearm pain and deformity.
There was no skin lesion or signs of compartment syndrome.

Fig 7.2.4-1a–b
a AP view.
b Lateral view.

Indication

Displaced both-bones forearm fractures are inherently unstable, and reduction and internal fixation is necessary to restore acceptable function. Nonoperative treatment has led to universally poor outcomes in these fractures.

Preoperative planning

Equipment

- LCP 3.5, 12 holes
- LCP 3.5, 16 holes
- 3.5 mm locking head screws (LHS)
- 3.5 mm cortex screws

(Size of system, instruments, and implants can vary according to anatomy.)

Patient preparation and positioning

Antibiotics: single dose 2nd generation cephalosporin
Thrombosis prophylaxis: none

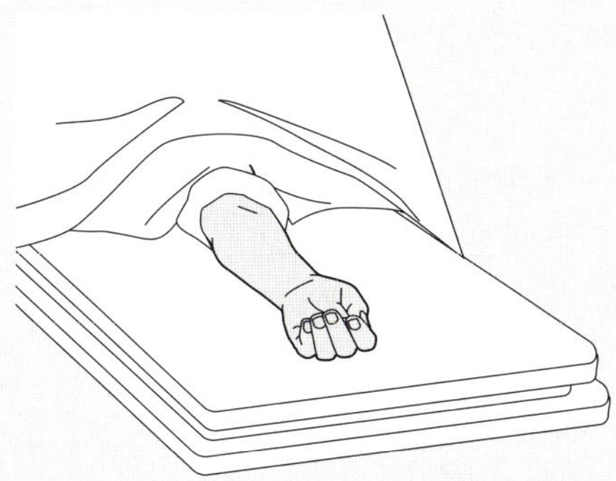

Fig 7.2.4-2 Position the patient supine on the table, with the extremity extended and supported on a hand table. A tourniquet is placed on the proximal arm. The extremity is prepped and draped free. General anesthesia is preferred so signs of compartment syndrome postoperatively are not ambiguous.

2 Surgical approach

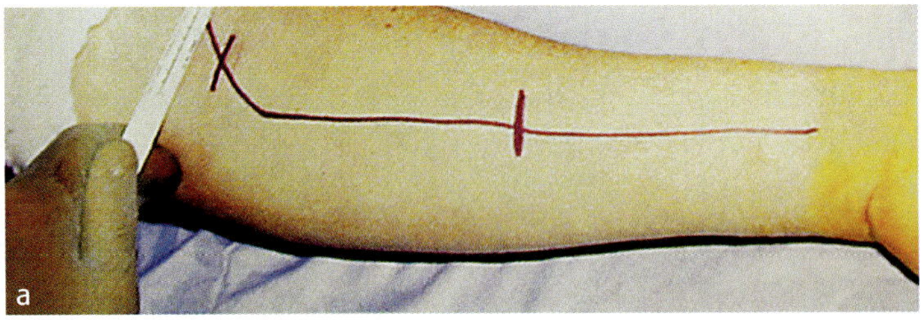

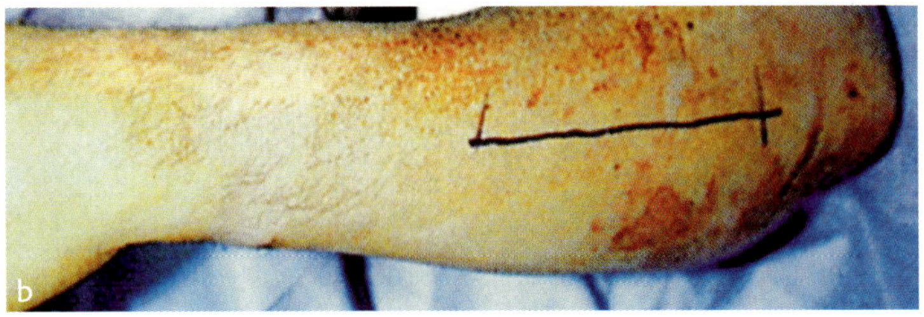

Fig 7.2.4-3a–b

a Use Henry's palmar approach for the midshaft radial fracture. Make a longitudinal incision directly over the fracture, and extend proximally or distally as needed.
Proximally, find the interval between the biceps and the brachioradialis muscles just distal to the elbow. Slightly distally, the dissection plane lies between the brachioradialis and the pronator teres muscles. In the midshaft, the internervous plane is between the brachioradialis and the flexor carpi radialis muscles. The radial artery runs with the muscle belly of the flexor carpi radialis muscle on the medial side of the wound. Find the superficial radial sensory nerve under the brachioradialis muscles laterally and protect it.
If proximal exposure is needed, reflect the insertion of the supinator muscles subperiosteally to protect the posterior interosseous nerve, and take care not to retract too vigorously. For deep exposure in the midshaft, reflect the pronator and flexor digitorum superficialis muscles subperiosteally. Distally, reflect the flexor pollicis longus and the pronator quadratus muscle subperiosteally to expose the volar surface of the radius.

b To expose the ulna, pronate the forearm and make an incision directly over the subcutaneous border of the ulna. The internervous plane lies between the flexor carpi ulnaris and extensor carpi ulnaris muscles.

3 Reduction and fixation

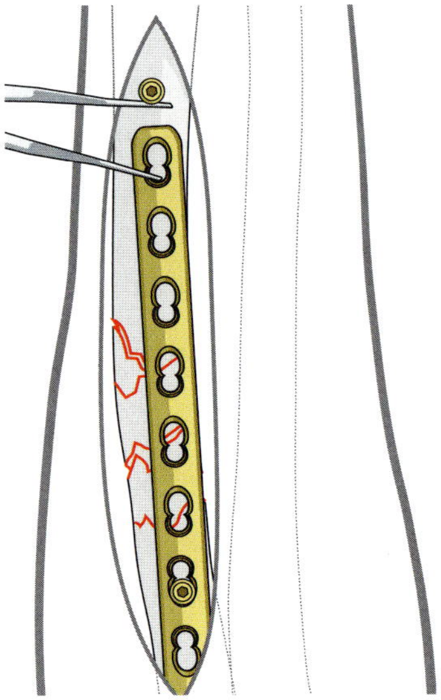

Fig 7.2.4-4 When comminution is present and a bridging technique will be used, do not expose and anatomically reduce each fracture fragment. Rather, attempt to restore length, rotation, and alignment of the bone. Address the more difficult fracture first, and stabilize it provisionally with a LCP 3.5 and reduction forceps. When one bone is adequately reduced, provisionally stabilize the other bone. Choose long plates of at least 10–12 holes. The most important aspect of reduction is to maintain the anatomical radial bow.
When fragments are overlapped and shortened, a temporary screw can be placed 1–1.5 cm from the end of the plate, and a laminar spreader is used to distract the fracture out to length.
With both bones provisionally reduced, insert 3.5 mm locking head screws in monocortical or bicortical fashion. Space out the screws and leave at least two holes open over the comminution.
Do not close the fascia of the forearm. Close only the subcutaneous tissue and skin over the suction drains.

4 Rehabilitation

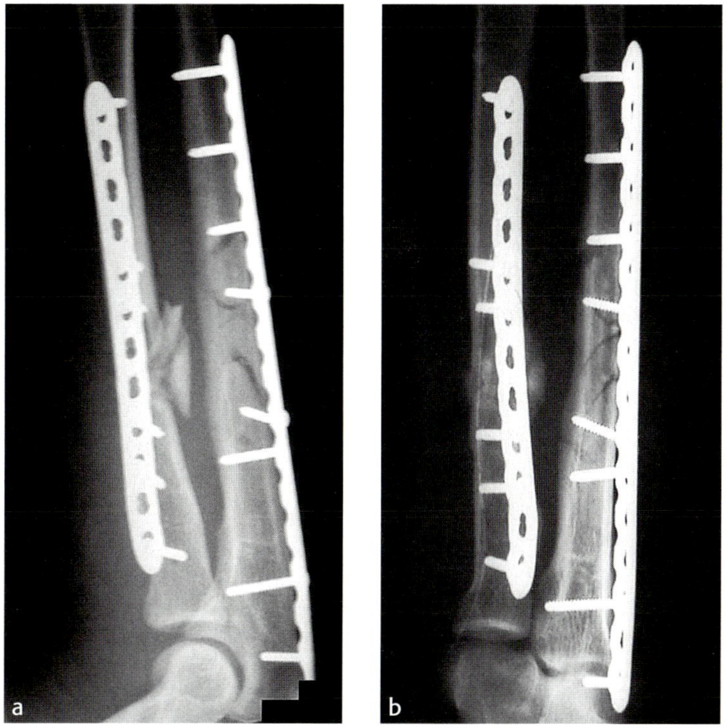

When stable fixation has been achieved in a reliable patient, plaster immobilization is not necessary.
Apply a loose dressing, elevate the extremity for 24 hours, and remove the drain.
Begin early physical therapy, including elbow, forearm, and wrist active exercises.

Fig 7.2.4-5a–b Fixation immediately postoperatively. Because these fractures are considered articular, anatomical restoration of length and alignment is required.
5 months postoperatively the patient had good forearm rotation and stable internal fixation. Significant callus has incorporated the radial comminution.
a AP view.
b Lateral view.

Implant removal

If the hardware becomes symptomatic, it may be removed after the fracture has healed. Controversy exists as to the minimum time required postoperatively, but we prefer at least 18 months.
Postremoval, the extremity must be protected in a splint. Activity should be limited for 3 months.

5 Pitfalls –

Approach
Many neurovascular structures are at risk during these two approaches. During the palmar approach to the radius, the radial artery runs on the surface of the supinator and pronator teres muscles. The superficial radial nerve runs under the brachioradialis muscles laterally, the posterior interosseous nerve runs through the origin of supinator muscle, and the median nerve emerges from the fibrous arch of the flexor digitorum superficialis muscle. When exposing the ulna posteriosly, the ulnar nerve is at risk during deep medial exposure of the ulna.

Reduction and fixation
The radial bow may easily be underestimated during reduction, and may be lost after provisional stabilization of the radius with clamps and a plate.
Fixation in the splinting method may be compromised by using plates that are too short.

Rehabilitation
The most common setback following open reduction and internal fixation is loss of supination and pronation.
Compartment syndrome may occur after forearm trauma.

6 Pearls +

Approach
During the palmar approach, careful dissection and subperiosteal muscle retraction will minimize neurovascular injury.
To prevent damage to the ulnar nerve through the posterior incision, raise the muscle masses subperiosteally. The nerve is only at risk if dissection strays into the muscle fibers. When proximal exposure is desired, the nerve can be identified before it passes through the two heads of the flexor carpi ulnaris muscle.

Reduction and fixation
Pay close attention to the restoration of the radial bow, and that the fracture ends do not slide medially or laterally or rotate under the plate during forearm manipulation, causing loss of reduction or straightening of the bow.

Rehabilitation
To optimize forearm motion, take care to restore the radial bow during the procedure, and initiate early supervised active exercises.
Postoperative compartment syndrome can be avoided by leaving the fascia open, using deep drains, and elevating the extremity to prevent further swelling.

7.3 Radius and ulna, distal

Cases

7 Radius and ulna

Author Daniel Rikli

7.3 Radius and ulna, distal

1 Incidence

The indication for internal fixation of distal radial fractures, the surgical approach (palmar, dorsal, combined palmar and dorsal), and the choice of implants must be based on a thorough analysis of the injury mechanism (patient history), the pathomechanics of the fracture (eg, Fernandez classification), the fracture pattern (conventional x-ray, x-ray in traction, CT scan), the quality of the bone, and the demands of the individual patient.

Special attention must be paid to the soft-tissue condition (open fracture, swelling, compartment syndrome, nerve injuries) and associated lesions at the level of the proximal carpal row (osseous or ligamentous) and the distal radioulnar joint. Analysis of the fracture under traction (ligamentotaxis) in the external fixator using conventional x-ray and CT facilitates understanding of the pathology and planning of the definitive operative strategy. Occult relevant ligament tears at the level of the proximal carpal row may be demonstrated under traction (disruption of Gilula's lines).

The three column model of the distal radius and ulna is of great help in planning internal fixation. All three columns should be stable (or stabilized by internal fixation) when early function commences.

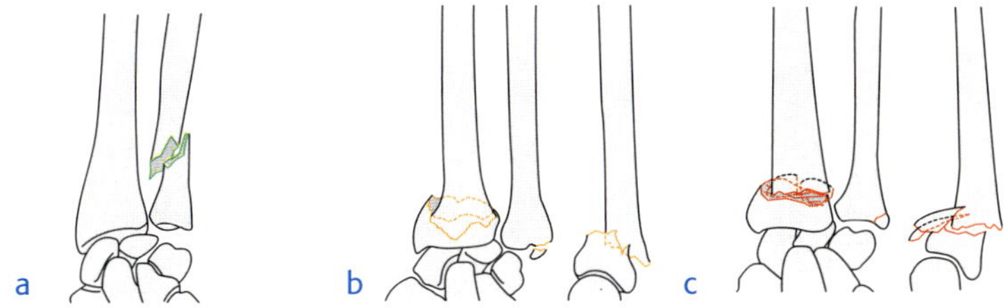

Fig 7.3-1a–c 23-A extraarticular fracture.
a 23-A1 ulna, radius intact
b 23-A2 radius, simple and impacted
c 23-A3 radius, multifragmentary

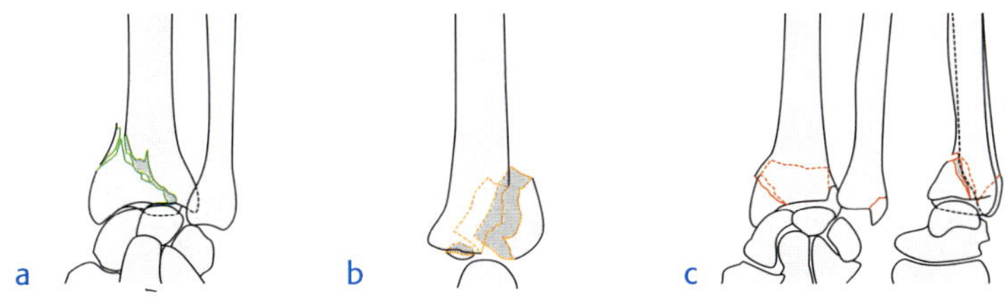

Fig 7.3-2a–c 23-B partial articular fracture.
a 23-B1 radius, sagittal
b 23-B2 radius, frontal, dorsal rim
c 23-B3 radius, frontal, volar rim

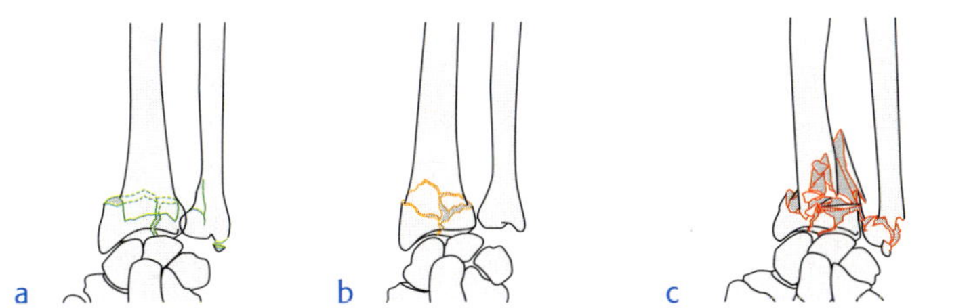

Fig 7.3-3a–c 23-C complete articular fracture of radius.
a 23-C1 articular simple, metaphyseal simple
b 23-C2 articular simple, metaphyseal multifragmentary
c 23-C3 articular multifragmentary

2 Classification

In addition to the Müller AO Classification, specific aspects regarding anatomical characteristics and trauma mechanics of the joint complexity are considered using the Fernandez classification.

Bending type fractures (Fernandez type I) with or without articular involvement respond to ligamentotaxis and are amenable to various treatment options (closed reduction and cast/

pinning, external fixation, palmar locking plate). Shear fractures (Fernandez type II) need a palmar buttress plate. Any impacted articular fragments must be addressed specifically. Axial compression fractures (Fernandez type III) usually need formal revision and reconstruction of the radiocarpal joint surface over a dorsal arthrotomy. The intermediate column is the key to the radiocarpal joint since the main pathology is at the level of the lunate facette (dorsoulnar/palmarulnar fragment). Avulsion injuries (Fernandez type IV) are fracture dislocations. Small osseous rim fragments and the radial styloid fracture correspond to osseous avulsion of the radiocarpal ligaments. These fragments and any purely ligamentous disruption must be addressed operatively. Early motion is not always feasible and immobilization of 6–8 weeks may be indicated to allow for ligamentous healing. Fractures with combinations of the above and / or diaphyseal involvement (Fernandez type V) should be treated according to the specific pathology. Relevant associated carpal ligament tears (Geissler type III and IV) should be addressed at the same time when treating the distal radial fracture.

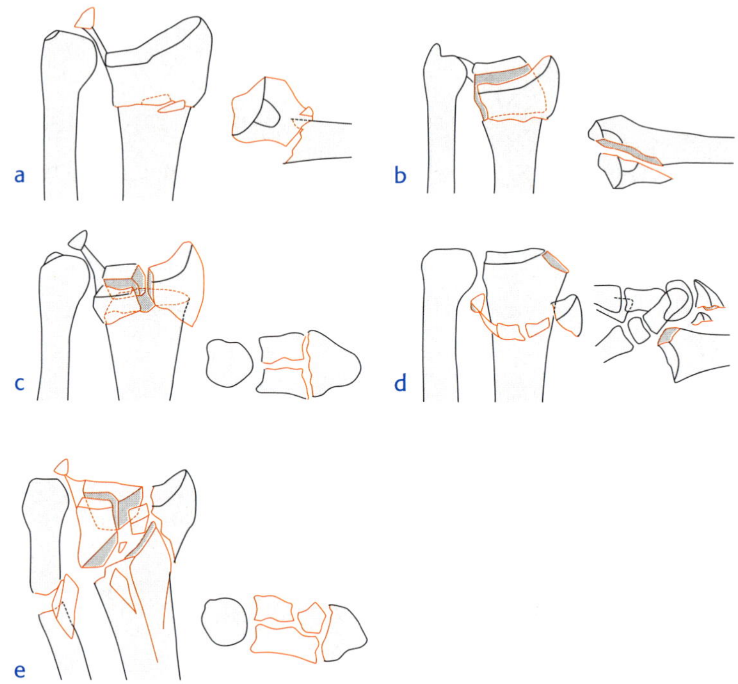

Fig 7.3-4a–e Fernandez classification.
a Type I bending fracture of the metaphysis
b Type II sharing fracture of the joint surface
c Type III compression fracture of the joint surface
d Type IV avulsion fractures, radiocarpal fracture, dislocation
e Type V combined fractures (I, II, III, IV); high velocity injury

3 Treatment methods

In simple fractures, eg, extraarticular, dorsally displaced Colles' type fracture, the treatment should be straightforward with a first and definitive measure to preclude repetitive manipulations. In more "complex" cases, eg, high-energy injuries, the application of a joint bridging external fixator as a first measure in the emergency situation may be advisable. This can be performed safely even by the less experienced surgeon in the emergency department. The soft-tissue injury can be treated.

Depending on fracture pattern, fracture fixation is to be performed by use of palmar, dorsal or combined dorsopalmar plating.

Locking palmar plates can be used in two "modes": either as a conventional "buttress plate" for Smith and reverse Barton type fractures or as an "angled blade plate" for dorsally displaced extra- and articular fractures. In the latter mode, the plate functions as an internal fixator and perfect adaptation of the plate to the bone is not mandatory. Today, many surgeons treat dorsally displaced bending type fractures (Colles') with palmar locking plates. A bone graft is not necessary.

Our rationale for dorsal plating follows the three column concept. Two plates are used to fix the radial and the intermediate column separately. Indications for dorsal double plating are: a displaced dorsoulnar fragment, impacted articular fragments that need formal revision, suspected or apparent associated lesions of the proximal carpal row and early corrective osteotomy of dorsally malunited fractures. The intermediate column is approached through the third extensor compartment and a limited dorsal arthrotomy is always performed. The radial column is approached by subcutaneous preparation between the skin flap and the retinaculum, the second and fourth compartment are left untouched. The first compartment is opened and the radial plate is slipped underneath the tendons to buttress the radial styloid.

Combined dorsal and palmar plates may be necessary for multifragmentary articular fractures. A hyperextended palmar articular fragment needs a palmar plate since this fragment cannot be controlled from the dorsal side. Hyperextended means: dorsal rotation of the fragment in the sagittal plane with no contact to the shaft and with comminution or extrusion of the fragment into the palmar soft tissue. If this palmar fragment is large and extends along the entire palmar rim including parts of the radial styloid, a palmar T-plate can be used. If the fragment is small, ie, a palmarulnar fragment, an L-plate is used to fix the fragment specifically. In these cases the radial column is buttressed separately with an S-plate from the palmar approach. An additional limited dorsal approach to the intermediate column is needed when the above mentioned situation is combined with a displaced dorsoulnar fragment and/or centrally impacted articular fragments at the level of the lunate facette. These fragments are reduced under direct control using a limited dorsal arthrotomy and then fixed with a contoured plate and locking head screws to support the radiocarpal joint surface.

Video 7.3-1

4 Implant overview

a b c d

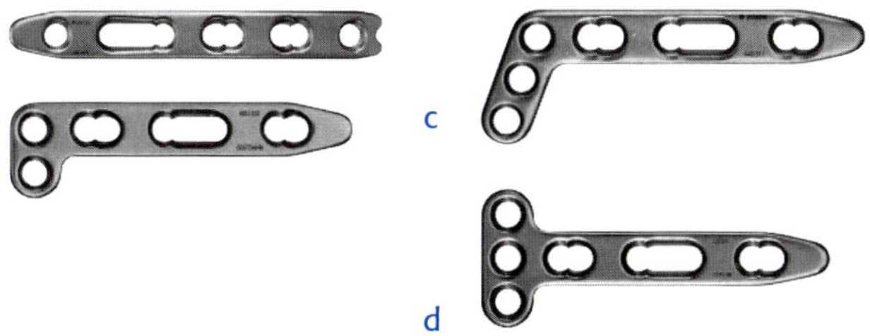

Fig 7.3-5a–d LCP distal radius plates 2.4, dorsal.
a LCP distal radius plate 2.4, straight
b LCP-L distal radius plate 2.4, right-angled
c LCP-L distal radius plate 2.4, oblique-angled
d LCP-T distal radius plate 2.4

a b

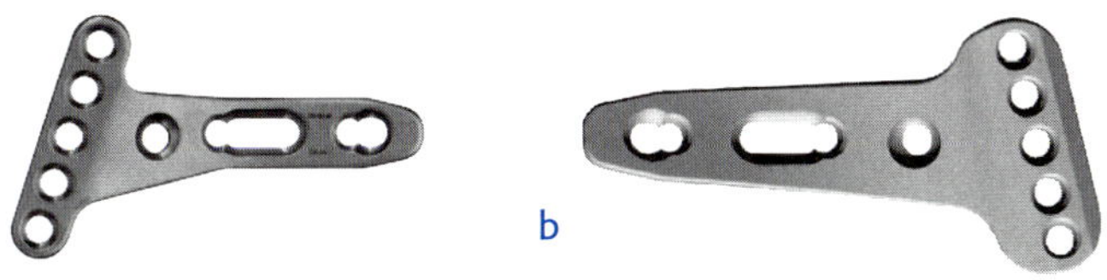

Fig 7.3-6a–b
a LCP distal radius plates 2.4, volar
b LCP distal radius plate 2.4, standard

5 Suggestions for further reading

Axelrod TS, McMurtry RY (1990) Open reduction and internal fixation of comminuted, intraarticular fractures of the distal radius. *J Hand Surg Am*; 15(1):1–11.

Fernandez DL (1993) Fractures of the distal radius: operative treatment. In: Heckmann JD, editor. Instructional Course Lectures: *Amer Acad Orthop Surg*; 42:73–88.

Fernandez DL, Jupiter JB (1995) Fractures of the Distal Radius. Berlin Heidelberg New York: Springer-Verlag.

Fernandez DL, Geissler WB, Lamey DM (1996) Wrist instability with or following fractures of the distal radius. In: Büchler U, editor. Wrist Instability. London: Martin Dunitz Ltd: 181–192.

Fernandez DL, Geissler WB (1991) Treatment of displaced articular fractures of the radius. *J Hand Surg Am*; 16 (3):375-384.

Geissler WB, Fernandez DL, Lamey DM (1996) Distal radioulnar joint injuries associated with fractures of the distal radius. *Clin Orthop*; (327):135–146.

Jupiter JB, Fernandez DL, Toh CL, et al (1996) Operative treatment of volar intra- articular fractures of the distal end of the radius. *J Bone Joint Surg Am*; 78(12):1817–1828.

Jupiter JB, Ring DC (2005) AO Manual of Fracture Management Hand an Wrist. Stuttgart and New York. Thieme-Verlag.

Rickli DA, Regazzoni P (1996) Fractures of the distal end of the radius treated by internal fixation and early function. A preliminary report of 20 cases. *J Bone Joint Surg Br*; 78(4):588–592.

Author Daniel Rikli

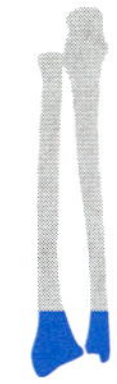

7.3.1 Extraarticular dorsally displaced distal radial fracture (Colles' fracture)—23-A3

1 Case description

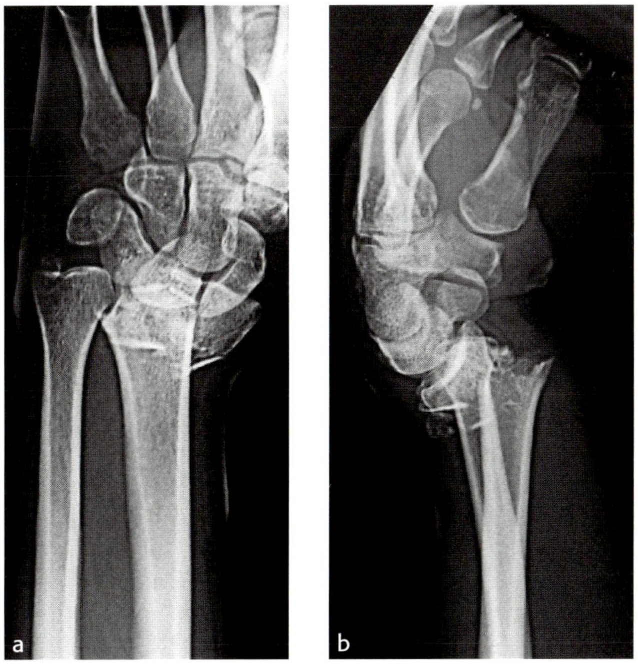

32-year-old man. Fall from bicycle. Extraarticular fracture of the distal radius with marked dorsal displacement of the distal fragment. Fracture of the tip of the ulnar styloid.

Fig 7.3.1-1a–b Injury x-rays.
a AP view.
b Lateral view.

Indication

Indication for reduction is evident. Restoration of angles and length is a prerequisite for functional recovery. Stable internal fixation allows for early motion and use of the extremity for unloaded activities.

Preoperative planning

Equipment
- LCP distal radius plate 2.4, 3 holes
- Locking head screws (LHS)

(Size of system, instruments, and implants can vary according to anatomy.)

Patient preparation and positioning
Position the patient supine on the table, with the extremity extended and supported on a hand table. Nonsterile pneumatic tourniquet is placed on the proximal arm. Prophylactic antibiotics optional.

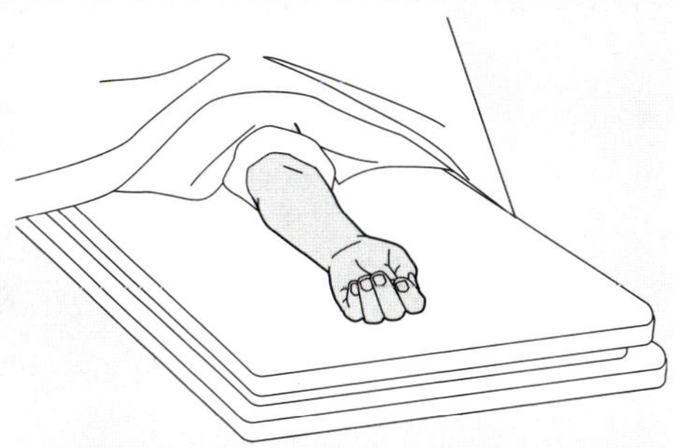

Fig 7.3.1-2 The patient is positioned supine on the table, with the limb extended and supported an a hand table.

2 Surgical approach

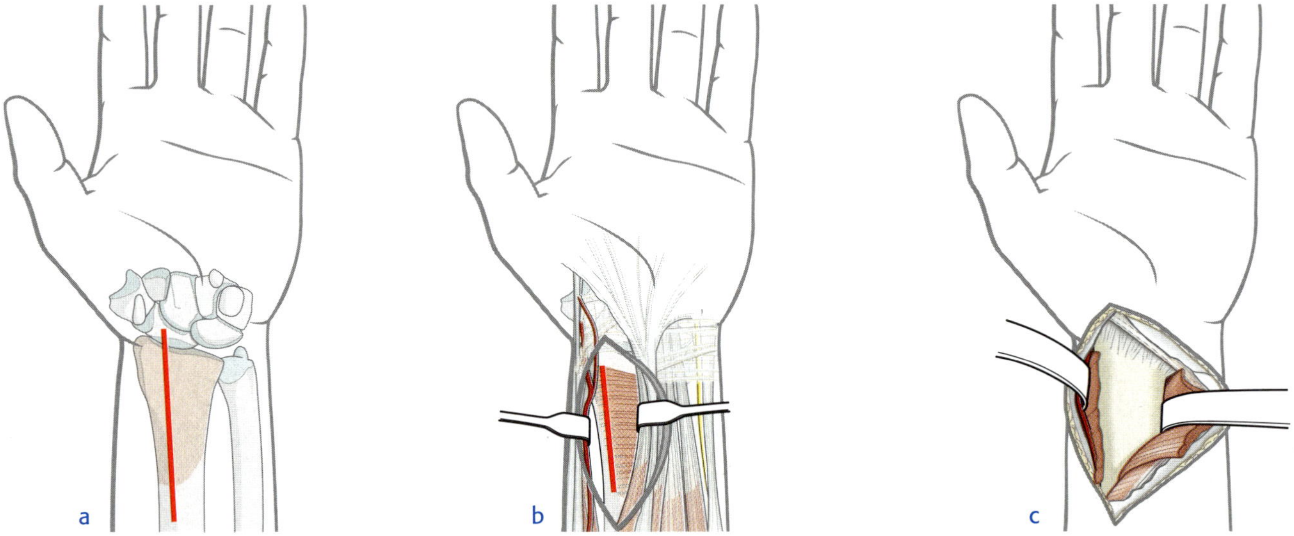

Fig 7.3.1-3a–c Henry's modified palmar approach to the distal radius. Straight incision between the radial artery and the tendon of the flexor carpi radialis muscle.

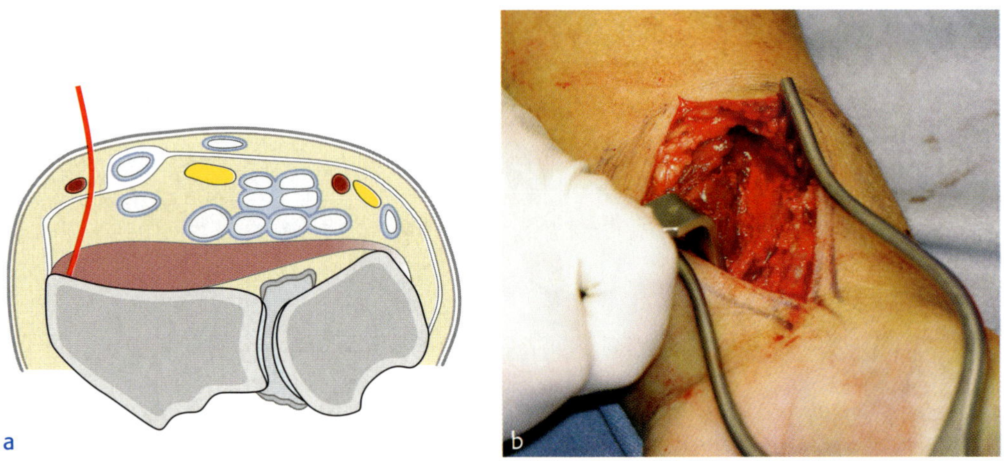

Fig 7.3.1-4a–b Dissection between the radial artery and the flexor carpi radialis tendon. The forearm fascia is divided and the pronator quadratus muscle is detached from the radial bony insertion. The fracture is visualized.

3 Reduction

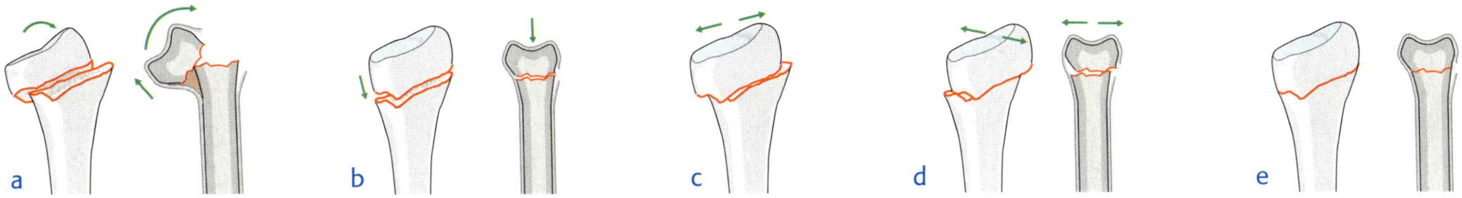

Fig 7.3.1-5a–d

- a The fracture is reduced manually.
- b Since the palmar cortex is of sufficiently good quality even in very osteoporotic bone, radial length
- c–d and axial alignment can be restored anatomically.
- e Manual reduction is usually sufficient to restore palmar tilt.

The distal fragment is pushed towards the plate by bringing the hand into flexion. Reduction is secured by inserting a first distal locking head screw in this position.

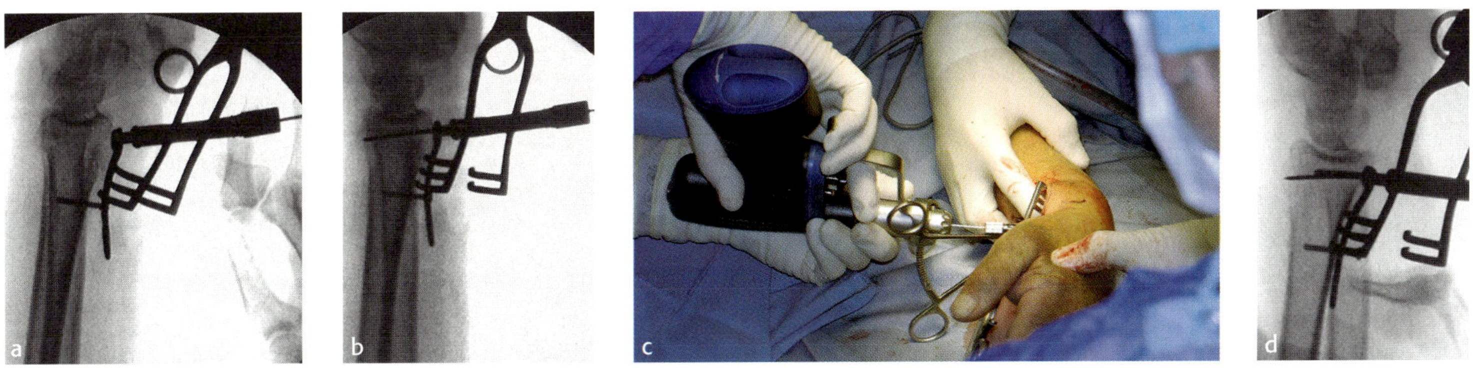

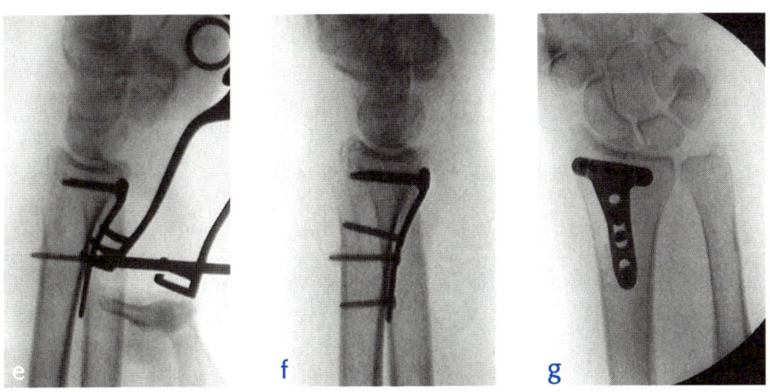

Fig 7.3.1-6a–g To correct the residual dorsal displacement and restore palmar tilt, the distal fragment can be reduced indirectly. The locking plate is fitted/equipped with the threaded drill sleeve and placed in position, where the drill sleeve and the radiocarpal joint line cover a dorsally open angle of 10°. A K-wire, an LHS, or both are used to fix the plate in this position. Note that the plate is now away from the radial shaft proximally. The shaft of the plate is reduced to the shaft of the radius manually and the distal fragment is thereby brought into the desired position of slight palmar flexion. The plate acts as an angled blade plate.

As an option, K-wires and Weber clamps can be used to temporarily hold the reduction.

4 Fixation

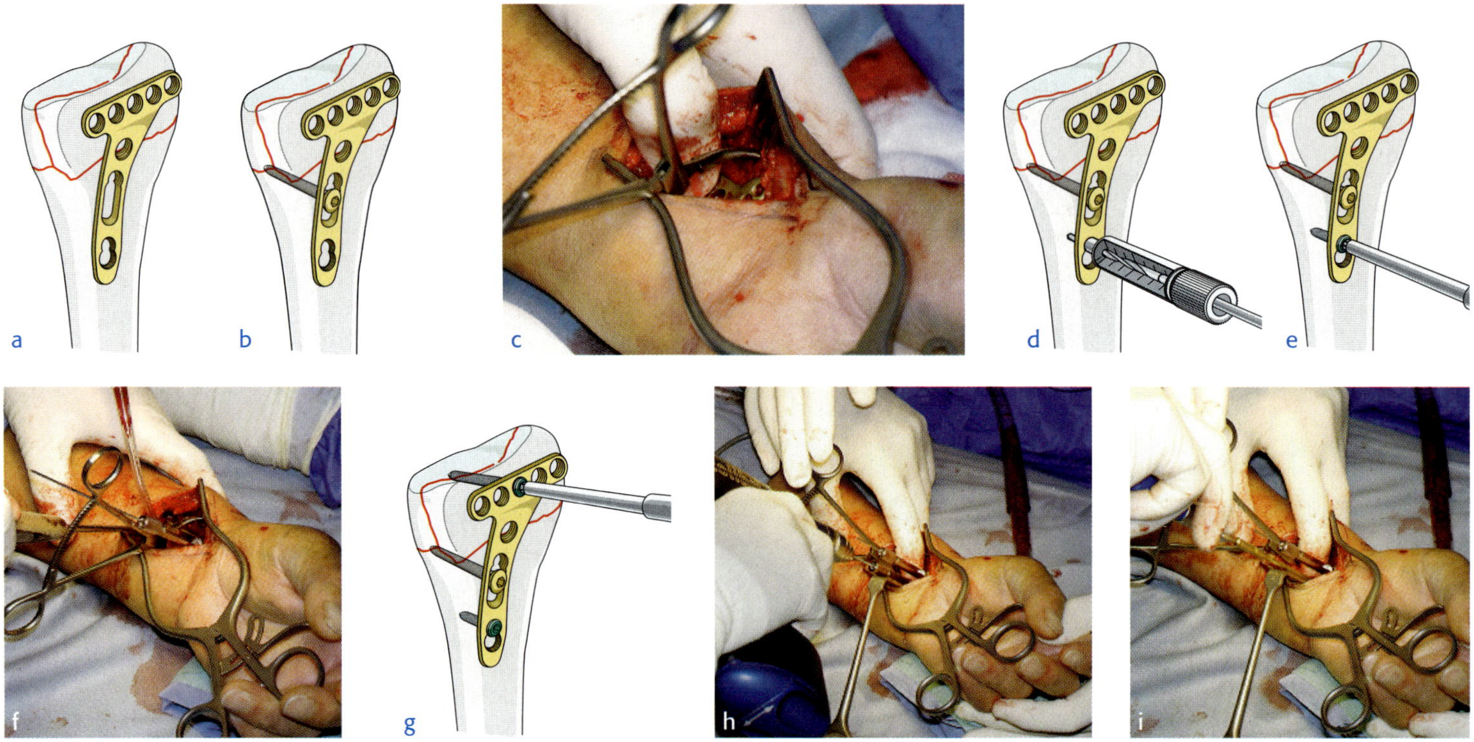

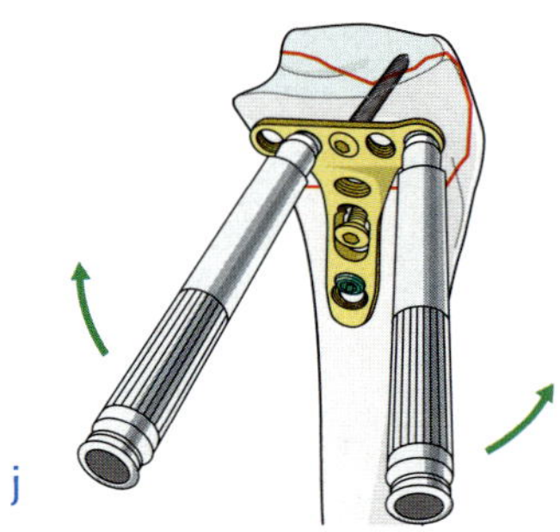

Fig 7.3.1-7a–l

a–c After manual reduction, the plate is placed in the correct position and fixed with a first cortex screw in the elongated plate hole in the radial shaft. Reduction and plate position are checked by fluoroscopy.

d–f As the correct plate position is determined and reduction is completed and secured using a K-wire (optional), the plate is definitively fixed with a second cortex or LHS in the most proximal hole of the plate.

g–j Internal fixation is completed by inserting the LHS in the distal part of the plate using the threaded drill guide. Care is to be taken when inserting the screws in order to obtain perfect purchase of the screw head in the threads of the plate.

4 Fixation (cont)

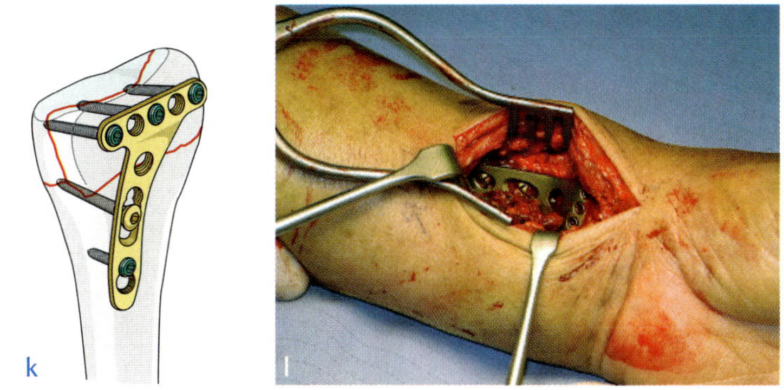

Fig 7.3.1-7a–l (cont)

k–l In osteoporotic bone insertion of five distal locking head screws is recommended. After documentation of the osteosynthesis by x-ray, the wound is closed and drained. A palmar or dorsal plaster splint is applied until the wound is healed.

5 Rehabilitation

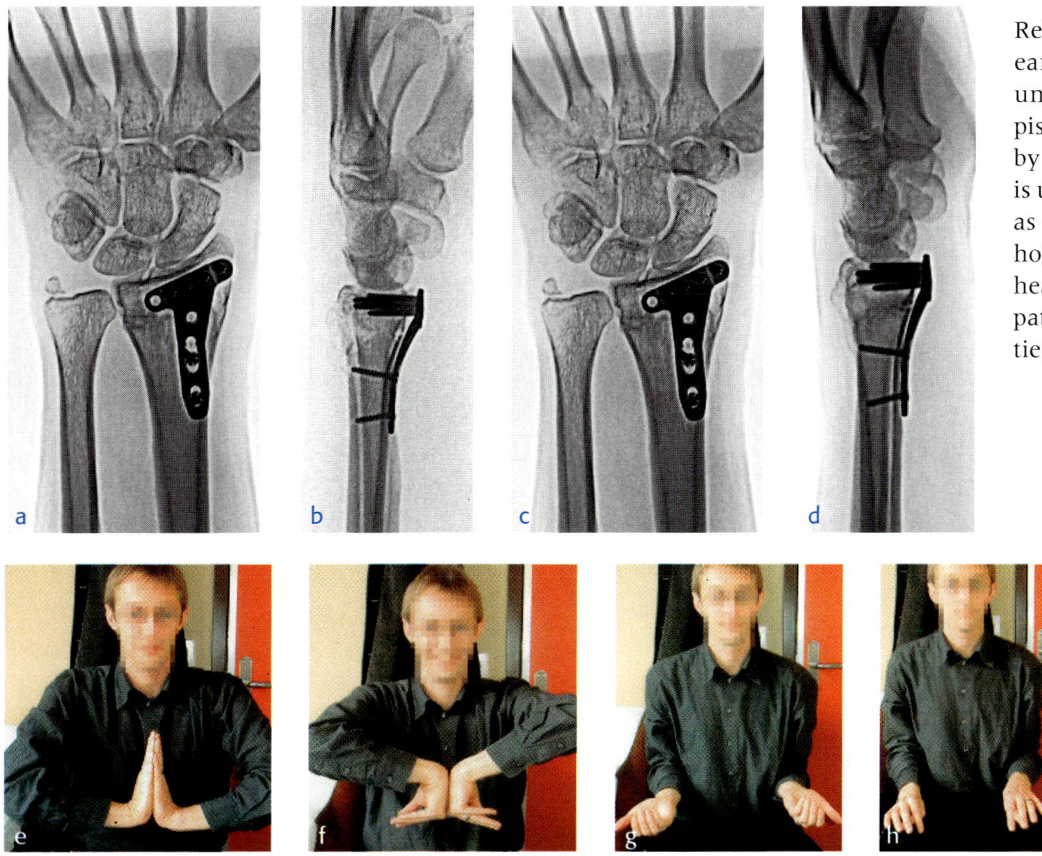

Rehabilitation consists of immediate early motion out of the plaster splint under the instruction of a physiotherapist. The plaster splint is later replaced by a removable velcro splint. The hand is used for unloaded daily activities such as eating, personal hygiene, tying a tie, holding paper. After six weeks fracture healing is documented by x-ray and the patient can usually start loaded activities.

Fig 7.3.1-8a–h

- a Postoperative x-ray after 1 week, AP view.
- b Postoperative x-ray after 1 week, lateral view.
- c Postoperative x-ray after 12 weeks, AP view.
- d Postoperative x-ray after 12 weeks, lateral view.
- e–h Functional results after 12 weeks.

6 Pitfalls –

Equipment

Fig 7.3.1-9 In some cases the radial "ear" of the T-arm of the plate should be bent back to avoid painful interference with the skin.

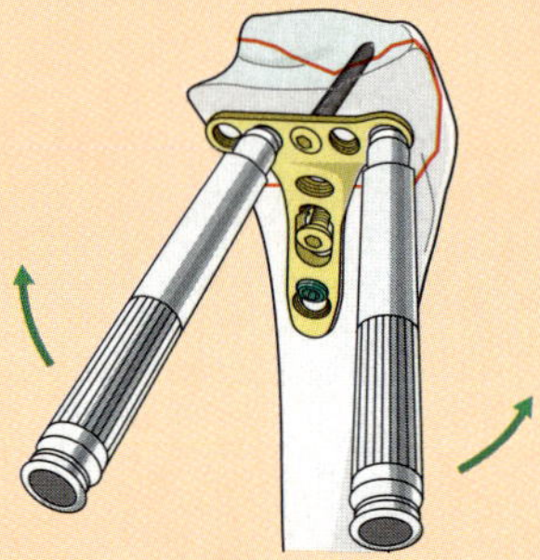

Reduction and fixation

Correct positioning of the plate must be checked by fluoroscopy to be sure that the radiocarpal joint is not penetrated by the distal LHS.

The LHS must be directed carefully in the correct direction in order to have perfect purchase of the screws heads in the plate hole. The screws must not be overtightened.

In very old people with osteoporotic bone and mental alteration the osteosynthesis should be protected by a closed plaster cast.

7 Pearls +

Equipment

Reduction and fixation

Fig 7.3.1-10a–b
Bone grafting is not necessary.

The technique is applicable also in osteoporotic bone.

A dorsally displaced Colles' fracture with simple, nondisplaced extension of the fracture into the radiocarpal joint can be treated in the same way. These injuries are usually caused by low energy bending forces and respond to manual ligamentotaxis for reduction.

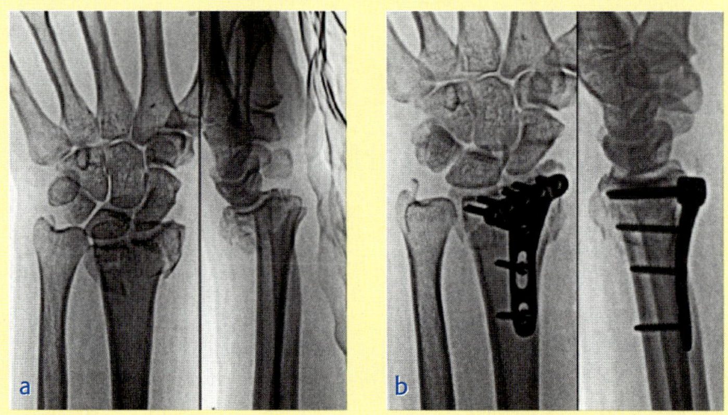

Author Christian Ryf

7.3.2 Extraarticular multifragmentary distal radial fracture—23-A3

1 Case description

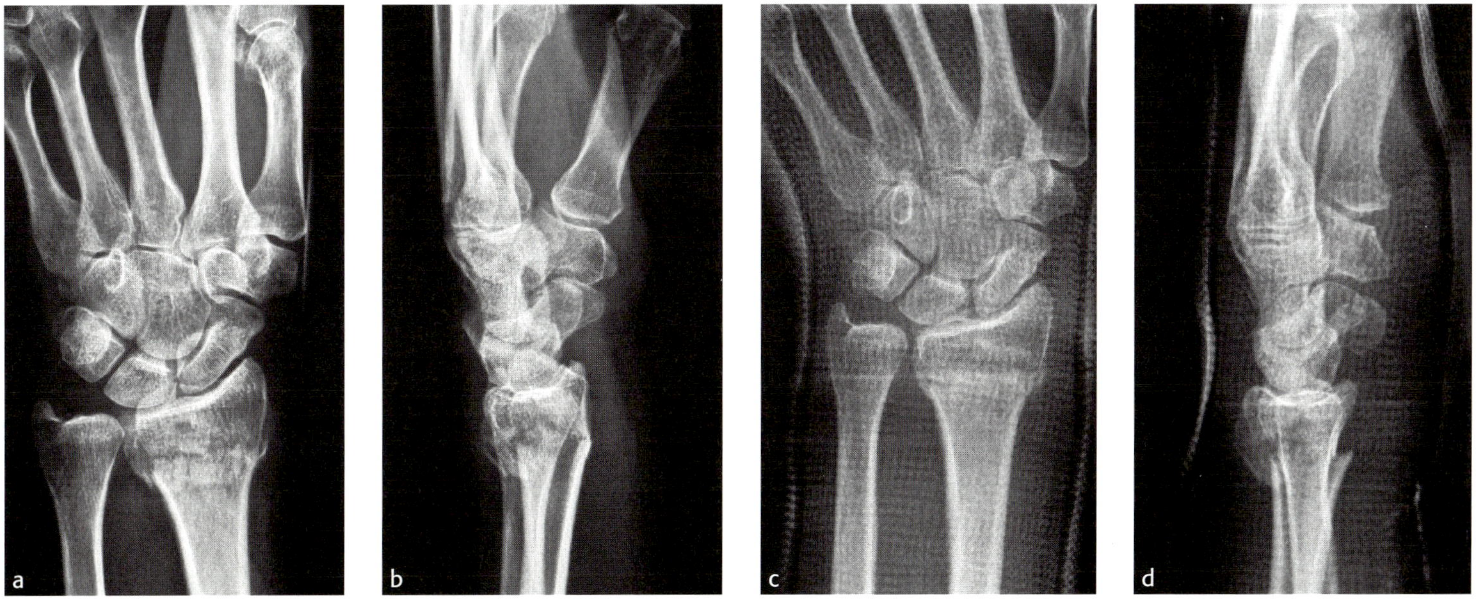

60-year-old woman fell while hiking and suffered a dorsally dislocated distal radial extraarticular fracture.

Fig 7.3.2-1a–d
- a Injury x-ray, AP view.
- b Injury x-ray, lateral view.
- c Fracture treated with cast, AP view.
- d Fracture treated with cast, lateral view.

Indication

Initially, the fracture was reduced closed and treated with a cast. In the further course the fracture dislocated, probably due to the multifragmentary zone dorsally. This is a clear indication for stabilization and plate osteosynthesis.
The palmar approach was preferred due to less critical anatomical structures.
The angular stable plate-screw combination offers a very good fixation, which can either be used dorsal or palmar.

Preoperative planning

Equipment

- LCP distal radius plate 2.4, 4 holes
- Locking head screws (LHS)

(Size of system, instruments, and implants can vary according to anatomy.)

Patient preparation and positioning

Antibiotics: single dose 2nd generation cephalosporin
Thrombosis prophylaxis: low-molecular heparin

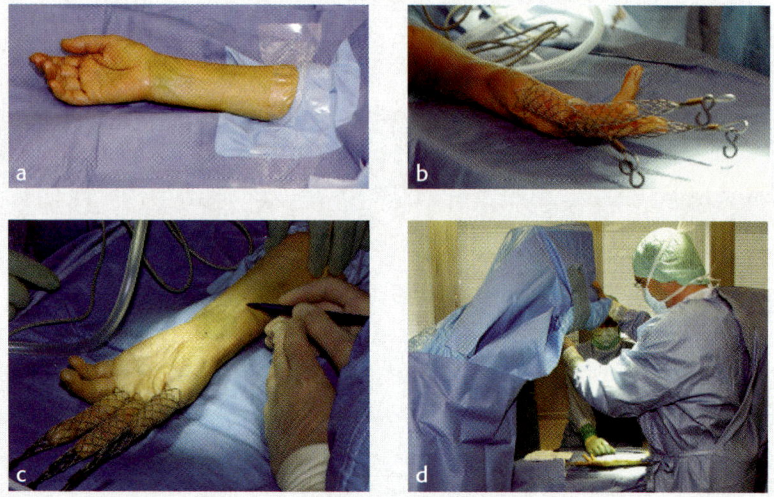

Fig 7.3.2-2a–d Patient in supine position, hand on hand table. Tourniquet. Extension of the forearm with finger traction.

- a Hand on hand table.
- b–c Finger traction.
- d Positioning of image intensifier.

2 Surgical approach

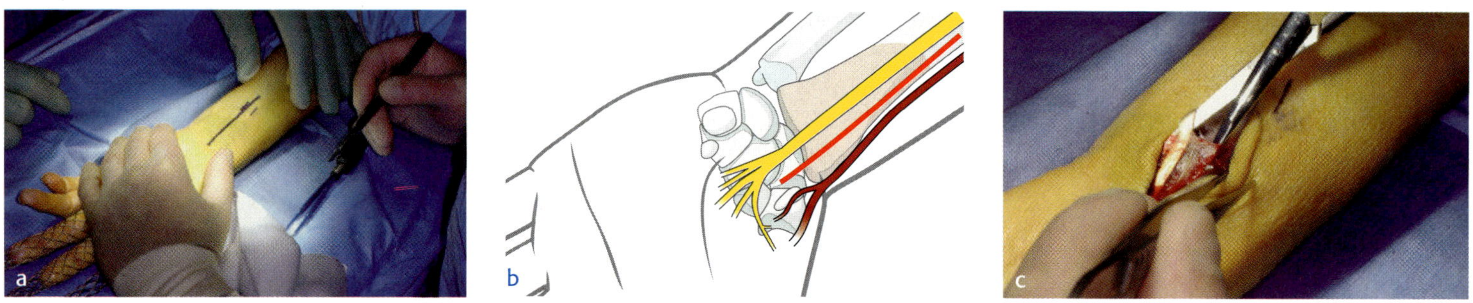

Fig 7.3.2-3a–f

- a–b Palmar approach: ulnar side of the palmaris longus tendon. Protection of the median nerve and the radial artery.
- c Retraction of the skin and exploration of the palmaris longus tendon.

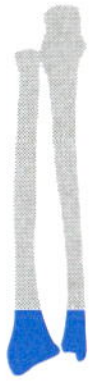

2 Surgical approach (cont)

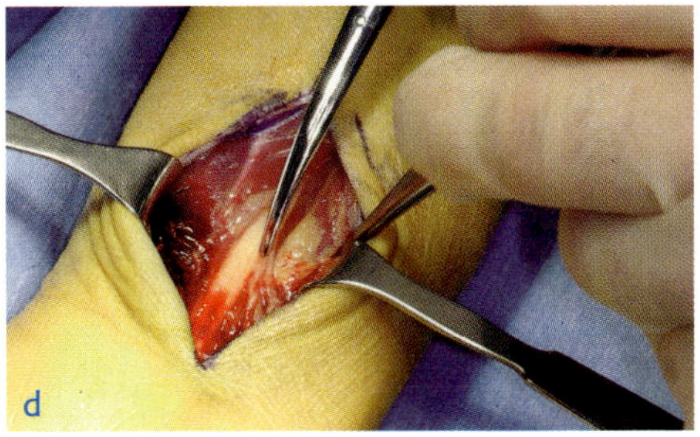

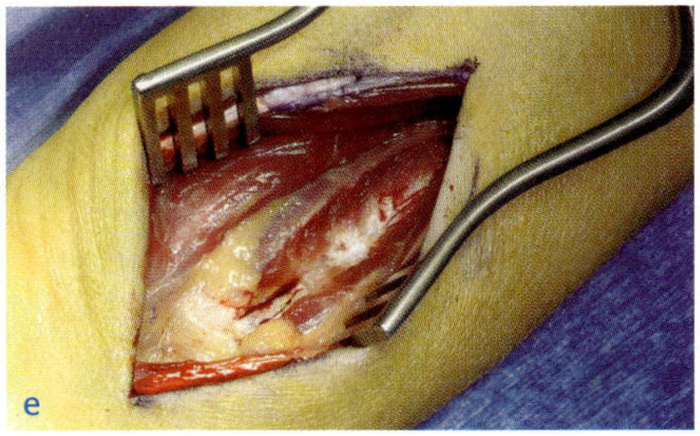

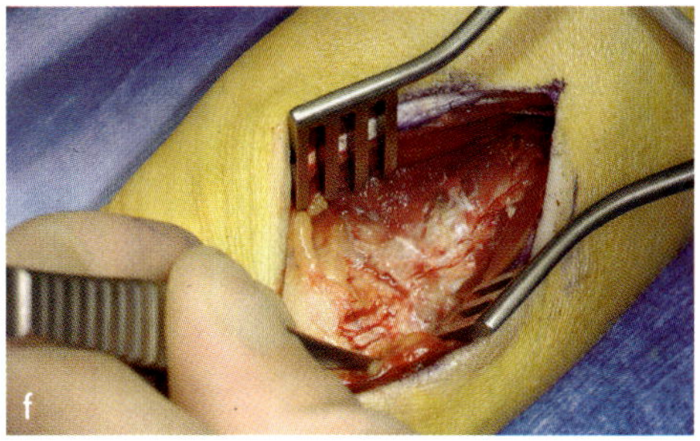

Fig 7.3.2-3a–f (cont)

d Inspection of the median nerve and protection of the palmar branches. The median nerve will be radially retracted.

e Incision of the pronator quadratus muscle.

f Exposure of the fracture zone.

3 Reduction

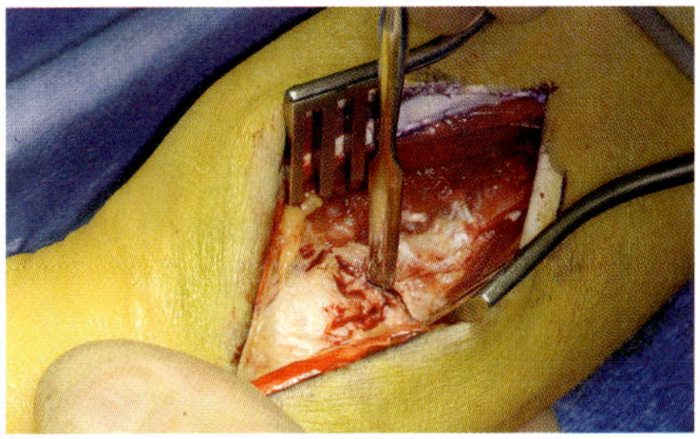

Fig 7.3.2-4 Reduction of the fracture with sharp hook and periosteal elevator.

4 Fixation

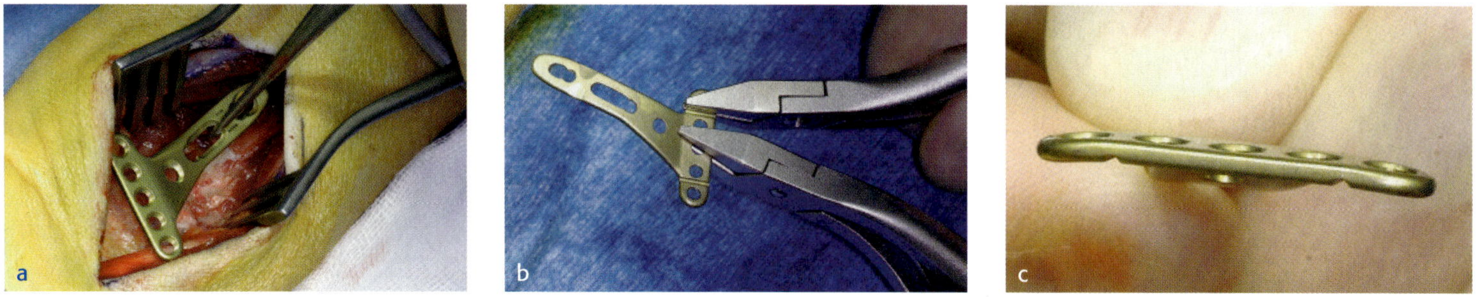

Fig 7.3.2-5a–p

a Positioning of the 4-hole LCP T-plate 2.4 in relation to the articular line and the fracture zone.

b–c Contouring of the T-part of the plate.

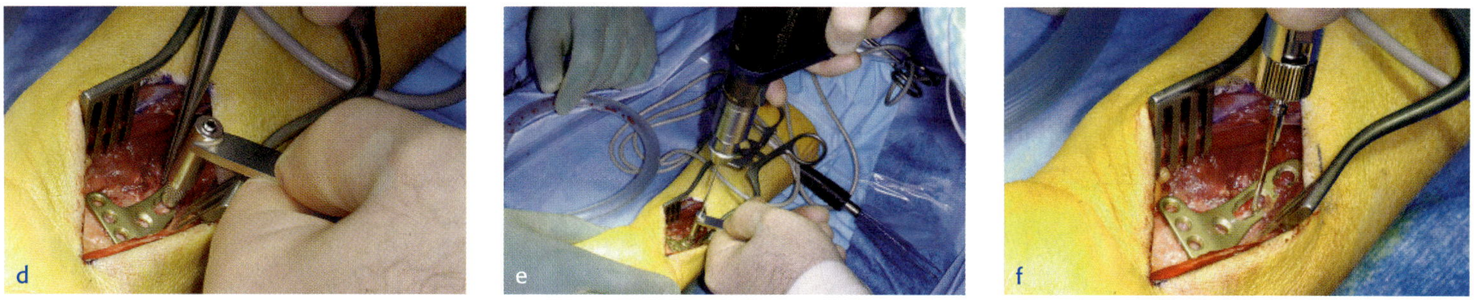

d–f The fixation starts with a cortex screw through the elongated plate hole. Predrilling the hole and measuring the length with the depth gauge.

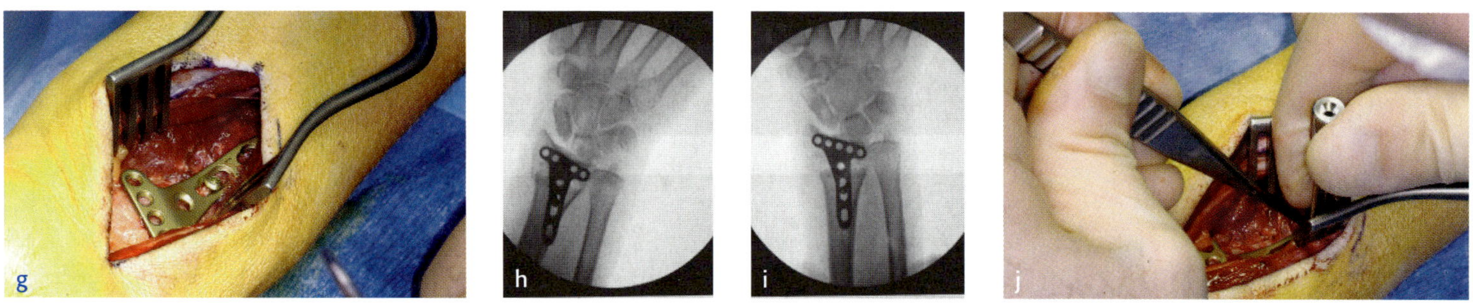

g Fixing the plate with a conventional screw to the radial shaft by tightening the screw not too much for further adjustments of the plate position.

h–j The definitive plate position is controlled with the image intensifier. Insert the drill guide in the most proximal hole (threaded part of the hole).

4 Fixation (cont)

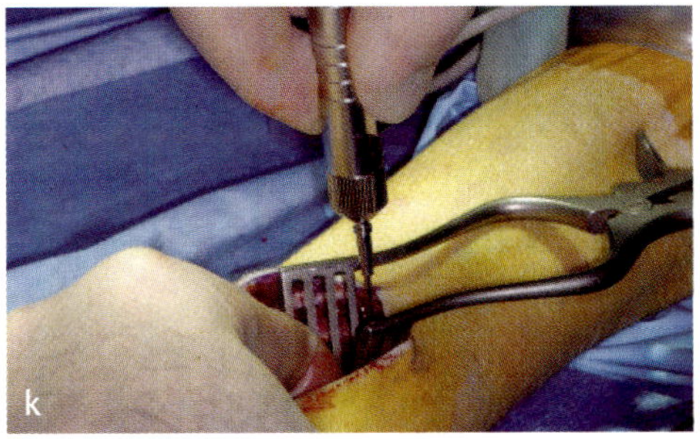
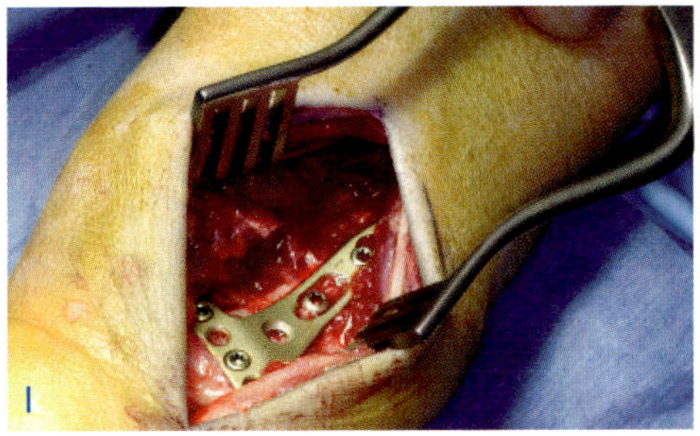
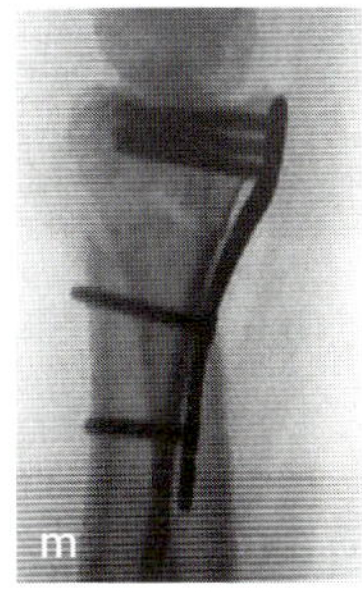

Fig 7.3.2-5a–p (cont)

k Measure the length of the hole for the locking head screw with depth gauge.

l–m Fixation of the articular block by inserting three locking head screws.

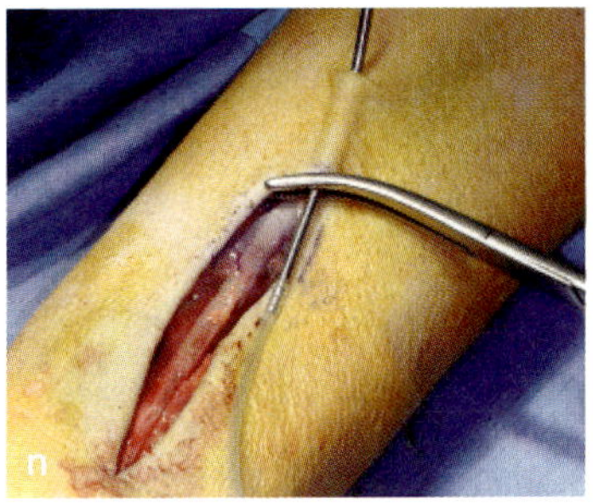
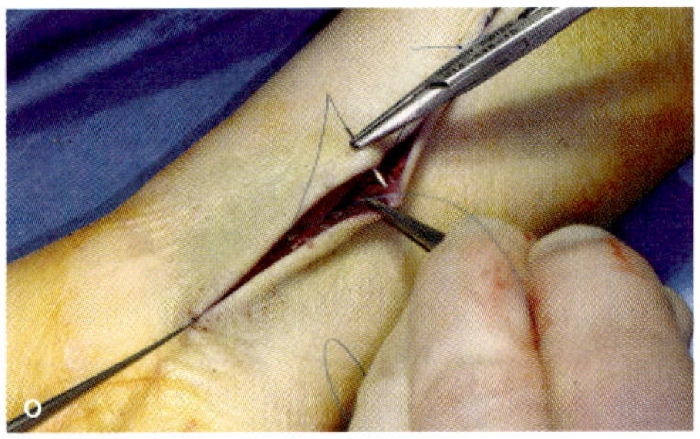
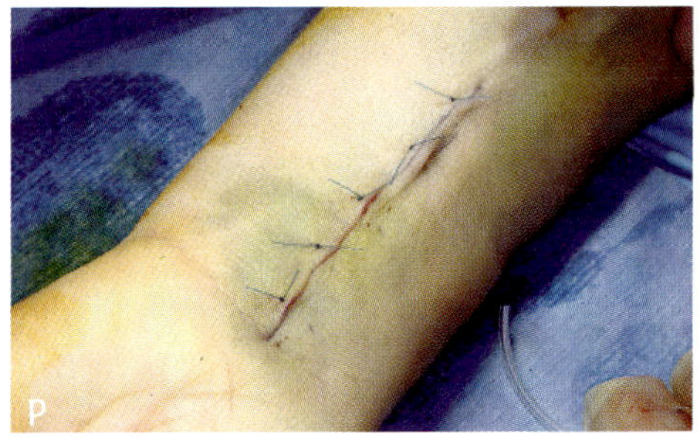

n Superficially inserted Manovac drainage

o–p Skin closure.

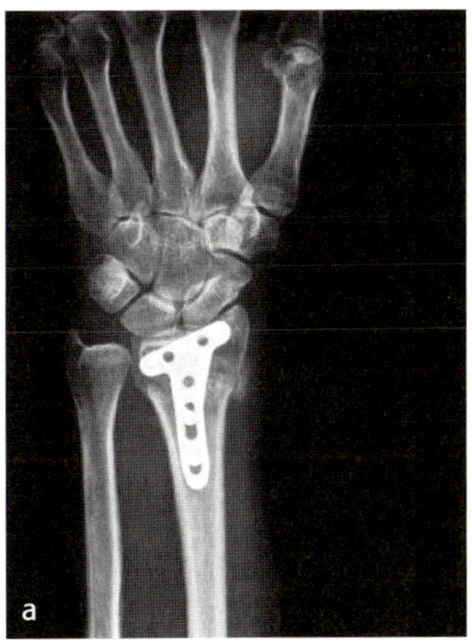
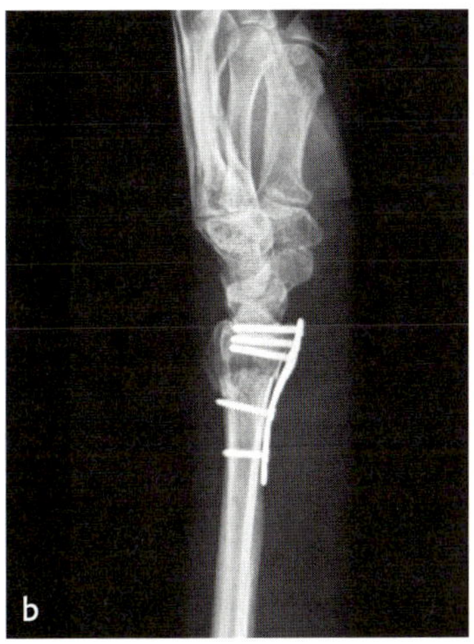

Fig 7.3.2-6a–b Postoperative x-rays after 4 weeks.

a AP view.

b Lateral view.

5 Rehabilitation

Additional immobilization: none, no weight bearing for 4 weeks.

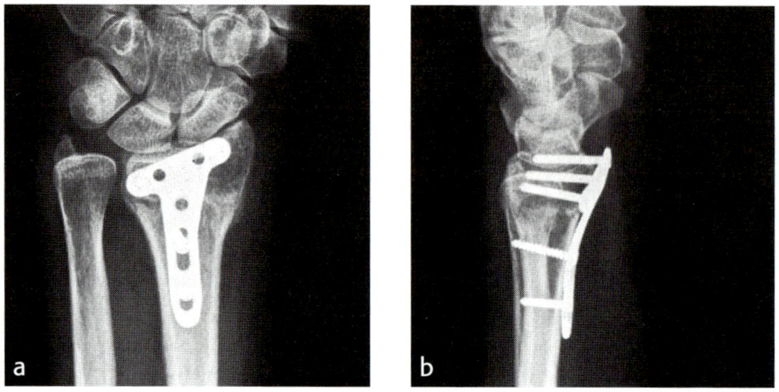

Fig 7.3.2-7a–b Postoperative x-rays after 6 months.
a AP view.
b Lateral view.

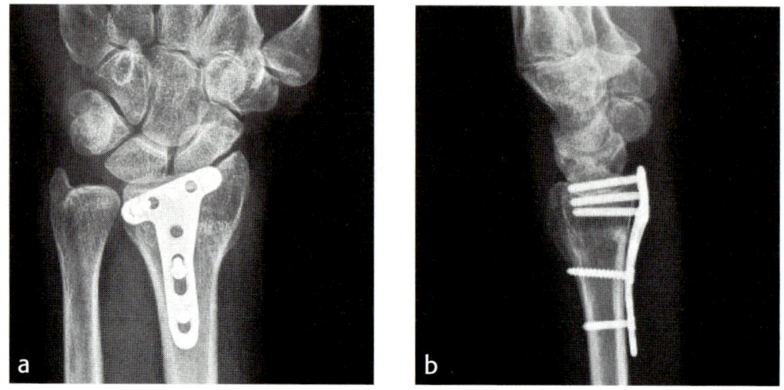

Fig 7.3.2-8a–b Postoperative x-rays after 12 months.
a AP view.
b Lateral view.

6 Pitfalls –

Approach

The radial artery and vein are present at the lateral edge of the wound and are at risk of injury.
If dissection strays medially, the median nerve may be encountered.

Reduction and fixation

Unstable, dorsally-angulated osteoporotic fractures may not be adequately stable following palmar plating alone. The dorsal angulation may be difficult to fully correct by direct methods.

Rehabilitation

Wrist range of motion may be diminished following distal radial fractures, particularly with intraarticular fractures.

7 Pearls +

Approach

Part of the approach entails carefully exposing the radial nerve to visualize its course, and gently retracting it laterally.
If dissection stays within the tendon sheath of the flexor carpi radialis muscle, the median nerve should not be in the operative field.

Reduction and fixation

To restore the anatomical 11° palmar tilt, the LCP may be used to aid reduction. Place the distal LHS in correct position in the epiphysis, leaving the proximal plate several millimeters off the bone. Clamp the proximal plate to the bone to achieve further palmar tilt.

Rehabilitation

To maximize rehabilitation potential, place the patient in a removable palmar wrist splint early and begin aggressive active range of motion exercises.

Authors Michael S Gardner, Dean L Lorich, David L Helfet

7.3.3 Partial articular distal radial fracture—23-B3

1 Case description

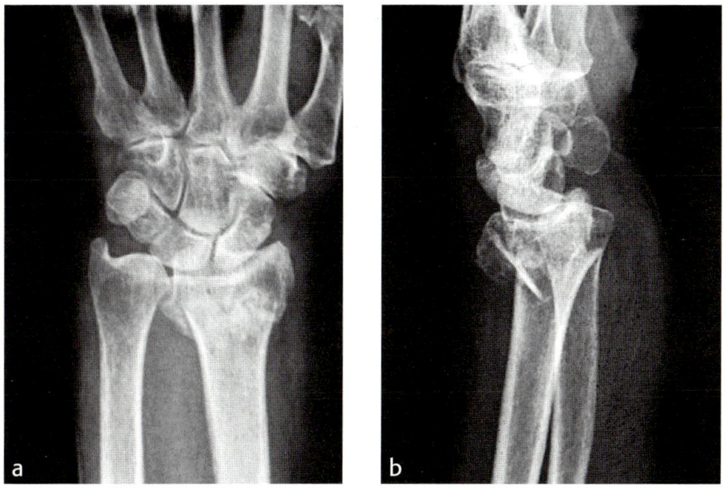

67-year-old woman (dominant right hand) slipped in a store and landed on her dorsiflexed right hand. She came to the emergency department complaining of pain and deformity. No neurological signs or skin compromise were present.

Fig 7.3.3-1a–b
a AP view.
b Lateral view.

Indication

The intraarticular displacement and impaction warrants anatomical reduction and fixation to minimize the risk of the development of osteoarthrosis.
In addition, the metaphyseal comminution makes this fracture highly unstable, and warrants internal stabilization to ensure anatomical alignment.

Preoperative planning

Equipment
- LCP distal radius plate 2.4, 2 holes
- Reconstruction plate 2.4, 7 holes
- 3.5 mm cortex screw
- Locking head screws (LHS)

(Size of system, instruments, and implants can vary according to anatomy.)

Patient preparation and positioning
Antibiotics: single dose 2nd generation cephalosporin
Thrombosis prophylaxis: none

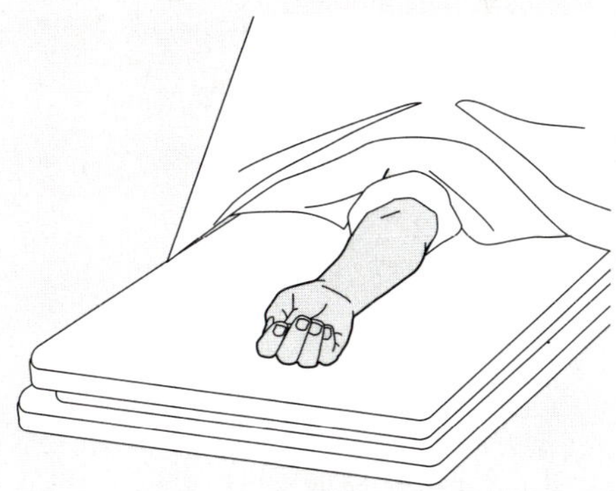

Fig 7.3.3-2 The patient is positioned supine on the table, with the limb extended and supported on a hand table. A tourniquet is placed on the proximal arm. The extremity is prepped and draped free.

2 Surgical approach

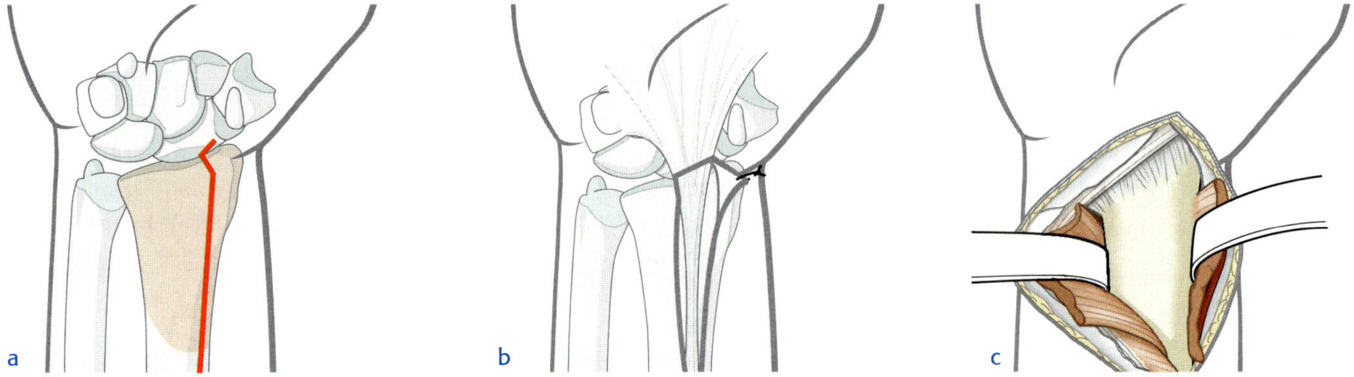

Fig 7.3.3-3a–c Make a longitudinal incision on the palmar forearm, 6–8 cm long, from the wrist crease proximally.

Dissect through the subcutaneous layer to identify the tendon sheath of the flexor carpi radialis muscle. In this position the radial artery will be lateral and is often visible in the surgical field. The median nerve is medial.

Expose the muscle fibers of the flexor carpi radialis muscle and retract them laterally. If proximal extension is needed, the flexor digitorum superficialis muscle will need to be retracted laterally as well.

Retraction of these muscles reveals the pronator quadratus muscle. Elevate this muscle subperiosteally and reflect it medially, exposing the volar surface of the distal radius.

Expose distally enough to visualize the palmar wrist capsule, taking care not to violate it.

In unstable, severely multifragmentary fractures, the surgeon may wish to apply a radial styloid plate to strengthen fixation. If this is necessary, reflect several slips of the brachioradialis tendon insertion while protecting the radial artery to allow exposure of the lateral side of the distal radius.

3 Reduction and fixation

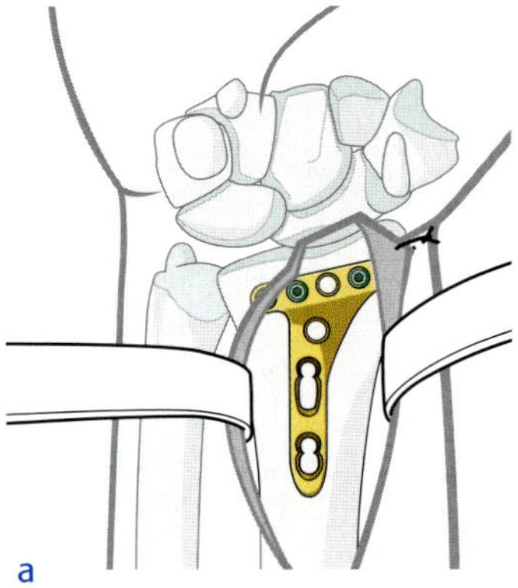

Fig 7.3.3-4a–b

a For the common dorsally-angulated and shortened distal radial fracture, the distal fragment needs to be disimpacted, palmarly flexed and tilted ulnarly. This can usually be accomplished through manual traction, flexion and ulnar deviation. Assess the accuracy of reduction on AP and lateral fluoroscopy.

Place the LCP distal radius plate 2.4 on the palmar surface of the distal fragment. Attach the threaded guide wires to use as a handle and slide the plate distally so it abuts on the palmar wrist capsule.

Use fluoroscopy to estimate the ideal plate placement. Place a cortex screw through the ovoid plate hole into the proximal fragment, and tighten it partially, grossly correcting the palmar flexion deformity.

Slide the plate to fine tune the length and reduction, and tighten the screw in the ovoid hole to press the plate onto the bone. Place a second cortex screw proximally to secure the plate and the reduction.

3 Reduction and fixation (cont)

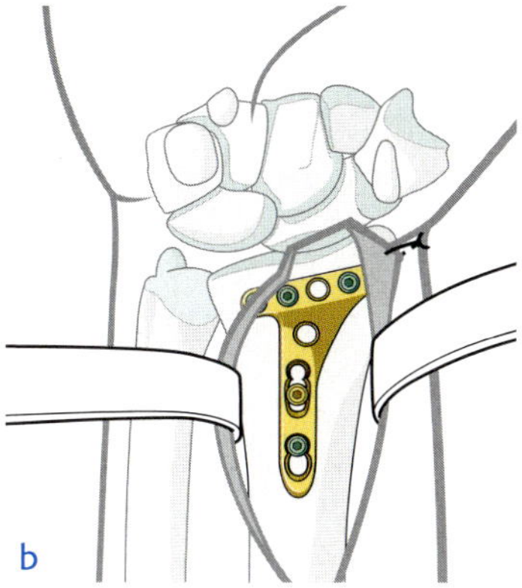

b

Fig 7.3.3-4a–b (cont) When metaphyseal comminution exists and the fracture is unstable, augment fixation on the radial column by contouring a 6- or 7-hole reconstruction plate 2.4 to the radial styloid. Release part of the brachioradialis muscle insertion for exposure.
First place a cortex screw at the apex of the fract ure into the proximal fragment to correct the radial inclination.
Stabilize the plate position by placing a second cortex screw proximally.

b With the radial inclination corrected, fine palmar tune volar flexion by wrist manipulation under fluoroscopic guidance. Place guide wires through the threaded drill guides into the distal fragment of the palmar plate.
After predrilling through the guides, place the LHS into the distal fragment.
Finally, return to the radial styloid plate. Insert a 2.4 mm cortex screw distally from radial to ulnar in between the previously placed palmar plate LHS.
Use a bone substitute to fill the void in the metaphyseal bone and add stability if necessary.
Release the tourniquet and obtain meticulous hemostasis. Ensure the radial vascular bundle has not been injured. Reapproximate the pronator quadratus muscle over the plate, and close the incision over a deep suction drain.

4 Rehabilitation

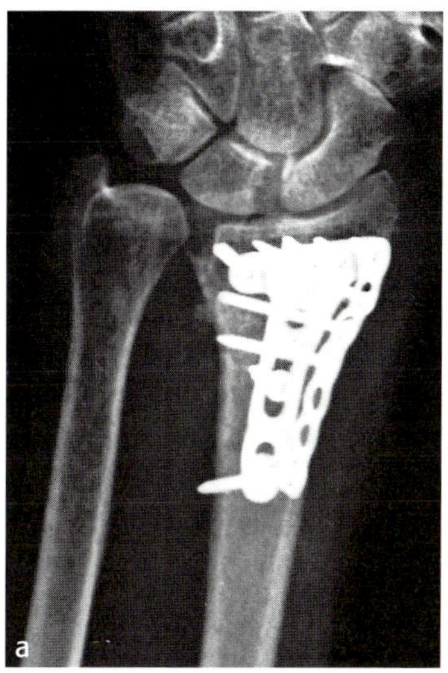

a

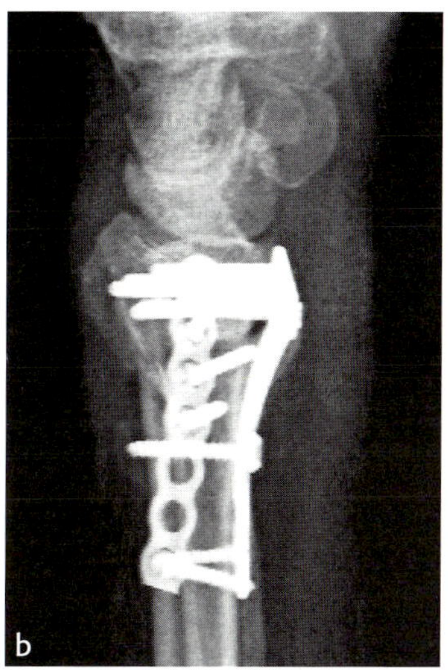

b

Place the forearm in a plaster splint and ace wrap and elevate the extremity.
Initiate physiotherapy immediately, including finger and elbow active and passive range of motion.
10–14 days postoperatively, remove the splint and check the wound. Place the patient in a removable wrist splint, and incorporate active wrist flexion, extension, supination, and pronation exercises into the therapy regimen.

Fig 7.3.3-5a–b Open reduction through a palmar approach and internal fixation with a palmar locking plate and radial styloid plate was performed. 4 months following surgery, the patient had excellent wrist range of motion and function.

5 Pitfalls –

Approach

The radial artery and vein are present at the lateral edge of the wound and are at risk of injury.

If dissection strays medially, the median nerve may be encountered.

Reduction and fixation

Unstable, dorsally-angulated osteoporotic fractures may not be adequately stable following palmar plating alone.

The dorsal angulation may be difficult to fully correct by direct methods.

Rehabilitation

Wrist range of motion may be diminished following distal radial fractures, particularly with intraarticular fractures.

6 Pearls +

Approach

Part of the approach entails carefully exposing the radial nerve to visualize its course, and gently retracting it laterally.

If dissection stays within the tendon sheath of the flexor carpi radialis muscle, the median nerve should not be in the operative field.

Reduction and fixation

To restore the anatomical 11° palmar tilt, the locking plate may be used to aid reduction. Place the distal locking head screws in correct position in the epiphysis, leaving the proximal plate several millimeters off the bone. Clamp the proximal plate to the bone to achieve further palmar tilt.

Rehabilitation

To maximize rehabilitation potential, place the patient in a removable palmar wrist splint early and begin aggressive active range of motion exercises.

Author Michael Wagner

7.3.4 Complete articular simple, metaphyseal simple distal radial fracture—23-C1

1 Case description

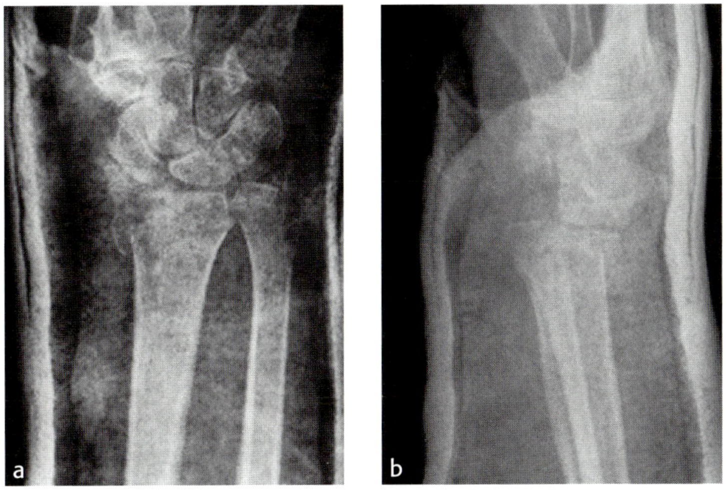

65-year-old woman fell and sustained injuries to the right wrist and the right ribs.

Fig 7.3.4-1a–b Fracture treated with cast.
a AP view.
b Lateral view.

Indication

C1-type fracture of the distal radius with dorsoulnar fragment and dorsal tilt. Failure of the primary conservative treatment attempt with reduction and cast application due to repeated dorsal tilting of the distal fragment.

Preoperative planning

Equipment

- LCP distal radius plate 2.4, 3 holes
- 2.4 mm locking head screws (LHS)
- 3.5 mm cortex screw
- 2.0 mm K-wire

(Size of system, instruments, and implants can vary according to anatomy.)

Patient preparation and positioning

Antibiotics: none
Thrombosis prophylaxis: low-molecular heparin

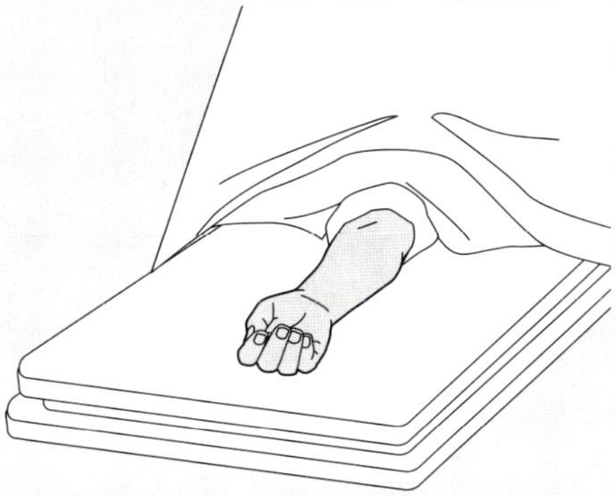

Fig 7.3.4-2 The patient is positioned supine on the table, with the limb extended and supported on a hand table.

2 Surgical approach

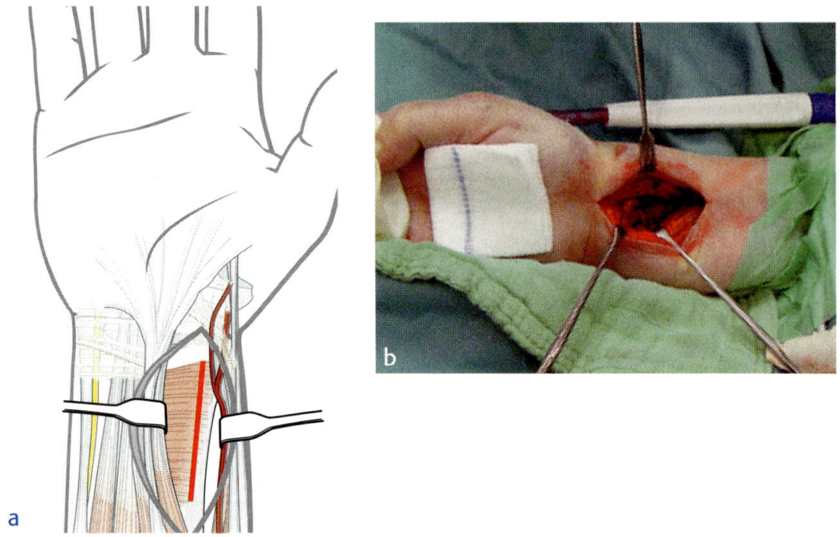

Fig 7.3.4-3a–b Palmar approach to the distal radius. Straight incision between the radial artery and the tendon of the flexor carpi radialis muscle.

3 Reduction and fixation

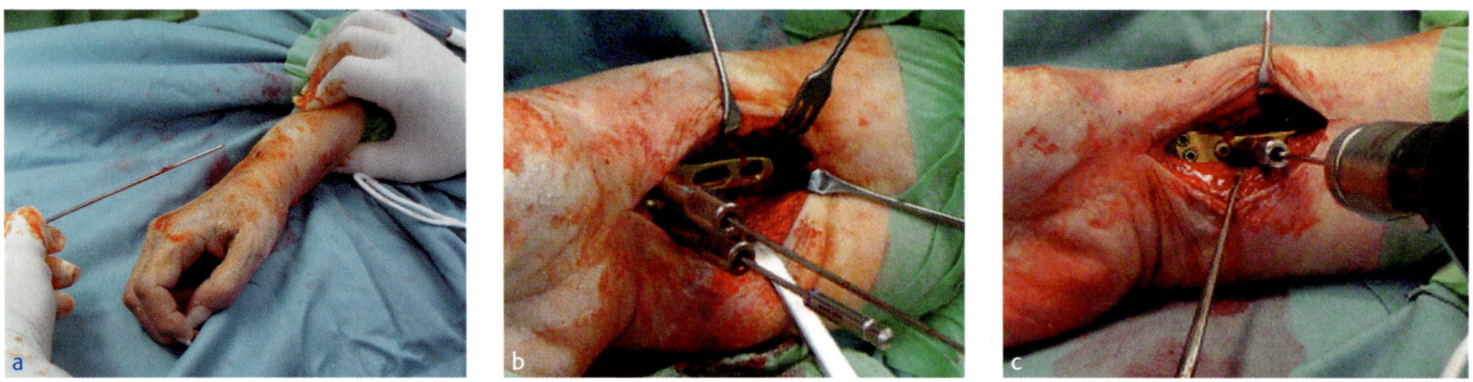

Fig 7.3.4-4a–c

a Direct percutaneous reduction with the aid of a 2.0 mm K-wire in the "Kaparandji" technique. One 2.0 mm K-wire is inserted from a dorsal direction through the fracture gap into the intramedullary space of the proximal shaft fragment. This reduction technique corrects the dorsal tilt of the distal fragment.

b Fixation of the plate to the distal fragment with a total of five LHS. Then definitive reduction with the aid of a cortex screw.

c Completion of osteosynthesis with LHS in the shaft fragment. Also the cortex screw (reduction screw) was changed to a LHS.

4 Rehabilitation

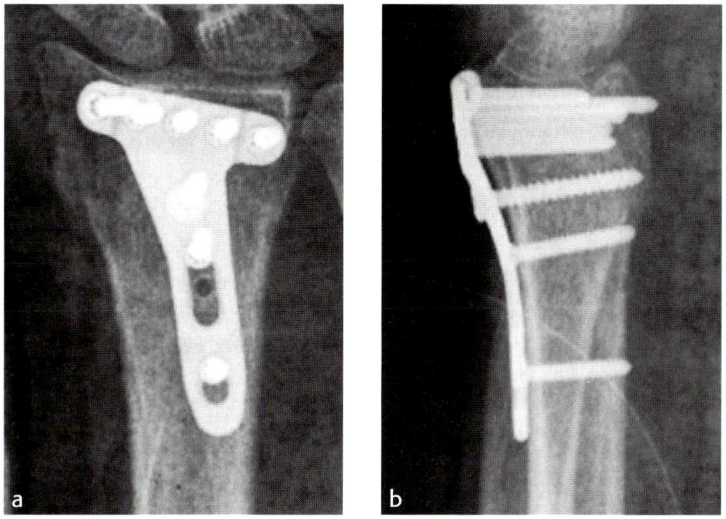

Fig 7.3.4-5a–b Postoperative x-rays after 1 day.
a AP view.
b Lateral view.

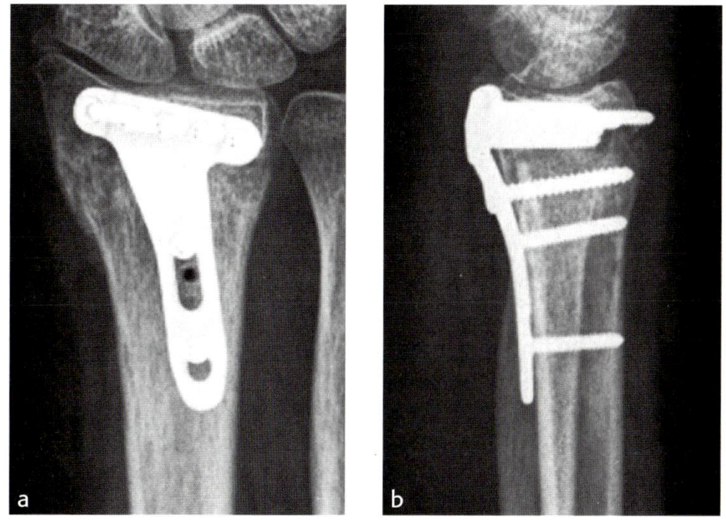

Fig 7.3.4-6a–b Postoperative x-rays after 4 weeks.
a AP view.
b Lateral view.

Postoperative immobilization in cast until suture removal.

5 Pitfalls –

Equipment
Fig 7.3.4-7 In some cases the radial "ear" of the T-arm of the plate should be bent back to avoid painful interference with the skin.

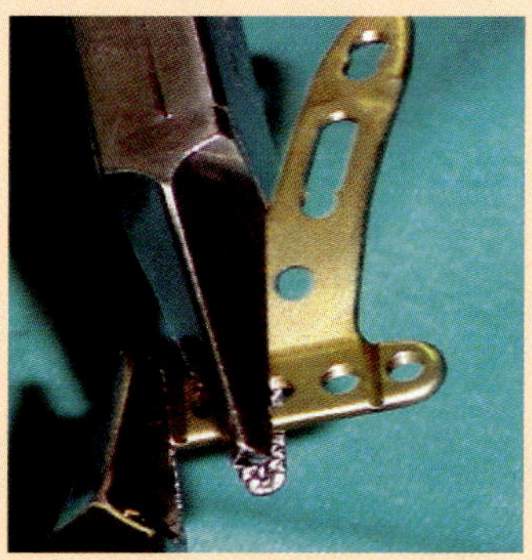

6 Pearls +

Equipment
The anatomically preshaped LCP may be used to aid reduction.

5 Pitfalls – (cont)

Reduction and fixation
Correct positioning of the plate must be checked with fluoroscopy in order not to penetrate the radiocarpal joint with the distal screws.

The LHS must be directed carefully in the correct direction in order to have perfect purchase of the screws in the plate. The screws must not be overtightened.

In very old people with osteoporotic bone and mental alteration the osteosynthesis should be protected by a plaster cast or splint.

6 Pearls + (cont)

Reduction and fixation
Most of the unstable, dorsally-angulated osteoporotic fractures may be treated by palmar plating with an angular stable screw plate device alone.

Bone grafting is not necessary.

The technique is applicable also in osteoporotic bone.

Author Daniel Rikli

7.3.5 Complex articular multifragmentary distal radial fracture—23-C3; dorsal double plating

1 Case description

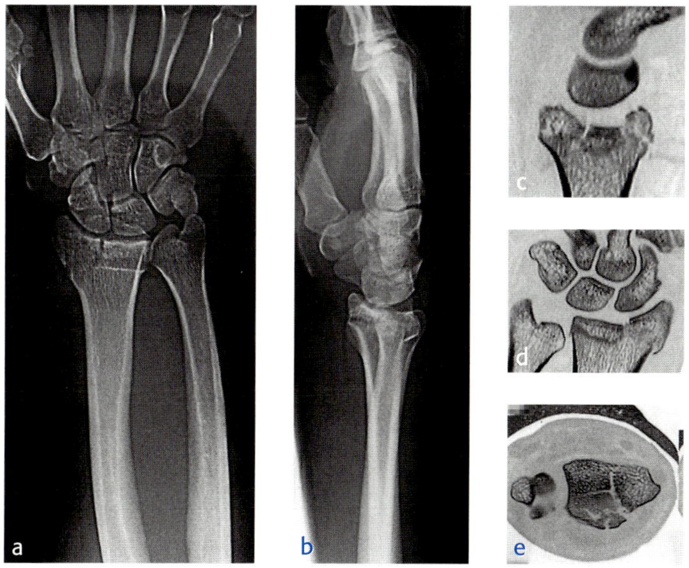

f

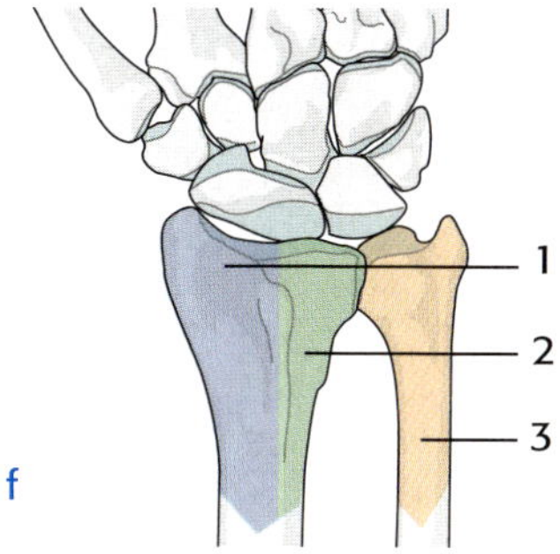

40-year-old patient fell from a ladder. Dorsally impacted intraarticular fracture of the distal radius. Intraarticular fracture of the distal radius with impaction of articular fragments into the metaphysis (23-C3), dorsal double plating.

Fig 7.3.5-1a–f
- a AP view.
- b Lateral view.
- c–e CT scans show slight impaction of the intermediate column.
- f Schematic representation of the distal radial columns: (1) radial column, (2) intermediate column, (3) ulnar column.

Indication

High energy axial forces lead to impaction of articular fragments into the metaphyseal cancellous bone. According to the three column model, the intermediate column (IC) is divided into two main fragments (dorso-ulnar, palmar-ulnar). The dorsoulnar fragment is centrally impacted. The radial styloid is separated (radial column RC). These articular fragments do not responsed to ligamentotaxis. Formal open revision is indicated to reconstruct the radiocarpal joint surface (IC) under vision. Additionally, this type of injury can be combined with a relevant ligamentous injury to the proximal carpal row. These ligaments can be revised during the dorsal approach by arthrotomy.

Preoperative planning

Equipment
- LCP distal radius plate 2.4, 6 holes
- LCP distal radius plate 2.4, 4 holes
- Small external fixator (optional)

(Size of system, instruments, and implants can vary according to anatomy.)

Patient preparation and positioning

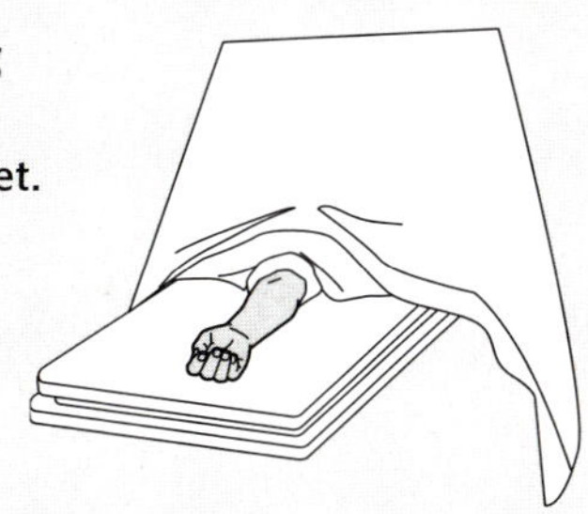

Fig 7.3.5-2 Supine forearm on hand table. Nonsterile pneumatic tourniquet. Prophylactic antibiotics optional.

2 Surgical approach

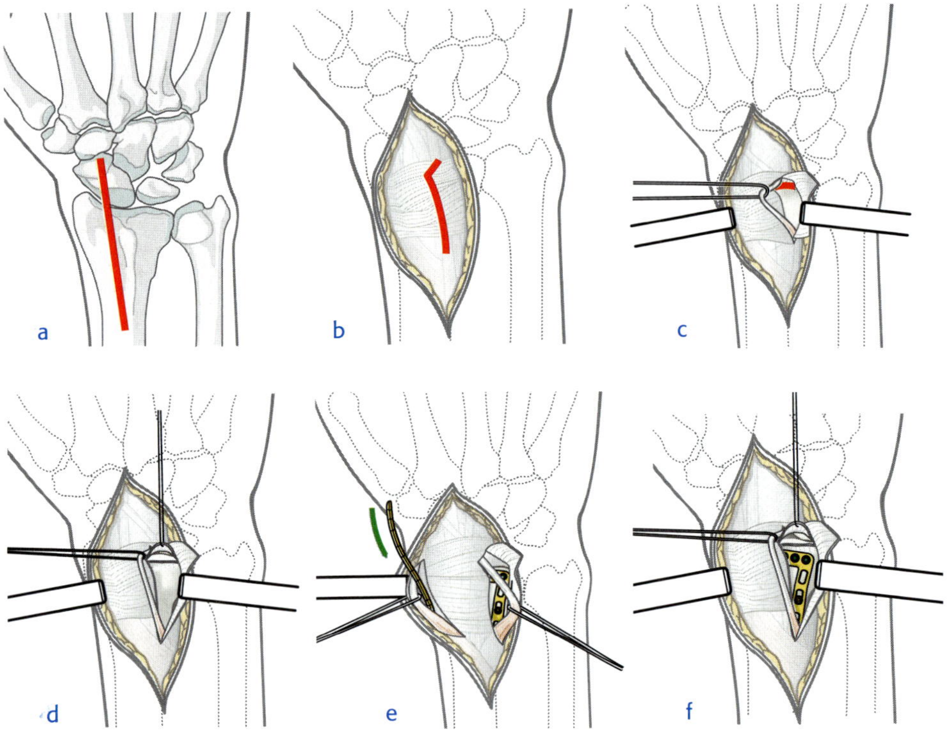

Fig 7.3.5-3a–f

a–d A straight dorsal incision is performed centered over the distal radius. The subcutaneous tissue is divided. To access the intermediate column, the extensor retinaculum is incised along the course of the extensor pollicis longus (EPL) tendon. The z-shape incision, as depicted, spares the distal portion of the tendon sheath to preserve the deflected course of the tendon and allows a flap drawn to be underneath the EPL tendon during closure in order to protect this tendon from the plate. The EPL tendon is freed and retracted with an eleastic thread. Preparation of the intermediate column is now strictly subperiosteal. The 2nd compartment is not touched.

e–f Access to the radial column: preparation between skin flap and retinaculum towards radial, take care of the superficial radial nerve which is always visible in the skin flap. The 1st compartment is incised and the abductor pollicis longus and extensor pollicis brevis tendons are freed enough for a S-plate to be slipped underneath in order to buttress the radial column. Note that the 2nd compartment is left untouched.

3 Reduction

A transverse arthrotomy exposes the radiocarpal joint surface at the level of the lunate facette and, partially, the scaphoid facette. The proximal carpal row can be revised for any ligamentous injury. The radiocarpal joint is now reconstructed under direct vision by levering the articular fragments towards the carpal row. Any step-off or gap should be eliminated. The dorsal cortical shells help to define length and serve as a buttress after reduction. Single fragments can optionally be fixed temporarily with small K-wires.

Distraction of the wrist using an external fixator is very helpful during reconstruction of the joint surface.

Reduction is checked by image intensification.

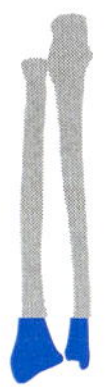

4 Fixation

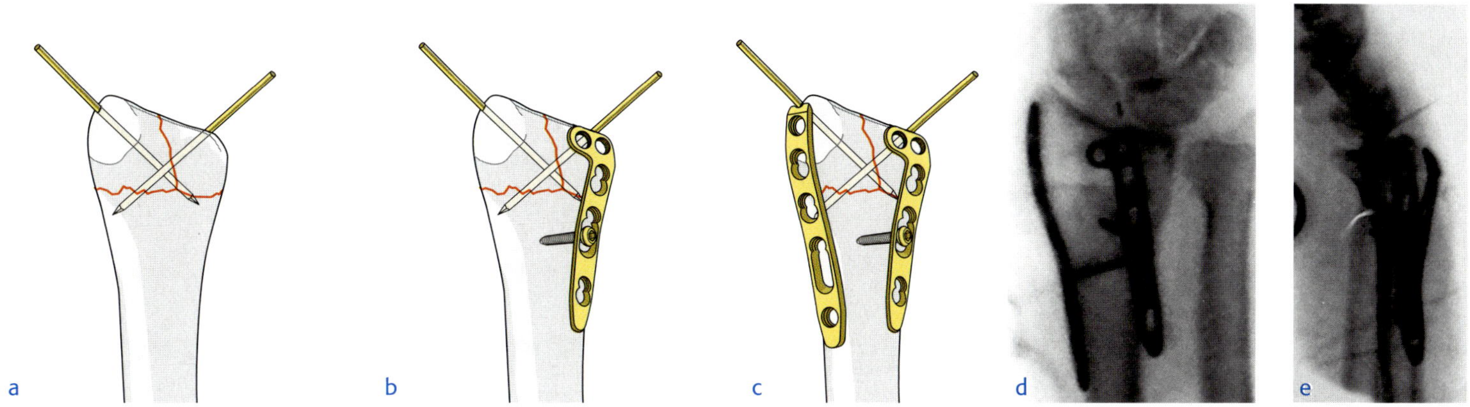

Fig 7.3.5-4a–e

a After reduction and preliminary fixation of the intermediate column an LCP L-plate or T-plate is chosen according to the anatomical configuration and need for fixation of fragments. The plate is precontoured, usually it has to be bent back at the distal end and twisted in itself. The plate is fixed with a first cortex screw in the elongated plate hole in the radial shaft.

b–e Now, the radial column is buttressed with a precontoured S-plate slipped underneath the tendons of the first compartment. The plate is fixed with a first cortex screw in the elongated plate hole in the radial shaft. Reduction and plate positioning is checked by fluoroscopy.

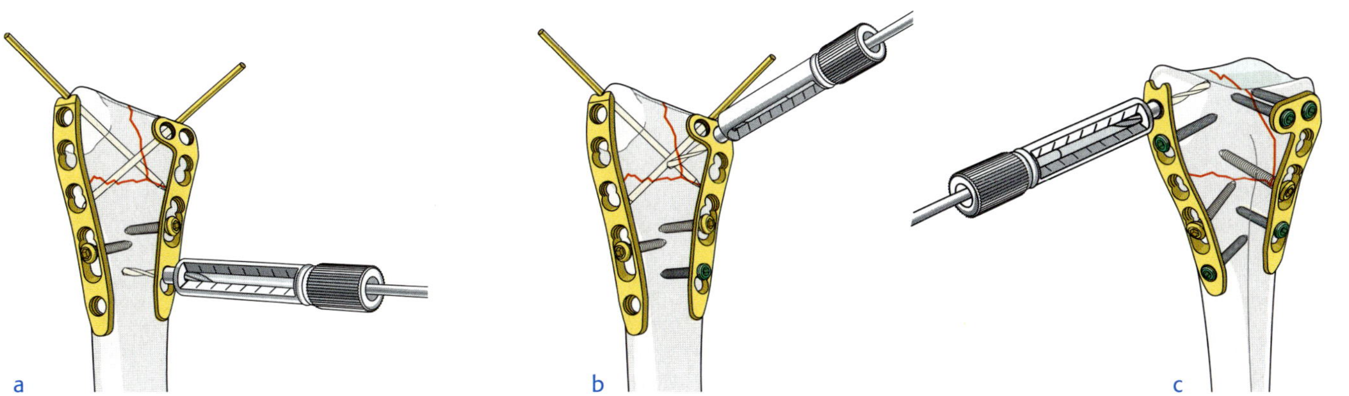

Fig 7.3.5-5a–e

a–c After correct reduction and plate positioning has been documented by fluoroscopy, the position of the plate is secured by applying a second cortex or locking head screw in the most proximal hole in the shaft. Only then is placement of the distal locking head screws started.

The distal locking head screws in the transverse part of the T- or L-plate support the radiocarpal joint surface. An additional bone graft to fill the metaphyseal defect is not required.

4 Fixation (cont)

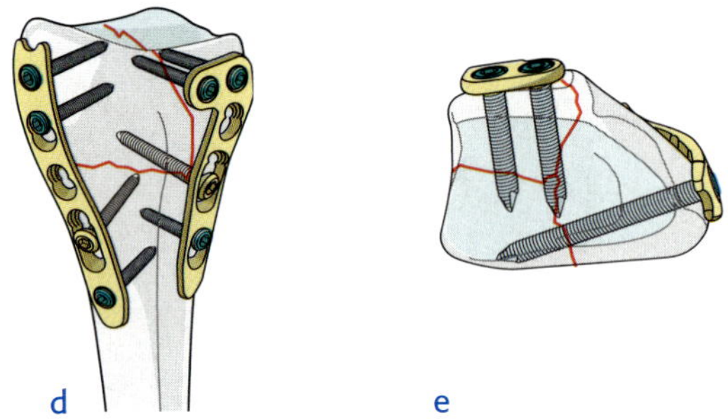

Fig 7.3.5-5a–e (cont)

d–e The wound is closed in layers. The EPL tendon is partially transposed subcutaneously by creating a retinaculum flap that covers the plate. Suction drainage is used. Only now is the external fixator, if applicable, withdrawn. A removable plaster splint is applied until the wound is clean and the pain has subsided.

5 Rehabilitation

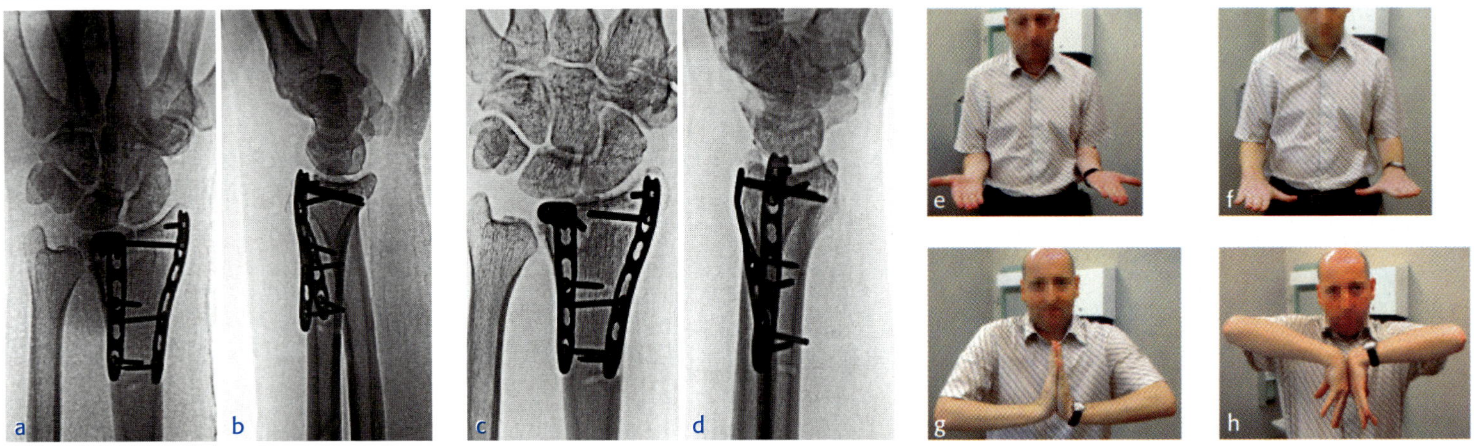

Fig 7.3.5-6a–h Early motion with assistance of a physiotherapist is started immediately. The plaster splint is changed to a removable velcro splint. The hand is used for unloaded daily activities such as eating, personal hygiene, tying a tie, holding paper. After 6 weeks fracture healing is documented by x-ray and the patient can usually start loaded activities.

6 Pitfalls –

Rotational deformities can be difficult to handle from a dorsal approach.
Hyperextended palmar articular fragments are difficult to control from an isolated dorsal approach. They usually need a palmar plate.
Centrally depressed fragments do not response to ligamentotaxis.

7 Pearls +

This concepts allows for early functional rehabilitation and helps to avoid dystrophy.
Bone graft is not necessary due to locking implants.
Injuries are usually caused by low energy bending forces and respond to manual ligamentotaxis for reduction.

Author Daniel Rikli

7.3.6 Complex articular distal radial fracture—23-C3

1 Case description

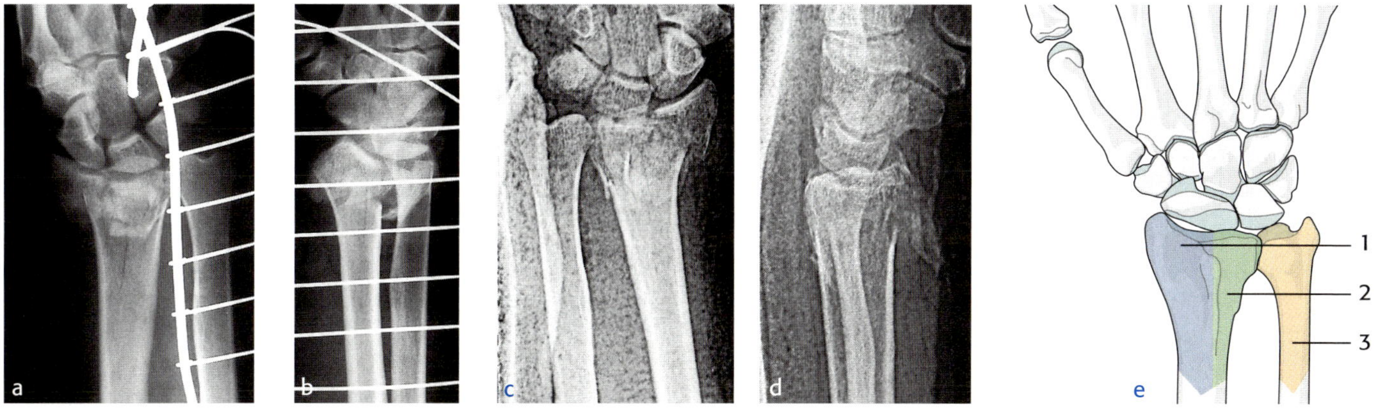

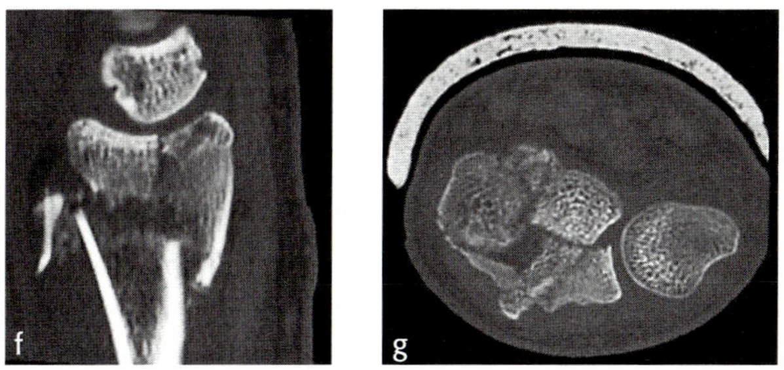

50-year-old patient fell skiing, referred three weeks after the accident. Complex intraarticular fracture of the distal radius (23-C3), combined palmar and dorsal approach and plate fixation.

Fig 7.3.6-1a–g
a–b AP and lateral view.
c–d AP and lateral view 3 weeks after the accident.
e Schematic representation of the distal radial columns: (**1**) radial column, (**2**) intermediate column, (**3**) ulnar column.
f–g CT scans show displaced radial column and the intermediate multifragmentary, displaced column with a step off in the radiocarpal and radioulnar joint.

Indication

Displaced radial column (RC). Intermediate column (IC), multifragmentary, displaced, step-off in the radiocarpal and radioulnar joint. Hyperextended palmarulnar fragment. Dorsoulnar fragment extruded. Extensive meta-/diaphyseal comminution. Avulsion of the tip of the ulnar styloid (ulnar column, UC).

Due to the hyperextended palmar-ulnar fragment and the displaced meta-/diaphyseal palmar fragment a palmar approach is necessary. The radial column can be controlled and buttressed separately with an S-plate from the palmar approach. Most probably an additional limited dorsal approach to reduce and buttress the dorsoulnar fragment will be needed.

Preoperative planning

Equipment
- LCP distal radius plates 2.4
- Locking head screws (LHS)
- Small external fixator (optional)

(Size of system, instruments, and implants can vary according to anatomy.)

Patient preparation and positioning
Antibiotics: cephalosporin
Thrombosis prophylaxis: low-molecular heparin

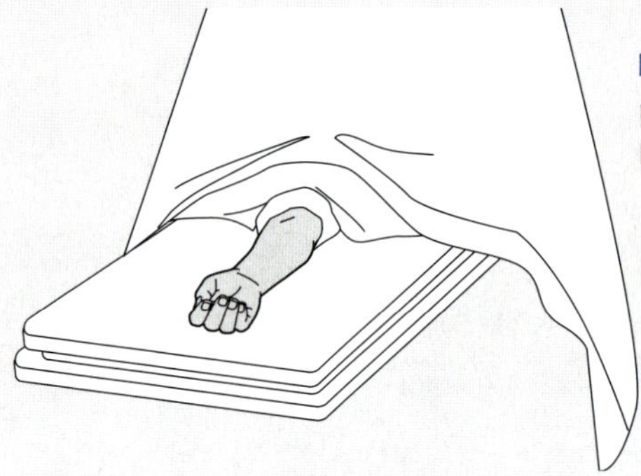

Fig 7.3.6-2 Supine positioning of patient with forearm on hand table. Nonsterile pneumatic tourniquet.

2 Surgical approach

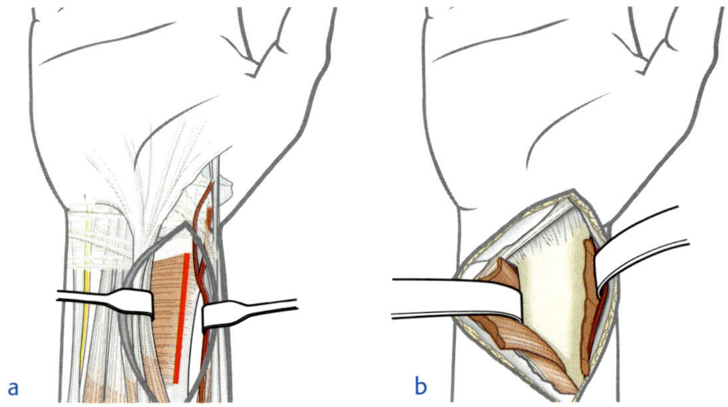

Fig 7.3.6-3a–b
a The surgical approach to the palmar side of the distal radius is described in case 3.7.1. It is developed first. The radial column can be approached using this approach by extending preparation around the radius and radial styloid. Occasionally, the insertion of the brachioradialis tendon has to be partially detached at the radial styloid in order to place the S-plate correctly.
b The surgical approach to the dorsal side of the distal radius is described in case 3.7.5. In cases where a combined palmar and dorsal approach is inevitable, the radial column should be reduced and buttressed from the palmar approach. The dorsal approach can then be limited to the intermediate column. A straight dorsal incision is performed and the retinaculum is incised along the course of the EPL tendon as described. Subperiosteal preparation develops access to the intermediate column. An arthrotomy is always performed in order to control reduction of the dorsoulnar fragment at the level of the radiocarpal joint and to revise the proximal carpal row for any additional ligamentous injuries. The 1st and 2nd compartment remain untouched.

3 Reduction and fixation

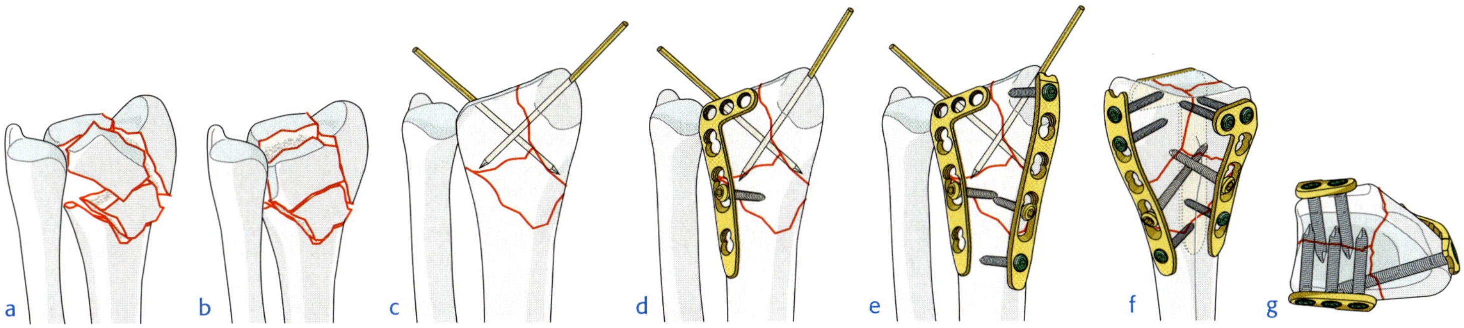

Fig 7.3.6-4a–g Reduction of the fragments is by direct manipulation. If necessary, the individual reduced fragments are fixed temporarily with K-wires. An external fixator for distraction during reconstruction is of particular help and is always used in such complex cases. Correct reduction must be checked by fluoroscopy before definitive fixation.
After reducing the individual fragments, the appropriate implants are chosen for definitive fixation the fracture. The intermediate column should be buttressed at the palmar aspect as well as dorsally by a separate locking L-plate. The radial column is buttressed from palmar using an S-plate. Starting on the palmar side by positioning the L- and the S-plates and fixing them provisionally with a conventional screw in the elongated plate hole in the radial shaft. This is checked by fluoroscopy. Then the dorsal incision is made to approach the intermediate column. After reducing the dorsoulnar fragment, the plate is positioned and temporarily fixed. After a check of reduction and plate position by fluoroscopy, the osteosynthesis is completed as described above.

4 Rehabilitation

Early motion is started immediately. The plaster splint is changed to a removable velcro splint. The hand is used for unloaded daily activities such as eating, personal hygiene, tying a tie, holding paper.

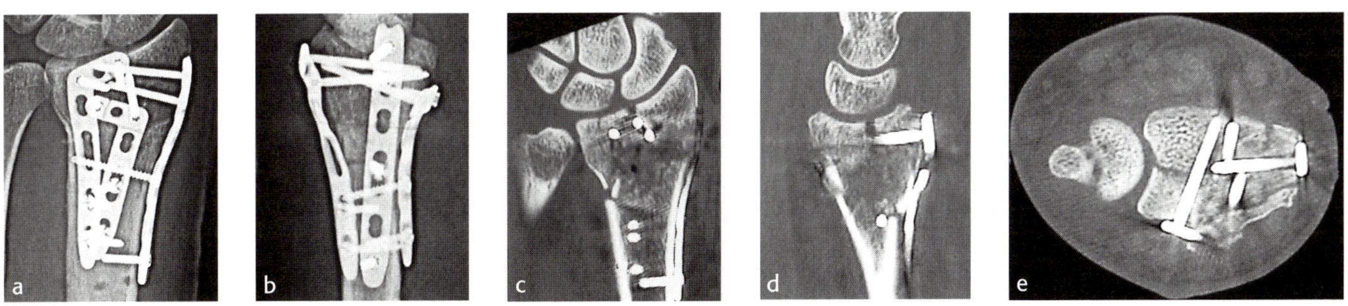

Fig 7.3.6-5a–e
a AP view.
b Lateral view.
c–e CT scans.

4 Rehabilitation (cont)

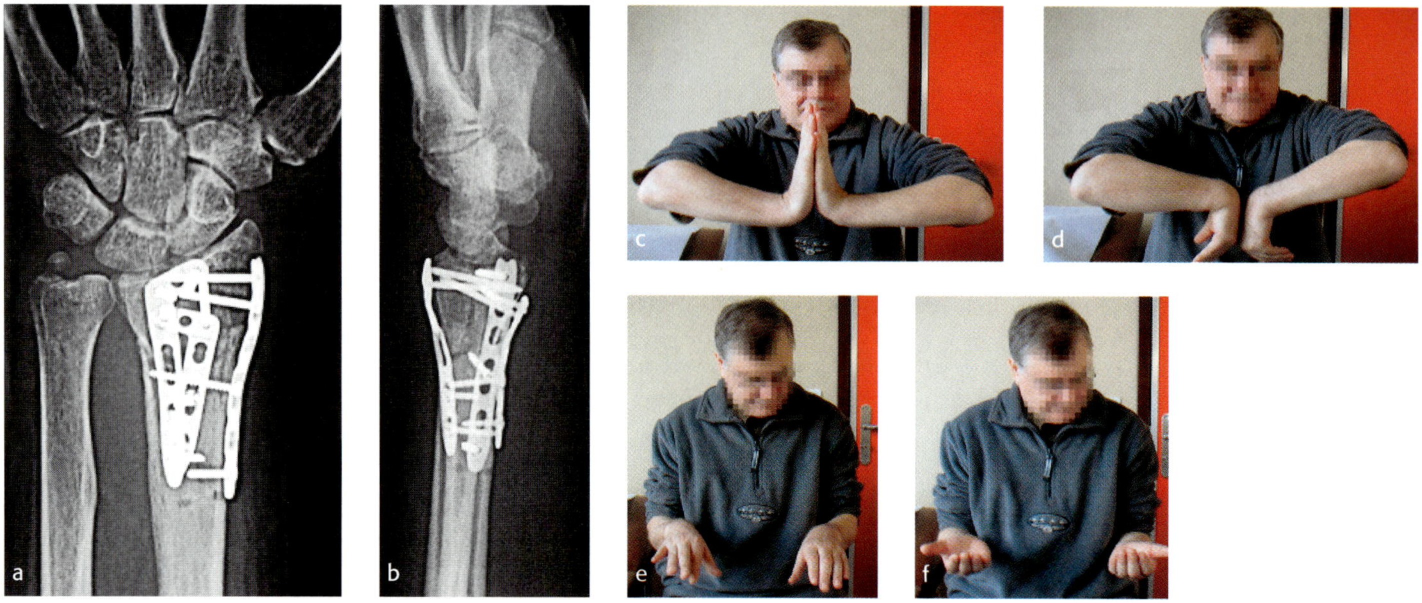

Fig 7.3.6-6a–f After 6 weeks fracture healing is documented with x-rays and the patient can start loaded activities.

5 Pitfalls –

Equipment

The surgeon must check the internal fixation for stability with image intensification in order to avoid secondary loss of fixation during early motion. If stability is not sufficient, external fixation or a plaster cast must be added for 4–6 weeks.

Care must be taken not to penetrate the radiocarpal and radioulnar joints with screws.

A CT scan and careful preoperative planning is mandatory.

6 Pearls +

Equipment

Do not hesitate to put these fractures in an external fixator as an emergency measure. X-rays with the hand in traction (ligamentotaxis) after mounting the external fixator simplifies interpretation of the fracture pattern dramatically.

The variety of the LCP distal radius plates 2.4 help to adapt the implants to the individual situation.

With the help of the CT scan, which is always performed after placing the external fixator, a strategy for definitive treatment according to the three column model is developed.

8 Pelvic ring and acetabulum

Cases

8 Pelvic ring and acetabulum

Author Tim Pohlemann

8.1 Pelvic ring and acetabulum

1 Incidence

Even with major advances in the treatment of pelvic and acetabular fractures, these injuries are still associated with several complications. Surgery is difficult and the observed clinical and radiological results are frequently less than satisfactory compared to injuries to the body.

By defining a specific injury type as "complex pelvic fractures" ("pelvic fracture with peripelvic soft-tissue injury, urogenital injury, holovisceral injury, muscle injury, or nerve injury") a group of patients under immediate vital threat was identified. The introduction of primary treatment algorithms for these patients, based on the principle of immediate emergency mechanical stabilization (external fixator/C-clamp) and subsequent surgical hemostasis in nonresponders (preferably by pelvic tamponade), led to constant improvements. The survival rate is now below 20% according to the German Multicenter Pelvic Study Group data (overall fatality after pelvic fractures: 5.9%).

For the other 90% of patients suffering from pure osteoligamentous injuries, a better understanding and usage of universal classification systems allows the setting of clear indication guidelines and standardized conventional surgical techniques for the various fracture patterns of pelvic ring injuries and acetabular fractures. The rate of long-term healing after anatomical surgical reconstruction improved to over 80%, even after C-type fractures including translational injuries to the posterior pelvic ring. Despite this progress, the rate of clinically excellent and good results for these injuries is still observed to be around 60%. This leads research to focus on the effect (on the quality of outcomes) of soft-tissue damage related to the injury and surgical intervention, an issue not currently being addressed.

2 Classification

The Müller AO Classification takes the pathomechanical aspects of stability or instability of the posterior arch of the pelvic ring into consideration. Acetabular fractures are classified separately.

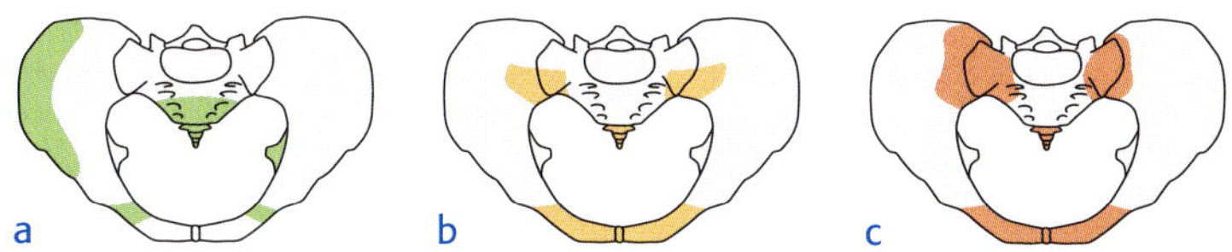

Fig 8.1-1a–c Müller AO Classification of pelvic ring fractures.
a 61-A Posterior arch intact, stable lesion
b 61-B Posterior arch disruption, incomplete, partially stable lesion
c 61-C Posterior arch disruption, complete, unstable lesion

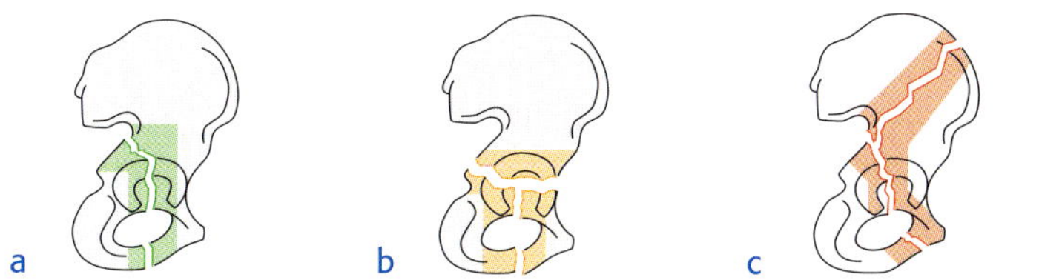

Fig 8.1-2a–c Müller AO Classification of acetabular fractures.
a 62-A Partial articular, one column
b 62-B Partial articular, transverse oriented
c 62-C Complete articular, both columns

3 Treatment methods

The introduction of locking technology increased the hope that there would be further improvement in the treatment modalities available to pelvic and acetabular surgery. A close review of the results presented over the last two years has shown that the LCP has the potential to improve treatment although reproducible improvements were found to be the result of enhanced preoperative visualization. The latter leads to a better understanding of the fracture pattern with subsequent standardization of primary evaluation, definitive diagnostics, classification, and surgical techniques.

Present efforts in the treatment of pelvic ring injuries are focused on closed and minimally invasive surgical techniques based on further advances in preoperative visualization and planning. The widespread use and acceptance of closed surgical techniques is still limited by the ability to perform and control reduction.

From outcome evaluation of larger series, it becomes clear that the standards of anatomical reduction and stable fixation with early mobilization still have to be met, even in cases of poor bone quality.

In the field of acetabular surgery the need for absolute anatomical reconstruction of the joint surfaces has been undisputed since the basic work by Letournel. Demographic changes lead to a rapidly increasing number of acetabular fractures in elderly patients, especially fractures of the anterior column and anterior column combined with posterior hemitransverse fractures and fractures of both columns. The value of primary total hip replacement in this patient group is still disputed with reports of unacceptable rates of early loosening. Therefore, an increasing number of surgical reconstructions of the acetabulum have to be performed within this age group. With the use of special techniques of stabilization, like locking compression plates and an adapted implant design, promising results can be achieved if disastrous secondary displacement after fixation failure can be avoided.

New special reconstruction plates with coaxial combination holes and better 3-D bending qualities support newer, minimally invasive techniques and will ease fracture treatment in situations with poor bone quality.

4 Implant overview

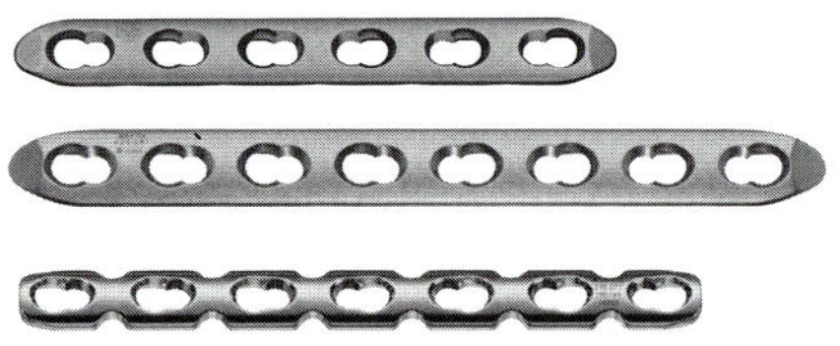

Fig 8-3a–c
a LCP 3.5
b LCP 4.5/5.0
c LCP reconstruction plate 3.5

5 Suggestions for further reading

Culemann U, Tosounidis G, Pohlemann T (2005) [Fractures of the accetabulum—treatment strategies and current diagnostics]. *Zentralbl Chir.;* 130(5):W58—71; quiz W72–73. German.

Culemann U, Tosounidis G, Reilmann H, et al (2004) [Injury to the pelvic ring. Diagnosis and current treatment options]. *Unfallchirurg;* 107(12):1169–1181; quiz 1182–1183. German.

Gansslen A, Pohlemann T, Krettek C (2005) [Internal fixation of sacroiliac joint disruption]. *Oper Orthop Traumatol;* 17(3):281–95. German.

Letournel E, Judet R (1981) *Fractures of the Acetabulum.* Berlin Heidelberg New York: Springer Verlag.

Pohlemann T, Gänsslen A, Hartung S (1998) *Beckenverletzungen / Pelvic injuries: Results of the German Multicenter Study Group.* Berlin Heidelberg New York: Springer Verlag.

Tile M, Burgess A, Helfet DL et al (1995) *Fractures of the Pelvis and Acetabulum.* Baltimore: Williams & Wilkins.

Tscherne H, Pohlemann T (1998) *Tscherne Unfallchirurgie. Pelvic and acetabulum.* Berlin Heidelberg: Springer Verlag.

Author Emanuel Gautier

8.1.1 Unstable pelvic ring fracture—61-C1

1 Case description

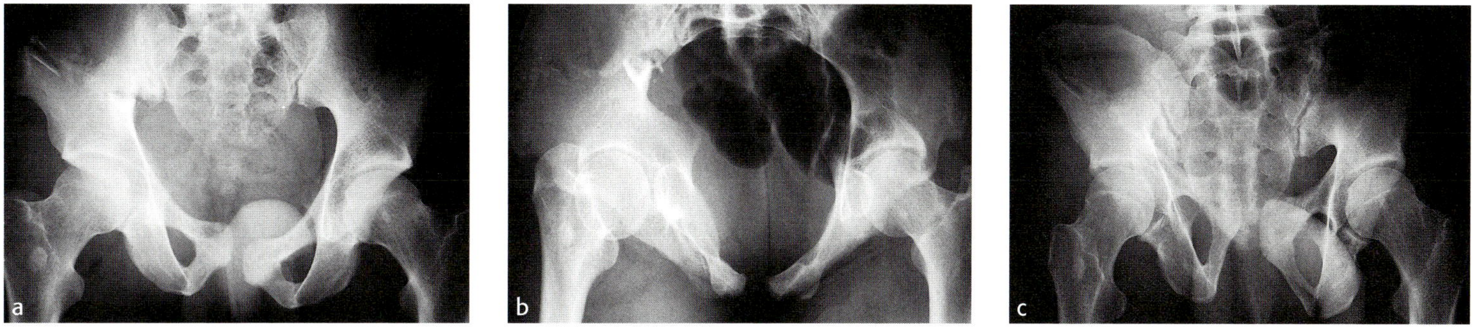

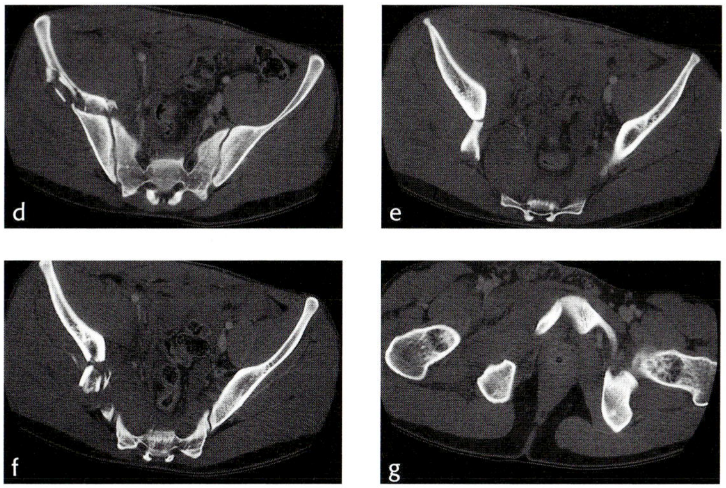

23-year-old man suffered a parachute injury (5 m fall). He sustained a pelvic ring injury with disruption of the pubic symphysis, a fracture of the ilium on the right side, and a stable, 2-level lumbar spine fracture.

Fig 8.1.1-1a–g
a AP view.
b Inlet view.
c Outlet view.
d–g CT scans show the multifragmentary fracture of the illium and an intercalated iliac fragment.

Indication

Indications for ORIF, anterior and posterior are:

- Instability of the anterior and posterior pelvic ring segments
- Asymmetry of the pelvic ring and true pelvis
- Intercalated fragment of the iliac wing

Preoperative planning

Equipment
- LCP reconstruction plate 3.5, 6 holes
- Reconstruction plate 3.5, 5 holes
- Locking head screws (LHS)
- 2.5 mm K-wire
- Pelvic reduction forceps (Faraboeuf)
- Pelvic reduction forceps (Jungbluth)

(Size of system, instruments, and implants can vary according to anatomy.)

Patient preparation and positioning
Antibiotics: cephalosporin
Thrombosis prophylaxis: low-molecular heparin

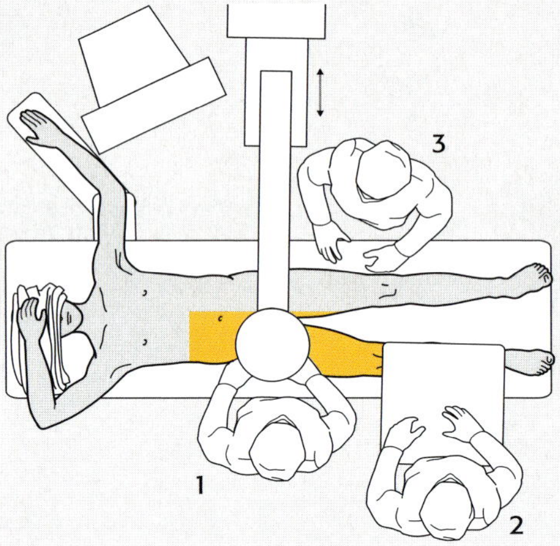

Fig 8.1.1-2 Patient in supine position with leg freely mobile on the injured side.

2 Surgical approach

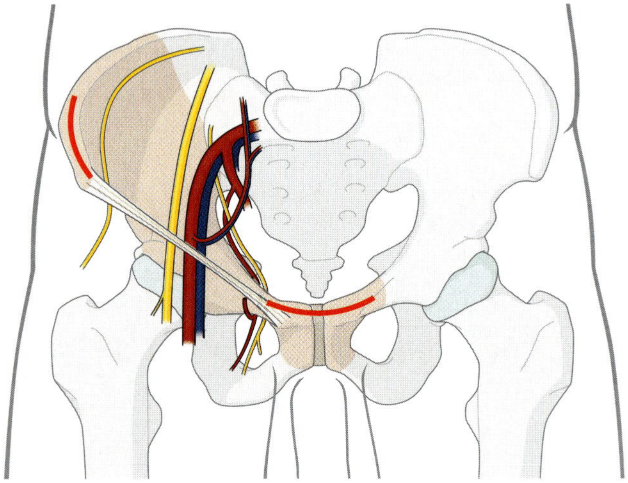

Fig 8.1.1-3 Modified Pfannenstiel approach with preparation of the symphysis and the pubic ramus dorsal to the rectus, without detachment of the rectus muscle.

Approach to the iliac ring through the first window of the ilioinguinal approach.

3 Reduction

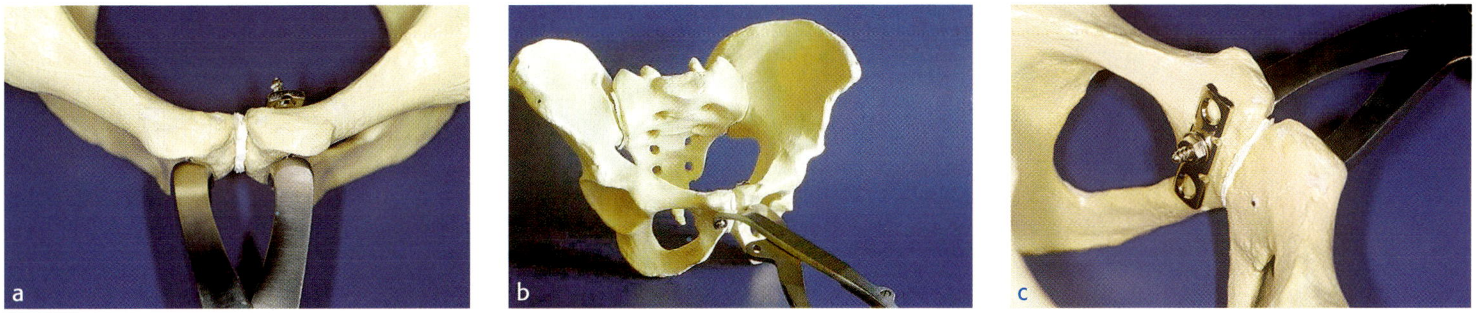

Possibilities for reduction of the symphysis:

- Pointed reduction forceps in both obturator foramen
- Matta technique
- Possibilities for reduction of the iliac ring: Faraboeuf forceps in the iliac crest

Fig 8.1.1-4a–c Reduction of the symphysis, according to Matta. The Jungbluth forceps are fixed on the unstable side with a 3-hole reconstruction plate 4.5. This allows a high pull on the pubic ramus without risk of screw pullout. Reduction of the ilium with the help of a Schanz screw inserted into the unstable side and used as a joystick, or with the aid of a Faraboef forceps.

4 Fixation

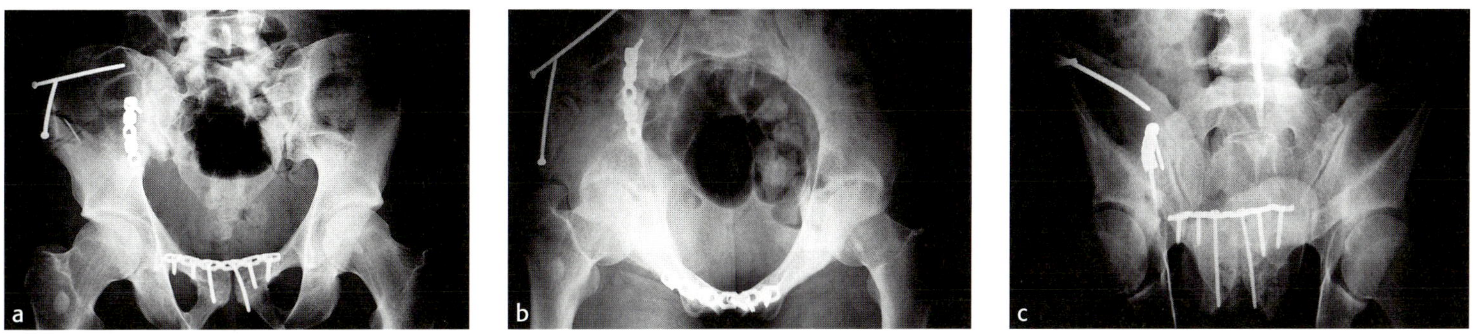

The symphyseal fracture is compressed by eccentric placement of cortex screws in the middle part of a 6-hole LCP reconstruction plate. Additional fixation of the plate to the pubic rami with LHS.
Fixation of the ilium is performed with two 3.5 mm cortex screws along the iliac crest and a 5-hole reconstruction plate close and parallel to the sacroiliac joint.

Fig 8.1.1-5a–c
a AP view.
b Inlet view.
c Outlet view.

5 Rehabilitation

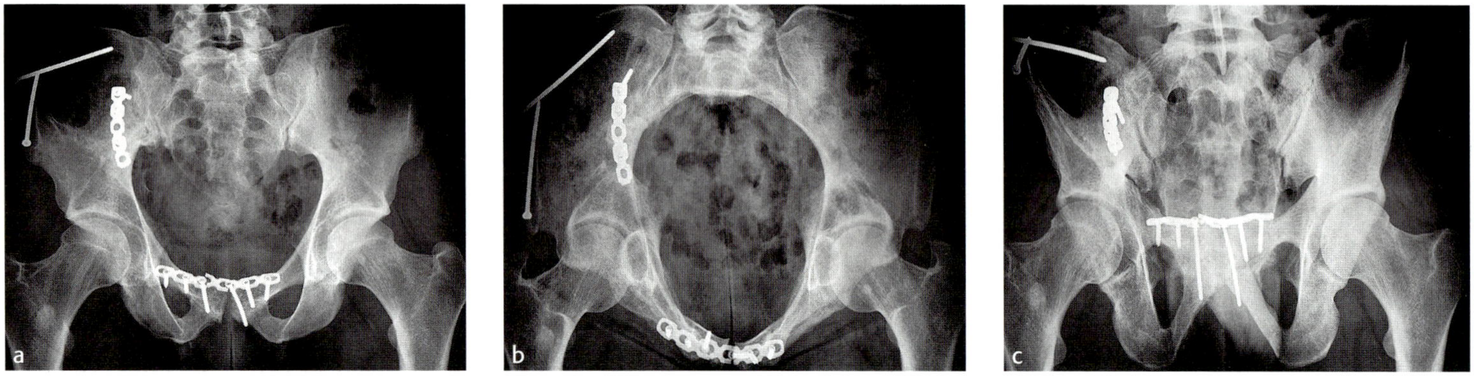

Fig 8.1.1-6a–c X-rays at one year show the consolidation of the fracture and rupture of the symphyseal plate.
a AP view.
b Inlet view.
c Outlet view.

The fracture was not additionally immobilized. 15 kg weight bearing for 6 weeks and full weight bearing after 12 weeks. Bone healing was seen after 12 weeks.

Implant removal

The patient was not keen to have the implants removed because he had no pain at all, even with the plate broken at two levels.

6 Pitfalls –

Reduction and fixation

In the posterior aspect of the pelvic ring a conventional reconstruction plate is used since it is not possible to insert an angular stable plate.

7 Pearls +

Reduction and fixation

Anterior symphyseal plating with LCP reconstruction plate is possible, enhancing the anchorage in the case of osteoporotic bone.

Authors Thomas J Hockertz, Andreas Gruner, Gabriele Streicher, Heinrich Reilmann

8.1.2 Symphysis avulsion plus transforaminal fracture of the sacrum—61-C

1 Case description

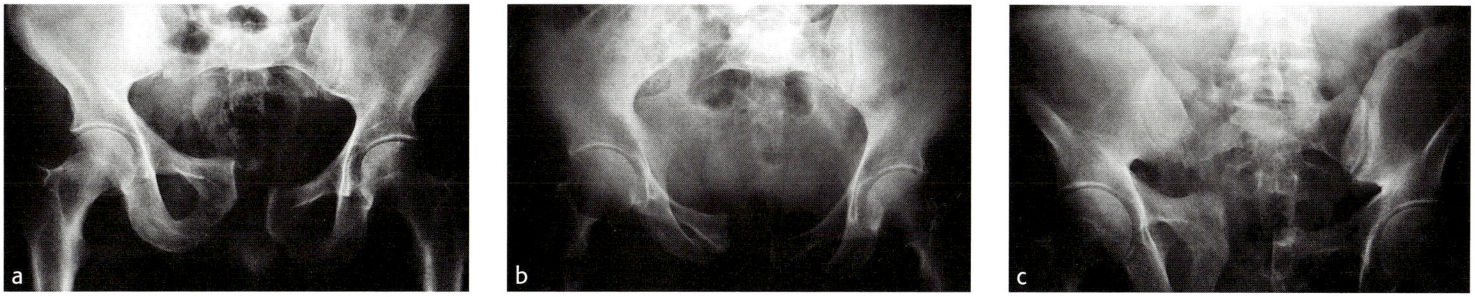

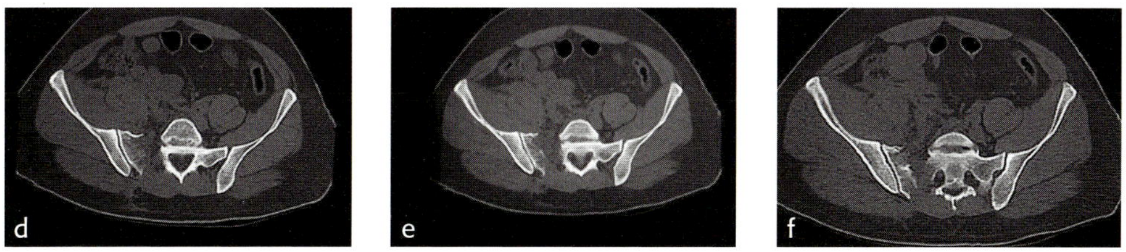

Fig 8.1.2-1a–f

a Preoperative overview of the pelvis.
b Preoperative view of the pelvic inlet.
c Preoperative view of the pelvic outlet.
d–f Preoperative CT scans.

46-year-old man with pelvic injury. Type of injury: high-energy trauma. Multiple trauma description: pelvic C-type fracture injury, wrist fracture (C2-fracture of the distal radius); concussion; multiple bruising.

Indication

Unstable C-type fracture. Protection of the plexus from the local osteosynthesis of the sacrum; early functional aftercare is possible.

Preoperative planning

Equipment

- LCP 4.5/5.0, 9 holes
- LCP 4.5/5.0, 4 holes
- LCP reconstruction plate 3.5, 3 holes
- Locking head screws (LHS)
- 4.5 mm cortex screws

(Size of system, instruments, and implants can vary according to anatomy.)

Patient preparation and positioning

Antibiotics: single dose 2nd generation cephalosporin
Thrombosis prophylaxis: low-molecular heparin

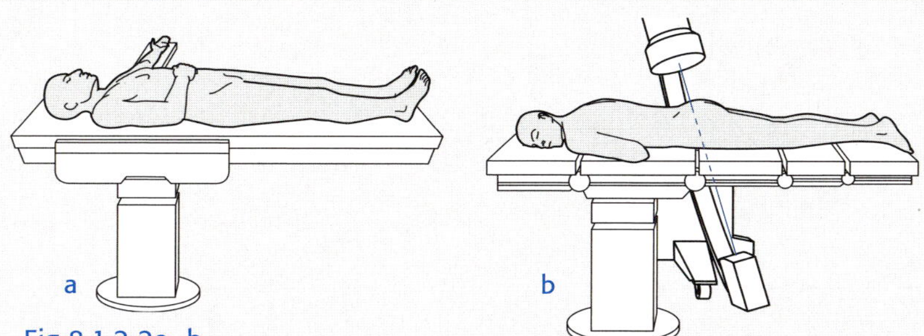

Fig 8.1.2-2a–b

a Stabilization of the symphysis with the patient in the supine position.
b Treatment of the dorsal pelvic ring in the prone position.

Preoperative planning (cont)

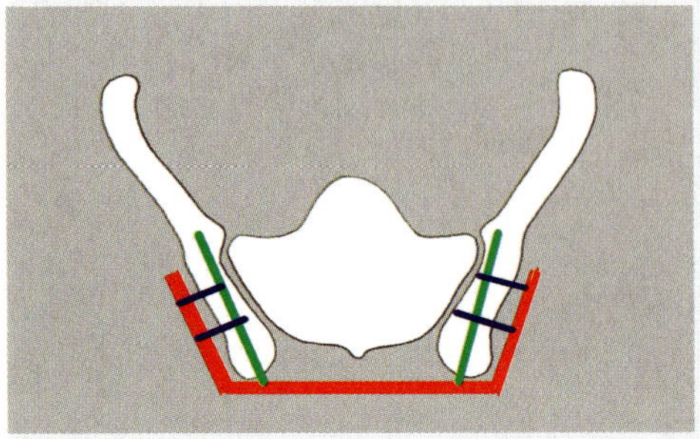

Fig 8.1.2-3 Sketch of preoperative planning. Positioning of the LCP (red), the cortex screws (green) and the LHS (blue).

2 Surgical approach

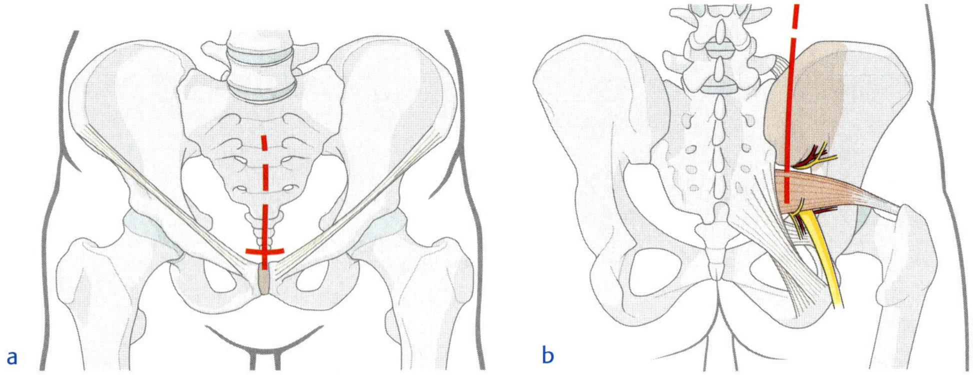

Fig 8.1.2-4a–b
a Approach to the pubic symphysis by horizontal Pfannenstiel type incision (7–12 cm).
b Posterior approach to the sacroiliac joint. The skin incision starts 1–2 fingerbreadths distal and lateral to the posterior superior iliac spine and runs in a straight line proximally (about 10–15 cm).

3 Reduction and fixation

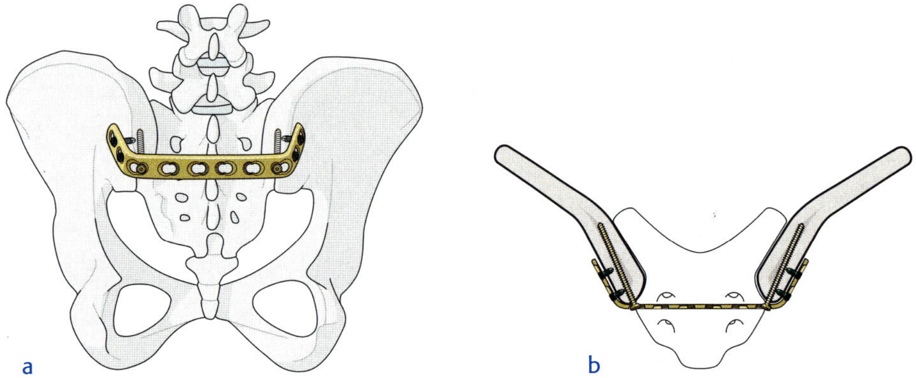

- Definitive reduction of the sacrum and local plate osteosynthesis.
- Protection of the osteosynthesis by bridging LCP according to internal fixator principles.
- Approximate reduction of the pelvis and stabilization of the avulsed symphysis by plate osteosynthesis in compression technique.

Fig 8.1.2-5a–b
a Position of the LCP on the posterior pelvis.
b Position of the LCP on the lateral pelvis.

3 Reduction and fixation (cont)

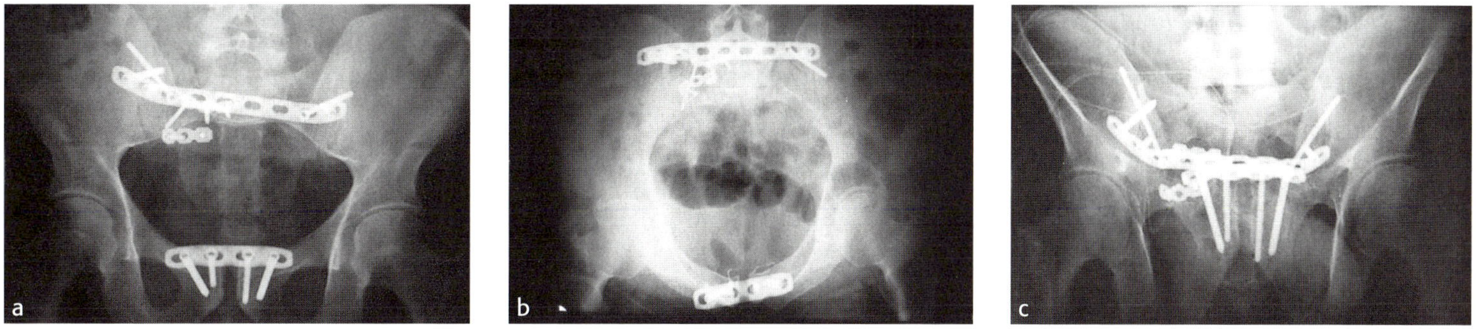

Fig 8.1.2-6a–c
a Postoperative overview of the pelvis.
b Postoperative overview of the pelvic inlet.
c Postoperative overview of the pelvic outlet.

4 Rehabilitation

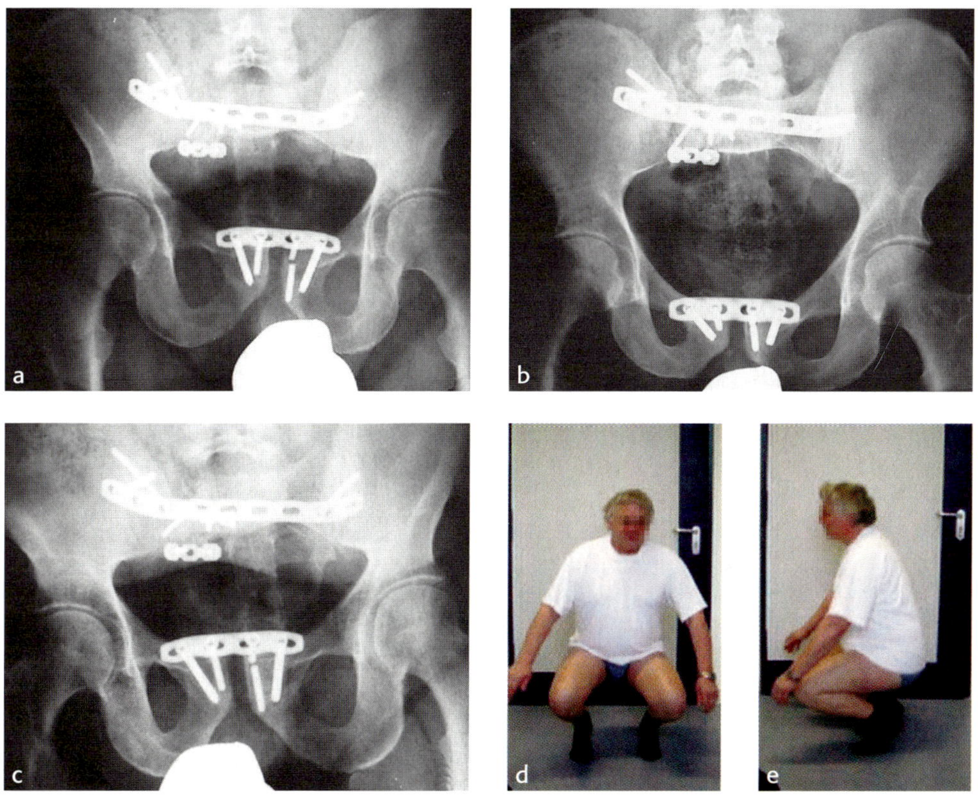

Weight bearing: 15 kg for 6 weeks; half body weight after 6 weeks; full weight bearing after 8 weeks.
Physiotherapy: from the second postoperative day.
Pharmaceutical treatment pain therapy with nonsteroid antiinflamatory drugs.

Fig 8.1.2-7a–e Postoperative x-rays after 5 months.
a AP view.
b Inlet view.
c Outlet view.
d–e Functional result.

Implant removal
Due to screw failure, the symphysis plate was removed after 8 months.

5 Pitfalls –

Equipment
It is difficult to determine the correct length of the LCP for posterior application and internal fixation.

Approach

Reduction and fixation
Due to the small incisions, difficult half-open reduction–only for experienced pelvic surgeons.

Rehabilitation

6 Pearls +

Equipment

Approach
Minimally invasive approach.

Reduction and fixation

Rehabilitation
Early mobilization is possible, therefore better functional outcomes.

No destruction of the sacroiliac joint since it is not in contact with screws.

Authors Tim Pohlemann, Ulf Culemann

8.1.3 Pelvic ring reconstruction–61-C1

1 Case description

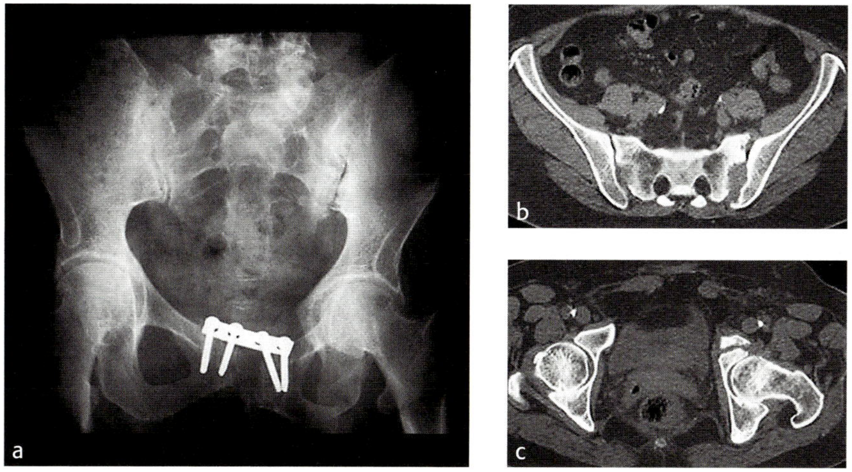

60-year-old woman with pseudarthrosis after complete pelvic ring injury in a car accident.
Type of injury: high-energy, monotrauma; closed fracture.

Fig 8.1.3-1a–c
a An x-ray taken 1 1/2 years after the car accident with the operative treatment of a complete pelvic ring fracture as shown.
b–c The CT scans demonstrate the nonhealing of the anterior and posterior pelvic ring fractures.

Indication

An unstable C-type fracture was misinterpreted as a B-type and operative stabilization was only performed for the anterior pelvic ring. The result after 1 1/2 years was a nonunion of the pelvic ring and pain because of the instability. The surgical treatment aimed to eliminate the dislocation of the anterior pelvic ring and the instability of the sacroiliac joint.

Preoperative planning

Equipment
- LCP reconstruction plates 3.5, 3 holes
- LCP reconstruction plates 3.5, 6 holes
- LCP 3.5, 4 holes
- 3.5 mm locking head screws (LHS)
- 3.5 mm cortex screws
- 7.0 mm cannulated screws
- Pelvic reduction forceps (optional)

(Size of system, instruments, and implants can vary according to anatomy.)

Patient preparation and positioning
Antibiotics: single dose 2nd generation cephalosporin for 10 days
Thrombosis prophylaxis: low-molecular heparin

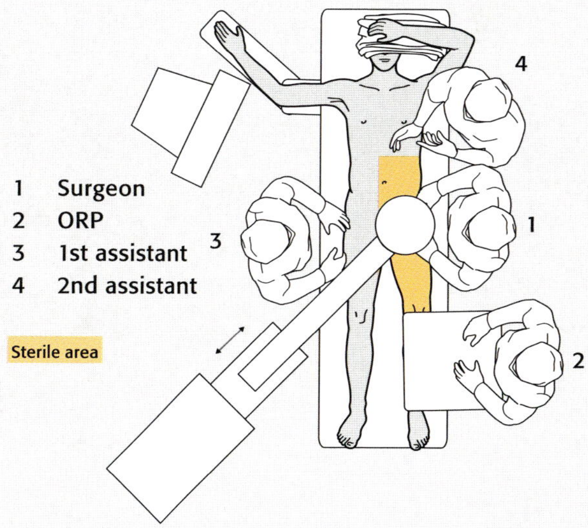

Fig 8.1.3-2 Patient in the supine position with the leg freely mobile.

2 Surgical approach

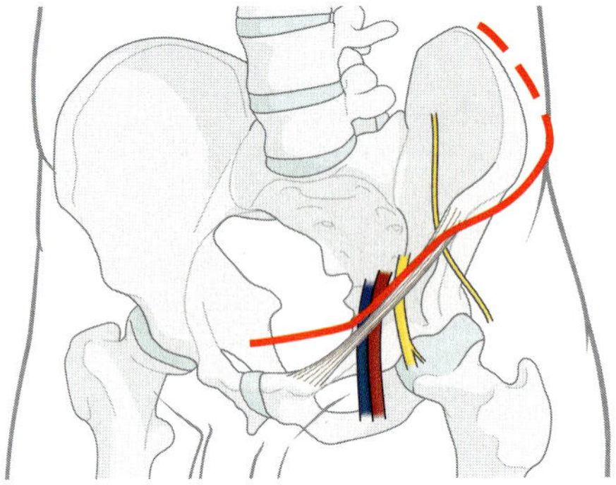

Fig 8.1.3-3a–h Ilioinguinal approach.
a Orientation points and skin incision.

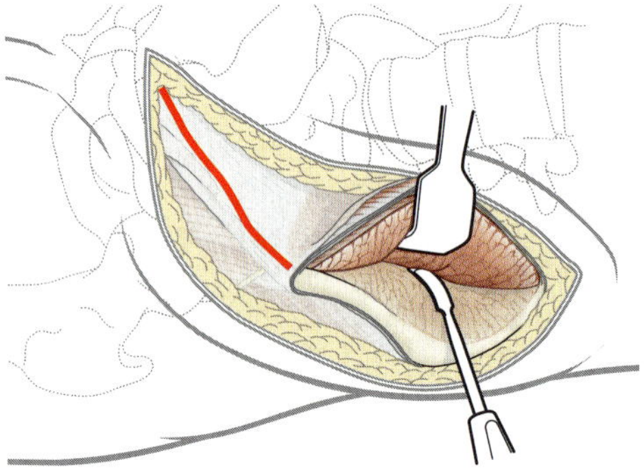

b Removal of iliac muscle from the iliac wing.

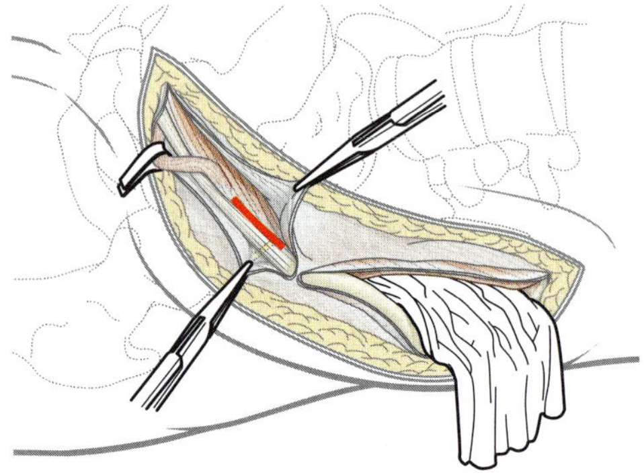

c Preparation of the muscular space.

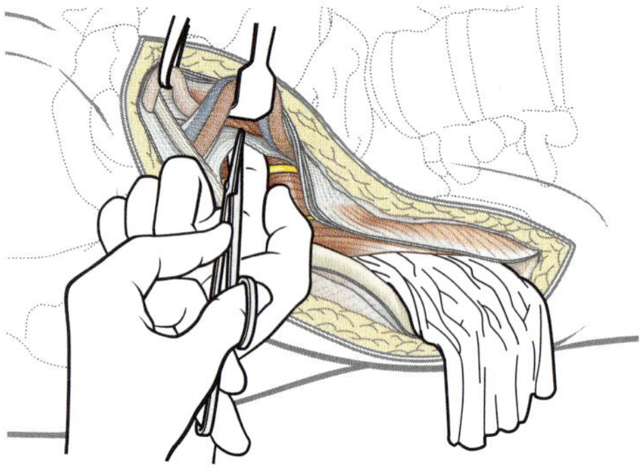

d Transection of the iliopectineal arch.

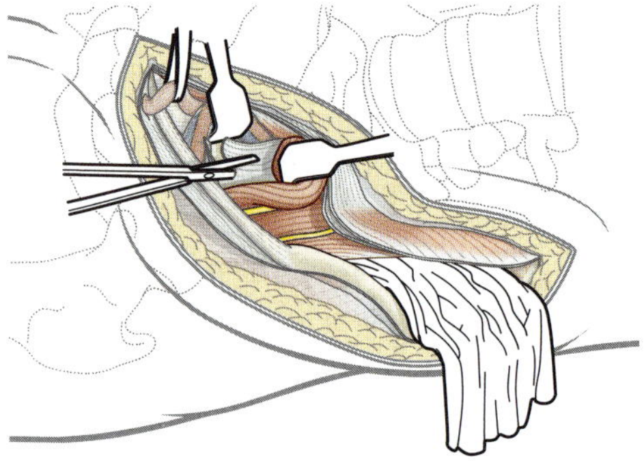

e Mobilization of the iliopsoas muscle from the posterior pectineal line.

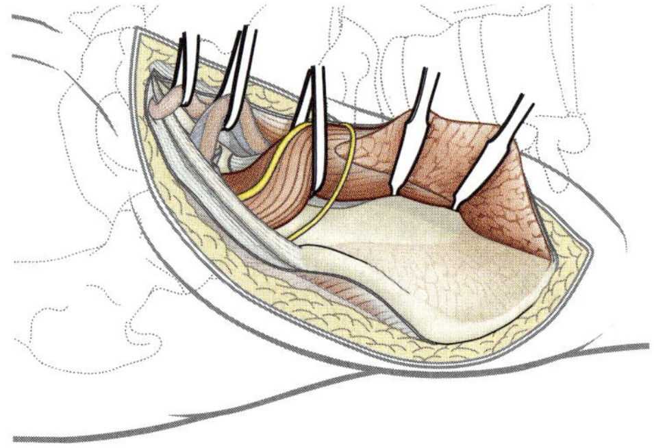

f First window of the ilioinguinal approach.

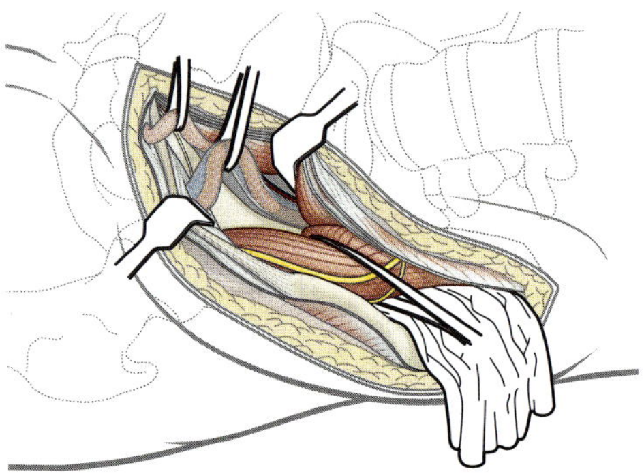

g Second window of the ilioinguinal approach.

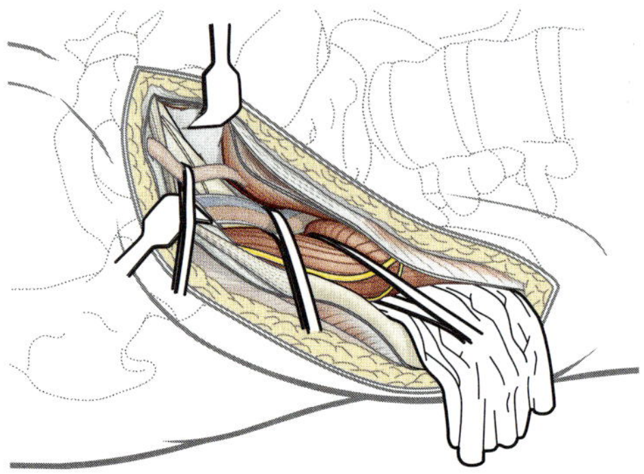

h Third window of the ilioinguinal approach.

3 Reduction and fixation

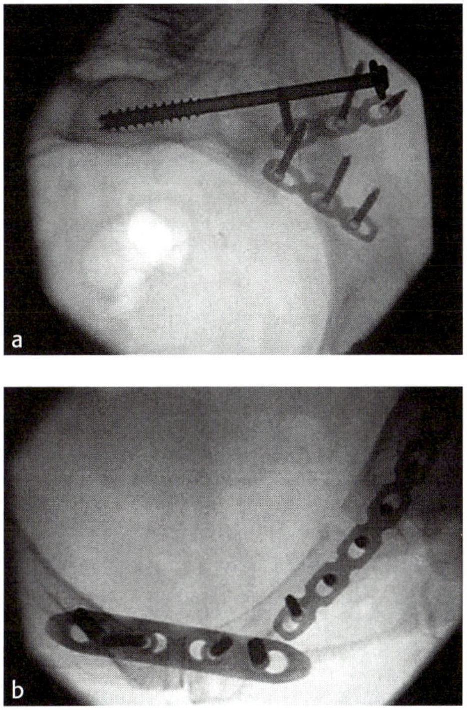

Fig 8.1.3-4a–b
a Dissection of the pseudarthrotic sacroiliacal joint, interposition of corticocancellous bone graft from the iliac crest and fixation by a 7.0 mm cannulated screw in combination with two LCPs.
b Anterior pelvic ring reconstruction.

Mobilization of the anterior part of the pseudarthrosis. Mobilization of the posterior part of the pseudarthrosis in open technique. Interposition of corticocancellous bone graft chip into the sacroiliac joint.

Arthrodesis of the sacroiliac joint by a 7.0 mm cannulated lag screw and two LCP reconstruction plates 3.5, 3 holes with self-tapping locking head screws and cortex screws.

Reduction of the anterior pelvic ring through the second and third window of the ilioinguinal approach and fixation with an LCP 3.5, 4 holes.

Fixation of the superior pubis rami and the symphysis with two LCP reconstruction plates 3.5, 6 holes.

4 Rehabilitation

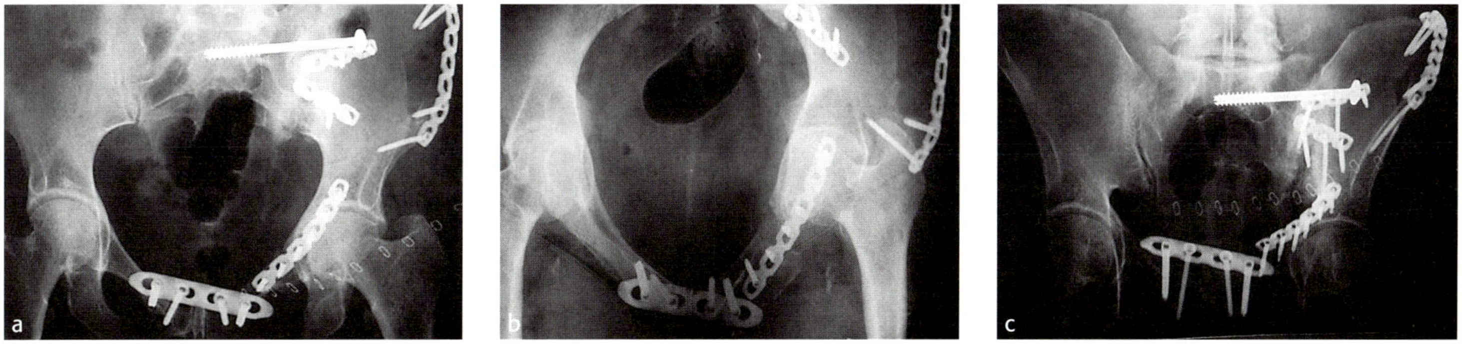

Weight bearing: 15 kg for 8 weeks; half-body weight after 12 weeks; full weight bearing after 16 weeks.
Physiotherapy: active and passive.
Pharmaceutical treatment: pain medication and antiphlogistics for 2 weeks.

Fig 8.1.3-5a–c Postoperative x-rays after 6 weeks.
a AP view.
b Inlet view.
c Outlet view.

4 Rehabilitation (cont)

Implant removal
Only necessary in cases of transfixation of the symphysis and/or sacroiliac joint.

5 Pitfalls –

Equipment
Full pelvic set with all reduction tools is needed.

Reduction and fixation
Axis of the locking head screws in the direction of the loading forces includes a high risk of pullout from the bone.

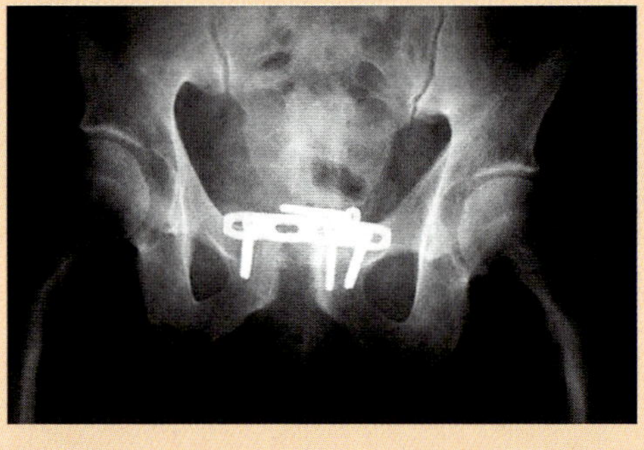

Fig 8.1.3-6
Pitfall because of the loading forces in the direction of the axis of the screws: pullout of the right cortex screw and the locking head screw from the bone, because of insufficient prebending of the plate.

6 Pearls +

Equipment
Reduction tools for arthrodesis.

Reduction and fixation
Prebending of the plate to prevent the screw axis being in the line of the loading forces.

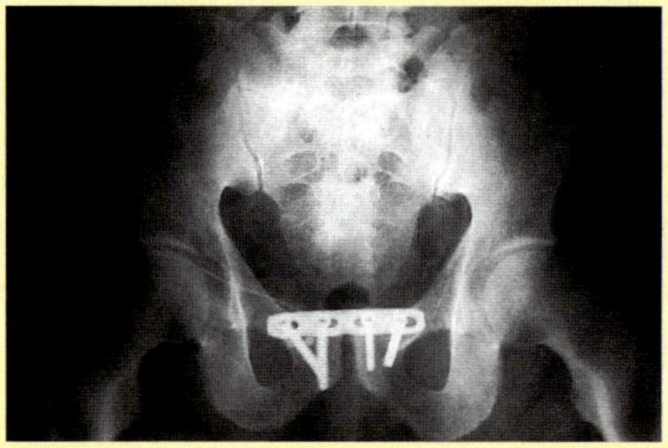

Fig 8.1.3-7
B-type fracture with rupture of the pubic symphysis. Postoperative control after fixation of the symphysis with LCP, locking head screws in the lateral holes, and cortex screws with compression in the middle part of the plate.

Authors Tim Pohlemann, Ulf Culemann

8.1.4 Pelvic ring and acetabular fracture—62-B3

1 Case description

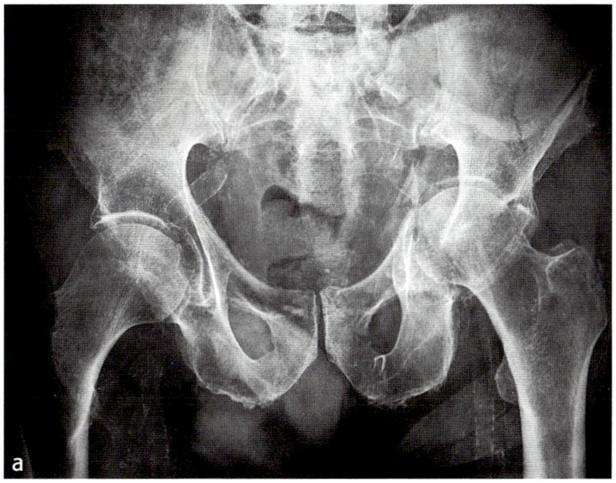

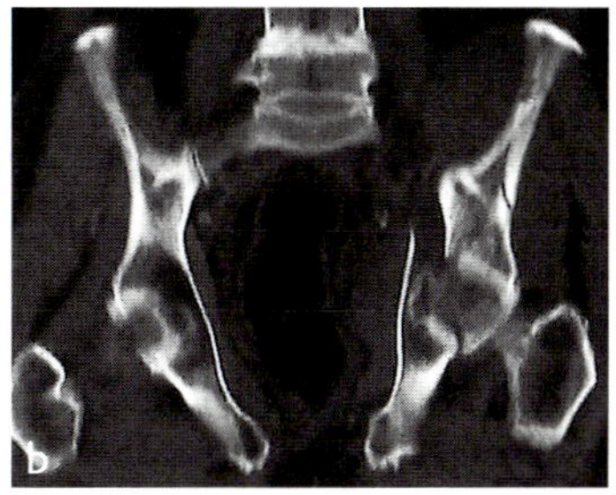

79-year-old woman with a fracture of the left pelvic ring and acetabulum. Low-energy, monotrauma; closed fracture.

Fig 8.1.4-1a–b
- a X-ray demonstrates a closed acetabular fracture on the left side with protrusion of the femoral head inside the pelvis.
- b The CT scan demonstrates the comminution of the domed part of the acetabular surface.

Indication

Typical fracture pattern of acetabular fractures in geriatric patients with fracture of the anterior column with posterior hemitransverse fracture. Incongruency of the joint requires reconstruction. Nonoperative treatment has the risk of early osteoarthrosis and/or nonunion. Primary total hip replacement (THR) is difficult due to the instability of the weight supporting fracture of the anterior column.

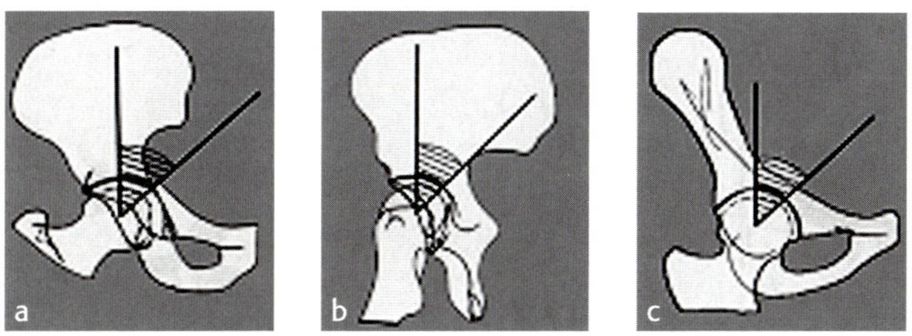

Fig 8.1.4-2a–c
- a AP view.
- b Ala view.
- c Obturator view.

Preoperative planning sketches: Roof arc measurements according to Matta to facilitate decision making for nonoperative/operative treatment.
The angle between a line perpendicular to the acetabular center and the first visible fracture line is over 45° in all three standard views (Fig 8.1.4-2), nonoperative treatment is possible.

Preoperative planning

Equipment
- LCP reconstruction plate 3.5, 3–4 holes
- Self-tapping locking head screws (LHS)
- 7.0 mm cannulated screw
- Additional pelvic reduction forceps

(Size of system, instruments, and implants can vary according to anatomy.)

Preoperative planning (cont)

Patient preparation and positioning
Antibiotics: single dose 2nd generation cephalosporin
Thrombosis prophylaxis: low-molecular heparin

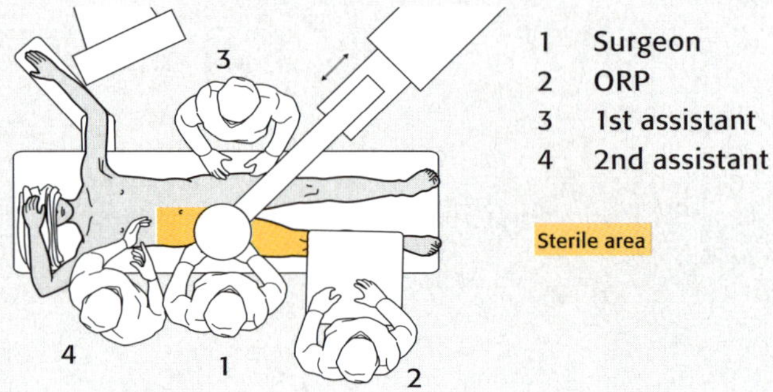

Fig 8.1.4-3 Patient in supine position with leg freely mobile.

2 Surgical approach

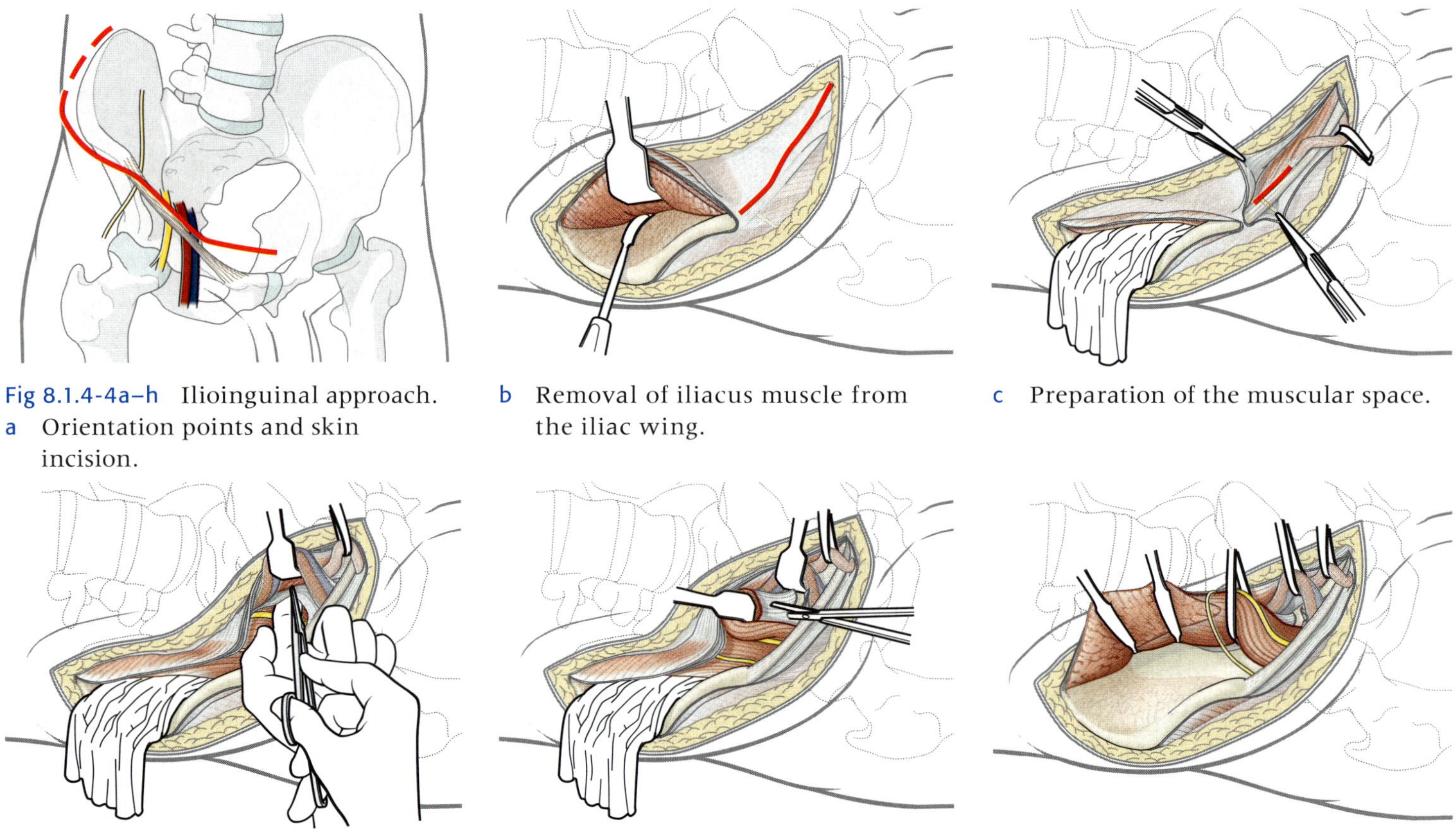

Fig 8.1.4-4a–h Ilioinguinal approach.
a Orientation points and skin incision.
b Removal of iliacus muscle from the iliac wing.
c Preparation of the muscular space.
d Transection of the iliopectineal arch.
e Mobilization of the iliopsoas muscle from the posterior pectineal line.
f First window of the ilioinguinal approach.

2 Surgical approach (cont)

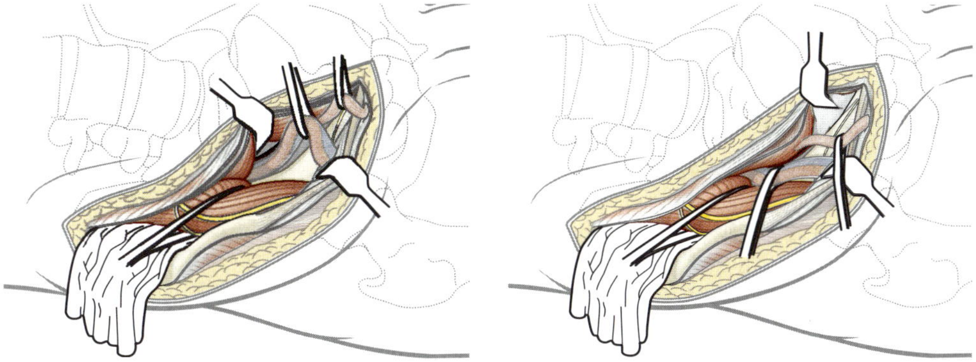

Fig 8.1.4-4a–h (cont)
g Second window of the ilioinguinal approach.
h Third window of the ilioinguinal approach.

3 Reduction and fixation

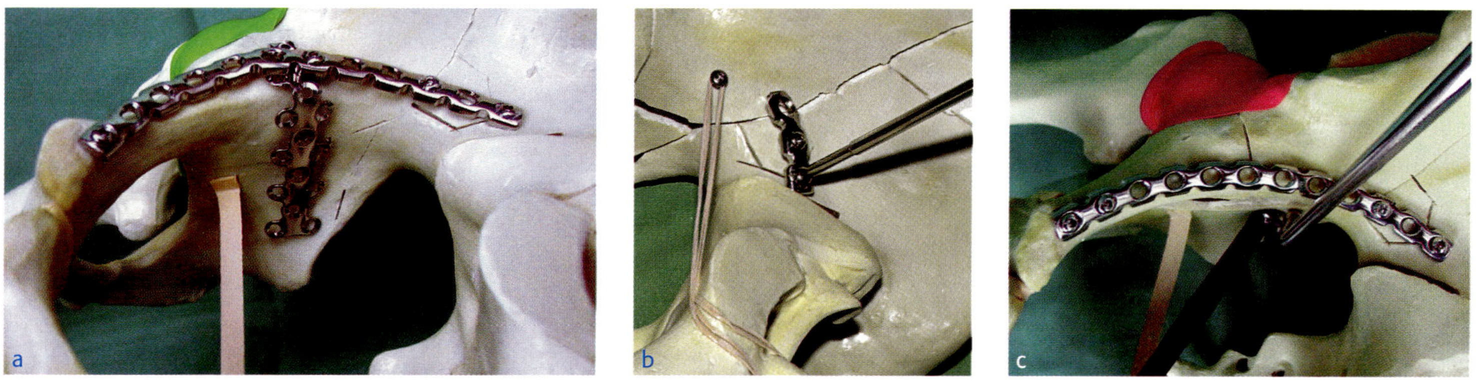

Fig 8.1.4-5a–c
a Anatomical reconstruction of the anterior column. Fixation with a prebent pelvic reconstruction plate.
b A stepwise reduction can be supported by special instruments like the "pushing-plate" described by Jeff Mast.
c Derotation of the posterior column and reduction with a collinear reduction clamp. Fixation with lag screws. In cases of poor bone quality, the use of additional locking head screws enhances overall stability.

4 Rehabilitation

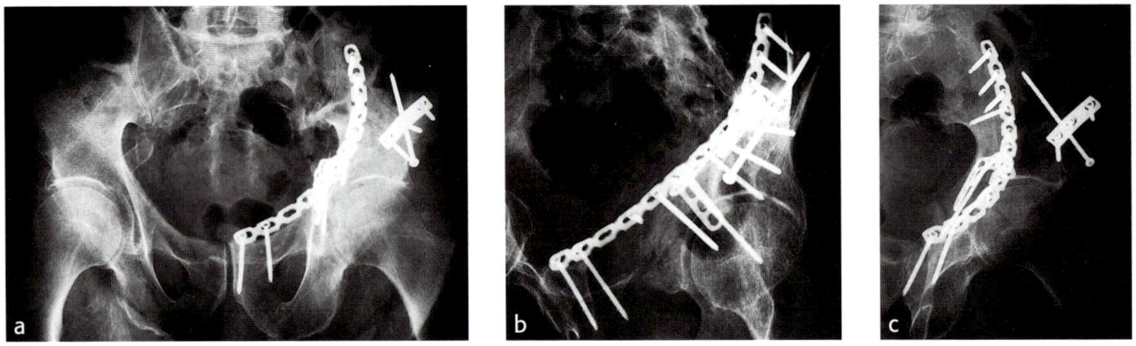

Fig 8.1.4-6a–c
Postoperative x-ray after 6 weeks.
a AP view.
b Obturator view.
c Ala view.

Implant removal
No implant removal if possible.

Weight bearing: 15 kg for 8 weeks; half body weight after 10 weeks; full weight bearing after 12 weeks.
Physiotherapy: functional postoperative treatment with active-assisted and continuous passive motion with physiotherapist as of the second postoperative day.
Pharmaceutical treatment: combination of painkillers and nonsteroidal antiphlogistics.

5 Pitfalls –

6 Pearls +

Approach
Explore the lateral femoral cutaneous nerve through the approach from 1 cm lateral to 4 cm medial of the anterior superior iliac spine.

Reduction and fixation
Fig 8.1.4-7 Control of all screws in the direction of the acetabulum with the image intensifier and/or 3-D CT scan intraoperatively.

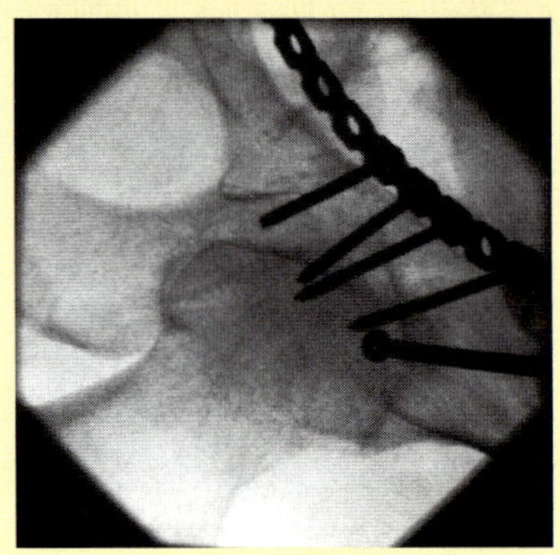

Author Emanuel Gautier

8.1.5 Acetabular fracture—62-B1

1 Case description

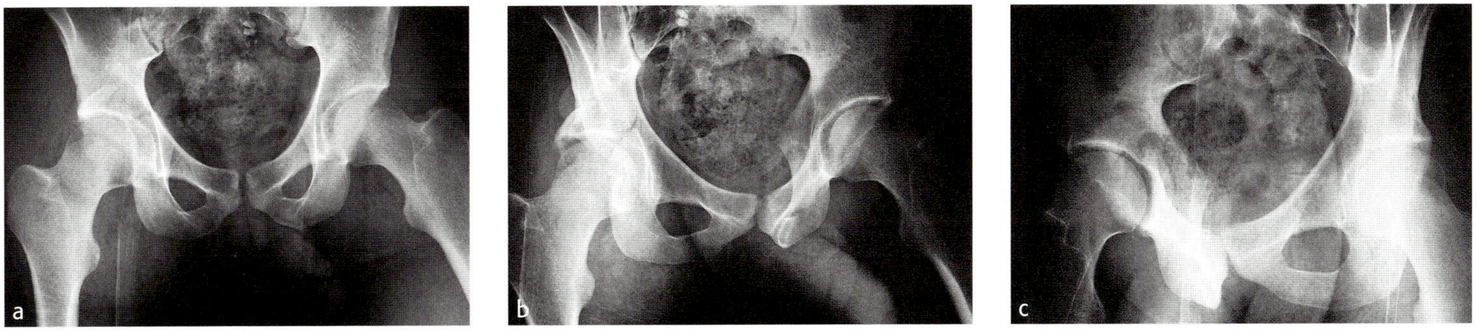

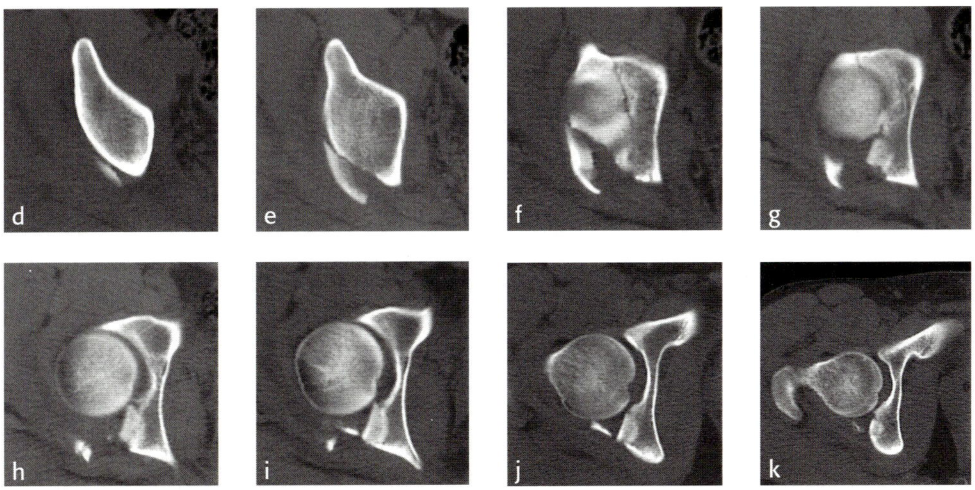

A 20-year-old man suffered a traumatic incident while driving his motorcycle, and sustained the following multiple injuries/fractures: right acetabulum (associated transverse and posterior wall fracture), left femoral shaft, right distal femur, right patella, open right lower leg, stable fracture of the first lumbar vertebra, ribs 3 to 10 on the right, and a rupture of the posterior crucila ligament on the right.

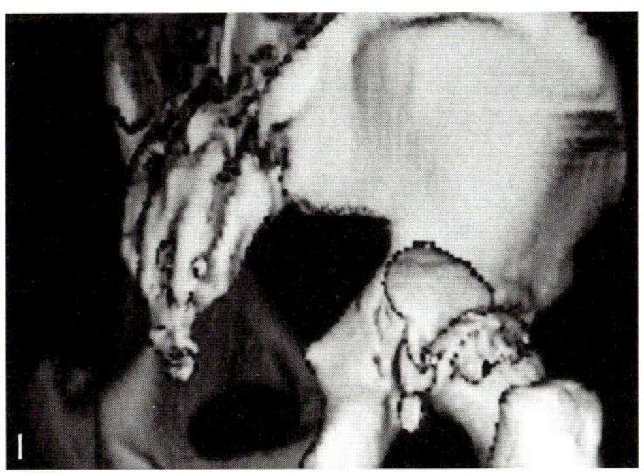

Fig 8.1.5-1a–l

- a AP view.
- b Obturator oblique view.
- c Iliac oblique view.
- d–k Transverse CT scans show the multifragmentary fracture of the posterior wall with marginal impaction and the undisplaced transverse fracture componet.
- l 3-D reconstruction.

Indication

To achieve congruity and containment of the hip, operative treatment is mandatory.

Preoperative planning

Equipment
- LCP reconstruction plate 3.5, 8 holes
- Reconstruction plate 3.5, 5 holes
- 3.5 mm locking head screws (LHS)
- 3.5 mm cortex screw
- Pelvic reduction forceps

(Size of system, instruments, and implants can vary according to anatomy.)

Patient preparation and positioning
Antibiotics: cephalosporin
Thrombosis prophylaxis: low-molecular heparin

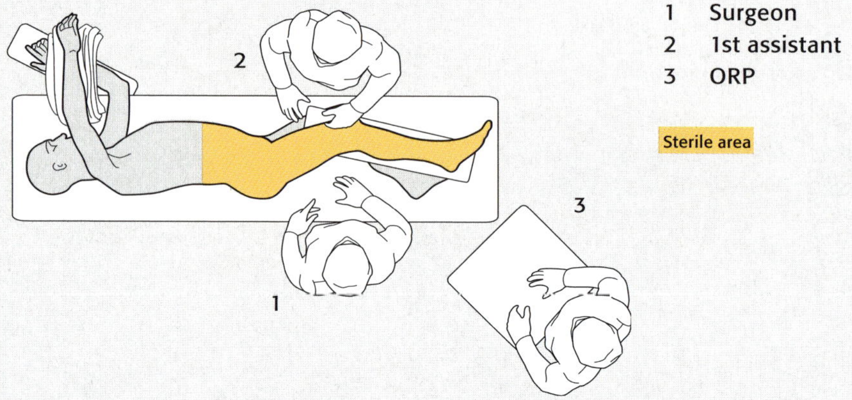

Fig 8.1.5-2 Lateral position on a standard operating table leg freely draped.

2 Surgical approach

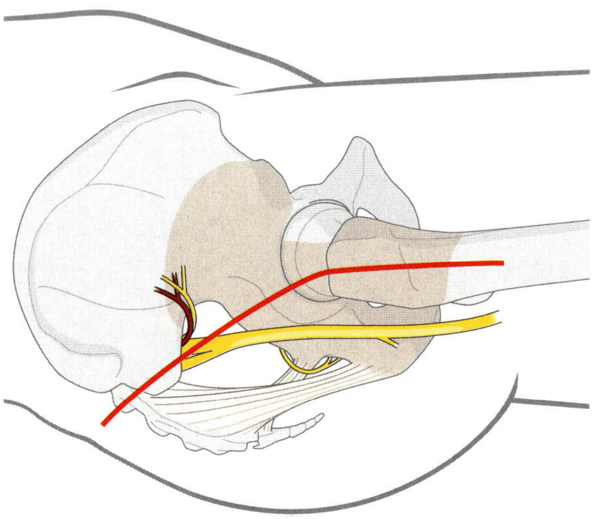

Fig 8.1.5-3 The fracture is approached via a Kocher-Langenbeck approach with a trochanteric flip osteotomy.

The angulated incision is centered over the greater trochanter. The tensor fascia lata and gluteus maximus muscle are split. The posterior borders of the gluteus medius and the vastus lateralis muscle are exposed and a flip osteotomy of the greater trochanter is performed.

Tenotomy of the piriform and of the obturator internus and gemelli muscles with partial elevation of the gluteus minimus muscle.

Capsulotomy of the hip joint should be performed without further devascularization of the fragments of the posterior wall. When surgical dislocation of the hip is needed, the intermedius muscle is detached anteriorly to allow anterior capsulotomy.

3 Reduction and fixation

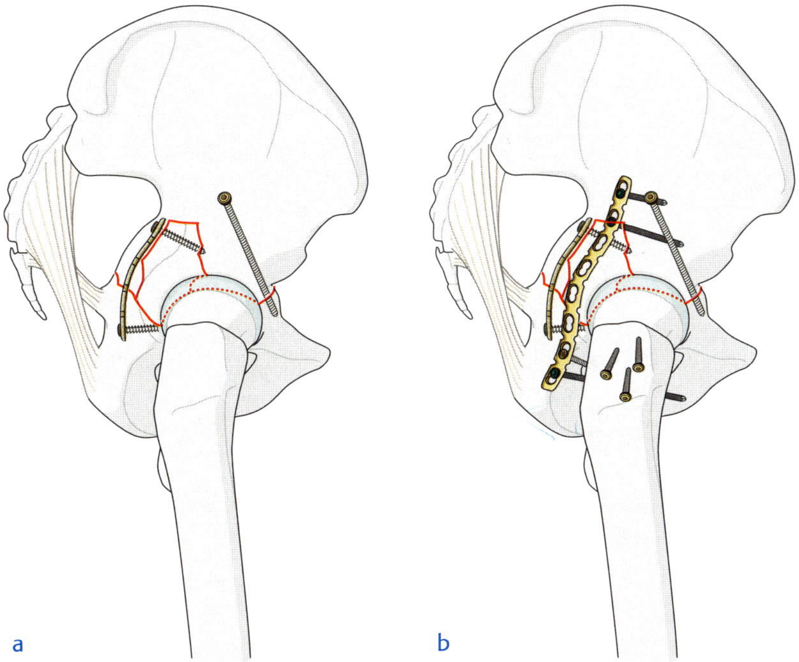

a b

Fig 8.1.5-4a–b Surgical dislocation of the hip. Stabilization of the transverse fracture compartment on the anterior part with a 3.5 mm cortex screw. Stabilization of the transverse fracture posteriorly with a 5-hole reconstruction plate with two screws. Elevation of the impacted fragment, and buttressing with a cancellous bone block taken from the trochanter. Reduction of the posterior wall with the ball spike with pointed ball tip, preliminary fixation with K-wires. Stabilization of the posterior wall with 8-holes 3.5 reconstruction plate with two screws in the supraacetabular area and two locking head screws in the ischium. The greater trochanter is fixed with three 3.5 mm cortex screws after suture of the joint capsule.

4 Rehabilitation

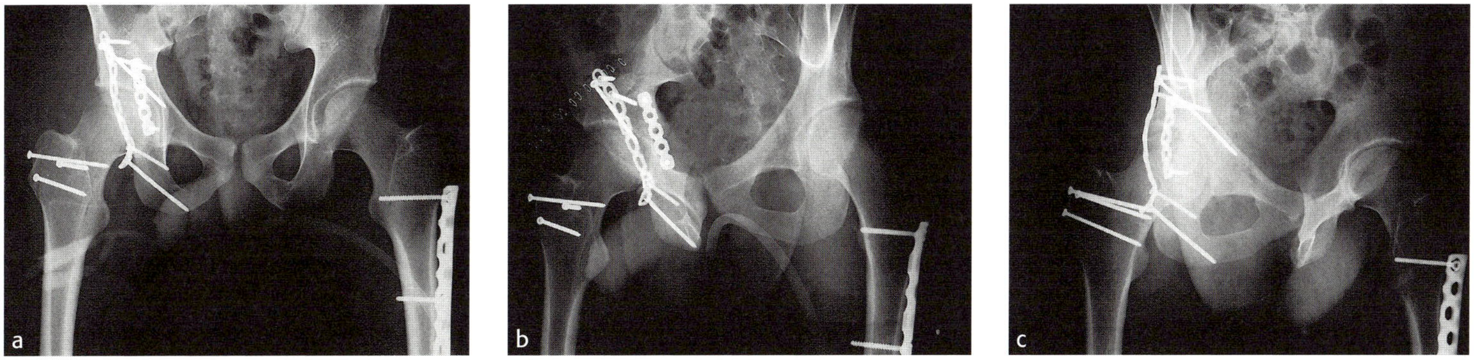

a b c

No flexion of the hip in the supine position and no flexion of the trunk (body) in the standing position to avoid loading of the posterior wall.
Bone healing and full weight bearing after 12 weeks.

Fig 8.1.5-5a–c Postoperative x-rays.
- a AP view after one week.
- b Iliac oblique view after one week.
- c Obturator oblique view after one week.

4 Rehabilitation (cont)

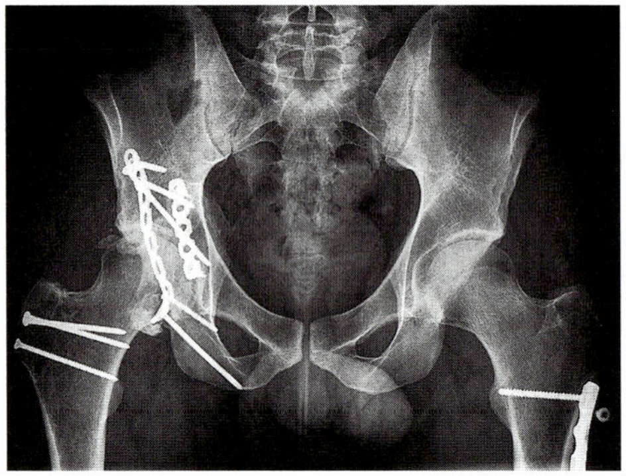

Fig 8.1.5-6 Follow-up x-ray after 3 1/2 years.

5 Pitfalls –

Approach
Danger of injury to the deep branch of the medial circumflex femoral artery during tenotomy and suture of the external rotators of the hip with the risk of avascular necrosis of the femoral head.

Reduction and fixation
The posterior wall fragment often needs additional fixation by means of 3.5 mm, 2.7 mm, or small fragment screws.

Impacted posterior wall fragments need elevation and buttressing using autologous bone.

6 Pearls +

Approach
The Kocher-Langenbeck approach provides a good view of the posterior column.
The enlargement of the standard Kocher-Langenbeck approach with the trochanteric flip osteotomy allows surgical dislocation of the hip and a complete view of the actebulum (from inside).

Reduction and fixation
Control of reduction of the transverse fracture component anteriorly and safe intraosseous, extraarticular screw placement into the anterior column with the femoral head dislocated laterally (in flexion and external rotation).

9.1 Femur, proximal

Cases

Case		Classification	Method	Implant used	Implant function	Page
9.1.1	Avulsion fracture of great trochanter		compression	LCP reconstruction plate 3.5	tension band plate	483
9.1.2	Extraarticular transcervical femoral neck fracture	31-B1	compression	LCP proximal femur plate 4.5	tension band plate and lag screw	487
9.1.3	Extraarticular intertrochanteric proximal femoral fracture	31-A1	compression and locked splinting	LCP proximal femur plate 4.5	compression plate and locked internal fixator	491
9.1.4	Femoral neck fracture; transverse intertrochanteric fracture; femoral shaft fracture	31-B2; 31-A3; 32-B2	compression and locked splinting	LCP proximal femur plate 4.5	compression plate and locked internal fixator	499
9.1.5	Proximal femoral osteolysis		locked splinting	LCP 4.5/5.0, broad	buttress plate	507
9.1.6	Congenital coxa vara with residual hip displasia		compression	LCP 3.5; LCP reconstruction plate 3.5	buttress plate	511

9 Femur

Author Emanuel Gautier

9.1 Femur, proximal

1 Incidence

Trochanteric fractures occur predominantly in geriatric patients; they are the most frequent fractures of the proximal femur. High demands are made on the mechanical stability of the internal fixation. The extracapsular fracture localization rarely compromises the vascularity of the femoral head and good postoperative results can generally be expected.

Femoral neck fractures are frequent in elderly patients. They may also occur in younger individuals after high-energy trauma. The intracapsular fracture localization highly compromises the vascularity of the femoral head. Undisplaced abduction fractures with valgus impaction may be stable enough not to require surgical procedure. Due to the danger of secondary displacement, stability should be checked regularly.

In femoral head fractures, additional lesions are to be considered. Therefore, concomitant femoral neck and acetabular fractures are frequent. The injury mostly occurs in car accidents. In such cases, hip dislocation has to be ruled out, otherwise a reduction has to be performed as soon as possible. In general, femoral head fractures require urgent treatment, anatomical reduction being mandatory.

2 Classification

According to the Müller AO Classification, fractures of the proximal femur are divided into three fracture types:

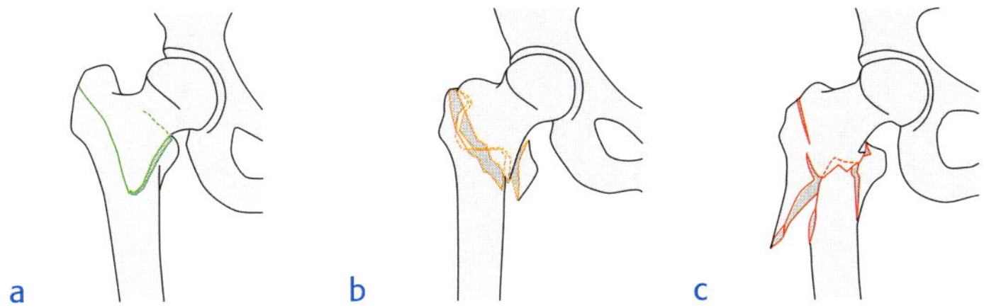

Fig 9.1.1a–c 31-A Extraarticular fracture, trochanteric area.
a 31-A1 pertrochanteric simple
b 31-A2 pertrochanteric multifragmentary
c 31-A3 intertrochanteric

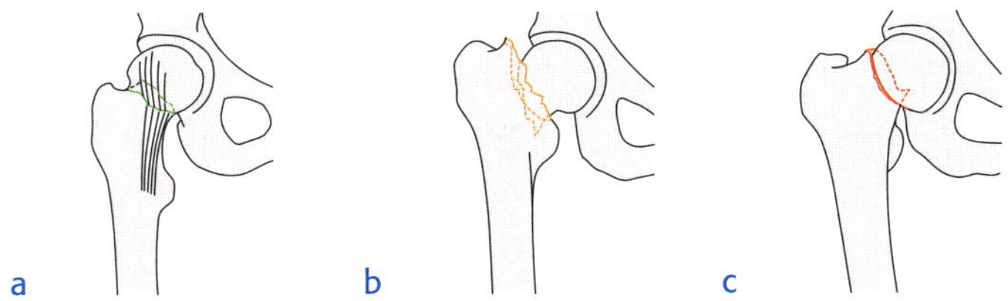

Fig 9.1-2a–c 31-B Extraarticular fracture, neck.
a 31-B1 subcapital, with slight displacement
b 31-B2 transcervical
c 31-B3 subcapital, displaced, nonimpacted

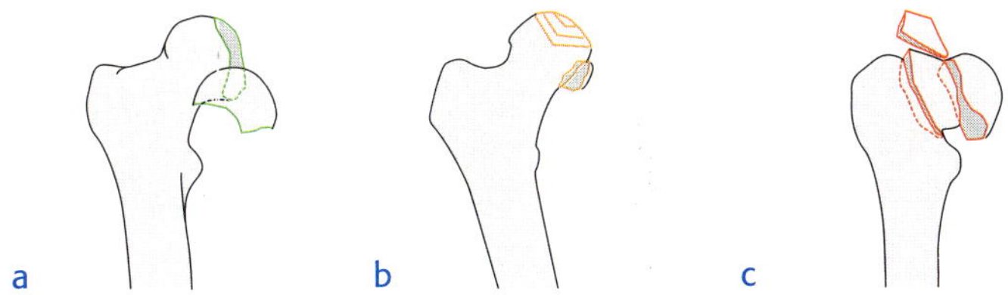

Fig 9.1-3a–c 31-C Articular fracture, head.
a 31-C1 split (Pipkin)
b 31-C2 with depression
c 31-C3 with neck fracture

3 Treatment methods

Mainly to be stressed is the concept of dynamic compression with the use of gliding femoral neck screws attached to an intra- or extramedullary implant along the femoral shaft.

Different implants with different mechanical characteristics are used to treat the fractures of the trochanteric area:

- Extramedullary implants with gliding femoral neck screw (DHS)
- Extramedullary implants with gliding femoral neck screw and gliding mechanism along the femoral shaft (DHS-Medoff)
- Intramedullary implants with gliding femoral neck screw (Gamma nail, PFN, Trochanteric nail)
- Extramedullary implants with nongliding blade in the femoral neck (95° condylar plate)

In elderly patients with poor bone quality, fixation relies mainly on gliding mechanisms along the femoral neck. Some concepts allow for secondary coaptation, impaction, and stabilization of the fracture in addition to gliding support for the femoral shaft. Thus, in the area of the proximal femur there is generally no need for stabilization using an internal fixator, with two exceptions, namely pathological fractures due to bone metastasis and intertrochanteric corrective osteotomies in children or adolescents.

4 Implant overview

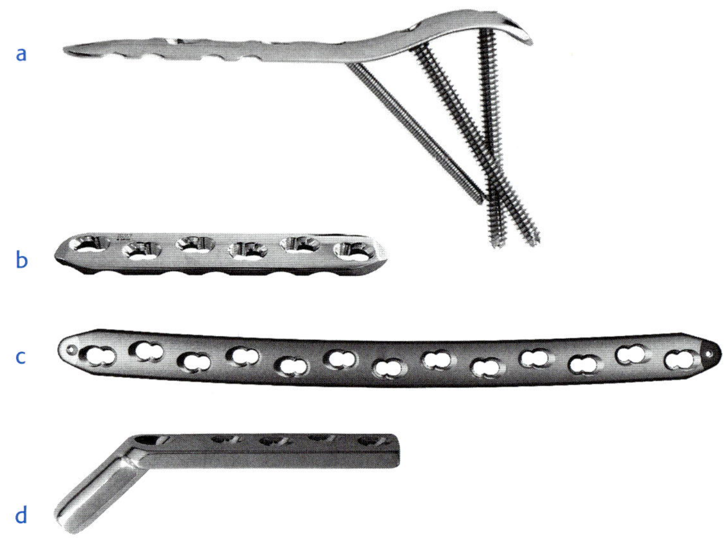

Fig 9.1-4a–d
a LCP proximal femur plate 4.5 (left and right version available)
b LCP 4.5/5.0, broad
c LCP 4.5/5.0, broad, curved
d LCP DHS

5 Suggestions for further reading

Davis TR, Sher JL, Horsman A, et al (1990) Intertrochanteric femoral fractures. Mechanical failure after internal fixation. *J Bone Joint Surg Br;* 72(1):26–31.

Larsson S, Friberg S, Hansson LI (1990) Trochanteric fractures. Influence of reduction and implant position on impaction and complications. *Clin Orthop Relat Res;* (259):130–139.

Schipper IB, Steyerberg EW, Castelein RM, et al (2004) Treatment of unstable trochanteric fractures. Randomised comparison of the gamma nail and the proximal femoral nail. *J Bone Joint Surg Br;* 86(1):86–94.

Adams CI, Robinson CM, Court-Brown CM, et al (2001) Prospective randomized controlled trial of an intramedullary nail versus dynamic screw and plate for intertrochanteric fractures of the femur. *J Orthop Trauma;* 15(6):394–400.

David A, Hüfner T, Lewandrowski KU, et al (1996) [The dynamic hip screw with support plate—a reliable osteosynthesis for highly unstable "reverse" trochanteric fractures?] *Chirurg;* 67(11):1166–1173.

Davison JN, Calder SJ, Anderson GH, et al (2001) Treatment for displaced intracapsular fractures of the proximal femur. A prospective, randomised trial in patients aged 65 to 79 years. *J Bone Joint Surg Br;* 83(2):206–212.

Parker MJ, Khan RJ, Crawford J, et al (2002) Hemiarthroplasty versus internal fixation for displaced intracapsular hip fractures in the elderly. A randomised trial of 455 patients. *J Bone Joint Surg Br;* 84(8):1150–1155.

Dreinhofer KE, Schwarzkopf SR, Haas NP, et al (1996) [Femur head dislocation fractures. Long-term outcome of conservative and surgical therapy.] *Unfallchirurg;* 99(6):400–409.

Asghar FA, Karunakar MA (2004) Femoral head fractures: diagnosis, management, and complications. *Orthop Clin North Am;* 35(4):463–472.

Siebenrock KA, Gautier E, Woo AKH, et al (2002) Surgical dislocation of the femoral head for joint debridement and accurate reduction of fractures of the acetabulum. *J Orthop Trauma;* 16(8):543–552.

Author Michael Wagner

9.1.1 Avulsion fracture of the great trochanter

1 Case description

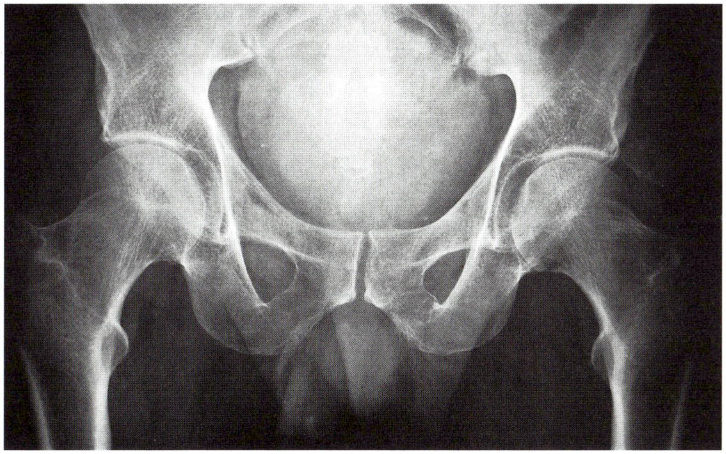

46-year-old man fell over on the street and landed on his left hip. Monotrauma. Closed fracture.

Fig 9.1.1-1 Avulsion fracture of the left greater trochanter. AP view.

Indication

Pain and muscular insufficiency of the pelvitrochanteric muscles due to a displaced avulsion fracture of the greater trochanter.

Preoperative planning

Equipment

- LCP reconstruction plate 3.5, 9 holes
- 3.5 mm locking head screws (LHS)
- 2.0 mm K-wires
- Cerclage wire

(Size of system, instruments, and implants can vary according to anatomy.)

Patient preparation and positioning

Antibiotics: none

Thrombosis prophylaxis: low-molecular heparin

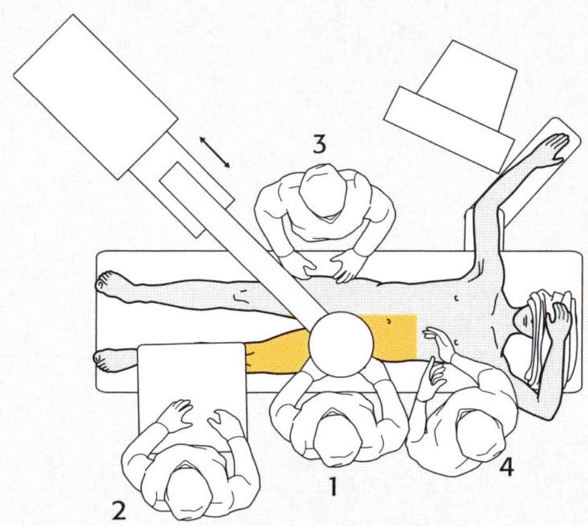

1 Surgeon
2 ORP
3 1st assistant
4 2nd assistant

Sterile area

Fig 9.1.1-2 Supine position on radiolucent operating table.

2 Surgical approach

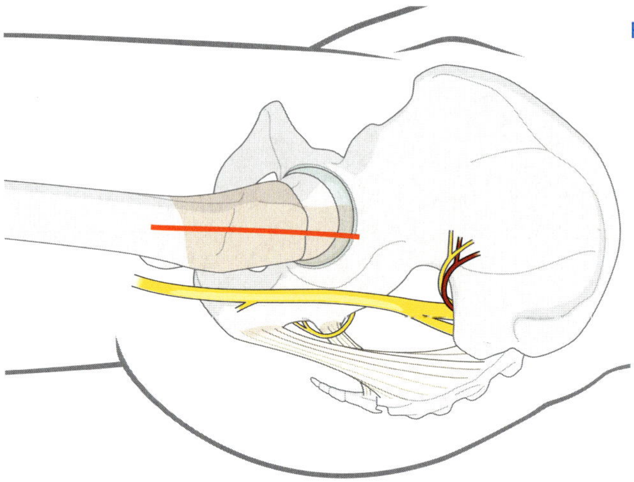

Fig 9.1.1-3 Straight lateral incision to the great trochanter.

3 Reduction and fixation

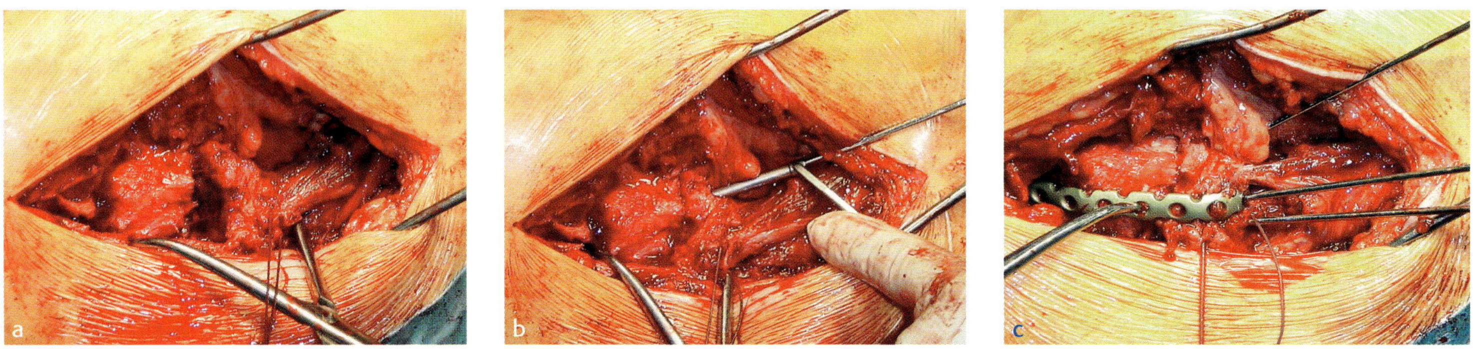

Fig 9.1.1-4a–c

a After division of the iliotibial tract, exposure of the displaced fracture. A strong thread is wrapped around the tip of the trochanteric fragment at the tendon insertion site and reduction is performed with pointed reduction forceps.

b Insert two 2.0 mm K-wires from the tip of the trochanter into the medullary cavity. They will be used later for tension band fixation.

c Preshaping of a 9-hole reconstruction LCP 3.5 to form a hook plate, whereby the hooked part will be placed around the tip of the trochanter (piriform fossa).

3 Reduction and fixation (cont)

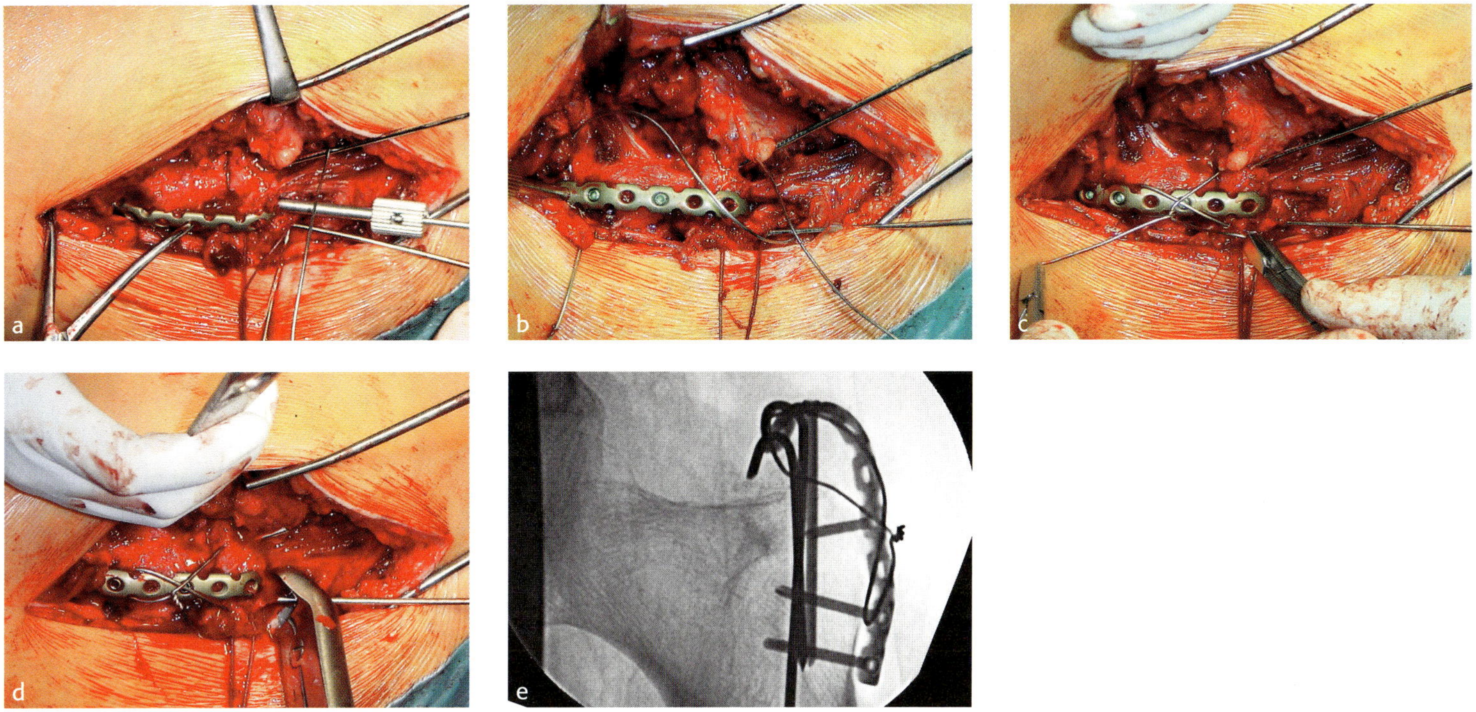

Fig 9.1.1-5a–e

- a After pretensioning the plate in a distal direction with the aid of the pointed reduction forceps, the reconstruction LCP is stabilized with a total of 4 monocortical LHS.
- b To achieve an additional tension band effect, the wire is wrapped around a distal locking head screw.
- c Tensioning of the cerclage wire.
- d The final construct.
- e Trochanteric tension band fixation and hook plate: intraoperative x-ray.

4 Rehabilitation

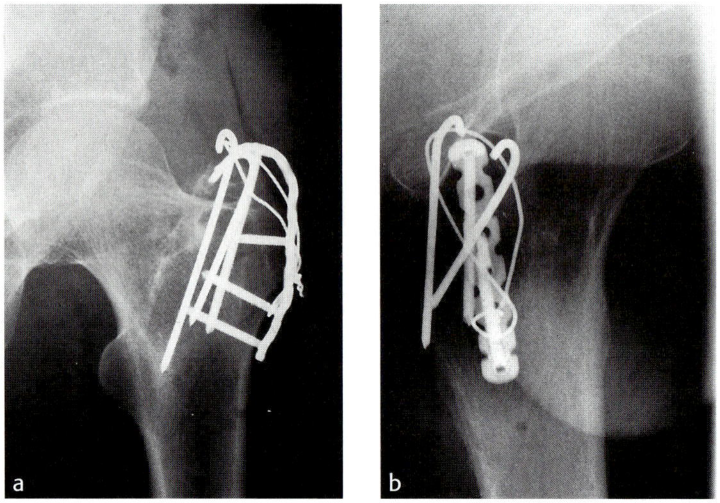

Full weight bearing after 2 weeks. Result of the follow-up investigation after 2 years: no pain, free function.

Fig 9.1.1-6a–b
Postoperative x-rays after 2 years.
a AP view.
b Lateral view.

Authors Michael J Gardner, Dean G Lorich, David L Helfet

9.1.2 Extraarticular transcervical femoral neck fracture—31-B1

1 Case description

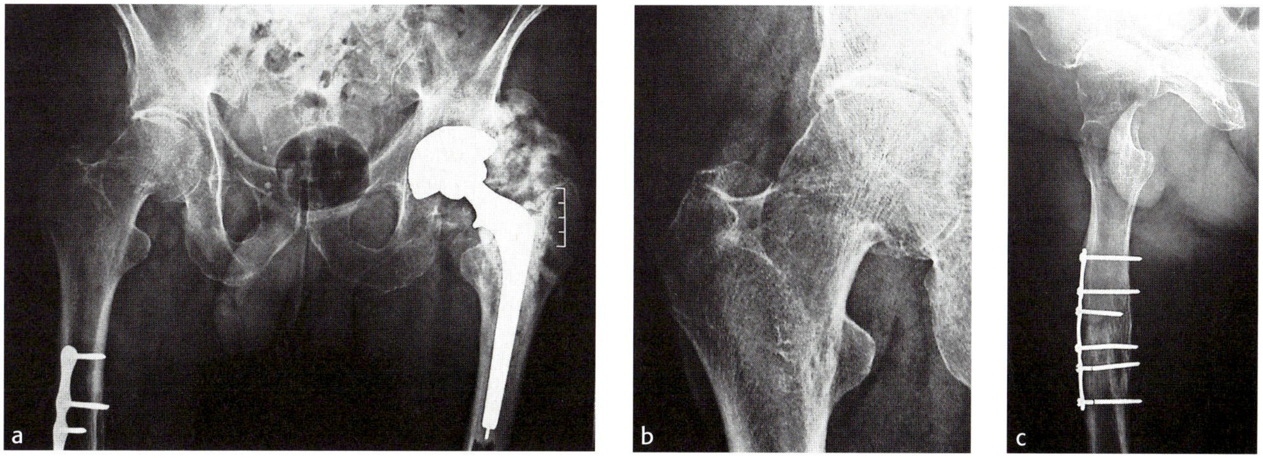

80-year-old active healthy man fell while walking, landed on his right side, sustained a femoral neck fracture with a slight varus and posterior angulation. There were no associated bony, soft-tissue, or neurovascular injuries. He had a history of a proximal femoral shaft fracture on the right side over 50 years previously, which had been treated with a plate. He also had a history of a femoral neck fracture of the left hip 3 years previously, which had been treated with cannulated screw fixation, which subsequently failed. He went on to salvage total hip arthroplasty, and developed mature heterotrophic ossification.

Fig 9.1.2-1a–c
a AP view.
b AP view detail.
c Lateral view.

Indication

This slightly displaced femoral neck fracture in an active patient requires reduction and fixation to attempt to retain the native femoral head and minimize the risk of osteonecrosis of the femoral head.

Preoperative planning

Equipment

- LCP proximal femur plate 4.5, 9 holes
- 5.0 mm and 7.3 mm locking head screws (LHS)
- 4.5 mm cortex screws
- 7.3 mm partially threaded cannulated screw

(Size of system, instruments, and implants can vary according to anatomy.)

Patient preparation and positioning

After intraoperative cultures have been taken, give antibiotics 2nd generation cephalosporins

Preoperative planning (cont)

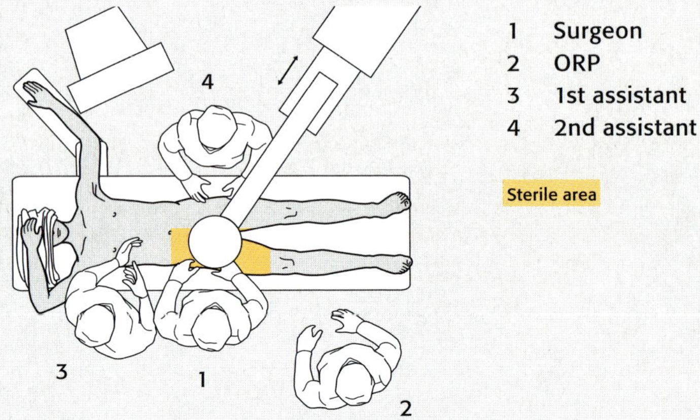

Fig 9.1.2-2 Supine position on radiolucent table or traction table.

2 Surgical approach

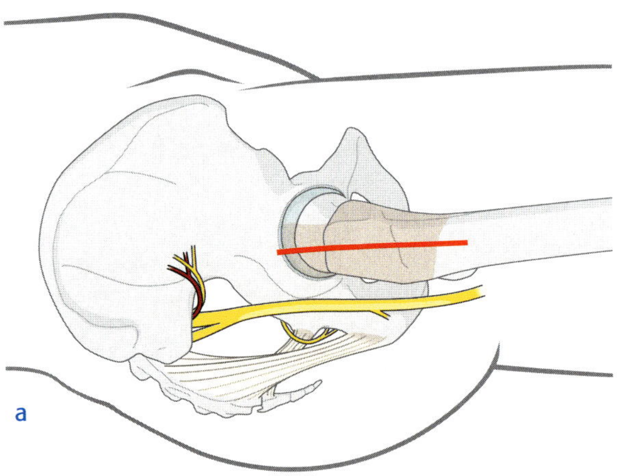

a

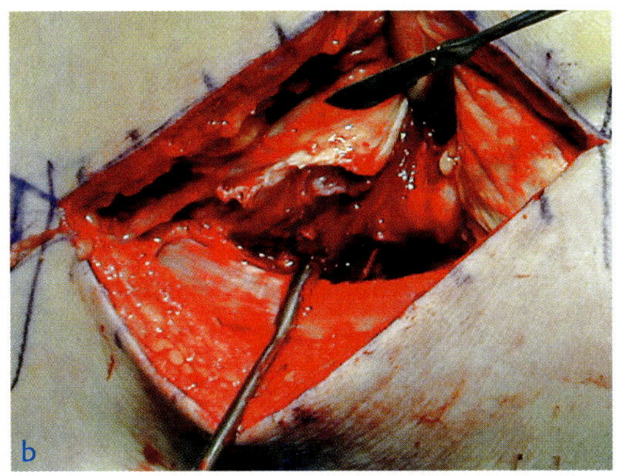

b

Fig 9.1.2-3a–b Prior to prepping and draping, the fracture should be meticulously reduced using closed manipulation with the aid of the traction table. Make a 10 cm incision along the proximal lateral thigh, starting at the greater trochanter distally. Dissect through the subcutaneous tissue and trochanteric bursa to expose the iliotibial band. Make an L-shaped incision in the iliotibial band to identify the vastus lateralis. Reflect the vastus lateralis from the vastus ridge to expose the proximal femur.

3 Reduction and fixation

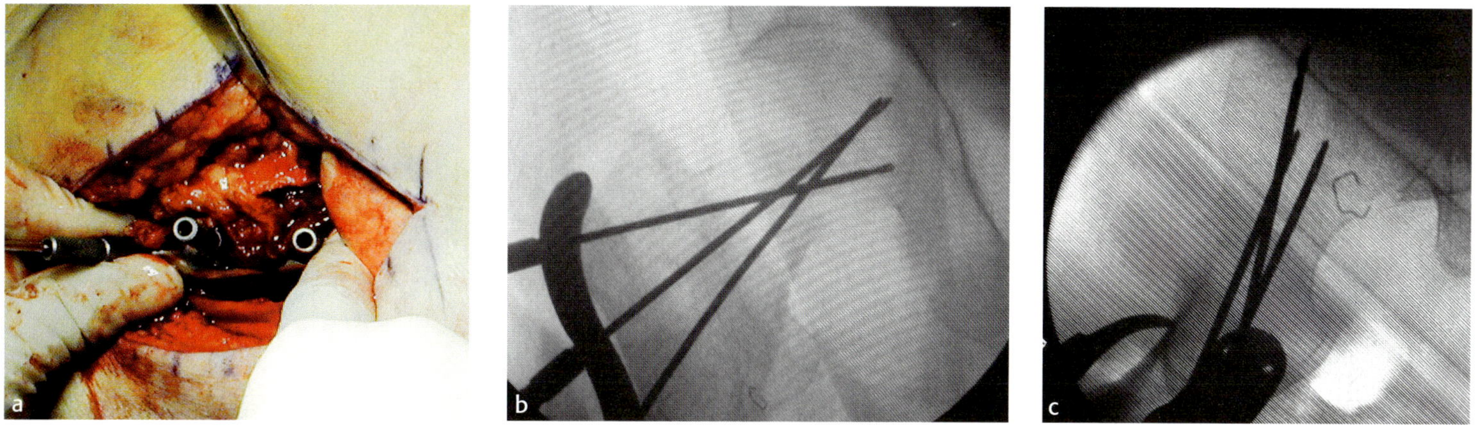

Fig 9.1.2-4a–c Initially, use the traction table to place axial traction on the injured leg. Use AP and lateral x-rays to visualize fracture reduction. Internally rotate the foot approximately 45–90° as necessary. Abduct the leg to correct varus alignment.

A ball-spike pusher may be placed through a stab incision and blunt dissection along the anterior femoral neck to correct posterior alignment. When appropriate position is obtained, slowly release axial traction to allow full contact of the femoral neck fragments.

Expose the proximal femur and place threaded guides in the plate to aid positioning and manipulation. Insert a guide wire in the 95° hole so that it runs approximately 1 cm below the piriform fossa. Ensure the wire is centered in the femoral neck and head on the lateral view. Place a cortex screw through a combination hole distally to secure the plate to the femoral shaft. Confirm that the 95° guide wire has remained in adequate position within the femoral head, and remove and reposition it if necessary. If indicated, place a 7.3 mm partially threaded cannulated screw outside the plate for additional fixation and to achieve initial compression.

Insert the guide wires through threaded guides into the 120° and 135° holes. Measure and insert the three corresponding locking head screws into the femoral head—7.3 mm (95°), 7.3 mm (120°), and 5.0 mm (135°). Secure the plate to the proximal femur through the distal screw holes using locking or nonlocking screws.

Reapproximate the vastus lateralis fascia laterally, suturing it to the plate if necessary. Insert a deep suction drain and close the wound in layers, repairing the iliotibial band incision.

4 Rehabilitation

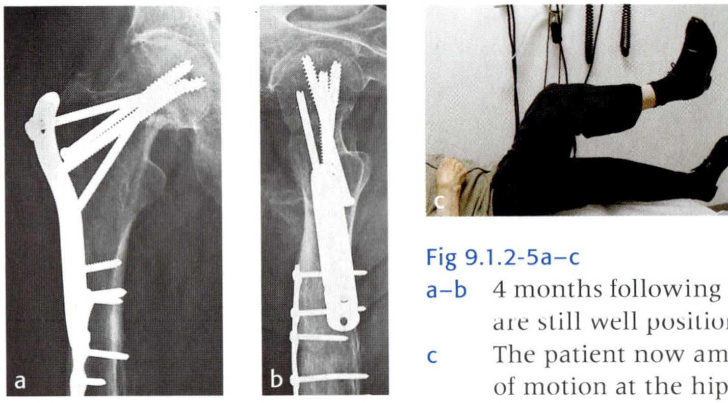

Fig 9.1.2-5a–c
a–b 4 months following locked plating of the right femoral neck, the implant and fracture are still well positioned.
c The patient now ambulates without difficulty or pain, and has good active hip range of motion at the hip.

Continue prophylactic antibiotics for 24 hours.
Initiate deep venous thrombosis (DVT) prophylaxis with low-molecular heparin and pneumatic foot pumps.
Mobilize the patient on the first postoperative day with physical therapy, using a regimen of 10 kg touchdown weight bearing for 6 weeks, increasing progressively to full weight bearing at 3 months.

5 Pitfalls –

Equipment
Currently, the 5.0 mm locking head screw system is available in maximum lengths of 95 mm, which may be too short for some patients.

Reduction and fixation
Often primarily the reduction maneuver is visualized on the AP x-ray, which may lead to inadequate reduction.

Rehabilitation
If weight bearing is advanced too quickly, fixation failure may occur.

It is often difficult to determine healing of the femoral neck.

6 Pearls +

Equipment
In particularly large patients, or in patients with long femoral necks, the screws may be too short. In this case, nonlocking screws or another device should be used.

Reduction and fixation
It is critical to pay close attention to the reduction on the lateral view. In the vast majority of cases, the proximal fragment is angled posteriorly, resulting an anterior apex position. Be sure to correct this position of malalignment. The major advantage of this device is that it maintains femoral neck length and hip anatomy.

Rehabilitation
The LCP proximal femur plate is optimally used in younger, mentally alert and fit patients who can reliably remain partially weight bearing for weeks. For elderly or demented patients, an alternative device that allows early full weight bearing may be preferable.

Closely monitor serial x-rays to assess change in screw position in the femoral head and evidence of healing of the femoral neck.

Authors Philip J Kregor, Erika J Mitchell

9.1.3 Extraarticular intertrochanteric proximal femoral fracture—31-A3

1 Case description

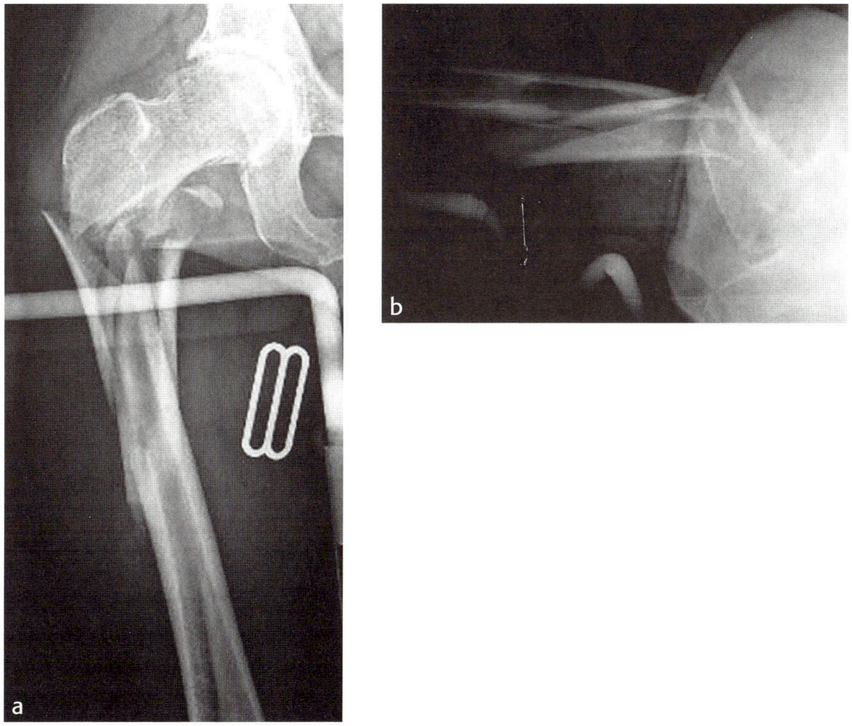

70-year-old woman fell down the stairs and sustained a fracture of her right proximal femur. Low-energy trauma, closed fracture.

Fig 9.1.3-1a–b
a AP x-ray of the right proximal femoral region. The x-ray depicted significant varus deformity and external rotation of the proximal femoral region. In addition, significant diaphyseal extension was seen with involvement of the lesser trochanter (mild osteoarthritis of the hip was also noted).
b Cross-table lateral of the proximal femur is usually difficult to obtain in this setting. Nonetheless, it gives helpful information. On this x-ray, one notes the significant flexion of the proximal fragment. In addition, no extension of fracture lines into the greater trochanter or piriform fossa region is noted.

Indication

This fracture represents a highly-displaced, proximal femoral fracture with deformity in an elderly, osteoporotic female. Nonoperative management would lead to significant deformity, inability to mobilize the patient, and a higher risk of nonunion. Surgical options for stabilization by internal fixation include an angled blade plate 95°, dynamic condylar screw 95°, cannulated trochanteric fixation nail or LCP proximal femur plate. The advantages of a 95° angled blade plate include avoidance of surgical insult to the abductors, but it does require a large surgical exposure. The cannulated trochanteric fixation nail avoids larger surgical exposures, but removes a relatively large amount of bone in the proximal femur and is also associated with surgical insult to the hip abductors.

Preoperative planning

Equipment

- LCP proximal femur plate 4.5, 14 holes
- 5.0 mm locking head screw (LHS)
- 7.3 mm LHS
- External fixator Schanz screws (5.0 and 6.0 mm) to help facilitate reduction
- Pointed reduction forceps (Weber forceps)

(Size of system, instruments, and implants can vary according to anatomy.)

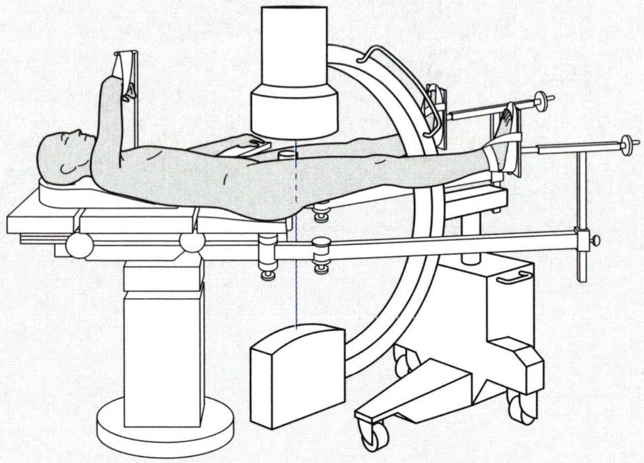

Fig 9.1.3-2 The patient is placed on a traction table. The foot is put in a well-padded boot, and the right lower extremity is in boot traction. For a high-energy fracture, right distal femoral traction may be applied, as a greater force for reduction may be needed. The left lower extremity lies in a well-leg holder, and the right arm is placed over padding of the chest.
The image intensifier is brought between the two legs and before preparation and drapeing, it is ensured that a good AP and lateral x-ray of the hip can be obtained. A small amount of traction was exerted.

Patient preparation and positioning

Antibiotics: cephalosporin
Thrombosis prophylaxis: low-molecular heparin

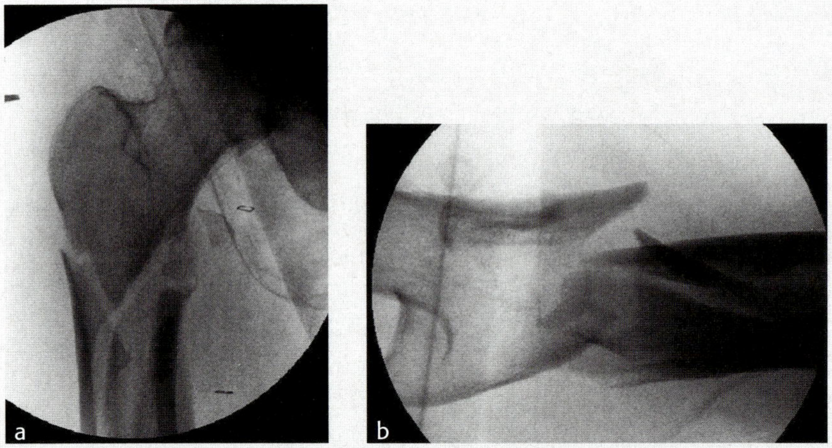

Fig 9.1.3-3a–b

a An AP x-ray of the proximal femur is noted under traction.

b Shows a cross-table lateral view of the proximal femur. There is still posterior displacement of the distal segment relative to the proximal segment, and a flexion deformity of the proximal segment. The piriform fossa region should also be examined at this point to see if there is any extension into this region. None was noted in this case.

2 Surgical approach

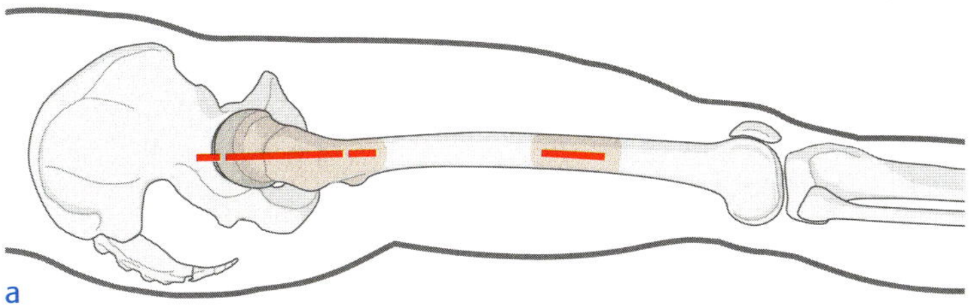

a

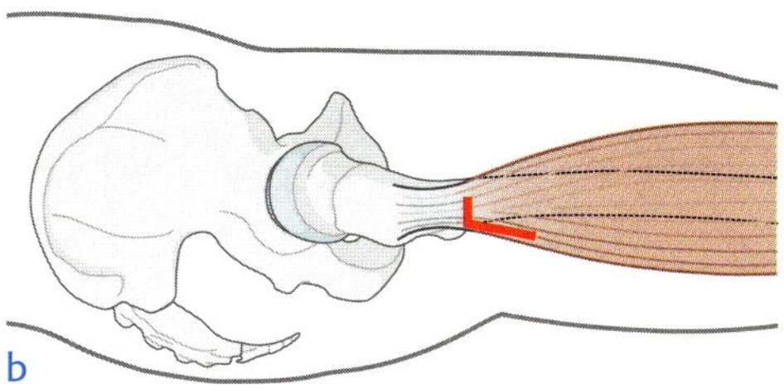

b

Fig 9.1.3-4a–b

a An 8–10 cm midline incision over the proximal aspect of the lateral femur is made, beginning approximately 1 cm cranial to the tip of the greater trochanter and continuing down the midlateral aspect of the femur. Sharp dissection is carried down through the skin and subcutaneous tissue to the level of the iliotibial band, which is incised.
A distal midline incision is made over the distal aspect of the plate, over approximately the distal 3 holes. This incision is analogous to the proximal incision over the proximal end of a 13-hole LISS fixator. It allows the surgeon to palpate the plate on the midlateral aspect of the femoral shaft. In addition the rotational relationship between the plate and the convex surface of the diaphyseal femur can be assessed and modified.

b An L-shaped incision in the vastus lateralis muscle is then made to detach the posterior 50% of the vastus lateralis from its origin.

3 Reduction and fixation

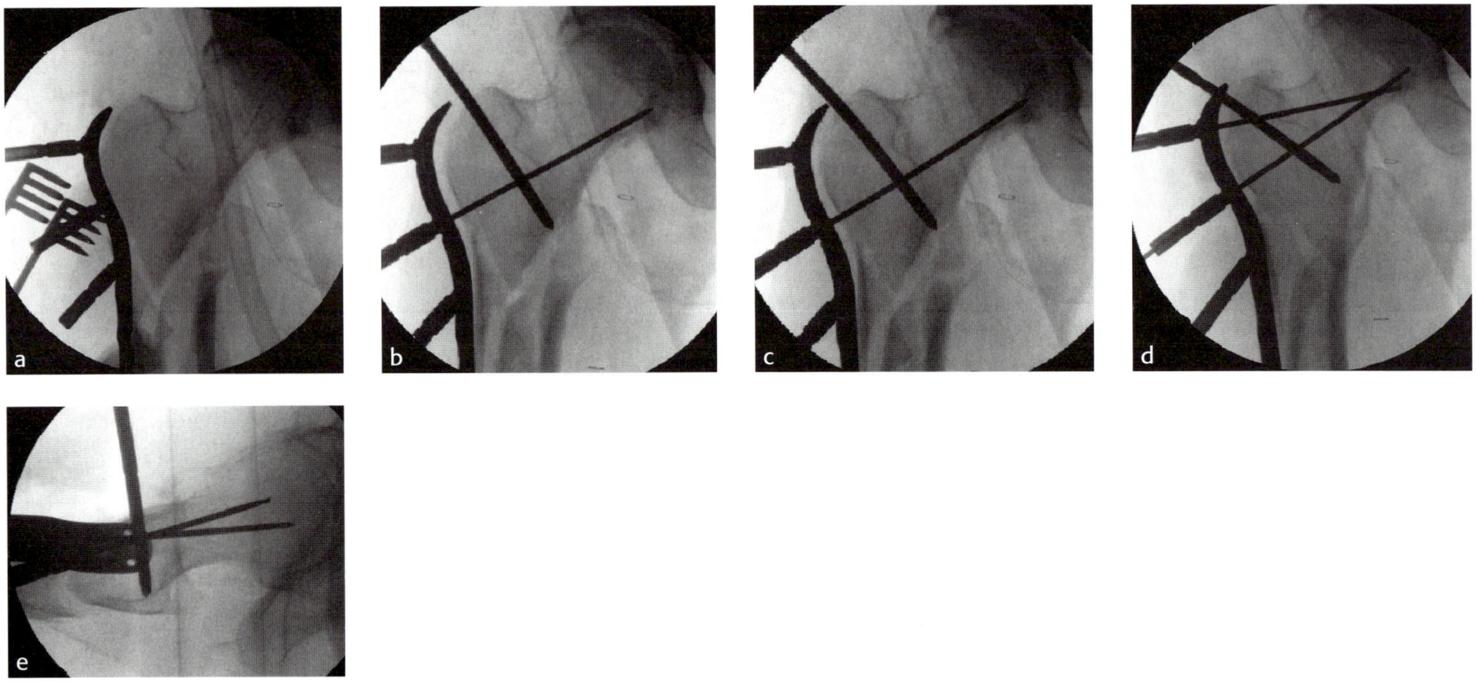

Fig 9.1.3-5a–e

a The LCP proximal femur plate is then inserted in a submuscular manner and an appropriate relationship to the proximal femur is established. Note the three sleeves for placement of 2.5 mm guide wires in the proximal femur. In preoperative planning, a 95° template of the plate on the opposite intact femur can predict where the first screw (7.3 mm) should be inserted into the proximal femur. The first screw of the plate is at a 95° angle to the long axis of the plate. The second screw (7.3 mm) is at an angle of 120°, and the third screw is at an angle of 135°. At this point the proximal femur was still in external rotation and in slight varus position.

b A Schanz screw is placed from the superior aspect of the greater trochanter from anterior to posterior. This Schanz screw is used to control external rotation and varus deformity. Care must be taken to ensure that the Schanz screw is not in the way of the eventual plate placement.

c The Schanz screw is used to correct a small amount of varus deformity.

d An additional guide wire is placed in the proximal femur (first drill guide) once the varus deformity has been corrected.

e Appropriate placement of the proximal guide wires (and hence eventual screws) must be confirmed via lateral image intensification view.

3 Reduction and fixation (cont)

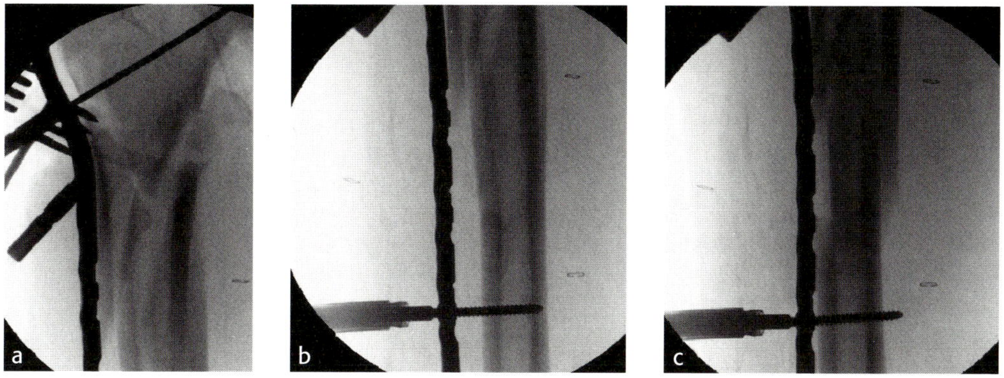

Fig 9.1.3-6a–c

a Medial translation of the distal segment is noted. However, appropriate length has been achieved.

b A bicortical cortex screw is used as a reduction device, bringing the femoral shaft to the plate. It should be noted that prior to doing this, an incision was made over the distal end of the plate to ensure that it is on the midlateral aspect of the femur. If this is the case, a guide wire is placed in the most distal hole to hold the plate on the midlateral aspect of the femur.

c Reduction of the femoral shaft to the plate.

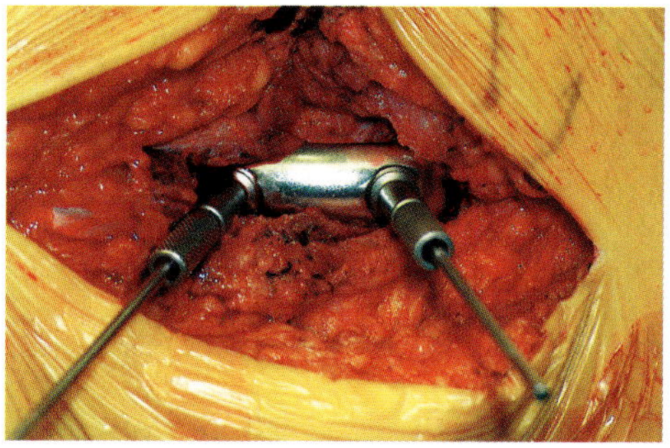

Fig 9.1.3-7 Intraoperative view of the proximal end of the fixator on the proximal femur. Note that no visualization of the fracture is seen, and no devitalization of the abductors occurs. Note that two 7.3 mm LHS, fully threaded, can then be placed over the two guide wires. Prior to this, the Schanz screw has been removed from the proximal femur. An additional third screw (5.0 mm) is then placed in the third hole. This should abut the first screw and act as a “kickstand” to prevent varus collapse of the first screw.

3 Reduction and fixation (cont)

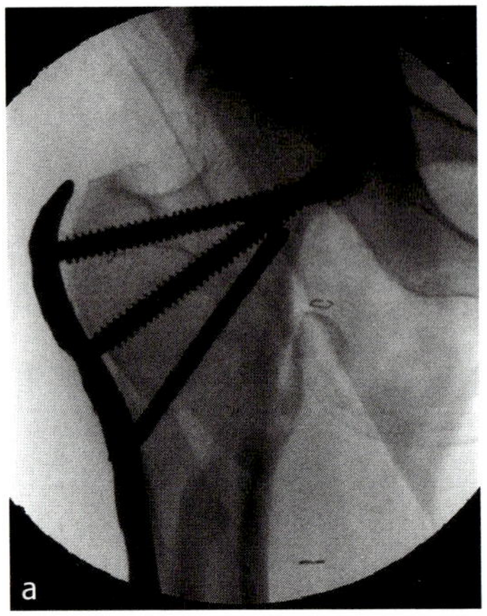

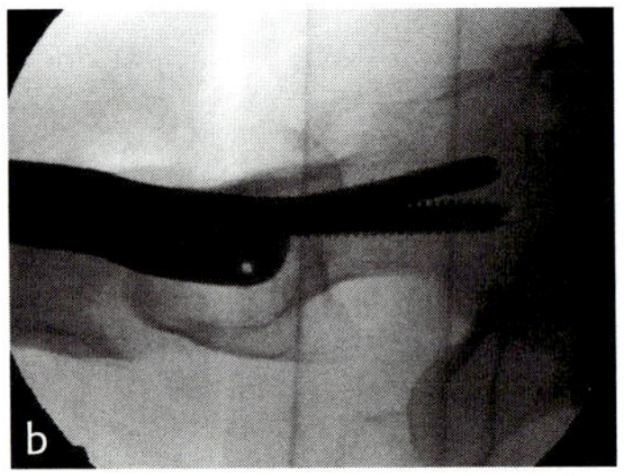

Fig 9.1.3-8a–b
a In this x-ray, the third screw is not of optimal length, and should be 5 mm longer.
b A lateral x-ray confirms appropriate placement of the three proximal screws in the femoral neck and head. It can also be utilized to determine the reduction in the lateral plane. Note that no attempt was made to reduce or fix the posterior butterfly fragment.

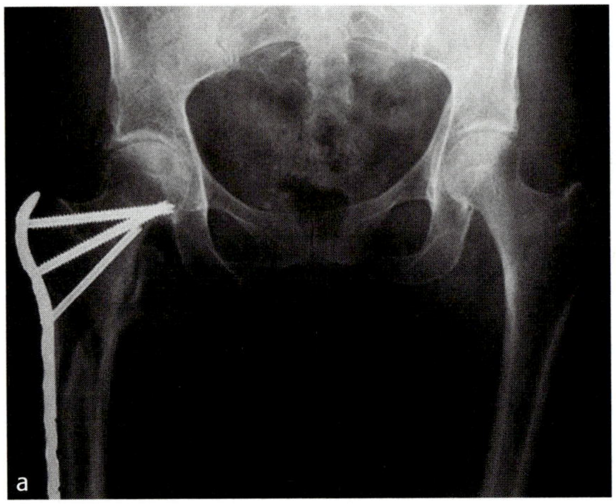

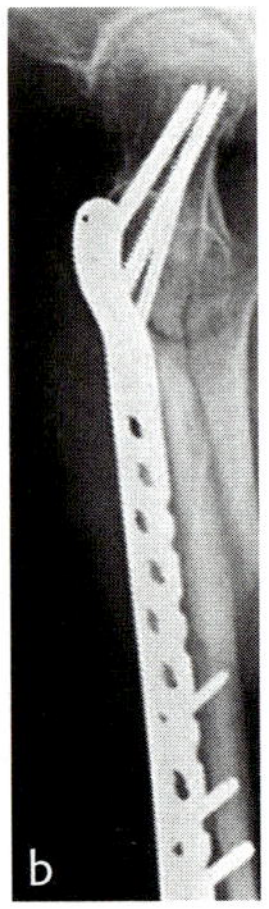

Fig 9.1.3-9a–b
a AP x-ray of postoperative reduction of the proximal femur. This x-ray was obtained postoperatively in the operating room with both legs in internal rotation. The surgeon should judge the reduction quality by looking at restoration of Shenton's line, comparison of the neck – shaft angle with the opposite site, and comparison of the morphology of the lesser trochanter to ascertain rotational profile (if the lesser trochanter is not involved).
b Postoperative lateral x-ray of the proximal femur, which demonstrates appropriate alignment of the proximal segment to the distal segment. Several locking head screws are placed in the distal segment due to the osteoporosis in this 70-year-old female.

4 Rehabilitation

Additional immobilization: No; braces are utilized.
Weight bearing: Half body weight after surgery. Full weight bearing after 6–8 weeks. It must be recognized in the geriatric osteoporotic individual that is it not possible for the patient to control weight bearing well. The patient has immediate range of motion of the hip and knee. Quadriceps femori and abductor muscles strengthening is emphasized.
Bone healing after 12 weeks.

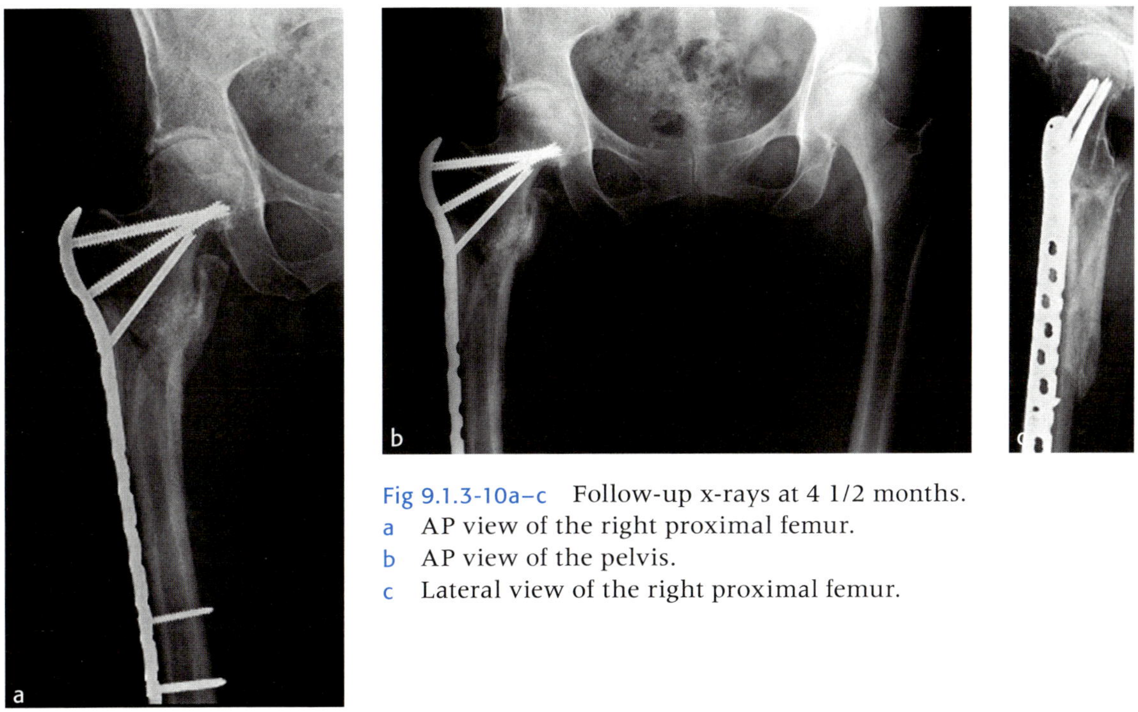

Fig 9.1.3-10a–c Follow-up x-rays at 4 1/2 months.
a AP view of the right proximal femur.
b AP view of the pelvis.
c Lateral view of the right proximal femur.

5 Pitfalls –

Equipment
Inability to obtain good AP and lateral views of the hip intraoperatively can make it difficult to assess appropriate guide-wire and screw placement.

Approach
Soft-tissue dissection to visualize the fracture is usually unnecessary and can lead to devitalization of the fracture.

Reduction and fixation
Failure to recognize or correct the external rotation and varus deformity of the proximal fragment will make it difficult to place the proximal screws appropriately and will also lead to malreduction.

It can be difficult to place and maintain a long plate on the midlateral aspect of the femur when placed using a submuscular approach. This can lead to malreduction if proximal fixation is performed before distal alignment of the plate is ensured.

6 Pearls +

Equipment
The image intensifier should be brought in prior to preparation and draping to ensure that good AP and lateral views can be obtained.

Approach
The vastus lateralis is elevated only enough to allow placement of the three proximal locking sleeves.

Reduction and fixation
Schanz screws in the greater trochanter or a Hohmann retractor placed posterior to the greater trochanter can be used to correct the deformity prior to placement of the proximal screws.

The proximal femur has been derotated and kicked out of varus by use of traction and with the aid of the Schanz pin placed in the proximal femur. It is then locked into position with two proximal guide wires. One bicortical screw has been placed just distal to the fracture. This screw can be used to bring the shaft to the plate for appropriate alignment.

A small incision is made over the distal aspect of the plate prior to definitive proximal fixation to ensure alignment on the midlateral femoral shaft. The plate is then held in place with a guide wire.

Authors Philip J Kregor, Erika J Mitchell

9.1.4 Femoral neck fracture—31-B2; transverse intertrochanteric fracture—31-A3; femoral shaft fracture—32-B2

1 Case description

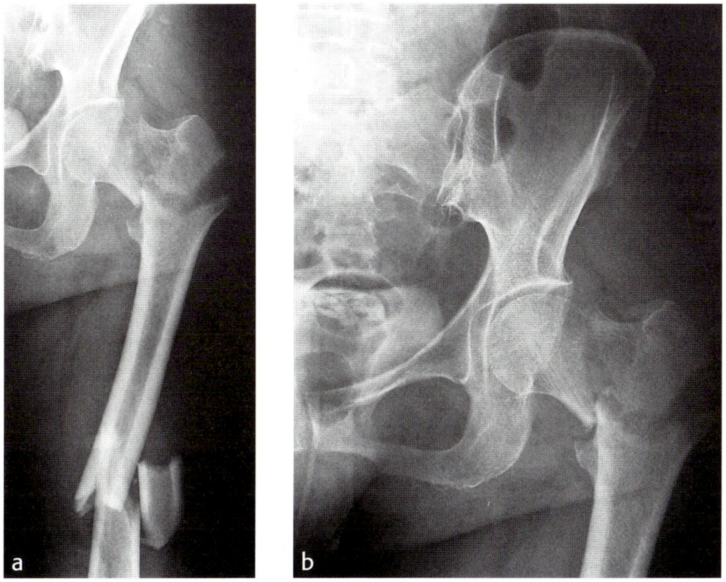

71-year-old woman who was involved in a motor vehicle collision and sustained multiple injuries: multiple facial fractures, left rib fractures, basilar skull fracture, left multifragmentary 8 cm open distal humeral fracture, left multifragmentary proximal ulnar fracture, left both-bone forearm fracture, and this complex proximal femoral fracture with associated femoral shaft fracture. The left lower extremity fracture consists of a vertical shear (Pauwels' classification grade III) femoral neck fracture, a transverse intertrochanteric fracture, and a diaphyseal femoral shaft fracture with separate wedge butterfly fragment laterally.

Fig 9.1.4-1a–b
a AP view of the diaphyseal femoral shaft fracture with separate wedge butterfly fragment laterally.
b X-ray of the vertical shear femoral neck fracture and the transverse intertrochanteric fracture.

Indication

This multilevel proximal femoral/femoral shaft injury in a polytraumatized elderly patient provides a clear indication for operative stabilization. It is recognized that a highly displaced Pauwels' classification type III femoral neck fracture in an elderly woman would ordinarily be an indication for an arthroplasty. However, the complex proximal femoral fracture, the associated distal femoral shaft fracture, as well as open wounds in the setting of a polytraumatized patient make the decision making for open reduction internal fixation versus arthroplasty not clear cut.

Possible options include:

1. Trochanteric nail placement after open reduction of the femoral neck fracture.
2. Hip arthroplasty or hemiarthroplasty with plate fixation of the distal femoral shaft fracture.
3. Open reduction internal fixation of the femoral neck fracture with fixation of the proximal femoral fracture and femoral shaft fractures with plate fixation.

Indication

Fig 9.1.4-2
The challenge in this case is to provide adequate fixation of the femoral neck fracture after appropriate reduction without disturbing the reduction by placing the implant utilized for fixation. There would be concern regarding displacement of the femoral neck fracture if the surgeon placed either an angled blade plate 95° or a trochanteric nail. For this reason, the LCP proximal femur plate 4.5 is ideal.

The three proximal screw holes are at the following angles: first proximal hole (7.3 mm cannulated screws) 95°, the second proximal hole (7.3 mm cannulated screws) 120°, and the third proximal hole (5.0 mm cannulated screws) 135°. The three proximal screws have conical and locking head options. Distally, LCP combination holes are present.

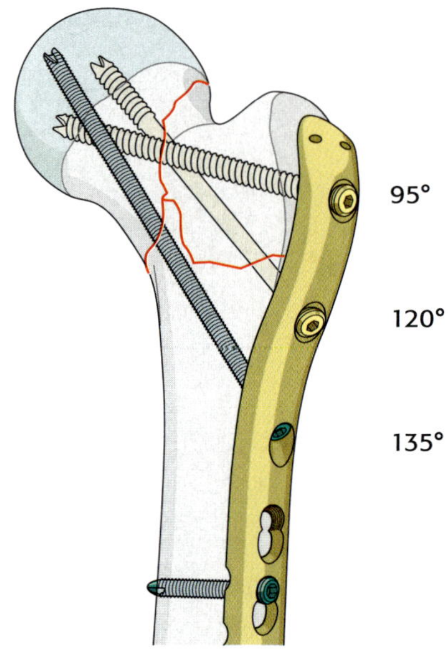

Preoperative planning

Equipment

- LCP proximal femur plate 4.5, 14 holes
- 4.5 mm locking head screws (LHS)
- 3.5 mm screws (for fixation of cortical fragments in the femoral neck).
- 4.0 mm and 5.0 mm Schanz screws
- K-wires
- Pointed reduction forceps (Weber clamps)

(Size of system, instruments, and implants can vary according to anatomy.)

Patient preparation and positioning

Antibiotics: first generation cephalosporin and aminoglycoside (secondary to open injury of the left distal humerus)
Thrombosis prophylaxis: low-molecular heparin for three weeks

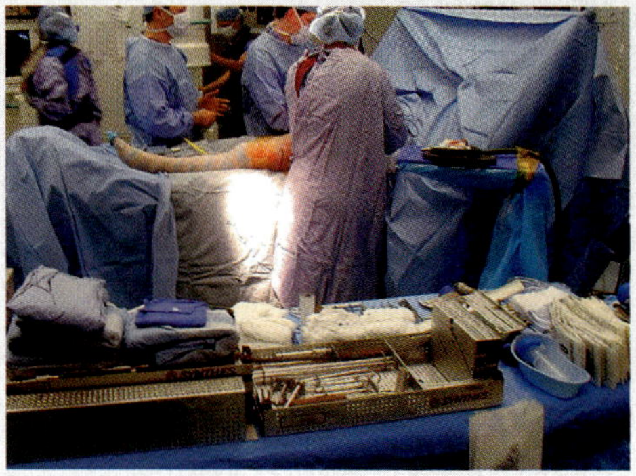

Fig 9.1.4-3 The patient is placed supine on a completely radiolucent table with a small bump underneath the left buttock. The entire left buttock area and left lower extremity is then prepped and draped free.

2 Surgical approach

The surgical approach for this case is a Watson-Jones approach for reduction and fixation of the proximal femoral fracture, followed by a closed reduction and submuscular plating of the femoral shaft fracture. A small incision is made over the fracture to manipulate the butterfly fragment into position.

A small distal skin incision is made over the distal femoral shaft. This is done to allow for palpation of the plate on the distal aspect of the femur. This also allows for placement of screws in the distal aspect of the femur.

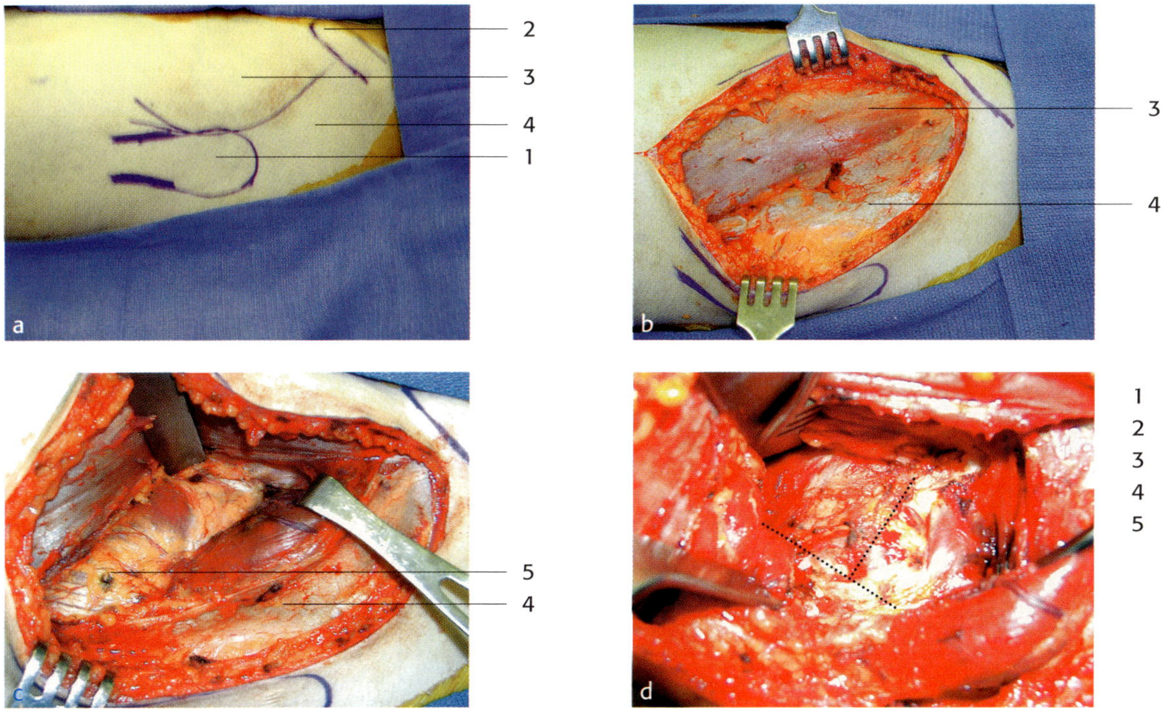

Fig 9.1.4-4a–d

a The Watson-Jones approach employs a curvilinear incision, which is centered over the anterior aspect of the greater trochanter. This incision begins approximately 4 cm distal to the iliac crest at approximately 3–4 cm posterior to the anterosuperior iliac spine.

b A fatty white stripe delineates the interval between the tensor of fasciae latae and the gluteus medius muscle. The interval is then split up to approximately 5 cm from the iliac crest.

c The vastus lateralis muscle is then reflected inferiorly, and the hip capsule is exposed. The fatty tissue on the anterior aspect of the hip capsule is removed.

d The dotted lines represent the T capsulotomy with the base at the intertrochanteric line.

3 Reduction and fixation

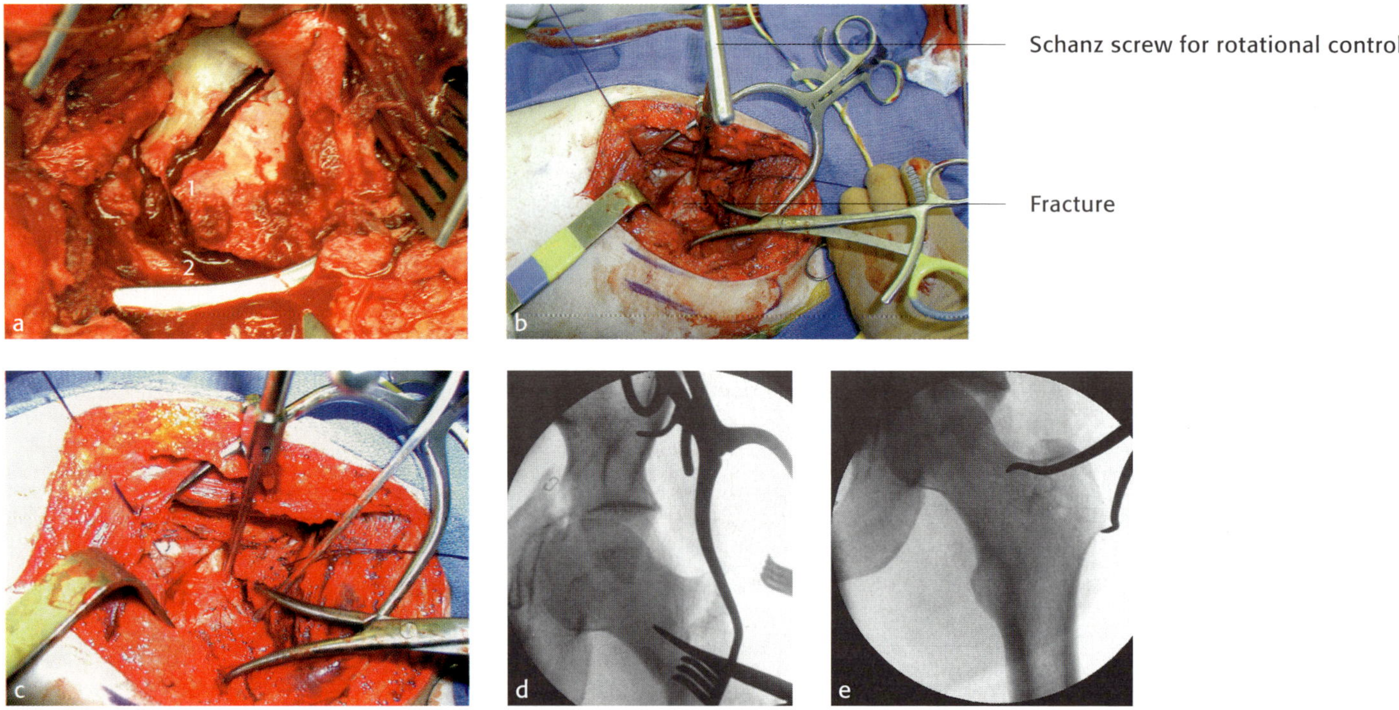

Fig 9.1.4-5a–e

a The Watson-Jones interval gives direct exposure of the vertical femoral neck fracture (1) and the intertrochanteric fracture (2). The key is to re-establish the medial cortex of the femoral neck and to obtain compression across the femoral neck.

b–e Reduction aids for the femoral neck fracture include: manual traction, a 4.0 mm Schanz screw in the femoral neck/head fragment for rotational control of this fragment, a 5.0 mm Schanz screw in the proximal femoral shaft, and large pointed reduction forceps. The pointed reduction forceps (Weber forceps) are extremely important in providing compression across the femoral neck fracture and for re-establishing the normal neck shaft angle. Often, a modified (straightened) tong of the Weber forceps is placed in the superior aspect of the femoral neck through a pilot hole and the other tong of the Weber forceps is placed on the lateral cortex of the proximal femur.
In this particular case, the anterior cortical piece in the inferomedial aspect of the femoral neck area is keyed back into position and a lag screw is placed from anterior to posterior.
Provisional fixation of the proximal femur is then employed and the LCP proximal femur plate is then slid down in a submuscular manner along the femoral shaft fracture.
Note: x-rays shown in this figure demonstrating reduction of the femoral neck are used for illustrative purposes and are not associated with the specific case under discussion.

3 Reduction and fixation (cont)

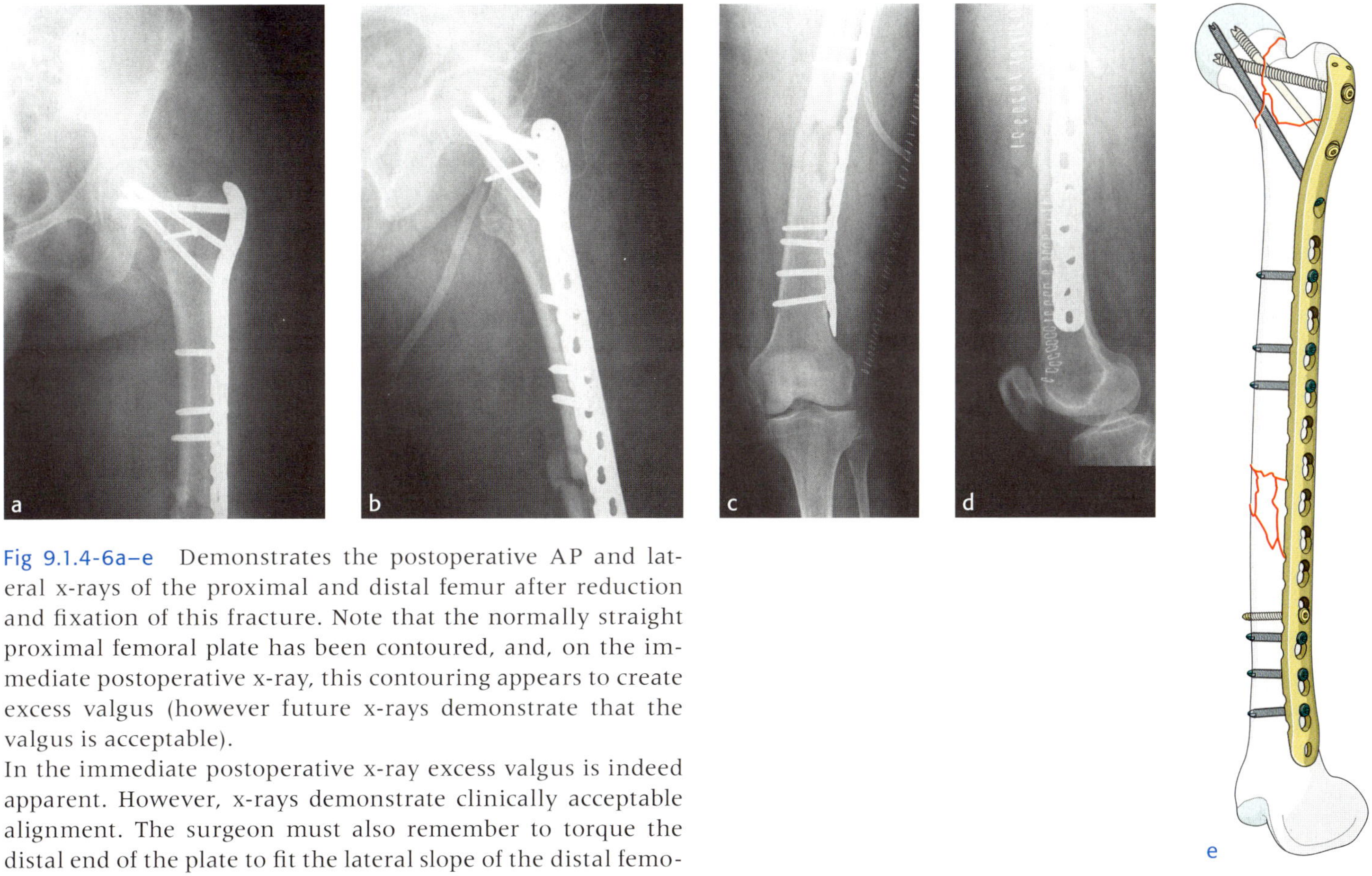

Fig 9.1.4-6a–e Demonstrates the postoperative AP and lateral x-rays of the proximal and distal femur after reduction and fixation of this fracture. Note that the normally straight proximal femoral plate has been contoured, and, on the immediate postoperative x-ray, this contouring appears to create excess valgus (however future x-rays demonstrate that the valgus is acceptable).
In the immediate postoperative x-ray excess valgus is indeed apparent. However, x-rays demonstrate clinically acceptable alignment. The surgeon must also remember to torque the distal end of the plate to fit the lateral slope of the distal femoral cortex.

4 Rehabilitation

The patient has immediate range of motion of her left hip and knee with quadriceps strengthening and abductor strengthening. Because of her complex left upper extremity injury, she was only able to go from bed to wheelchair for the first 14 weeks. After that time, progressive weight bearing was allowed. She was full weight-bearing by week 16.

4 Rehabilitation (cont)

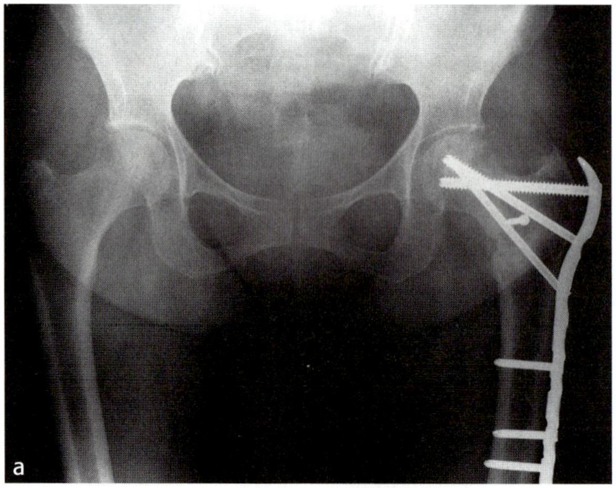
a

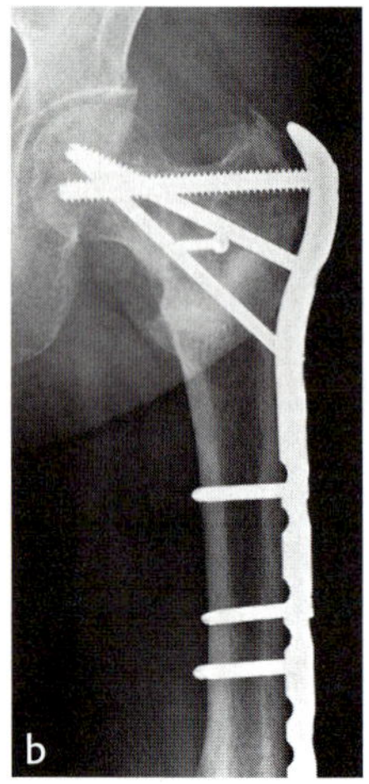
b

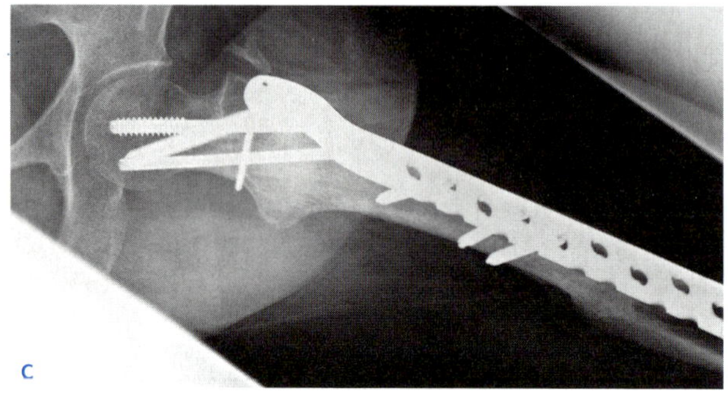
c

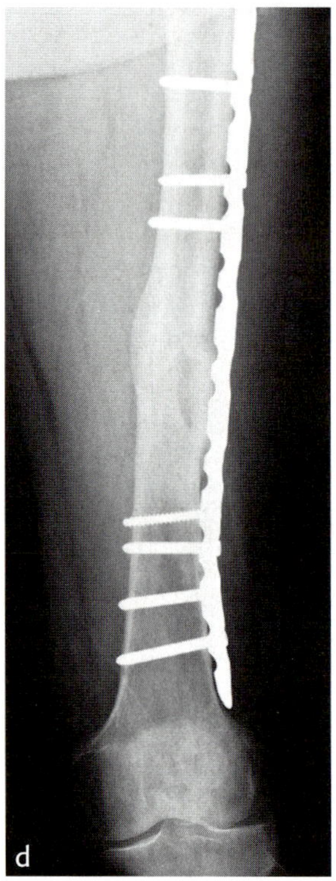
d

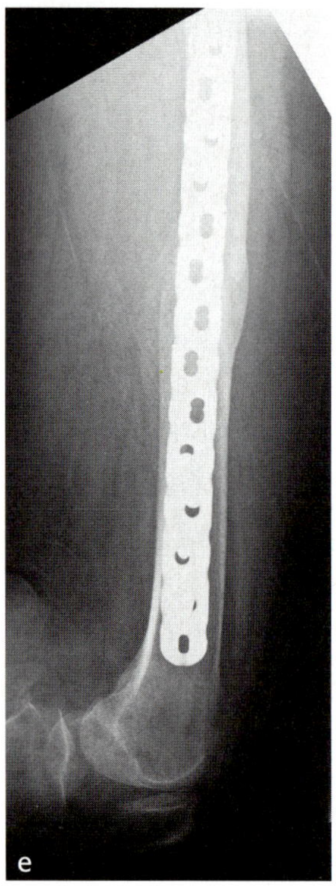
e

Fig 9.1.4-7a–e Postoperative x-rays after 1 year. She has a completely normal hip, no signs of left lower extremity shortening, slight clinical valgus (approximately 3°).

- a AP view pelvis.
- b AP view left proximal femur.
- c Lateral view left distal femur.
- d AP view left distal femur.
- e Lateral view left distal femur.

5 Pitfalls –

Equipment

The placement of the LCP proximal femur plate 4.5 on the proximal femur is critical to the placement of the screws and must be checked both on the AP and lateral x-rays.

When utilizing a long LCP proximal femur plate 4.5 or any plate placed in a submuscular manner, the appropriate valgus and slight internal rotational twist on the distal aspect of the plate should be effected.

Approach

The common mistake is to enter into the muscle belly of either the tensor fasciae latae or the gluteus medius.

If the T-component of the capsulotomy in the hip joint is not centered over the midportion of the femoral neck, this can make exposure suboptimal.

Reduction and fixation

The major pitfall with open reduction and internal fixation of the femoral neck fracture is lack of complete visualization of the medial aspect of the femoral neck. This is important because this must be completely restored. In addition, it is imperative that the femoral neck fracture be compressed for ultimate stability. Finally, a pitfall would be for displacement of the femoral neck fracture with the implant utilized for fixation.

6 Pearls +

Equipment

Careful placement of the LCP proximal femur plate 4.5 in terms of distal cranial placement and in terms of anteversion can make relatively large changes in the placement of the screws. As long as this is controlled radiographically, screw placement can be ideal.

Utilization of intraoperative saw-bone models for the distal femur may be helpful in judging the contouring of the distal aspect of the fixator. In addition, utilization of image intensification views of the distal femur compared with the contouring of the fixator may be helpful.

Approach

Careful delineation of the fatty white strip between the tensor fascia lata and the gluteus medius muscle will ensure proper development of the interval.

With a small amount of traction on the leg, either by manual traction or with a traction table, image intensification of the center of the femoral neck is helpful.

Reduction and fixation

If the Watson-Jones approach is appropriately made, good visualization of the entire femoral neck is possible. The surgeon can key in separate cortical fragments, and then compress the fracture as noted in this case via Weber forceps. Rotational control of the two fragments is made possible via Schanz screws in either the proximal segment or the distal segment. Utilization of the LCP proximal femur plate 4.5 will allow for nonaggressive placement of the implant in the proximal femur. In addition, nonlocking screws may be placed which are partially threaded. They allow compression. In this case one such partially threaded cancellous bone lag screw is used.

5 Pitfalls – (cont)

A common pitfall in the submuscular fixation of the femoral shaft fracture is failure to recreate the anterior curvature of the femoral shaft.

Rehabilitation
Stiffness of the knee or hip can be problematic in this complex fracture.

6 Pearls + (cont)

Bumps of 8, 10, and 12 towels rolled up in elastic bandage may be utilized on the posterior aspect of the leg to help recreate the normal anterior curvature of the femoral shaft. Slight changes in the placement or size of the bump can make large changes in the sagittal plane reduction.

Rehabilitation
Aggressive range of motion of the hip and knee is possible postoperatively secondary to the good stability afforded by the LCP proximal femur plate 4.5.

Author Michael Wagner

9.1.5 Proximal femoral osteolysis

1 Case description

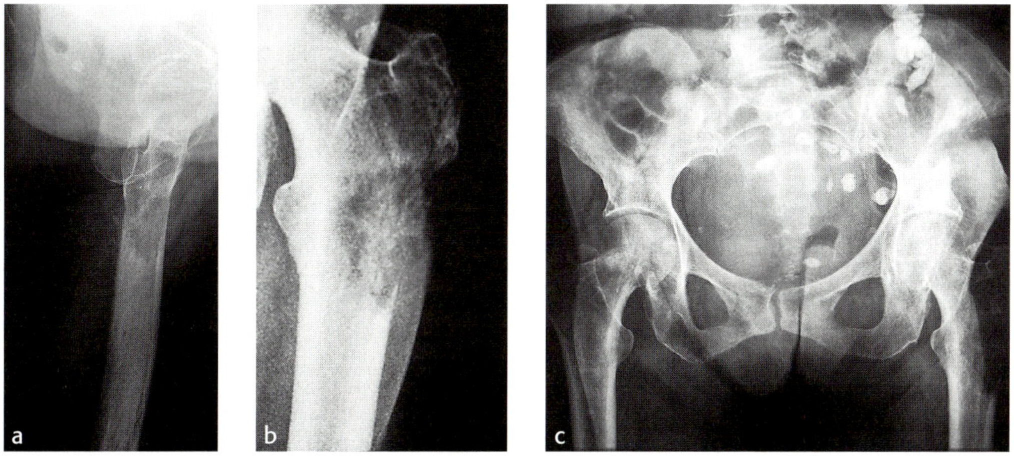

62-year-old woman pathological osteolysis of the left proximal femur with mamma tumor, threatened fracture, and pain. Generalized bone metastases in the lumbar spine and pelvis, additional hepatal and pulmonary secondary metastases.

Fig 9.1.5-1a–c
a AP view.
b AP view detail.
c Lateral view.

Indication

Threatened fracture of the proximal femur with pathological osteolysis. Palliative stabilization in order to allow the patient to be mobilized with as little pain as possible.

Preoperative planning

Equipment

- LCP 4.5/5.0, broad, 17 holes
- Locking head screws (LHS)
- 2.0 mm K-wires

(Size of system, instruments, and implants can vary according to anatomy.)

Patient preparation and positioning

Antibiotics: 4th generation cephalosporin
Thrombosis prophylaxis: low-molecular heparin

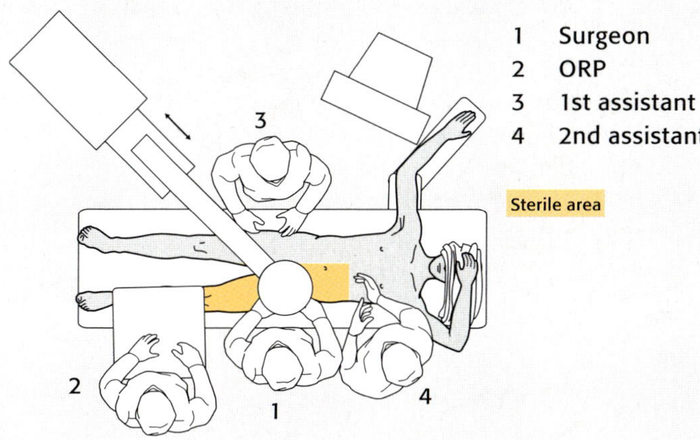

Fig 9.1.5-2 Supine position on radiolucent operating table.

2 Surgical approach

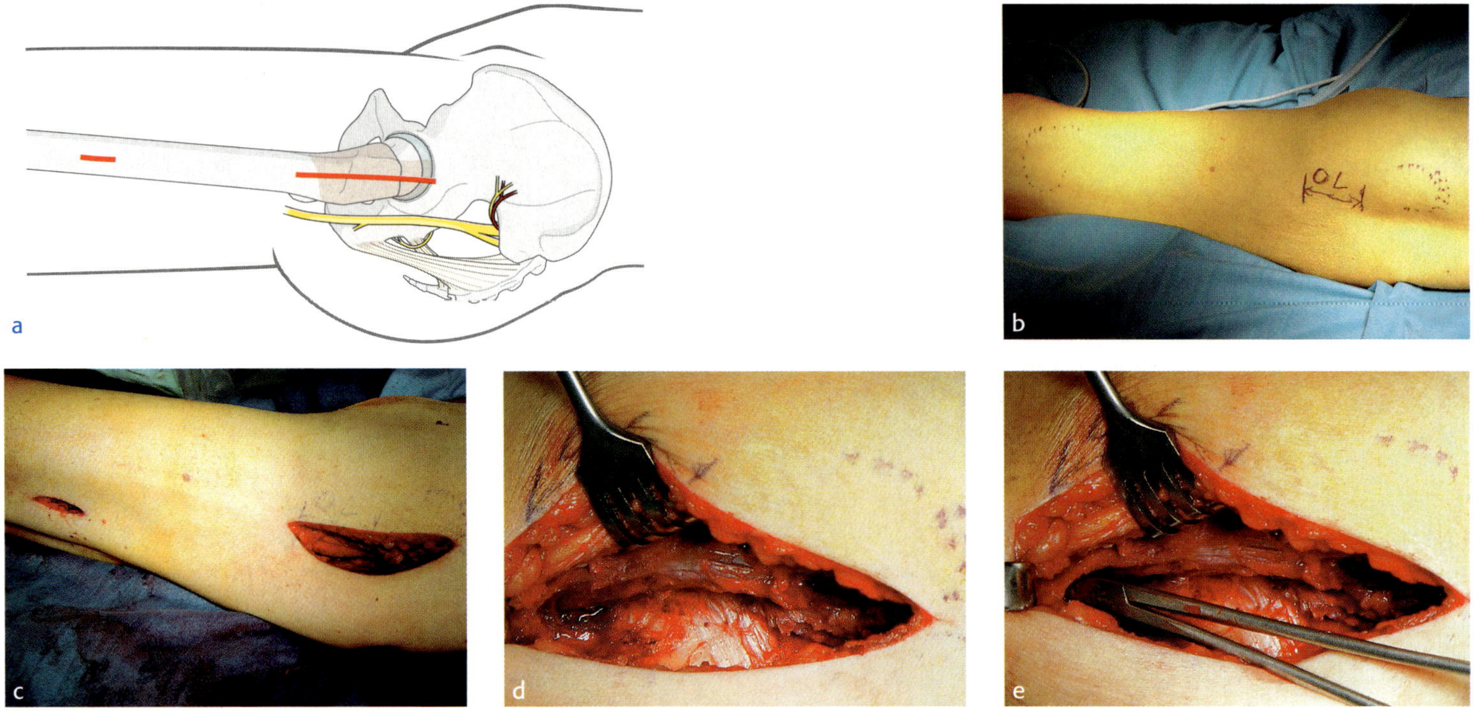

Fig 9.1.5-3a–e
- a Lateral approach to the proximal femur and additional lateral approach to the midshaft.
- b Preoperative marking of landmarks and osteolysis zone.
- c Lateral incision to the proximal femur and predefined distal end of the plate in the midshaft of the femur.
- d Following splitting of the fascia and mobilization of the rectus vastus lateralis, the metastasis is revealed.
- e Submuscular tunneling for preparation of the epiperiosteal space prior to plate insertion in a proximal to distal direction.

3 Reduction and fixation

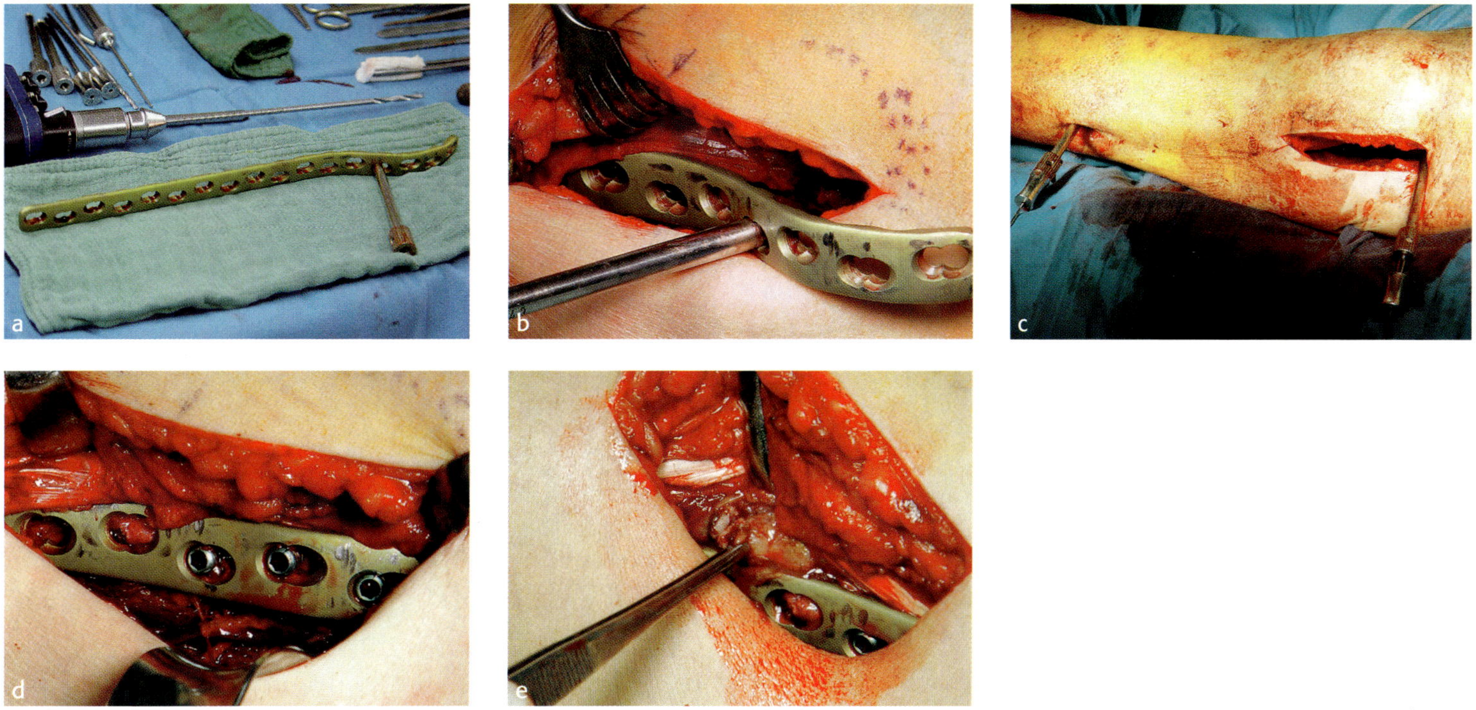

Fig 9.1.5-4a–e

a Prebending of the broad LCP 4.5/5.0 to fit to the anatomy of the proximal femur. A threaded drill sleeve is used as a handle.

b The plate is inserted submuscularly, with the aid of the threaded drill sleeve, into the epiperiosteal space in a proximal to distal direction.

c After screwing in a second drill sleeve at the distal end of the plate and applying two guiding sleeves for 2.0 mm K-wires, temporary fixation of the plate with the aid of two K-wires and control using the image intensifier.

d Subsequent proximal fixation with three self-tapping LHS. Prebending of the plate allows them to run in a converging direction.

e The points of the tweezers are pointing to the tumor tissue in the area of the proximal femur.

Fixation of the broad LCP proximally with four self-drilling and distally with four self-drilling, self-tapping LHS.

4 Rehabilitation

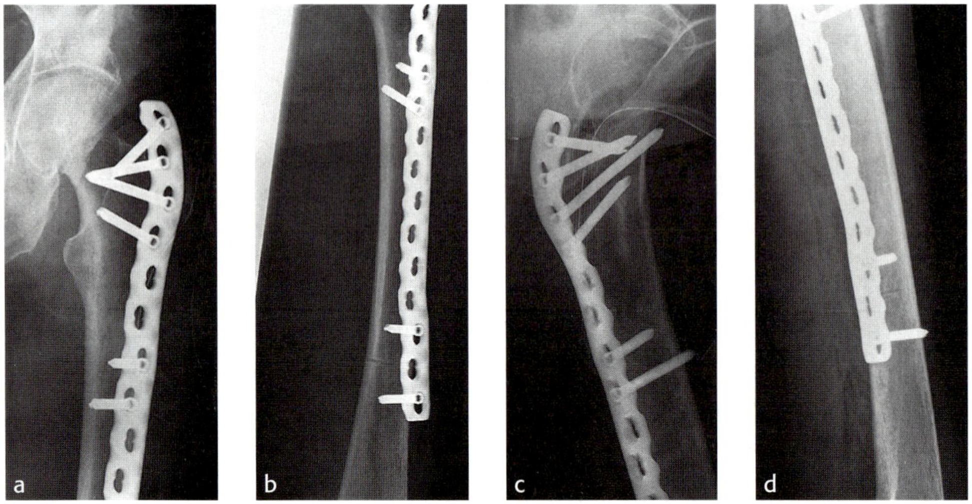

Mobilization with full weight bearing from day 1 postoperatively.

Fig 9.1.5-5a–d Postoperative x-rays
a AP view.
b Distal end of the plate in AP view.
c Lateral view.
d Distal end of the plate in lateral view.

5 Pitfalls –

Equipment

Reduction and fixation

6 Pearls +

Equipment
The LCP proximal femur 4.5 is an alternative implant.

Reduction and fixation
MIPO provides a good option for the palliative stabilization of the proximal femur, in order to prevent a threatened fracture and to allow the patient to be mobilized despite the osteolysis. Due to the additional metastases it was decided to refrain from resection of the bone metastases.

Authors Emanuel Gautier, Roland P Jakob

9.1.6 Congenital coxa vara with residual hip dysplasia

1 Case description

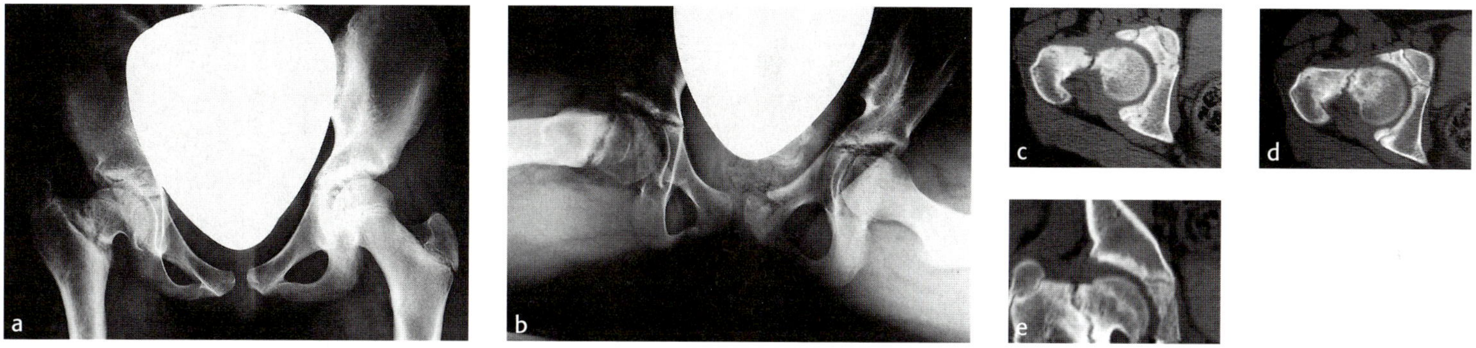

Fig 9.1.6-1a–e
a AP view shows coxa vara with nonunion of the femoral neck.
b Dunn view shows a high retrotorsion of the right femur.
c–e CT scans confirm the nonunion.

This patient was operated at the age of 7 for a fatigue fracture of the femoral neck on the right side. She presented with congenital coxa vara with pseudarthrosis of the femoral neck, retrotorsion of the proximal femur, and residual hip dysplasia.

Indication

The indication for a triple pelvic osteotomy is given due to the residual hip dysplasia to restore normal acetabular index and femoral head coverage.

An intertrochanteric osteotomy is indicated for two reasons:

1) Restore the anatomy of the proximal femur (by valgization and derotation)
2) Decrease the bending load on the neck nonunion by valgization osteotomy.

Preoperative planning

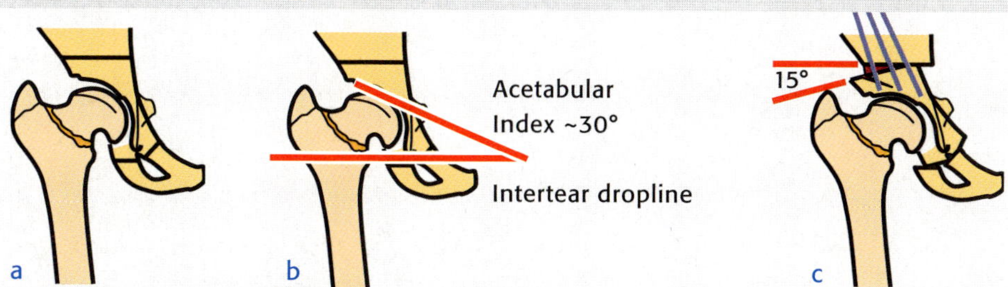

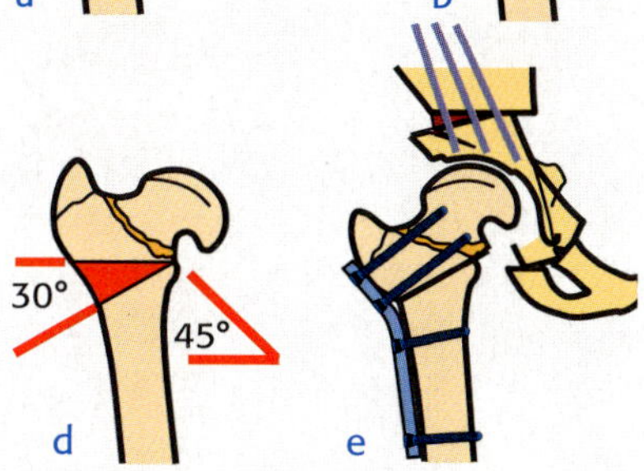

Fig 9.1.6-2a–e
a–c Planning of the triple osteotomy of the hip.
d–e Planning of the intertrochanteric osteotomy of the femoral neck.

Preoperative planning (cont)

Equipment
- LCP 3.5, 7 holes
- LCP reconstruction plate 3.5, 5 holes
- Locking head screws (LHS)
- 2.5 mm K-wires
- Instruments to perform the triple pelvic osteotomy

(Size of system, instruments, and implants can vary according to anatomy.)

Patient preparation and positioning
Antibiotics: cephalosporin
Thrombosis prophylaxis: no

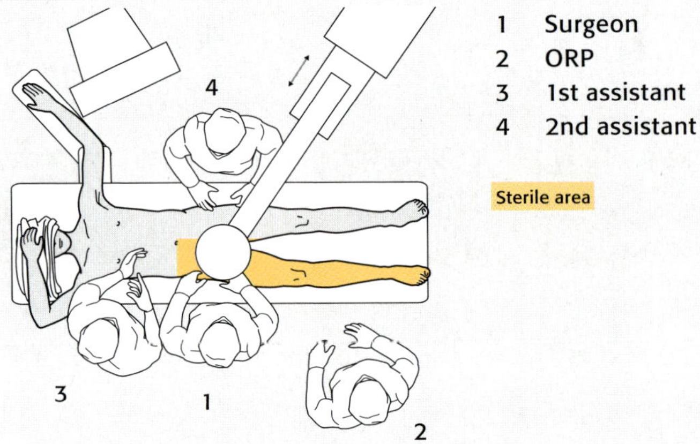

Fig 9.1.6-3 Supine position on radiolucent operating table, leg draped freely.

2 Surgical approach

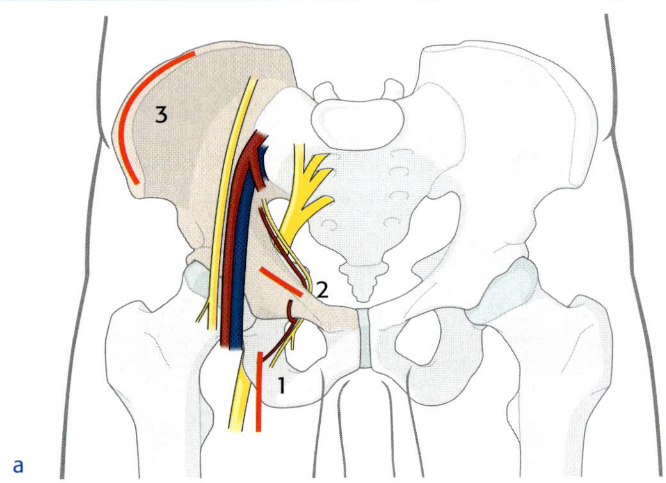

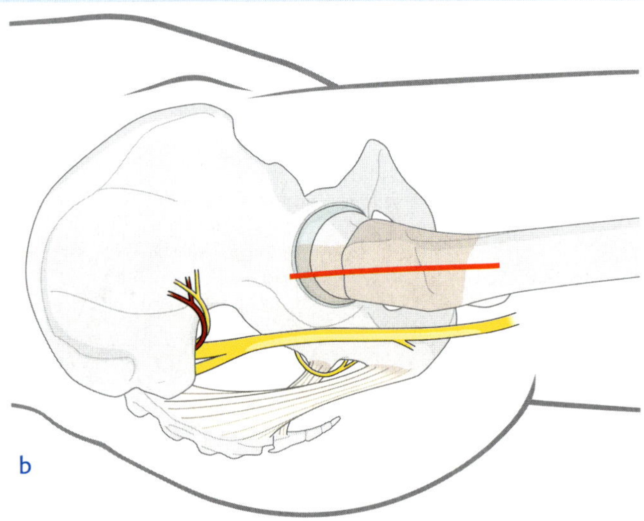

Fig 9.1.6-4a–b
a The triple pelvic osteotomy is performed using three approaches: (1) Ludloff approach for the osteotomy of the ischium, (2) a partial ilioinguinal approach to perform the osteotomies of the superior pubic ramus, and (3) the approach to the illium.
b Anterolateral approach to the hip to perform the intertrochanteric correction osteotomy.

3 Reduction and fixation

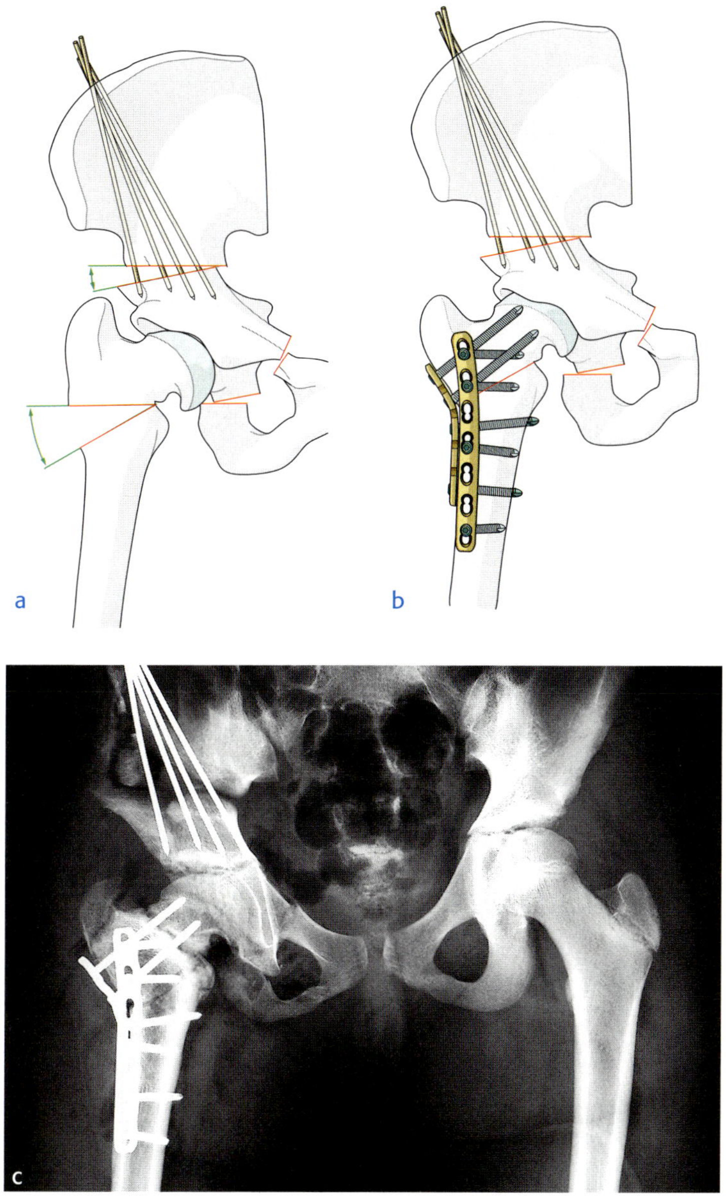

Fig 9.1.6-5a–c

a Preliminary fixation of the triple pelvic osteotomy with two 2.5 mm K-wires. After correction, definitive stabilization with K-wires.

b Lateral fixation with a 5-hole 3.5 LCP with two proximal locking head screws passing through the pseudarthrosis of the femoral neck. Additional anterior fixation with a 7-hole LCP using locking head screws.

c Postoperative x-ray.

4 Rehabilitation

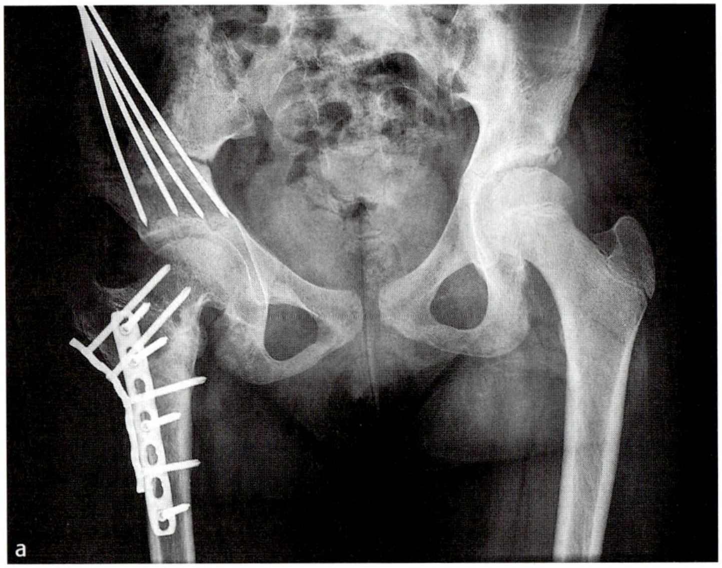

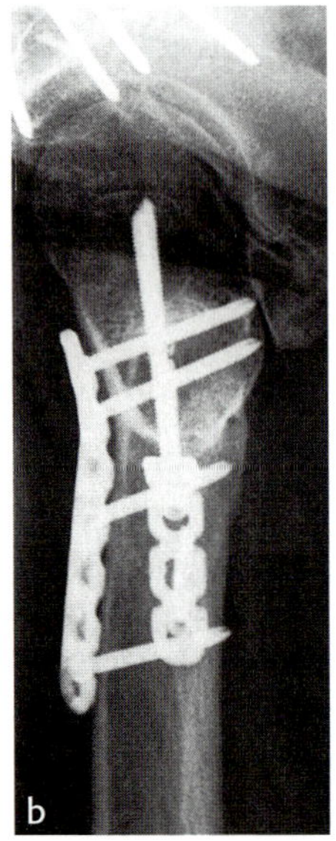

Additional immobilization with pelvis and leg splint for three months. K-wires were removed after 4 months. Weight bearing: 15 kg for 4 weeks, full weight bearing after 4 months.

Fig 9.1.6-6a–b Postoperative x-ray after 18 weeks showing healing of the intertrochanteric osteotomy and the pelvic osteotomy.
a AP view.
b Axial view.

5 Pitfalls –

Equipment
The LCP 3.5 in titanium is difficult to remove.

Reduction and fixation

6 Pearls +

Equipment
One should consider the use of steel implants.

Reduction and fixation
Very stable fixation of the femoral osteotomy with two plates, one laterally, one anteriorly.

9.2 Femur, shaft

Cases

9 Femur

Author Michael Wagner

9.2 Femur, shaft

1 Incidence

Some characteristic signs such as axial deviation, shortening, abnormal function and pain, clinical diagnosis of femoral shaft fractures, including subtrochanteric fractures, are obvious.

Clinical examination has to integrate soft-tissue involvement. Due to dense soft-tissue wrapping, open fractures are less common. Neurovascular deficiencies are to be detected immediately. Standard x-ray examinations consist of views in two planes, including joints to rule out additional ipsilateral fractures of the femoral neck or tibial head.

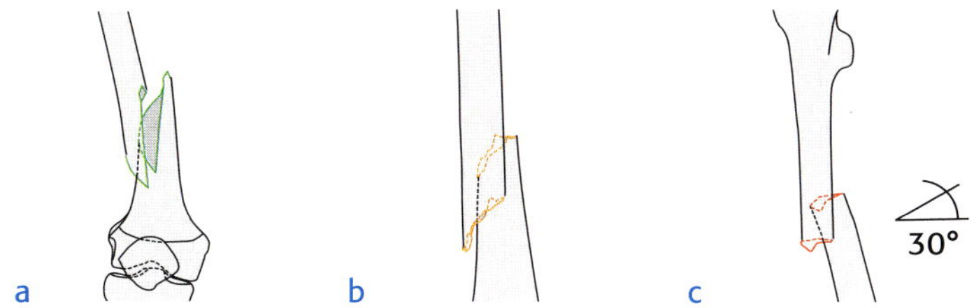

Fig 9.2-1a–c 32-A simple fracture.
a 32-A1 spiral
b 32-A2 oblique (> 30°)
c 32-A3 transverse (< 30°)

2 Classification

The shaft area includes the subtrochanteric region. The Müller AO Classification considers simple, wedge and complex fractures. Additionally, soft-tissue damage has to be taken into account.

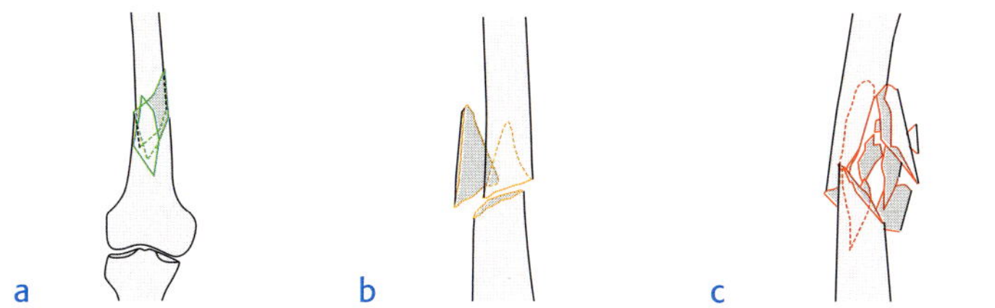

Fig 9.2-2a–c 32-B wedge fracture.
a 32-B1 spiral wedge
b 32-B2 bending wedge
c 32-B3 fragmented wedge

3 Treatment methods

Different methods of closed reduction are practicable such as manual traction or distraction using a traction table or a Schanz screw-assisted distractor. To facilitate the intramedullary nailing procedure, a short nail may be used as a "joystick" to handle the proximal fragment. Ligamentotaxis may be effective in the reduction of complex fractures.

Just a small longitudinal incision of about 3–5 cm is recommended for antegrade femoral nailing and placed approximately 12–15 cm proximal to the tip of the greater trochanter.

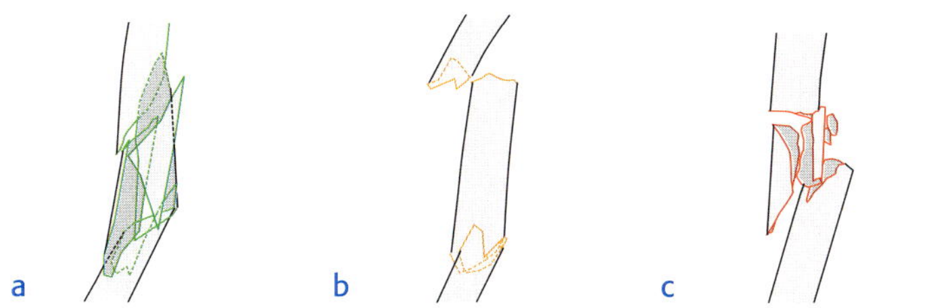

Fig 9.2-3a–c 32-C complex fracture.
a 32-C1 spiral
b 32-C2 segmental
c 32-C3 irregular

In conventional plating a large skin incision is made on the lateral side of the thigh extending from the greater trochanter to the lateral femoral condyle. Fracture exposure follows the fascia lata splitting and retracting of the vastus lateralis muscle along the intermuscular septum down to the linea aspera. Preferably, the perforating vessels should be preserved. In comparison, less invasive plating procedures require an insertion point restricted to a 3–5 cm skin incision, usually placed anterolaterally at the level of the lateral femoral condyle. Following indirect fracture reduction, the submuscular dissection for plate insertion along the shaft of the femur is prepared using an elevator. Screws are inserted percutaneously using small separate incisions.

Reduction has to consider length and alignment (ante- recurvatum deformity, varus, valgus and rotation). Approximate reduction is the key to achieving correct length in simple fractures. Draping of the uninjured side facilitates intraoperative control and comparison of length, alignment and rotation.

Video 9.2-1

The choice of implants depends on a number of factors such as the condition of the patient, fracture pattern and location, size of the medullary canal and soft-tissue conditions. Further aspects may be presence of other implants, personal experience and preference and availability of implants, instruments and intraoperative imaging.

Depending on different conditions, intramedullary nailing remains overall the treatment of choice in femoral shaft fractures. Plate osteosynthesis is applicable for special indications, for example, in combined femoral shaft and femoral neck fractures, polytrauma and correction osteotomy.

The open plating technique with broad access to the fracture is as adequate as semi- closed procedures with indirect reduction and less invasive operative techniques.

In open plating technique, possible devitalization of fracture fragments by attempts at anatomical reduction has to be taken into consideration. Therefore, precise reduction and rigid fixation by interfragmentary compression should only be performed to treat simple fractures. Otherwise, a blood-supply saving procedure, leaving the fracture area untouched and bridged by a long plate, is to be favored.

In subtrochanteric fractures, especially in those without a medial bone buttress, plate fatigue is likely. Bone grafting may become necessary to optimize static conditions.

In general, different implants are suitable for subtrochanteric fracture treatment such as condylar plates, dynamic condylar screws (DCS), proximal femoral nails (PFNA) and solid femoral nails (UFN) using the spiral blade device. Moreover, intramedullary nailing is recommended in diaphyseal fractures. In type A and type B midshaft fractures the universal or the new cannulated nail inserted after reaming of the medullary cavity and using the interlocking technique is advisable. In comparison, complex type C midshaft fractures and fractures of the proximal and distal third may be stabilized using the solid or cannulated intramedullary nail. In exceptional cases, plating may be indicated using the broad LC-DCP 4.5, the long condylar plates, the dynamic condylar screw, the broad 4.5/5.0 LCP, the LCP proximal femur plate, the LCP-DF or the LISS-DF.

Today, in plate osteosynthesis for subtrochanteric fractures, indirect reduction procedures and less invasive operative techniques are preferred to avoid unnecessary limitation of the blood supply to the fragment. Bone grafting may occasionally be useful, even in complex multifragmented fractures.

As a rule, simple fractures can be anatomically reduced and stably fixed by the principles of absolute stability with interfragmentary compression while multifragmentary cases are preferably treated by indirect reduction and bridge plating.

Bridge plating with minimal access can be performed using the plates mentioned above, the LISS-DF (less invasive stabilization system), or the LCP-DF.

In unstable fracture patterns or in cases of poor bone stock, subtrochanteric fractures can be treated with the proximal femoral nail (PFN).

In cases of severe soft-tissue injury, temporary external fixation is recommended as well as unreamed or minimally reamed intramedullary nailing. The external fixator minimizes local and systemic interference and is therefore recommended in severely polytraumatized patients. To avoid the obvious risk of pin-track infection, secondary stable internal fixation should be performed within 1–2 weeks.

Immediate start of physiotherapeutic postoperative care is essential. Ambulation may be delayed due to the patient's overall condition, concomitant injuries and patient compliance. Primary partial weight bearing (10–15 kg) should be possible without exception. Depending on fracture pattern and type of fixation, subsequent management and increasing load have to be judged on an individual basis.

4 Implant overview

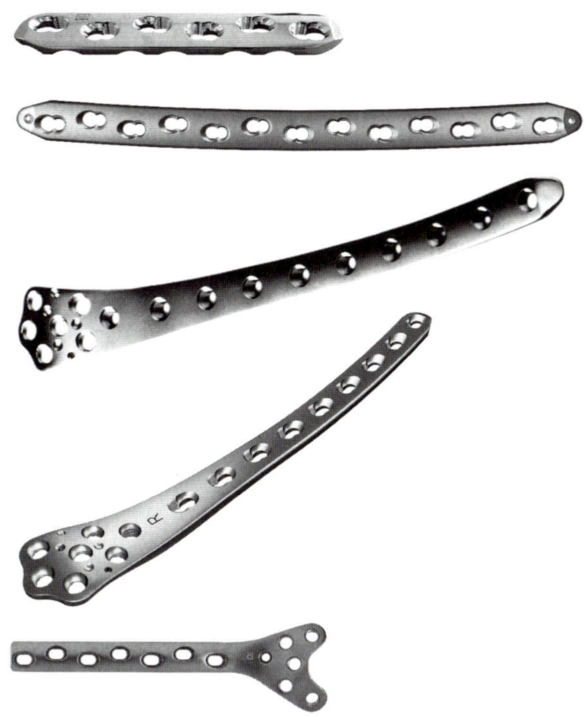

Fig 9.2-4a–e
- a LCP 4.5/5.0, broad
- b LCP 4.5/5.0 broad, curved
- c LISS-DF 5.0 (left and right version available)
- d LCP-DF 4.5/5.0 (left and right version available)
- e LCP condylar plate 4.5/5.0 (left and right version available)

5 Suggestions for further reading

Bone LB, Johnson KD, Weigelt J, et al (2004) Early versus delayed stabilization of femoral fractures: a prospective randomized study. *Clin Orthop Relat Res*; (422):11–16.

Roberts CS, Pape HC, Jones AL, et al (2005) Damage control orthopaedics: evolving concepts in the treatment of patients who have sustained orthopaedic trauma. *Instr Course Lect*; 54:447–462. Review.

Pape HC, Hildebrand F, Pertschy S, et al (2002) Changes in the management of femoral shaft fractures in polytrauma patients: from early total care to damage control orthopedic surgery. *J Trauma*; 53(3):452–461; discussion 461–462.

Pape HC, Grimme K, Van Griensven M, et al (2003) EPOFF Study Group. Impact of intramedullary instrumentation versus damage control for femoral fractures on immunoinflammatory parameters: prospective randomized analysis by the EPOFF Study Group. *J Trauma*; 55(1):7–13.

Stephen DJ, Kreder HJ, Schemitsch EH, et al (2002) Femoral intramedullary nailing: comparison of fracture-table and manual traction. a prospective, randomized study. *J Bone Joint Surg Am*; 84-A(9):1514–1521.

Farouk O, Krettek C, Miclau T, et al (1999) Minimally invasive plate osteosynthesis: does percutaneous plating disrupt femoral blood supply less than the traditional technique? *J Orthop Trauma*; 13(6):401–406.

Agus H, Kalenderer O, Eryanilmaz G, et al (2003) Biological internal fixation of comminuted femur shaft fractures by bridge plating in children. *J Pediatr Orthop*; 23(2):184–189.

Kinast C, Bolhofner BR, Mast JW, et al (1989) Subtrochanteric fractures of the femur. Results of treatment with the 95 degrees condylar blade-plate. *Clin Orthop Relat Res*; (238):122–130.

Authors Emanuel Gautier, Marc Lottenbach

9.2.1 Spiral wedge femoral shaft fracture—32-B1

1 Case description

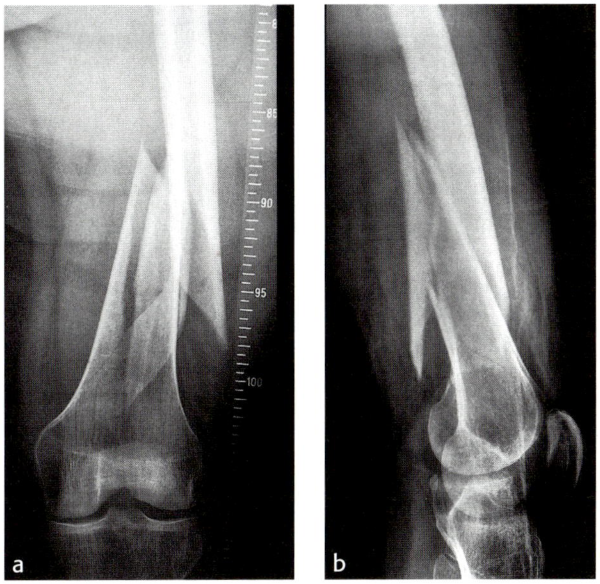

56-year-old female was involved in a ski accident and fractured her left femur.

Fig 9.2.1-1a–b The x-rays show a spiral fracture of the distal femoral shaft with a posterior wedge.
a AP view.
b Lateral view.

Indication

This unstable femoral shaft fracture is an absolute indication for osteosynthesis. In this distal femoral shaft fracture, the LISS osteosynthesis with locking head screws allows good anchorage of the plate in the condylar fragment, even in cases of osteoporosis.

Preoperative planning

Equipment

- LISS-DF, 13 holes
- 5.0 mm locking head screws (LHS)
- 1.6 mm K-wires

(Size of system, instruments, and implants can vary according to anatomy.)

Patient preparation and positioning

Antibiotics: single dose 2nd generation cephalosporin for 48 hours.
Thrombosis prophylaxis: low-molecular heparin.
In addition, the patient is treated with antiosteoporotic medication.

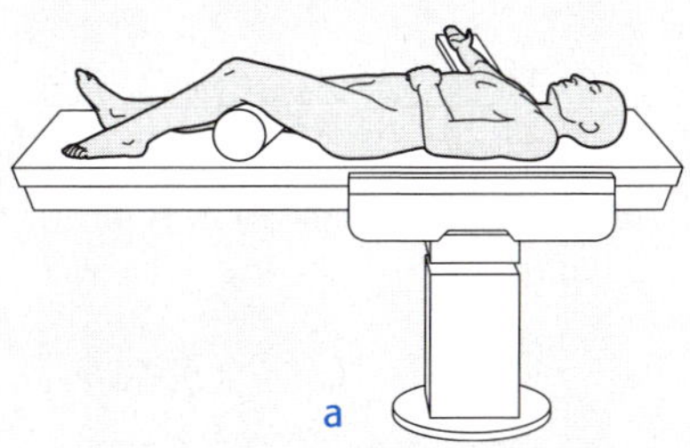

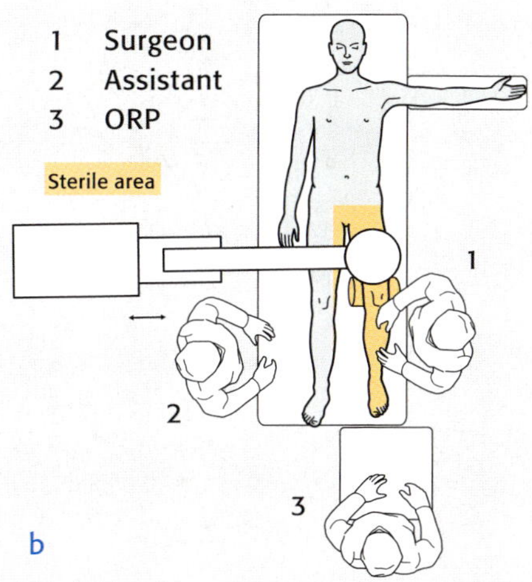

Fig 9.2.1-2a–b
a Supine position on a standard operating table.
b The image intensifier is placed on the contralateral side.

2 Surgical approach

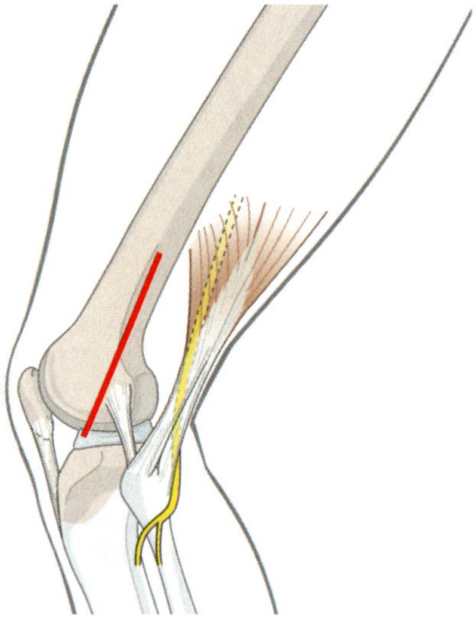

Fig 9.2.1-3 Short lateral skin incision curved toward the tibial tuberosity with a lateral arthrotomy.

3 Reduction and fixation

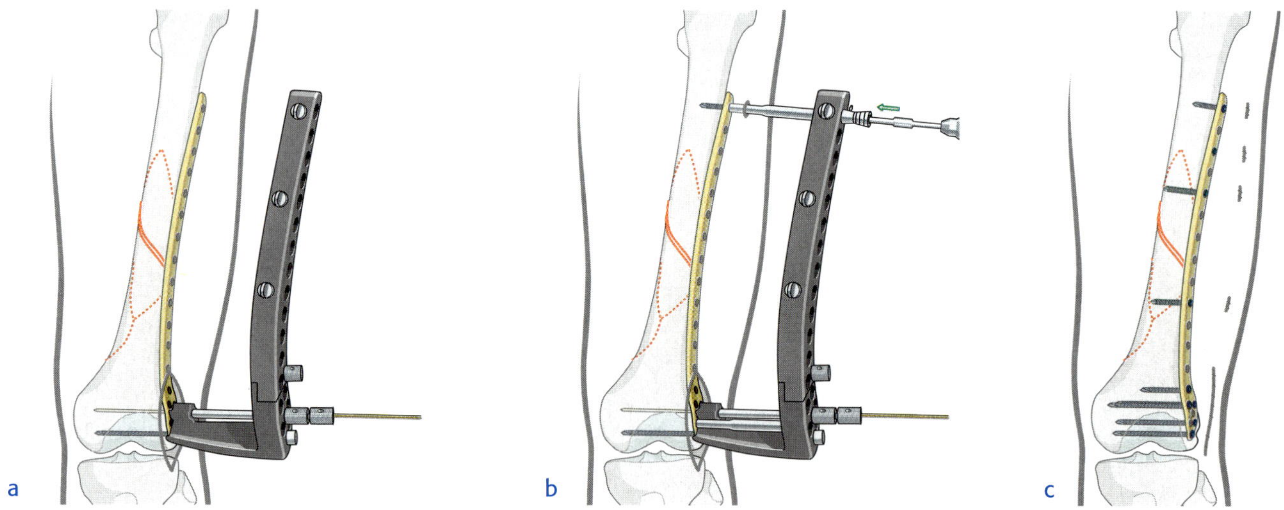

Fig 9.2.1-4a–c

- a The fracture is reduced by manual traction. The plate is inserted with the help of the aiming device in MIPO technique. First the plate is fixed distally with a locking head screw. Care is given to align the plate properly with respect to the axis of the femur in the lateral view.
- b Plate position is assessed by image intensification, followed by fixation with a second screw distally, and insertion of the proximal and distal screws.
- c Wound closure and definitive osteosynthesis.

4 Rehabilitation

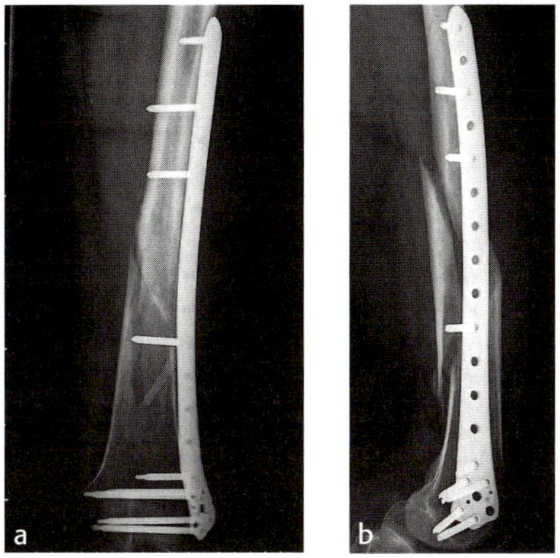

Fig 9.2.1-5a–b Postoperative x-rays after 8 weeks showing correct alignment in both planes.
a AP view.
b Lateral view.

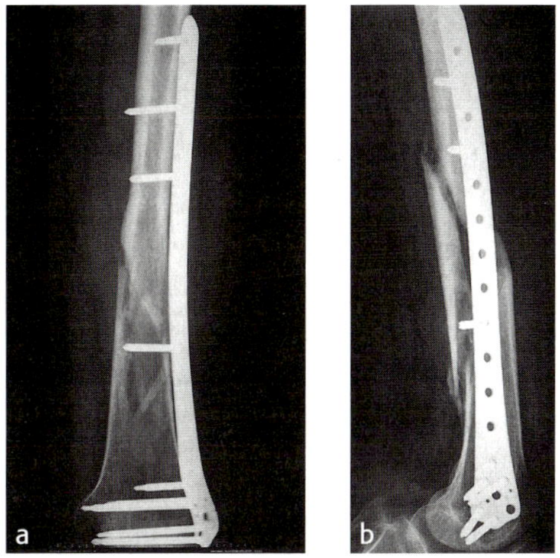

Fig 9.2.1-6a–b Postoperative x-rays after 12 weeks showing integration of the wedge fragment into the callus.
a AP view.
b Lateral view.

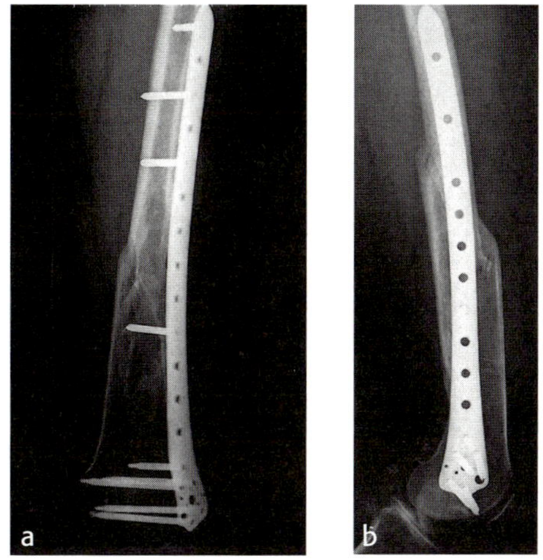

Fig 9.2.1-7a–b Postoperative x-rays after 15 months.
a AP view.
b Lateral view.

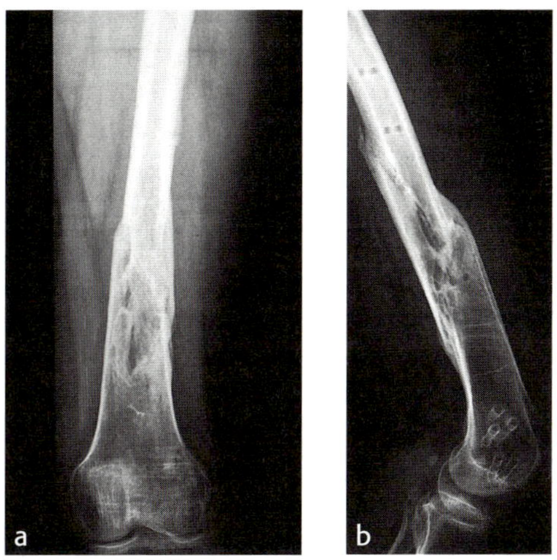

Fig 9.2.1-8a–b Postoperative x-rays after 18 months.
a AP view.
b Lateral view.

Implant removal
If the fracture has healed and the hardware becomes symptomatic, hardware may be removed through a similar approach at a minimum of 18 months.

5 Pitfalls –

Reduction and fixation

Reduction and plate position have to be checked by the image intensifier.

Control of reduction is difficult and only clinically possible (internal-external rotation of the flexed hip)

Danger of creating an extensional malalignment (recurvation).

6 Pearls +

Reduction and fixation

No-touch reduction technique with preservation of the bone vascularity is possible.

Indirect reduction technique without exposure of the fragments.

Submuscular insertion of the plate.

Rapid integration of the wedge fragment into the callus.

Author Michael Wagner

9.2.2 Spiral wedge femoral shaft fracture—32-B1

1 Case description

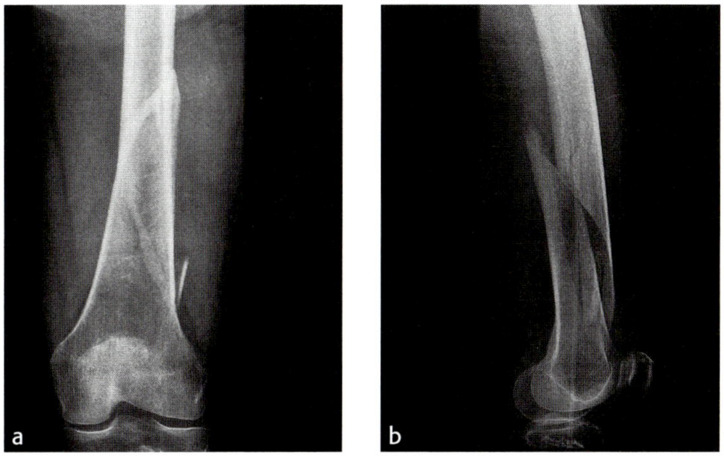

68-year-old woman had a domestic fall and sustained a femoral shaft injury.

Fig 9.2.2-1a–b
a AP view.
b Lateral view.

Indication

Unstable spiral fracture of the femoral shaft with fracture fissures extending into the condylar block. Given this fracture pattern, nail fixation with transverse locking would be extremely difficult and sufficient anchorage uncertain in osteoporosis.

Preoperative planning

Equipment

- LCP 4.5/5.0, broad, 17 holes
- Self-tapping locking head screws (LHS)
- 2.0 mm K-wire
- Schanz screw and T-handle to be used as a joystick
- Soft-tissue retractor

(Size of system, instruments, and implants can vary according to anatomy.)

Patient preparation and positioning

Antibiotics: single dose 2nd generation cephalosporin
Thrombosis prophylaxis: low-molecular heparin

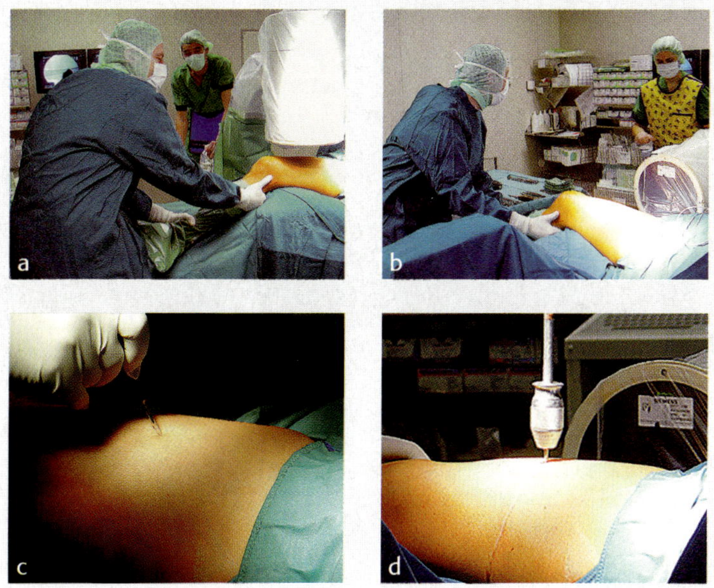

Fig 9.2.2-2a–d
a Supine position with flexed knee (45°) with support.
b The possibility of closed indirect reduction by manual traction and external support is evaluated by image intensifier before starting the incision.
c–d To reduce the displacement in the sagittal plane use a joystick in the proximal fragment (near the fracture zone).

2 Surgical approach

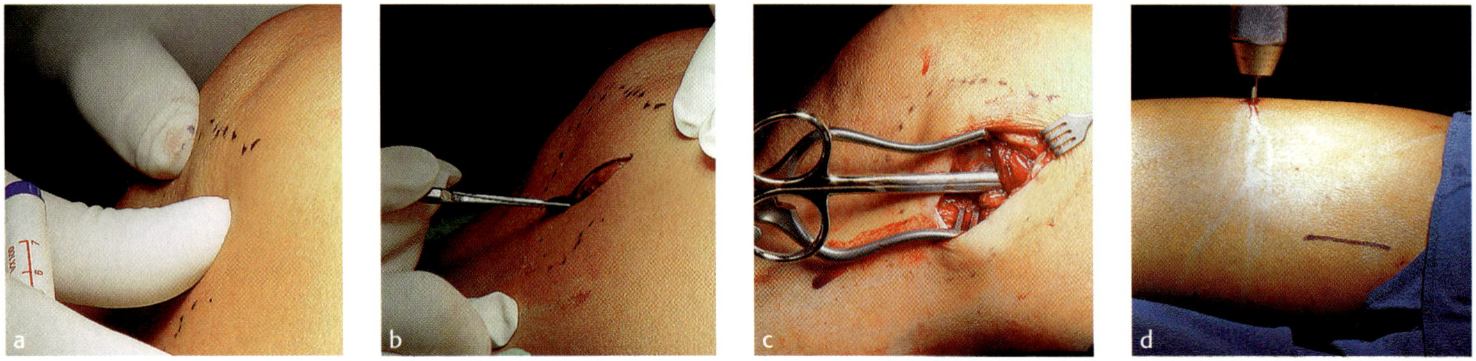

Fig 9.2.2-3a–d
Minimally invasive approach:

- a Find the landmarks on the distal lateral femoral condyle.
- b Mark and make a short incision on the lateral femur condyle.
- c Divide the iliotibial tract in the direction of its fibers and open the epiperiosteal space beneath the vastus lateralis of the quadriceps femoris.
- d Planned proximal incision.

3 Reduction and fixation

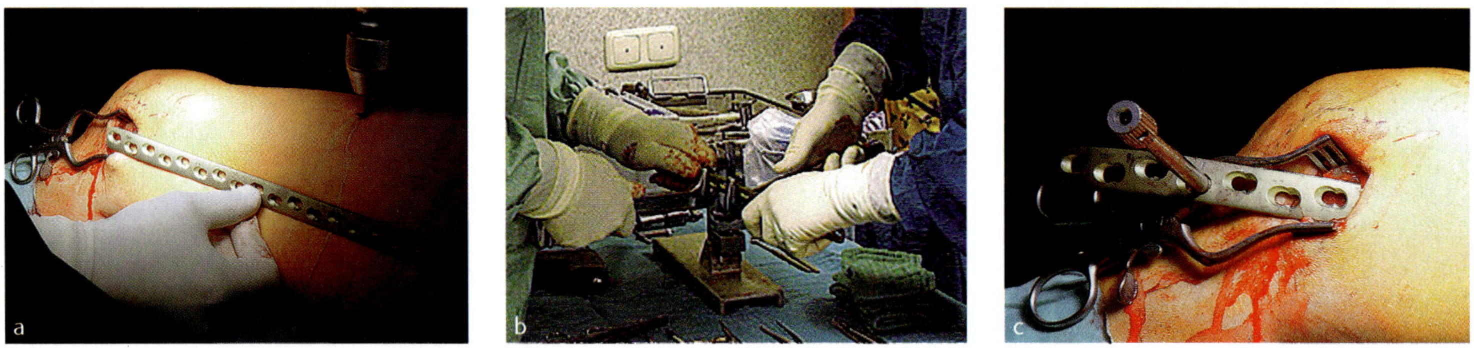

Fig 9.2.2-4a–c
Reduction with manual longitudinal traction (under image intensifier control).
Anterior insertion of the Steinmann pin with T-handle into the proximal fragment (joystick).

- a Measure for plate length.
- b Bend the LCP with the help of the bending press and bending irons.
- c Submuscular slide-insertion of the plate from distal to proximal–whereby a drill sleeve acts as a handle.

3 Reduction and fixation (cont)

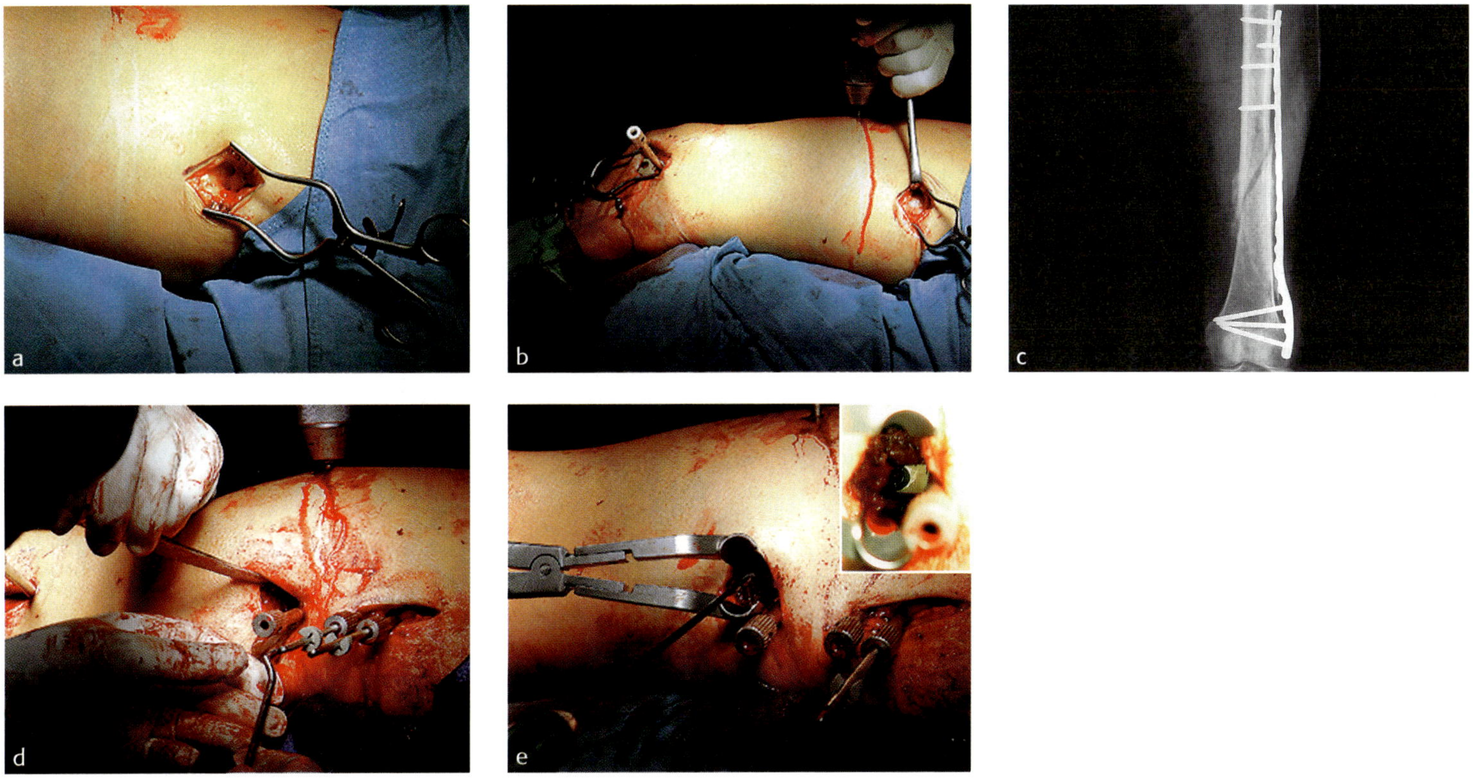

Fig 9.2.2-5a–e

- a Identify and achieve visibility of the proximal end of the plate through the most proximal incision.
- b Preliminary fixation of the plate proximally and distal insertion of a 2.0 mm K-wire. Use the image intensifier to check the position of the plate.
- c Distal fixation of the plate with three self-tapping locking head screws. These screws will be positioned convergently because of the bends in the contoured plate. The longest screws possible are inserted in the metaphyseal region.
- d A total of four locking head screws are required for the proximal fixation. The screws are inserted through an additional incision.
- e The soft-tissue retractor is helpful. The fourth screw is inserted proximally through an additional incision. A speculum is used to obtain a better view of the plate hole without dissection.

3 Reduction and fixation (cont)

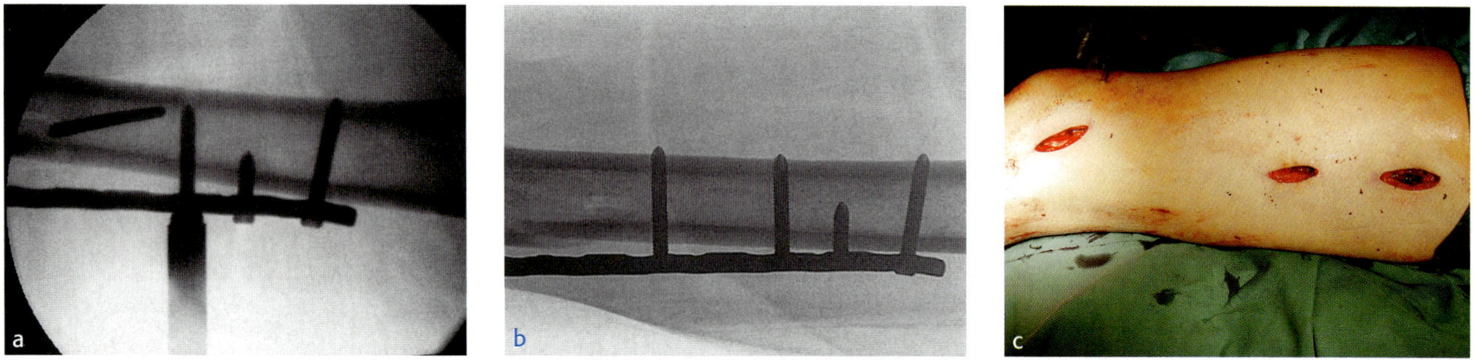

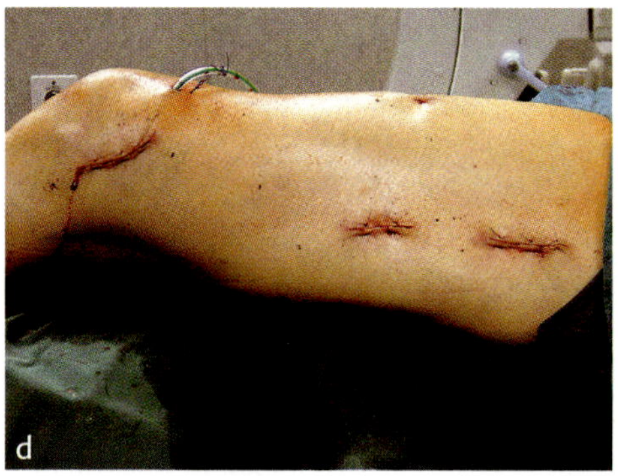

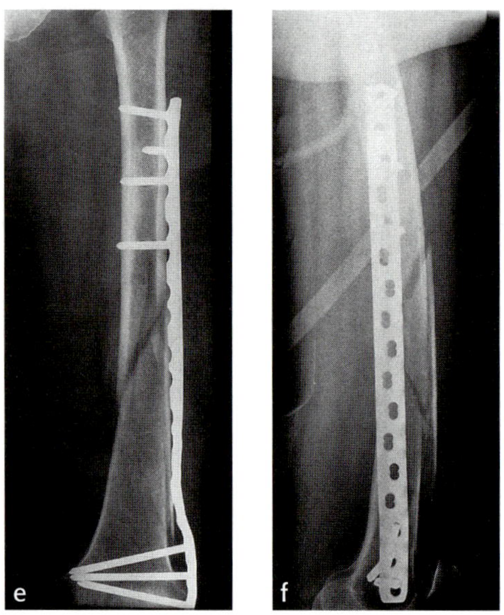

Fig 9.2.2-6a–f

- a Since the plate was initially not properly seated on the bone in the proximal region, the method of fine-tuning was applied whereby all the screws are disengaged from the plate, the proximal fragment is drawn towards the plate using the screw holding sleeve, and the screws are then screwed back into the plate holes.
- b The two most proximal screws will be positioned divergently due to the bend at the proximal end of the plate.
- c Incisions after completion of plate fixation.
- d Redon drains with subsequent skin closure.
- e–f Postoperative x-rays, AP and lateral view. Three screws are inserted bicortically because of the osteoporotic condition of the bone (increased rotational stability).

4 Rehabilitation

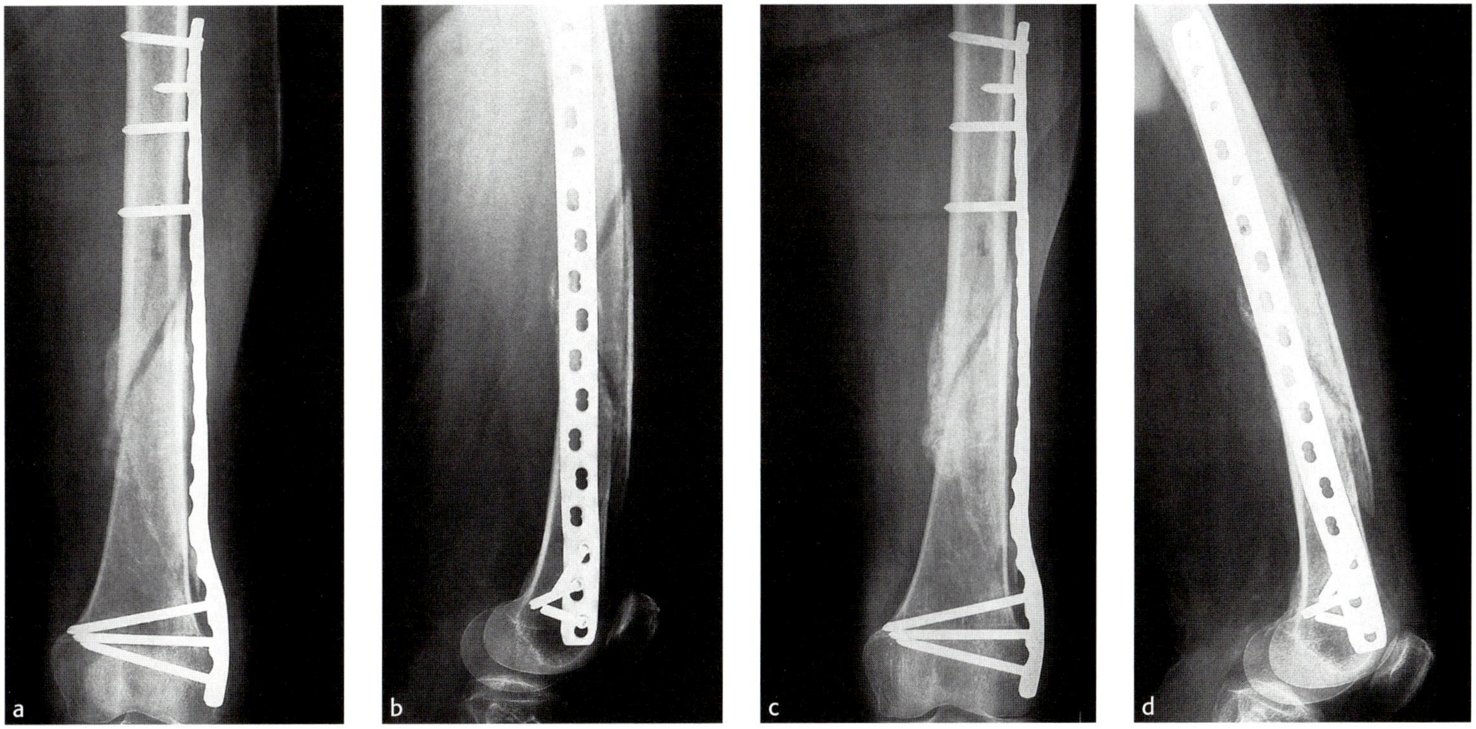

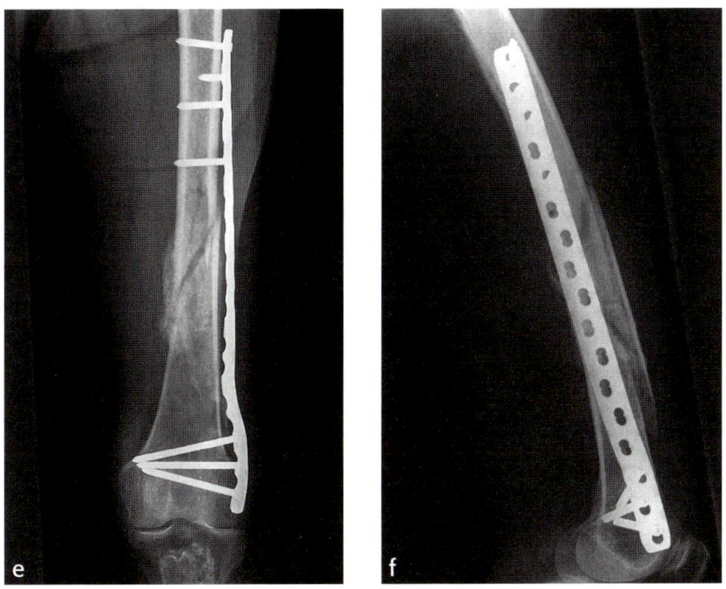

Fig 9.2.2-7a–f Mobilization with walker, rollator, or underarm crutches and half body weight (elderly patient).

a–b 8 weeks—callus formation, fracture gap only indistinctly visible, start of full weight bearing.

c–d 4 months—clearly apparent increase in callus formation.

e–f 18 months—bone consolidation.

5 Pitfalls –

Equipment

Correct positioning of a long straight plate is not easy. A curved long plate fits the antecurvature of the femur better.

Reduction and fixation

Fig 9.2.2-8 The plate has no contact with the bone in the proximal region. Use the method of fine-tuning to correct improper position of the plate.

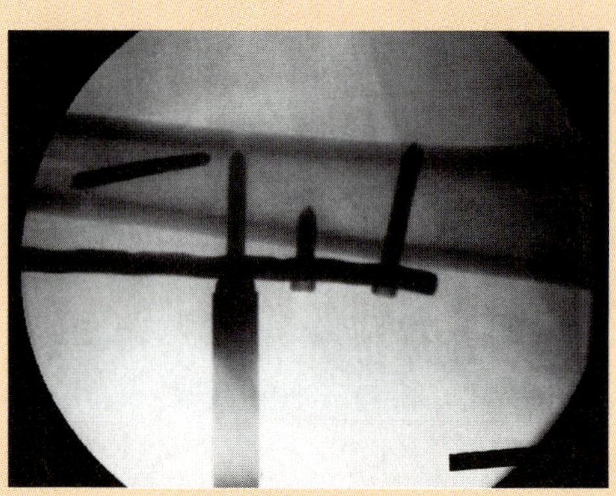

6 Pearls +

Equipment

Fig 9.2.2-9 The long broad 4.5/5.0 LCP is also available as a curved version. This plate fits the anatomical shape of the femur better.

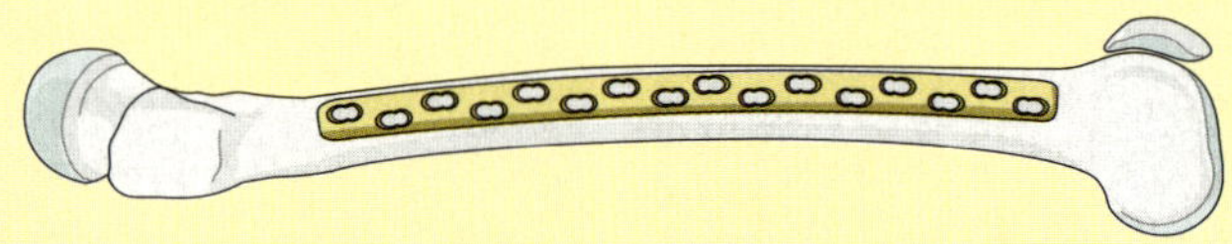

Reduction and fixation

The soft-tissue retractor is a very helpful instrument to protect the soft tissues.

Authors Michael Schütz, Norbert P Haas

9.2.3 Complex spiral femoral shaft fracture—32-C1

1 Case description

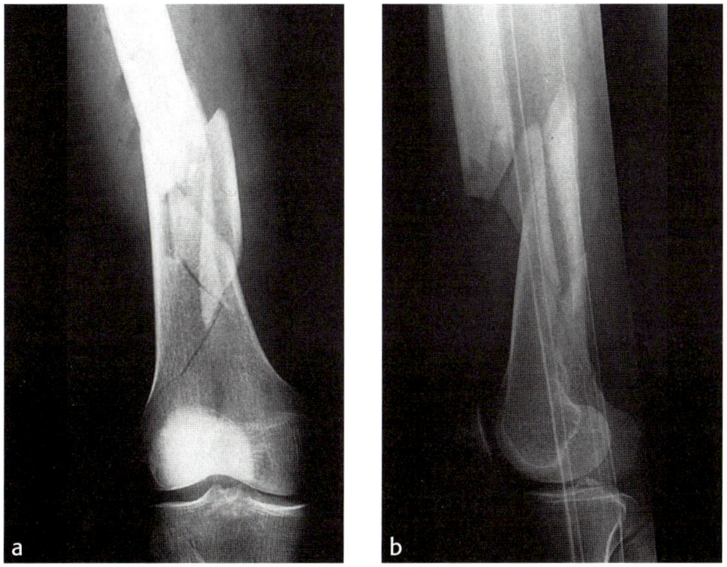

67-year-old woman suffered a distal femoral monotrauma when she fell off her motorbike (32-C1). The patient was operated immediately after diagnosis.

Fig 9.2.3-1a–b
a AP view.
b Lateral view.

Indication

This is a clear indication for reduction of the fracture in axis, length, and rotation to allow early functional treatment. In this case, a LISS-DF, 13 holes, to be inserted in minimally invasive technique, was chosen for fracture stabilization.

Preoperative planning

Standard x-rays of the knee and femur were sufficient in this case for preoperative planning. A sketch is made taking into account the soft-tissue injury and the radiological analysis. This sketch should contain the stabilization procedure with implant length and screw positioning (at least four in the proximal fragment). Free screw holes should also be planned to allow biomechanical motion of the implant.

Patient preparation and positioning
Antibiotics: 2nd generation cephalosporin
Thrombosis prophylaxis: low-molecular heparin

Equipment
- LISS-DF, 13 holes
- 5.0 mm locking head screws (LHS)
- 2.0 mm partially threaded K-wires

(Size of system, instruments, and implants can vary according to anatomy.)

The patient is positioned on the radiolucent table, allowing image intensification of the whole femur. This has to be checked before the operation. The uninjured leg must be extended and lowered (about 30° hip extension) to allow lateral image intensifier projection.

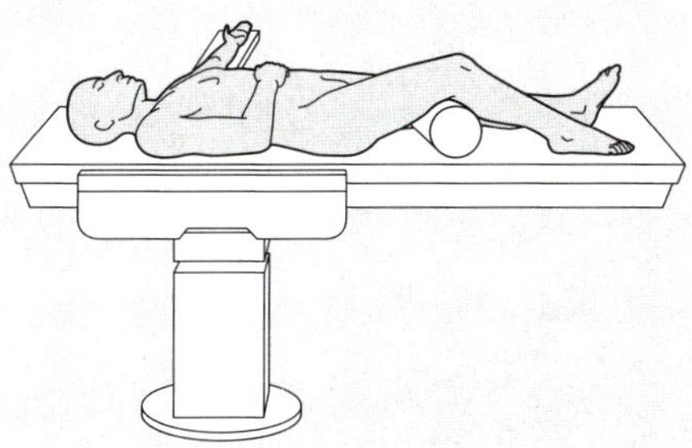

Fig 9.2.3-2 Supine position, knee joint flexed to approximately 30°.

2 Surgical approach

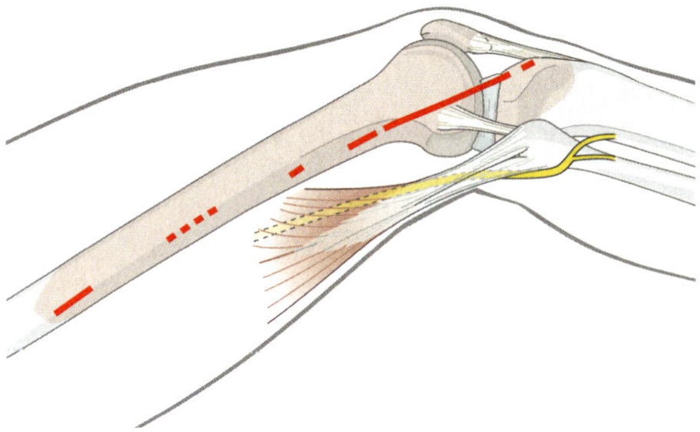

Fig 9.2.3-3 Lateral approach to the distal femur and additional small incisions in the region of the femoral shaft.

3 Reduction and fixation

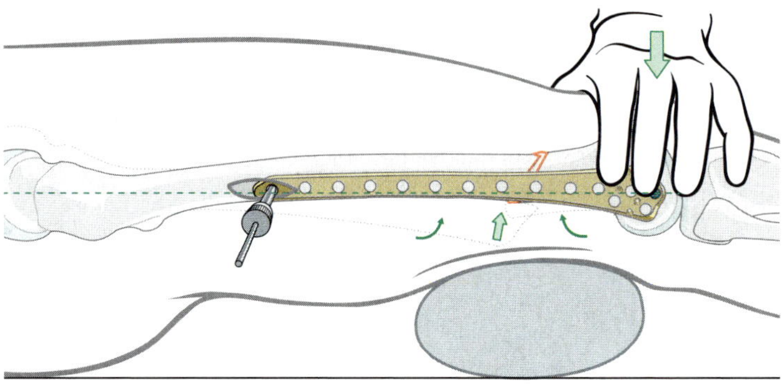

a

Fig 9.2.3-4a–b

a Anatomical reduction of the fracture by longitudinal traction paying attention to leg length, axis, and rotation. The fracture is temporarily fixed with two percutaneously inserted K-wires. They must not interfere with implant positioning. The reduction can be supported with towel rolls. Alternatively, an external fixator or distractor can maintain the reduction. The metaphyseal fracture fragments are not touched during this minimally invasive procedure. A further minimal adjustment of the reduction can be achieved using the implant itself.
The 13 hole LISS-DF is inserted with the aid of the insertion guide and is introduced under the vastus lateralis.
Estimated placement of the LISS on the lateral condyles. The LISS has to be positioned parallel to the condyles to prevent irritation of the iliotibial tract. The proximal trocar is applied. Fixation of the implant with proximal and distal K-wires. The distal K-wire should be parallel to the joint surface. The anatomically prebent implant now maintains the reduction.

3 Reduction and fixation (cont)

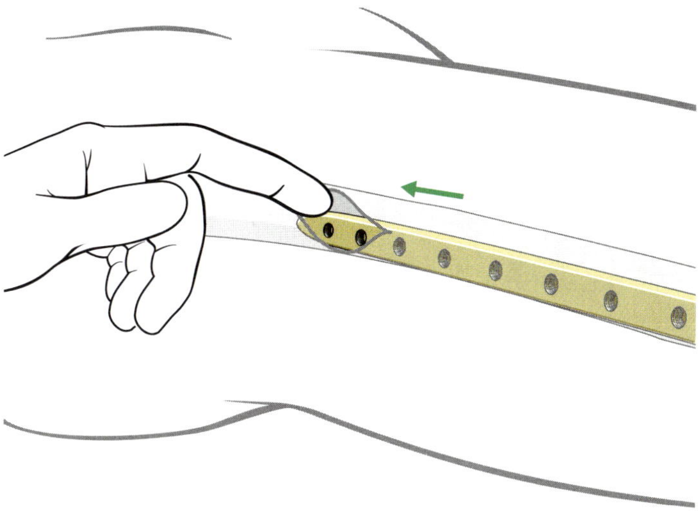

b

Fig 9.2.3-4a–b (cont)

b It is recommended that a 3 cm long incision be made proximally to verify the position of the plate. In this case, the anterior aspect of the femur was palpated and the implant was advanced towards the finger.

If the fracture is now reduced correctly in axis, rotation, and length, the first locking head screw can be inserted distally and should be parallel to the articular surface.
The distractor is applied proximally and a correction of about five degrees can be achieved. A monocortical locking head screw is inserted percutaneously into the adjacent hole.
The reduction and the position of the plate are assessed clinically and by image intensification (axis, length, rotation). The remaining locking head screws are inserted in accordance with the preoperative plan.
The insertion guide is removed and the wound is closed.

4 Rehabilitation

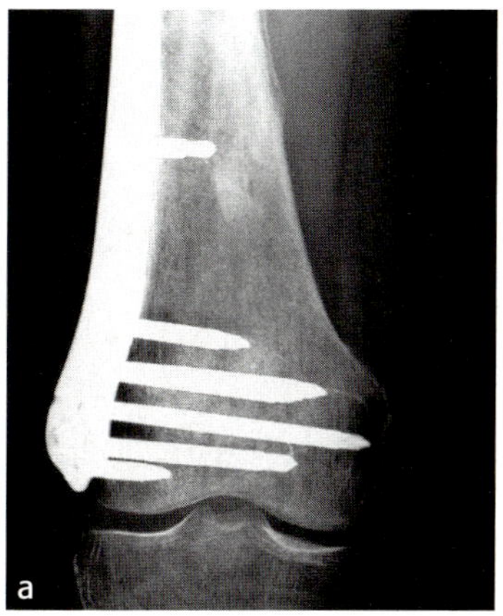

a

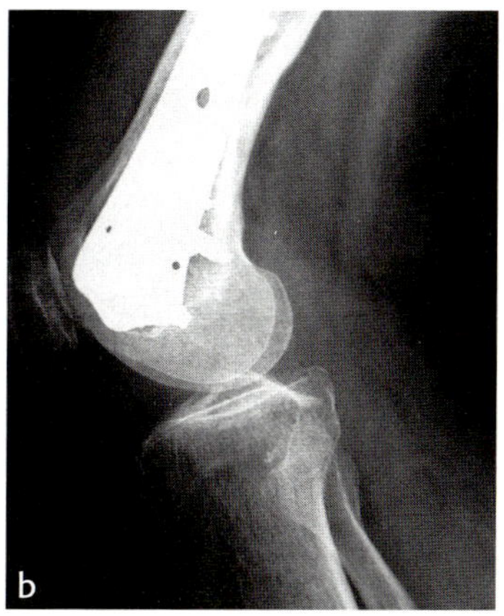

b

Apply sterile dressings.
Gentle active and passive motion exercises begin immediately on day 1 postoperatively.
The use of the continuous passive motion machine is highly recommended.
Mobilization with partial weight bearing as soon as the general and local condition of the patient allows it. Increased weight bearing after 4 weeks, full weight bearing after 6 weeks.

Fig 9.2.3-5a–b Follow-up x-rays after 5 months.
a AP view.
b Lateral view.

4 Rehabilitation (cont)

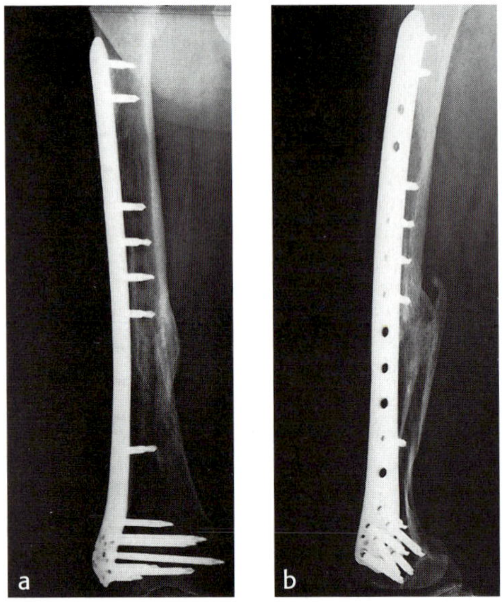

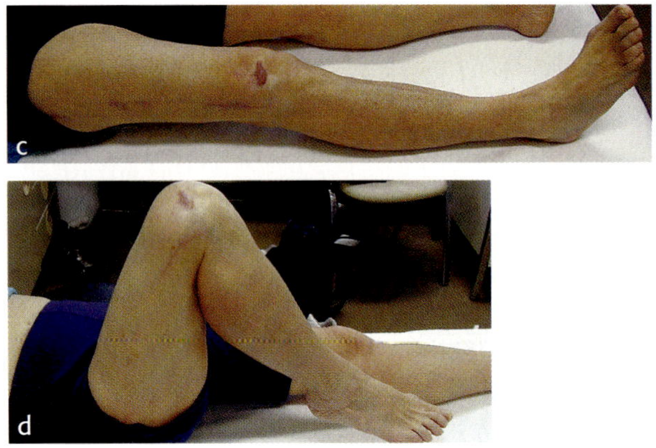

Fig 9.2.3-6a–d
Postoperative x-rays after 12 months.
a AP view.
b Lateral view.
c–d Functional result.

Implant removal

After definitive consolidation (2 years after surgery) and on the request of the patient, the implant was removed.

5 Pitfalls –

Approach

A too extensive exposure of the metaphyseal fracture zone may damage the blood supply to the bone fragments.

Reduction and fixation

Incorrect positioning of the implant in relation to the shaft may lead to early implant loosening.
Incorrect positioning of the implant in relation to the distal fragment may lead to soft-tissue irritations.
A too short implant increases the risk of implant loosening.
A too stable implant fixation increases the risk of implant failure.

Rehabilitation

Prolonging physiotherapy may lead to a decreased range of knee motion.

6 Pearls +

Approach

Indirect reduction technique for extraarticular fractures.

Reduction and fixation

Careful control of implant position using direct and indirect control mechanisms (visualization, palpation, and image intensification).
The use of long implants and few screws is necessary to allow implant motion and better stress distribution.

Rehabilitation

Careful early active and passive physiotherapy is essential for good joint function.

Authors Thomas J Hockertz, Gabriele Streicher, Andreas Gruner, Heinrich Reilmann

9.2.4 Simple spiral femoral shaft fracture, implant failure—32-A1

1 Case description

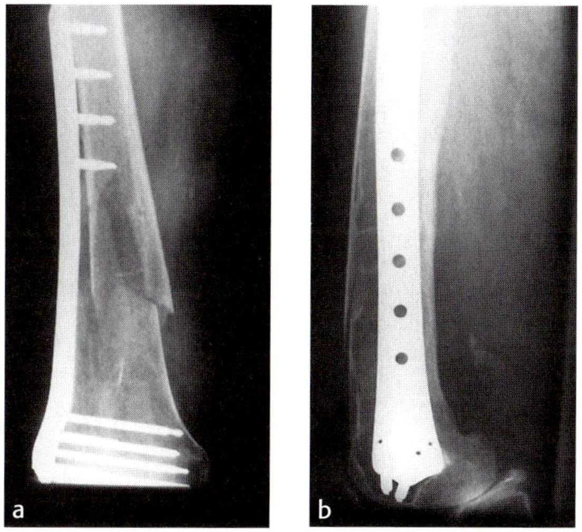

75-year-old man with fracture of the distal third of the femoral shaft. Cause of injury unknown.
Type of injury: low-energy trauma, monotrauma, closed fracture, severe osteoporosis.

Fig 9.2.4-1a–b
a AP view after primary treatment.
b Lateral view after primary treatment.

Indication

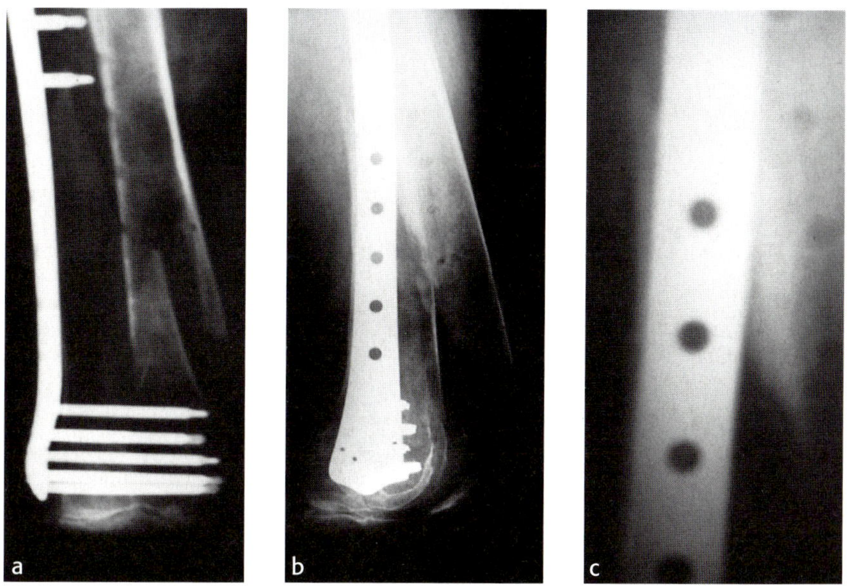

Instability, pain, and blood loss after plate breakthrough at the femur (emergency situation). Treatment to provide stability.

Fig 9.2.4-2a–c
a Protrusion of LISS in AP view.
b Protrusion of LISS laterally.
c Protrusion of LISS; close up.

Preoperative planning

Equipment
- LISS-DF, 13 holes
- 5.0 mm locking head screws (LHS)
- "Selvage ring"

(Size of system, instruments, and implants can vary according to anatomy.)

Patient preparation and positioning
Antibiotics: single dose 2nd generation cephalosporin
Thrombosis prophylaxis: low-molecular heparin

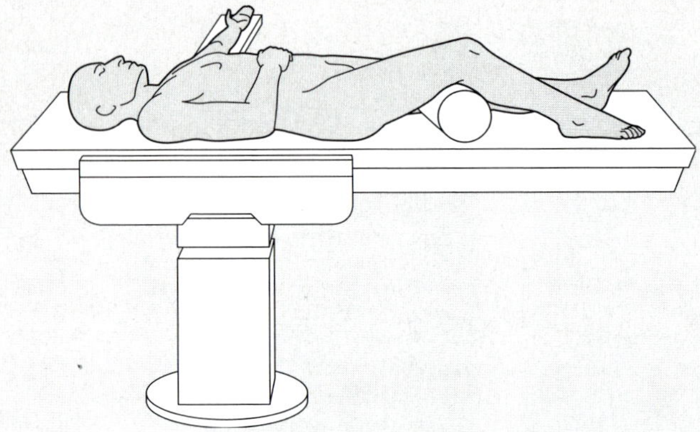

Fig 9.2.4-3 Supine position with elevation of the injured leg, support the knee with a towel roll.

2 Surgical approach

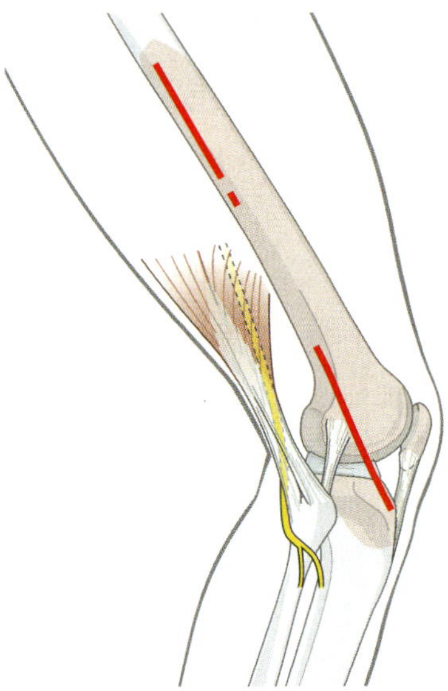

Fig 9.2.4-4 Lateral incision over the lateral femoral condyle and longitudinal division of the iliotibial tract.
Preparation of the plate bed with an elevator starting distally and working in a proximal direction along the lateral femoral shaft.
Incision over the proximal end of the plate after slide-insertion of the implant.

3 Reduction and fixation

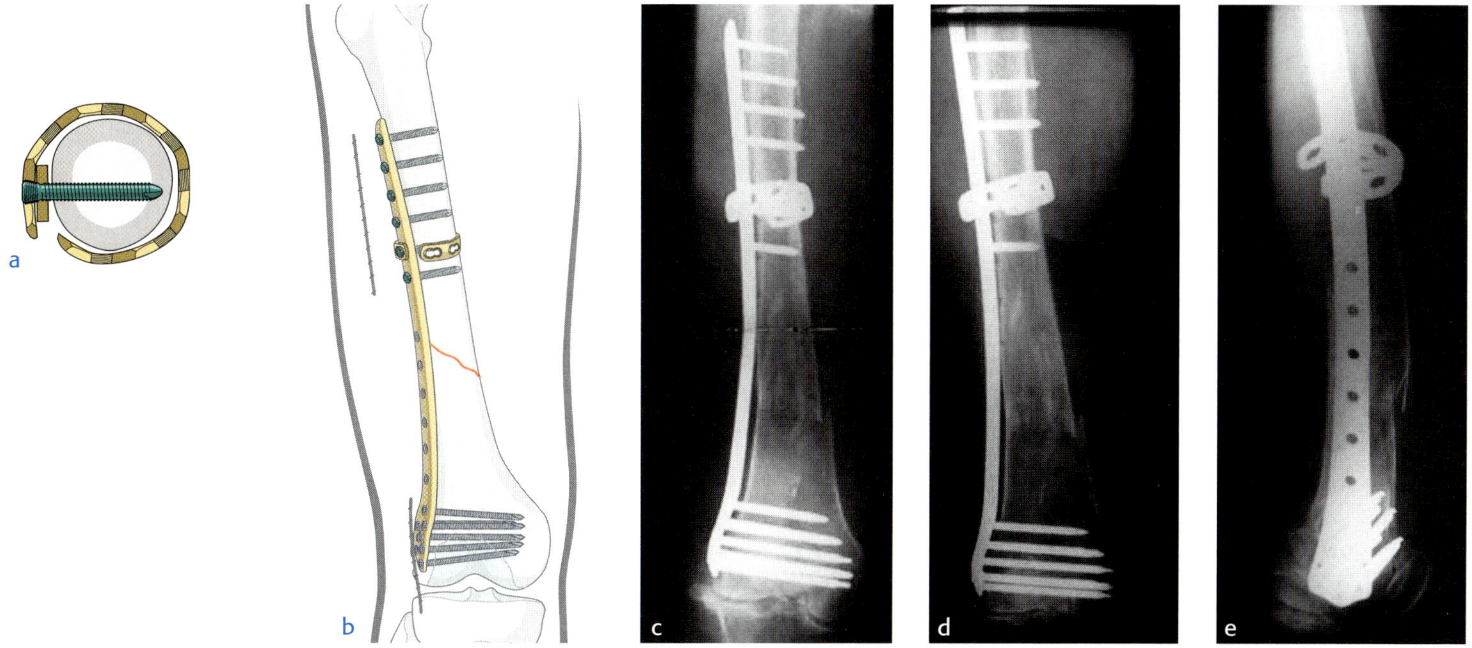

Fig 9.2.4-5a–e Approximate reduction under longitudinal traction and alignment of the axis of the injured leg.
Positioning of the plate to the bone and temporary fixation with K-wires.
Precise reduction prior to definitive fixation of the plate with the insertion guide.

After definitive reduction and plate positioning has been achieved, insert the screws alternately in the distal and proximal holes. In the shaft bicortical self-tapping LHS are used.
To secure the proximal fragment and plate position, mount a "selvage ring" after precontouring and adapting it to the femoral diameter. Fixation of the ring with two locking head screws.

4 Rehabilitation

No additional immobilization.
Weight bearing: 15 kg for 8 weeks; full weight bearing after 8 weeks.
Physiotherapy: from the third postoperative day.
Pharmaceutical treatment: nonsteroid antiinflammatory drugs.

Implant removal
Implant removal after 24 months. If the implant is causing symptoms, it can be removed. The implant can be left in place in elderly patients.

5 Pitfalls –

Reduction and fixation

Fig 9.2.4-6 Special feature of this case: fracture line running longitudinally that joined up the individual holes—cause uncertain.

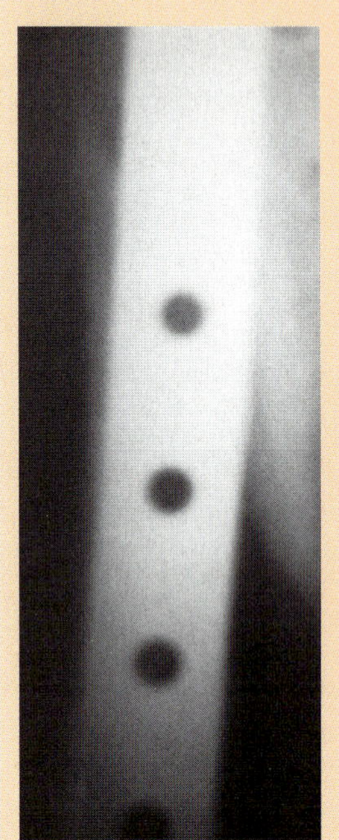

Monocortical fixation in osteoporotic bone and a too short internal fixator can lead to implant failure.

6 Pearls +

Reduction and fixation

Fig 9.2.4-7a–b This “selvage ring” developed by Hockertz helps to gain control over difficult situations at a revision operation. A short narrow LCP 4.5/5.0 is used to create this individual device. Alternatively cerclage wire with wire mounts can be used (see case 9.2.9). Also bicortical LHS (self tapping) are recommended in osteoporotic bone.

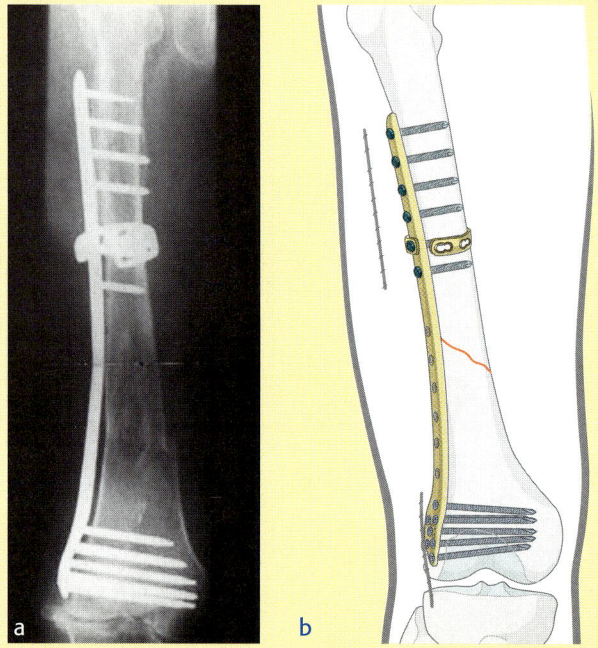

Author Michael Wagner

9.2.5 Subtrochanteric fracture of the proximal femoral shaft after osteomyelitis—32-A1

1 Case description

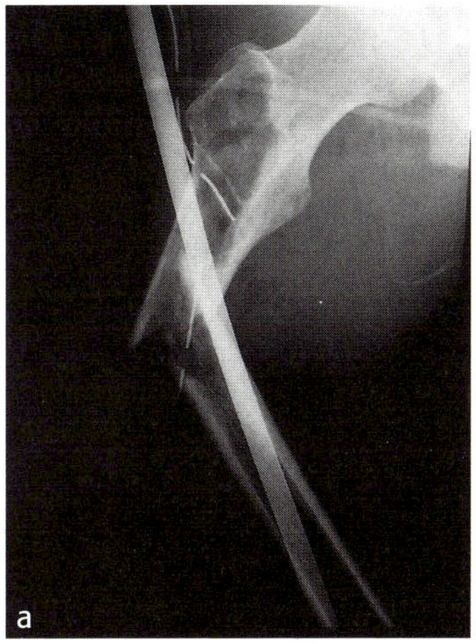

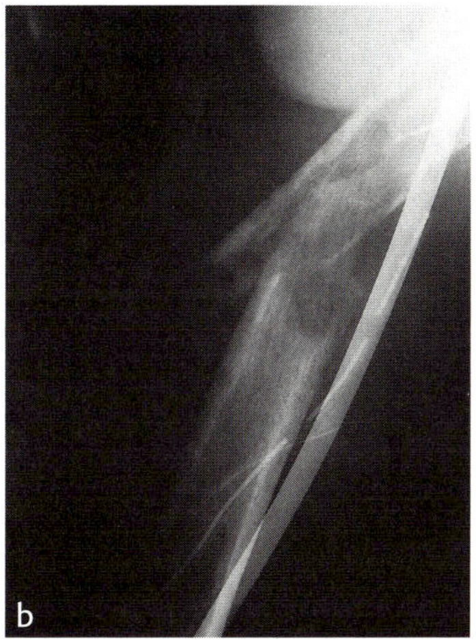

33-year-old man with subtrochanteric fracture of the right proximal femoral shaft after fenestration of the femoral shaft due to hematogenic osteomyelitis. Postoperative fracture in the infected region of the femur occurred due to the degradation and fenestration of the cortex.

Fig 9.2.5-1a–b
a AP view.
b Detail of AP view.

Indication

Unstable subtrochanteric shaft fracture in the osteomyelitic zone is a clear indication for operative stabilization that will facilitate mobilization of the patient. Stabilization with an external fixator is possible but uncomfortable for the patient. There is the additional risk of pin-track infection because the required period of fixation is long. Intramedullary nailing is no option because of the osteomyelitis. Stabilization with a locked internal fixator provides adequate stability and can be applied even in the presence of infection.

Preoperative planning

Equipment

- LCP 4.5/5.0, broad, curved, 16 holes
- 5.0 mm locking head screws (LHS)
- 2.0 mm K-wires
- Screw hole insert

(Size of system, instruments, and implants can vary according to anatomy.)

Patient preparation and positioning

Antibiotics: 3rd generation cephalosporin
Thrombosis prophylaxis: low-molecular heparin

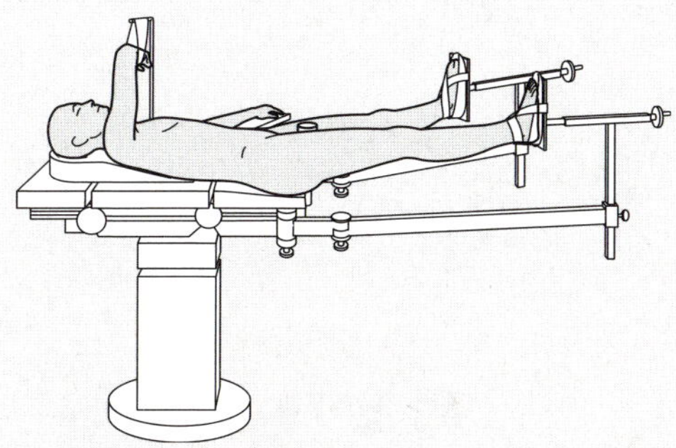

Fig 9.2.5-2
Supine position on traction table.

2 Surgical approach

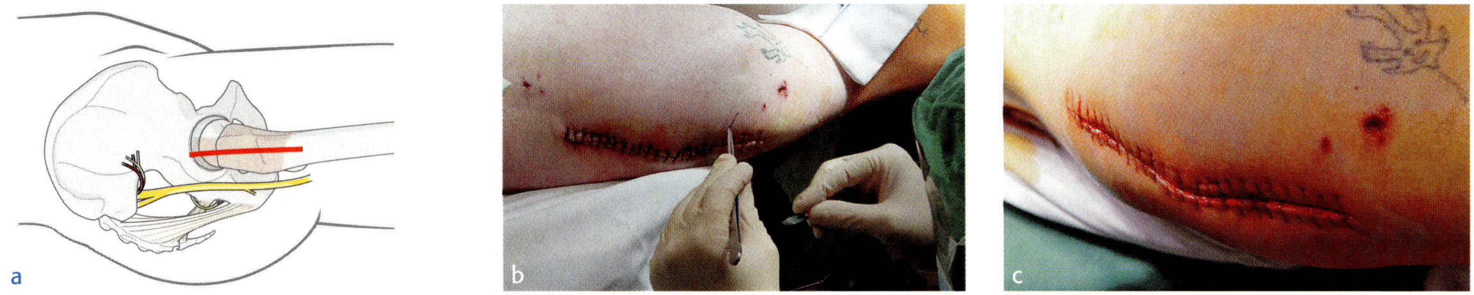

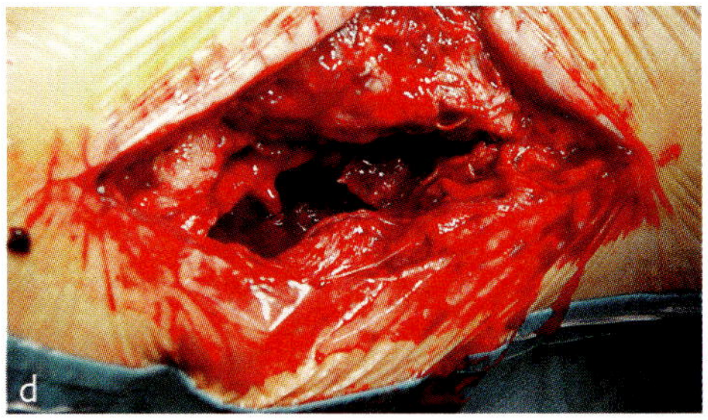

The surgical approach was dictated by the incisions of the first operation.

Fig 9.2.5-3a–d

- a Lateral approach to the proximal femoral shaft.
- b–c In a first step, the sutures from the previous operation were removed (fenestration of the bone due to osteomyelitis).
- d Debridement and irrigation of the surgical wound and the infected fracture.

3 Reduction and fixation

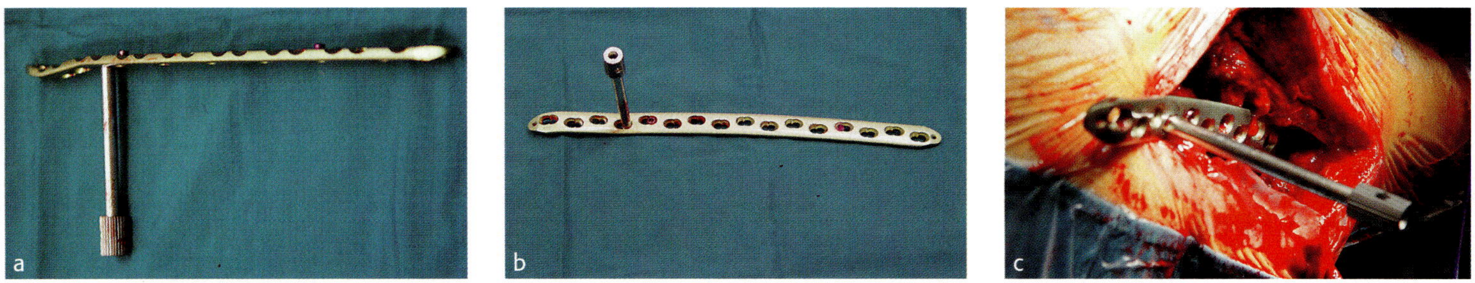

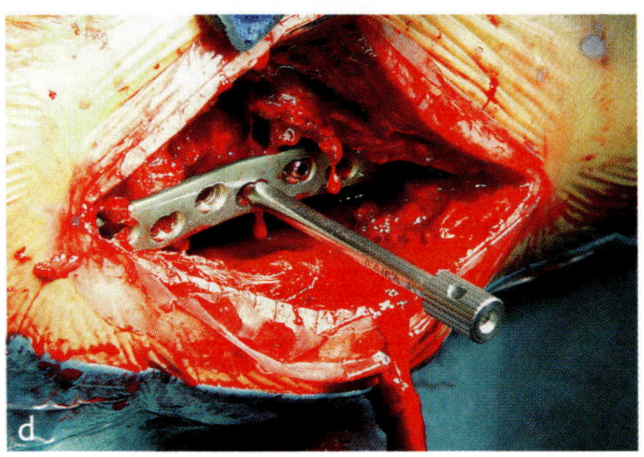

Reduction by means of traction table and assessment by image intensification.

Fig 9.2.5-4a–h

- a–b Prebending of the proximal end of a broad curved 16-hole LCP 4.5/5.0 in order to adapt it to the lateral anatomy of the trochanter.
  Insertion of the screw hole inserter in the 5th hole from the proximal end and in the 4th hole from the distal end to prevent compression of the periosteum after plate fixation.
- c–d Insertion of the plate from proximal to distal into the epiperiosteal space under the lateral femoral vastus lateralis. A threaded LCP drill guide can be used as a handle.

3 Reduction and fixation (cont)

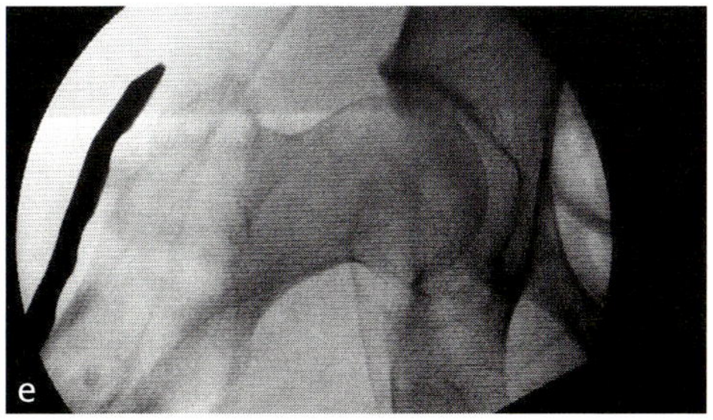

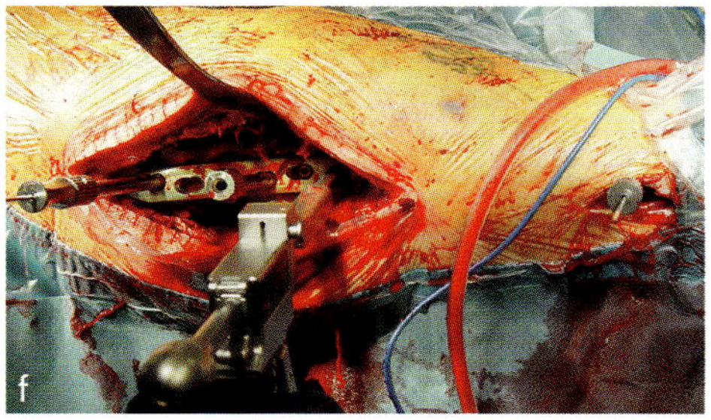

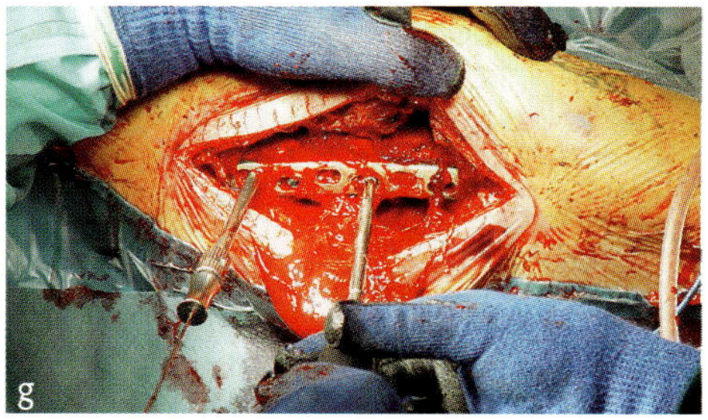

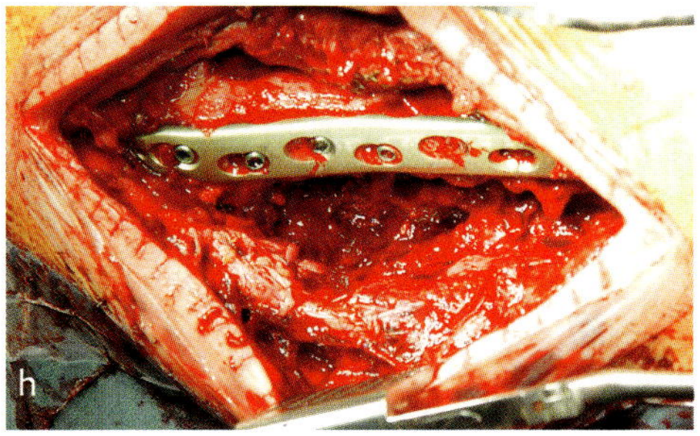

Fig 9.2.5-4a–h (cont)
- e Check plate position on the image intensifier.
- f Temporary proximal and distal fixation by insertion of K-wires into the most proximal and most distal plate holes and reduction of the fracture with the help of the collinear reduction forceps.
- g Fixation of the plate with bicortical locking head screws proximally and distally.
- h Fixation of the proximal fragment with a total of four locking head screws whereby the screws will be angled in different directions due to the anatomy of the proximal femur.

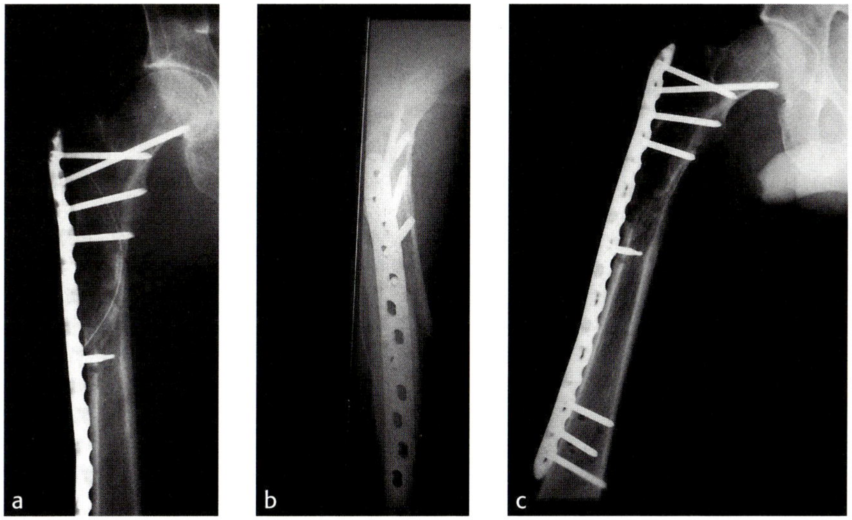

Fig 9.2.5-5a–c Postoperative x-rays show the reduction of the fragments and the fixation of the proximal part of the plate with four LHS, whereby the second screw has been inserted so that it lies close to the thick medial cortex of the femoral neck. The distal fragments are fixed by means of three bicortical LHS at the distal end of the plate and by one self-drilling, self-tapping LHS adjacent to the fracture.

3 Rehabilitation

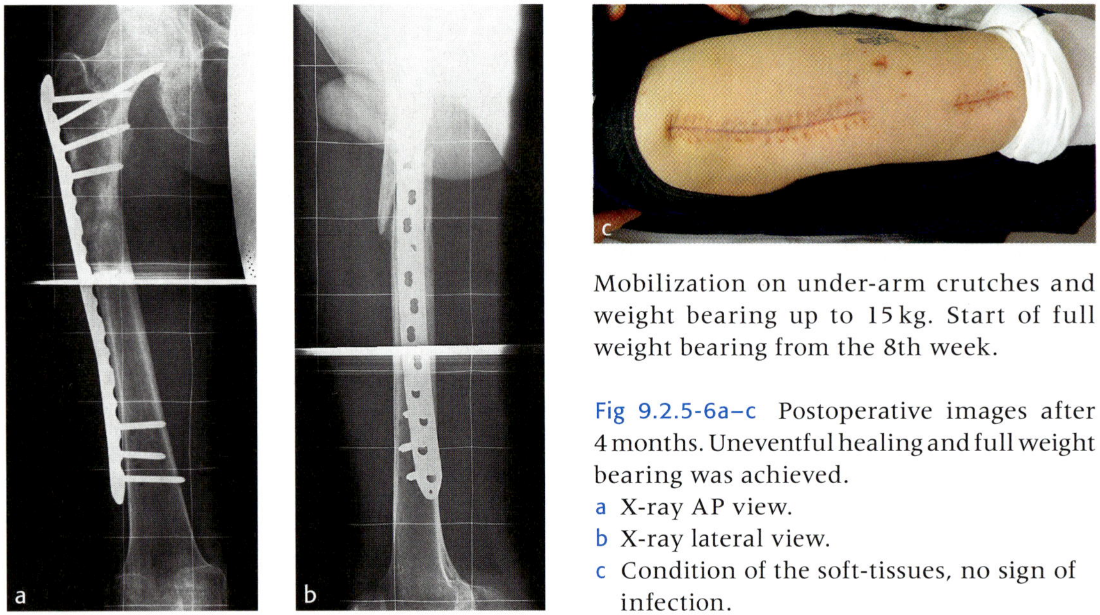

Mobilization on under-arm crutches and weight bearing up to 15 kg. Start of full weight bearing from the 8th week.

Fig 9.2.5-6a–c Postoperative images after 4 months. Uneventful healing and full weight bearing was achieved.

a X-ray AP view.

b X-ray lateral view.

c Condition of the soft-tissues, no sign of infection.

5 Pitfalls –

Reduction and fixation

6 Pearls +

Reduction and fixation

The internal fixator is a noncontact plate and causes only minimal damage to the periosteal blood supply. For this reason, it can be applied at low risk in situations of bone infection, especially if the indication for an external fixator is poor. Long LHS offer adequate anchorage in the metaphyseal region and act as an "individual" blade plate.

Author Reto Babst

9.2.6 Simple spiral femoral shaft fracture, periprosthetic—32-A1

1 Case description

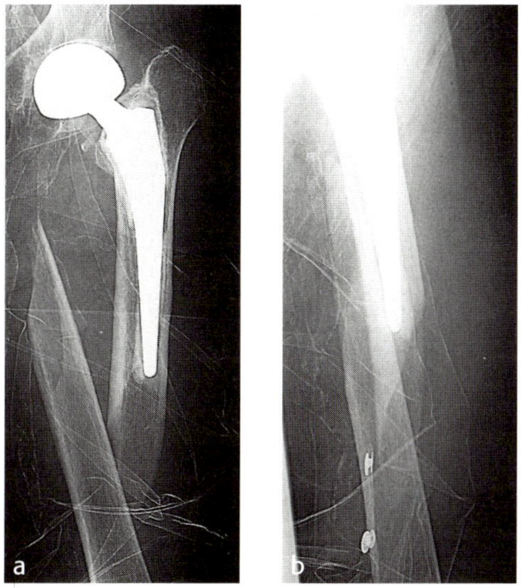

91-year-old woman. Low impact fall at home. Displaced spiral fracture distal to a clinically stable cemented hemiarthroplasty with severe osteopenia. The patient has limited walking capacity and lives in a nursing home.

Fig 9.2.6-1a–b
a AP view.
b Lateral view.

Indication

Relevant displacement of this spiral femoral fracture. Even though the hemiarthroplasty has radiological signs of instability, the patient, who had limited walking capacity, had no pain before the fall. Operative treatment in this frail old lady aimed at a minimally invasive procedure, which would allow for rapid mobilization at least in a wheelchair. Nonoperative treatment with traction is associated with prolonged bedrest and not an option in elderly patients.

Preoperative planning

Equipment

- LCP 4.5/5.0, broad, 22 holes
- 5.0 mm locking head screws (LHS)
- Large distractor, push-pull distractor
- Hohmann retractor
- Collinear reduction clamp

(Size of system, instruments, and implants can vary according to anatomy.)

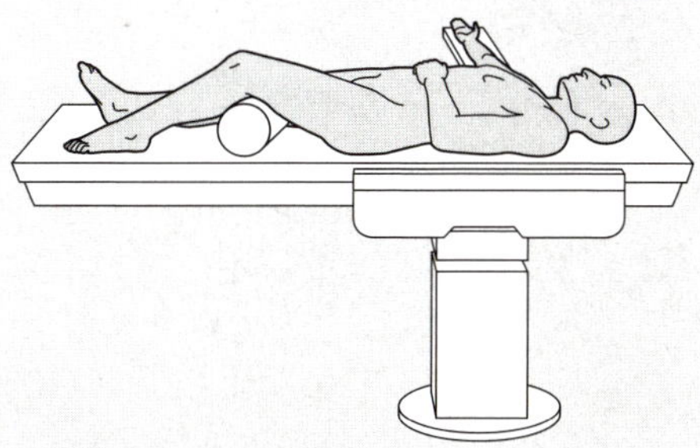

Fig 9.2.6-2
The fractured leg is placed with the knee flexed at 20–30°, whereas the uninjured leg is placed on a leg holder.
Mark the center of the femoral head and the center of the ankle joint for intraoperative alignment control with the cable method.
Alternatively both legs are draped free on a radiolucent table for intraoperative comparison of the femoral axis in respect to the uninjured leg.

Patient preparation and positioning

Antibiotics: single dose 2nd generation cephalosporin
Thrombosis prophylaxis: low-molecular heparin

2 Surgical approach

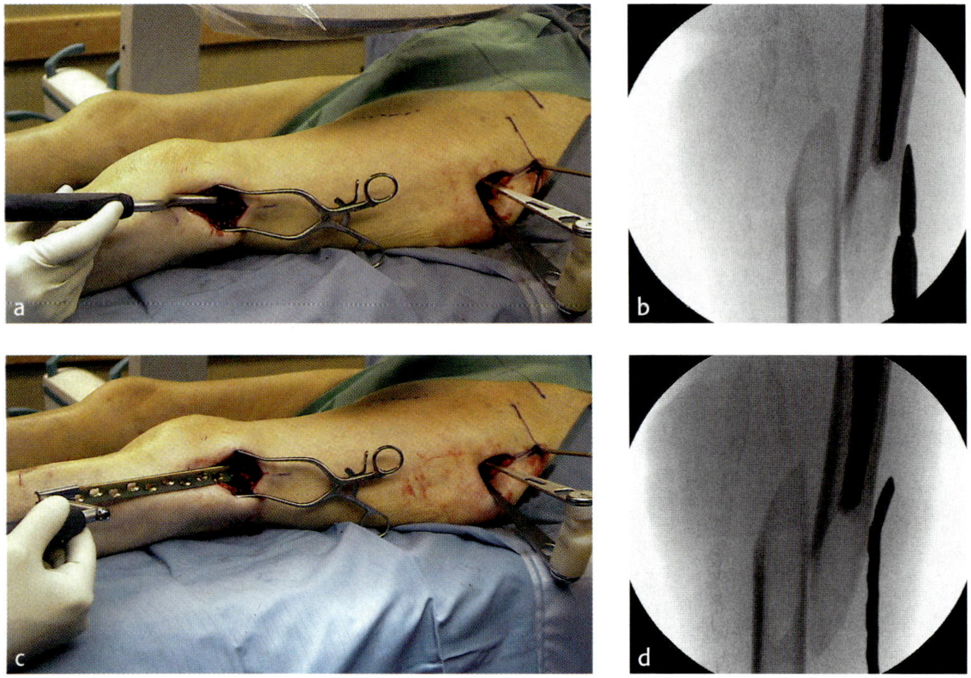

Fig 9.2.6-3a–d

a–b Two incisions are made, one in the middle aspect of the lateral condyle, the other one in the region of the future end of the plate. Preoperative planning for plate length is mandatory and plate length is marked on the skin. After distal and proximal incisions (transmuscular approach proximally) and positioning the proximal shaft of the femur between two Hohmann retractors, the femoral end of the plate can be seen and palpated. An epiperiosteal rasp prepares the tunnel for the LCP.

c–d The plate is then inserted with a plate holder along the femoral shaft and directed between the two proximal Hohmann retractors.

3 Reduction and fixation

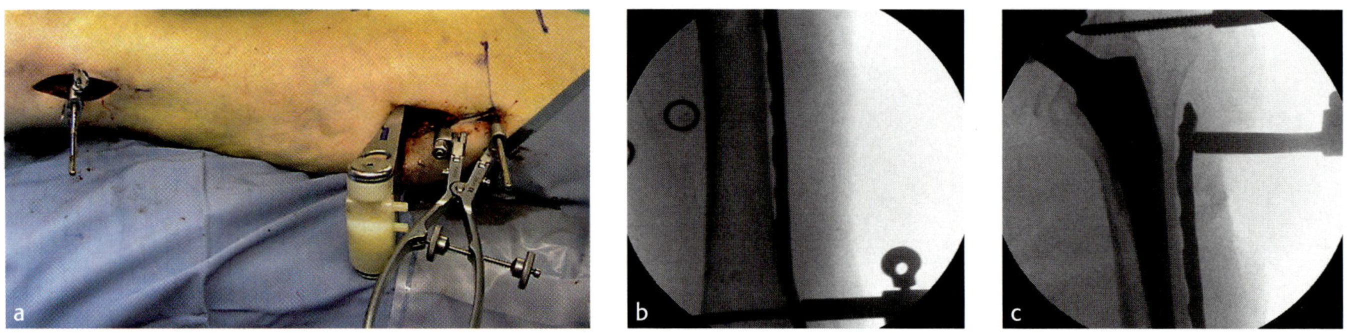

Fig 9.2.6-4a–c The plate is fixed distally with a Schanz screw and pressed against the shaft using a sleeve of the large distractor. A push-pull clamp is mounted on a Schanz screw, which has been inserted into the last hole at the proximal plate end.

3 Reduction and fixation (cont)

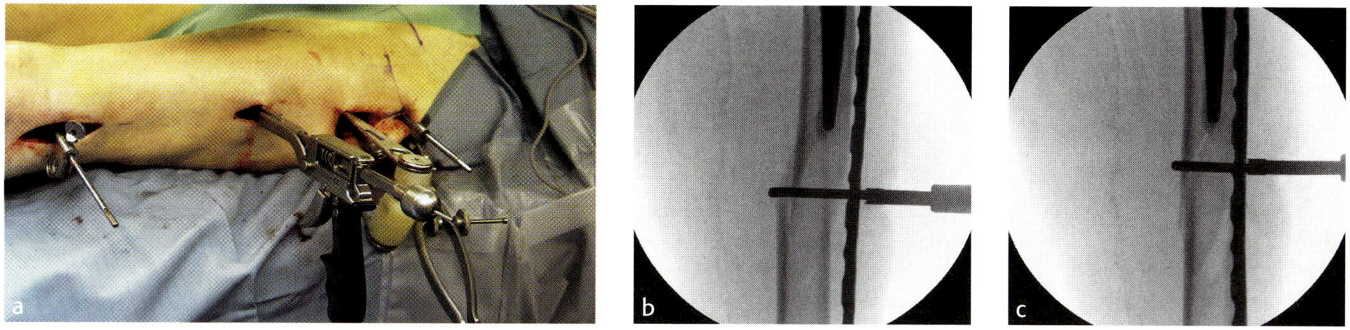

Fig 9.2.6-5a–c
a–c With the push-pull distractor used in this case, the fracture is indirectly reduced against the plate. Final reduction is achieved directly using the collinear reduction forceps.

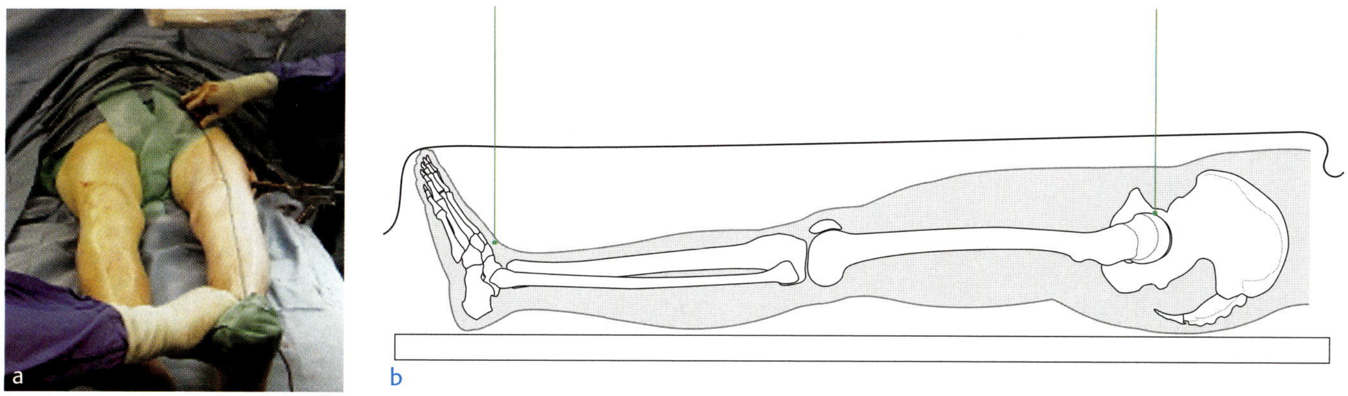

Fig 9.2.6-6a–c
a–b Before definitive fixation of the plate, reduction is controlled by the cable method.
c After percutaneous fixation with screws, wound closure with suction drains completes the procedure.

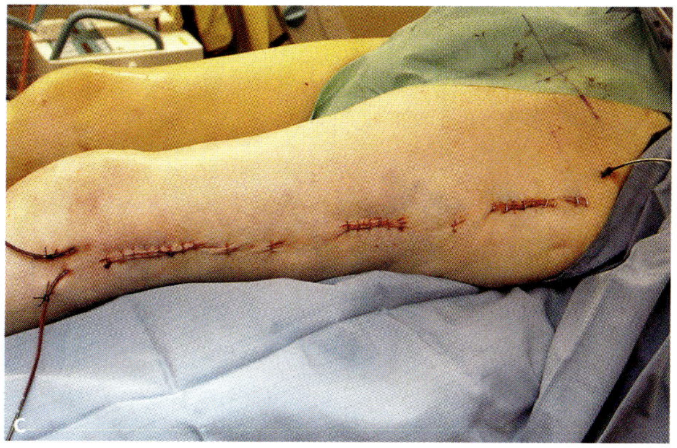

4 Rehabilitation

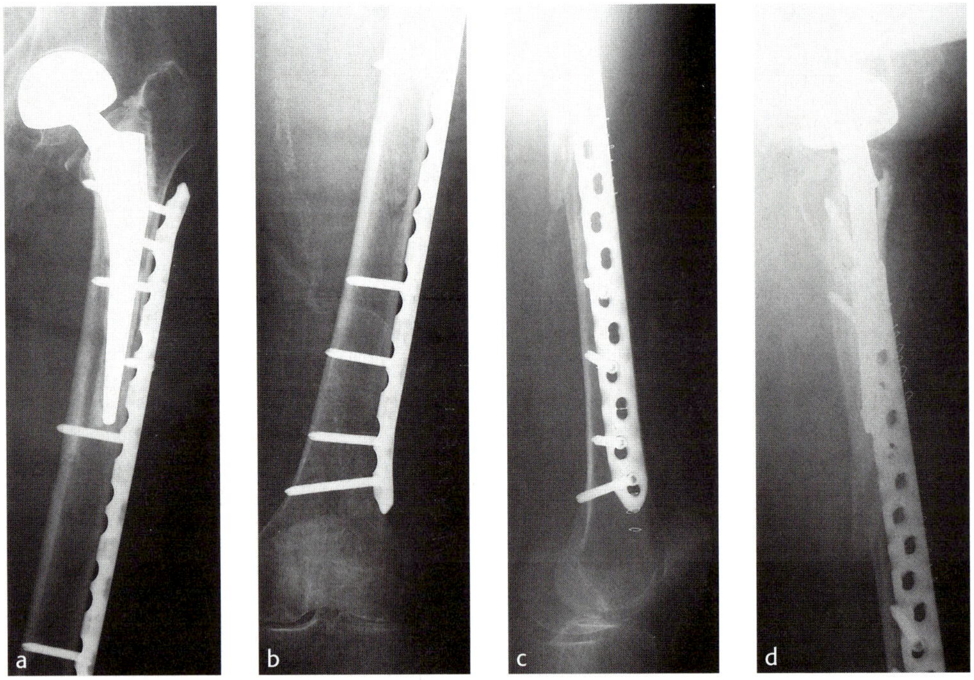

Physiotherapy: continuous passive motion beginning the first postoperative day without limitation except pain.
Mobilization with partial weight bearing for 8–10 weeks depending on the x-ray 6 weeks postoperatively.
Pharmaceutical treatment: medication depending on the postoperative pain.
Implant removal after 18–24 months if symptomatic.

Fig 9.2.6-7a–d Postoperative x-rays 1 year after surgery. The fracture shows secondary bone healing with callus formation due to the bridge plating principle in this simple fracture pattern. Uneventful healing and full weight bearing was achieved.

5 Pitfalls –

Reduction and fixation
Malunion is easily achieved using MIPO, therefore all precautions should be taken to reduce this risk, eg, cable method, contralateral uninjured leg, intraoperative x-ray.

The distal position of the plate is critical, it should not be closer than one centimeter from the articular joint line anteriorly and distally otherwise irritation of the iliotibial tract may become a problem. The correct position of the plate in the proximal part is of the same importance otherwise the screws do not gain adequate purchase and will tear off.

6 Pearls +

Reduction and fixation
Indirect reduction of the bone with an external fixator or a large distractor or the push-pull clamp to the submuscular slide-insertion plate after applying traction manually, helps to reduce the risk of malunion.

Positioning of two K-wires to control correct plate position distally and visual and digital control through the small proximal incision can help to prevent incorrect plate placement.

Reduction control with the cable method and/or both legs draped free for intraoperative comparison of the femoral axis and rotation.

Author Reto Babst

9.2.7 Simple spiral femoral shaft fracture, periprosthetic—32-A1

1 Case description

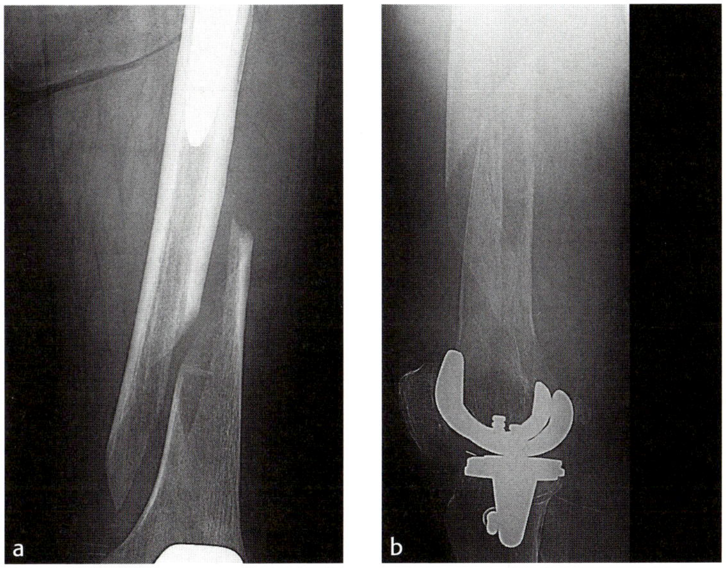

89-year-old woman. Low impact fall at home. Displaced spiral fracture between a stable noncemented total hip and a non-constrained total knee arthroplasty in a severe osteopathic patient.

Fig 9.2.7-1a–b
a AP view.
b Lateral view.

Indication

Relevant displacement with impossibility to mobilize the patient. Conservative treatment with traction or splints is associated with prolonged bed rest which is deleterious for older age patients.

Preoperative planning

Equipment

- LISS-DF, 13 holes
- 5.0 mm self-drilling, self-tapping locking head screws (LHS)
- LISS periprosthetic screws
- Large distractor
- Collinear reduction clamp
- Hohmann retractors

(Size of system, instruments, and implants can vary according to anatomy.)

Patient preparation and positioning

Antibiotics: single dose 2nd generation cephalosporin
Thrombosis prophylaxis: low-molecular heparin

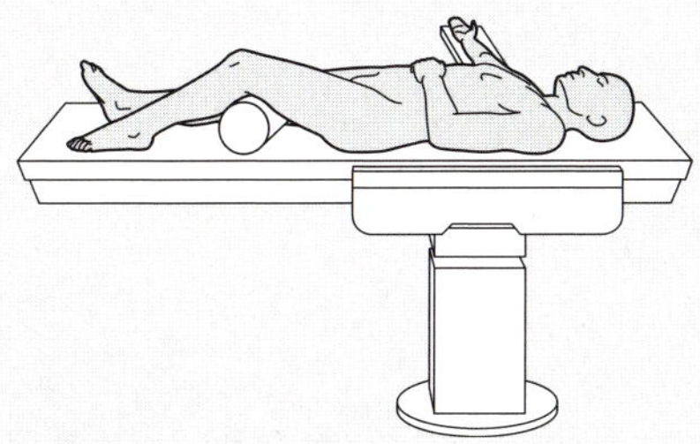

Fig 9.2.7-2 The fractured leg is placed with the knee flexed at 20–30°, whereas the uninjured leg is on a leg holder or straight on the table. Mark the center of the femoral head and the center of the ankle joint for intraoperative alignment control with the cable method. Alternatively both legs are draped free on a radiolucent table for intraoperative comparison of the femoral axis in respect to the uninjured leg.

2 Surgical approach

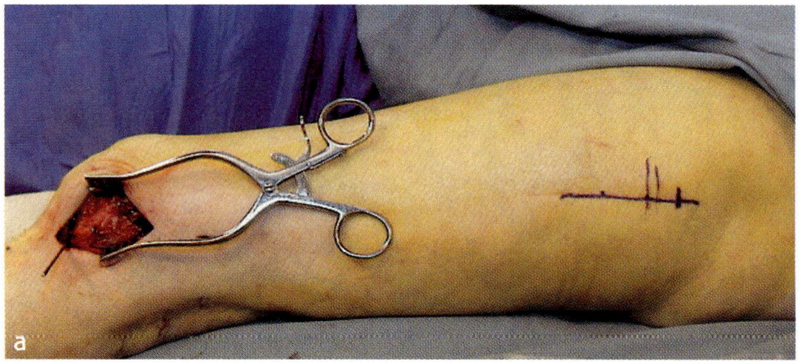
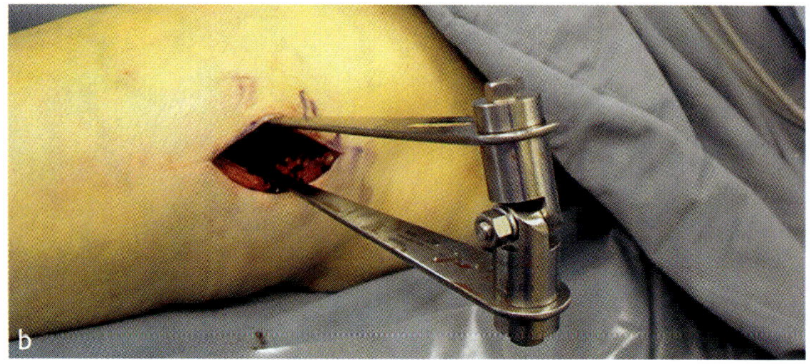

Fig 9.2.7-3a–b
a Two incisions are made, one in the middle aspect of the lateral condyle, the other one in the region of the future end of the plate. Preoperative planning of the plate length and marking on the skin are recommended.
b The proximal incision is transmuscular and the femoral shaft becomes visible between two Hohmann retractors, which are held by a mounted "Hohmann holder".

3 Reduction and fixation

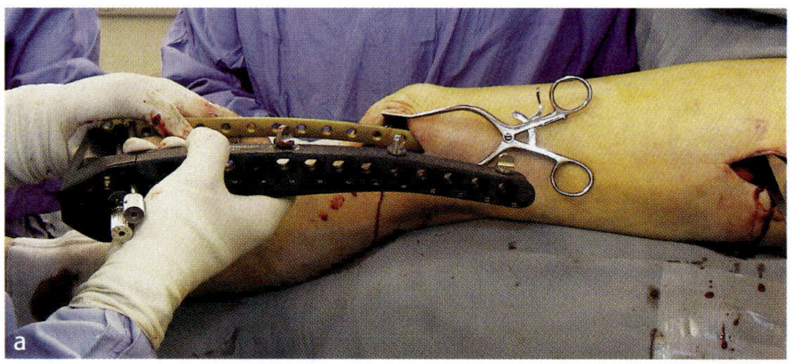
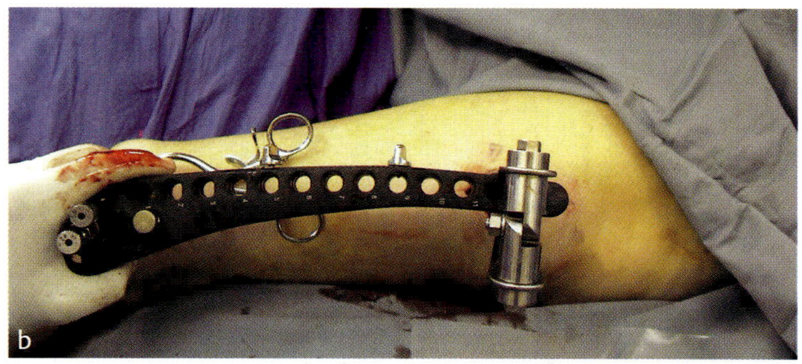
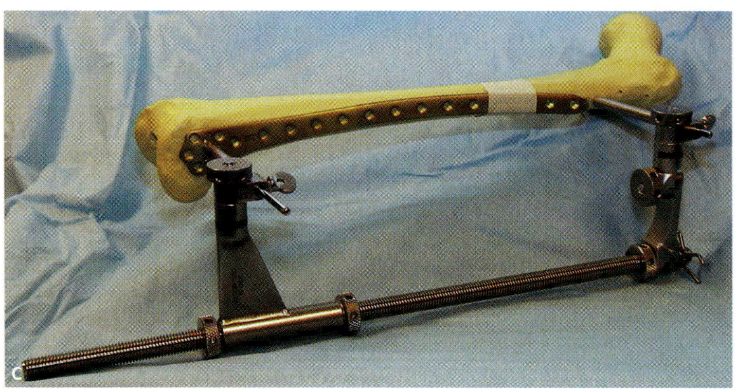

Fig 9.2.7-4a–c
a The LISS with the insertion guide is inserted distally.
b It glides along the femoral shaft and is then directed between the two Hohmann retractors proximally.
c With manual traction or a large distractor the insertion guide has to be removed and the large distractor has to be mounted with one Schanz screw through the distal middle hole and the other proximal one, proximal to the end of the plate.

3 Reduction and fixation (cont)

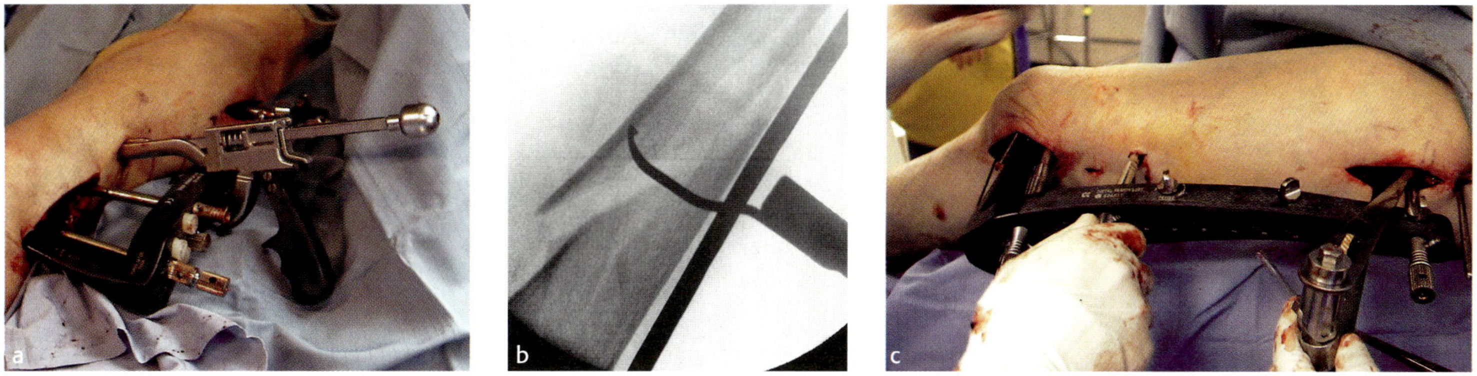

Fig 9.2.7-5a–c

- a After indirect reduction of the fracture against the plate by traction with the large distractor, direct percutaneous reduction is achieved with the collinear reduction clamp.
- b X-ray control for axis and rotation. The plate is fixed with two LHS in the proximal and distal fragment. The distractor is then removed and the insertion guide is fixed again to allow for easy percutaneous plate fixation.
- c The screws are then placed through the insertion guide. Screws in this case are all applied in a monocortical fashion. Of the five proximal screws, the two most proximal screws are periprosthetic screws.

4 Rehabilitation

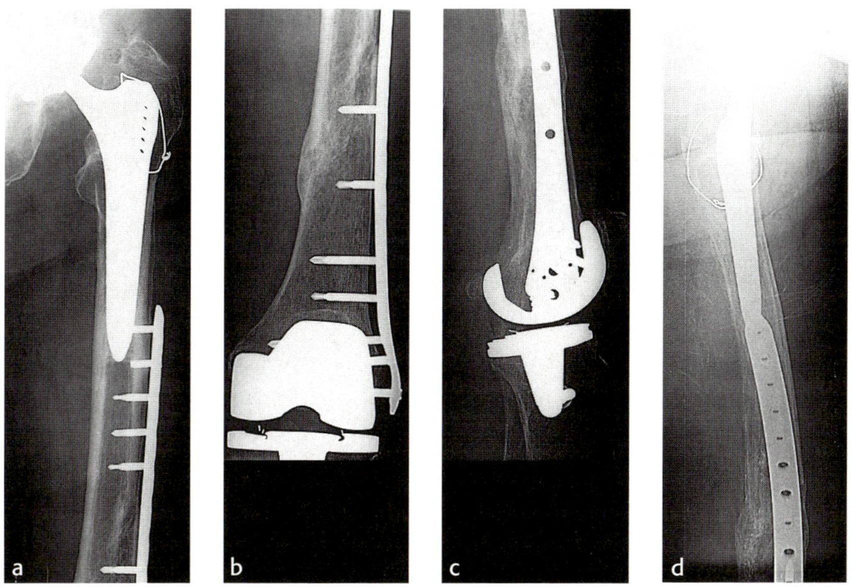

Physiotherapy: continuous passive motion beginning the first postoperative day without limitation except pain.

Mobilization with partial weight bearing for 8–10 weeks depending on the x-ray 6 weeks postoperatively.

Pharmaceutical treatment: pain medication depending on the postoperative pain.

Implant removal 18–24 months if symptomatic.

Fig 9.2.7-6a–d Postoperative x-ray 1 year after the operation. The fracture shows secondary bone healing with callus formation due to the splinting method in this simple fracture pattern. Uneventful fracture healing and full weight bearing was achieved.

5 Pitfalls –

Reduction and fixation

Fig 9.2.7-7 Malunion is easily achieved in MIPO, therefore all precautions should be taken to reduce this risk (eg, cable method, contralateral uninjured leg, intraoperative x-ray).

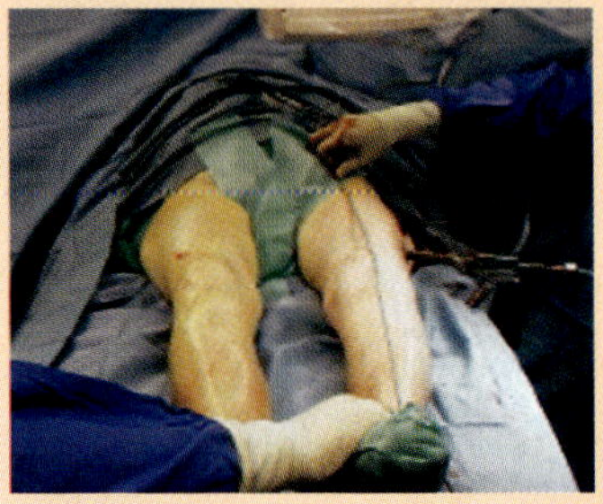

The distal position of the plate is critical, it should not be closer than one centimeter from the articular joint line anteriorly and distally otherwise irritation of the iliotibial tract may become a problem. The correct position of the plate in the proximal part is of the same importance otherwise the screws do not gain adequate purchase and will tear off.

6 Pearls +

Reduction and fixation

Fig 9.2.7-8 Indirect reduction with an external fixator or with a large distractor through the distal plate hole to the submuscular slide-insertion plate after applying traction manually, helps to reduce the risk of malunion.

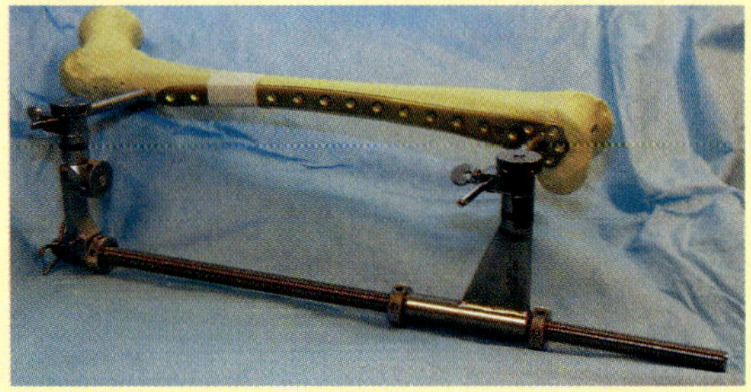

Positioning of two K-wires to control correct plate position distally and visual and digital control through the small proximal incision can help to prevent incorrect plate placement.

Fig 9.2.7-9a–b Direct percutaneous reduction is achieved with the collinear reduction clamp.

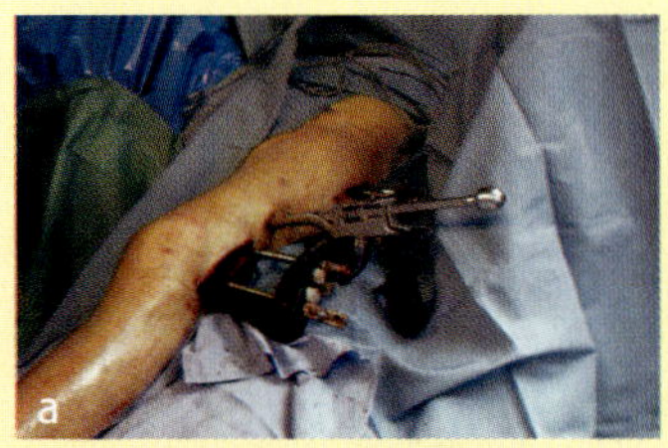

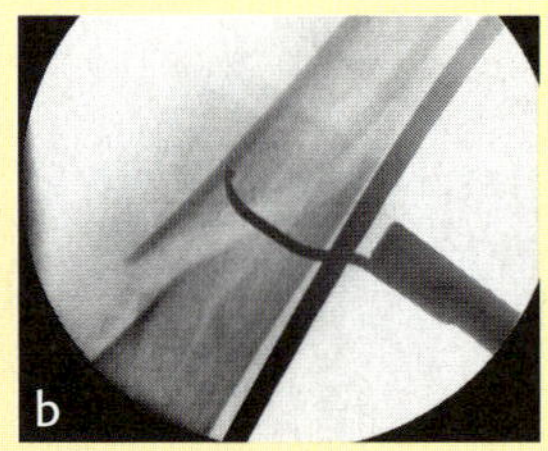

Authors Andreas Gruner, Thomas J Hockertz, Gabriele Streicher, Heinrich Reilmann

9.2.8 Femoral shaft fracture, periprosthetic—32-A1

1 Case description

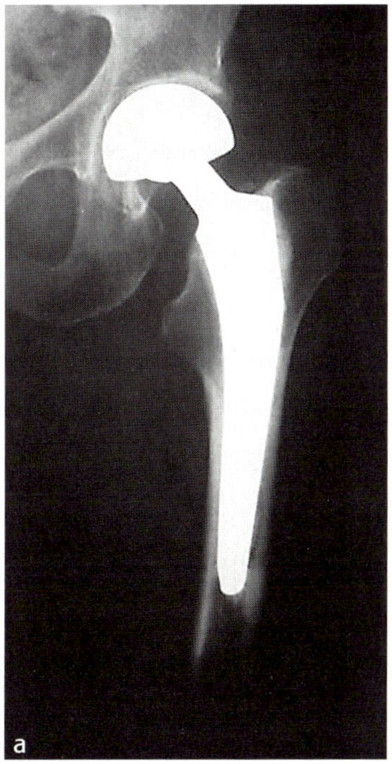

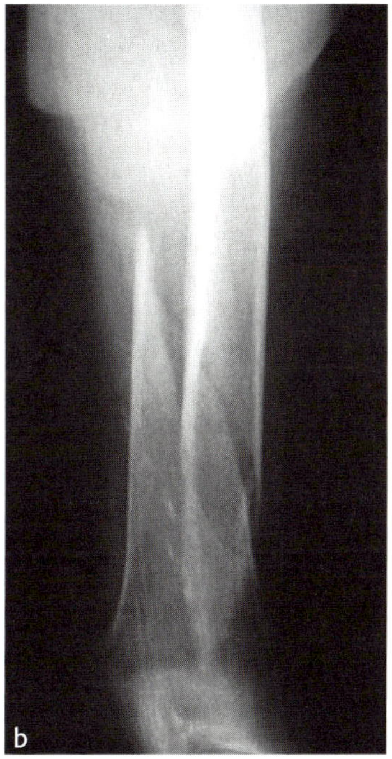

89-year-old man fell on the way to the bathroom at the old people's home and injured his left femur.
Type of injury: low-energy trauma, monotrauma, closed fracture.

Fig 9.2.8-1a–b
a AP view.
b Detail AP view.

Indication

Periprosthetic fracture of the left femur with implanted cemented semi-hip arthroplasty. No clinical or radiological signs of loosening. Before the accident the patient was mobile without crutches and without symptoms.

Preoperative planning

Equipment

- LISS-DF, 13 holes
- 5.0 mm self-drilling, self-tapping locking head screws (LHS)
- LISS periprosthetic screws
- 2.0 mm K-wires

(Size of system, instruments, and implants can vary according to anatomy.)

Patient preparation and positioning

Antibiotics: cephalosporin
Thrombosis prophylaxis: low-molecular heparin

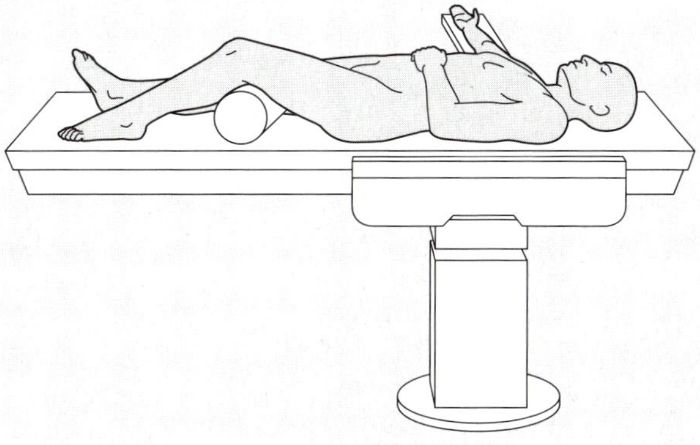

Fig 9.2.8-2 Supine position, the leg is free draped for intraoperative mobility, elevation of the injured limb, and flexion of the knee joint at approximately 30°, lower the contralateral leg for better intraoperative x-ray assessment, cushion the distal femur of the injured leg, eg, with a towel roll.

2 Surgical approach

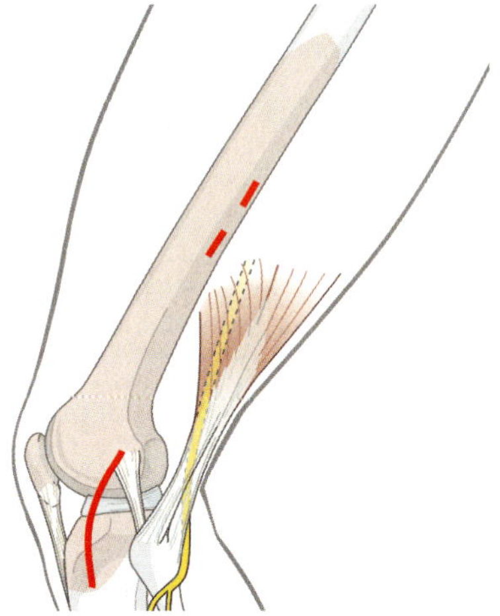

Fig 9.2.8-3 Skin incision from Gerdy's tubercle in a proximal direction. Divide the iliotibial tract in the direction of its fibers and dissect to the periosteum while retracting the vastus lateralis. Additional small incisions for proximal fixation.

3 Reduction and fixation

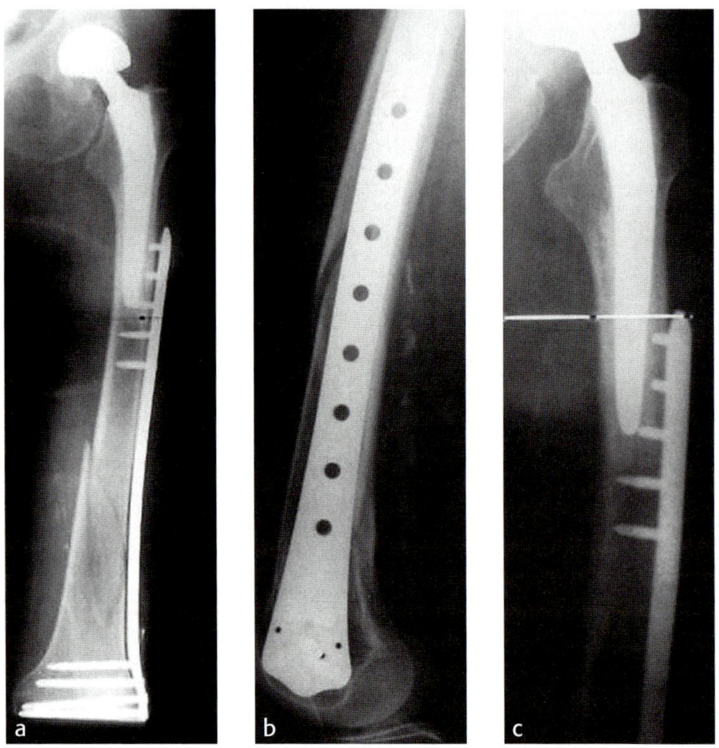

Fig 9.2.8-4a–c Approximate reduction of the fracture and the longitudinal axis by applying axial tension with the knee flexed to approx-imately 30° to relax the gastrocnemius.

Prepare the plate bed from distal to proximal by epiperiosteal tunneling with a long bone rasp under the vastus lateralis muscle.

Select the appropriate plate length under image intensifi-cation and insert the implant into the plate bed; make an incision at the proximal end of the plate to complete the correct positioning of the LISS.

Stabilize the implant by inserting K-wires proximally and distally through the implant and check plate position in two planes.

Precise reduction of the shaft fragments with the pulling device.

Insert the screws alternately in the distal and proximal holes starting distally, determine screw length according to Tab 3-2, chapter 3, whereby the special prosthesis drill with limited drill depth and the special periprosthetic screws should be used proximally once the stem of the prosthesis is in position. This avoids collision with prosthetic components and any associated thread stripping in the cortex.

4 Rehabilitation

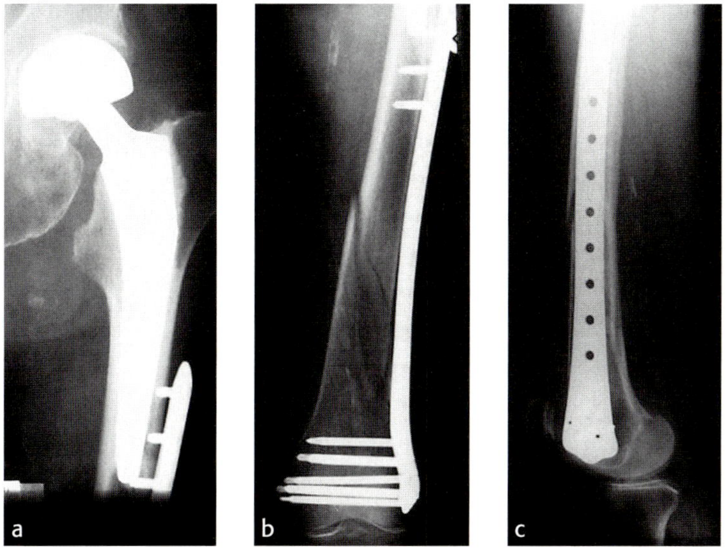

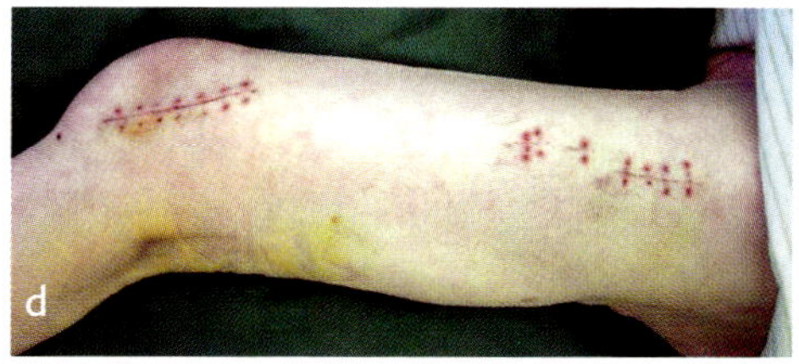

Weight bearing: 15 kg for 2 weeks; half body weight after 4 weeks; full weight bearing after 6 weeks.
Physiotherapy: from 2nd postoperative day and continuous passive motion.
Pharmaceutical treatment: pain therapy and nonsteroid anti-inflamatory drugs.

Fig 9.2.8-5a–d
a–c Postoperative x-rays after 1 week.
d Clinical picture after 1 week.

5 Pitfalls –

Equipment
Incorrect plate length: when inserting short monocortical periprosthetic screws it is especially important to ensure that there is adequate anchorage in the cortex.
The prosthesis must be firmly seated.

Approach
Inadequate preparation of the distal femur and, consequently, plate positioning too far anteriorly or posteriorly and risk of trapping the iliotibial tract.

Reduction and fixation
Displacement of the manual reduction and axis, incorrect screw length and abutment of the LISS screws before head locking is achieved. Consequent thread stripping.

Rehabilitation
Immobilization for too long time.

6 Pearls +

Equipment
Monocortical anchorage in the LISS shaft in the region of the prosthesis bed.

Approach

Reduction and fixation
Anchorage is possible in the presence of endoprostheses with shaft components or correction endoprostheses.
Use of periprosthetic screws.

Rehabilitation
Partial weight bearing cannot always be achieved with elderly patients.

Author Michael Wagner

9.2.9 Spiral femoral shaft fracture, periprosthetic—32-A1

1 Case description

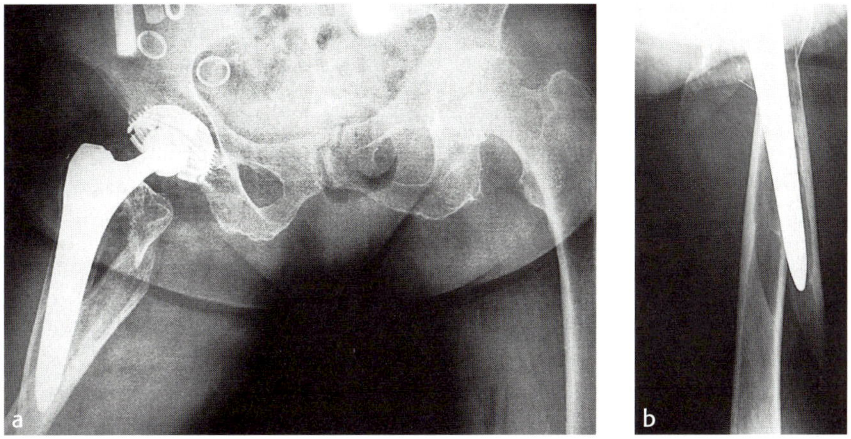

93-year-old woman fell at home. Displaced spiral fracture distal to a clinically stable uncemented hip arthroplasty with severe osteopenia.

Fig 9.2.9-1a–b
a AP view.
b Lateral view.

Indication

Relevant displacement of the spiral femoral shaft fracture. Even though the arthroplasty has radiological signs of instability, operative treatment with a minimally invasive procedure, which allows for rapid mobilization, was indicated in this frail old woman. Another operative option is to change the unstable femoral stem of the prosthesis to a longer revision stem with additional cerclage wire. Nonoperative treatment with traction is associated with prolonged bedrest and is not an option in elderly patients.

Preoperative planning

Equipment
- LCP 4.5/5.0, broad, 16 holes
- Locking head screws (LHS)
- Cerclage wires
- Wire mounts
- Pelvic reduction forceps

(Size of system, instruments, and implants can vary according to anatomy.)

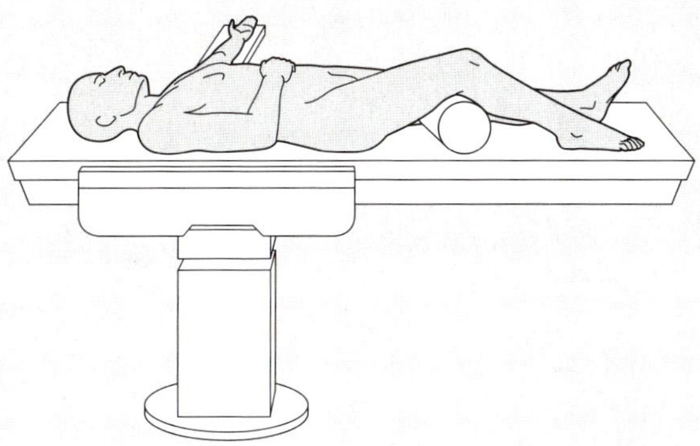

Fig 9.2.9-2 The fractured leg is placed with knee flexed at 20–30°, whereas the uninjured leg is placed straight on the table.

2 Surgical approach

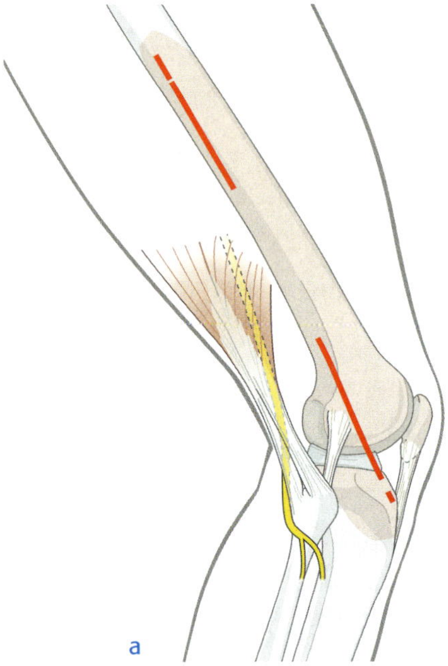

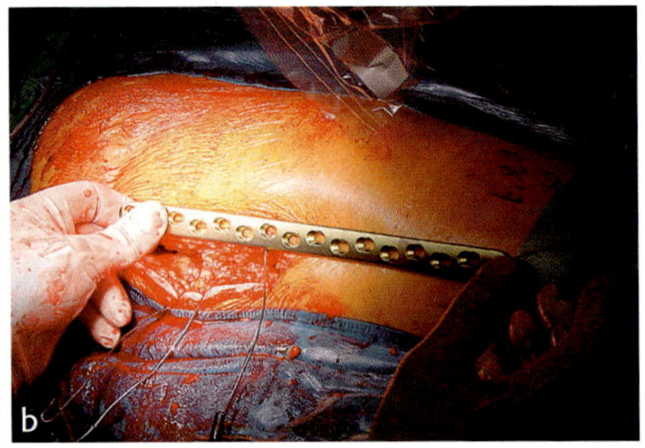

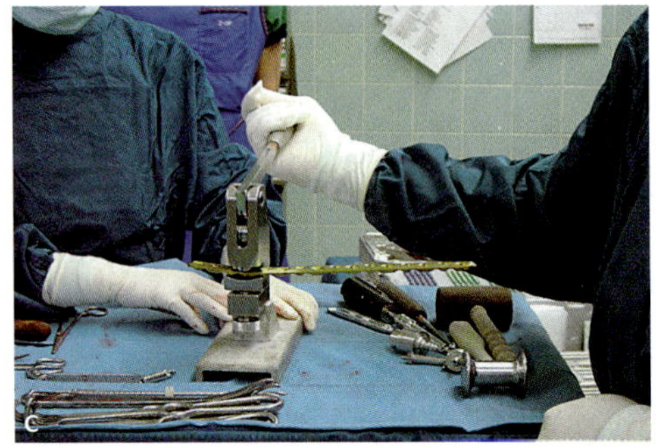

Fig 9.2.9-3a–c

a Two incisions are chosen, one on the lateral side of the proximal femur, the other one in the region of the future distal end of the plate.

b–c Preoperative planning for plate length is mandatory. The plate is chosen in the appropriate length and prebent to the lateral aspect on the femoral shaft. After making distal and proximal incisions (transmuscular approach proximally) and positioning of two cerclage wires around the shaft of the femur, a third cerclage wire is inserted at the level of the fracture distal to the prosthetic stem.

3 Reduction and fixation

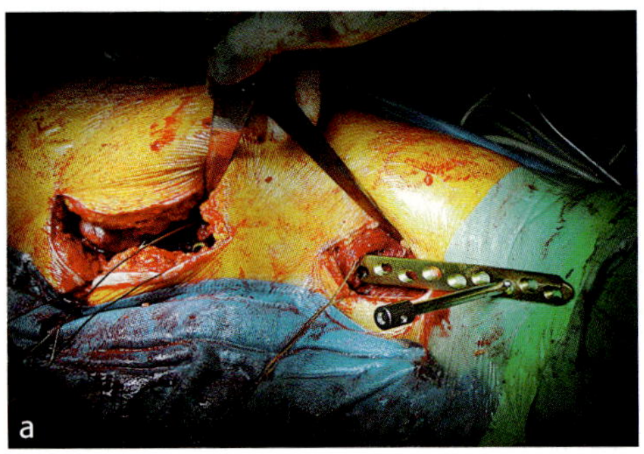

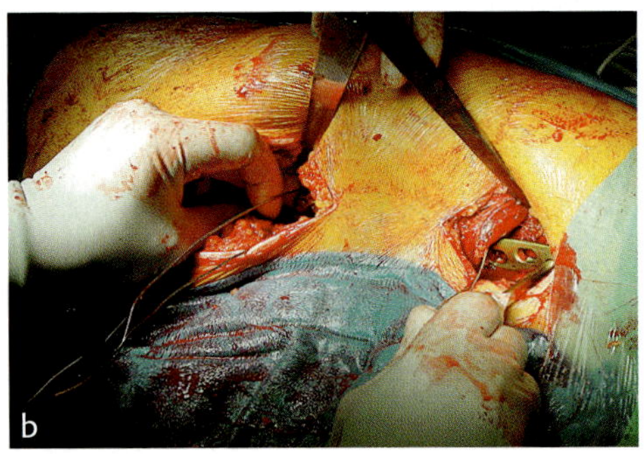

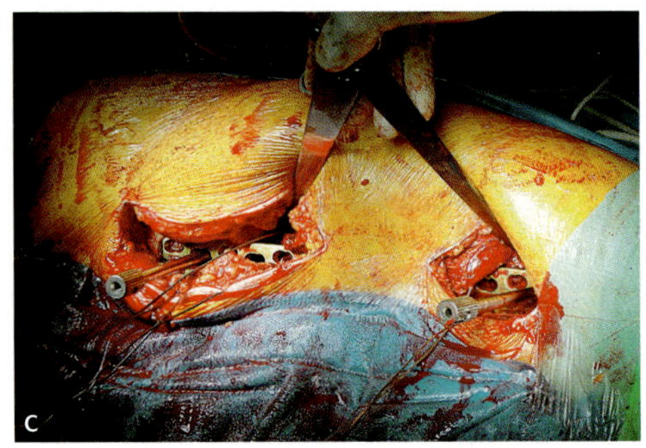

Fig 9.2.9-4a–k

a The plate is inserted along the femoral shaft from distal to proximal.
A threaded drill sleeve is fixed in the distal part of the plate and used as a handle.

b The end of the plate can be seen and palpated through the proximal incision. This allows correct positioning of the plate on the lateral aspect of the femur.

c Preliminary multiple cerclage wires were led around the femur and the plate.

3 Reduction and fixation (cont)

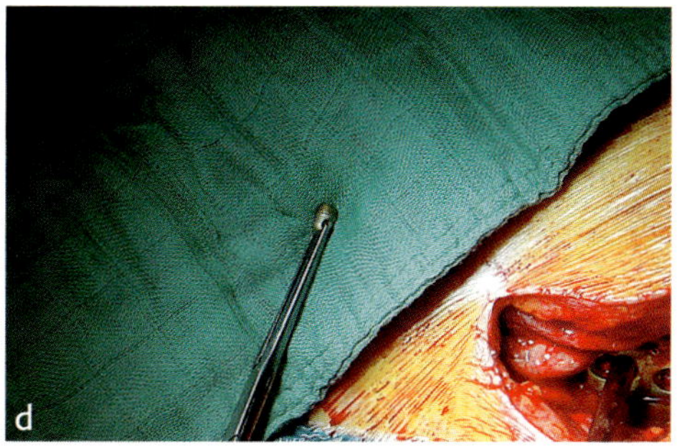

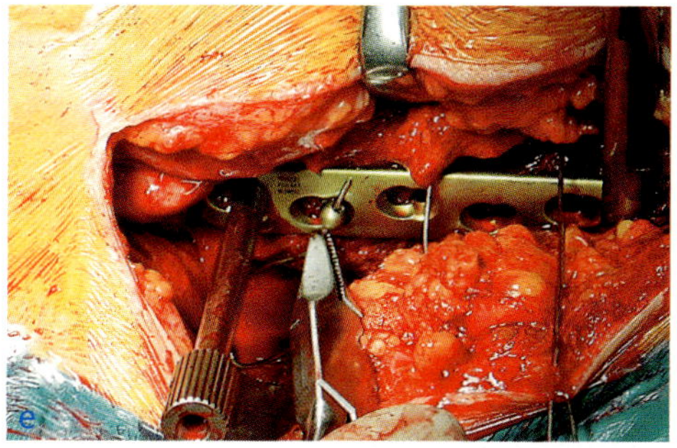

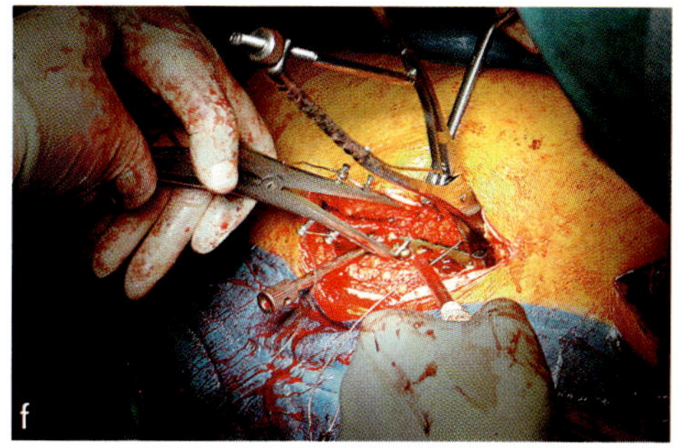

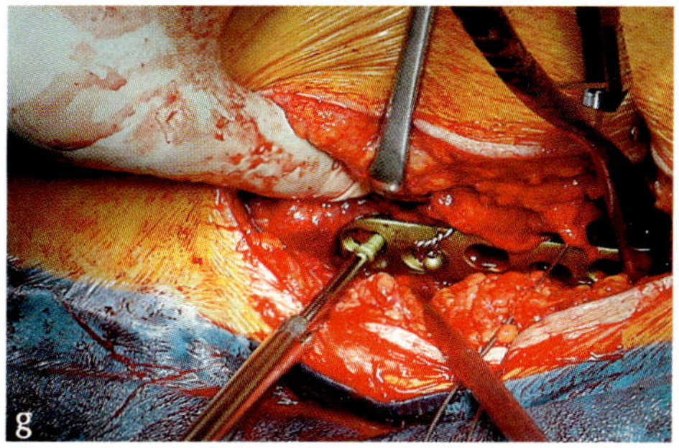

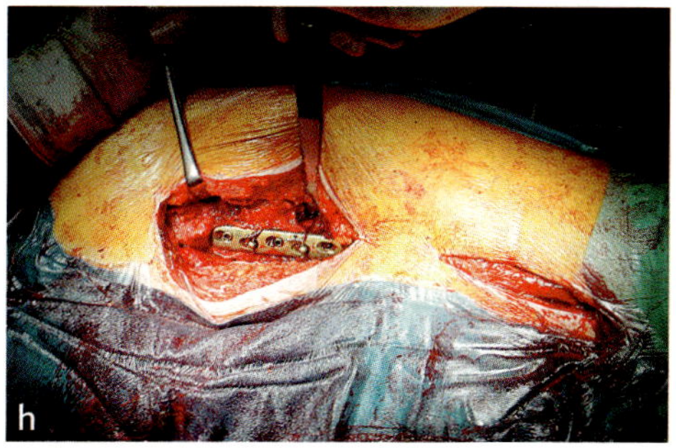

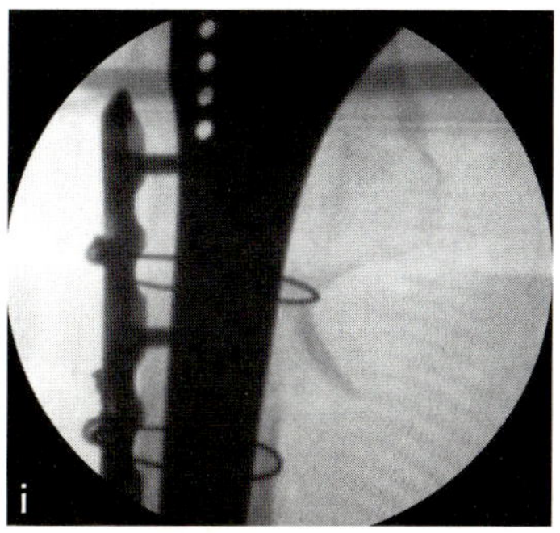

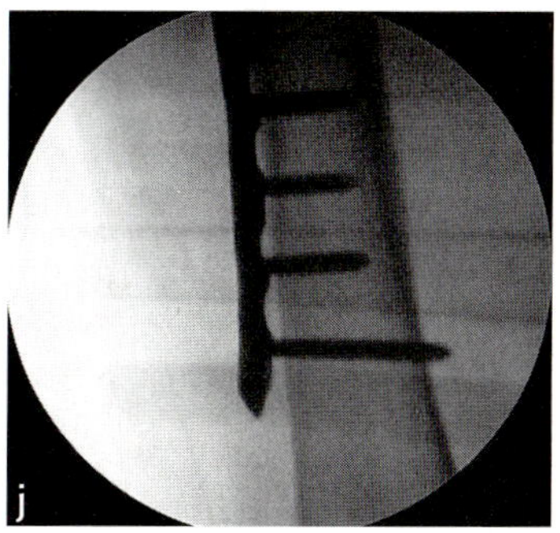

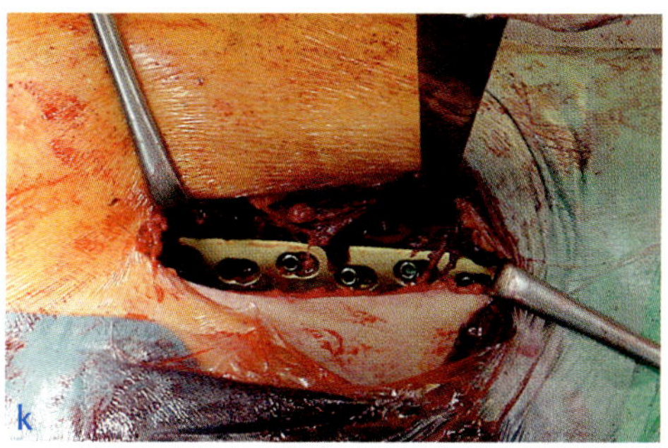

Fig 9.2.9-4a–k (cont)

- d A clamp or a screwdriver with screw holder sleeve is used to hold the wire mount.
- e The wire mounts were inserted in the conical, threaded part of the combination hole and the cerclage wires were pushed through the holes.
- f Reduction starts by simultaneous manual traction, direct reduction with reduction forceps, and tightening the cerclage wires with the cerclage tightening forceps.
- g Fixation of the proximal fragment with a self-tapping LHS in the most proximal hole. In the second proximal hole the cerclage wire through the wire mount is seen.
- h Further proximal fixation of the plate with one additional LHS and one wire mount in the third and fourth proximal plate holes.
- i Intraoperative image intensifier control of the fracture reduction and the proximal fracture fixation.
- j Intraoperative image intensifier control of the distal plate fixation.
- k Distal plate fixation with four LHS, three of them monocortically.

4 Rehabilitation

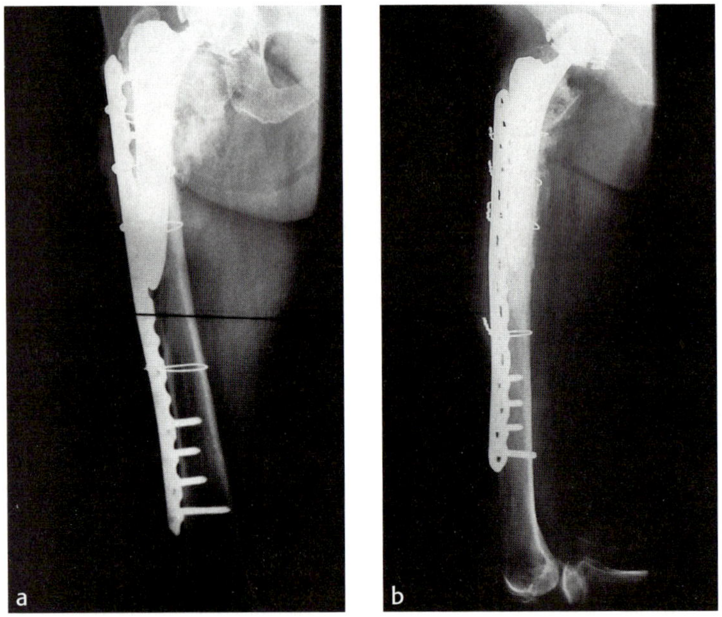

Physiotherapy: continuous passive motion beginning on the first postoperative day without limitation except pain.
Mobilization with partial weight bearing for 8–10 weeks depending on the x-rays 6 weeks postoperatively.
Pharmaceutical treatment: pain medication depending on postoperative pain.

Fig 9.2.9-5a–b
Postoperative x-rays 3 months after the operation. The fracture shows good bone healing with callus formation due to the bridging plate principle in this simple fracture pattern. The cerclage wires are necessary for reduction and proximal plate fixation and do not disturb indirect bone healing.
a AP view.
b Lateral view.

5 Pitfalls –

Reduction and fixation
Malunion is easily achieved using MIPO, therefore every precaution should be taken to reduce this risk (eg, cable method, contralateral uninjured leg, intraoperative x-ray).

The proximal fixation of the plate in a periprosthetic femoral fracture is critical. In the case of a bulky stem, only short monocortical LHS can be used.

6 Pearls +

Reduction and fixation
Direct reduction with cerclage wires and reduction clamps is a simple technique to the submuscular slide-insertion plate after applying traction manually, and helps to reduce the risk of malunion.
Singular cerclage wires do not prevent indirect bone healing

Wire mounts prevent cerclage wires from moving proximally or distally and helps to fix the LCP.

Cerclage wires through wire mounts are helpful for reduction and fixation

9.3 Femur, distal

Cases

9 Femur

Author Michael Schütz

9.3 Femur, distal

1 Incidence

The incidence of distal femoral fractures is 12 per 100,000 population and accounts for 6–7% of all femoral fractures. These fractures occur predominantly in two age groups: younger patients between 20 and 35 years of age and elderly patients.

The younger patients are mostly male and sustain a distal femoral fracture as a result of high-velocity traumas, generally car or motorbike accidents, whereby the fracture occurs as a consequence of direct application of force to the flexed knee joint. Road traffic accidents are involved in over 50% of the fracture cases. Over 30% of these patients are polytraumatized. Additional injuries to the affected limb are frequent.

A well known pathomechanism in road-traffic accidents is the socalled "dashboard injury", whereby an impact on the flexed knee joint forces the patella back in between the femoral condyles like a wedge. This explains the combined injuries of patellar fractures and intraarticular distal femoral fractures. When forces act on the longitudinal axis of the leg with the knee joint in extension, the tibial plateau is pressed against the condyles. This leads to a supracondylar femoral fracture and possibly splits the condylar block and the femoral shaft.

The second age peak occurs in patients, mostly female, between the ages of 60 and 75 years. The incidence of distal femoral fractures even rises to 170 per 100,000 population for patients older than 85 years. The type of accident in this patient group is predominantly a low-energy trauma. There is often a tendency for fractures to be due to an osteoporotic bone structure.

According to the literature and our own observations, patients who have sustained a distal femoral fracture will have a concomitant fracture of the patella in 10–15% of cases, a patellar ligament instability requiring treatment in 20–30% and further bone lesions of the ipsilateral leg in 20–25% of cases. The "floating knee" is a very specific injury pattern. This combina-

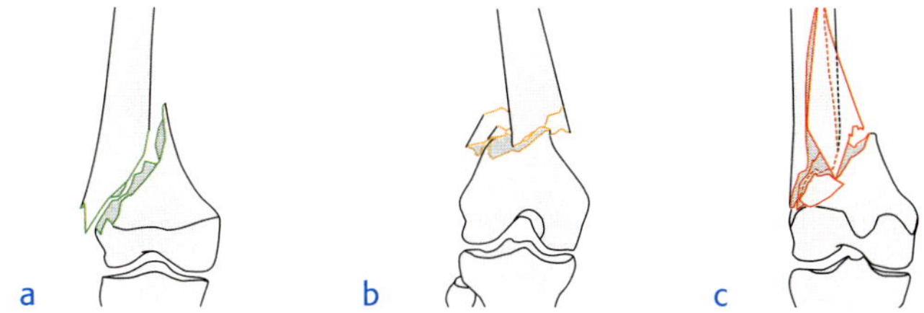

Fig 9.3-1a–c 33-A Extraarticular fracture.
a 33-A1 simple
b 33-A2 metaphyseal wedge and/or fragmented wedge
c 33-A3 metaphyseal complex

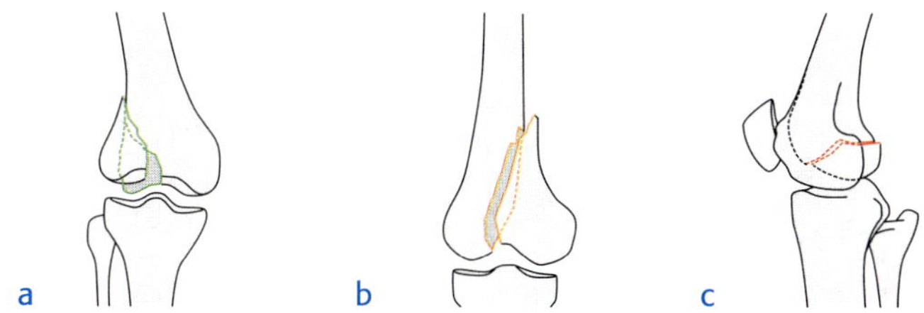

Fig 9.3-2a–c 33-B Partial articular fracture.
a 33-B1 lateral condyle, sagittal
b 33-B2 medial condyle, sagittal
c 33-B3 frontal

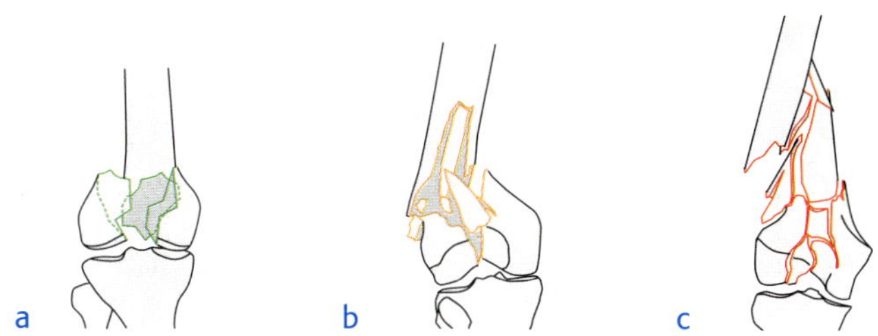

Fig 9.3-3a–c 33-C Complete articular fracture.
a 33-C1 articular simple, metaphyseal simple
b 33-C2 articular simple, metaphyseal multifragmentary
c 33-C3 articular multifragmentary

tion of a distal femoral fracture with a proximal tibial fracture is diagnosed in approximately 5% of all patients with distal femoral fractures. In contrast, concomitant vessel and nerve injuries are relatively rare (<5%) but must nevertheless always be assessed and excluded. Concomitant injuries tend to be rare in elderly patients affected by a low-energy trauma.

Injury	Incidence
Polytrauma	44%
Closed soft-tissue injuries	20%
Open fractures	24–40%
Nerve and vessel injuries	3%
Ligamentous injuries	10–19%
Damage to the meniscus	4%
Cartilaginous injuries (flake fractures)	7%
Patellar fractures	4–19%
Chain injuries to the ipsilateral limb	17–27%
Injuries to the contralateral limb	10–13%

Tab 9.3-1 Injury patterns and concomitant injuries in distal femoral fractures.

2 Classification

A number of different classifications are available for distal femoral fractures, eg, Stewart, Neer, Seinsheimer or Schatzker and Lambert. The Müller AO Classification (Fig 9.3-1, Fig 9.3-2, Fig 9.3-3) has proven its worth and has become well established.

The advantage of the Müller AO Classification is that it permits precise fracture categorization and a prognosis for each type of injury as well. The 5-digit alphanumeric code incorporates fracture site and type based on a comprehensive evaluation. With its subdivisions regarding type A, B and C this classification takes into account essential considerations concerning therapeutic procedure and prognosis. The degree of fracture severity increases from type A to C and from subgroup 1 to 3 as the prognosis worsens in terms of unsuccessful healing.

3 Treatment methods

Distal femoral fractures today are treated operatively almost without exception, whereby a broad spectrum of different operative techniques and implants is available. Regardless of these differences, the aim of treatment remains the same. Treatment should lead to an optimal restoration of the joint surfaces and correct axial alignment of the distal fragment in relation to the shaft permitting early functional, cast- free rehabilitation.

Although the operative treatment of distal femoral fractures was not well recommended up to the 1960s, a first case series of 112 patients was published by the AO in 1970 documenting clearly improved outcomes obtained by operative treatment. In almost 75% of the cases the outcome was found to be good or very good. This was a significant progress compared to the data published in the 1960s by Stewart and Neer who had achieved a satisfactory result in only 50% of patients treated surgically. Further publications reporting on improved outcomes after operative treatment were published in quick succession.

For a long time, the aim of treatment was the anatomical reconstruction of all fragments, including the metaphyseal region, and high primary stability. This was achieved by extensive exposure of the fracture site and by insertion of numerous independent lag and plate screws. A potential complication of such excessive procedures, namely disturbed fracture healing, was handled by use of extensive primary bone graft, a procedure that was performed in up to 86% of the published cases.

Today, "biological" osteosynthesis and indirect reduction techniques without anatomical reduction of every individual fragment permit better conservation of the bone-to-soft- tissue connections in nonarticulating regions and ensure higher fragment vascularization. The "rediscovered" relevance of iatrogenic soft-tissue trauma and the influence of blood supply to the fragments led to new concepts in terms of surgical techniques: MIPO—minimally invasive percutaneous plate osteosynthesis, TARPO transarticular joint reconstruction and indirect plate osteosynthesis and finally new extramedullary implants. It was proven experimentally that minimally invasive approaches caused less iatrogenic damage to the blood supply and led to increased restitution. Very good results were also obtained under clinical conditions.

The surgeon has to consider a multiplicity of factors when choosing the most appropriate operative procedure: fracture type, concomitant injuries, bone quality, general condition of the patient, his own experience and that of the operating team, logistic prerequisites, and regional preferences. A preoperative drawing is indispensable to detail the fracture pattern, to plan the reduction, and to choose type and size of the implant. It is also important to anticipate unforeseen local circumstances and to consider alternative surgical procedures.

Extraarticular distal femoral fractures can be treated by extra- or intramedullary techniques. In general, it is preferable to perform indirect reduction and minimally invasive stabilization. Therefore, extramedullary treatment makes use of angular stable implants (condylar plate, DCS, or internal fixator). For intramedullary procedures, antegrade and retrograde nailing techniques are available. Partially intraarticular fractures (type B fractures) are stabilized by screw fixation. In cases of exceptionally poor bone quality, a protective plate osteosynthesis or an internal fixator may become necessary. Even completely intraarticular fractures can be stabilized by using extra- or intramedullary techniques. Sufficient anchorage in the distal fragment is a decisive factor for the choice of the implant. Today, the locked internal fixator is the standard implant in cases of severe comminution, open fracture with excessive bone loss or in a very small distal fragment.

4 Implant overview

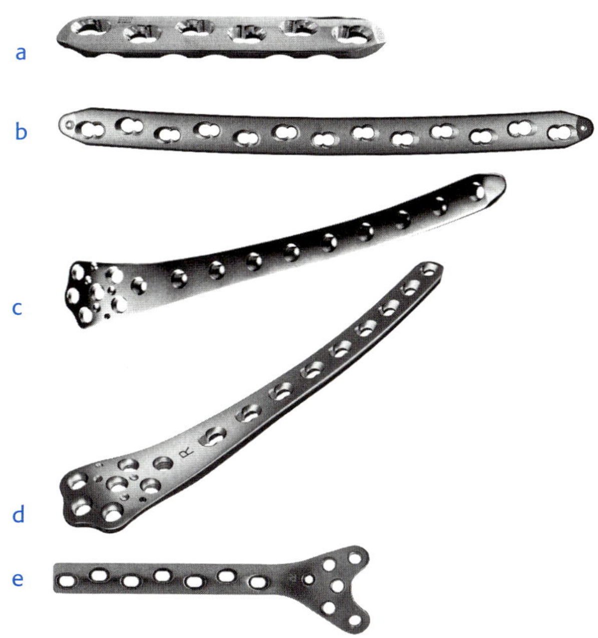

Fig 9.3-4a–e
a LCP 4.5/5.0, broad
b LCP 4.5/5.0 broad, curved
c LISS-DF 5.0 (left and right version available)
d LCP-DF 4.5/5.0 (left and right version available)
e LCP condylar plate 4.5/5.0 (left and right version available)

5 Suggestions for further reading

Babst R, Hehli M, Regazzoni P (2001) [LISS tractor. Combination of the "less invasive stabilization system" (LISS) with the AO distractor for distal femur and proximal tibial fractures.] *Unfallchirurg;* 104(6):530–535.

Krettek C, Schandelmaier P, Tscherne H (1996) [Distal femoral fractures. Transarticular reconstruction, percutaneous plate osteosynthesis and retrograde nailing]. *Unfallchirurg;* 99(1):2–10.

Stocker R, Heinz T, Vecsei V (1995) [Results of surgical management of distal femur fractures with joint involvement]. *Unfallchirurg;* 98(7):392–397.

Baumgaertel F, Gotzen L (1994) [The "biological" plate osteosynthesis in multi-fragment fractures of the para-articular femur. A prospective study.] *Unfallchirurg;* 97(2):78–84.

Bolhofner BR, Carmen B, Clifford P (1996) The results of open reduction and internal fixation of distal femur fractures using a biologic (indirect) reduction technique. *J Orthop Trauma;* 10(6):372–377.

Ostrum RF, Geel C (1995) Indirect reduction and internal fixation of supracondylar femur fractures without bone graft. *J Orthop Trauma;* 9(4):278–284.

Fankhauser F, Gruber G, Schippinger G, et al (2004) Minimal-invasive treatment of distal femoral fractures with the LISS (Less Invasive Stabilization System): a prospective study of 30 fractures with a follow up of 20 months. *Acta Orthop Scand;* 75(1):56–60.

Schuetz M, Mueller M, Krettek C, et al (2001) Minimally invasive fracture stabilization of distal femoral fractures with the LISS: a prospective multicenter study. Results of a clinical study with special emphasis on difficult cases. *Injury;* 32(Suppl 3):SC48–54.

Syed AA, Agarwal M, Giannoudis PV, et al (2004) Distal femoral fractures: long-term outcome following stabilisation with the LISS. *Injury;* 35(6):599–607.

Krettek C, Miclau T, Grün O, et al (1998) Intraoperative control of axis, rotation and length in femoral and tibial fractures—technical note. *Injury;* 29(Suppl3):29–39.

Danziger MB, Caucci D, Zecher SB, et al (1995) Treatment of intercondylar and supracondylar distal femur fractures using the GSH supracondylar nail. *Am J Orthop;* 24(9):684–690.

Iannacone WM, Bennett FS, DeLong WG Jr, et al (1994) Initial experience with the treatment of supracondylar femoral fractures using the supracondylar intramedullary nail: a preliminary report. *J Orthop Trauma;* 8(4):322–327.

Moed BR, Watson JT (1995) Retrograde intramedullary nailing, without reaming, of fractures of the femoral shaft in multiply injured patients. *J Bone Joint Surg Am;* 77(10):1520–1527.

Herscovici D Jr, Whiteman KW (1996) Retrograde nailing of the femur using an intercondylar approach. *Clin Orthop Relat Res;* (332):98–104.

David SM, Harrow ME, Peindl RD, et al (1997) Comparative biomechanical analysis of supracondylar femur fracture fixation: locked intramedullary nail versus 95-degree angled plate. *J Orthop Trauma;* 11(5):344–350.

Firoozbakhsh K, Behzadi K, DeCoster TA, et al (1995) Mechanics of retrograde nail versus plate fixation for supracondylar femur fractures. *J Orthop Trauma;* 9(2):152–157.

Maier DG, Reisig R, Keppler P, et al (2005) [Post-traumatic torsional differences and functional tests following antegrade or retrograde intramedullary nailing of the distal femoral diaphysis.] *Unfallchirurg;* 108(2):109–117.

Author Michael Wagner

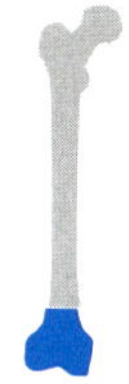

9.3.1 Extraarticular distal femoral fracture—33-A2

1 Case description

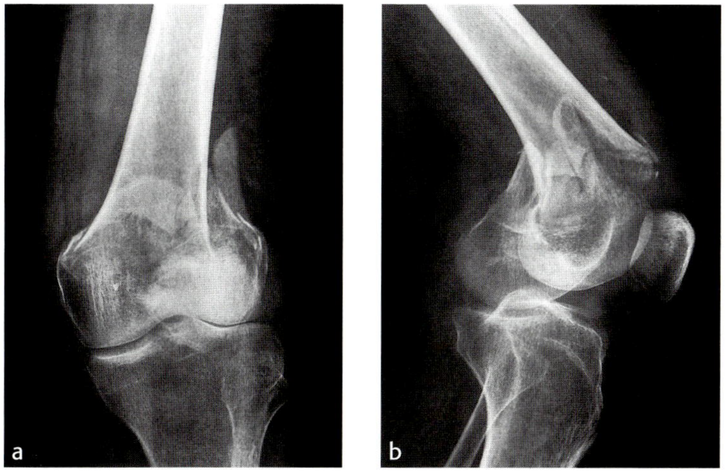

48-year-old man stumbled and fell in the street sustaining a closed fracture of his left distal femur.

Fig 9.3.1-1a–b
a AP view.
b Lateral view.

Indication

Unstable displaced fracture of the left distal femur with multiple fragmentation of the bending wedge. The indication to operate and the choice of implant arise from the very small distal fragment as this small joint fragment must be securely stabilized.

Preoperative planning

Equipment

- LCP-DF, 9 holes
- 5.0 mm locking head screws (LHS)
- 2.0 mm K-wires
- Small reduction table

(Size of system, instruments, and implants can vary according to anatomy.)

Patient preparation and positioning

Antibiotics: none
Thrombosis prophylaxis: low-molecular heparin

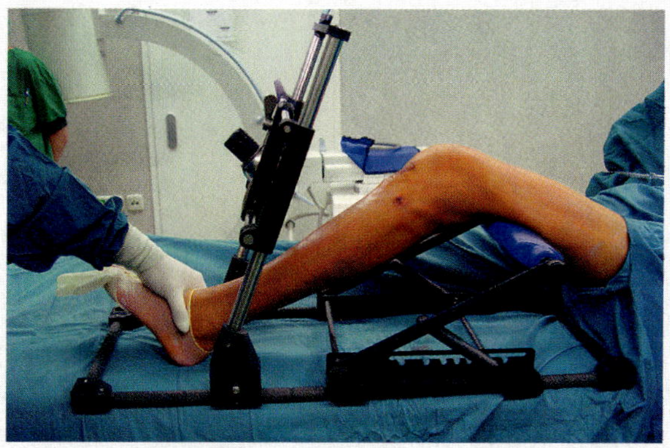

Fig 9.3.1-2—Supine position and reduction on the small reduction table.

2 Surgical approach

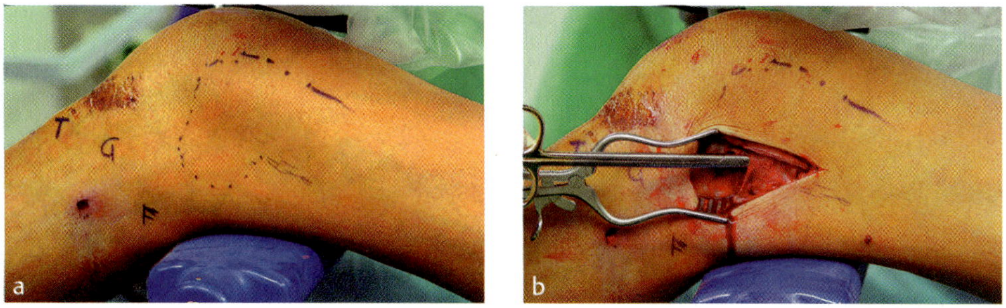

Fig 9.3.1-3a–b Lateral extraarticular approach to the distal femur. A straight incision is made over the lateral femoral condyle. After division of the iliotibial tract, the epiperiosteal space beneath the vastus lateralis is prepared.

3 Reduction and fixation

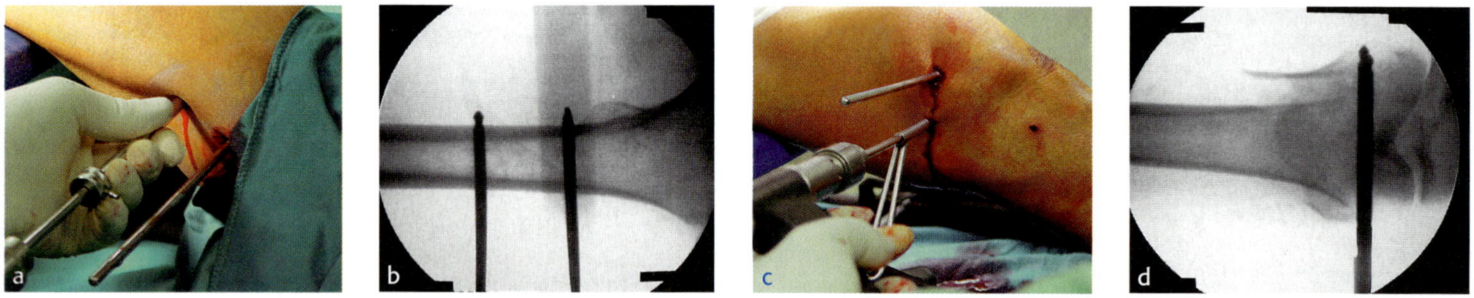

Fig 9.3.1-4a–o

a–b In a first step two 5.0 mm Schanz screws are inserted into the proximal femur from the lateral aspect through two stab incisions.

c–d Two more Schanz screws are inserted into the small distal fragment from the medial aspect.

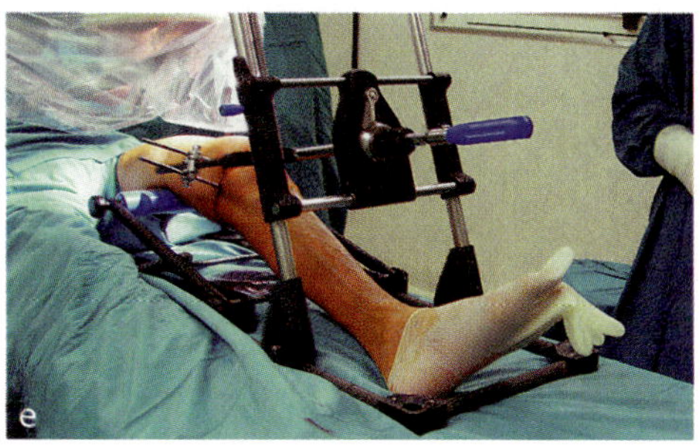

e These Schanz screws are connected to the small reduction table by means of universal clamps.

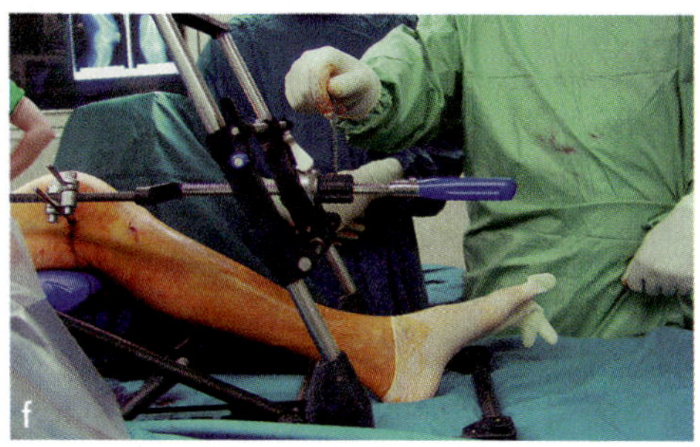

f Closed reduction follows using the small reduction table.

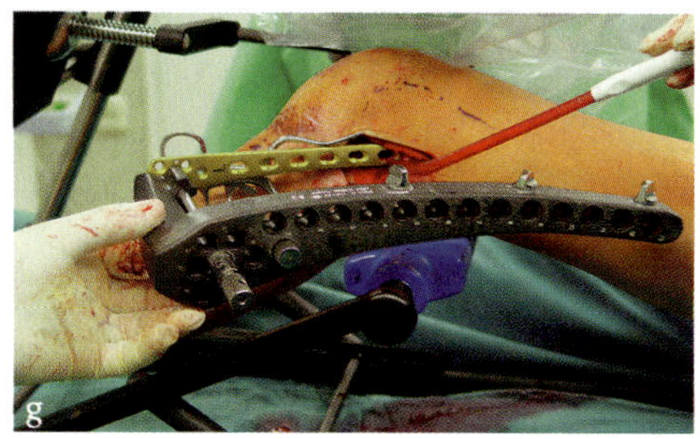

g After mounting the insertion guide on the LCP-DF, the plate is inserted into the epiperiosteal space from distal to proximal.

3 Reduction and fixation (cont)

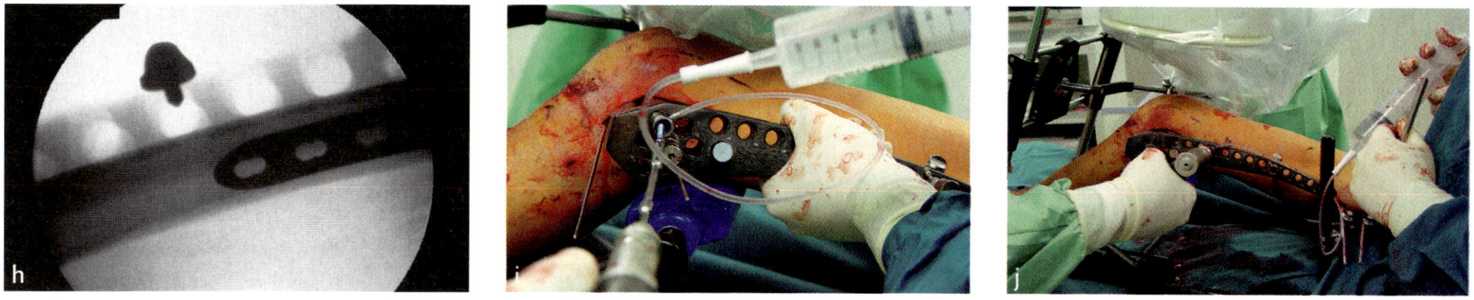

Fig 9.3.1-4a–o (cont)

h Assessment of plate position with the image intensifier.

i–j Temporary fixation of the plate to the bone with K-wires and insertion of self-drilling, self-tapping LHS through the drill guide of the insertion guide.

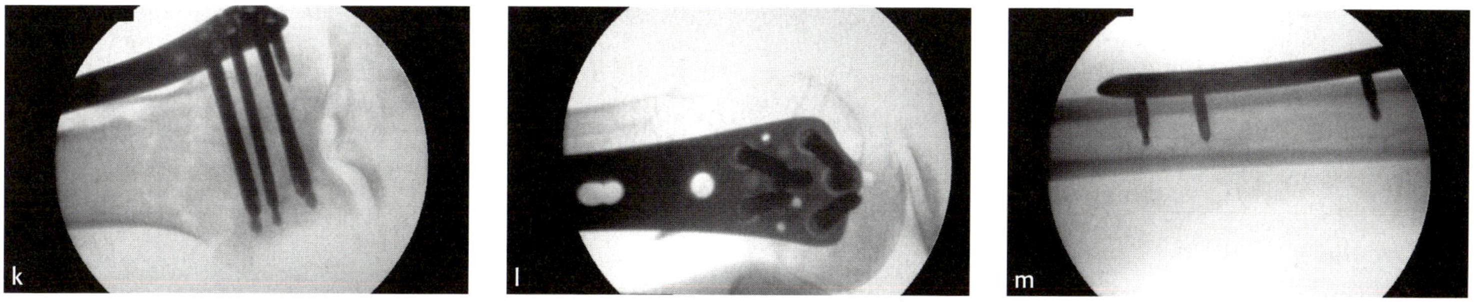

k–m Intraoperative x-ray imaging after insertion of the LHS. The plate is fixed to the shaft with four monocortical self-drilling, self-tapping LHS, and to the distal segment with six LHS.

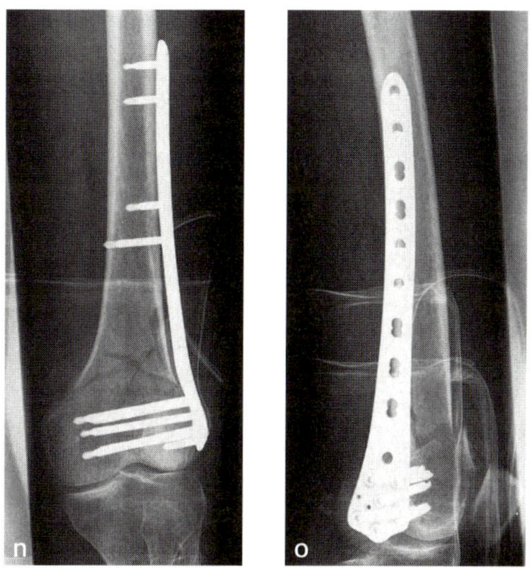

n Postoperative x-ray, AP view.

o Postoperative x-ray, lateral view.

4 Rehabilitation

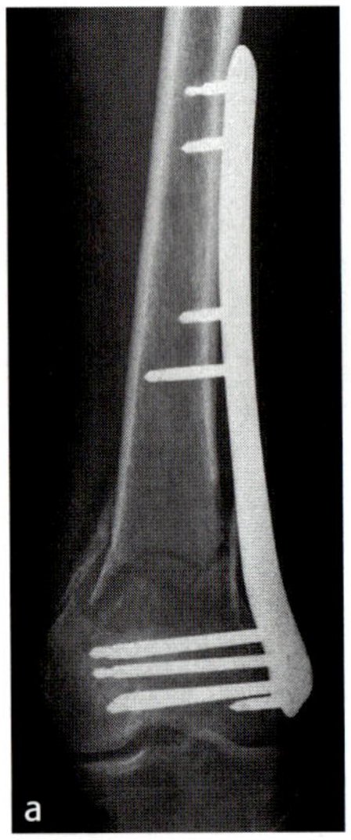

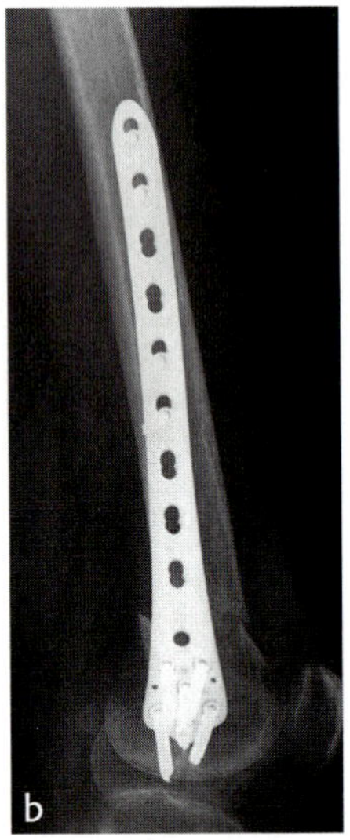

Partial weight bearing for 4 weeks up to 20 kg; full weight bearing after 6 weeks.

Fig 9.3.1-5a–b Postoperative x-ray imaging after 6 weeks.
a AP view.
b Lateral view.

5 Pitfalls –

Reduction

Indirect reduction of this very distal femoral fracture is difficult and requires additional instruments such as the large distractor or small reduction table and possibly use of the joystick technique.

Fixation

Particular attention needs to be paid to exact positioning of the implant on the lateral side of the femur.

6 Pearls +

Reduction

The small reduction table is a useful device for indirect reduction of femoral fractures.

Fixation

Angular stable, anatomically precontoured plates enable the stable fixation of fractures, especially of very small distal fragments and permit implant insertion in a minimally invasive technique.

Authors Gabriele Streicher, Thomas J Hockertz, Andreas Gruner, Heinrich Reilmann

9.3.2 Supracondylar femoral fracture with joint involvement—33-C2

1 Case description

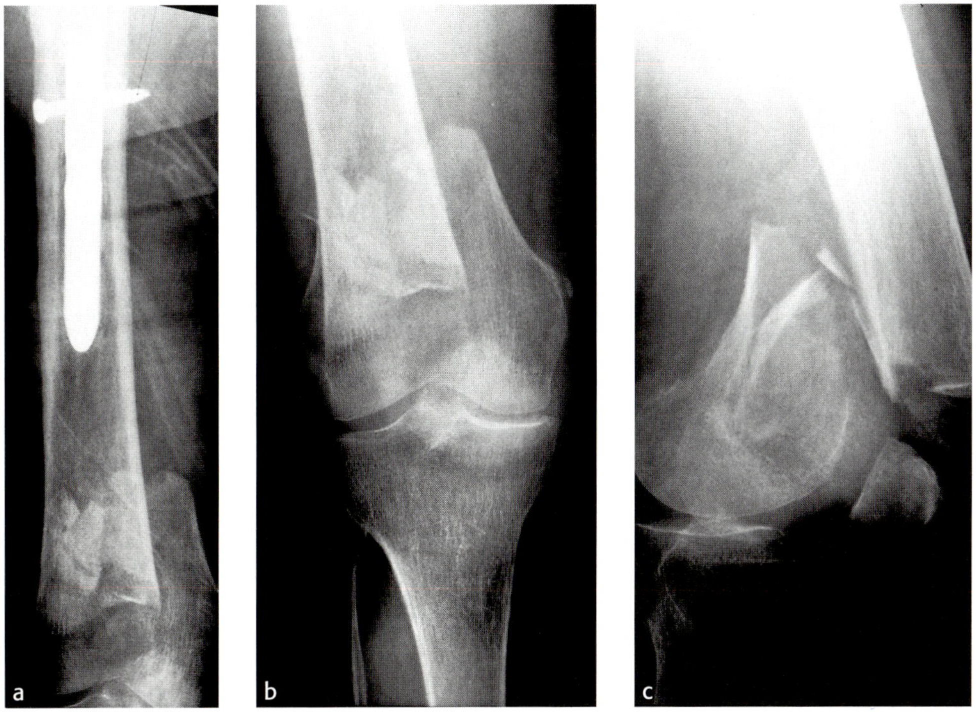

85-year-old woman who fell out of bed at the old people's home and sustained a supracondylar distal femoral fracture with joint involvement. Proximal femoral nail in place, inserted to treat an earlier femoral fracture adjacent to the hip. Type of injury: low-energy, monotrauma, closed fracture.

Fig 9.3.2-1a–c
a AP view.
b Detailed AP view.
c Lateral view.

Indication

Fracture of the right femur with implanted proximal femoral nail. Previous femoral fracture adjacent to the hip joint clinically and radiologically healed. The patient was mobile before the accident without crutches and without any symptoms.

Preoperative planning

Equipment

- LISS-DF, 9 holes
- 5.0 mm self-drilling, self-tapping locking head screws (LHS)
- 6.5 mm cancellous bone screw with washer
- LISS periprosthetic screws
- 2.0 mm K-wires

(Size of system, instruments, and implants can vary according to anatomy.)

Patient preparation and positioning

Antibiotics: single dose 2nd generation cephalosporin
Thrombosis prophylaxis: low-molecular heparin

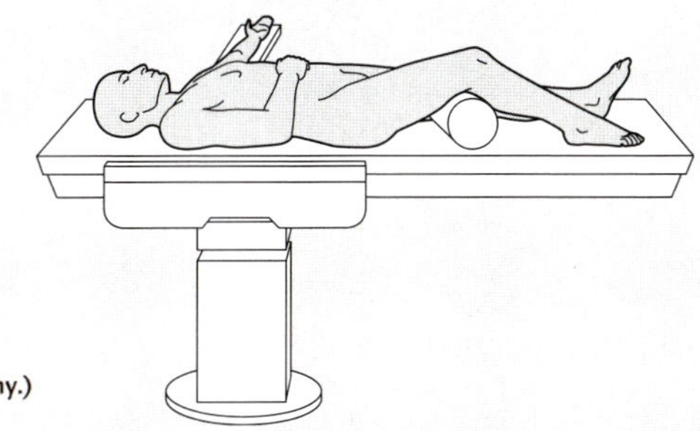

Fig 9.3.2-2 Supine position, the leg is free-draped for intraoperative mobility, elevation of the injured limb and flexion of the knee joint at approximately 30°, lower the contralateral leg for better intraoperative x-ray assessment, cushion the distal femur of the injured leg, eg, with a towel roll, and position the image intensifier on the opposite side.

2 Surgical approach

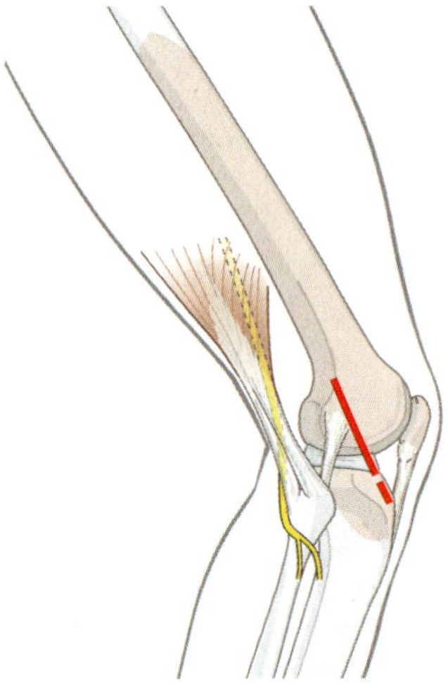

Fig 9.3.2-3 Anterolateral parapatellar skin incision extending in a proximal direction for better control of the reduction of joint fragments and restoration of the femoral condyles.
Divide the iliotibial tract in the direction of its fibers and dissect to the periosteum.

3 Reduction and fixation

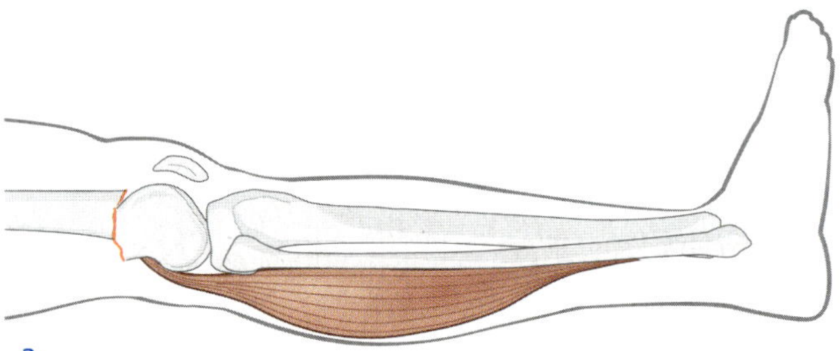

a

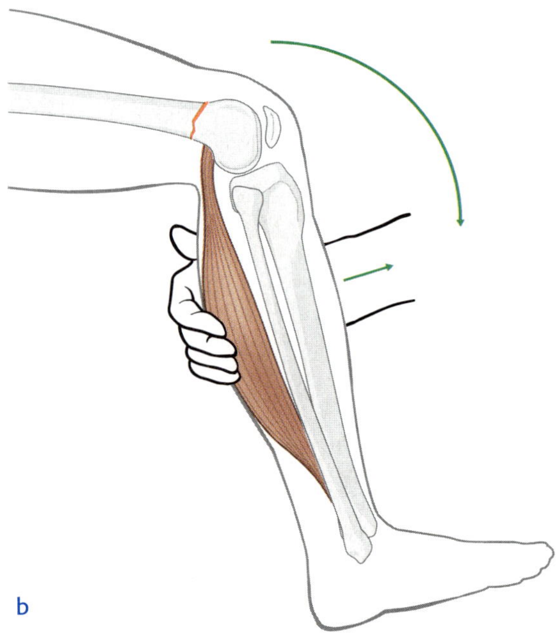

b

Fig 9.3.2-4a–b
a Approximate reduction of the fracture and the longitudinal axis by applying axial tension with the knee flexed to approximately 30° to relax the gastrocnemius muscle.
b Reduction of the condylar and joint components of the distal femur by transverse compression and temporary K-wire fixation. The anterolateral approach permits adequate assessment of the joint surfaces.

3 Reduction and fixation (cont)

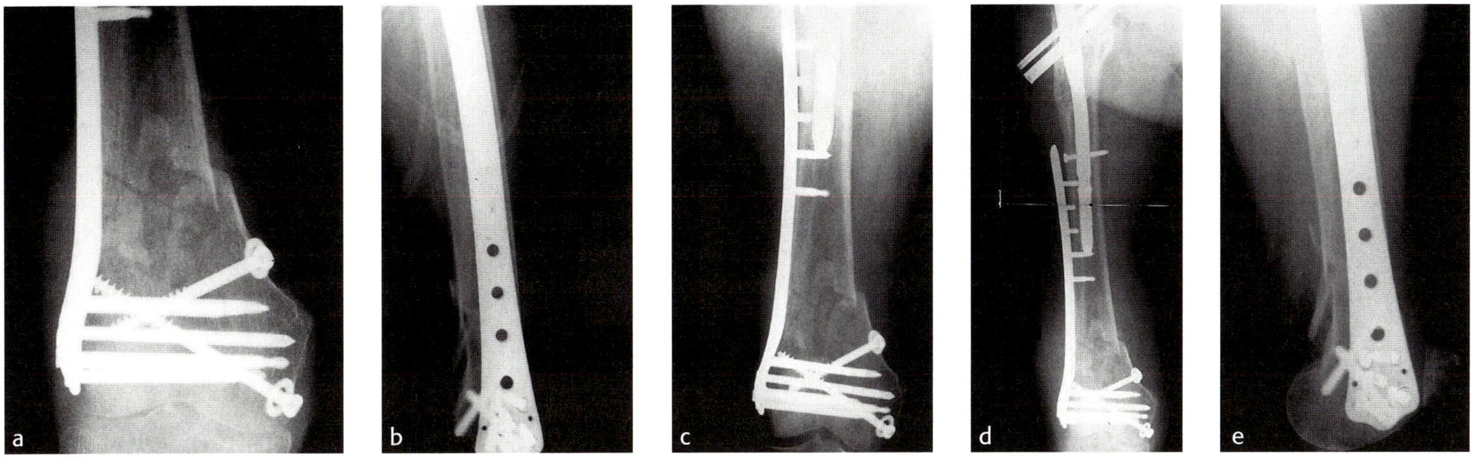

Fig 9.3.2-5a–e Osteosynthesis of the distal femur to stabilize the supracondylar and joint fractures. Make a stab incision medially and, after predrilling, insert a 6.5 mm cancellous bone screw with washer. Remove the temporary K-wires. Prepare the plate bed by epiperiosteal tunneling from distal to proximal under the vastus lateralis with a long bone rasp.
Identify the appropriate length of plate under image intensification and slide the implant into the plate position. Make an incision at the proximal end of the plate to complete the osteosynthesis. Elevate the distal fragment out of its recurvature position from the dorsal side using the elevator.
Stabilize the implant on the proximal and distal sides by inserting K-wires and check plate position in two planes.
Precise reduction of the shaft fragments with the pulling device.
Insert the screws alternately in the distal and proximal holes starting distally, determine screw length according to Tab 3-2.
The special prosthesis drill with limited drill depth and the special LISS periprosthetic screws are used in this case because of the intramedullary load carrier, and to avoid stripping of the screw thread in the cortex.

4 Rehabilitation

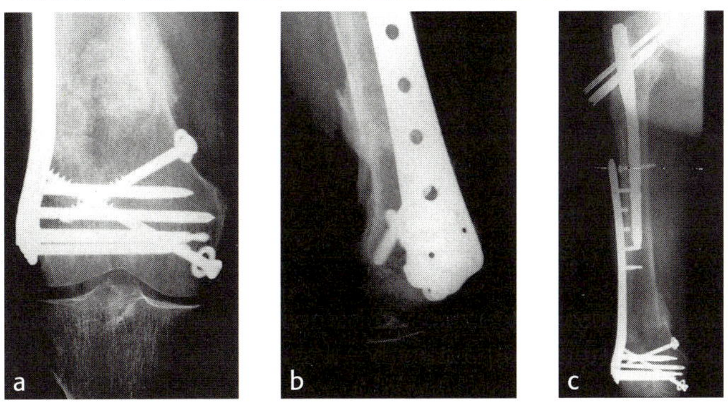

Weight bearing: 15 kg for 4 weeks; half-body weight after 4 weeks, full weight bearing after 8 weeks.
Physiotherapy: from the second postoperative day and continuous passive motion.
Pharmaceutical treatment: pain therapy and nonsteroid antiinflammatory drugs.

Fig 9.3.2-6a–c Postoperative x-rays after 6 months.

4 Rehabilitation (cont)

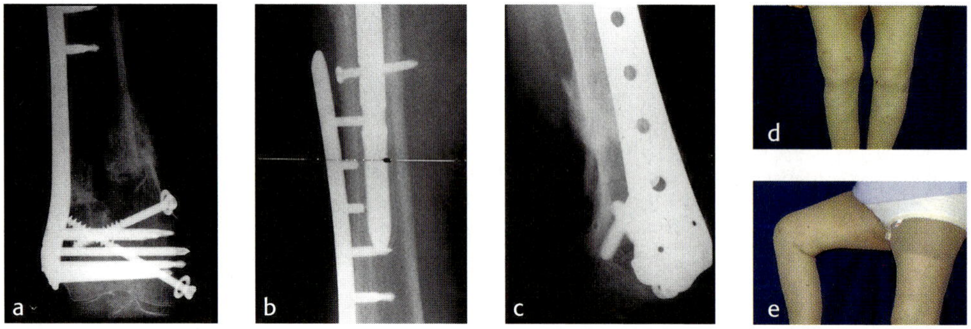

Fig 9.3.2-7a–e
a–c Postoperative x-ray after 6 months.
d–e Clinical pictures after 10 months.

5 Pitfalls –

Equipment
Incorrect plate length: When inserting short monocortical periprosthetic screws it is especially important to ensure that there is adequate anchorage in the cortex.

Approach
Inadequate preparation of the distal femur and, consequently, plate positioning too far anteriorly or posteriorly and risk of trapping the iliotibial tract.

Reduction and fixation
Loss of manual reduction and axial alignment, incorrect screw length especially in the region of the nail with abutment of the LISS screws before head locking was achieved. Consequent thread stripping.

Rehabilitation
Immobilization for too long.

6 Pearls +

Equipment
Monocortical anchorage of the LISS shaft in the region of the implant bed.
Use of periprosthetic LHS.

Approach
Permits implant positioning and simultaneous reduction and control of the joint fracture.

Reduction and fixation
In multifragmentary C-type fractures the LISS-DF is the most useful implant for fracture treatment. The locked internal fixator is especially helpful in osteoporotic bone.

Rehabilitation
Partial weight bearing cannot always be achieved with elderly patients. Full weight bearing was just possible in this case.

Author Christoph Sommer

9.3.3 Intraarticular distal femoral fracture—33-C2

1 Case description

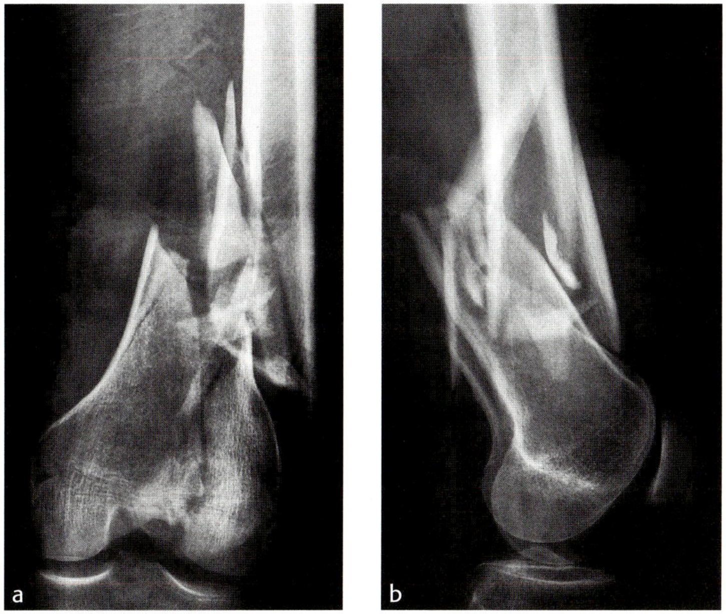

53-year-old man suffered a motorcycle injury. He had an open, intraarticular fracture of the left distal femur (Gustilo type II, 33-C2.3). The condyles were fractured slightly on the lateral side of the midline with a small intermediate fragment. The patient also suffered a displaced distal radial fracture.

Fig 9.3.3-1a–b
a AP view.
b Lateral view.

Indication

This injury is an absolute indication for immediate operative stabilization of the fracture as well as debridement and jet lavage of the soft tissue. The LISS-DF is an ideal implant with which to stabilize the fracture. Alternatively, a DCS, a condylar plate, or a conventional plate system could be used. The intermediate fragment, placed in the intercondylar notch, would tend to be regarded as a contraindication for retrograde nailing.

Preoperative planning

Equipment

- LISS-DF, 13 holes
- 5.0 mm locking head screws (LHS)
- 3.5 mm cortex screws
- Large distractor

(Size of system, instruments, and implants can vary according to anatomy.)

Patient preparation and positioning

Antibiotics: single dose 2nd generation cephalosporin
Thrombosis prophylaxis: low-molecular heparin

1 Surgeon
2 ORP
3 1st assistant
4 2nd assistant

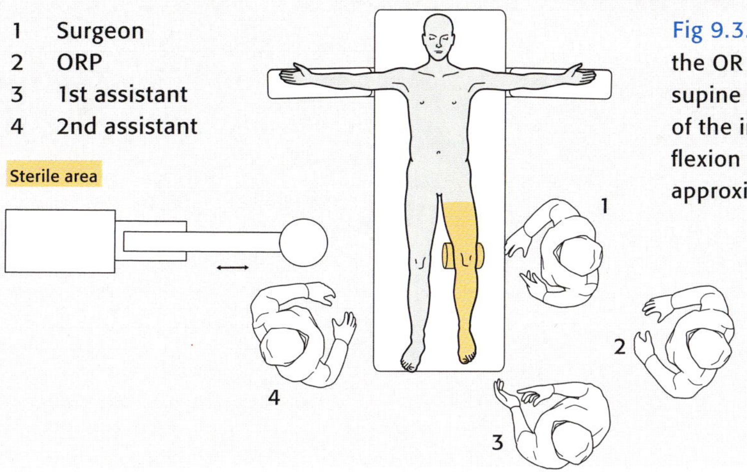

Fig 9.3.3-2 Position of the OR team. Patient in supine position, elevation of the injured leg, and flexion of the knee joint to approximately 30°.

2 Surgical approach

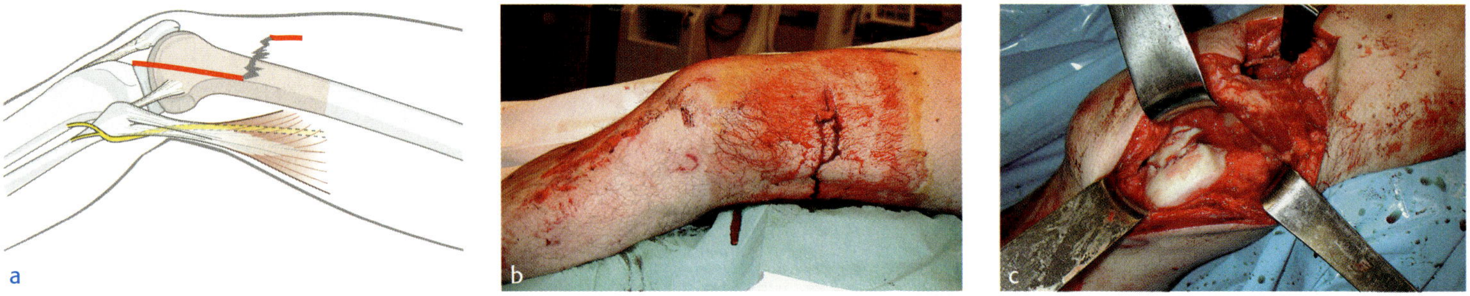

Fig 9.3.3-3a–c

a–b The wound at the anterolateral apsect is intergrated in the parapatellar approach.

c The joint is opened by a parapatellar arthrotomy just lateral to the vastus lateralis. The central part of the quadriceps tendon had been cut by the sharp edge of one of the metaphyseal fracture fragments. A clear view of the fracture zone and the soft tissue is possible after jet lavage.

3 Reduction and fixation

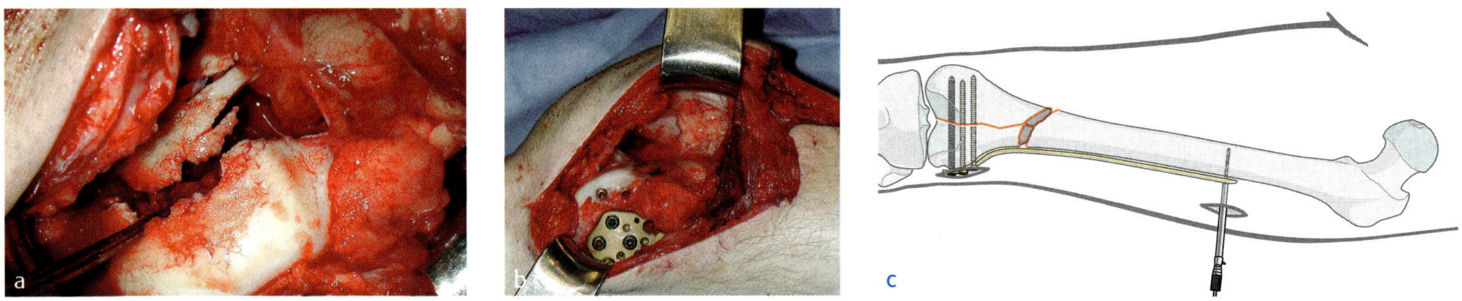

Fig 9.3.3-4a–c

a–b The joint block is reduced and held with the help of pelvic reduction forceps inserted laterally through the incision and medially percutaneously technique. The intermediate fragment is maneuvered into position. Preliminary fixation with K-wires follows and two 3.5 mm cortex screws are inserted ventrally and subchondrally. The LISS-DF, 13-hole plate is then inserted under the vastus lateralis in a proximal direction. The plate is held distally in the correct position with the center of the plate between the anterior and middle third of the lateral condyle.

After temporary fixation with K-wires at its distal end, the position is then controlled with image intensification. The most distal screw must be inserted strictly parallel to the joint surface. To determine the screw direction, a K-wire is inserted through a drill sleeve under image intensification. If the K-wire is parallel to the joint surface, one locking head screw is inserted. The meta- and diaphyseal zones are reduced and held in correct length and rotation by manual traction or with the help of a large distractor or external fixator.

c A small incision is made over the most proximal hole. A drill sleeve is inserted and the plate is brought into proper position over the bone. The plate must be in a central position over the bone before drilling. A hole is drilled bicortically with a 4.3 mm drill bit. The drill bit is then left in the bone to maintain temporary reduction.

3 Reduction and fixation (cont)

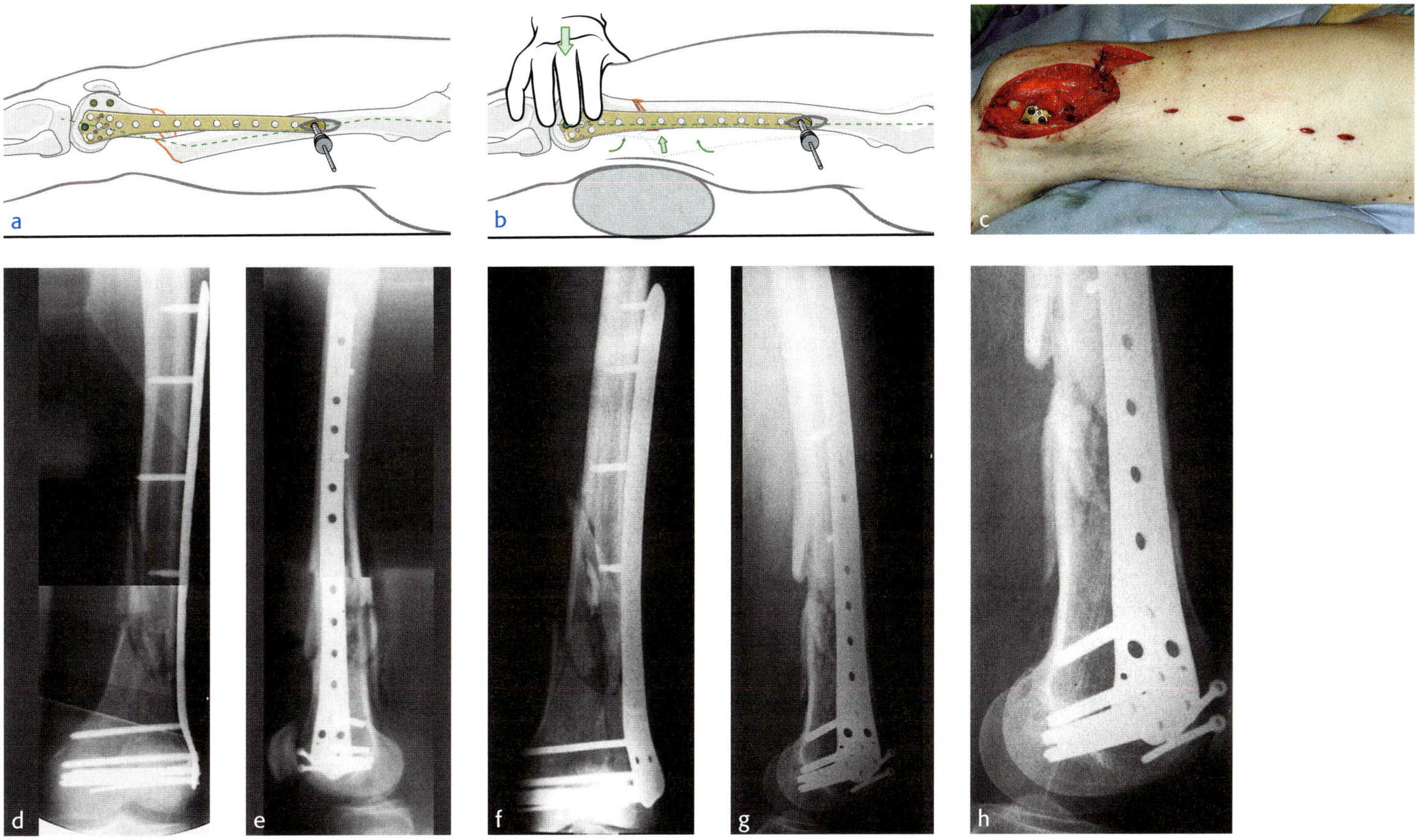

Fig 9.3.3-5a–h

- a In a lateral view, slight retrocurvature is apparent in the extended knee position.
- b This can be corrected by placing a towel roll under the fracture and by applying counterpressure.
- c Once the correct position has been confirmed, at least four to five LHS are inserted into the joint block and there should be anchorage in at least four cortices on the proximal side. This means insertion of at least four monocortical self-tapping, self-drilling LHS (with insertion guide) or bicortical self-tapping LHS (without insertion guide). If the bone is osteoporotic, at least six to eight cortices should be used. The central cut in the quadriceps tendon is then sewn together.
- d–e The intraoperative x-rays show correct axial alignment in both planes. Six cortices are used proximally (two monocortical and two bicortical LHS).
- f–h The joint is reduced without any step-off; interfragmentary compression is maintained by lag screws. The intermediate metadiaphyseal fracture zone is not touched; this zone is bridged with a locked internal fixator in splinting method.

4 Rehabilitation

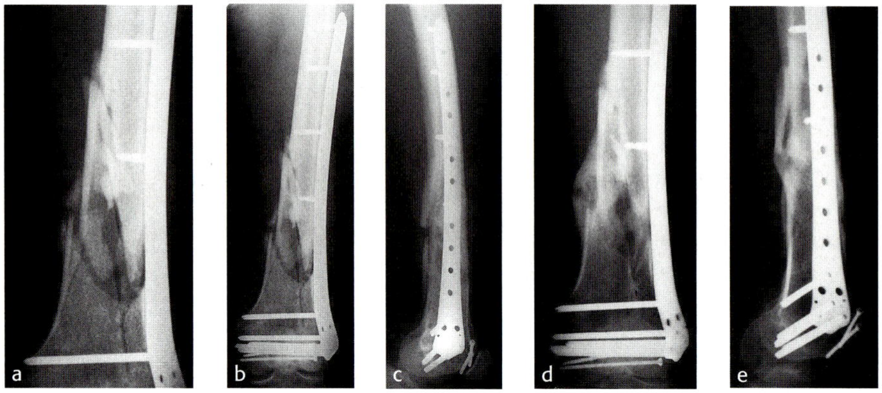

Fig 9.3.3-6a–e

a–c The patient is instructed to practise early functional training with partial weight bearing (10 kg) for 6 weeks, then half body weight bearing until 3 months after the operation. The control x-rays show early callus formation in the meta- and diaphyseal zones. The intraarticular fracture is radiologically consolidated. The patient can start full weight bearing at this point. The further course of healing was uneventful.

d–e After 1 year the fracture showed a complete callus bridge and the start of remodeling.

Implant removal

The plate was removed after 14 months because of a slight irritation of the iliotibial tract over the distal end of the LISS plate.

5 Pitfalls –

Equipment

Approach

The minimally invasive approach to bridging the metadiaphyseal fracture zones is associated with a high risk of postoperative malalignment (if not done properly).

Reduction and fixation

To avoid postoperative axial or rotational malalignment, intraoperative x-ray control must be performed. The fractured leg has to be compared with the healthy leg (pre- or intraoperatively).

Rehabilitation

Irritation of the iliotibial band over the distal end of the LISS plate.

6 Pearls +

Equipment

The LISS-DF or LCP-DF is the ideal implant for minimally invasive surgery of C-type fractures of the distal femur. The plate need not be bent.

Approach

The minimally invasive procedure conserves the blood supply of the supracondylar and diaphyseal zones by preserving more of the perforator vessels (compared to an open approach).

Reduction and fixation

The reduction can be performed over the anatomically precontured plate (with or without insertion guide) using an appropriate technique. LHS provide high stability mainly in osteoporotic bone in cases without medial bone contact.

Rehabilitation

Early functional treatment can be performed even in osteoporotic bones. Full weight bearing is possible before complete consolidation of the fracture.

Author Christoph Sommer

9.3.4 Intraarticular distal femoral fracture with multifragmentary fracture of the patella—33-C2

1 Case description

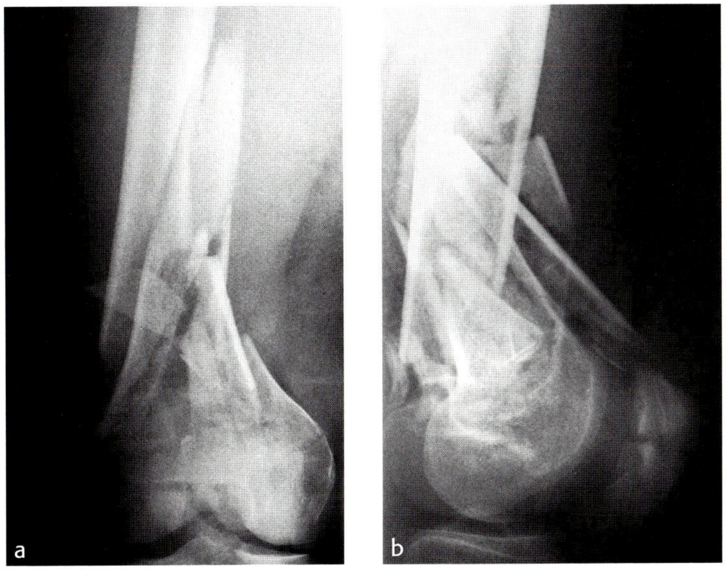

40-year-old man fell asleep while driving a car and collided with a tree. He suffered several fractures of his lower limbs. On his left side, he had a Gustilo type I open patellar fracture and a fracture of the tibial head. These injuries are not described here.

He also suffered a Gustilo type II open intraarticular femoral fracture (33-C2.3) with multifragmentary fracture of the patella on the right leg. No neurovascular damage.

Fig 9.3.4-1a–b
a AP view.
b Lateral view.

Indication

In this open fracture situation, the indication for emergency stabilization and debridement with lavage is clear. Because the fracture is very distal, an osteosynthesis system with locking head screws, for example, a LISS-DF or LCP, would be ideal. In a highly contaminated situation, a temporary joint-bridging external fixator with definitive reconstruction in a second or third stage would have been preferred.

Preoperative planning

Equipment

- LCP 4.5/5.0, broad, 15 holes
- Locking head screws (LHS)
- 6.5 mm cancellous bone screw
- Large distractor

(Size of system, instruments, and implants can vary according to anatomy.)

Patient preparation and positioning

Antibiotics: single dose 2nd generation cephalosporin
Thrombosis prophylaxis: low- molecular heparin

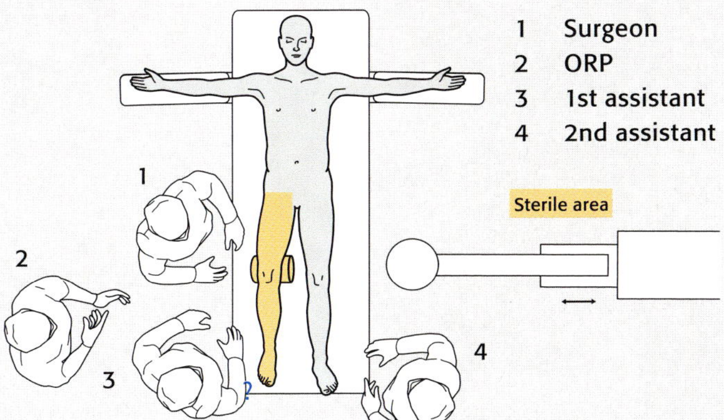

Fig 9.3.4-2 Supine position, the leg is free draped for intraoperative mobility, elevation of the injured limb and flexion of the knee joint at approximately 30°.

2 Surgical approach

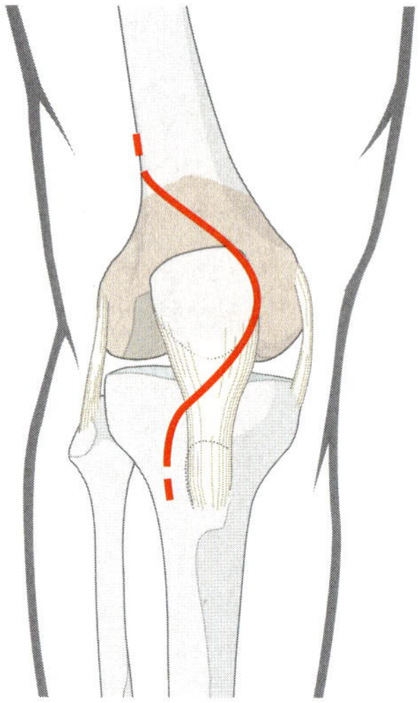

Fig 9.3.4-3 A parapatellar, lateral, vertical approach is planned. But, because the soft tissue is traumatized medially, the wound is excised and the medial incision is enlarged cranially and caudally in a lateral direction. This specific approach is performed through the patellar fracture and involves incision of the lateral retinaculum horizontally. The superior parts of the patella are held cranially and the inferior parts caudally. The articular part of the femoral fracture can now be addressed under maximal flexion of the knee joint. At the level of the proximal end of the plate, a small lateral approach along the anterior border of the lateral intramuscular septum is performed for precise lateral placement of the plate. This second approach is far distant from the metadiaphyseal fracture zone which is not opened.

3 Reduction and fixation

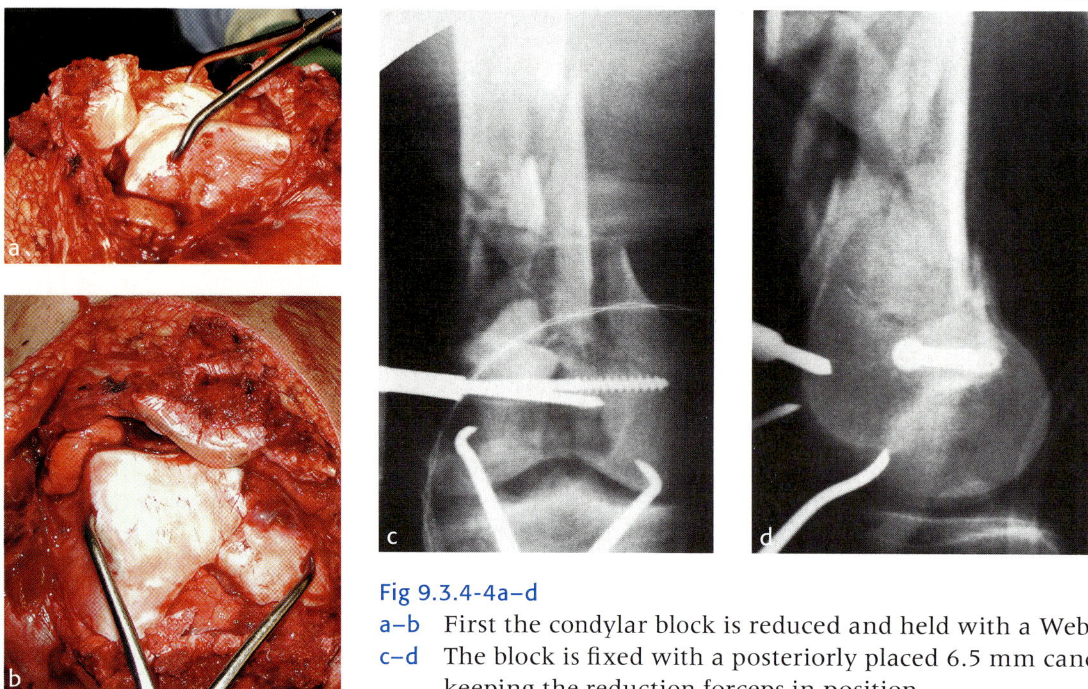

Fig 9.3.4-4a–d
a–b First the condylar block is reduced and held with a Weber forceps.
c–d The block is fixed with a posteriorly placed 6.5 mm cancellous bone screw (lag screw), keeping the reduction forceps in position.

3 Reduction and fixation (cont)

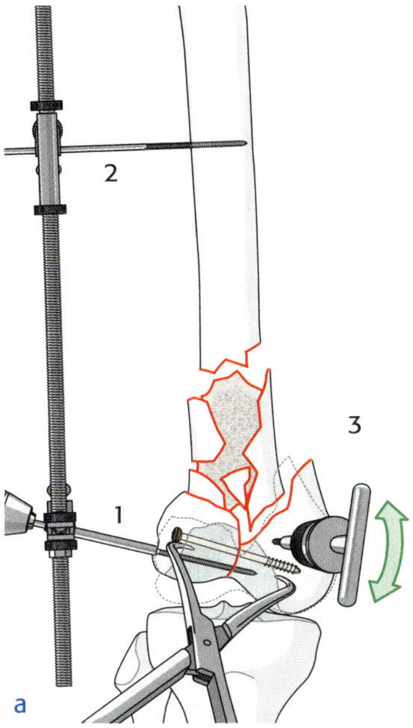

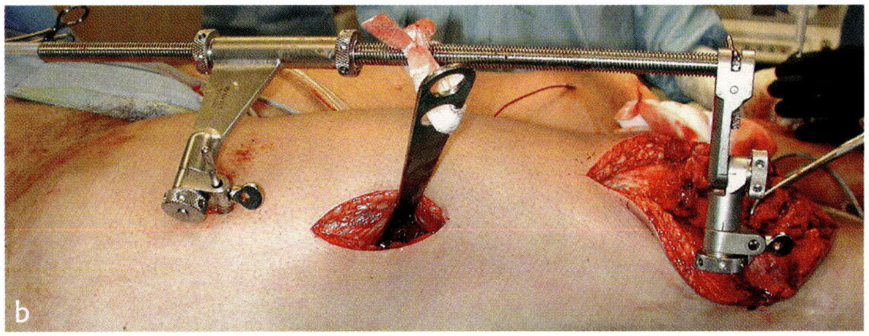

Fig 9.3.4-5a–b The alignment of the condylar block to the diaphysis is performed with the aid of the large distractor. The first Schanz screw is inserted into the condylar block in a lateral to medial direction (1), the second one into the proximal femoral shaft (2). With the help of a T-handle connected to the distal Schanz screw over the loosely attached distractor clamp, the fracture is reduced into correct varus-valgus position. With a third Schanz screw inserted into the condylar block from anterior to posterior, the fracture can be reduced in correct anterior-posterior position (3). After correct alignment, the distractor clamps are tightened onto the Schanz screws. Finally, the length is adjusted using the distractor. Comparison with the healthy leg and/or observation of the fracture fragments under image intensification help identify the correct length. It is important to examine both ante- and retrocurvature of the leg by image intensification in the lateral view.

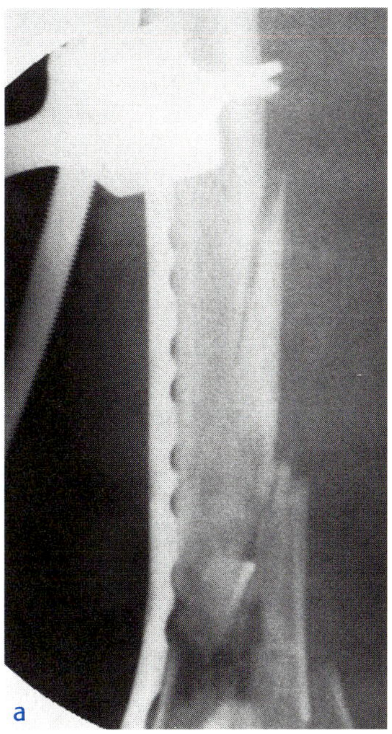

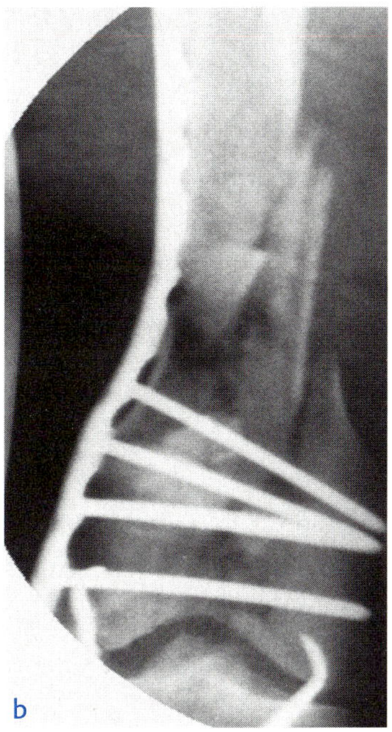

Fig 9.3.4-6a–b Once correct alignement has been achieved, a bent, broad LCP 4.5/5.0 is inserted under the vastus lateralis. The plate is fixed with at least three to four LHS in the condylar block. The proximal position of the plate is examined via the proximal incision (a LISS-DF, LCP-DF, locking condylar plate, or curved, broad LCP 4.5/5.0 might be a better alternative).

3 Reduction and fixation (cont)

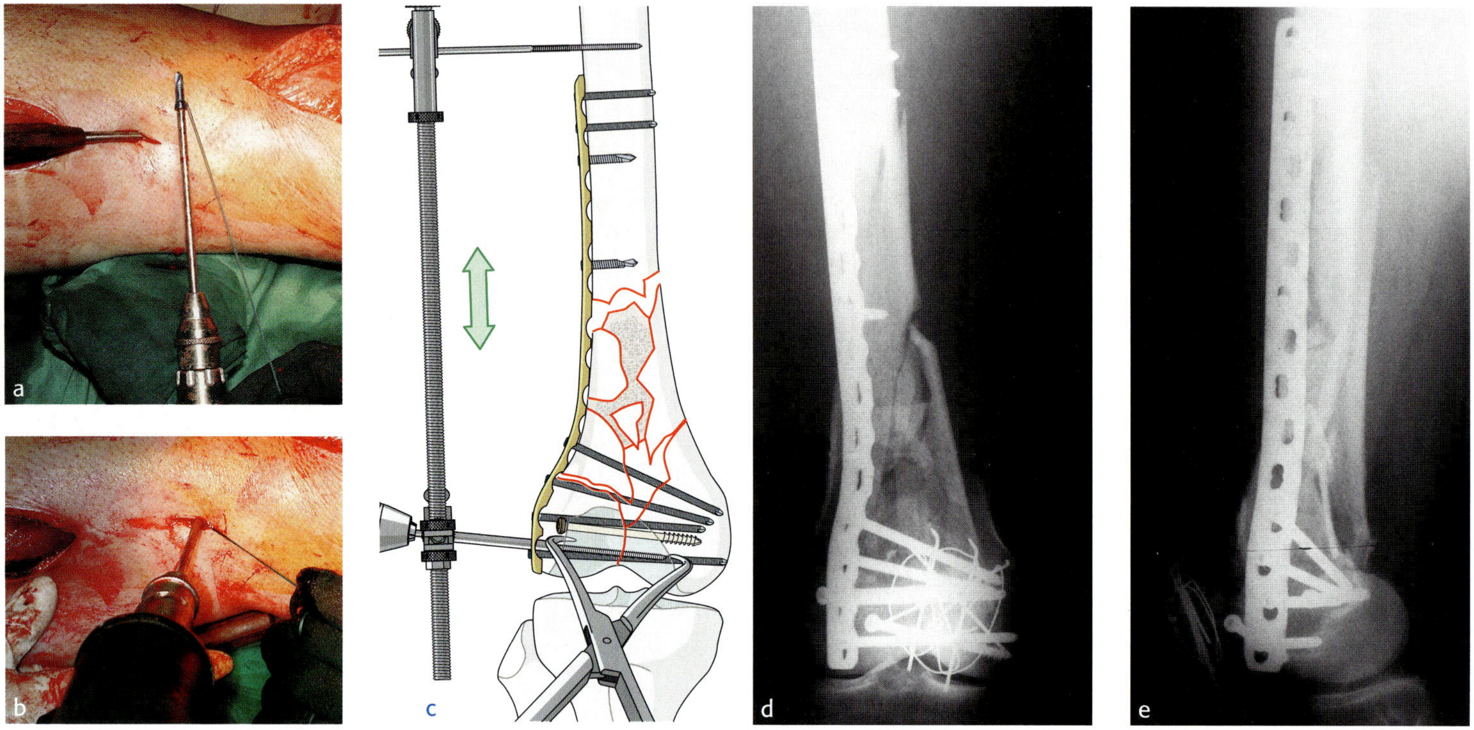

Fig 9.3.4-7a–e

a–c With the plate centrally positioned, one to two bicortical LHS are inserted. Further LHS, possibly monocortical screws, are inserted via small incisions, as required. Threads are fixed to the heads of the screws and held under tension to avoid losing the screws in the soft tissue.

d–e Now the multifragmented patella is reconstructed by tension band wiring. The postoperative x-rays show correct bridging of the fracture zone and correct axial alignment of the leg as well as anatomical joint surface reconstruction.

4 Rehabilitation

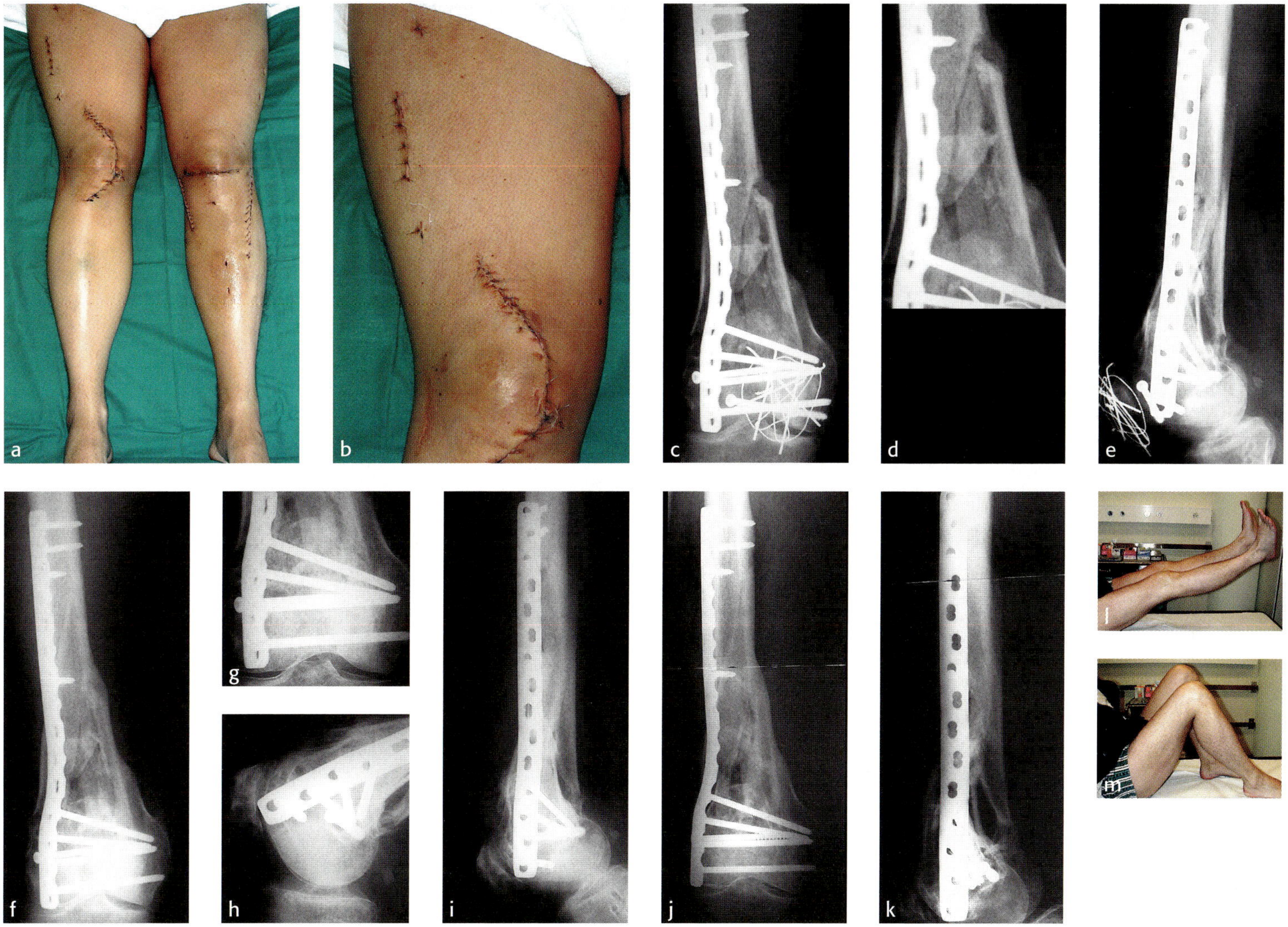

Fig 9.3.4-8a–m

a–b Early functional treatment of the fracture is done with the help of a continuous passive motion machine. The soft tissue shows no irritation 6 days after the operation. For the first month, the patient was mobilized in a wheelchair, then with four-point mobilization and half body weight bearing on both sides.

c–e After 3 months, the consolidation of the fracture was advanced and full weight-bearing was allowed.

f–i After 6 months the callus was circular.

j–m After 1 year and implant removal at the patella, the femoral fracture was fully consolidated and partial remodeling of the distal fracture on the right side could be seen. Clinically, the function of the knee joint was quite good with good extension and considerable flexion.

4 Rehabilitation (cont)

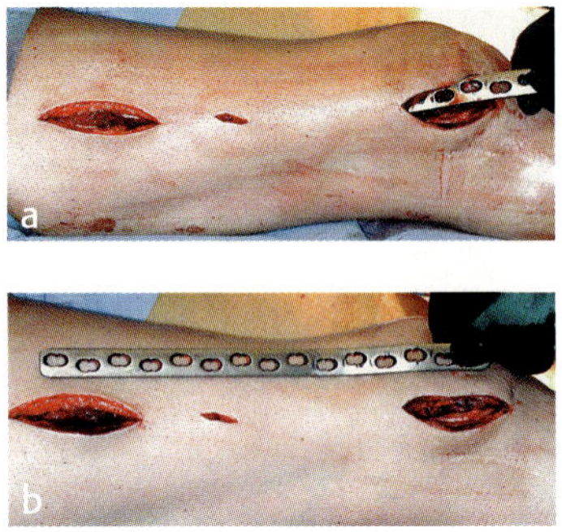

Implant removal

Fig 9.3.4-9a–b Due to irritation of the iliotibial tract, the plate was removed 13 months after the operation.

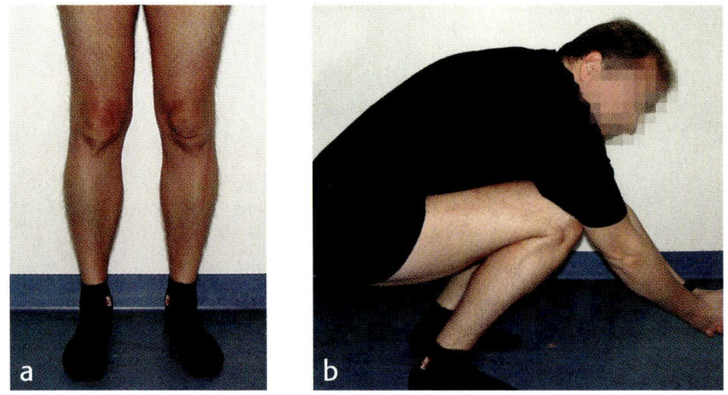

Fig 9.3.4-10a–b 3 years after the operation there is practically full flexion with correct axial alignment of both legs. The patient intentionally lost 20 kg by pursuing regular sporting activities (walking, biking).

5 Pitfalls –

Equipment
The LCP 4.5 can only be used if the condylar block is big enough to hold three to four screws. If the fracture is more distally, a LISS-DF, LCP-DF, locking condylar plate would be a better alternative.

Approach
The plate could end up in an eccentric position on the femoral shaft if the proximal approach is insufficient.

Reduction and fixation
If the condylar block is very short, distal fixation of the plate would be insufficient. Also, the proximal screws might pull out if the plate was eccentrically positioned or if monocortical screws were used in osteoporotic bone.

Rehabilitation
Too early full weight bearing could bend the plate (mainly in bilateral fractures).

6 Pearls +

Equipment
The LCP system allows the combination of locking head screws and cortex screws (compression or lag screws), as required.

Approach
A minimally invasive approach conserves the blood supply to the metaphyseal and diaphyseal fracture zones.

Reduction and fixation
The large distractor is a good aid for the reduction of complex fractures of the distal femur, mainly in very muscular patients.

Rehabilitation
Early functional treatment is essential for the healing of complex knee joint fractures.

Author Emanuel Gautier

9.3.5 Complete articular multifragmentary distal femoral fracture—33-C3

1 Case description

62-year-old man was involved in a high-energy frontal car collision. He sustained multiple injuries including splenic rupture, rupture of the liver in segment III, bilateral intraarticular distal femoral fractures, lower leg fracture, talus fracture and cuneiform fracture on his left side, open olecranon fracture and open ulna fracture, and a malleolar fracture on his right side. The pubic bone was fractured on both sides. The patient had an additional traumatic peroneal nerve lesion on his right side.

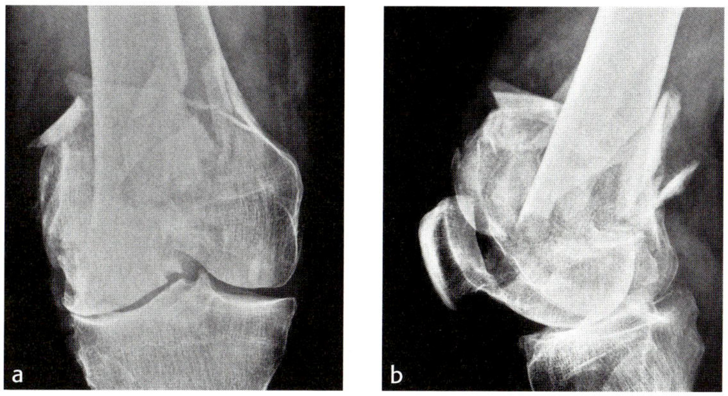

Fig 9.3.5-1a–b
a AP view showing a distal intraarticular femoral fracture. The articular fragments seem to be only slightly displaced. There is evidence of preexisting femorotibial osteoarthritis mainly in the lateral compartment.
b Lateral view showing the metaphyseal comminution, the short condylar fragment medially and laterally, and the oblique fracture line of the lateral condyle in the frontal plane (33-B3 Hoffa type configuration).

Indication

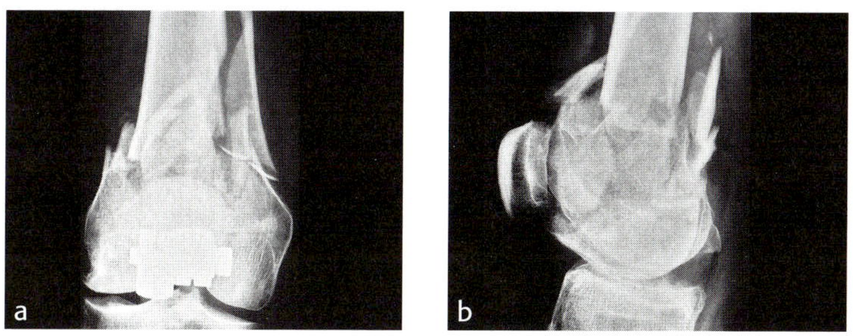

Initially the distal femoral fracture was stabilized in this emergency situation with a knee-bridging external fixator. The definitive treatment of the fracture was performed 3 1/2 weeks after injury after the cardio-pulmonary situation had become stable.

Fig 9.3.5-2a–b
a AP view.
b Lateral view.

Preoperative planning

Equipment
- LISS-DF, 13 holes
- 5.0 mm locking head screws (LHS)
- 2.7 mm cortex screws
- Large distractor
- 1.6, 2.0, 2.5 mm K-wires
- Pelvic reduction forceps

(Size of system, instruments, and implants can vary according to anatomy.)

Patient preparation and positioning
Antibiotics: single dose 2nd generation cephalosporin

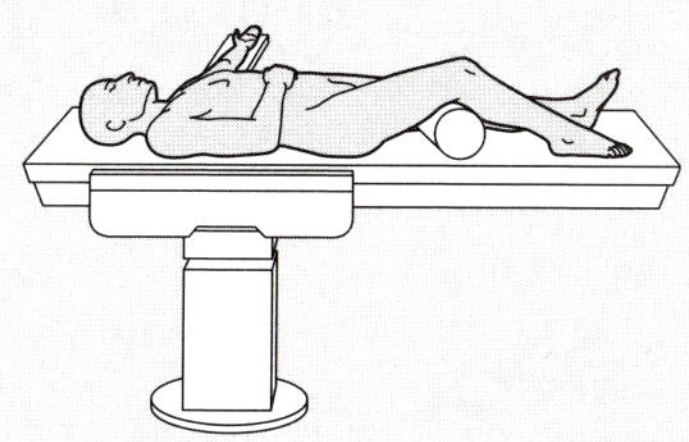

Fig 9.3.5-3 Supine position without pneumatic tourniquet.

2 Surgical approach

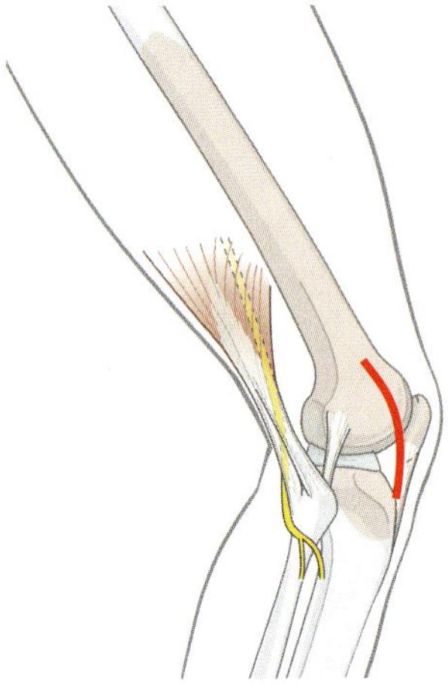

Fig 9.3.5-4 Arthrotomy was performed via a lateral approach.

3 Reduction and fixation

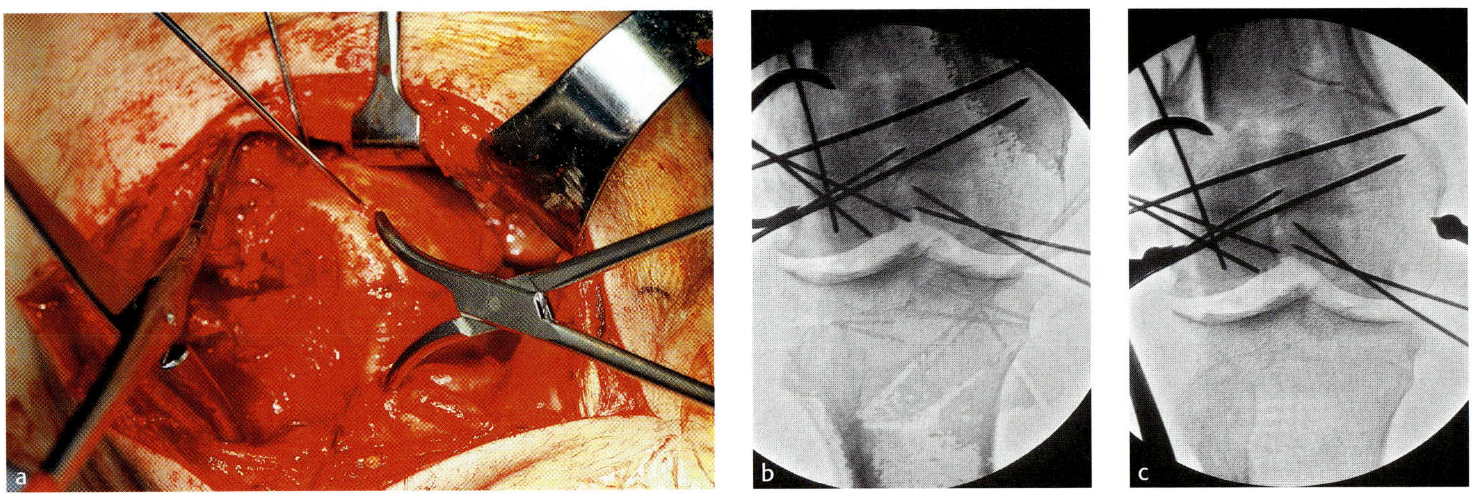

Fig 9.3.5-5a–g

a The joint fragments are reduced directly with the pointed reduction forceps. On the lateral border of the femoral condyle some osteophytes are visible.

b The fragments are initially fixed with K-wires: from laterally and percutaneously from medially. The image intensifier shows correct reduction of the lateral femoral condyle, but a gap between the medial and the lateral condyles at the intercondylar groove is still present. This gap is closed later on using pelvic reduction forceps.

c The reduction is completed with the help of the pelvic reduction forceps. The forceps are inserted percutaneously at the medial aspect. Definitive fixation of the femoral condyles is performed using 2.7 mm lag screws.

3 Reduction and fixation (cont)

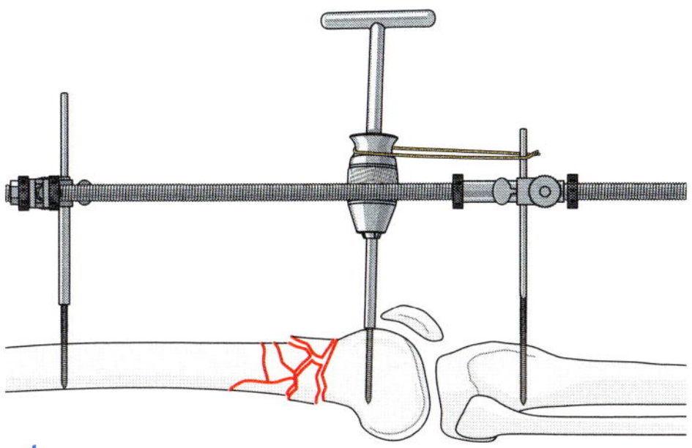

d

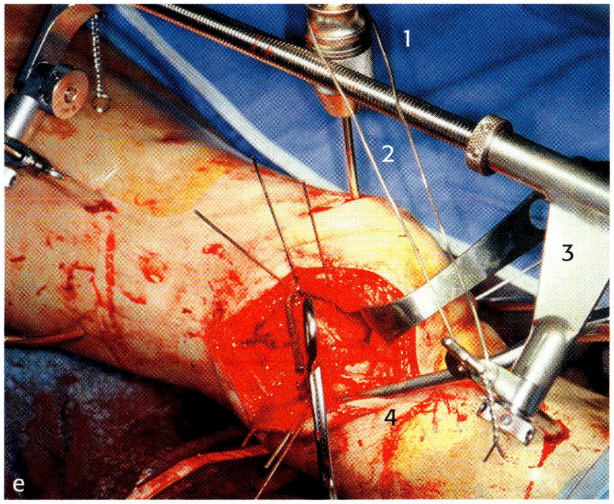

e

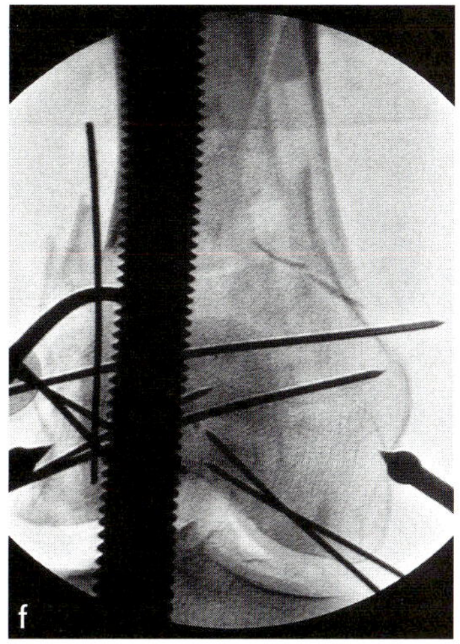

f

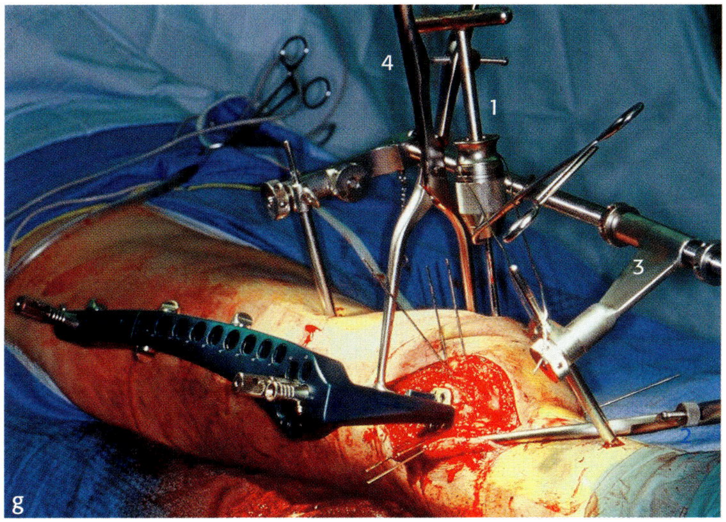

g

Fig 9.3.5-5a–g (cont)

d Due to the pull of the gastrocnemius, the distal fragment has a tendency to be displaced into extension at the metaphyseal fracture area.
To avoid this, the knee is brought into full extension, and the distal femoral fragment is stabilized in this position to the tibia using either an external fixator or temporary cerclage wire around a Schanz screw inserted in the distal femur and the proximal tibia.

e Showing the intraoperative situation with all reduction tools in position: The Schanz screw with the T-handle (**1**) and the cerclage wire around it (**2**) a second Schanz screw inserted into the proximal tibia is utilized to hold the distal femoral fragment in full extension with respect to the knee joint. The large femoral distractor (**3**) aligns the femoral shaft to the tibial shaft and the pelvic reduction forceps (**4**).

f The reduction is now assessed by image intensifier.

g The LISS plate can be inserted once the insertion guide has been mounted. One screw is inserted distally into the articular block and the implant is adjusted with respect to flexion and extension. Two screws are then inserted proximally. Further monocortical screws are used on the proximal fragment and locking head screws are inserted into the articular block.

4 Rehabilitation

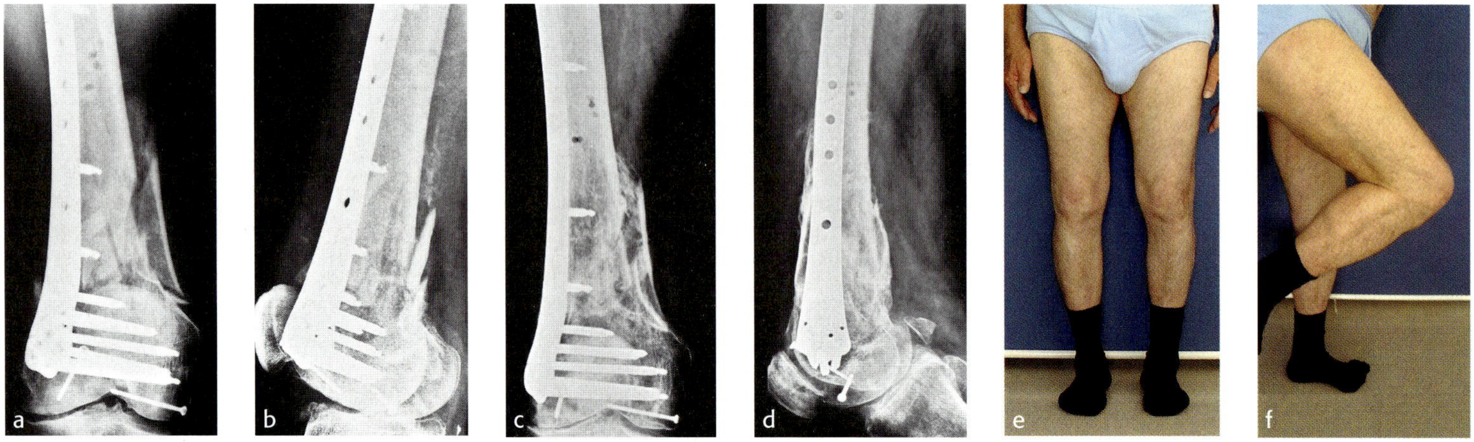

The fracture was not additionally immobilized. Weight bearing was not possible for this polytraumatized patient. For the first 4 months, the patient was only transferred from the bed to the wheelchair. Today, the patient works fulltime as a craftsman.

Fig 9.3.5-6a–f

a–b AP and lateral view showing correct anatomical reduction of the articulation as well as correct alignment of the femoral shaft and the articular block in both planes.

c–d At 5 months postoperatively, the multifragmentary metaphyseal area has healed. The x-rays show integration of the fragments into the bridging callus on the medial and the posterior aspect of the femur.

e–f Clinical result at 6 years. The axis of the leg is correct. The mobility of the right knee joint for flexion-extension is 100°–5°–0° (120°–0°–0° on the left). The limited mobility of the right knee is at least partially due to the preexisting osteoarthritis.

5 Pitfalls –

Reduction and fixation

Improper alignment of the femoral shaft and the articular block. The most frequent deformity is a flexion deformity at the fracture site leading to an extension deficit at the knee joint.

Difficulty of proper plate positioning in the proximal part.

6 Pearls +

Reduction and fixation

Direct reduction technique for the fractures of the femoral condyles.

Indirect (no-touch) reduction technique to properly align the femoral shaft with respect to the distal femoral fragment.

Rapid integration of multifragmentary metaphyseal fragments into the bridging callus.

Authors Michael Schütz, Norbert P Haas

9.3.6 Open complete articular multifragmentary distal femoral fracture—33-C3

1 Case description

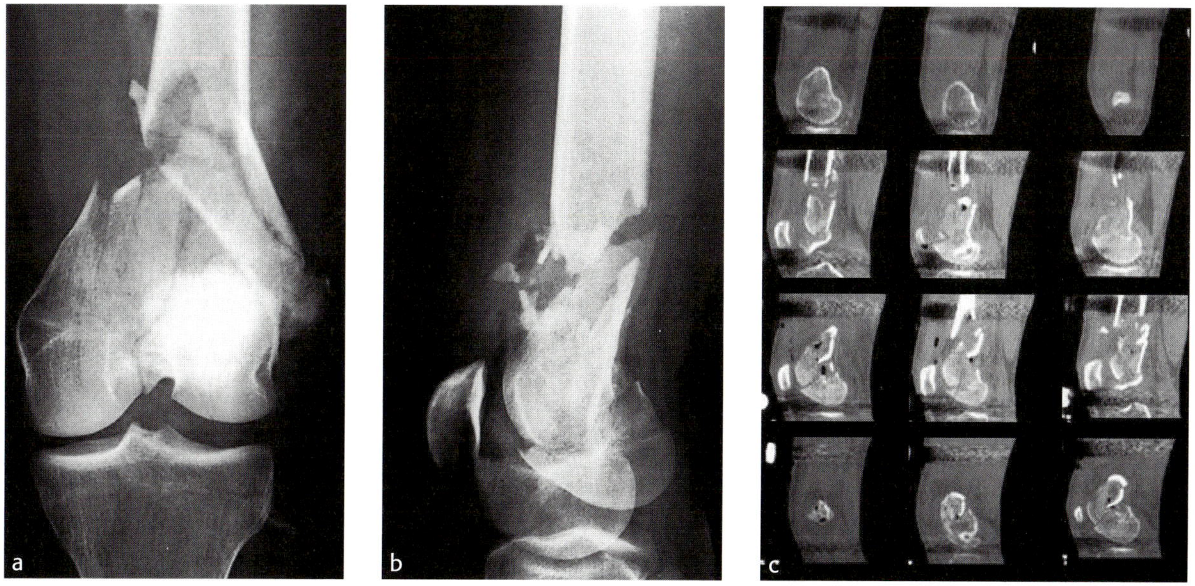

Fig 9.3.6-1a–c
a AP view.
b Lateral view.
c CT scans.

23-year-old woman sustained a bilateral femoral fracture, a foot injury, and a blunt thorax trauma in a motorbike accident. The femoral fracture on the right side was a closed distal femoral fracture with soft-tissue injury. The fracture on the left side was a Gustilo type IIIA fracture with metaphyseal bone loss (33-C3). To treat this injury pattern, debridement of the open fracture and closure with synthetic wound covering and stabilization of the fractures with an external fixator was performed immediately the same night. After further diagnosis of the distal femur with CT scan, the patient was operated on again on the following day. After intramedullary nailing of the femoral fracture on the right (not illustrated), the left femur was operated.

Indication

Indubitably, there is a clear need for osteosynthesis of a third degree open distal femoral fracture. The timing of the osteosynthesis depends on the pattern of injuries that the patient has sustained. Wound debridement and application of an external fixator should be carried out. In this case, the correct positioning of the external fixator is essential for secondary reduction and implant placement. In this specific case, the external fixator was applied to the anterior aspect. The definitive treatment of the fracture depends on several factors relating to the injury pattern and also the available infrastructure. To achieve the best result, the correct reduction of the articular surfaces is essential.

Preoperative planning

A conventional x-ray of the whole femur and a CT scan are necessary to plan the operation. Taking into account the soft-tissue injuries and the radiological analyses, a sketch is made to determine implant length, position of the screws, and approach. The implant length of the external fixator must allow the placement of at least four screws in the proximal fragment. For biomechanical reasons, some holes must be left unoccupied to allow for micromotion of the plate. In this case, a LISS-DF, 9 holes was chosen.

Equipment
- LISS-DF, 9 holes
- 5.0 mm self-drilling, self-tapping locking head screws (LHS)
- 3.5 mm cortex screws
- 2.0 mm K-wires

(Size of system, instruments, and implants can vary according to anatomy.)

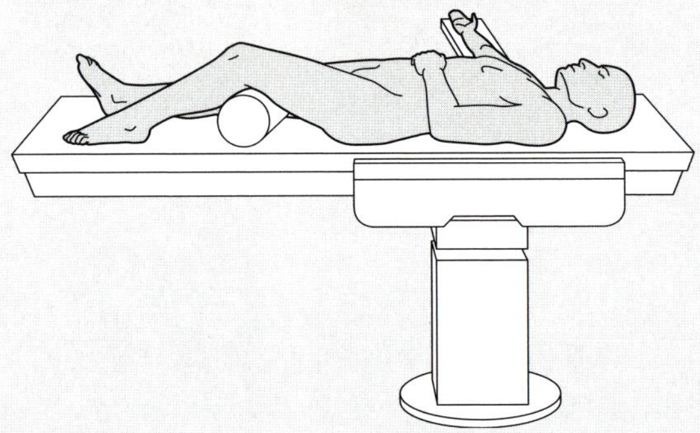

Fig 9.3.6-2 Supine position, knee joint flexed to approximately 30°.

Patient preparation and positioning
Antibiotics: cephalosporin
Thrombosis prophylaxis: low-molecular heparin

The patient is positioned on the x-ray table. X-ray of the entire femur must be possible. The uninjured leg should be extended and lowered (about 30° hip extension) to allow lateral x-ray projection. The injured leg is flexed to 30° at the knee joint, but must also allow flexion up to 60° to relieve the gastrocnemius muscles. This can also be achieved by using sterile drapes. The sterile covering must allow full motion of the leg. It may be helpful to uncover both legs when treating very complex fractures in order to achieve correct adjustment and comparison of length and rotation.

2 Surgical approach

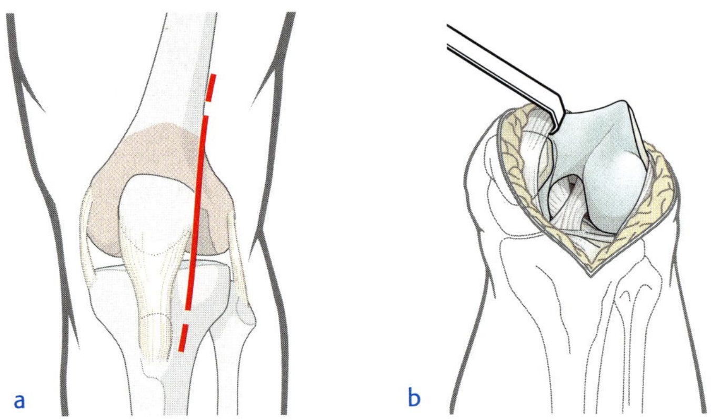

Fig 9.3.6-3a–b In the case presented here, a lateral parapatellar approach with inclusion of the soft-tissue injury was chosen.

3 Reduction and fixation

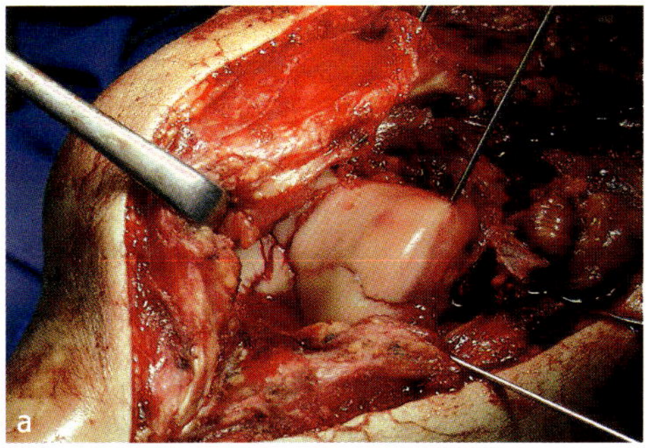

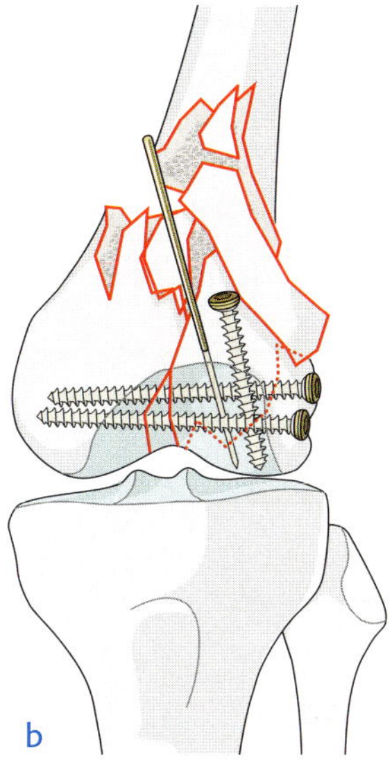

b

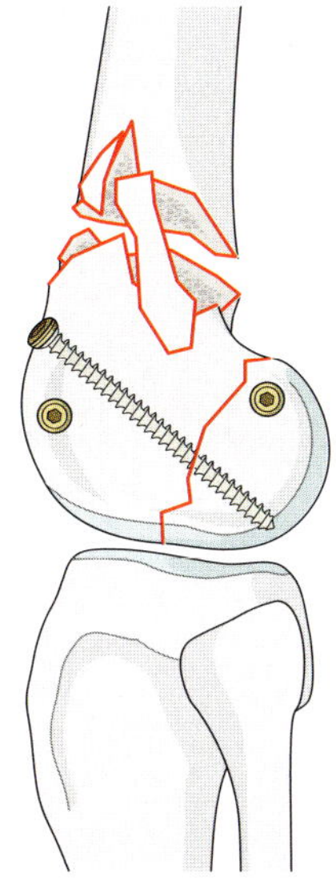

c

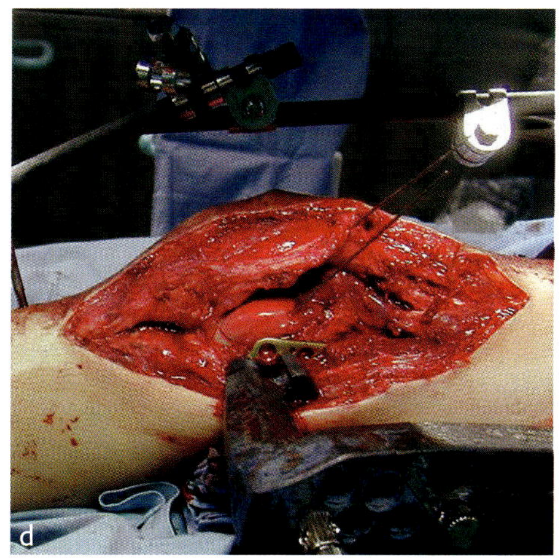

Fig 9.3.6-4a–g

- a Anatomical reduction of the intraarticular fracture with the help of the pointed reduction forceps. The reduction is temporarily fixed with 2.0 mm K-wires.
- b The joint block is fixed with an isolated 3.5 mm lag screw. The fracture alone determines the positions of the screws. Now the joint block is reduced taking into account length, axis, and rotation and using the external fixator on the anterior aspect to manipulate the fragments. Slight adjustments are made by inserting a K-wire into the joint block and using it as a joystick. The reduction is maintained in alignment with an elevator (antecurvature, retrocurvature). The metaphyseal fracture zone should not be touched and anatomical reduction is not necessary. The reduction is temporarily fixed with two K-wires inserted through the joint block into the diaphysis. The K-wires should not interfere with the implant placement. If an insufficient reduction persists, the implant can be adjusted to make slight corrections.
- c–d The LISS-DF, 9 holes is inserted under the vastus lateralis using the insertion guide. The LISS plate must be parallel to the condyles to prevent an irritation of the iliotibial tract. The most proximal hole is connected to the plate with a trocar. The implant is temporarily fixed with 2.0 mm K-wires inserted proximally and distally. The distal K-wire must be parallel to the condyles in the anteroposterior projection. In this position, the anatomically prebent implant should match the bone.

3 Reduction and fixation (cont)

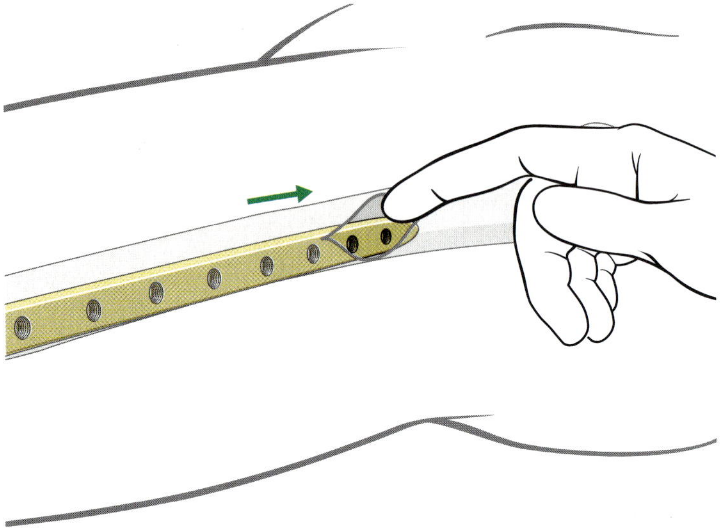

e

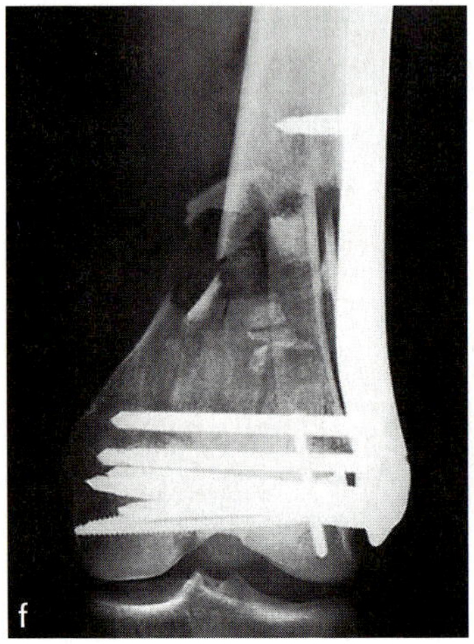

f

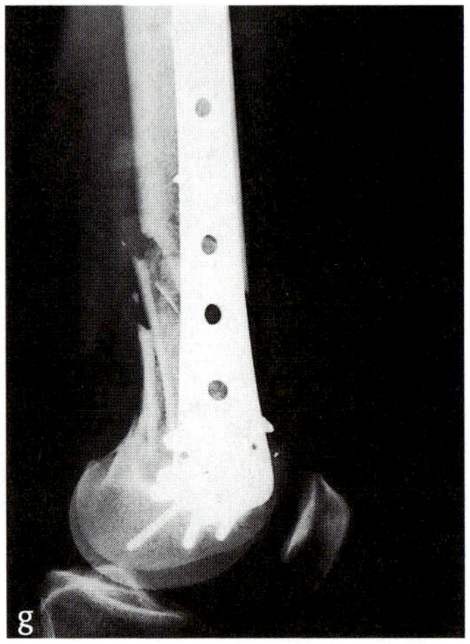

g

Fig 9.3.6-4a–g (cont)

e It is recommended that a 3 cm long incision be made proximally to verify the position of the plate. In the described procedure, the anterior aspect of the femur was palpated and the implant was advanced toward the finger. As soon as the reduction is anatomically correct, locking head screws are inserted into the distal fragment. The insertion of a K-wire is recommended to determine screw length and to avoid collision with a previously inserted lag screw. The screw can then be inserted through the trocar. This screw should also be parallel to the condyles in the AP projection.
A first proximal monocortical locking head screw is inserted. The reduction and the position of the plate are controlled clinically and by image intensification (axis, length, rotation). The remaining locking head screws are inserted in accordance with the preoperative plan.
The insertion guide is removed and the wound is closed.

f Intraoperative x-ray, AP view.

g Intraoperative x-ray, lateral view.

4 Rehabilitation

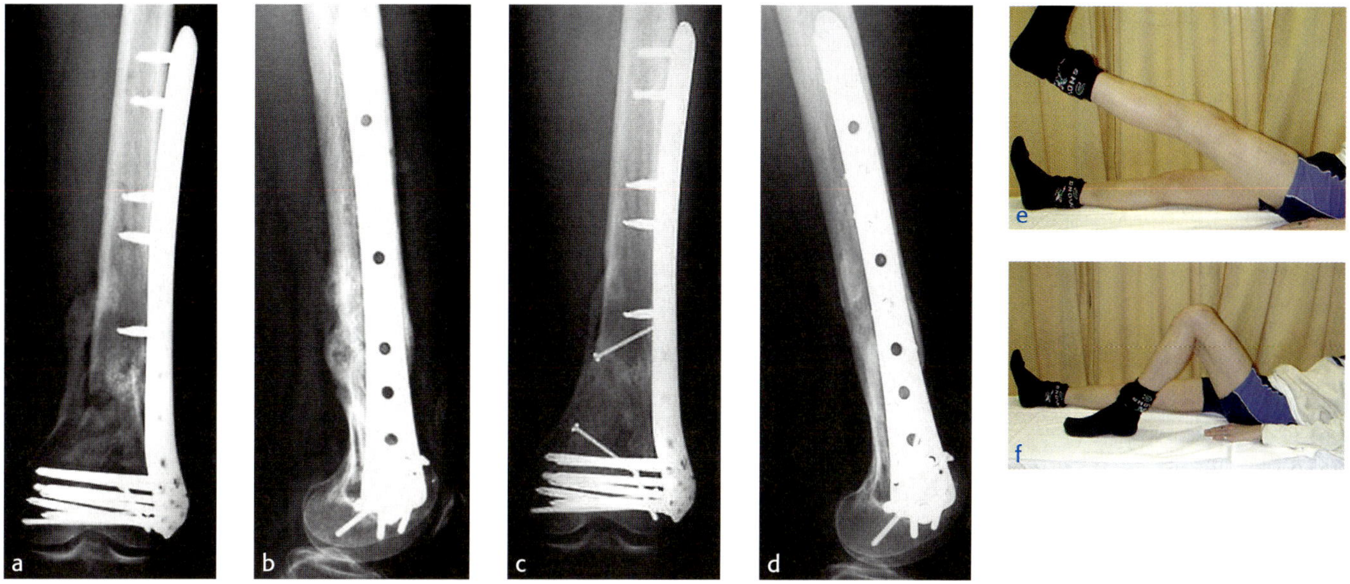

Gentle active and passive motion begins immediately on day 1 postoperatively. The use of the continuous passive motion machine is highly recommended. Mobilization with partial weight bearing as soon as the general and local condition of the patient allows it.

Fig 9.3.6-5a–f
a–b Postoperative x-rays after 9 weeks.
c–d 6 months after the initial operation, a bone defect on the medial side still persisted. Secondary cortico-cancellous bone grafting and screw fixation was necessary.
e–f Functional pictures 18 months postoperatively.

4 Rehabilitation (cont)

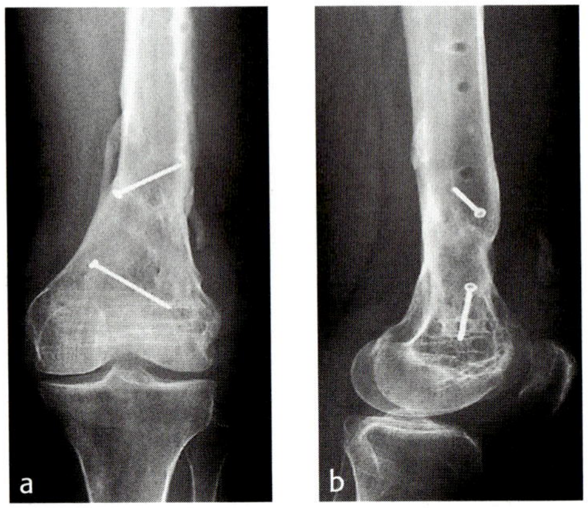

Implant removal

Fig 9.3.6-6a–b 3 years after the accident there was definitive bone healing in this young patient, but the implant had to be removed because of irritation of the iliotibial tract.

5 Pitfalls –

Approach
Too extensive exposure of the metaphyseal fracture zone may damage the blood supply of the bone fragments.

Reduction and fixation
Incorrect positioning of the implant in relation to the shaft may lead to early implant loosening.

Incorrect positioning of the implant in relation to the distal fragment may lead to soft-tissue irritations.

A too short implant increases the risk of implant loosening.

A too stiff implant fixation increases the risk of implant failure.

Rehabilitation
Late physiotherapy may lead to intraarticular adhesions and joint stiffness.

6 Pearls +

Approach
Open reduction of the intraarticular fracture component combined with an indirect reduction technique for the complex metaphyseal component.

Reduction and fixation
Careful control of implant position using direct and indirect control mechanisms (visualization, palpation, and image intensification).

The use of long implants and few screws is necessary to allow implant elasticity and better stress distribution (splinting method is an elastic fracture fixation).

Rehabilitation
Careful early active and passive physiotherapy is essential for good joint function.

Author Philip J Kregor

9.3.7 Open complete intraarticular multifragmentary distal femoral fracture—33-C3

1 Case description

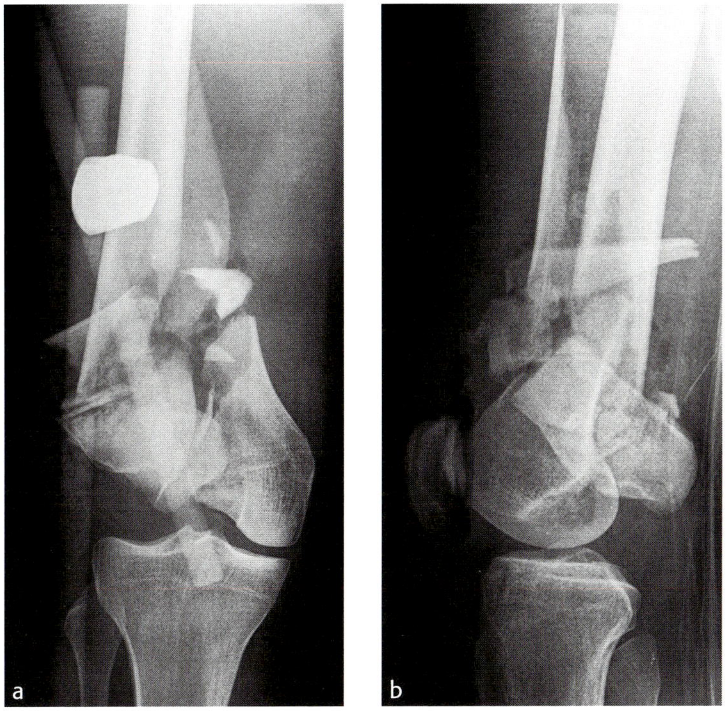

Fig 9.3.7-1a–b

a AP x-ray of the distal femur after the spanning external fixator was placed about the femur. It demonstrates a supracondylar/intercondylar femoral fracture with probable complex articular injury (Müller AO Classification 33-C3). The femur length has been restored with the use of the external fixator.

b Lateral x-ray showing typical hyperextension deformity of the distal femur and significant posterior displacement of cortical fragments. Because of the posterior displacement of the fragments, a possible vascular injury should be suspected. An ankle-ankle index (AAI) was performed and was found to be 0.98, which is not suggestive of an arterial injury.

22-year-old man, polytrauma with bilateral pneumothorax requiring bilateral chest tubes, grade III right hepatic lobe laceration, right acetabular fracture and open right distal femur fracture, Gustilo type II (5 cm open anterolateral wound over metaphyseal region, with muscle exposed).

Initially the patient was hemodynamically unstable and not able to proceed to the operating room. Therefore, in the intensive care unit under sterile preparation and draping, the 5 cm open incision about the right distal anterolateral thigh was debrided. The bone ends were curetted and debrided and the wound lavaged. A spanning external fixator was placed. A sterile dressing and splint were applied.

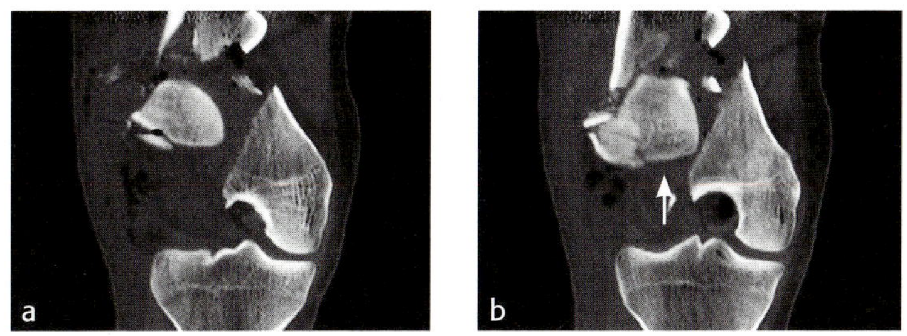

Fig 9.3.7-2a–b

a Anterior frontal plane reconstruction CT scan of the right distal femur. This demonstrates that the medial aspect of the femoral condyle has no significant articular injury but that there is a significant displacement of the lateral femoral condyle.

b More posteriorly placed frontal plane reconstruction of the right distal femur. This demonstrates an intraarticular split of the lateral femoral condyle (arrow).

Indication

Indications for operative stabilization of this distal femoral fracture include:
- polytraumatized patient,
- open fracture,
- severe articular injury with significant displacement,
- unstable supracondylar/intercondylar femoral fracture.

Preoperative planning

Equipment
- LISS-DF, 13 holes
- 5.0 mm locking head screws (LHS)
- 2.0 mm cortex screws
- 2.7 mm cortex screws
- 5.0 and 6.0 mm external fixator Schanz screws
- Pointed reduction forceps (with Weber clamp)
- Large pelvic reduction forceps

(Size of system, instruments, and implants can vary according to anatomy.)

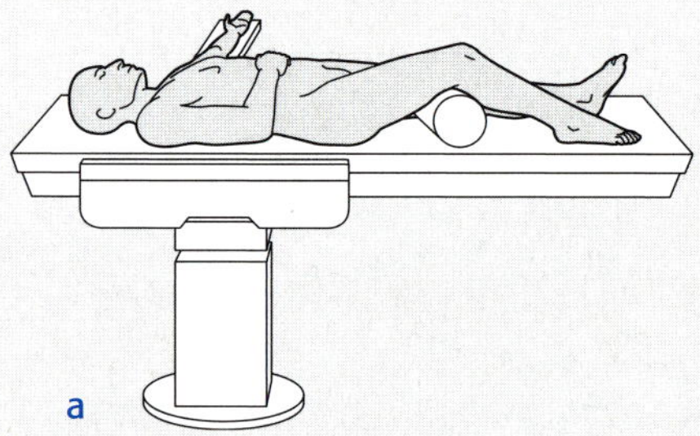

a

Patient preparation and positioning
Antibiotics: cephalosporin, aminoclycoside
Thrombosis prophylaxis: low-molecular heparin

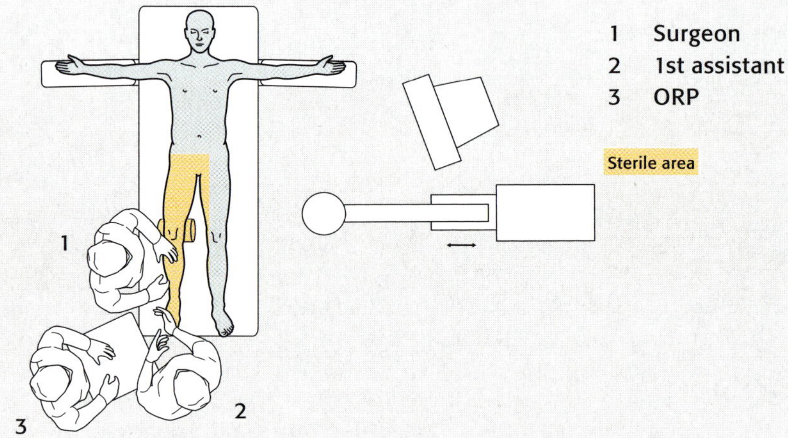

b

Fig 9.3.7-3a–b
a The patient is placed supine on a completely radiolucent table. The bilateral upper extremities and left lower extremity are secured and appropriately padded. A bump is placed underneath the left side of the pelvis in order to tilt the pelvis approximately 20° (as a result, at the end of the case, the foot should be externally rotated 5–10°).
In the preoperative period, the hip rotational profile of the right side was determined so that this could be checked and compared with the operative side postoperatively.

b The image intensifier is brought in from the opposite side of the table. The 1st assistant stands at the end of the radiolucent table to provide manual traction.

2 Surgical approach

The patient had a distal femoral fracture (33-C3) with a complex articular involvement of the lateral femoral condyle. No Hoffa fracture (frontal plane split) in the distal femoral condyles was noted. In addition, the patient had a 5 cm anterolateral wound over the distal femur which had previously undergone irrigation and debridement. This wound is now extended in both a proximal and distal direction and transformed into a modified lateral parapatellar approach for appropriate visualization of the articular surface of this C3 injury.

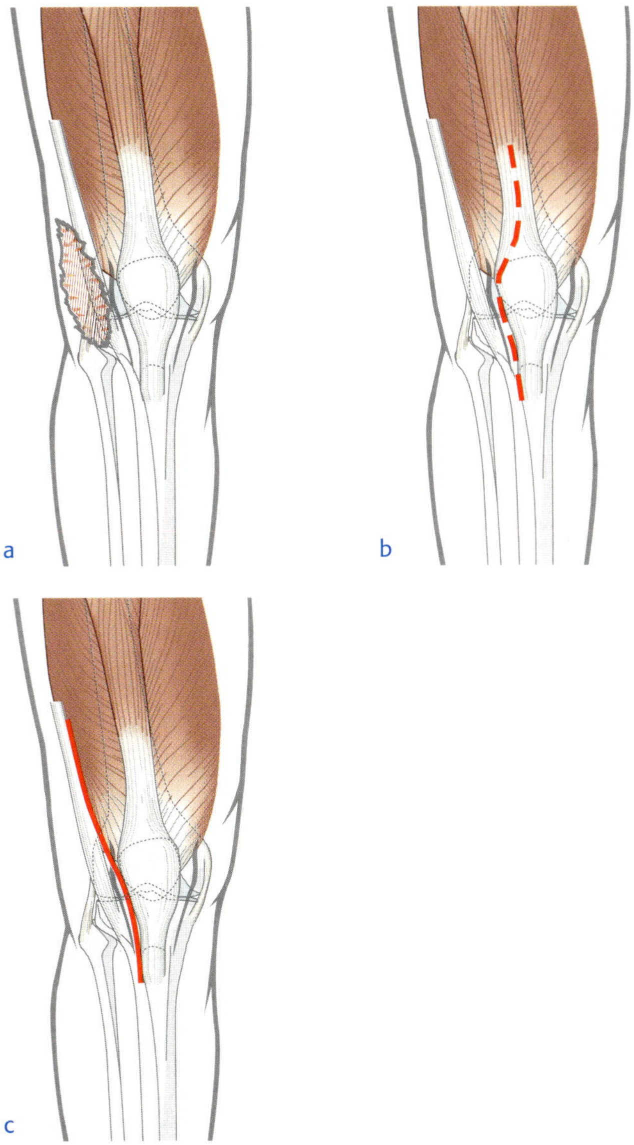

Fig 9.3.7-4a–c

- a Schematic drawing of the wound over the distal aspect of the right distal femur.
- b Schematic drawing of the normal lateral parapatellar approach to the distal femur. In general the quadriceps tendon is divided in its mid substance (or slightly lateral to its mid substance) and a cuff of tissue approximately 8 mm is left on the lateral aspect of the patella.
- c In this particular case secondary to the injury to the lateral aspect of the quadriceps, the surgical approach is modified so as not to penetrate the mid substance of the quadriceps tendon but rather remain lateral to the quadriceps femori.

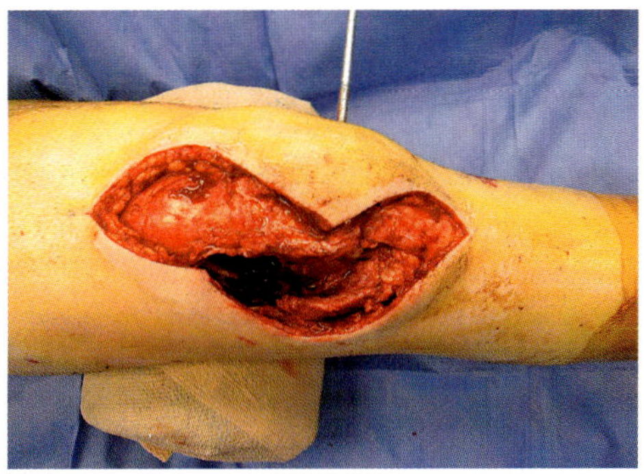

Fig 9.3.7-5 Intraoperative image of the surgical approach to the distal femur. A supracondylar bump of 10 towels has been placed posteriorly to the supracondylar region and a 6.0 mm Schanz screw has been placed in the medial femoral condyle for purposes of articular surface reduction.
Note that the exposure is lateral to the quadriceps femori and that the quadriceps tendon is not disrupted.

3 Reduction and fixation

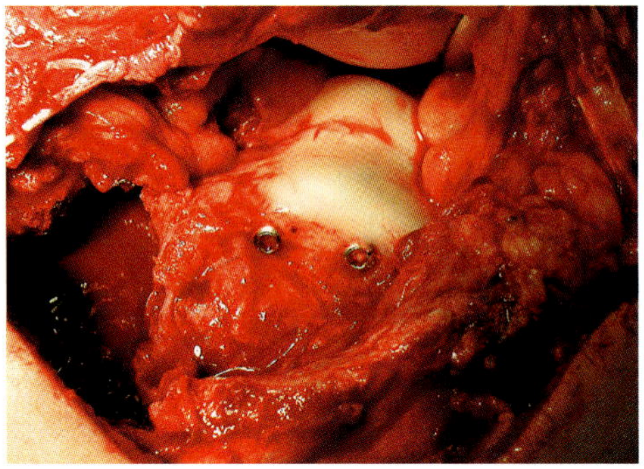

Fig 9.3.7-6 Visualization of the articular surface of the distal femur is possible through the lateral parapatellar approach. The articular surface of the distal femur is reduced with the aid of:

1. Complete relaxation of the patient.
2. A 6 mm Schanz screw in the medial femoral condyle to act as a reduction aid.
3. Pointed reduction forceps from the medial femoral condyle to the lateral femoral condyle.
4. Provisional K-wire fixation of the lateral femoral condyle to the medial femoral condyle.

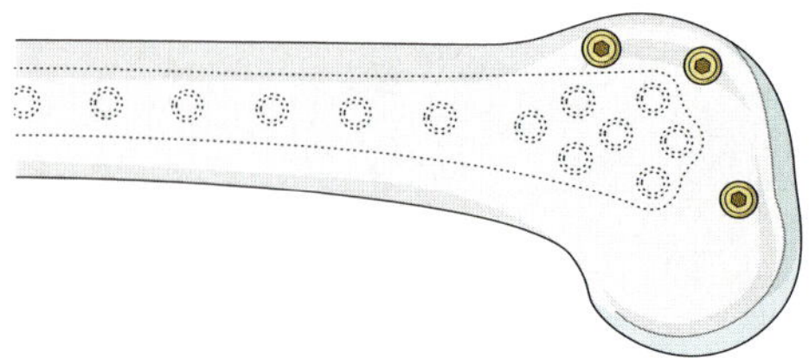

Fig 9.3.7-7 Here, three 3.5 mm lag screws from lateral to medial have been placed. The screws are at the periphery of the distal femoral condyle.

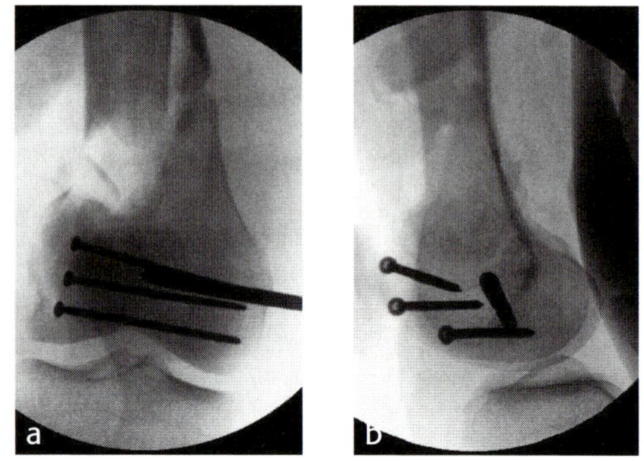

Fig 9.3.7-8a–b Direct visualization of the articular surface is utilized to judge the reduction. Image intensification is generally not relied upon. However, intraoperative x-rays do demonstrate appropriate reduction of the articular surface (AP and lateral).

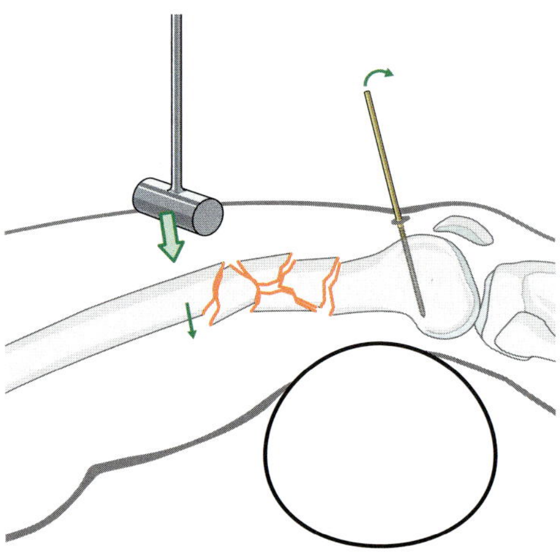

Fig 9.3.7-9 The next step after appropriate articular surface reconstruction is to "learn the fracture." That is, the closed reduction of the metaphyseal/diaphyseal component of the fracture is viewed under image intensification, and judged in the AP and lateral planes. The image intensifier unit is brought in from the opposite side of the table and the closed reduction of the metaphyseal/diaphyseal component of the fracture is achieved through a combination of:

- complete relaxation of the patient,
- towel bumps placed posteriorly in the supracondylar region,
- manual traction,
- manipulation of the distal femoral fragment using Schanz screws. A screw placed from medial to lateral can be used to control varus/valgus angulation. A Schanz screw placed from anterior to posterior can correct the hyperextension deformity.
- A mallet can be used to exert force on the anteromedial aspect of the distal aspect of the femoral shaft fragment, as long as this proximal fragment is adducted and flexed.

3 Reduction and fixation (cont)

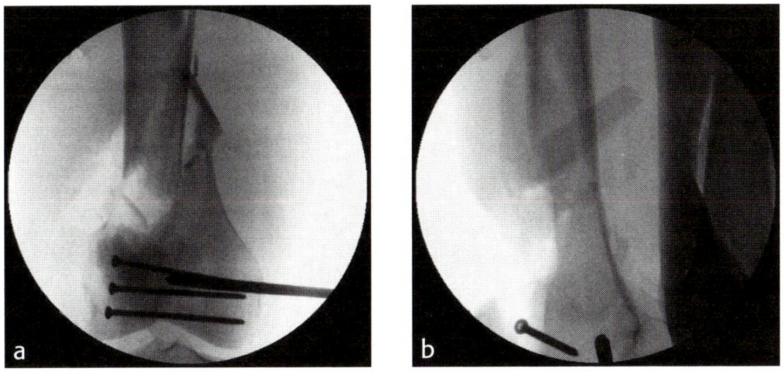

Fig 9.3.7-10a–b AP and lateral x-rays of the distal femur are obtained and the image intensifier is used to scan the distal femur in both AP and lateral projections to learn of any deformity and to check reduction.

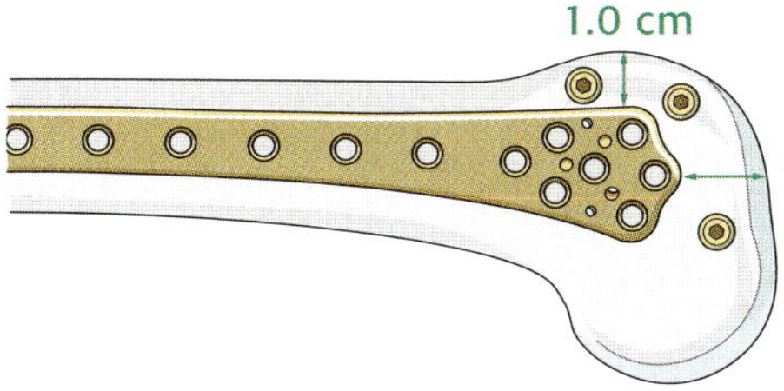

Fig 9.3.7-11 After the articular reduction and fixation has been completed, the fracture is "learned" under image intensification guidance, and appropriate reduction of the metaphyseal/diaphyseal component of the fracture is obtained and maintained via manual traction, the LISS fixator is inserted. The LISS fixator is slid in a submuscular manner beneath the vastus lateralis. Tactile sensation of the tip of the fixator is utilized as the fixator is being passed in a cranial direction. The appropriate relationship of the fixator to the distal end of the femur is then established. In general, the anterior aspect of the fixator is approximately 1 cm posterior to the anterior aspect of the femoral condyles and the distal end of the fixator is approximately 1.5 cm from the distal aspect of the femoral condyle.

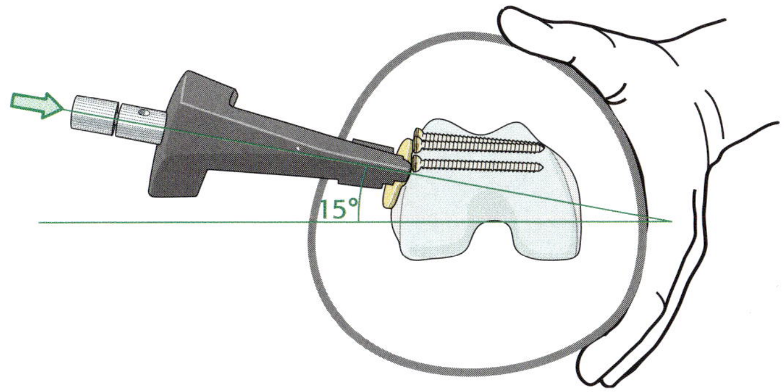

Fig 9.3.7-12 Often, the fixator is passed slightly more cranially than needed. The fixator is then pushed slightly distally, and allowed to settle back on the femoral condyles. The insertion guide for the LISS is then raised approximately 10–15° and counterpressure by the surgeon's left hand is exerted on the medial aspect of the femoral condyle.
At this point, with the femoral LISS/distal femoral condylar block relationship established, a guide wire is placed through hole A. If the appropriate varus/valgus has been established, and if the guide wire is not bent, the guide wire should be parallel to the joint surface.

Next, appropriate length and rotation are established through manual traction and/or use of the Schanz screws in the distal femoral condyle. After this has been accomplished, a guide wire is placed in the most proximal hole through the previous connecting bolt.

Next, several locking head screws may be placed in the distal femoral block. Especially with placement of the first LHS, care must be taken to ensure that the LISS fixator is pressed against the femoral condyles, as the LHS will tend to push away the bone.

3 Reduction and fixation (cont)

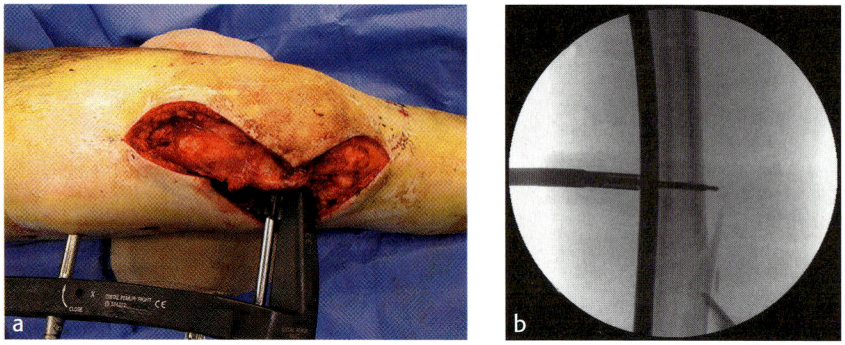

Fig 9.3.7-13a–b Then, a pulling device ("whirlybird") is utilized to bring the diaphysis to the femoral LISS.
Multiple LHS are then placed through the insertion guide proximally and distally.

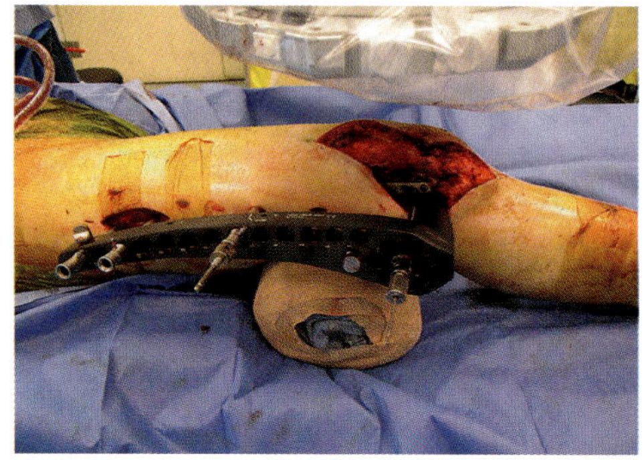

Fig 9.3.7-14 Note that a proximal incision has been made to palpate the fixator on the midlateral aspect of the femur.

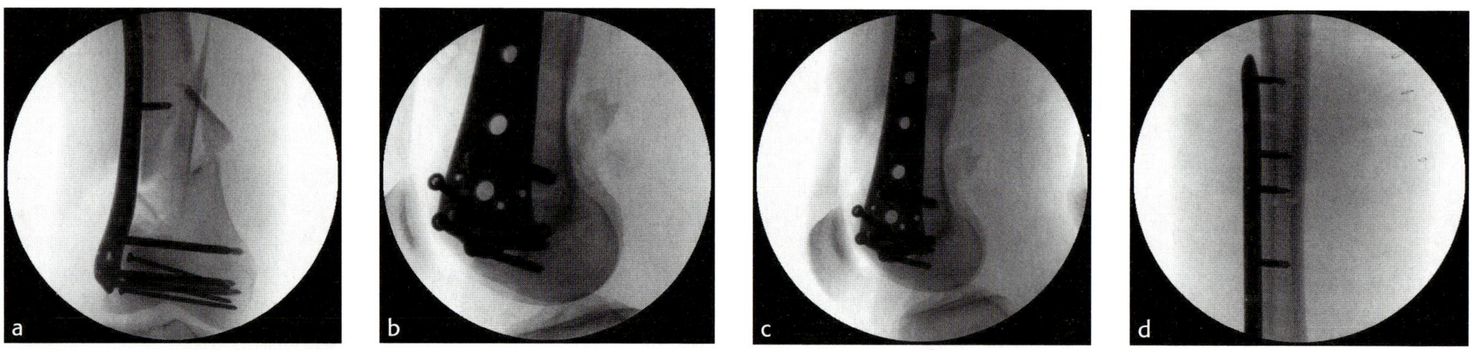

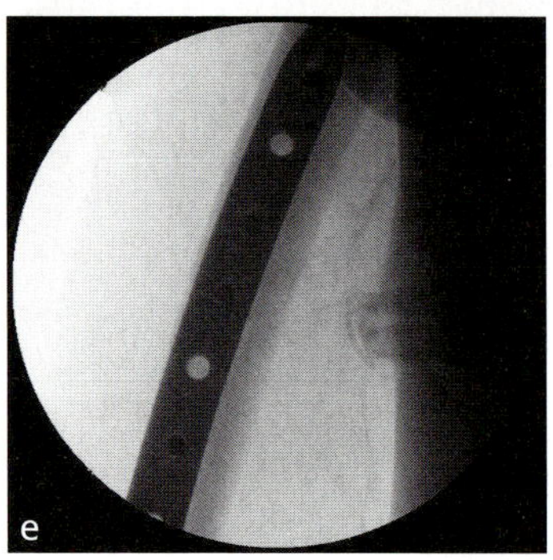

Fig 9.3.7-15a–e Intraoperative x-rays confirm that the fixator is in the appropriate position distally and proximally.

4 Rehabilitation

The patient is allowed 10 kg weight bearing for 10 weeks. Aggressive immediate range of motion is begun with physiotherapy. Quadriceps strengthening exercises are also emphasized. At 10 weeks, progressive weight bearing is allowed, with the goal of ambulation with cane by weeks 12–14 postoperatively. No braces are utilized.

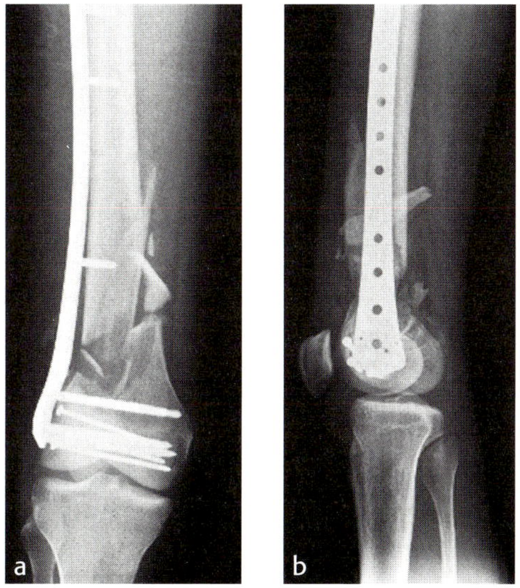

Fig 9.3.7-16a–b 3 weeks postoperative x-rays.

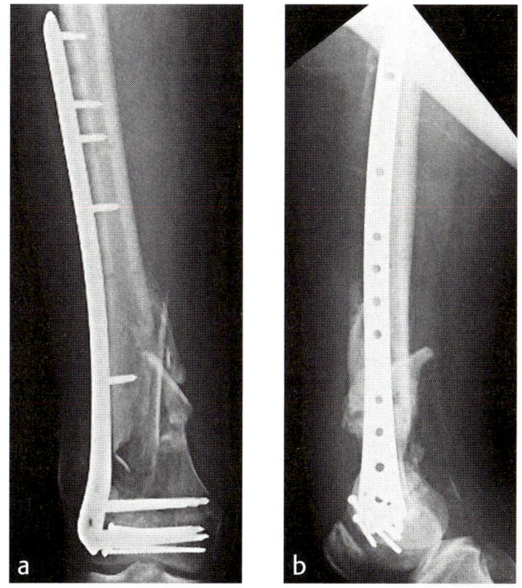

Fig 9.3.7-17a–b Callus formation at 10 weeks.

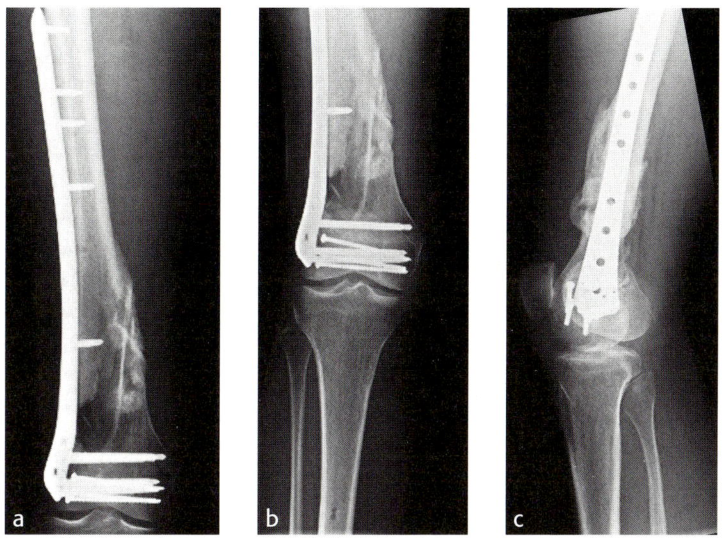

Fig 9.3.7-18a–c Follow-up x-rays after 7 months.

5 Pitfalls –

Approach
Improper division of the quadriceps tendon proximally: this leads to poor quality of wound closure.

Reduction and fixation

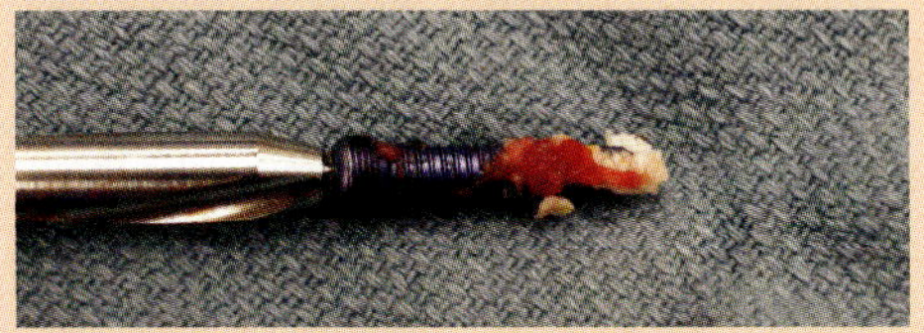

Fig 9.3.7-19 Screw plugging with bone in case of a very thick cortex.

Postoperative deformity of valgus.

Postoperative deformity of external rotation of the distal femur.

Screws are too long on the medial aspect of the femur.

LISS fixator incorrectly positioned on the proximal femur.

Rehabilitation
Knee stiffness.

6 Pearls +

Approach
The surgeon should visualize the medial and lateral aspect of the quadriceps tendon well and then divide the tendon in its midline (or slightly lateral to it).

Reduction and fixation
In self-drilling, self-tapping LHS, the flutes of the screw can become filled with bone. The surgeon "feels" this when the screw does not advance easily. The screw should be withdrawn, and the flutes cleaned. The screw will then advance easily. Special self-drilling, self-tapping LHS with a long drilling tip are available.

Long-leg x-rays of the femur will alert the surgeon to the deformity. This can be corrected by a change in the vector of manual traction or utilization of a Schanz screw from medial to lateral in the distal femoral block.

If the pelvis is tilted 20°, the foot should be rotated 5–10° during reduction and externally fixation. A careful assessment of the postoperative rotational profile should be compared with the opposite side.

It should be remembered that the medial aspect of the distal femur slopes approximately 25°. Therefore anterior screws should appear "short" on the AP x-ray.

Especially with a 13-hole LISS, an incision is made proximally (over holes 12 and 13) to palpate the proximal end of the plate. This ensures that the fixator is on the midlateral aspect of the femur and that proper rotation of the fixator is carried out.

Rehabilitation
Immediate, aggressive range of motion is mandatory in all cases. No braces are utilized.

Authors Thomas J Hockertz, Andreas Gruner, Gabriele Streicher, Heinrich Reilmann

9.3.8 Periprosthetic distal femoral fracture with implanted total knee endoprosthesis—33-A2

1 Case description

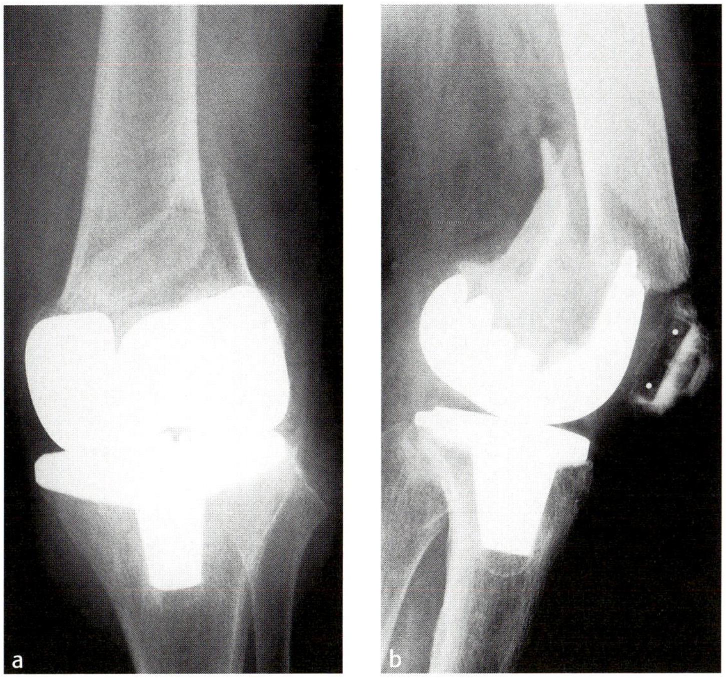

81-year-old woman who tripped on the curb when walking down the street, fell and broke her left femur.
Type of injury: low-energy trauma, monotrauma, closed fracture.

Fig 9.3.8-1a–b
a AP view.
b Detail AP view.

Indication

Periprosthetic fracture of the left femur with implanted cemented knee arthroplasty. No clinical or radiological signs of loosening. Before the accident the patient was mobile without crutches and without symptoms.

Preoperative planning

Equipment

- LISS-DF, 5 holes
- 5.0 mm self-drilling, self-tapping locking head screws (LHS)
- 2.0 mm K-wires

(Size of system, instruments, and implants can vary according to anatomy.)

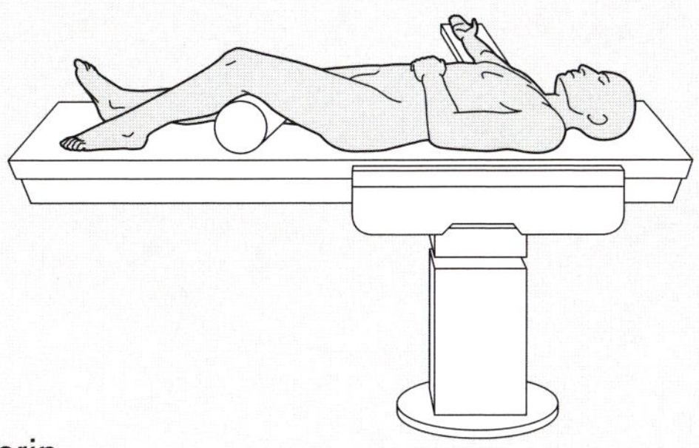

Fig 9.3.8-2 Supine position, the leg is free draped for intraoperative mobility, elevation of the injured limb and flexion of the knee joint at approximately 30°. Lower the contralateral leg for better intraoperative x-ray assessment, cushion the distal femur of the injured leg, eg, with a towel roll.

Patient preparation and positioning

Antibiotics: single dose 2nd generation cephalosporin
Thrombosis prophylaxis: low-molecular heparin

2 Surgical approach

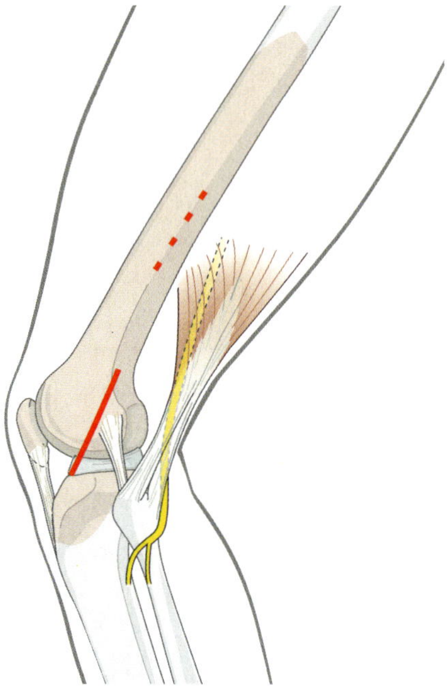

Fig 9.3.8-3 Skin incision from Gerdy's tubercle in a proximal direction. Divide the iliotibial tract in the direction of its fibers and dissect to the periosteum while retracting the vastus lateralis.

3 Reduction and fixation

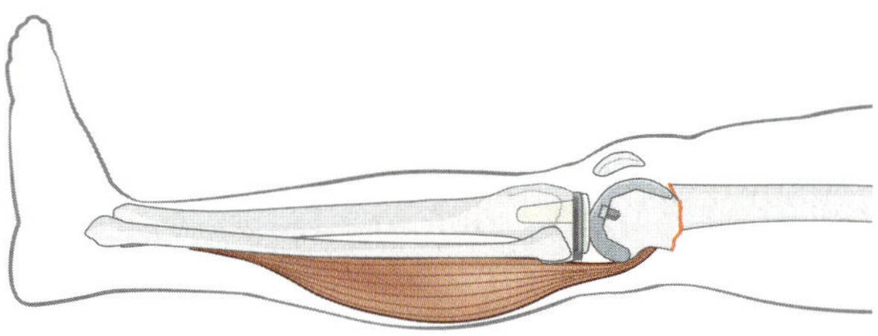

a

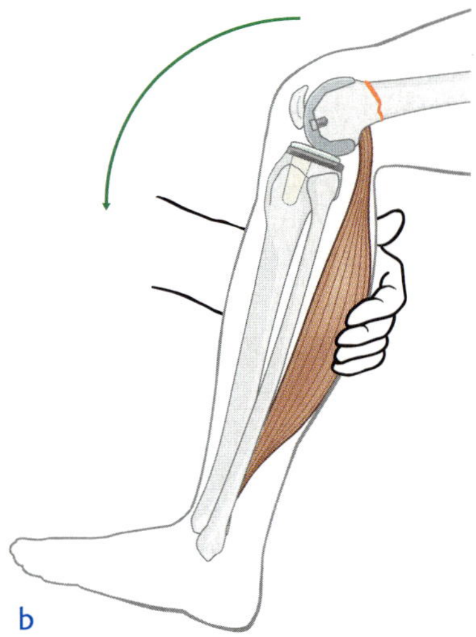

b

Fig 9.3.8-4a–b
a Approximate reduction of the fracture and the longitudinal axis by applying axial tension with the knee flexed to approximately 30° to relax the gastrocnemius.
b From the posterior aspect, elevate the distal fragment from its tilted position in recurvature with the elevator or by employing a Schanz screw inserted anterolaterally as a joystick.

3 Reduction and fixation (cont)

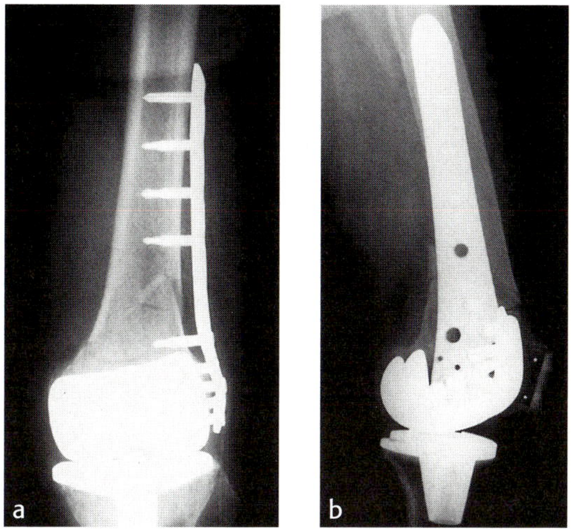

Fig 9.3.8-5a–b Prepare the plate bed from distal to proximal by epiperiosteal tunneling under the vastus lateralis muscle with a long bone rasp.
Select the appropriate plate length under image intensification and insert the implant into the plate bed. Make an incision at the proximal end of the plate to complete the procedure.
Stabilize the implant on the proximal and distal sides by inserting K-wires and check plate position in two planes.
Precise reduction of the fragments with the pulling device, which pulls the fragment to the LISS plate.
Insert the screws alternately in the distal and proximal holes starting distally, determine screw length according to Table 3-2, whereby screw length is measured distally using K-wires in the presence of an implanted prosthesis. This avoids interference with prosthesis components and any associated stripping of the screw thread.

4 Rehabilitation

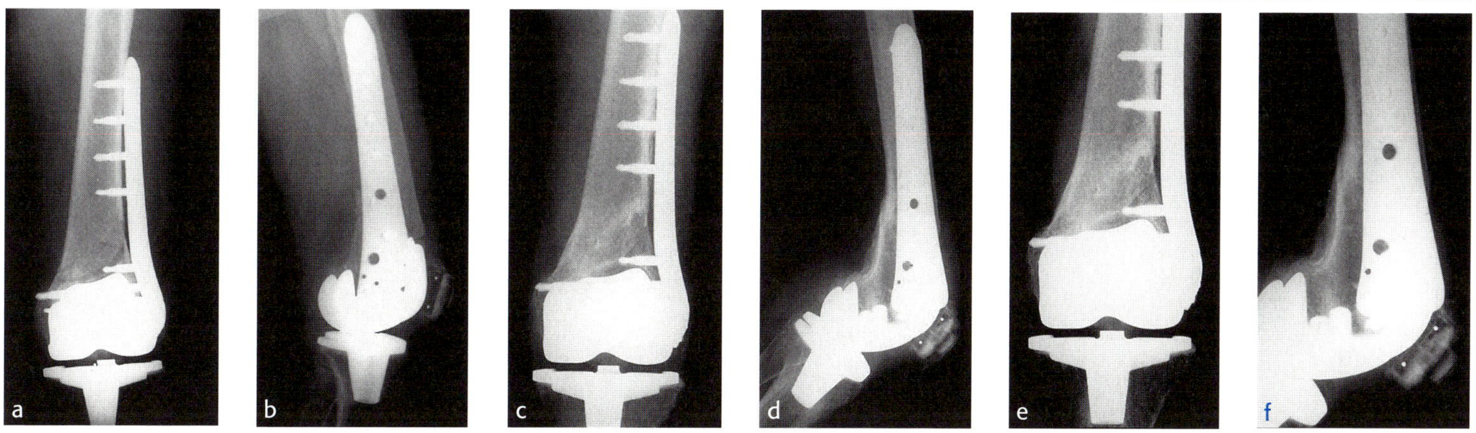

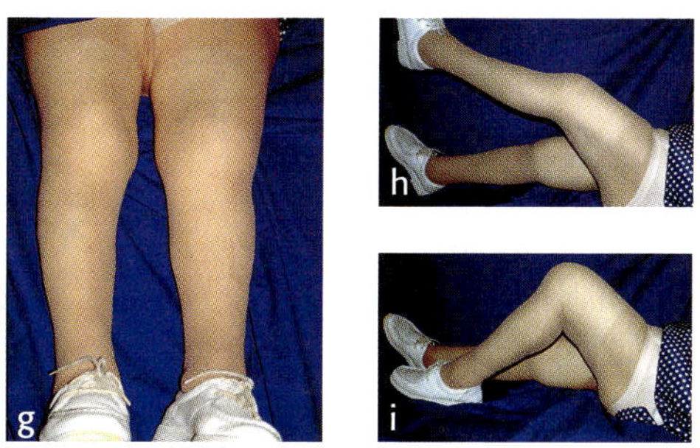

Weight bearing: 15 kg for 2 weeks, half body weight after 4 weeks, full weight bearing after 6 weeks.
Physiotherapy: from the second postoperative day and continuous passive motion.
Pharmaceutical treatment: pain therapy and nonsteroid antiinflammatory drugs.

Fig 9.3.8-6a–i
a–b Postoperative x-rays after 6 weeks.
c–d Postoperative x-rays after 12 weeks.
e–f Postoperative x-rays after 18 weeks.
g–i Clinical pictures after 18 weeks.

5 Pitfalls –

Equipment
Incorrect plate length so that not enough locking head screws can be inserted into the shaft. The LISS-DF must be properly seated.

Approach
Inadequate preparation of the distal femur and, consequently, plate positioning too far anterior or posterior and risk of trapping the iliotibial tract.

Reduction and fixation
Loss of manual reduction and axial alignment, incorrect screw length and abutment of the screws before head locking is achieved. Consequent thread stripping.

Rehabilitation
Immobilization for too long.

6 Pearls +

Equipment
Good control over implant positioning due to a closed system and predetermined screw positioning via stab incisions.

Approach
Minimally invasive approach, fragments retain their soft-tissue attachments.

Reduction and fixation
Anchorage possible in the presence of endoprostheses with shaft components or correction endoprostheses.

Rehabilitation
Partial weight bearing cannot always be achieved with elderly patients. In this case, immediate full weight bearing was permitted.

Author Philip J Kregor

9.3.9 Bilateral open supracondylar femoral fractures above total knee arthroplasties—33-A3

1 Case description

67-year-old woman was involved in a motor vehicle collision and sustained a left intertrochanteric hip fracture and bilateral open supracondylar femoral fractures above total knee arthroplasties. She was initially hemodynamically unstable. After appropriate resuscitation, she was taken to the operating room and had fixation of her intertrochanteric hip fracture utilizing a dynamic hip screw. She had irrigation and debridement of her open 6 cm wounds on both the right and left lower extremities. She subsequently had spanning external fixators placed across her knee joint.

The patient was brought back to the operating room on postinjury day two for definitive treatment of her distal femoral fractures.

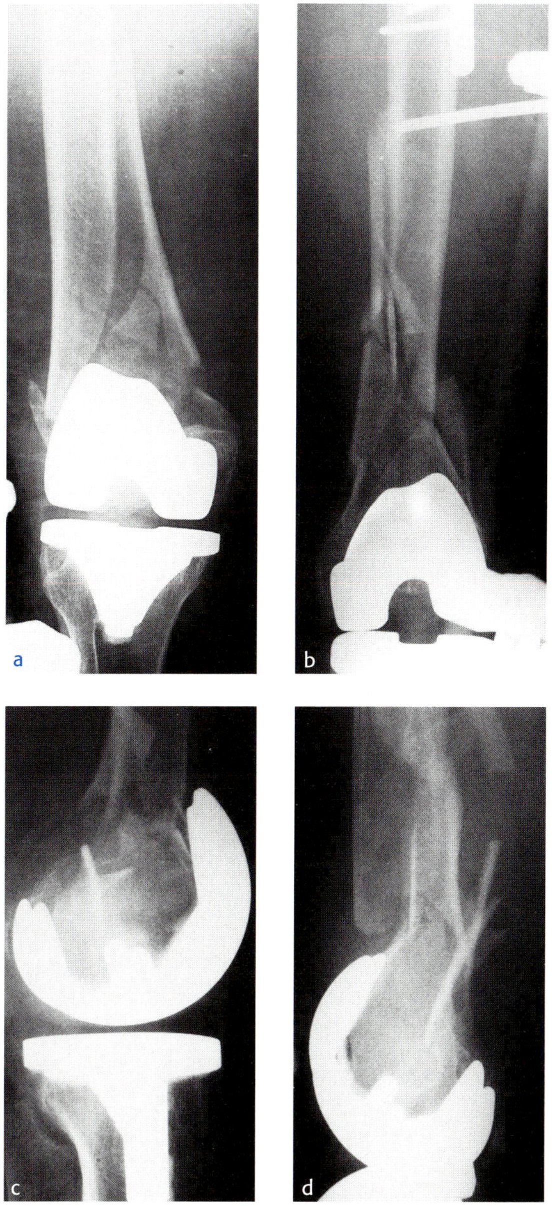

Fig 9.3.9-1a–d
- a–b AP x-rays of both the right and left supracondylar femur fractures above the total knees. Both are characterized by short distal segments and comminution in the metaphyseal region.
- c The lateral x-ray of the right distal femur. Note that the distal femoral block is quite short, but that it is well fixed to the femoral component.
- d The lateral x-ray of the left distal femur. The distal femoral block is well fixed to the femoral component of the total knee arthroplasty.

Indication

Indications for operative stabilization of this distal femoral fracture include:
- Polytraumatized patient,
- Open fracture,
- Displaced supracondylar femoral fractures above total knee arthroplasties.

While nonoperative treatment of nondisplaced or minimally displaced fractures above total knee arthroplasties can be considered, both of these fractures demonstrated significant instability.

Preoperative planning

Equipment
- LISS-DF, 13 holes, left
- LISS-DF, 13 holes, right
- 5.0 mm self-drilling, self-tapping locking head screws (LHS)
- K-wires

(Size of system, instruments, and implants can vary according to anatomy.)

Patient preparation and positioning
Antibiotics: cephalosporin and aminoglycoside (secondary to the open nature of the fracture)
Thrombosis prophylaxis: low-molecular heparin

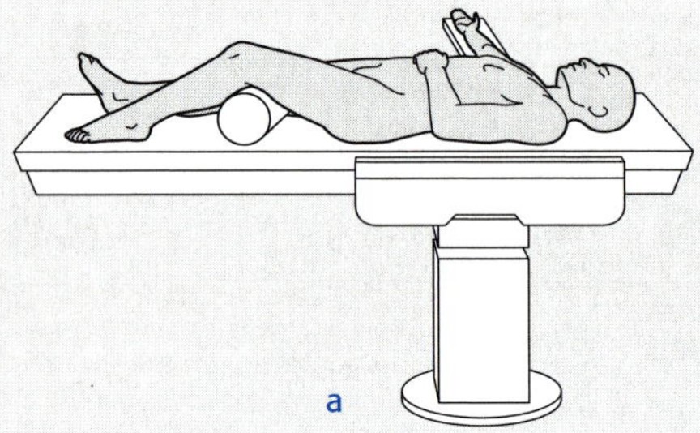

a

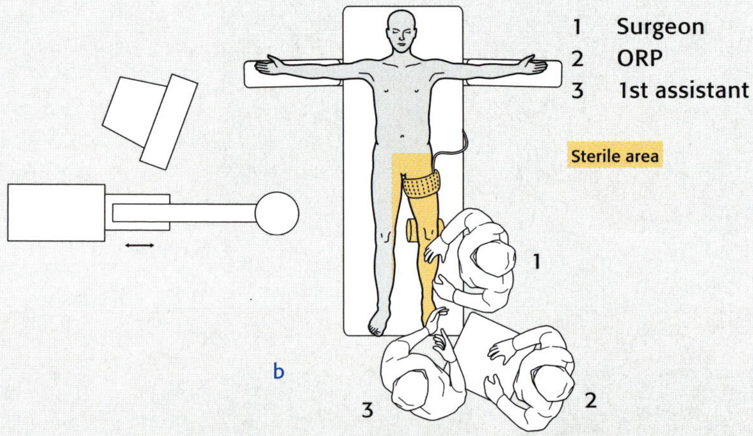

b

Fig 9.3.9-2a–b The patient is placed supine on a completely radiolucent table.

a A bump was placed underneath the left side of the pelvis in order to tilt the pelvis approximately 20° (as a result, at the end of the case, the foot should be externally rotated approximately 5–10°).

b The image intensifier is brought in from the opposite side of the table. The surgeon is standing. First assistant is at the end of the radiolucent table to provide manual traction.

The left lower extremity will be addressed first. In order not to confuse the rotational profile of the bilateral lower extremities, they are operated on one at a time. Reversed positions for the right lower extremity.

2 Surgical approach

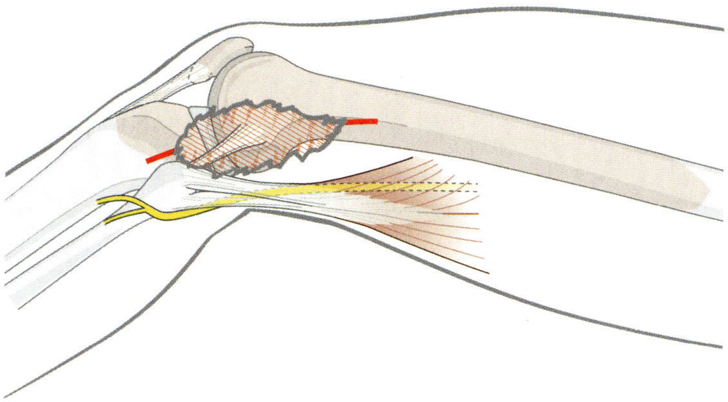

The patient initially had a repeat irrigation and debridement of the distal femoral fracture. This consisted of aggressive debridement of the subcutaneous tissue and quadriceps musculature that had been devitalized due to the fracture. In addition, curettage of the bone fragments was also performed. Finally, copious irrigation with 6 liters of pulsatile lavage was then carried out. After this, the left lower extremity was prepped again and was once again draped out.

Fig 9.3.9-3 The open distal femoral wound was extended both proximally and distally. It was initially on the lateral aspect of the distal femur.

3 Reduction and fixation

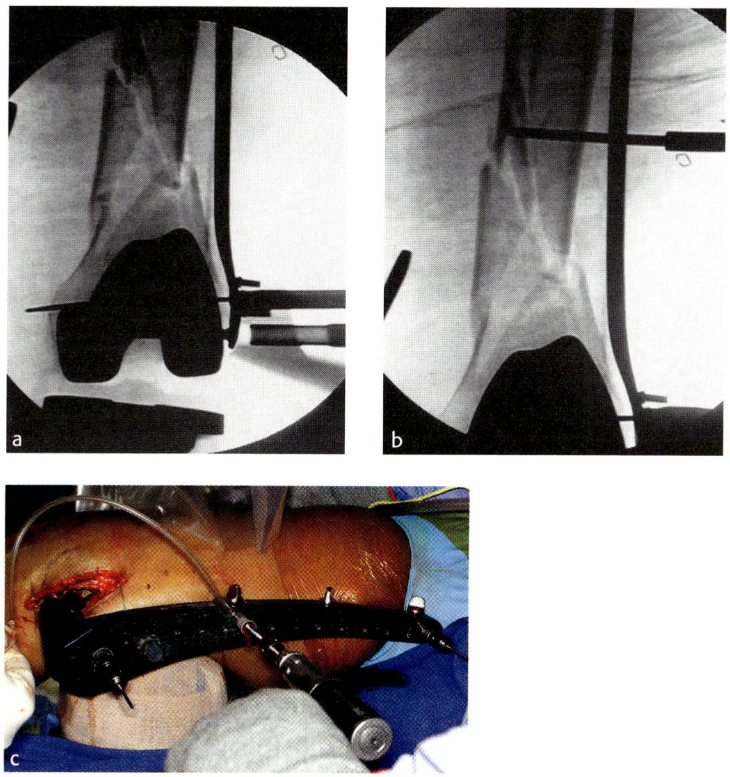

The LISS fixator is then slid in a submuscular manner through the distal femoral wound.

Fig 9.3.9-4a–c

a This x-ray shows the LISS fixator slid up along the midlateral aspect of the femur with the distal guide wire being placed through a drill sleeve in the insertion guide for the LISS fixator. Note that the guide wire should be parallel with femoral component. Note also that the distal aspect of the proximal segment is adducted. It was also noted to be slightly flexed.

b A mallet placed on the anterior aspect of the distal component of the femoral shaft was then used to reduce the anterior translation of the distal segment of the distal shaft and a "whirlybird" device (pulling device) was then used to bring the femoral shaft to the LISS fixator.

c Intraoperative image of the supracondylar bump posterior to the distal aspect of the femur. Note the surgical approach.

3 Reduction and fixation (cont)

As is detailed in case 9.3.7, several additional steps of LISS fixation of this distal femur fracture are carried out:
Before the "whirlybird" is utilized, an incision over holes 12 and 13 is then made to palpate the LISS fixator on the femur. This is done to ensure that the LISS is on the midlateral aspect of the femur and that appropriate rotation of the LISS fixator is made.
As with any LISS fixation, the fracture had been learned before the LISS fixator was slid in. It is especially important to learn the sagittal plane reduction.

Several distal locking head screws are then placed through the insertion guide into the distal femoral component and multiple monocortical locking head screws are placed in the proximal aspect of the femur.
Usually in osteoporotic cases, such as this, five to six distal locking head screws and five to six proximal locking head screws are utilized.

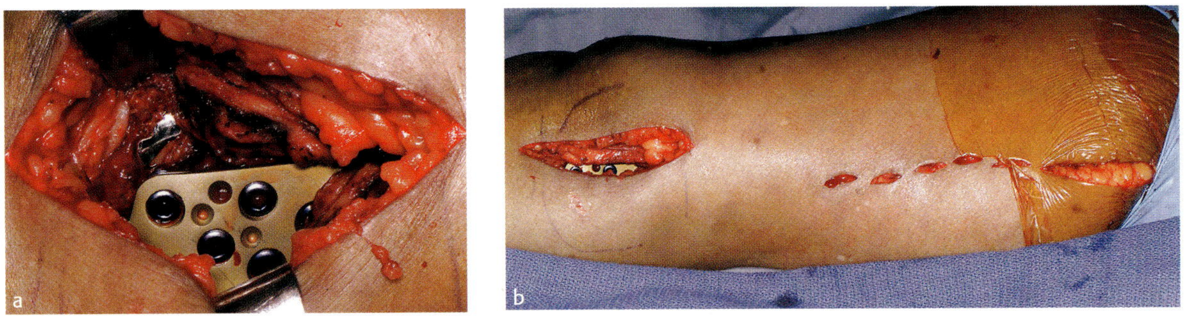

Fig 9.3.9-5a–b
a The LISS fixator after the insertion guide has been removed. Note that in this case the fixator is brought quite distal to ensure adequate fixation of the distal femoral block.
b Intraoperative image showing the distal femoral incision, the proximal femoral incision, and multiple percutaneous incisions for placement of the monocortical shaft screws.

4 Rehabilitation

The patient was bed to wheelchair for 12 weeks. She had morbid obesity which made ambulation difficult. At 12 weeks, she began ambulation with a walker. She converted to a cane at 20 weeks postoperatively. Immediate range of motion exercises were begun postoperatively. Her final range of motion was 0–90° bilaterally. This was the same as before the injury. Full weight bearing after 14 weeks.

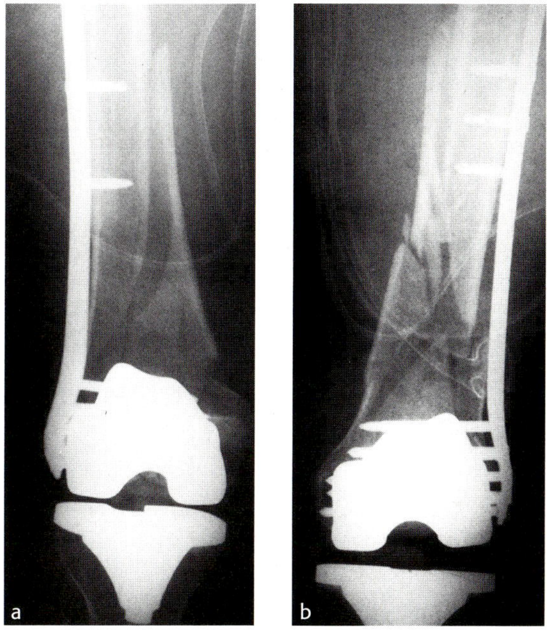

Fig 9.3.9-6a–b Postoperative AP x-rays of both the right and left lower extremities.

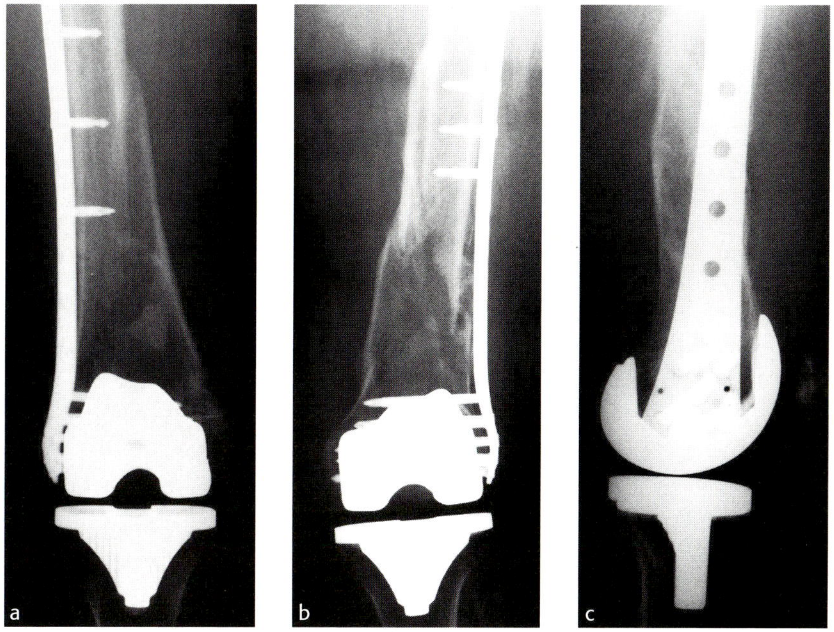

Fig 9.3.9-7a–c

a–b Follow-up x-rays after 5 months. Significant callus formation is seen.

c Lateral x-ray of the left distal femur demonstrates consolidation.

5 Pitfalls –

Surgical approach
Devitalization of the metaphyseal/diaphyseal component of the fracture may lead to delayed union or nonunion.

Reduction and fixation
Gaining distal fixation in a short segment with osteoporotic bone can be difficult. In addition, the femoral component of the total knee arthroplasty may make the placement of certain screws impossible.

The common deformity seen with placement of the distal femoral LISS is that of external rotation and valgus deformity.

Rehabilitation
Stiffness of the knee.

6 Pearls +

Surgical approach
The surgeon must strive to leave soft-tissue attachments intact in the metaphyseal/diaphyseal area. No attempt is made to reduce or visualize comminution.

Reduction and fixation
The LISS fixator should be brought relatively distal on the femoral condyle. It is slightly more distal than in a nonarthroplasty case. A good cross table lateral of the distal femoral block will also allow the surgeon to plan the placement of the LISS fixator in the appropriate position to optimize the number of screws in the distal femoral block. This may require placing the LISS fixator slightly more anterior or posterior than the usual placement. Visualization of the femoral component of the total knee arthroplasty.

The external rotation deformity can be carefully controlled for by placing the pelvis at approximately a 20° tilt. In doing so, the foot should be approximately 10° externally rotated at the end of the case.

Utilizing the image intensifier to scan up and down this femur can be very advantageous to discern any slight valgus deformity.

If a valgus deformity is noted, it can be corrected by:
- Manual traction in a slight varus direction,
- placing a "whirlybird" (pulling device) into the proximal aspect of the distal femoral block,
- utilizing a 6.0 mm Schanz screw through a small stab incision on the medial aspect of the distal femoral block and utilizing this Schanz pin as a reduction device.

Rehabilitation
Immediate range of motion of the knees is begun.
No braces are utilized.

Author Ronald van Heerwaarden

9.3.10 Double osteotomy for valgus leg deformity due to lateral compartment knee osteoarthritis

1 Case description

37-year-old woman, direct knee trauma 20 years ago. Previous surgery: arthrotomy 20 years ago (unknown), total lateral meniscectomy 6 years ago, partial medial meniscectomy, recently. Progressive valgus leg deformity after initial trauma increased after lateral meniscectomy. Knee pain during weight bearing and at rest, instability due to valgus and loss of motion.
Examination: valgus leg alignment, antalgic gait pattern, knee range of motion: 90/15/0, knee swelling, contracted valgus deformity.

Deformity: valgus leg alignment of 16° in standing position. Extension deficit 15°. No associated transverse plane deformities.

X-rays: Grade 4 OA lateral compartment (Ahlback grading), grade 1 OA medial compartment.

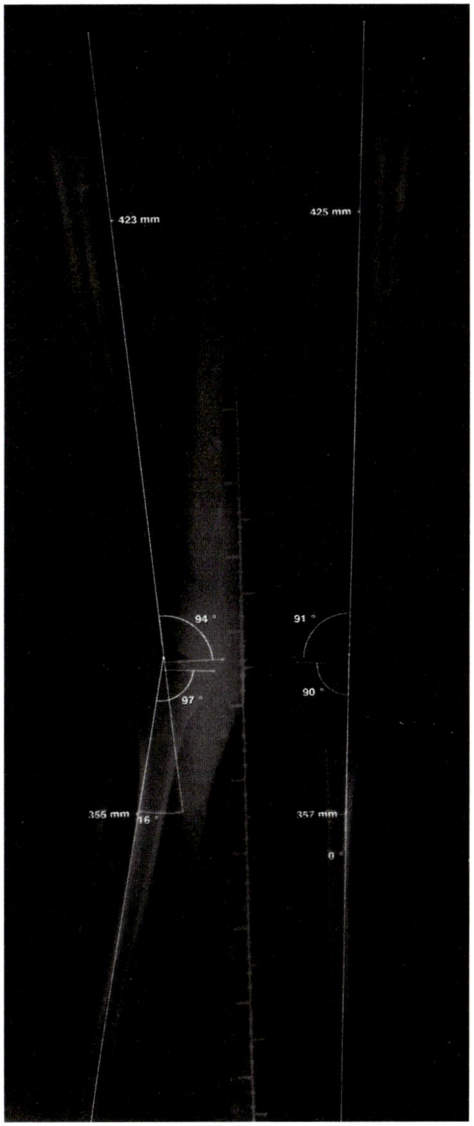

Fig 9.3.10-1 Standing x-rays both legs.

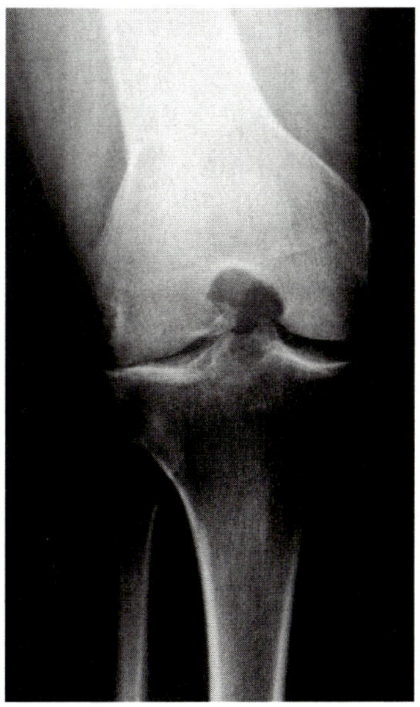

Fig 9.3.10-2 45° flexion weight bearing AP view (Rosenberg-view).

Deformity analysis

1. Full leg weight-bearing x-ray: weight-bearing line through lateral compartment. Tibiofemoral angle: 16° valgus, no associated sagittal plane bone deformities of femur and tibia.

2. Deformity analysis (according to Paley):

Conclusion

Lateral compartment osteoarthritis, single plane 16° valgus deformity, bone deformity localized in the femur 5° (LPFA + mLFDA) and proximal medial tibia 10° (MPTA). Associated medial joint line opening 2° (JLCA).

Angle	Patient	Normal
Lateral proximal femoral angle (LPFA)	86°	90°
Mechanical lateral distal femoral angle (mLDFA)	86°	88°
Medial proximal tibial angle (MPTA)	97°	87°
Lateral distal tibial angle (LDTA)	89°	89°
JLCA	4°	2°

Indication for osteotomy

Progressive symptomatic lateral compartment osteoarthritis with progressive valgus deformity causing gait abnormalities and symptoms at other joints. Range of motion impaired by contracted valgus deformity and joint compartment obliteration.
Nonoperative treatment (medication, infiltration, shoe inlays, brace treatment) had failed.

Preoperative planning

Planning of deformity correction

Goals

1. Leg alignment correction to neutral or slight varus alignment to unload the lateral compartment for pain improvement and normalization of gait.
2. Range of motion improvement with restoration of full extension.

Methods

1. Double osteotomy: 10° medial closing wedge osteotomy of the proximal tibia to normal MPTA and 5° lateral opening wedge osteotomy of the distal femur with insertion of bone wedge material taken from the proximal tibia. As 2° of valgus deformity is due to medial joint line opening (JLCA: 4°) no overcorrection is necessary to create slight varus alignment.
2. Intraarticular resection of osteophytes in the intercondylar notch and release of contracted lateral capsule.

Preoperative planning (cont)

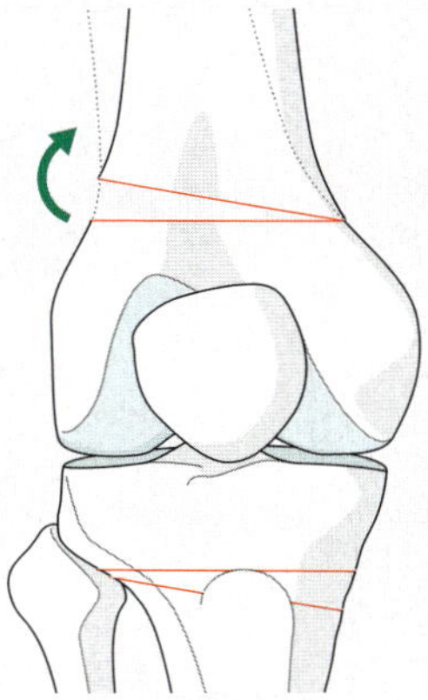

Fig 9.3.10-3 Planning of double osteotomy. Double osteotomy of 15° will create slight varus alignment with normal knee joint line orientation. Intraarticular release aimed at improvement of range of motion

Equipment

- LISS-DF, 5 holes
- Locking head screws (LHS)
- Tomofix tibial head plate, medial, proximal, 4 holes
- Sawguide
- Rigid whole leg alignment bar
- Simple ruler (for measurement of osteotomy gap)

(Size of system, instruments, and implants can vary according to anatomy.)

Patient preparation and positioning

Prophylactic antibiotics: single dose 2nd generation cephalosporin

Thrombosis prophylaxis: low-molecular heparin

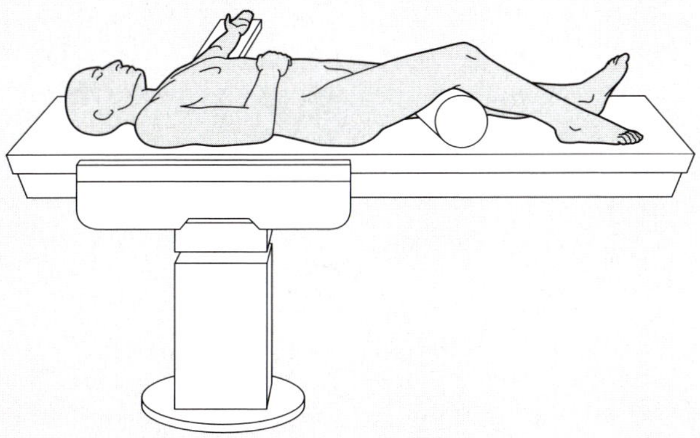

Fig 9.3.10-4 Supine position. Whole leg freely moveable and accessible with the image intensifier. Full leg draped free. Sterile or nonsterile pneumatic tourniquet high on the femur.

2 Surgical approach

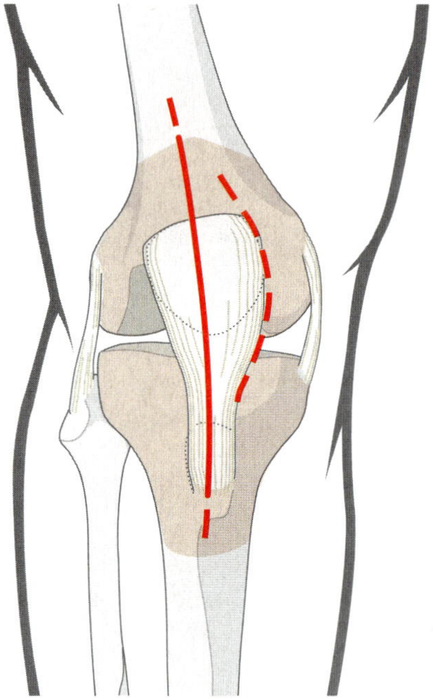

Existing scar of previous arthrotomy extended distally to expose the proximal, medial part of the tibia. Small arthrotomy to remove osteophytes in the notch of the lateral compartment. Closure of arthrotomy.

Tibial approach: blunt Hohmann retractor positioned posteriorly (subperiosteally) on the tibia, cranial of the pes anserinus tendons, and retractor exposing the anterior part of the tibia.

Femur approach: blunt Hohmann retractor positioned posteriorly (subperiosteally) on the femur and sharp Hohmann retractor positioned anteriorly on the femur.

Fig 9.3.10-5 Standard longitudinal approach with medial parapatellar capsular incision (Payer) used because of the scar from the previous arthrotomy, and anticipated total joint replacement in case of progressive OA in the future.

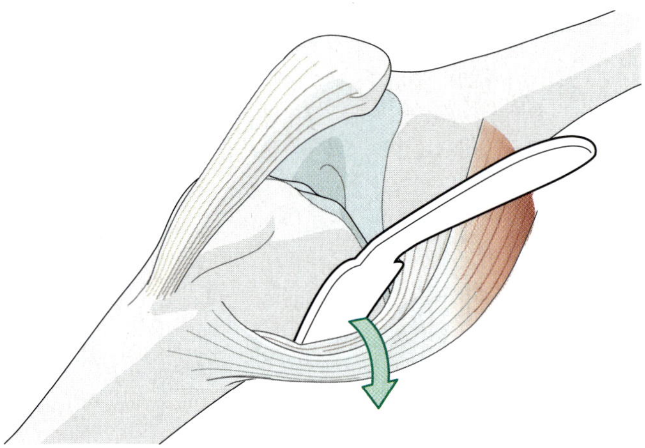

Fig 9.3.10-6 Medial approach to the medial proximal tibia and retractor.

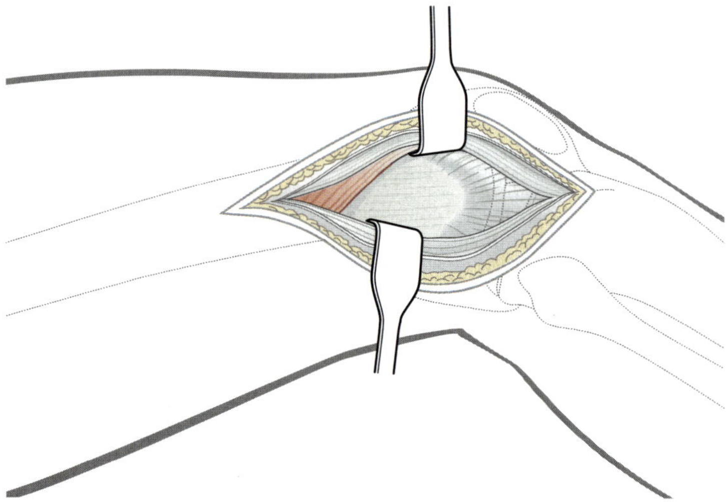

Fig 9.3.10-7 Lateral approach to the femur through a longitudinal incision.

3 Closing wedge tibial osteotomy

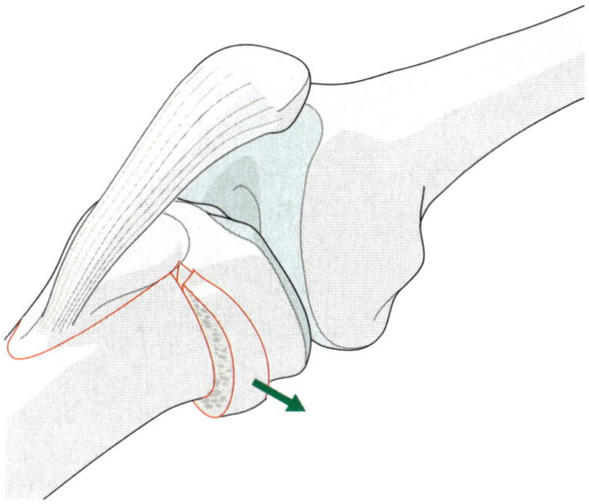

Fig 9.3.10-8 Osteotomy direction. Distally tuberosity osteotomy in the area of planned wedge removal. Tibial osteotomy: oblique starting medially and ending in the lateral proximal tibia approximately 1 cm inside the lateral cortex.

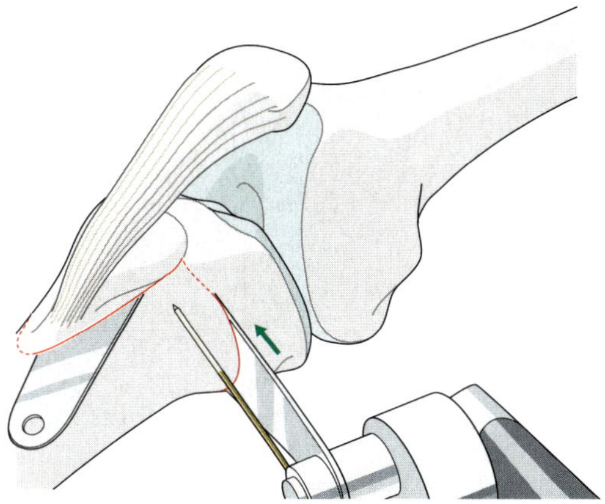

Fig 9.3.10-9 The distal tuberosity osteotomy is made and a small saw blade is positioned in the osteotomy to protect the tuberosity during the tibial osteotomy.
For precise wedge planning K-wire positioning at the planned correction angle and an aiming device, or a combined aiming and sawguide, is helpful. The sawguide is positioned over the planned osteotomy area and fixed to the bone with K-wires under image intensifier control.

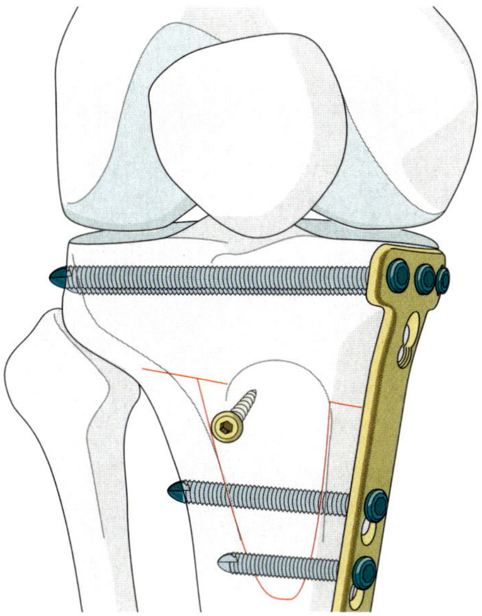

Fig 9.3.10-10 Both saw cuts are made with a new saw blade under intense rinsing with retractors protecting anterior and posterior soft tissues. Wedge removal and closure of the tibial osteotomy.

Plate fixation. Subcutaneous plate positioning over the soft tissues with proximal bicortical fixation with three LHS and distal fixation with one bicortical LHS and three monocortical LHS. A lag screw is used to fix the tuberosity osteotomy.

4 Open wedge femur osteotomy

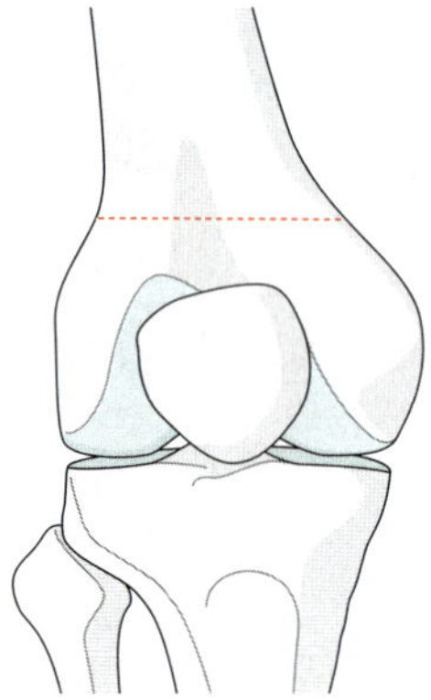

Fig 9.3.10-11 Osteotomy direction. Positioning of blunt Hohmann retractor subperiosteally posteriorly on the distal femur and anteriorly on the distal femur. Femur osteotomy: oblique starting lateral and ending in the medial femur condyle just inside the medial cortex. Saw direction and saw depth is verified with a K-wire under image intensifier control.

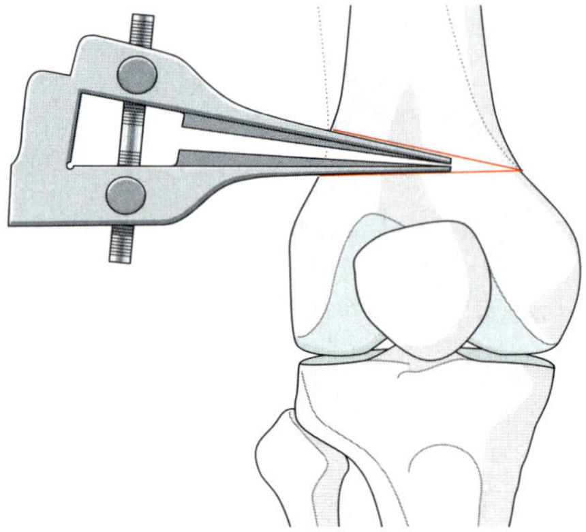

Fig 9.3.10-13 Opening of the wedge with a calibrated wedge spreader and correction to neutral leg alignment is checked with a rigid alignment bar. The size of the opened wedge is measured with a ruler.

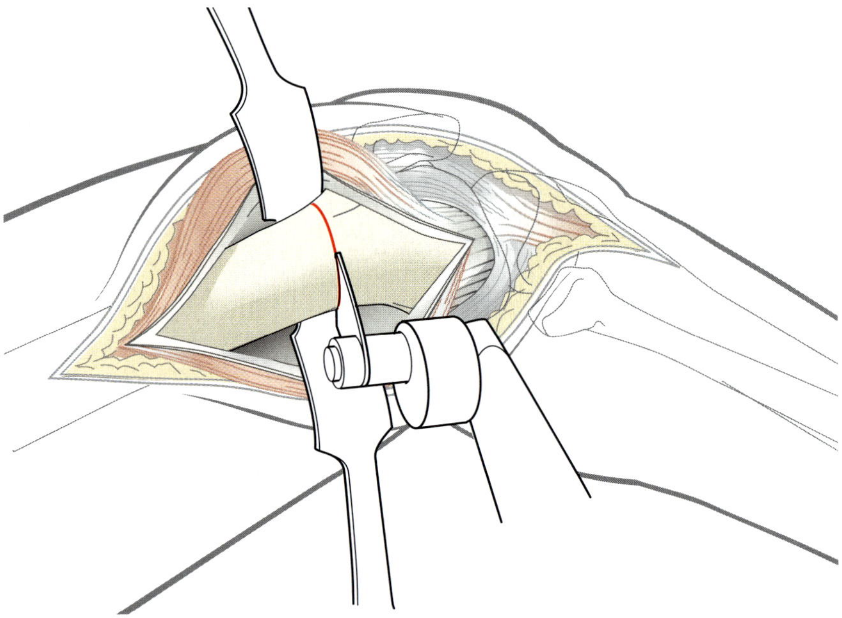

Fig 9.3.10-12 A saw cut is made under intense rinsing with retractors protecting anterior and posterior soft tissues.

4 Open wedge femur osteotomy (cont)

Removal of wedge spreader, positioning of a bone spreader and opening of the wedge to the size previously measured with the ruler. Part of the bone wedge removed from the proximal tibia is now inserted into the gap prepared.

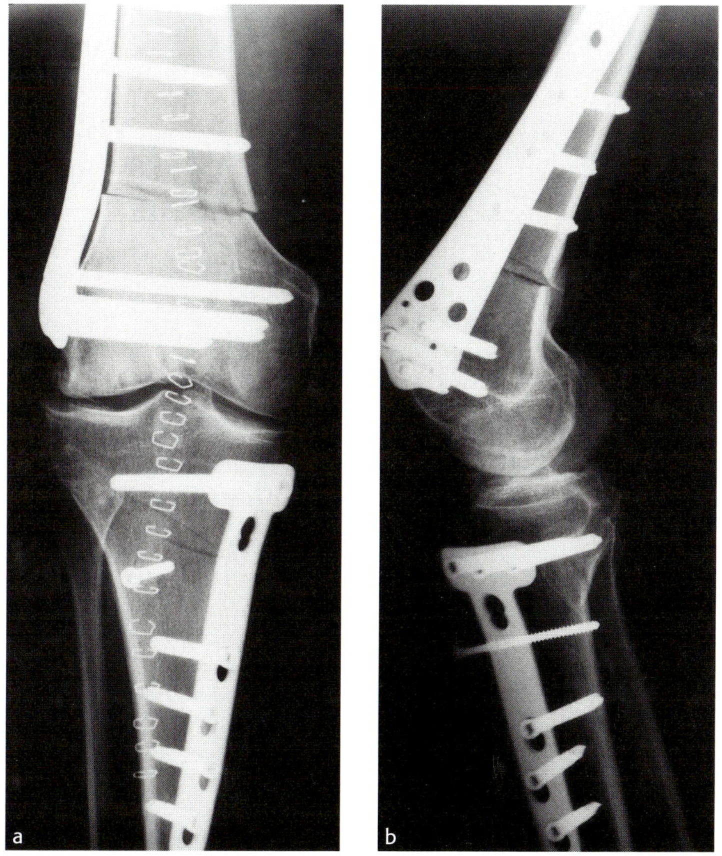

Fig 9.3.10-14a–b Fixation of the LISS-DF plate proximally with three bicortical locking head screws and distally with four locking head screws.

5 Rehabilitation

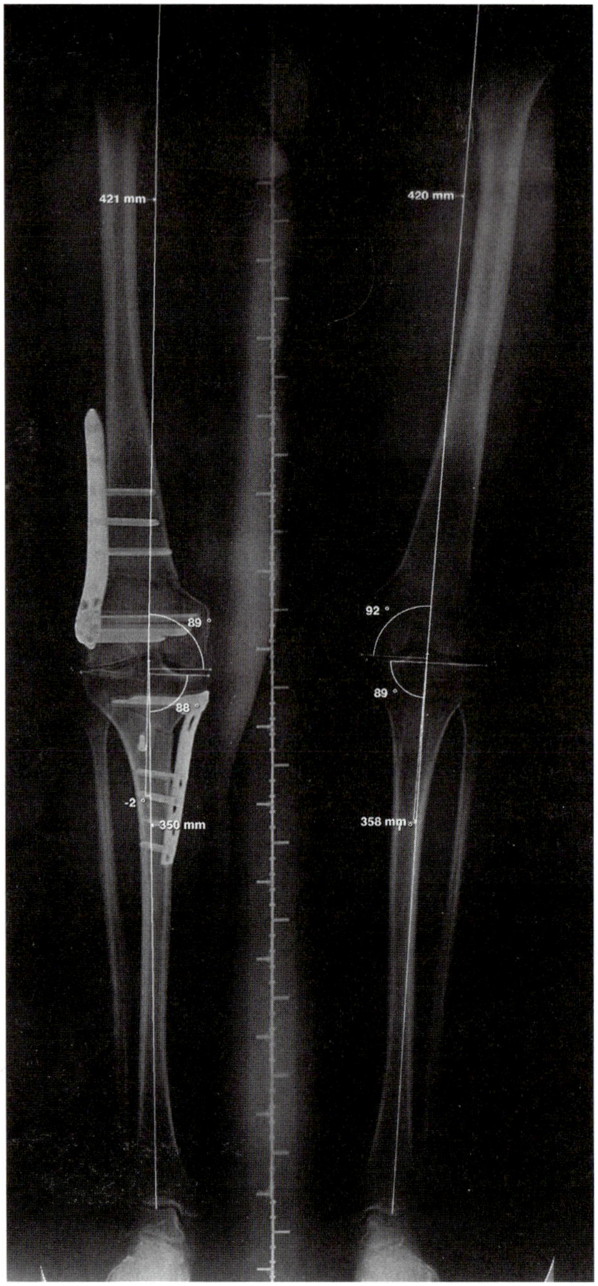

Fig 9.3.10-15 Leg alignment postoperatively.

No additional immobilization.

Weight bearing: 15 kg with two elbow crutches until 6–8 weeks postoperatively. After that, full weight bearing depending on bone healing.

Physiotherapy: from 1st postoperative day functional postoperative treatment with active assisted movement with a physiotherapist, active extension and flexion to 90° allowed. After wound healing, active flexion and extension as tolerated.

Pharmaceutical treatment: pain medication if needed, antithrombotic medication

X-rays to evaluate bone healing after 6 weeks, 12 weeks, 24 weeks, and 1 year.

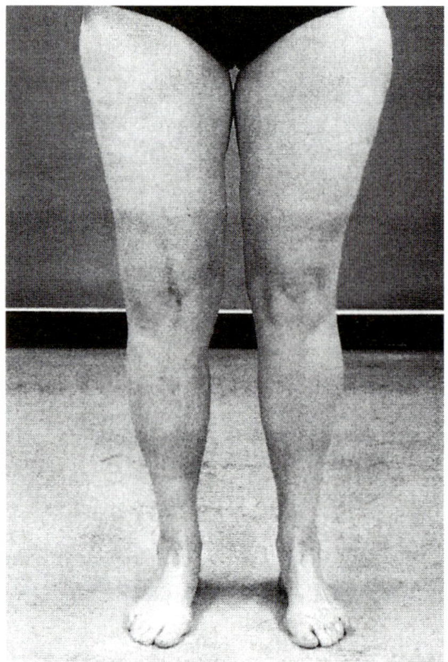

Fig 9.3.10-16 Leg alignment postoperatively at 3 months. Neutral leg alignment. Knee range of motion 115-0-0.

5 Rehabilitation (cont)

Implant removal one year postoperatively through the existing scars if the implants are disturbing the patient (after full consolidation).

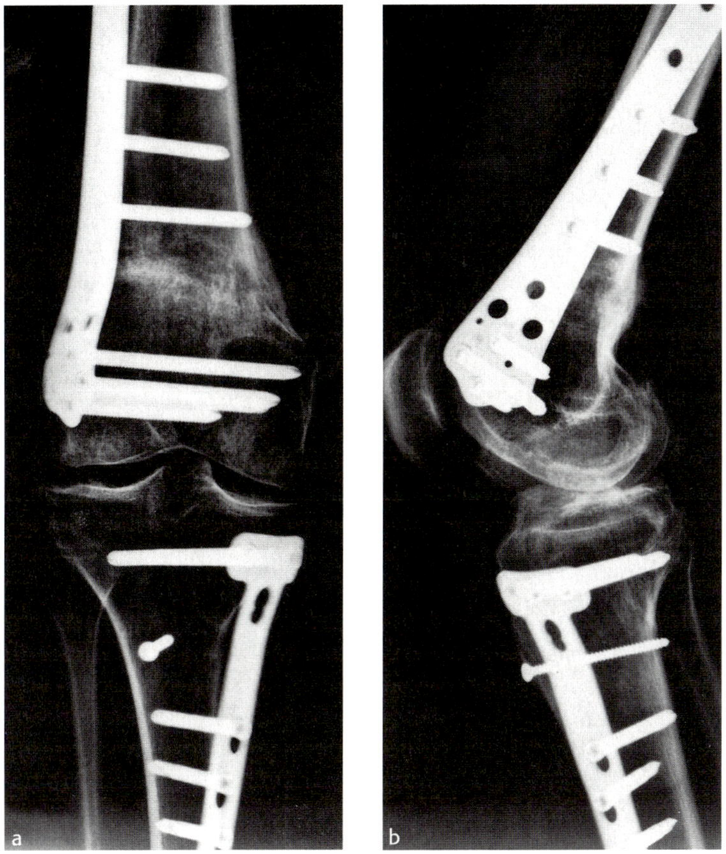

Fig 9.3.10-17a–b X-rays after full consolidation.
a AP view.
b Lateral view.

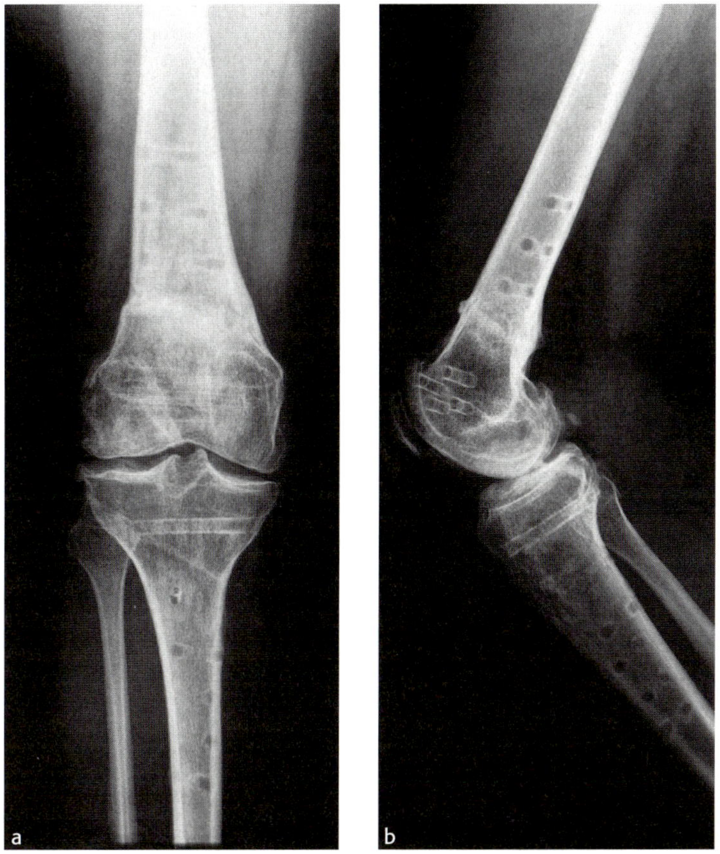

Fig 9.3.10-18a–b X-rays after implant removal.
a AP view.
b Lateral view.

6 Pitfalls –

Planning

Deformities of the proximal femur and distal tibia may exaggerate the bone deformity measured at the distal femur and proximal tibia. Ligament laxity at the knee joint may add to the whole leg deformity.
Planning of osteotomies without taking into account the joint line obliquity may produce shear forces at the knee joint.

Range of motion and angular correction constraints

Intra- and extraarticular constraints to range of motion may prevent joint motion and deformity correction specifically in contracted deformities. Osteophytes in the notch and at the intercondylar eminence may mechanically constrain an angular correction.

Osteotomy and fixation

Osteotomy must be preferably incomplete (intact lateral cortex on the tibia and medial cortex on the femur) for maximum construct stability of the osteotomy and plate fixation.

7 Pearls +

Planning

Deformity analysis of the whole leg will reveal bone deformities at proximal and distal parts of the bones as well as ligament laxities due to abnormality of the joint line congruence angle. Osteotomy corrections that aim to restore the normal values of the tibia and femur will reveal the need to perform a double osteotomy and will prevent excessive joint line obliquity.

Range of motion and angular correction constraints

Intra- and extraarticular capsular release will enlarge range of motion and enhance deformity correction in contracted deformities. Removal of osteophytes in an arthroscopic or open procedure will remove these restraints to angular correction.

Osteotomy and fixation

In case of fracture of the contralateral cortex, compression can be exerted on this cortex by a lag screw positioned in the combihole next to the osteotomy and by additional bicortical screw fixation.

10.1 Tibia and fibula, proximal

Cases

Cases (cont)

Case		Classification	Method	Implant used	Implant function	Page
10.1.10	Complete articular multifragmentary proximal tibial fracture and avulsion fracture of the fibular head	41-C3	compression and locked splinting	LCP T-plate 4.5/5.0	lag screws and locked internal fixator and protection plate	673
10.1.11	Inversed Y-fracture of the tibial head with impression of the anterolateral joint surface	41-C3	compression and locked splinting	LCP L-plate 4.5/5.0	lag screws and locked internal fixator and protection plate	677

10 Tibia and fibula

Author Michael Wagner

10.1 Tibia and fibula, proximal

1 Incidence

Fractures of the tibial plateau are increasing in incidence because of their relationship to sports and traffic accidents (4.83% of the total).

Tibial plateau fractures are fractures occurring above the tibial tuberosity and involving the tibial condyles. They represent 1% of all fractures overall but are more common in the elderly, comprising 8% of all fractures in that population. Tibial plateau fractures are articular fractures most commonly involving the lateral plateau.

The frequency of tibial plateau fractures is higher in older women than in older men, because of the greater incidence of osteoporosis in women.

When they occur in younger patients, most of these fractures are due to high-energy trauma. The most common mechanism is a strong valgus force coupled with axial loading, which subsequently drives the femoral condyles into the tibial plateau, producing the fracture. These injuries are sometimes referred to as "car bumper injuries," because the most common setting in which they occur is when the bumper of a car strikes the lower leg.

While high-energy trauma is the rule in tibial plateau fractures in the young, the elderly may sustain fatigue and stress fractures of the tibial plateau with minimal or even no identified trauma. These fractures are usually the result of compressive forces acting on osteoporotic bone. In fact, any hemarthrosis of the knee occurring in an elderly person should be assumed to be a tibial plateau fracture until proven otherwise.

Fractures of the tibial plateau are commonly accompanied by damage to the collateral ligaments, a fact easily explained by examining the major mechanisms of injury. Avulsion fractures of the lateral tibial plateau are accompanied by a concurrent ACL rupture in 75% to 100% of cases. This special type

2 Classification

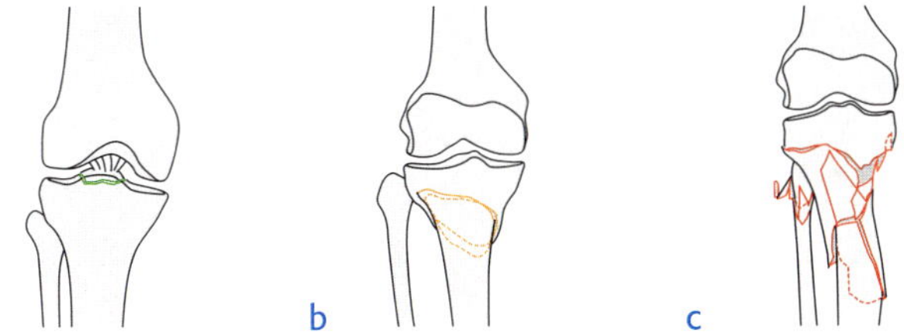

a b c

Fig 10.1-1a–c 43-A Extraarticular fractures.
a 41-A1 Avulsion
b 41-A2 Metaphyseal simple
c 41-A3 Metaphyseal multifragmentary

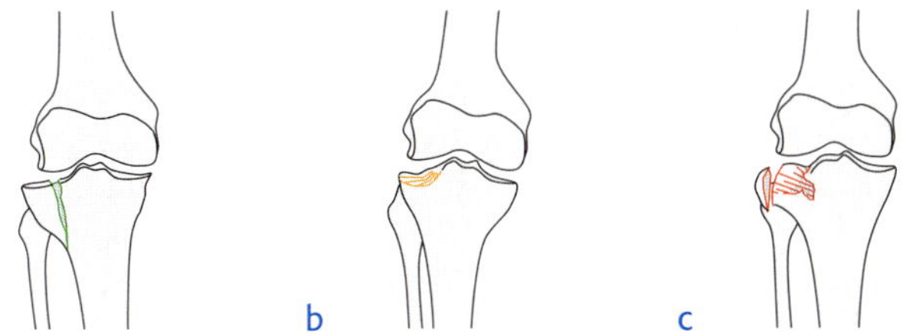

a b c

Fig 10.1-2a–c 43-B Partial articular fractures.
a 41-B1 Pure split
b 41-B2 Pure depression
c 41-B3 Split-depression

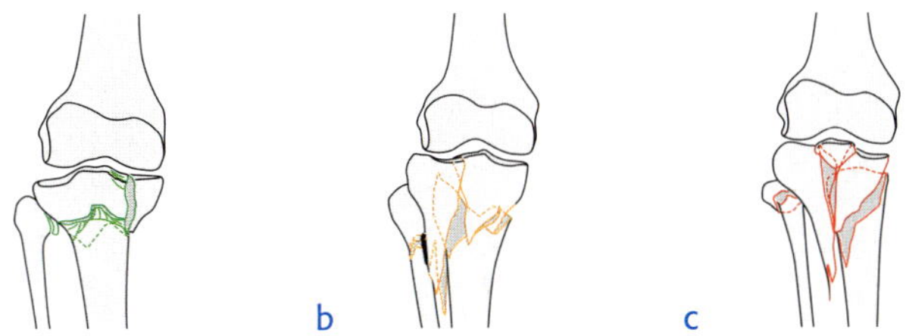

a b c

Fig 10.1-3a–c 43-C Complete articular fractures.
a 41-C1 Articular simple, metaphyseal simple
b 41-C2 Articular simple, metaphyseal multifragmentary
c 41-C3 Articular multifragmentary

of tibial plateau fracture usually occurs in sporting events and is due to mechanisms of injury that produce knee flexion, excessive internal rotation, and varus stress.

3 Treatment methods

The aims of surgery are:
- to restore articular congruity, joint stability, and the original knee axis;
- to provide fracture stability allowing for early painfree movement of the knee and mobilization of the patient;
- to obtain full functional recovery as the long term goal;
- to avoid posttraumatic arthritis.

Anatomical reduction and complete restoration of the height of both tibial plateaus should be attempted in all instances. This may be difficult with bone loss, in severely displaced AO type C fractures, or when delayed reconstruction is necessary.

Nonoperative treatment. In undisplaced fractures, nonoperative treatment may be a safe alternative. This principle may also be of value for aged and bedridden patients. Varus/valgus stability on physical examination indicates that limb alignment will be assured upon fracture healing. Patients who present with a low risk of developing arthritis may also be good candidates for nonoperative treatment.

Extraarticular fractures (41-A)

Most of these fractures benefit from operative stabilization even if not greatly displaced or unstable. Different methods have been described, but due to the short proximal segment and the biomechanical problems described above, plates providing angular stability are preferred; they can usually be applied with minimal or no exposure of the fracture focus. Early reports about the clinical use of the LISS plate and LCP have shown promising results regarding fracture union, infection rate and secondary loss of reduction. The fracture must be reduced before fixation. This is achieved with the help of the large distractor and reduction clamps placed on the main fracture fragments through small incisions. Sometimes, additional lag screws or a medial plate are needed to stabilize isolated fragments.

Timing in fractures with severe soft-tissue damage is critical because there is a high risk of wound healing problems. To avoid this, external fixation as a primary temporary stabilization is performed. The fixation frame may bridge the knee joint or is placed on the tibial plateau allowing knee motion. After soft tissue conditioning, the external frame is replaced by internal fixation. As an alternative, the hybrid external fixator may be applied.

Intramedullary nailing

Conventional intramedullary nails are not really suited to the stabilization of proximal tibial fractures. Some new nail designs, eg, the expert tibia nail have up to five interlocking options proximally. Furthermore, the proximal locking screw can be fixed in position by the blocking end cap, thus providing angular stability. The proximal fracture must be reduced before nail insertion.

Articular fractures

Lateral plateau—split fractures (41-B1)

Pure split fractures (41-B1) may be treated by immediate lag screw fixation. In order to ascertain that no further displacement has occured, arthroscopic control may be useful. Two large cancellous screws with washers are used for fixation. A third screw with a washer is recommended in an antiglide position.

Lateral plateau—pure impaction fracture (41-B2)

If available, intraoperative CT scanning is to be preferred to ascertain complete reduction and secure fixation with screws.

Lateral plateau—split-depression fractures (41-B3)

Fixation is best achieved by a plate. Lag screws may be inserted independently and/or through the plate. These fractures are also good indications for the LISS, or special plates that a low “rafting” of screws to support the impacted joint surface

Medial plateau fractures (41-B2.2/B3.2)

Reduction may be obtained with the large “King Kong” forceps percutaneously and even the insertion of screws and /or a buttress plate may be done through small incisions posteromedially.

Bicondylar fractures (41-C)

Many of these fractures will require an initial joint-spanning external fixator while the soft tissues settle.

Percutaneous reduction with a large forceps may be attempted in pure split fractures. ORIF should be performed to achieve anatomical reduction and stable fixation. Plates providing angular stability (Tibia LISS plate or LCP) appear to be especially suited for these more complex type C2 and C3 fractures. The anatomic proximal tibial locking plate can be used as a buttress, usually does not require contouring and can provide angular stability. Initial lag-screw fixation of the articular block prior to plate application is essential, while any metaphyseal or diaphyseal comminution may be bridged with a long locking plate.

4 Implant overview

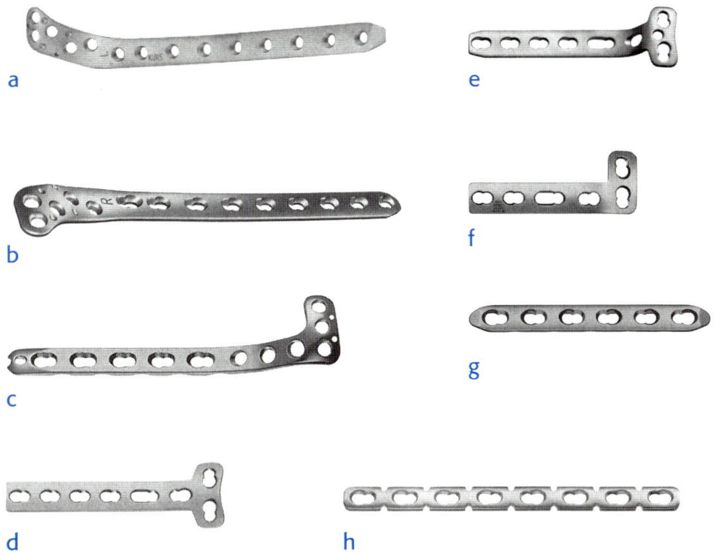

Fig 10.1-4a–h
- a LISS-PLT 5.0 (left and right version available)
- b LCP-PLT 4.5/5.0 (left and right version available)
- c LCP proximal tibial plate 4.5/5.0 (lateral left and lateral right version available)
- d LCP T-plate 4.5/5.0
- e LCP T-buttress plate 4.5/5.0
- f LCP L-buttress plate 4.5/5.0 (left and right version available)
- g LCP 4.5/5.0, narrow
- h LCP reconstruction plate 4.5/5.0

5 Suggestions for further reading

Bennett WF, Browner B (1994) Tibial plateau fractures: a study of associated soft tissue injuries. *J Orthop Trauma;* 8:1838. 8(3):183–188.
Cole PA, Zlowodzki M, Kregor PJ (2003) Compartment pressures after submuscular fixation of proximal tibia fractures. *Injury;* 34(Suppl 1-A):436.
Tscherne H, Lobenhoffer Ph (1993) Tibial plateau fractures. *Clin Orthop;* 292:87–100.
Shepard L, Abdollahi K, Lee J, et al (2002) The prevalence of soft tissue injuries in nonoperative tibial plateau fractures as determined by magnetic resonance imaging. *J Orthop Trauma;* 16:628–631.
Chan P, Klimkiewicz J, Lucketti W, et al (1997) Impact of CT scan on treatment plan and fracture classification of tibial plateau fractures. *J Orthop Trauma;* (11):484–489.
Brophy D, O'Malley M, Lui D, et al (1996) MR imaging of tibial plateau fractures. *Clin Radiol;* 51(12):873–878.
Yacoubian SV, Nevins RT, Sallis JG, et al (2002) Impact of MRI on treatment plan and fracture classification of tibial plateau fractures. *J Orthop Trauma;* 16:632–637.
Weber WN, Neumann CH, Barakos JA, et al (1991) Lateral tibia rim (Segond) fractures: MR imaging characteristics. *Radiology;* 180-3:731–734.
Bai B, Kummer FJ, Sala DA, et al (2001) Effect of articular step-off and meniscectomy on joint alignment and contact pressures for fractures of the lateral tibial plateau. *J Orthop Trauma;* 15:101–106.
Martinez A, Sarmento A, Latta LL (2003) Closed fractures of the proximal tibia treated with a function brace. *Clin Orthop;* 417:293–302.
Georgialis G (1994) Combined anterior and posterior approaches for complex tibial plateau fractures. *J Bone Joint Surg [Br];* 76(2):285–289.
Duwelius PJ, Rangitsch MR, Colville MR, et al (1997) Treatment of tibial fractures by limited internal fixation. *Clin Orthop;* 339:47–57.
Russell T, Leighton R, Bucholz R, et al (2004) The gold standard in tibial plateau fractures? A multicentre randomized study of bone graft versus Alpha-BSM. Presented at OTA Meeting, Hollywood, Florida.
Gosling T, Schandelmaier P, Müller M, et al (2005) Single lateral locked screw plating of bicondylar tibial plateau fractures. *Clin Orthop Relat Res*; 439:207–214.
Court-Brown CM, McBirnie J (1995) The epidemiology of tibial fractures. *J Bone Joint Surg [Br]*; 77:417–421.
Hansen M, Rommens PM (2002) The proximal extraarticular tibial fracture. *Unfallchirurg*; 105:851–872.
Schutz M, Kaab MJ, Haas N (2003) Stabilization of proximal tibial fractures with the LISS System; early clinical experience in Berlin. *Injury*; 34(Suppl 1-A):30–35.
Wagner M (2003) General principles for the clinical use of the LCP: *Injury*; 34(Suppl 1-B):31–45.
Bono CM, Levine RG, Rao JP, et al (2001) Nonarticular proximal tibia fractures: treatment options and decision making. *J Am Acad Orthop Surg*; 9-3:176–186.
Roberts CS, Dodds JC, et al (2003) Hybrid external fixation of proximal tibia: strategies to improve frame stability. *J Orthop Trauma*; 17:415–420.
Cole JD (1998) Intramedullary fixation of proximal tibia fractures. *Techniques in orthopaedics*; 13:27–37.
Krettek C, Miclau T, Schandelmaier P, et al (1999) The mechanical effect of blocking screws („Poller screws") in stabilizing tibia fractures with short proximal or distal fragments after insertion of small diameter intramedullary nails. *J Orthop Trauma*; 13:550–553.
Buchko G, Johnson D (1996) Arthroscopy assisted operative management of tibial plateau fractures. *Clin Orthop*; 332:29–36.
Biyani A, Reddy NS, Chaudhury J, et al (1995) The result of surgical management of displaced tibial plateau fractures in the elderly. *Injury*; 26-5:291–295.
Stevens DG, Beharry R, McKee MD, et al (2001) The long-term functional outcome of operatively treated tibial plateau fractures. *J Orthop Trauma*; 15:312–320.
Honkonen S (1995) Degenerative arthritis after tibial plateau fractures. *J Orthop Trauma*; 9:273–277.

Authors Michael J Gardner, Dean G Lorich, David L Helfet

10.1.1 Postoperative nonunion after extraarticular metaphyseal multifragmentary proximal tibial fracture—41-A3

1 Case description

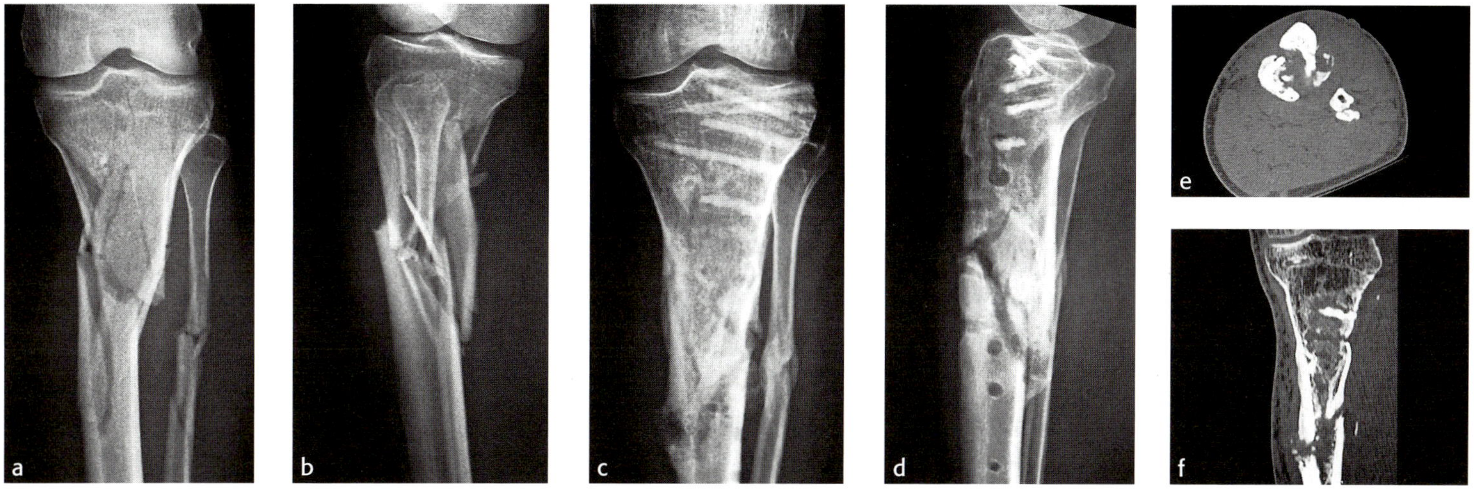

Fig 10.1.1-1a–f
a–b Extraarticular proximal tibial and fibular fracture.
c–d Following treatment with a LISS plate, the implant was removed 9 months later and revealed a nonunion.
e–f To further characterize the nonunion pattern, a CT scan was obtained and confirmed lack of bony bridging.

50-year-old construction worker, with a significant smoking history, fell 5 meters from scaffolding. Sustained a multifragmentary fracture of the proximal tibia and fibula. Other injuries included contralateral 2nd and 3rd metatarsal and cuneiform fractures and an L3 burst fracture without retropulsion of the fragments into the spinal canal or neurologic symptoms.
The soft-tissue envelope had significant swelling. Moderate ecchymosis was present. There were no signs of compartment syndrome or evidence of neurological or vascular injury. He was treated initially with a LISS plate, and 9 months postoperatively he complained of persistent pain along the distal extent of the plate.
A CT scan was obtained and he was diagnosed with a nonunion.

Indication

Absence of complete healing 9 months postoperatively requires take down of the nonunion and revision open reduction, internal fixation, and bone grafting to stimulate fracture healing.

Preoperative planning

Equipment

- LCP proximal tibial plate 4.5/5.0, 11 holes
- LCP reconstruction plate 3.5, 6 holes
- Locking head screws (LHS)
- Threaded 2.0 mm K-wires
- Pelvic reduction forceps
- Synthetic bone substitute

(Size of system, instruments, and implants can vary according to anatomy.)

Patient preparation and positioning

After intraoperative cultures have been taken, give antibiotics; 2nd generation cephalosporins

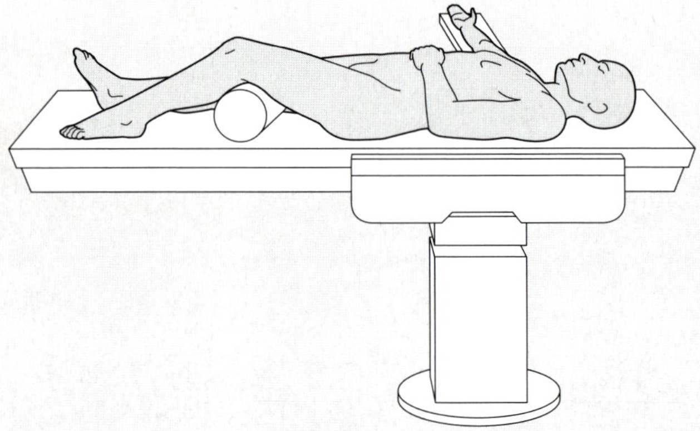

Fig 10.1.1-2 Position the patient supine on the operating room table. Place a tourniquet on the upper thigh. Prepare and drape the leg free and place a towel roll under the knee. Position the image intensifier to ensure adequate AP and lateral views.

2 Surgical approach

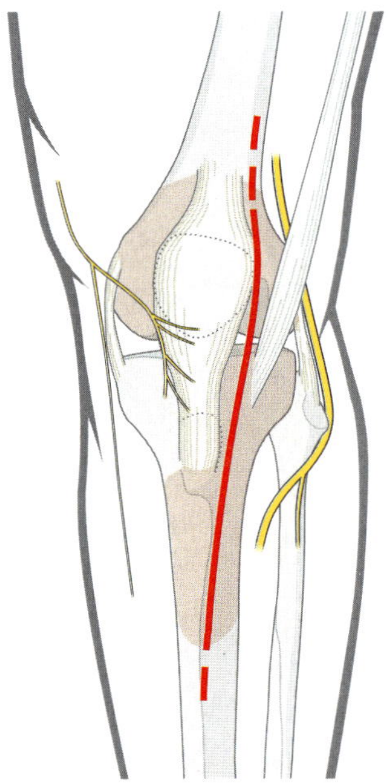

Fig 10.1.1-3 Use the same incision as was used previously—make a straight incision over the lateral proximal tibia extending distally approximately 10 cm.
Raise full-thickness flaps down to the fascia.
Follow the investing fascia of the anterior compartment medially to the tibial crest, and sharply elevate the entire compartment from the anterolateral tibial surface without violating the compartment.
Remove the previous implant and debride the fibrous nonunion back to bleeding bone surfaces.

3 Reduction and fixation

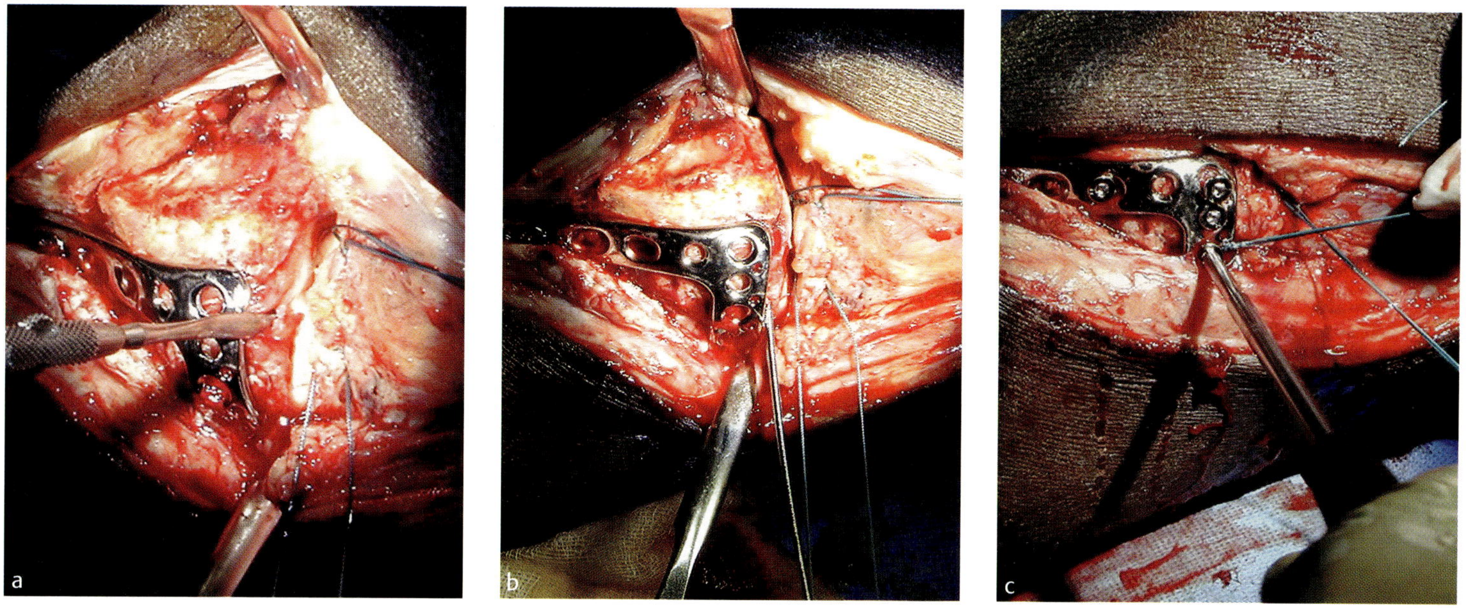

Fig 10.1.1-4a–c Attempt to manually reduce the fracture under image intensification guidance.

Often, the fibula will be healed and will impede reduction of the tibia. In this case, make a separate lateral incision over the previous fibula fracture site. Connect drill holes with an osteotome to make an oblique osteotomy.

Ensure the tibia can be reduced and compressed under direct visualization.

Place a long LCP proximal tibial plate over the lateral surface of the tibia. Use a cortex screw for compression first and secure it proximally to the bone, then use locking head screws in the proximal limb of the plate. Use a reduction clamp to reduce the distal fragment to the lateral plate to restore proper axis and alignment in the coronal plane.

Next, place a straight 3.5 locking reconstruction plate on the anterior surface of the tibia, and secure it distally with a 3.5 mm cortex screw to indirectly reduce the fracture in the sagittal plane.

Use a large pointed reduction forceps from the distally fixed anterior plate to the lateral plate which has been fixed proximally to compress across the fracture site.

With the fracture reduced, use lag screws through the anterior plate and eccentric cortex screws through the lateral plate to apply additional compression. Place another cortex screw in the anterior plate distal to the fracture site, and space out locking head screws at the ends of the plate.

Finally, place one or two locking head screws percutaneously in the distal end of the lateral plate for definitive fixation.

Pack the nonunion site with demineralized bone matrix mixed with bone graft.

Close wounds over suction drains, and apply a soft bulky dressing with a locked hinged knee brace.

Place the patient in a plaster short leg splint and knee immobilizer.

4 Rehabilitation

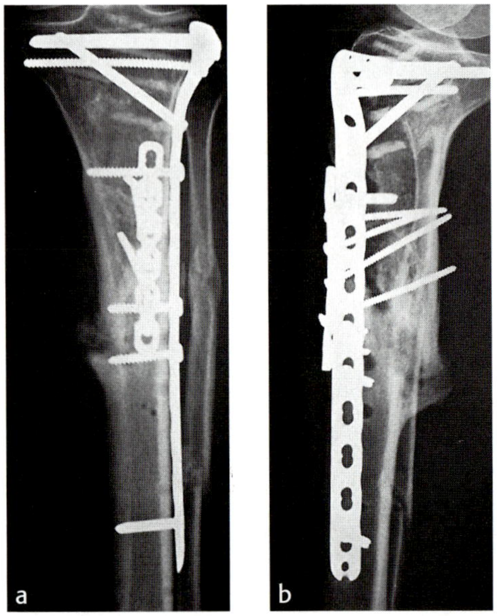

Postoperatively, initiate low-molecular weight heparin for deep venous thrombosis prophylaxis.
Continue antibiotic therapy for 24–48 hours until cultures are negative.
Apply a hinged knee brace locked in extension initially for patient comfort, which may be unlocked while the patient is in bed.
On day 1 or 2 postoperatively, begin passive and active assisted range of motion and quadriceps strengthening exercises supervised by a physical therapist.
The patient should be kept touch-down weight bearing for at least 6 weeks, and progressed slowly to full weight bearing over the next 8–12 weeks.
When quadriceps control returns, the brace may be discontinued.

Fig 10.1.1-5a–b 4 months following open reduction, nonunion takedown, revision plating, and bone grafting, the fracture shows signs of healing.

Implant removal

If the implant is prominent, consider removing the fixation at least 18–24 months after the procedure. Protected weight bearing and bracing should be instituted for 6–8 weeks following removal.

5 Pitfalls –

Equipment
The locking head screw heads may become jammed in the screw holes during insertion.

Reduction and fixation
When inserting a screw into hole 10 or higher (more distal from the plateau), the superficial peroneal nerve may be injured.
The anterior tibial vessels may be tented by the distal tip of the plate.

Rehabilitation
Fractures about the knee, particularly nonunions in which knee motion may have been limited for prolonged periods, are often associated with some degree of arthrofibrosis.

6 Pearls +

Equipment
Insert the first 2/3 of the screw under power and seat the screw using a torque-limited screwdriver.

Reduction and fixation
When using a plate longer than 10 holes, always protect the superficial peroneal nerve or visualize the bone prior to screw insertion. Make sure the distal tip of the plate is flush on the bone to prevent damage to the anterior tibial artery and vein.

Rehabilitation
Initiate passive and active motion as soon as possible, and instruct the patient on the importance of their active role.

Author Christoph Sommer

10.1.2 Tibial plateau fracture—41-B3 and spiral wedge proximal tibial shaft fracture—42-B1

1 Case description

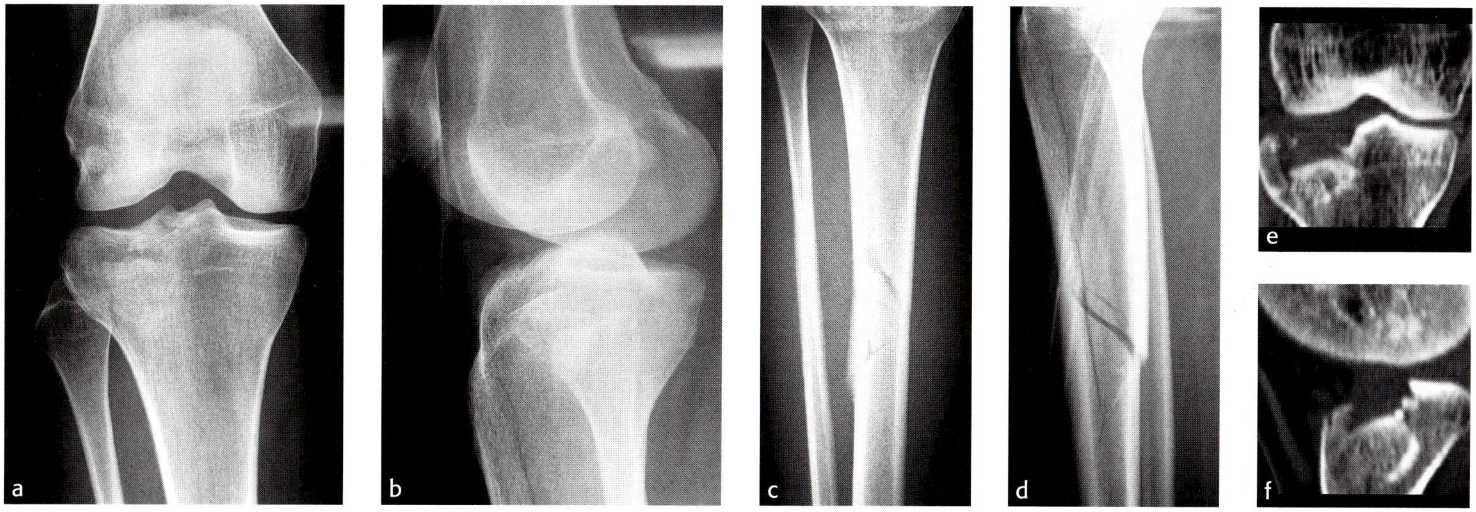

31-year-old woman skier with a torsion valgization trauma of her right lower leg. A combination injury with tibial plateau fracture (41-B3.1) and fracture of the proximal tibial shaft can be seen on the x-ray (wedge fracture, spiral wedge middle section). No soft-tissue injury.

Fig 10.1.2-1a–f
- a AP view of the tibial plateau fracture.
- b Lateral view of the tibial plateau fracture.
- c AP view of the proximal tibial shaft fracture.
- d Lateral view of the proximal tibial shaft fracture.
- e–f A CT scan was obtained for more precise diagnosis and showed a 1–1.5 cm impaction of the anterolateral articular surface.

Indication

The indication for an operative procedure is clear. The impacted joint fracture is treated by open reduction, cancellous bone grafting, and screw osteosynthesis. The shaft fracture on its own would be ideal for a nail osteosynthesis, but since this is a combination fracture, stabilization with a LISS-PLT is ideal. The same approach can be used for both fractures. A nail osteosynthesis would not be ideal because the articular lag screws could interfere with the nail and a second incision would be necessary.

Preoperative planning

Equipment
- LISS-PLT, 13 holes
- 5.0 mm self-tapping locking head screws (LHS)
- 3.5 mm cortex screws
- K-wires

(Size of system, instruments, and implants can vary according to anatomy.)

Patient preparation and positioning
Antibiotics: single dose 2nd generation cephalosporin
Thrombosis prophylaxis: low-molecular heparin

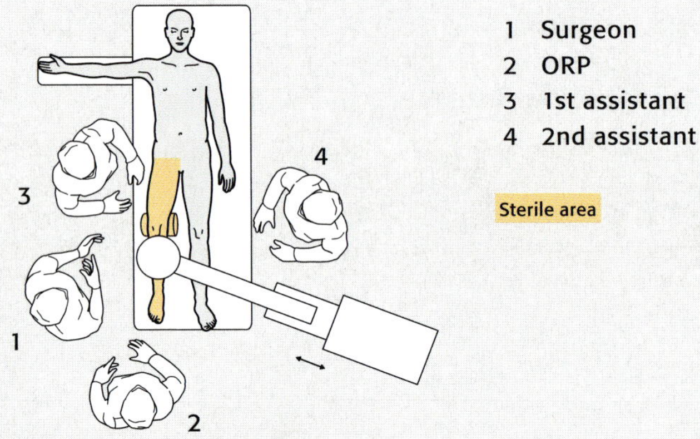

Fig 10.1.2-2 The entire leg is prepared and draped under sterile conditions, including the iliac crest so that cancellous bone can be harvested. The injured leg is extended but is supported below the knee with a metal triangular block or large towel roll, which can be removed as the situation requires.

2 Surgical approach

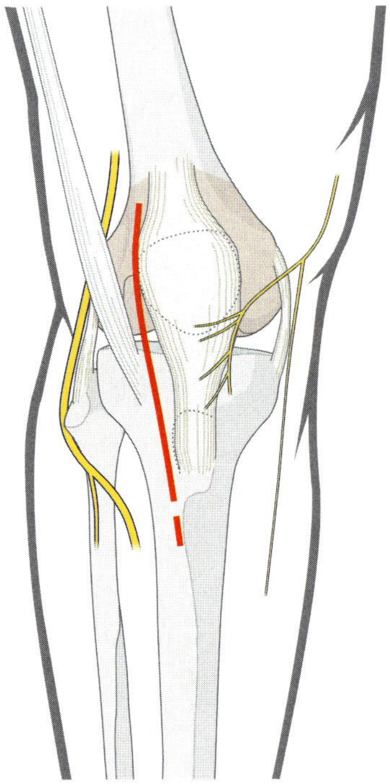

Fig 10.1.2-3 At the level of the tibial head a 6–7 cm long incision arching in an anterior direction is made. The iliotibial tract is divided and detached at Gerdy's tubercle. A submeniscal arthrotomy in the first 2/3 is performed. A good overview of the fracture can be obtained by lifting the meniscus. The meniscal tear is sewn together and lifted cranially with threads.

3 Reduction and fixation

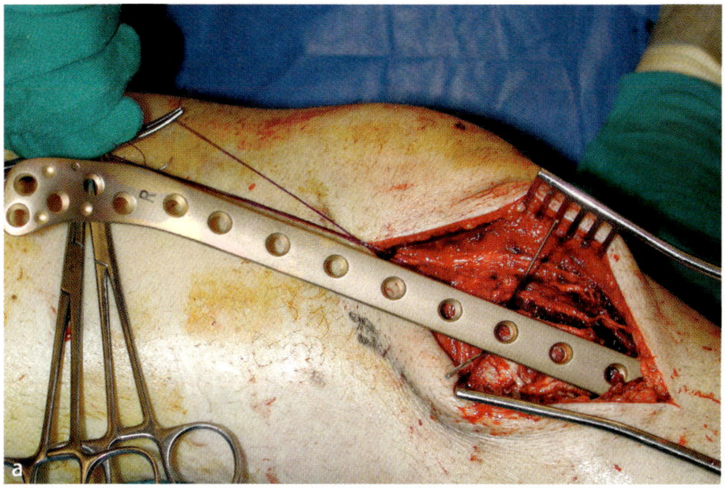

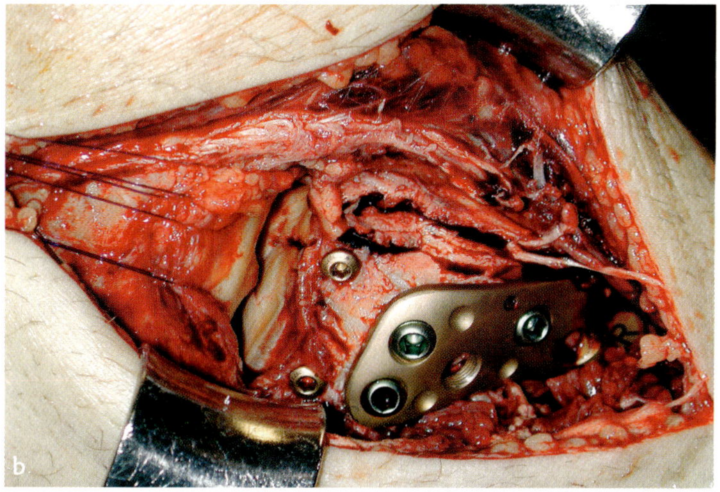

Fig 10.1.2-4a–f First the sagittal fracture split of the lateral plateau is opened by use of a blunt instrument.
After this, the impacted joint fragment can be lifted to the level of the medial joint surface. In the case of a large defect, it should be filled with cancellous bone graft or bone substitute.
The sagittal fracture split is now closed with a medial percutaneously inserted reduction forceps (large Weber forceps or pelvic reduction forceps) and temporarily retained with a K-wire.
After image intensification control, the plateau fracture can be fixed with two 3.5 mm lag screws, inserted close to the articular surface and compressing the lateral wall to the reduced central fragment and medial plateau. Another screw can be inserted from anterior to posterior to provide additional support.

A 13-hole LISS-PLT stabilizes the diaphyseal fracture. The plate is inserted under the anterior tibial muscle either with the insertion guide or by hand.
The reduction of the fracture in this case is easily achieved by manual traction and slight rotational movement on the lower leg. Alternatively, percutaneously inserted reduction forceps can be used (large Weber forceps, reduction forceps). These forceps are best applied after the plate has been inserted and checked under image intensification. Otherwise the reduction forceps can obstruct the insertion of the plate.
The LISS plate is fixed cranially with a locking head screw in one of the two most proximal screw holes. This screw has to be parallel to the articular surface (in AP view).

3 Reduction and fixation (cont)

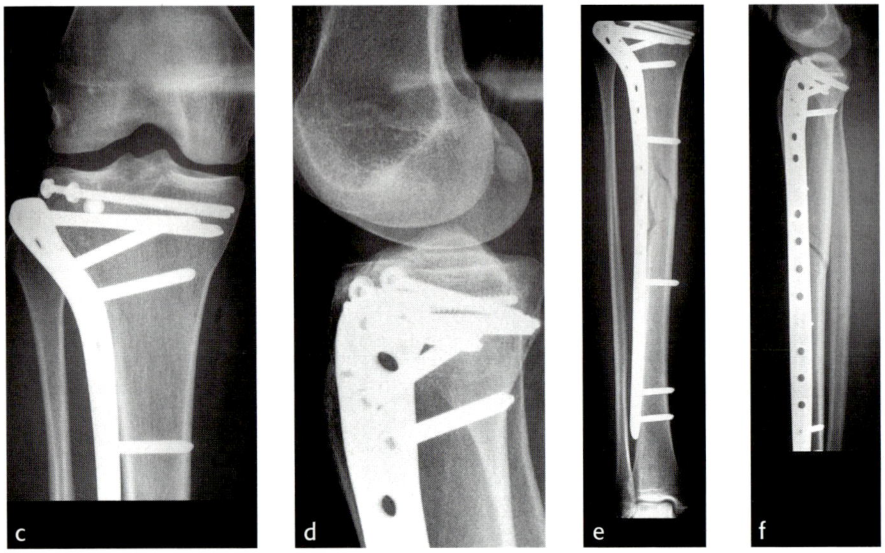

Fig 10.1.2-4a–f (cont) When correct rotational and longitudinal alignment has been achieved, the most distal plate hole is occupied with an LHS to stabilize this position. If the insertion guide is used, self drilling, self-tapping LHS are inserted in the shaft area. If the insertion guide is not being used, bicortical self-tapping LHS are preferred.

At this point an ante- or retrocurvature can still be corrected and therefore examination by image intensifier (lateral view) is carried out.

Depending on the bone quality, the plate is fixed in the tibial head area with four to five LHS. Four to six cortices are used for shaft fixation (four to six monocortical screws or two to three bicortical screws).

4 Rehabilitation

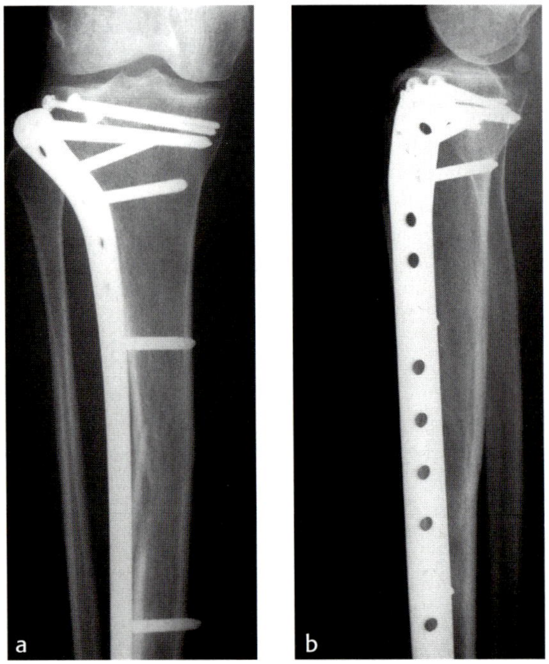

Mobilization started on the third postoperative day with functional treatment. Initial weight bearing was 10–15 kg for 6 weeks, then 30 kg for another 6 weeks. Full weight bearing started after the third month. After 16 months the control x-rays showed good consolidation of the fracture and identical position of the implant. The plate was removed after one year because the patient complained of a slight irritation of the iliotibial tract at the upper part of the plate.

Fig 10.1.2-5a–b X-rays after 16 months showing good consolidation of the fracture.

a AP view.

b Lateral view.

5 Pitfalls –

Equipment

Approach
The anterior tibial artery and the deep peroneal nerve are endangered by drill insertion of the distal percutaneous screws.

Reduction and fixation
If a simple shaft fracture is not precisely reduced, a delayed or nonunion can occur.

Rehabilitation
Noncompliance with early full weight bearing can result in a redislocation of the tibial plateau with collapse of the elevated fragment.

6 Pearls +

Equipment
LISS (or alternativly the LCP-PLT) is an ideal implant for the stabilization of combined injuries of the tibial head and the proximal or mid tibial shaft.

Approach
Both fracture components (partly open tibial plateau, partly percutaneous tibial shaft) can be treated via this small incision.

Reduction and fixation

Rehabilitation
Functional treatment is possible without restriction.

Author Christoph Sommer

10.1.3 Lateral tibial plateau fracture with two additional displaced osteochondral plateau fragments—41-B3

1 Case description

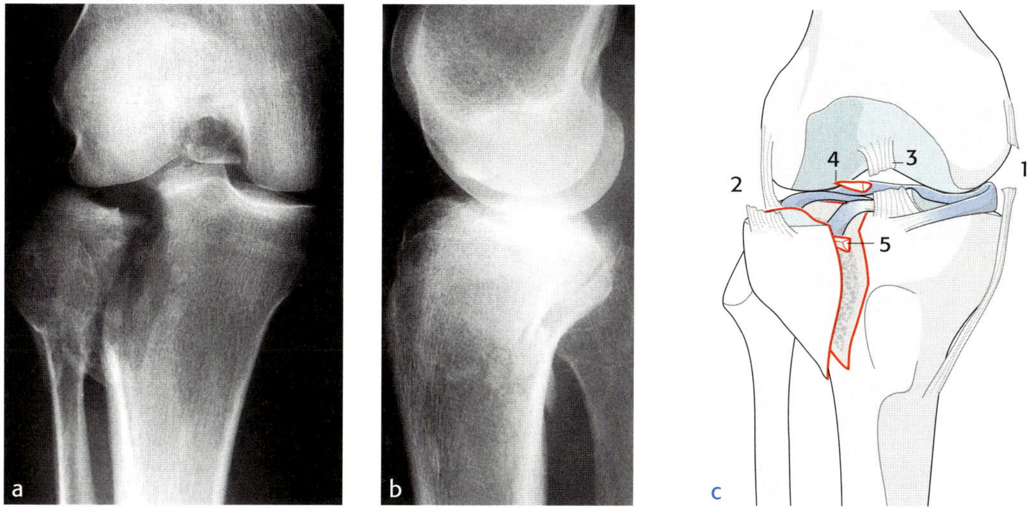

1 Femoral rupture of the MCL
2 Complete rupture of the lateral meniscus
3 Complete rupture of the ACL
4 Small osteochondral fragment
5 Small osteochondral fragment

Fig 10.1.3-1a–c
a AP view.
b Lateral view.
c Drawing of the injured structures.

39-year-old woman suffered a valgization and external rotation trauma while skiing. The x-ray showed a lateral tibial plateau fracture with two additional displaced osteochondral plateau fragments, one situated between the condyles .
The fracture is a 41-B3.1 (partial articular fracture, split depression laterally). Because of the high velocity, an additional ligament component has to be considered. Intraoperative inspection and stability testing after osteosynthesis show the full extent of the damage. Complete rupture of the lateral meniscus and interposition into the fracture zone as well as rupture of the meniscotibial ligaments. The medial collateral ligaments (MCL) and the posterior oblique ligaments (POL) have been completely torn out of the femoral compartment. There is intraligamentous tear of the anterior cruciate ligament (ACL).

Indication

This injury is a clear indication for open reduction of the fracture and treatment of knee damage. A preoperative MRI would show the whole extent of the injury. The preferred approach is the standard anterolateral approach and submeniscal arthrotomy with open reduction under visual control and a lateral supporting osteosynthesis. A medial approach may be required to treat the other knee injuries.

Preoperative planning

Equipment
- LCP T-plate 4.5/5.0, 3 holes
- 5.0 mm self-tapping locking head screws (LHS)
- 6.5 mm cancellous bone screws
- 4.5 mm cortex screws
- K-wires
- Instruments for capsule-ligament fixation

(Size of system, instruments, and implants can vary according to anatomy.)

Patient preparation and positioning
Antibiotics: single dose 2nd generation cephalosporin
Thrombosis prophylaxis: low-molecular heparin

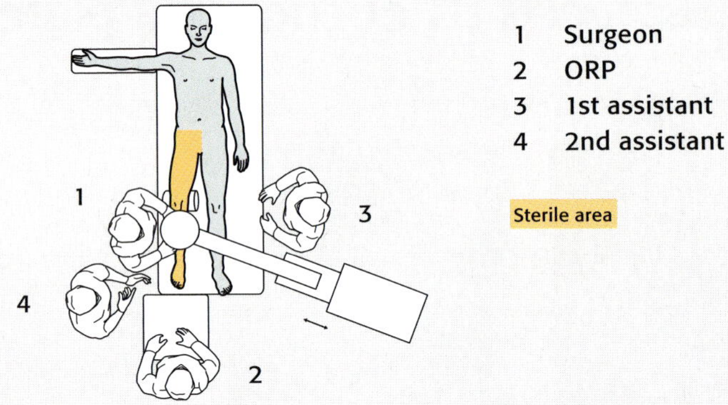

Fig 10.1.3-2 The entire leg is prepared and draped under sterile conditions, including the iliac crest so that cancellous bone can be harvested. The injured leg is extended but is supported below the knee with a metal triangular block or large towel roll, which can be removed as the situation requires.

2 Surgical approach

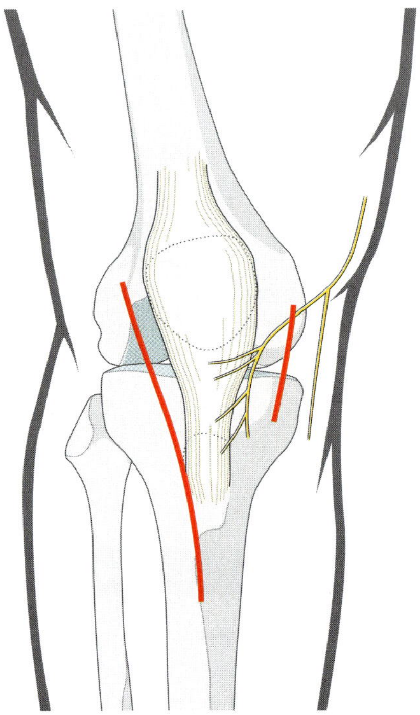

Fig 10.1.3-3 An anterolateral standard approach is performed and the iliotibial tract is divided at the level of the joint. The tract is detached from the lateral tibial head. Additional small medial approach for MCL repair.

3 Reduction and fixation

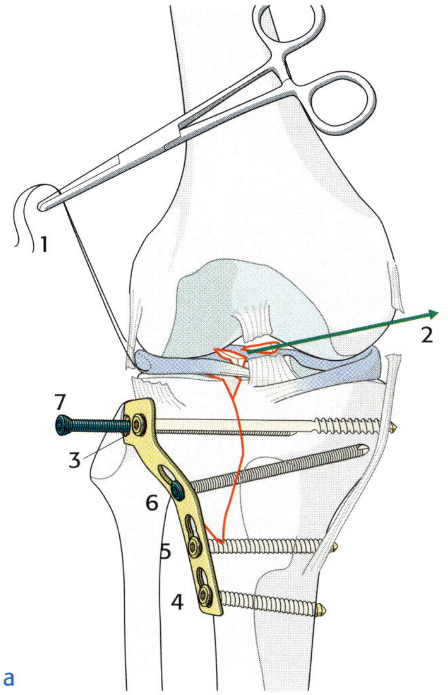

a

1 The meniscus is held cranially by some threads
2 The osteochondral fragments are removed
3 6.5 mm cancellous bone screw for compression
4 Cortex screw 4.5 mm
5 Cortex screw 4.5 mm
6 Self-tapping LHS 5.0 mm
7 Self-tapping LHS 5.0 mm

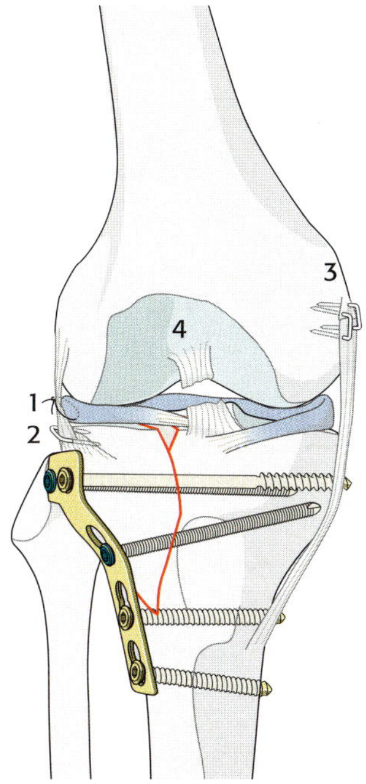

b

1 Knot
2 Refixation of the meniscotibial ligament with a staple
3 Revision and refixation of the MCL with two staples
4 ACL not reconstructed

Fig 10.1.3-4a–b

a The anterior tibial compartment is opened approximately 4 cm. At this point, the rupture of the meniscotibial ligament is already visible. After the lateral plateau fragment has been lifted to the side, the meniscus can be seen deep in the fracture zone. The meniscus is reduced and held cranially by some threads for better visibility of the tibial plateau. The joint is rinsed through the fracture zone under valgus stress. The two small osteochondral fragments from the lateral tibial plateau are too small to be fixed and are removed. The main bone fragment is reduced with the pelvic reduction forceps, which are inserted medially through a small incision. The fracture is temporarily stabilized with K-wires and the reduction is checked under image intensification. A 3-hole LCP T-plate 4.5/5.0 is bent and placed on the anterolateral aspect. The first screw to be inserted is a 6.5 mm cancellous bone lag screw with long thread to compress the fracture zone. Further fixation of the plate distally follows with the insertion of two 4.5 mm cortex screws (sufficient in good bone quality). For the definitive fixation of the compressed fracture zone, two 5.0 mm self-tapping LHS are inserted proximally. These screws should be as long as possible without penetrating the opposite cortex to prevent an irritation of the pes anserinus.

b Inspection of the intercondylar region shows the intraligamentous rupture of the ACL. The stability of the knee joint is checked after osteosynthesis and a medial instability is discovered. The MCL has to be refixed. A medial approach and small incision at the level of the knee joint is performed. The approach is anterior to the pes anserinus. The MCL is treated by open reduction and fixed with two staples to the femoral part. With this intervention, the stability is clearly improved. The ACL cannot be sutured and an ACL replacement should not be performed in this acute situation. It can be considered at a later stage after consolidation of the fracture if there is symptomatic knee instability.

3 Reduction and fixation (cont)

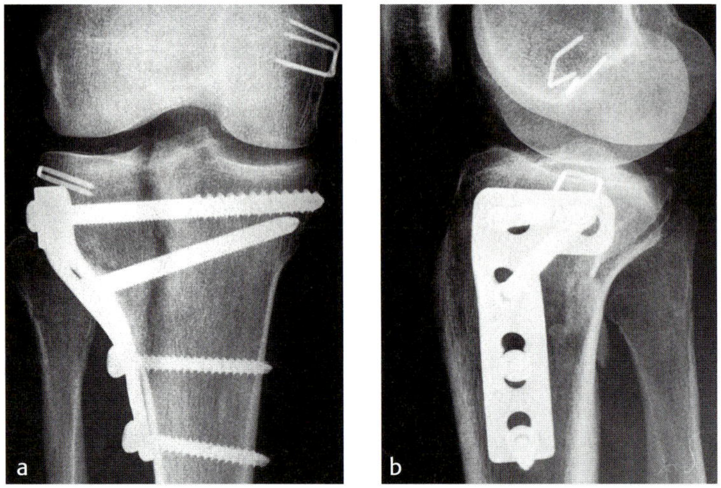

Fig 10.1.3-5a–b The postoperative x-rays confirmed the anatomical reconstruction of the lateral tibial plateau with a small centrolateral defect (due to the two missing osteochondral fragments). The medial ligament staple fixation and the lateral capsule fixation can be seen.

4 Rehabilitation

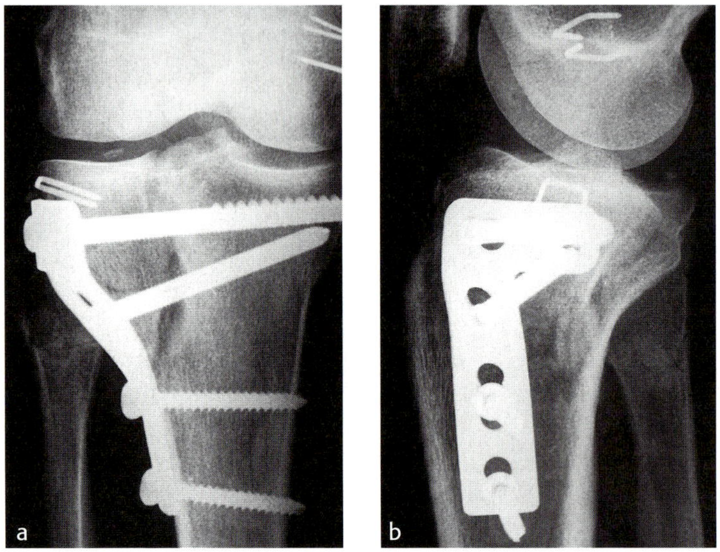

Fig 10.1.3-6a–i

a–b The knee was immobilized with a removable splint for 4 weeks. Mobilization began on the third day with 10–15 kg weight bearing. Active movement and strengthening of the quadriceps and hamstring muscles were practised. After 6 weeks the fracture showed endosteal consolidation.

4 Rehabilitation (cont)

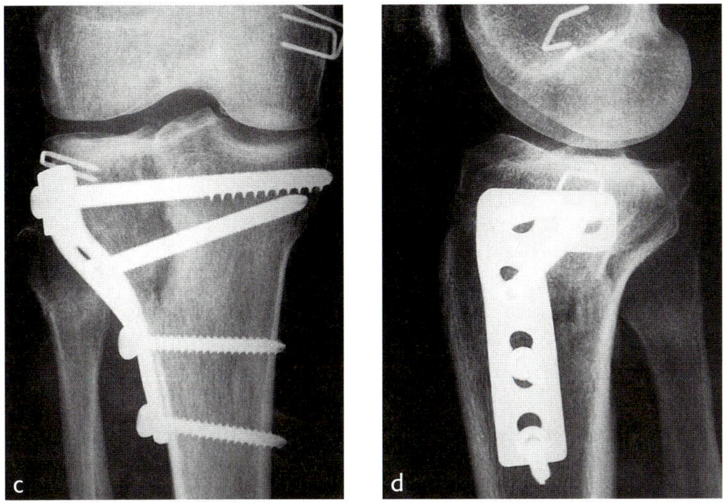

Fig 10.1.3-6a–i (cont)

c–d The fracture was further consolidated after 3 months and full weight bearing began.

e–i After 7 months the fracture was completely consolidated with a normal knee joint space. At this time, the patient showed normal knee joint movement and no sign of instability. An ACL replacement was not necessary, the prepatellar scar originates from an earlier patellar fracture and osteosynthesis.

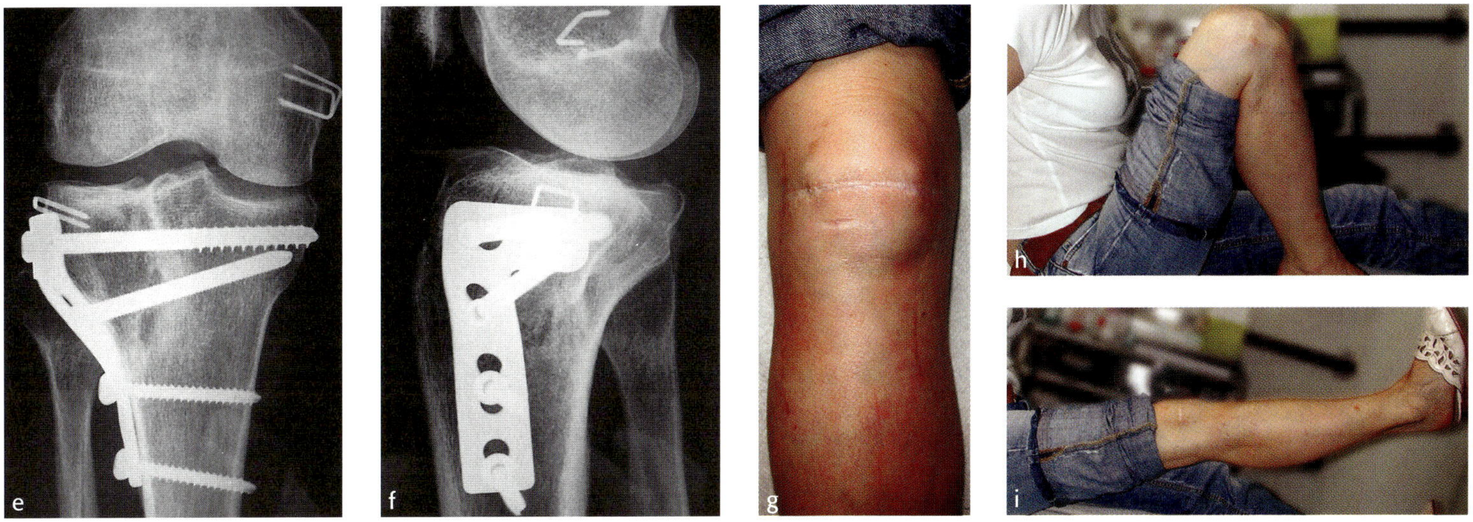

5 Pitfalls –

Equipment

Approach
An anterolateral standard approach bears few risks. A double approach anterolaterally and medially can be associated with the risk of skin necrosis. Careful handling of the soft tissue is essential.

Reduction and fixation

Rehabilitation
Failure to immobilize the knee joint endangers the fixation of the ligaments, particularly the medial ligaments. Specific, guided, active movement out of the splint is necessary to prevent knee stiffness.

6 Pearls +

Equipment
LCP is an ideal implant for this indication, angular stability would not be required in good bone quality.

Approach
Even difficult displaced fractures can be treated with the help of these two small incisions.

Reduction and fixation
With persisting instability after correct osteosynthesis, the reconstruction of the capsule and ligaments is required.

Rehabilitation

Author Christian Ryf

10.1.4 Partial articular proximal tibial fracture with split-depression—41-B3

1 Case description

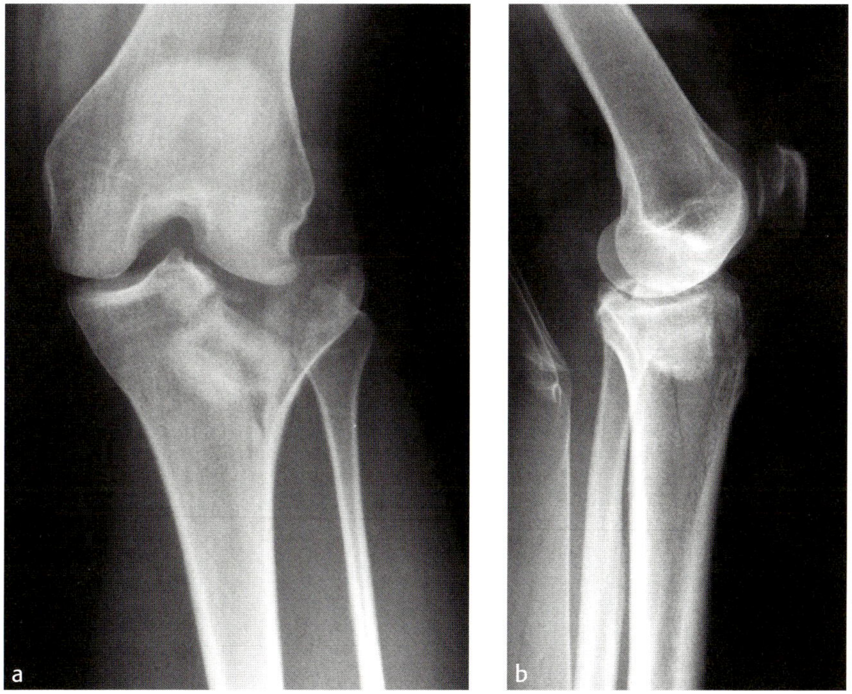

34-year-old woman fell while skiing and sustained a proximal articular lateral tibial fracture.

Fig 10.1.4-1a–b
a AP view.
b Lateral view.

Indication

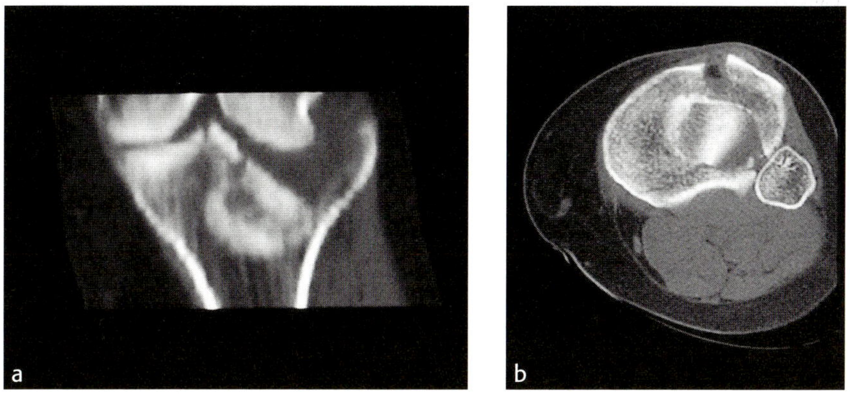

After initial radiological and CT scan analyses, regression of swelling and no indication for a compartment syndrome, the fracture was operated on. With this articular fracture and dislocation of the lateral tibial joint surface, the indication for operative treatment was clear.

Fig 10.1.4-2a–b CT scans.

Preoperative planning

Equipment

- LISS-PLT, 5 holes
- 5.0 mm self-tapping locking head screws (LHS)
- 6.5 mm cancellous bone screws
- 2.0 mm K-wires

(Size of system, instruments, and implants can vary according to anatomy.)

Patient preparation and positioning

Antibiotics: 4th generation cephalosporin

Thrombosis prophylaxis: low-molecular heparin

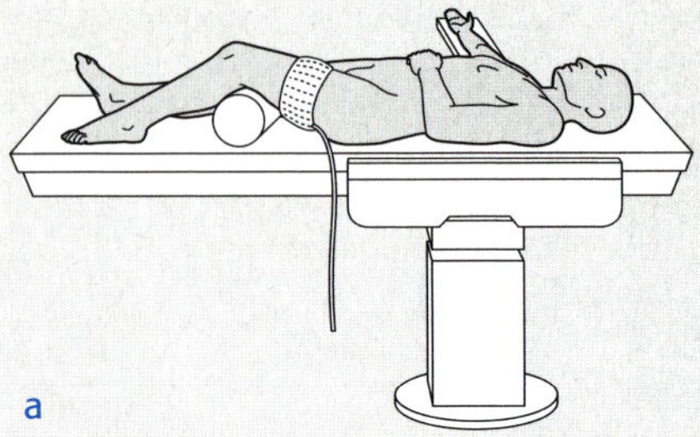

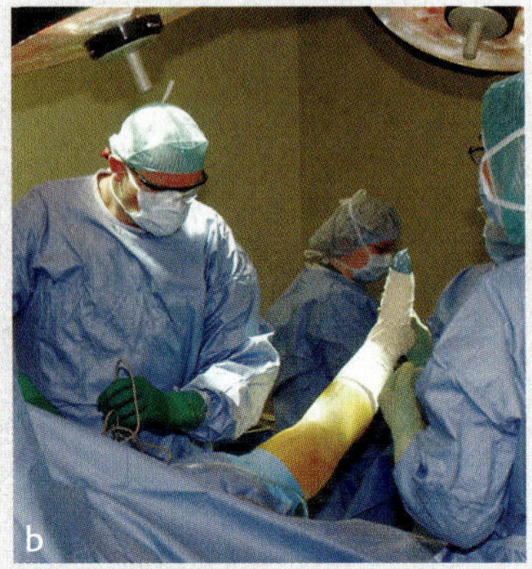

Fig 10.1.4-3a–b Supine position with elevation of the injured limb and flexion of the knee joint to approximately 30°. Tourniquet on the femur.

2 Surgical approach

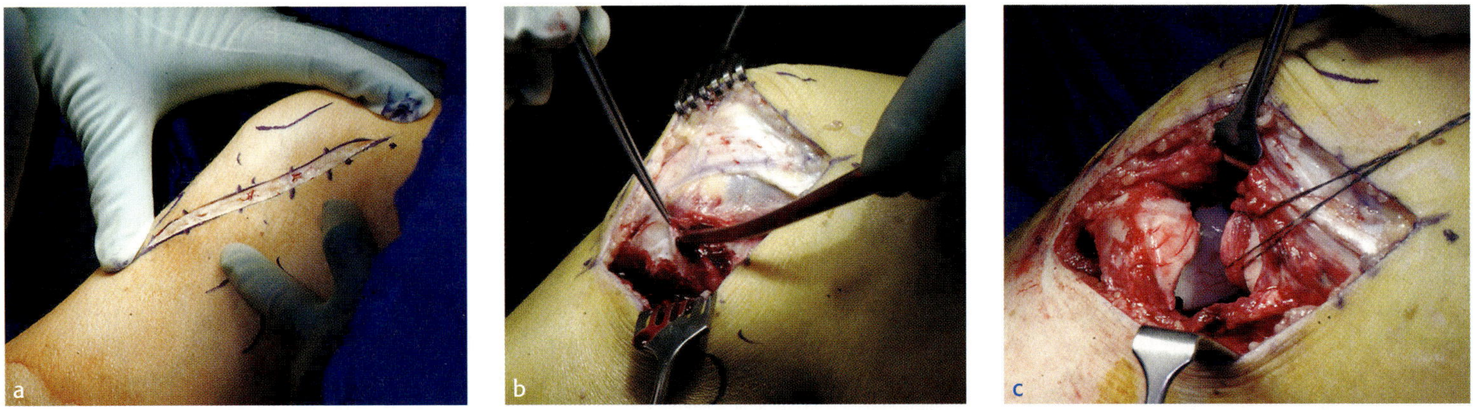

Fig 10.1.4-4a–c

a All the palpable structures are marked. Incision lateral to the patellar edge.

b The iliotibial tract is split and partially detached from the lateral tibial head. The joint is now opened.

c The lateral meniscus is presented and dislocated cranially.

3 Reduction and fixation

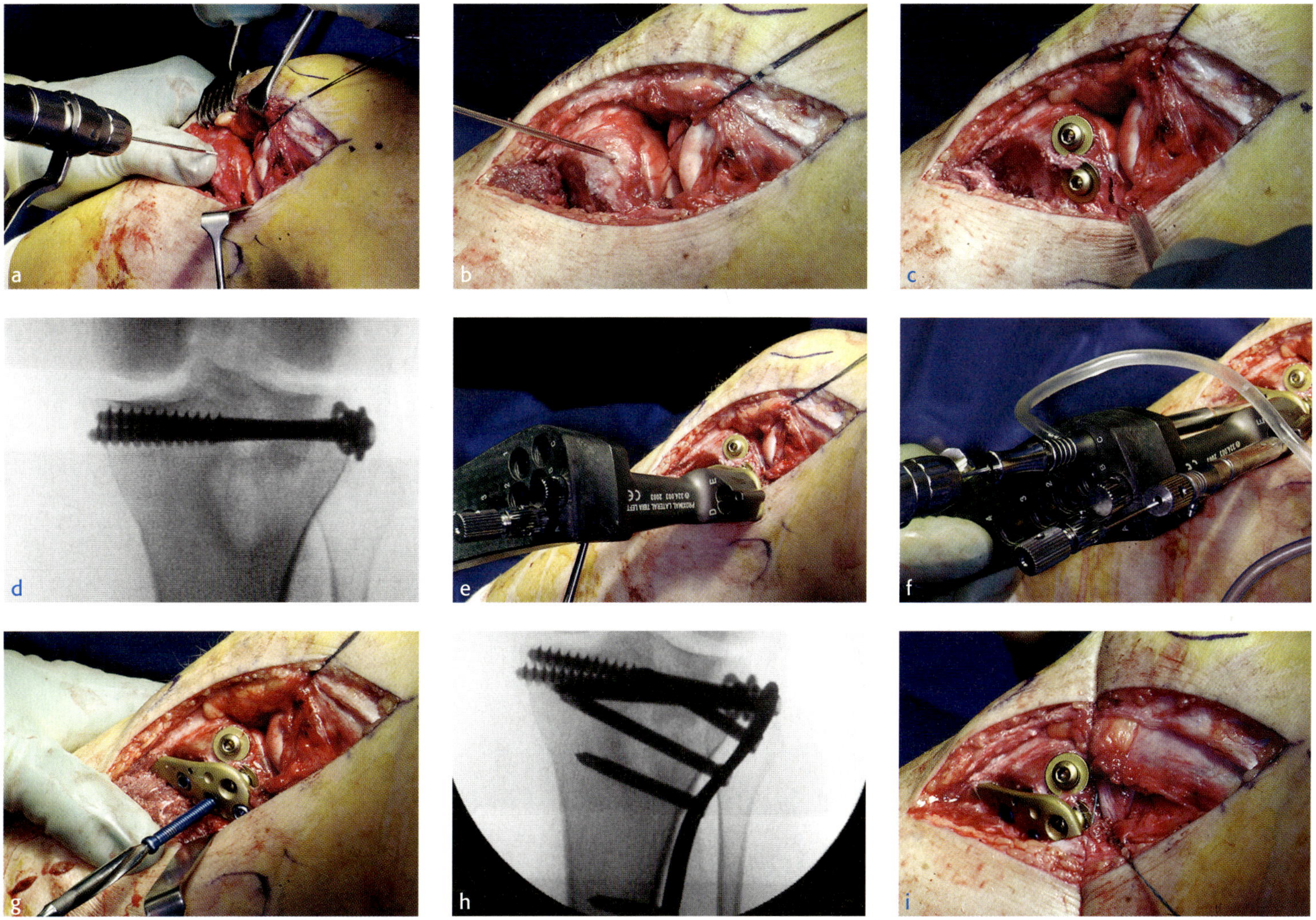

Fig 10.1.4-5a–i

- a Reduction of the lateral fragment with a chisel.
- b Preliminary fixation of the reduced fragment with K-wires.
- c–d The reduced lateral fragment is definitively fixed with two cancellous bone screws with washers inserted from lateral to medial. These two subchondral screws must be parallel to the joint surface.
- e–f To achieve a stable osteosynthesis, a LISS plate is inserted submuscularly and preliminarly fixed with two K-wires proximally and distally.
- g–h The proximal fixation follows. Four LHS are inserted for this purpose. Four monocortical LHS are inserted distally.
- i Removal of the insertion guide and refixation of the meniscus.

4 Rehabilitation

Additional immobilization: none, partial weight bearing and therapy with the continuos passive motion machine.
Weight bearing: 15 kg for 6 weeks; half body weight after 8 weeks; full weight bearing after 10 to 12 weeks.

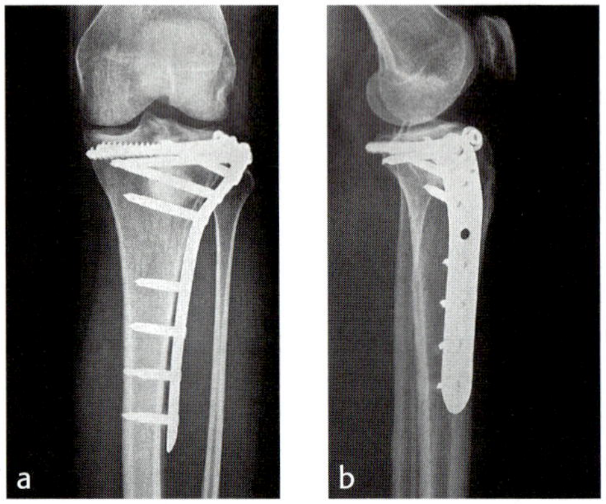

Fig 10.1.4-6a–b Postoperative x-rays after 6 weeks.
a AP view.
b Lateral view.

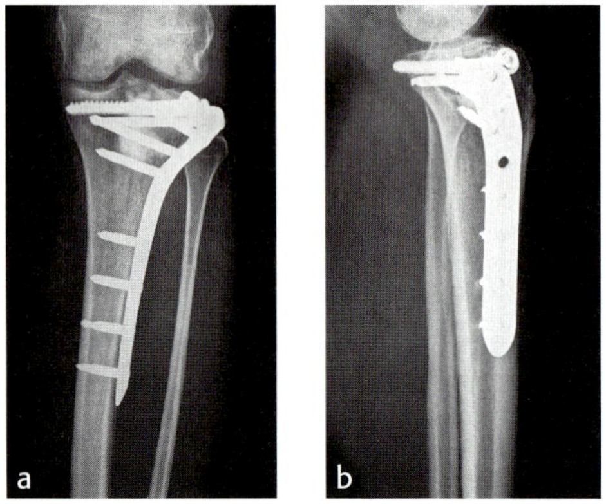

Fig 10.1.4-7a–b Postoperative x-rays after 3 months.
a AP view.
b Lateral view.

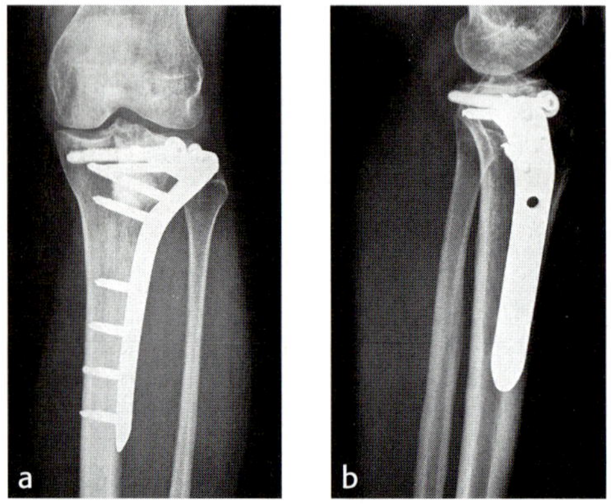

Fig 10.1.4-8a–b Postoperative x-rays after 8 months.
a AP view.
b Lateral view.

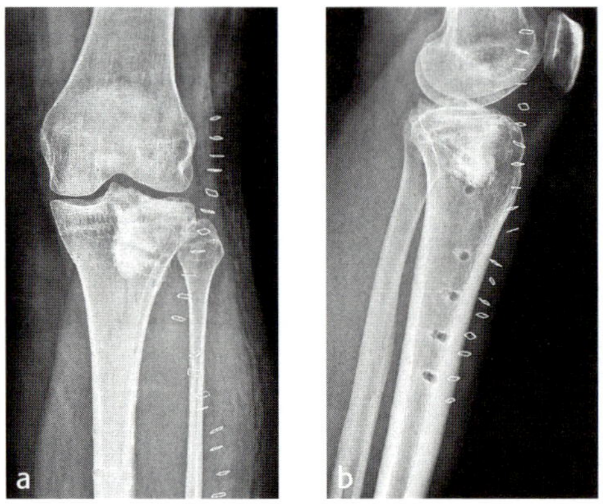

Fig 10.1.4-9a–b X-rays after implant removal.
a AP view.
b Lateral view.

Implant removal
Implant removal after 18 months.

Author Christoph Sommer

10.1.5 Partial articular, dislocated tibial head fracture with split-depression—41-B3

1 Case description

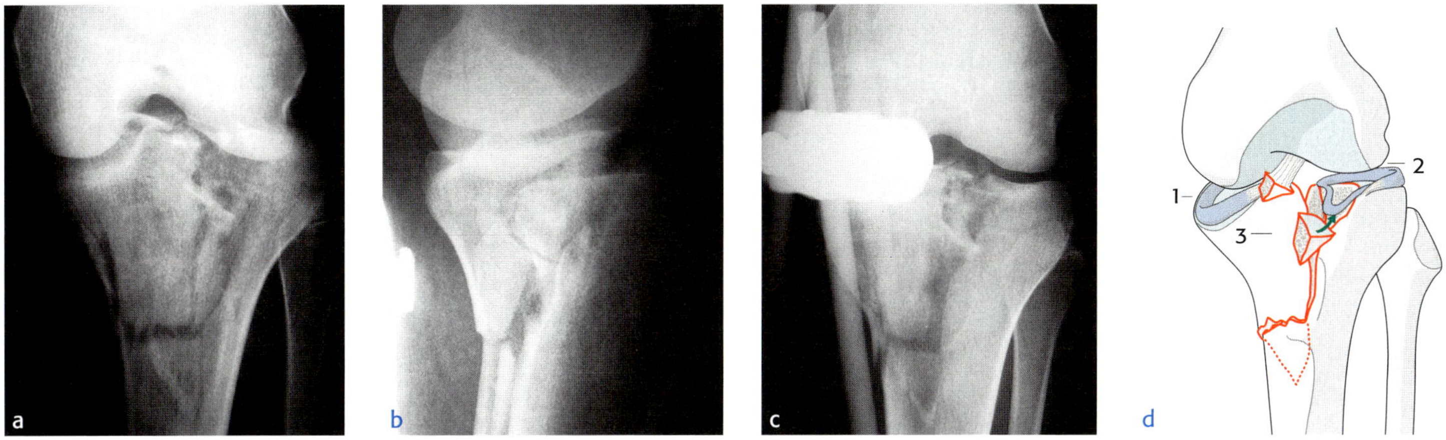

29-year-old skier with massive valgization trauma of her left knee. Severe soft-tissue swelling and the beginning of compartment syndrome. Radiologically, a tibial head dislocation fracture was identified as a 41-B3.3 (partial articular fracture split-depression, involving the tibial tubercles and one of the surfaces). Closed reduction and fixation with an external fixator bridging the joint had been performed in a smaller hospital. A conventional radiological examination with the reduced joint and a CT scan was performed at our hospital. Two joint fragments were pushed into the metaphysis. The tubercles of the intercondylar eminence had sustained multifragmentary fracture. Anterior crucial ligament (ACL) damage and injury to the lateral meniscus due to the dislocation of the lateral joint had to be assumed.

Fig 10.1.5-1a–d
a AP view initial x-ray.
b Lateral view initial x-ray.
c AP view after preliminary fixation with external fixator.
d The damage as verified intraoperatively. Distal avulsion of the anterior cruciate ligament (ACL) (1). Backed handle rupture of the lateral meniscus (2). Impacted centrolateral joint fragment (impediment to reduction, if not reduced as a first step) (3).

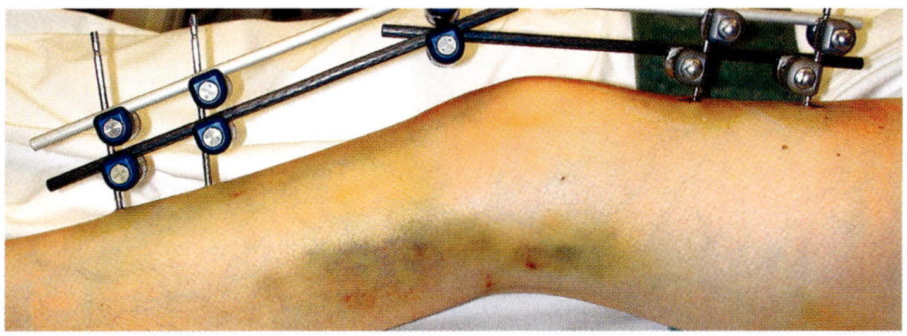

Fig 10.1.5-2 7 days after initial treatment, normal soft-tissue condition and reduced danger of compartment syndrome; the moment is ideal for definitive internal fixation.

Indication

This case presents a clear indication for an osteosynthesis. The specific partial joint fracture, with the combination of intact lateral condyle and impacted posterolateral articular fragments, is one of the most difficult fractures to treat. A minimally invasive technique is unlikely to be successful. In addition, injury to the lateral knee ligaments and lateral meniscus is probable. The posteromedial approach is ideal for buttressing the displaced medial condyle with a plate, but this approach does not allow fixation of the meniscus nor reduction of the impacted joint fragments. Therefore, as a first step, an anterolateral approach must be preferred. This allows the refixation of the menisco-ligamentous structure as well as the reduction of the impacted joint fragment. This is followed by a limited posteromedial, extraarticular approach for reduction and plate fixation of the main medial condyle.

Preoperative planning

Equipment

- LCP T-plate 4.5/5.0, 5 holes
- 5.0 mm self-tapping locking head screws (LHS)
- 4.5 mm cortex screw
- K-wires
- Pelvic reduction forceps
- Large distractor
- Aiming device for transosseous ACL fixation

(Size of system, instruments, and implants can vary according to anatomy.)

Patient preparation and positioning

Antibiotics: single dose 2nd generation cephalosporin

Thrombosis prophylaxis: none

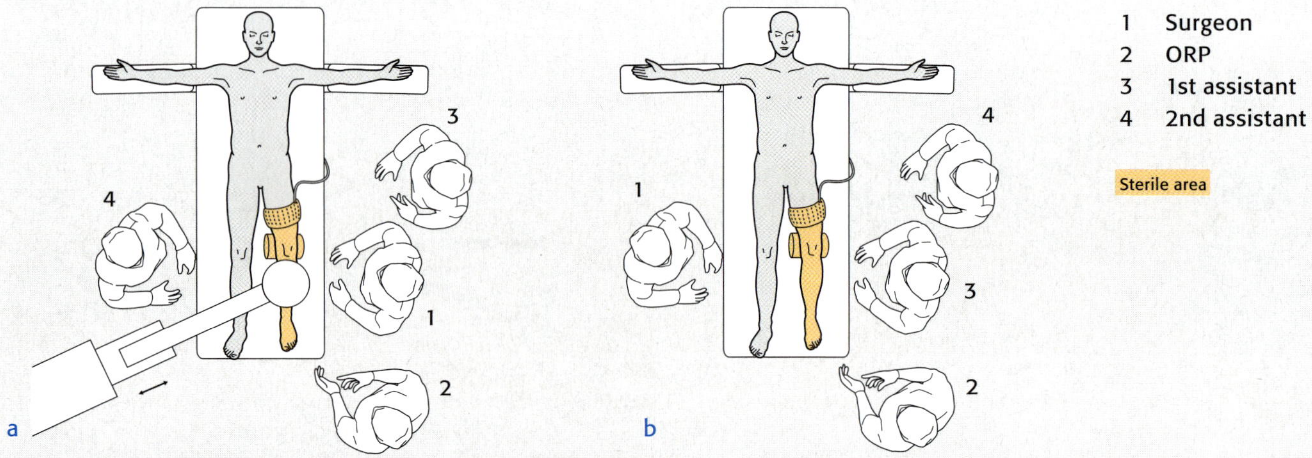

Fig 10.1.5-3a–b Positioning follows two phases:

a Lateral approach, the surgeon stands on the lateral side, the whole leg and iliac crest are accessible, image intensifier on the opposite side.

b Medial approach, the surgeon and the second assistant change to the opposite side, the rest stays in place.

2 Surgical approach

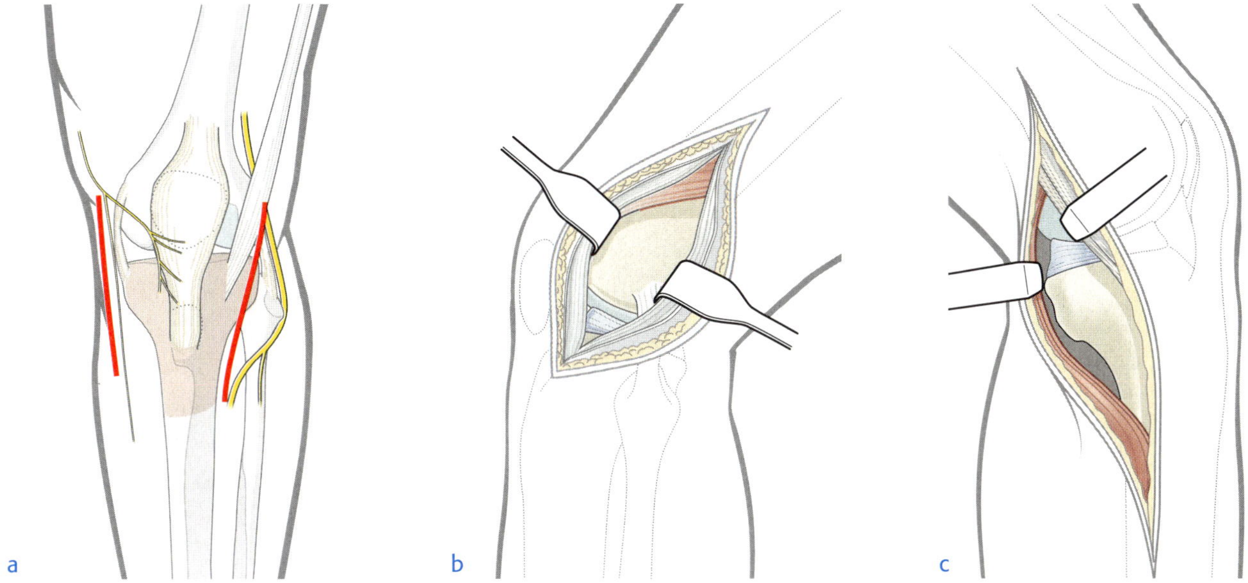

Fig 10.1.5-4a–c
a Surgical field.
b The anterolateral incision begins above the knee joint and extends for approximately 5–6 cm in a distal direction.
c The posteromedial incision begins at the joint space and runs distally (extraarticular approach).

3 Reduction and fixation

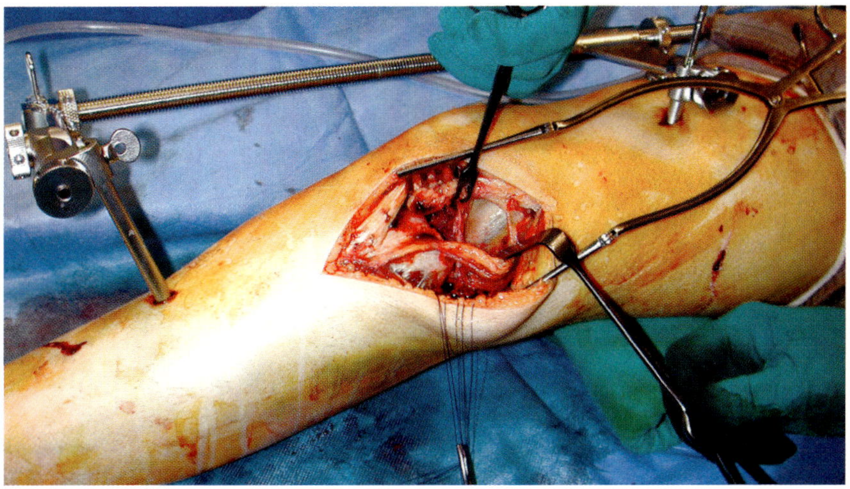

Fig 10.1.5-5 First the anterior external fixator is partially removed and the large distractor is fixed onto two Schanz screws that were left in situ. A towel is placed under the knee which is positioned at 20–30° flexion. Anterolateral approach and division of the iliotibial tract follows.

3 Reduction and fixation (cont)

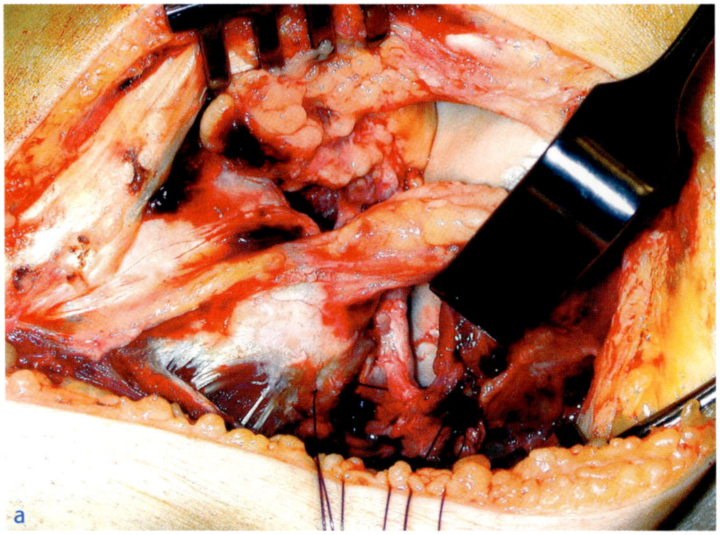

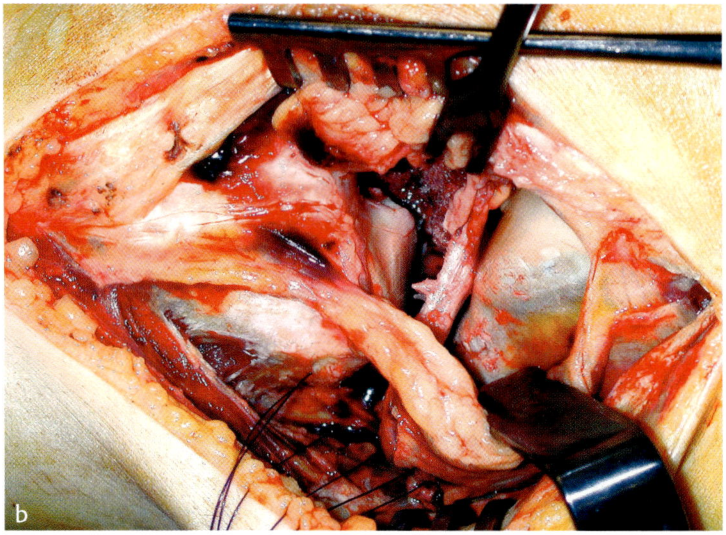

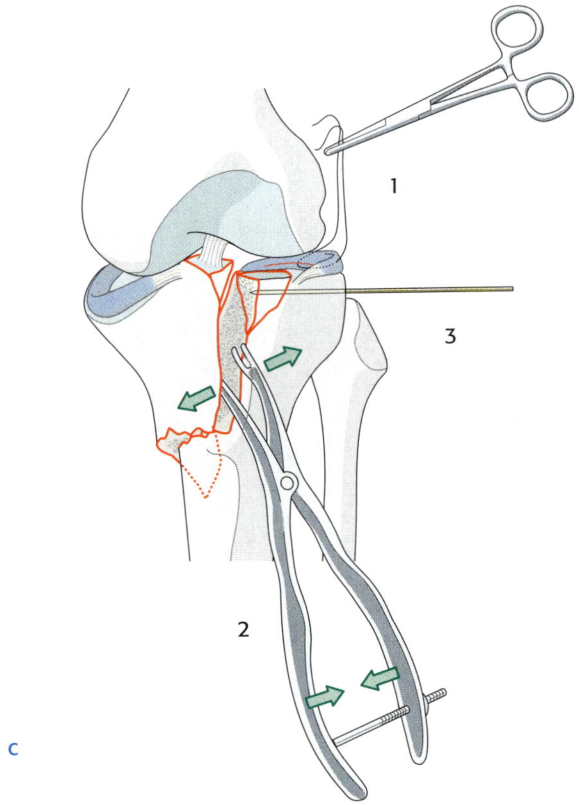

Fig 10.1.5-6a–c

a After the submeniscal transverse arthrotomy, the ruptured menisco-tibial ligaments are visible.

b An additional anterolateral capsulotomy for a better overview of the fracture and the intercondylar eminence is performed.

c The lateral meniscus shows a backed handle rupture from front to back with interposition of the ruptured medial part into the fracture gap. It has to be reduced and fixed with prepared threads (**1**). Through the anterolateral capsulotomy, the main fracture gap is opened with a bone spreader (**2**). The two impacted osteochondral fragments are identified. The smaller fragment is too small for refixation and therefore removed. The large fragment is held and correctly positioned with the aid of a K-wire (used as a joystick) and temporarily fixed with another 1.6 mm K-wire inserted from lateral through the intact condyle (**3**). This second K-wire should not penetrate the fragment entirely, nor touch or interfer with the main medial condylar fragment, which will be reduced later.

3 Reduction and fixation (cont)

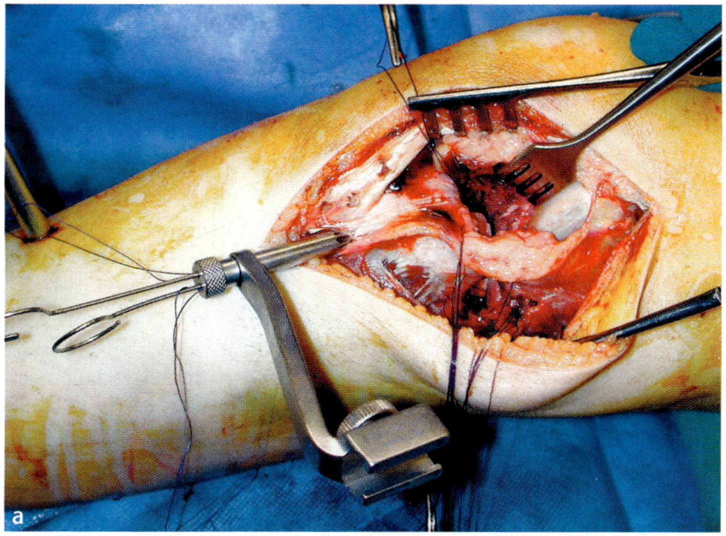

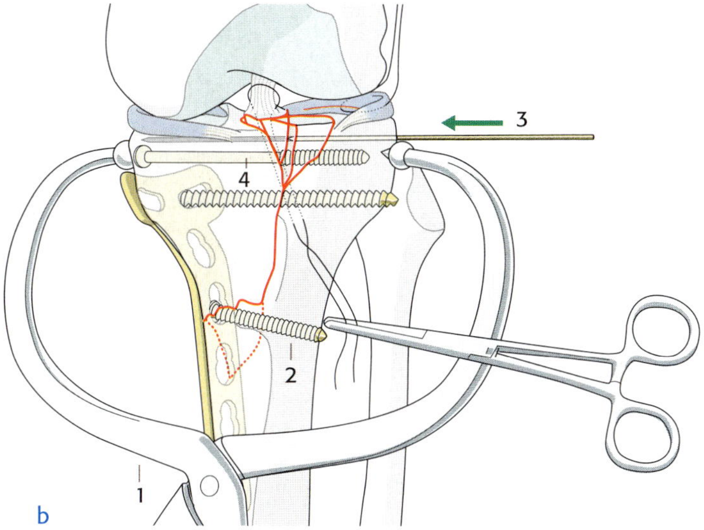

Fig 10.1.5-7a–d

a As a next step, the large anterior eminential fragment, to which the ACL adheres, is encircled by a thick nonresorbable thread. With the help of the drill guide, two 2.0 mm holes are drilled parallel from the anterior aspect into the fracture zone. The threads can now be pulled through the holes in an anterior direction allowing the reduction of the tubercle. The thread is not yet knotted.

b The team of surgeons changes sides. Now the posteromedial approach is made 10 cm distal to the joint while conserving the great saphenous vein and the saphenous nerve. The fracture zone is entered from behind the pes anserinus and the MCL towards the posteromedial tibial border. Only a small amount of periosteum is detached to show the reference lines for visual control. The reduction is managed with the pelvic reduction forceps placed on the posteromedial and anterolateral aspects near the joint (**1**).

Fine reduction can be achieved either using large K-wires as joysticks or with the LCP T-plate 4.5/5.0. The plate is slightly twisted and adapted to the posterior edge. The first screw is a 4.5 mm cortex screw inserted immediately distal to the fracture line (**2**). A persisting displacement can be reduced directly over the plate. After examining the reduction under image intensification, the threads from the eminence can be knotted tightly pulling the eminence into the fracture gap. An additional K-wire can support the reduction (**3**). Definitive compression is obtained with a lag screw from posteromedial to anterolateral. This screw has to be placed close to the articular surface, preventing a malrotation of the main medial condylar fragment. Depending on the position of the plate, this lag screw can be placed through a plate hole or independently (as in this case) (**4**).

3 Reduction and fixation (cont)

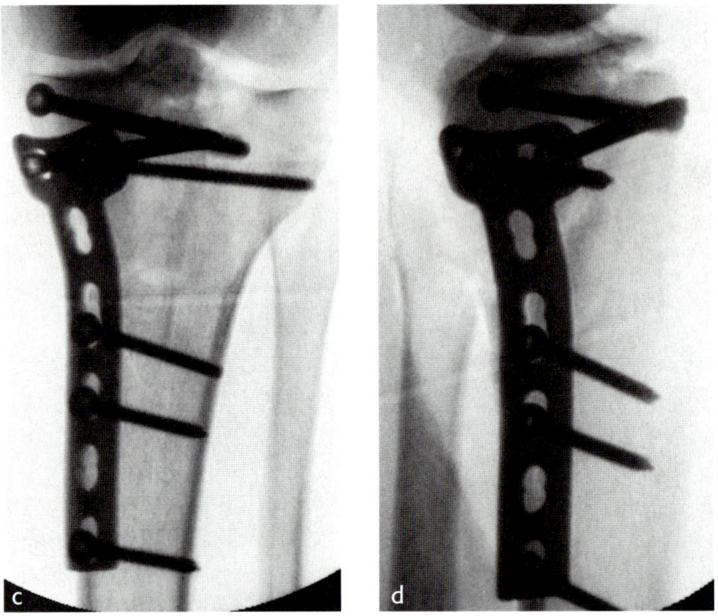

Fig 10.1.5-7a–d (cont)
c–d After removal of the pelvic reduction forceps another lag screw can be inserted subchondrally. The final fixation is achieved by inserting an angular stable 5.0 mm self-tapping locking head screw into the joint block and two cortex screws (only in good bone quality) or locking head screws (osteoporotic bone) into the shaft. At the end of the operation, x-ray assessment shows correct reduction of the tibial head with ideal positioning of the posteromedial plate and the 4.5 mm lag screw just under the fracture line. The eminence is slightly raised (2–3 mm) on the lateral view.

4 Rehabilitation

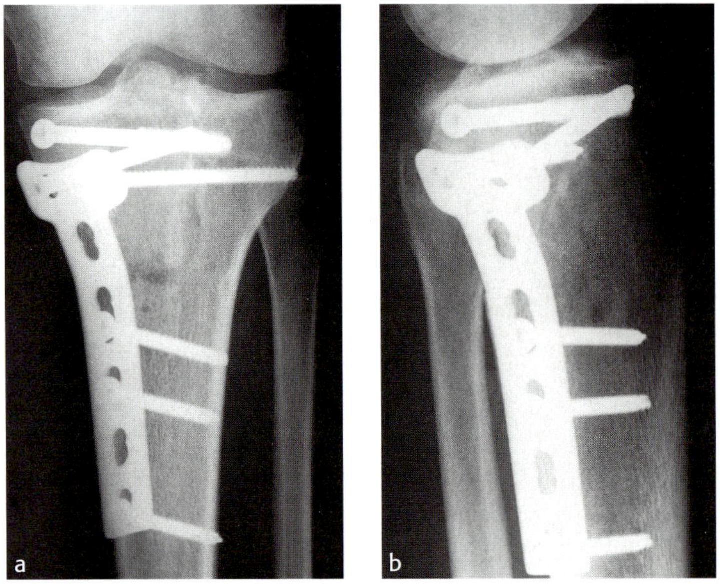

Mobilization began on the third postoperative day with a removable knee brace to protect the damaged ligaments of the knee. Initially 10–15 kg weight bearing and after 6 weeks half body weight.

Fig 10.1.5-8a–b The fracture was nearly completely consolidated after 3 months. At that time full weight bearing was started and tolerated without complaints.

4 Rehabilitation (cont)

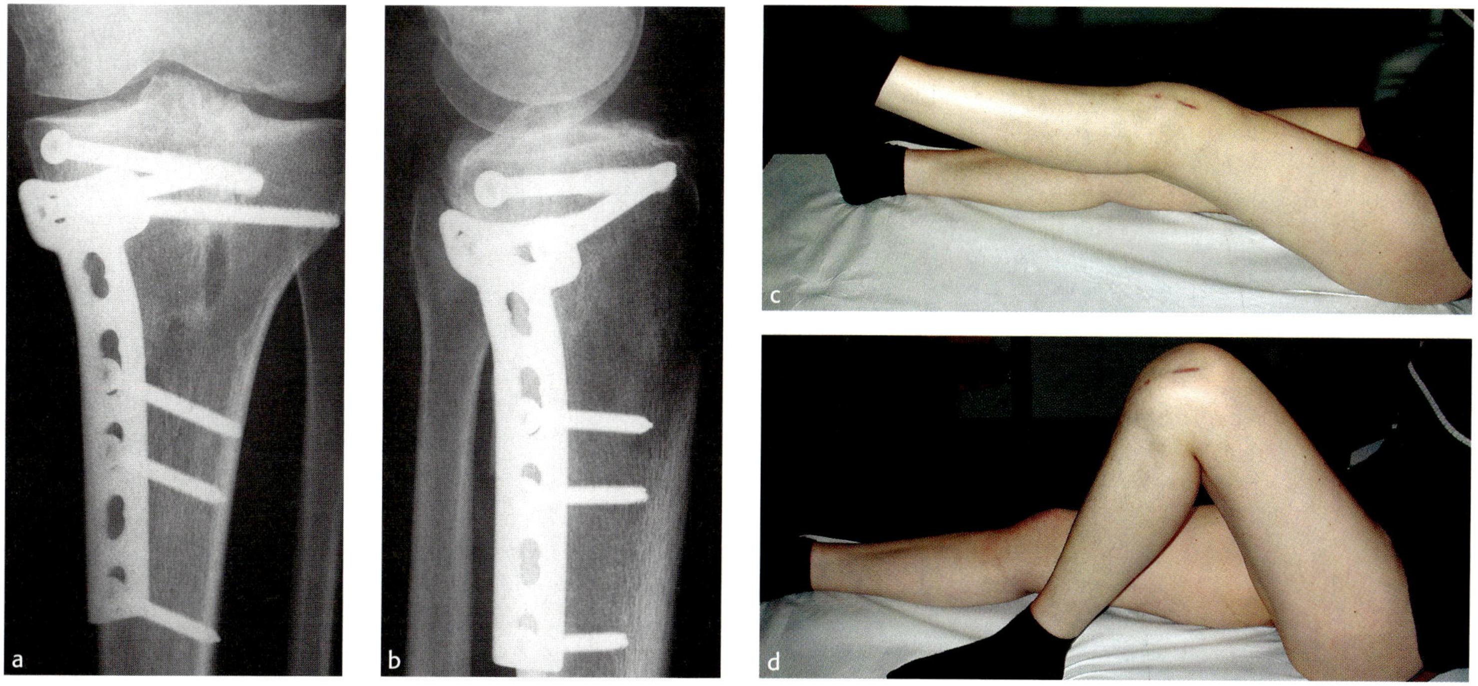

Fig 10.1.5-9a–d

a–b After 9 months the fracture is no longer visible, even the initially slightly elevated tibial spine shows a smooth ingrowth with good remodeling.

c–d At this time, there was good knee function with a slight active extension deficit of 10° but passive full extension.

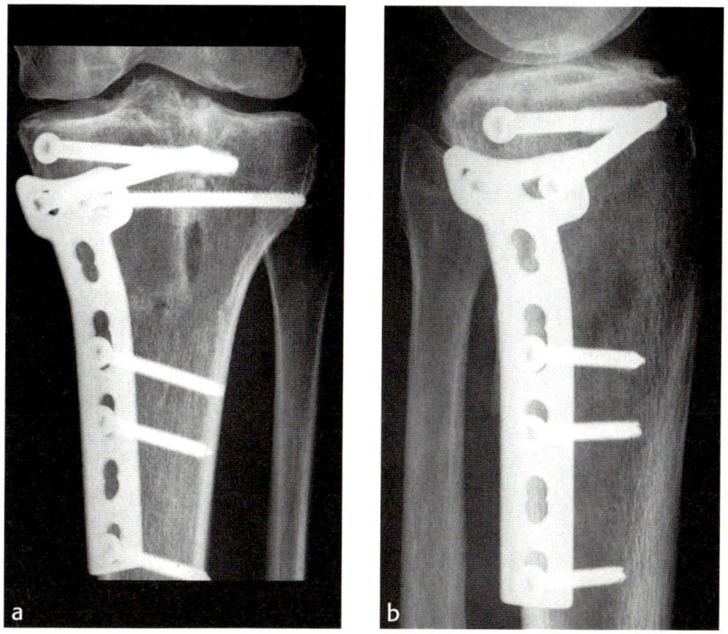

Fig 10.1.5-10a–b After 16 months the remodeling process was completed leaving a small defect in the metaphyseal part. The joint space was normal and identical in both knees without any sign of secondary arthrosis. The patient had no complaints and showed good activity. The knee was stable in all directions.

5 Pitfalls –

Approach
The double approach, ie, anterolateral and posteromedial, can endanger the soft tissue. A broad anterior soft-tissue bridge is necessary.

Reduction and fixation
A posteromedial approach would be insufficient for adequate treatment of this injury, which is very difficult to handle. The impacted lateral fragments, which would jeopardize correct reduction, could not be reduced and fixed with this approach only. Also the injured meniscus could not be treated. An anterolateral approach for reduction of the articular and meniscal fragments is absolutely mandatory before the medial condyle can be reduced.

Rehabilitation
Early full weight bearing could lead to secondary displacement and chronic instability of the joint (the eminence could pull out).

6 Pearls +

Approach
The anterolateral and posteromedial double approach is ideal to treat this complex fracture. The soft-tissue bridge is not endangered if it is broad enough. This approach provides a good overview over the fracture and offers ideal positioning of the posteromedial plate.

Reduction and fixation

Rehabilitation
A stable osteosynthesis and stable fixation of the anterior eminence allows early functional treatment.

Authors Andreas Gruner, Thomas J Hockertz, Gabriele Streicher, Heinrich Reilmann

10.1.6 Complete articular proximal tibial fracture—41-C1 with long spiral fracture of the shaft—42-A1

1 Case description

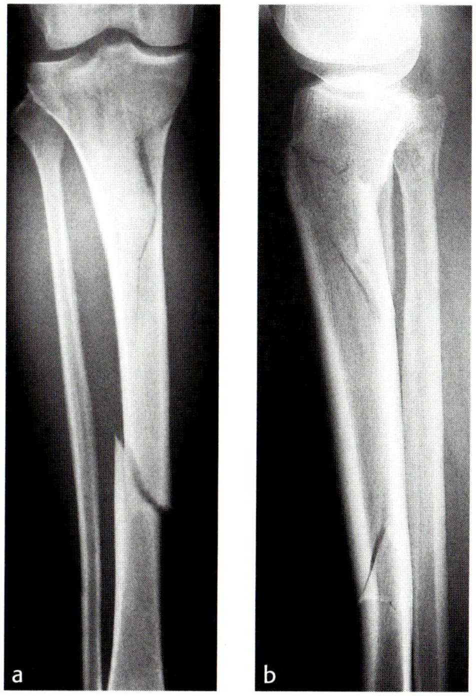

60-year-old woman with injury to the right tibia.
Type of injury: monotrauma, closed fracture.

Fig 10.1.6-1a–b
a AP view.
b Lateral view.

Indication

Multifocal fracture of the right tibia; no important axial malalignment due to the accident, the fracture included fracture of the tibial head plus torsion fracture of the tibial shaft extending to the transition area from the mid to the distal third. The patient was 60 years old at the time of the accident and adipose. Operative treatment was required to reconstruct the joint surfaces and to preserve knee joint function and axis of the tibia.

Preoperative planning

Equipment

- LISS-PLT, 13 holes
- 5.0 mm self-drilling, self-tapping locking head screws (LHS)
- 2.0 mm K-wires
- 6.5 mm cancellous bone screws

(Size of system, instruments, and implants can vary according to anatomy.)

Patient preparation and positioning

Antibiotics: 2nd generation cephalosporin
Thrombosis prophylaxis: low-molecular heparin

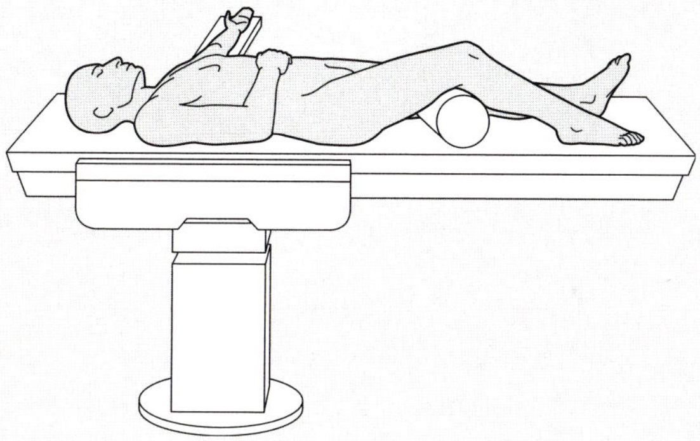

Fig 10.1.6-2 Supine position with elevation of the injured limb and flexion of the knee joint to approximately 30°, lowering of the contralateral leg for better intraoperative x-ray assessment, cushioning of the distal femur of the injured limb, eg, with a towel roll.

2 Surgical approach

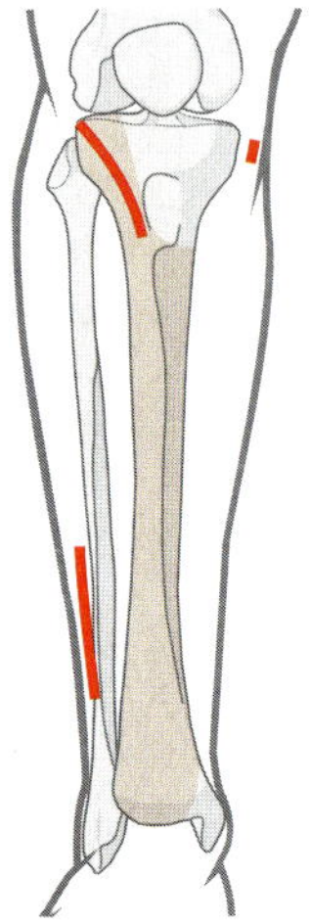

Fig 10.1.6-3 Hockey-stick incision approximately 5 cm long from Gerdy's tubercle extending in a distal direction, and dissection to the periosteum.

3 Reduction and fixation

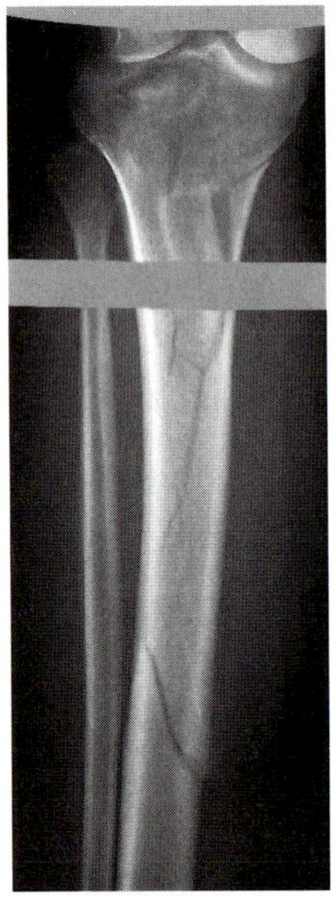

Fig 10.1.6-4
Approximate reduction of the joint surfaces by tension ad axim and tap out the collapsed joint surface components from the distal side to restore joint congruency, temporary fixation by subchondral insertion of K-wires.
Secure reduction by inserting cancellous bone screws from the medial side and parallel to the joint surface through a stab incision after predrilling.
Prepare the plate bed from proximal to distal epiperiosteally in the compartment of the anterior tibialis muscle with a long bone rasp, taking special care when crossing the distal fracture zone.
Determine correct plate length under image intensification and slide the implant into the plate bed.

3 Reduction and fixation (cont)

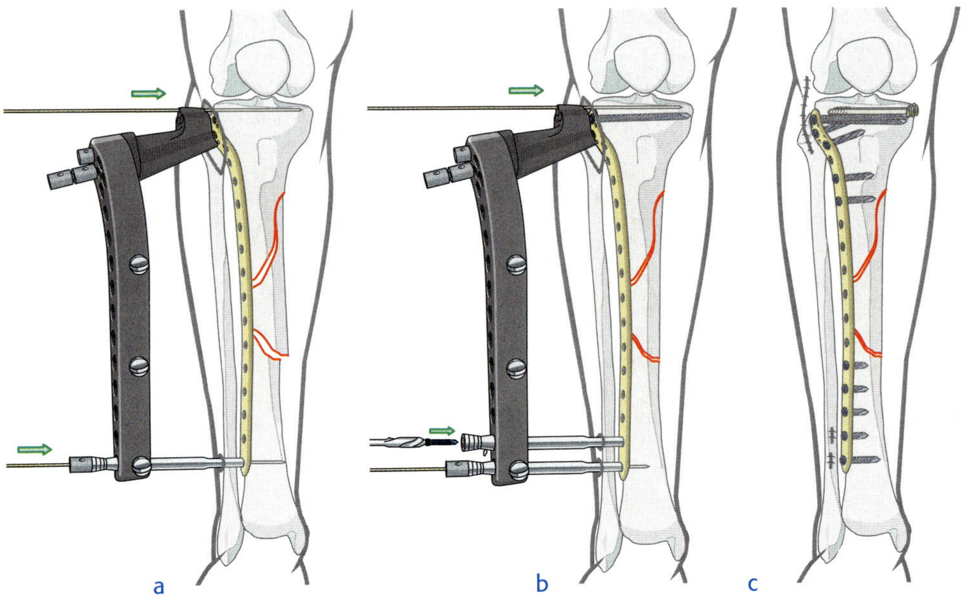

Fig 10.1.6-5a–c
Stabilize the implant temporarily with K-wires and check plate position in two planes.
Precise reduction of the fragments with the pulling device.
Insert the screws alternately in the distal and proximal holes starting proximally, determine screw length according to Tab 3-2; chapter 3).

4 Rehabilitation

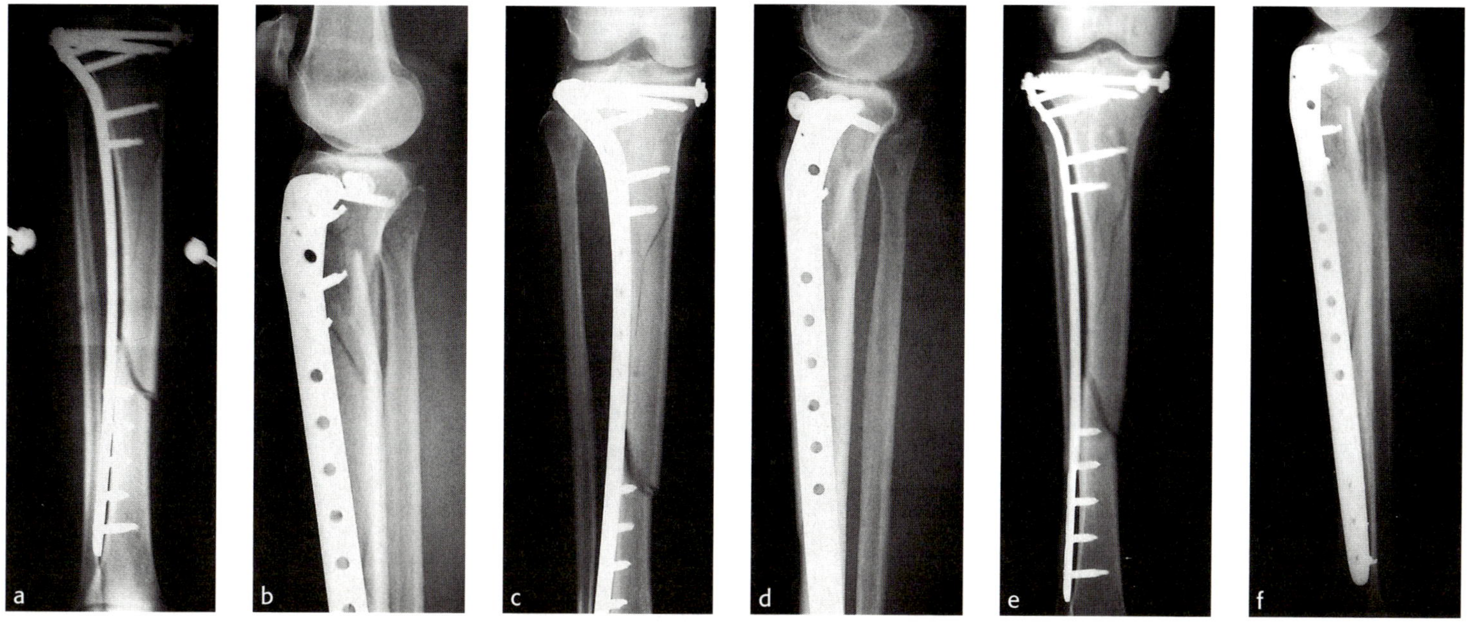

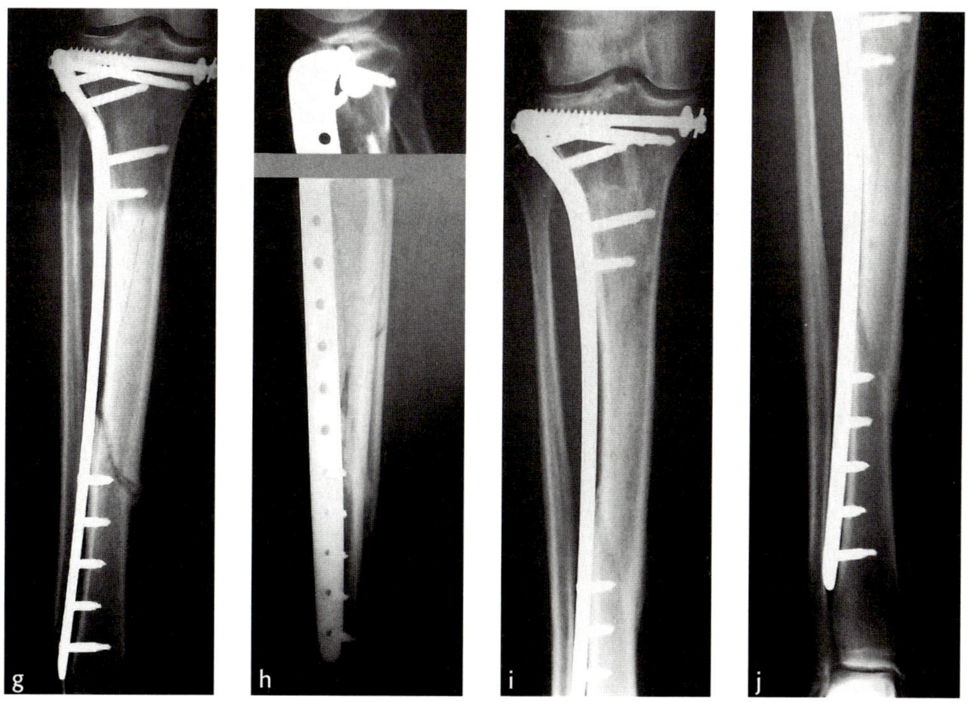

Weight bearing: half body weight until 6 weeks, full weight bearing after 6 weeks.
Physiotherapy: from the second postoperative day and continuous passive motion.
Pharmaceutical treatment: pain therapy and nonsteroid antiinflammatory drugs.

Fig 10.1.6-6a–j Postoperative x-rays.
a–b After 1 week.
c–d After 2 weeks.
e–f After 1 month.
g–h After 3 months.
i–j After 1 year.

4 Rehabilitation (cont)

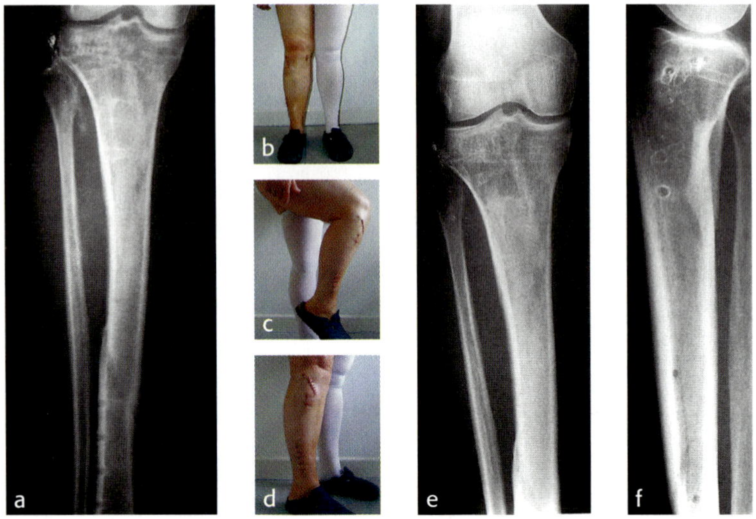

Implant removal

After 16 months. Reason for implant removal: mechanical irritation of the implant bed proximally. Technique for implant removal: removal of screws through stab incision and removal of the LISS via the original proximal approach.

Fig 10.1.6-7a–f

a After implant removal.

b–d Functional pictures after implant removal.

e–f X-rays 6 months after implant removal.

5 Pitfalls –

Equipment

Length of plate too short and, consequently, too few screws in the distal fragment.

Approach

Inadequate preparation of the tibial head leads to incorrect plate positioning (too far posterior or too far anterior).

Reduction and fixation

Pull-out of the pulling device due to osteoporosis or a reduction distance that was too long, incorrect length of the cancellous bone screws for the tibial head—irritation of the LISS bed/or inadequate anchorage.

Rehabilitation

Premature full weight bearing with joint involvement.

6 Pearls +

Equipment

Facility to bridge a multifocal fracture with one implant and good positioning due to the insertion guide.

Approach

Reduction and fixation

Primary restoration of the joint block and reconstruction of the joint surface, subsequent connection to the shaft fragment

Rehabilitation

Early mobilization with partial/full weight bearing.

Authors Michael Schütz, Norbert P Haas

10.1.7 Simple articular proximal tibial fracture with metaphyseal comminution—41-C2

1 Case description

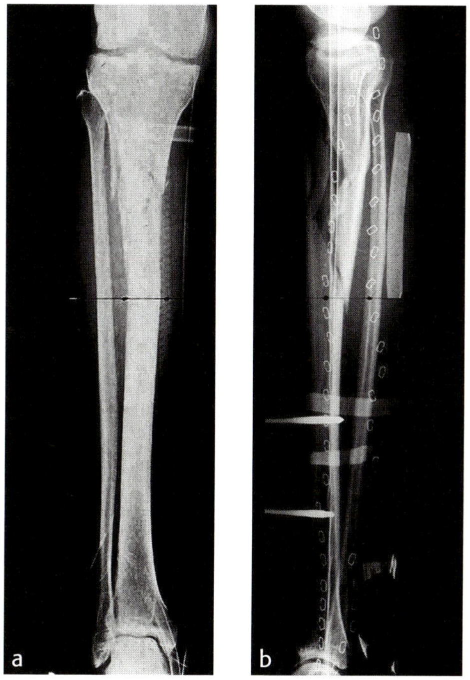

56-year-old man suffered multiple injuries as the result of a road traffic accident, including a type 41-C2 fracture of the proximal tibia radiating into the diaphysis. The fracture was initially stabilized with an external fixator because the patient's general condition was critical and relieving incision was performed to avert imminent compartment syndrome.

Fig 10.1.7-1a–b
a AP view.
b Lateral view.

Indication

Nondislocated, simple articular fracture with a complex metaphyseal multifragmentary fracture. It is essential to achieve stable fixation of the articular fracture with bridging of the metadiaphyseal zone and early functional rehabilitation being careful to avoid joint contractures.

Preoperative planning

Equipment
- LISS-PLT, 13 holes
- 5.00 mm self-drilling, self-tapping locking head screws (LHS)
- 7.0 mm cannulated cancellous bone screws
- 2.0 mm K-wires

(Size of system, instruments, and implants can vary according to anatomy.)

Patient preparation and positioning
Antibiotics: single dose 2nd generation cephalosporin
Thrombosis prophylaxis: low-molecular heparin

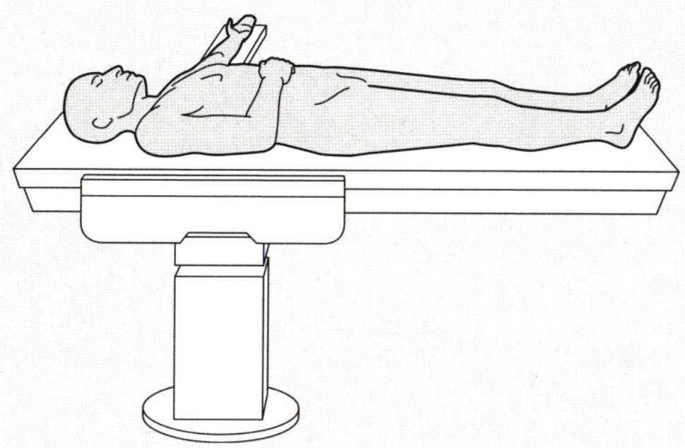

Fig 10.1.7-2 Supine position.

2 Surgical approach

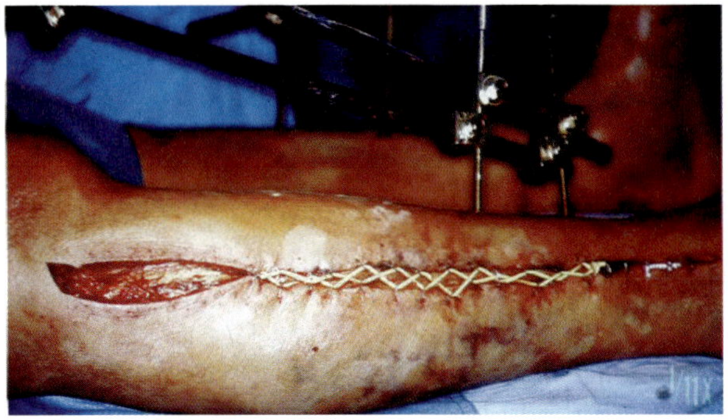

The proximal part of the surgical approach is used in this operation to access the compartments.

Fig 10.1.7-3 The proximal insertion of the anterior tibial muscle is detached sparingly. It is recommended that part of the muscle fasciae be left on the bone to facilitate reinsertion later. The muscle is carefully retracted with the bone rasp.

3 Reduction and fixation

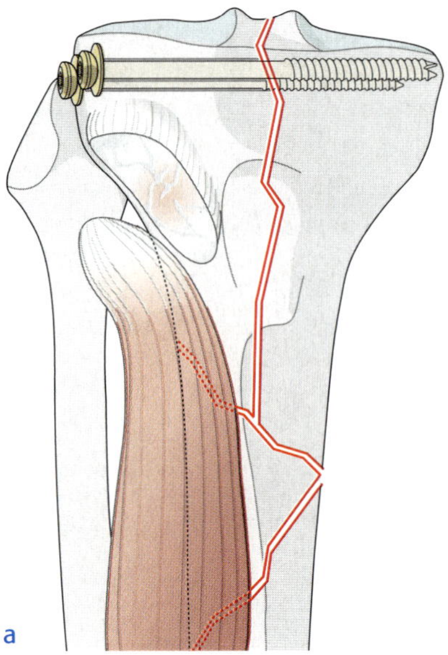

a

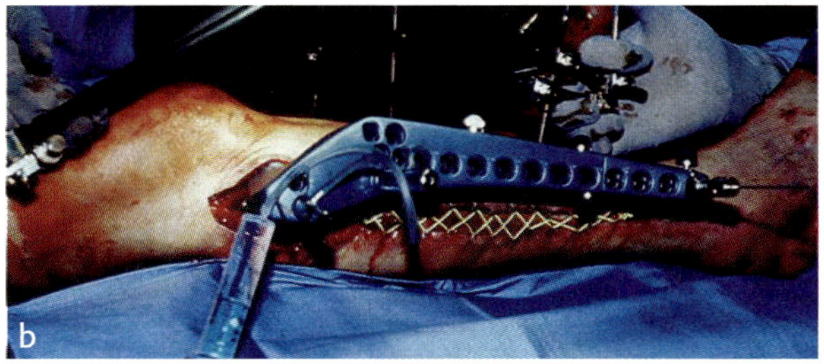

b

Fig 10.1.7-4a–d

a Screw fixation of the tibial head in closed technique with two 7.0 mm cannulated cancellous bone screws with a 32 mm thread is performed first. Washers are used to prevent the screw heads from sinking into the bone. Axial, rotational, and length alignment is checked with the aid of the external fixator that was applied in this first operation.

b Submuscular insertion of the 13-hole LISS-PLT along the lateral tibia with the help of the insertion guide. Alignment with the tibial head. Stab incision over the most distal plate hole, insertion of the connecting trocar between the insertion guide and the implant.
Palpation of correct implant position on the shaft. This is possible on the tibial ridge without extending the incision because of the minimal soft-tissue coverage. Temporary fixation of the proximal and distal connecting bolts with partially threaded 2.0 mm K-wires.

3 Reduction and fixation (cont)

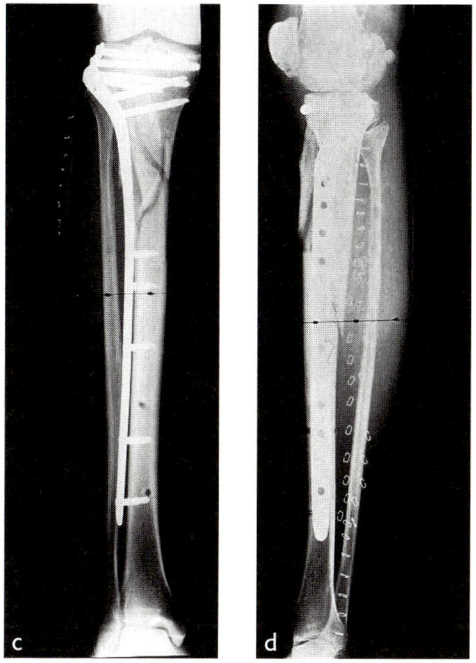

Insertion of the first LHS close to the joint so that it is situated beneath the cancellous bone screws and parallel to the joint surface.
The alignment of the diaphysis is finely adjusted in the anteroposterior plane with the aid of the external fixator and stabilized. Axial, rotational, and length alignments are reassessed clinically and radiologically.
The remaining locking head screws are then inserted.
The method of locked splinting fixation over a longer diaphyseal distance is recommended in order to benefit from the advantages of a biomechanically elastic fracture fixation.
The insertion guide is dismantled and the external fixator is removed. Reinsertion of the fasciae just beyond the proximal end of the implant. Wound closure by layers.

Fig 10.1.7-4a–d (cont)
c Postoperative x-ray, AP view.
d Postoperative x-ray, lateral view.

4 Rehabilitation

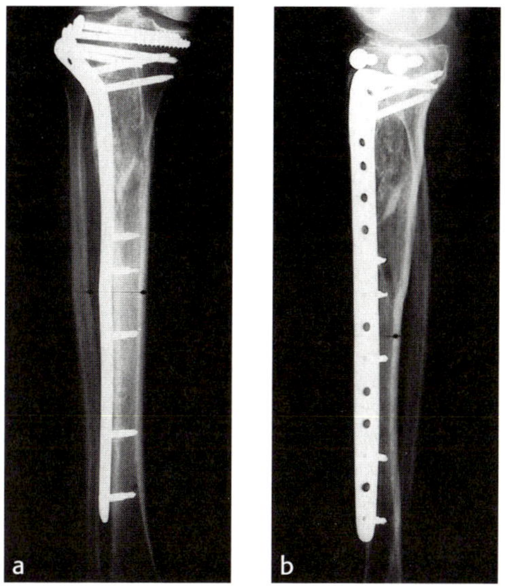

Apply sterile dressings.
Physiotherapy: gentle active and passive range of motion immediately on day one postoperatively.
The use of the continuous passive motion machine is highly recommended.
Mobilization with partial weight bearing as soon as the general and local condition of the patient allows it.

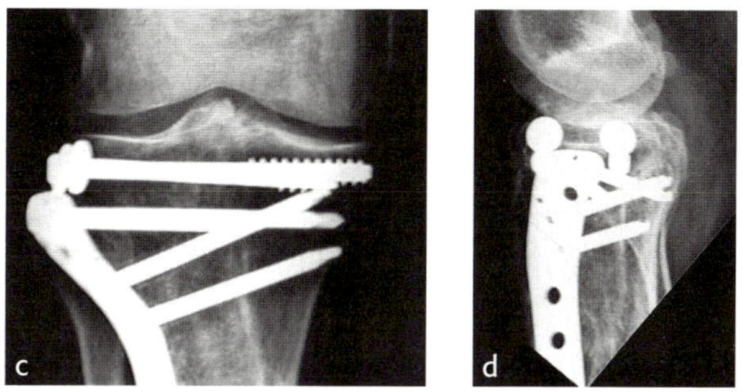

Fig 10.1.7-5a–d
Postoperative x-rays after 12 months.
a AP view.
b Lateral view.
c AP detail view.
d Lateral detail view.

4 Rehabilitation (cont)

Implant removal
It may be necessary to remove the implant if the proximal part of the plate is causing irritation.

5 Pitfalls –

Approach
Too extensive exposure of the metaphyseal fracture zone may damage the vascularity of the bone fragments.

Reduction and fixation
Incorrect positioning of the implant on the shaft may lead to early implant loosening. Incorrect positioning of the implant on the lateral tibial head may lead to soft-tissue irritations.

A too short implant increases the risk of implant loosening.

A too rigid implant fixation increases the risk of implant failure.

Rehabilitation
Prolonging physiotherapy may lead to intraarticular adhesions and joint stiffness.

6 Pearls +

Approach
Open, direct reduction of the articular fracture component, but indirect reduction techniques for a complex metaphyseal component.

Reduction and fixation
Precise, anatomical reduction and interfragmentary compression, of the articular fracture with lag screws.

Alignment and splinting of the multifragmentary metaphyseal fracture.

Careful control of implant position using direct and indirect control mechanisms (palpation, and image intensifier).

Use of longer implants for the locked splinting method. Some plate holes in the region of the diaphysis should be left unoccupied so that the fixation has a better stress distribution.

Rehabilitation
Careful early active and passive physiotherapy.

Author Christopher W Geel

10.1.8 Articular multifragmentary proximal tibial fracture—41-C3

1 Case description

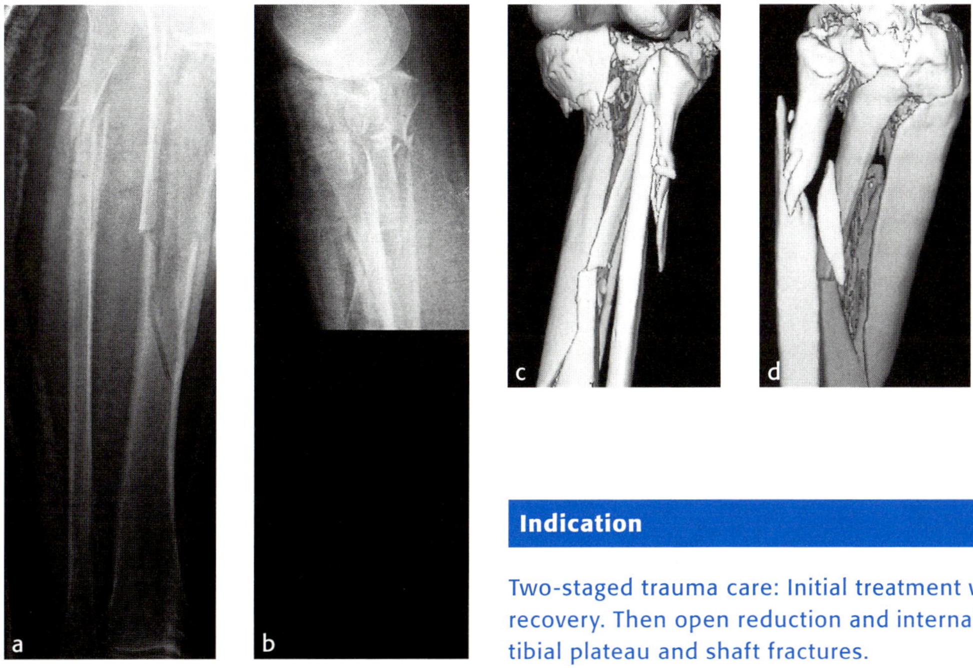

59-year-old woman fell and broke her right proximal tibia.

Fig 10.1.8-1a–d
a AP view.
b Lateral view.
c–d 3D CT scan.

Indication

Two-staged trauma care: Initial treatment with spanning external fixator until soft-tissue recovery. Then open reduction and internal fixation (ORIF) of multifragmentary, articular tibial plateau and shaft fractures.

Preoperative planning

Equipment

- LCP proximal tibial plate 4.5/5.0, 12 holes
- Locking head screws (LHS)
- 6.5 mm cancellous bone screws
- K-wires
- Pointed reduction forceps

(Size of system, instruments, and implants can vary according to anatomy.)

Patient preparation and positioning

Antibiotics: cephalosporin
Thrombosis prophylaxis: low-molecular heparin

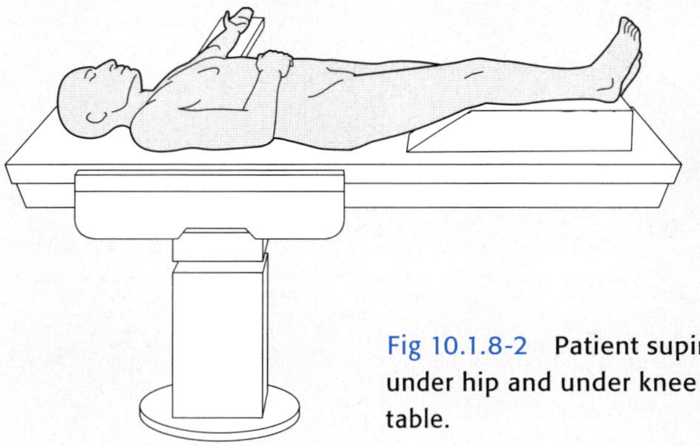

Fig 10.1.8-2 Patient supine with bump under hip and under knee on radiolucent table.

2 Surgical approach

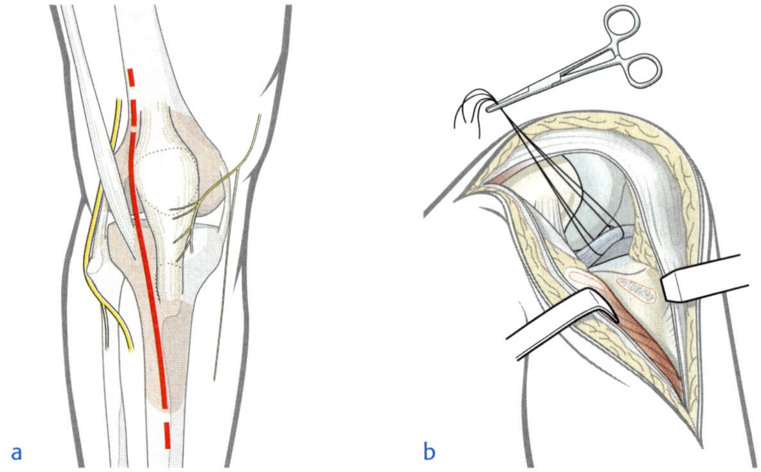

Fig 10.1.8-3a–b Curvylinear anterior parapateller lateral incision. Parapatellar lateral arthrotomy. Elevation of lateral meniscus. Incision of peroneal muscle compartment in an L-shape fashion.

3 Reduction and fixation

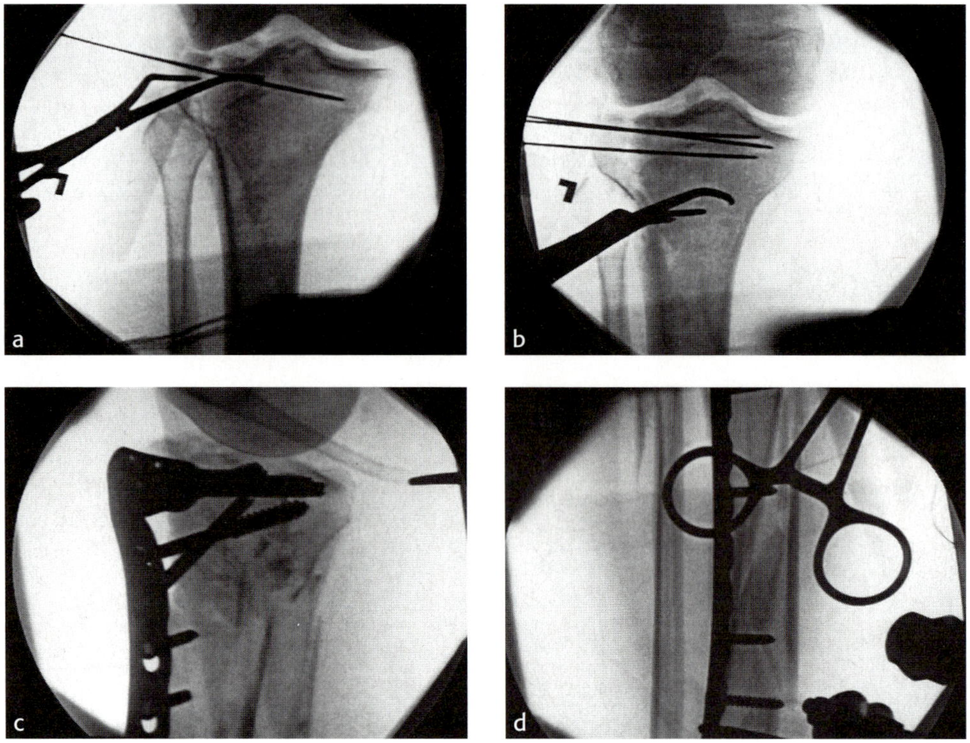

Fig 10.1.8-4a–d

- a–b Preliminary fixation of the reduced joint surface with K-wires and two pointed reduction forceps using the external fixator as an indirect reduction tool.
  Verify reduction with image intensifier.
- c 12-hole LCP proximal tibia plate 4.5/5.0 is adjusted to the lateral plateau and is used as a reduction tool for the metaphyseal-diaphyseal junction: push-pull principle.
- d Fixation proximally first to restore the joint surface and the tibial condyles.

3 Reduction and fixation (cont)

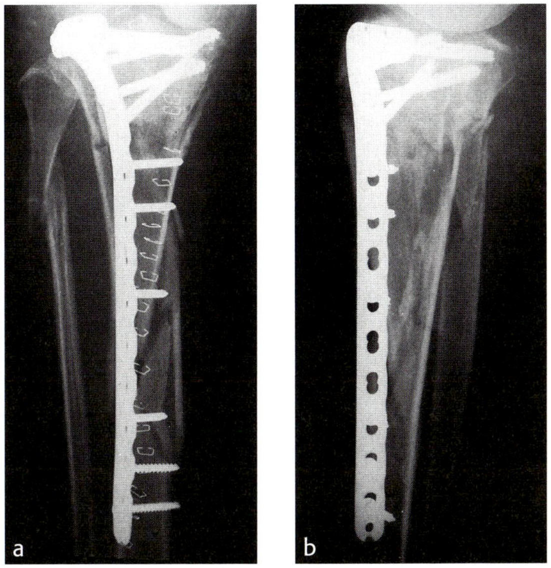

Fig 10.1.8-5a–b Fixation of the diaphysis to the plate after verifying the correct position of the plate in AP and lateral image intensifier views.

4 Rehabilitation

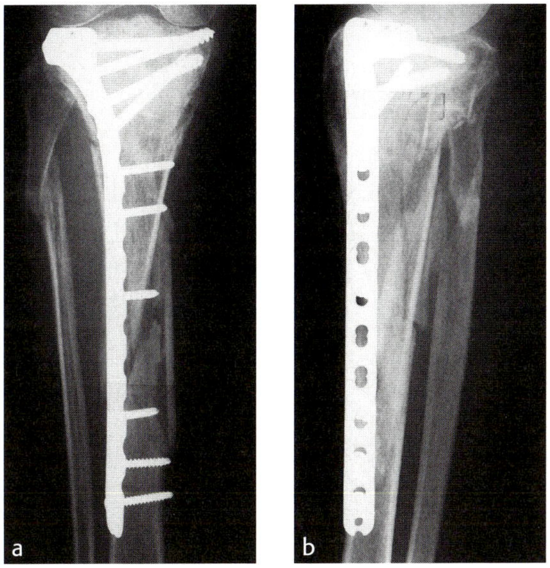

Weight bearing: 15 kg for 4 weeks; half body weight after 9 weeks; full weight bearing after 14 weeks.
Physiotherapy: Range of motion exercise of the ankle and knee joints to be started on day one postoperatively.

Fig 10.1.8-6a–b Postoperative x-rays after 6 weeks.
a AP view.
b Lateral view.

4 Rehabilitation (cont)

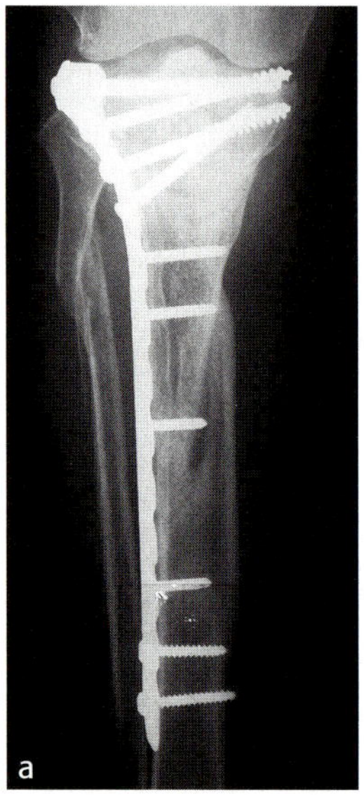

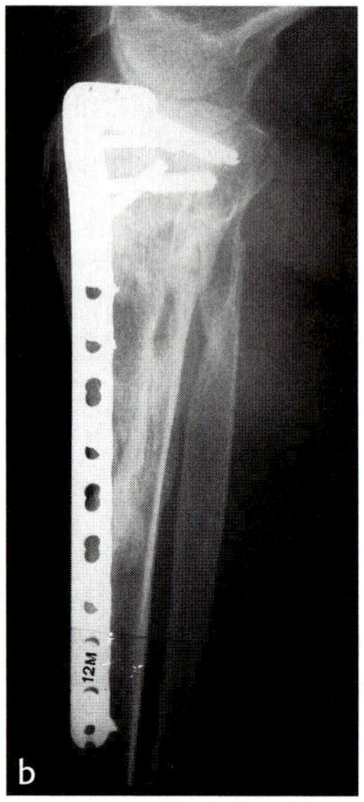

Fig 10.1.8-7a–b Postoperative x-rays after 12 months.
a AP view.
b Lateral view.

Bone healing after 12 weeks.

5 Pitfalls –

Equipment

Rehabilitation

Cartilage is crumbled and crushed but more than 50% of this injured surface is covered by meniscus.

6 Pearls +

Equipment

Fig 10.1.8-8a–b Image intensifier as preoperative planning is helpful with so-called traction views because it allows assessment and efficacy of indirect reduction using an external fixator or a large distractor.

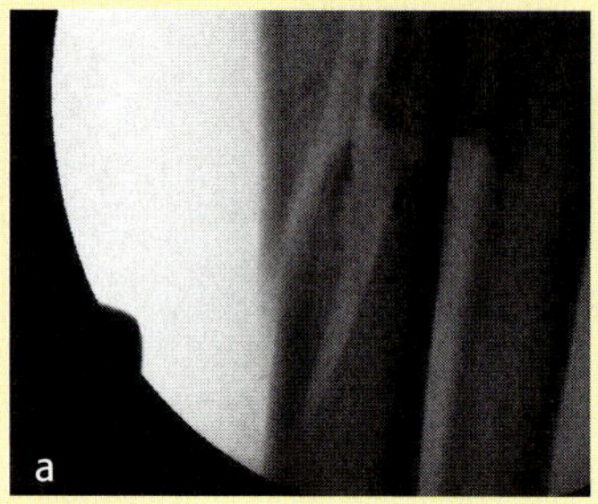

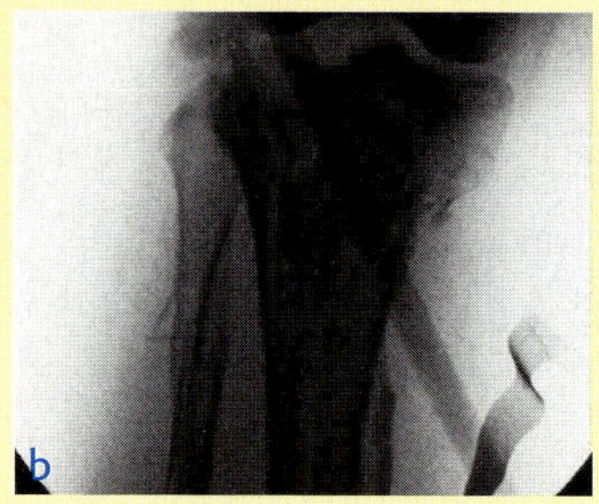

Rehabilitation

Authors Gabriele Streicher, Thomas J Hockertz, Andreas Gruner, Heinrich Reilmann

10.1.9 Articular multifragmentary proximal tibial fracture—41-C3

1 Case description

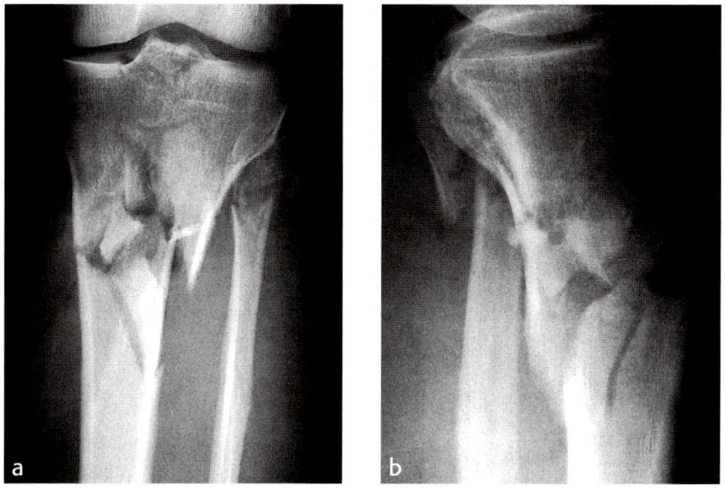

52-year-old man with injury to the tibial head. Type of injury: high-energy trauma, monotrauma, open fracture Gustilo type II.

Fig 10.1.9-1a–b
a AP view.
b Lateral view.

Indication

Proximal articular multifragmentary fracture of the tibial head with obvious dislocation (41-C3), unstable joint fracture with involvement of the proximal third of the tibia. Operative treatment is indicated to reconstruct the joint surfaces and preserve knee joint function.

Preoperative planning

Equipment
- LISS-PLT, 9 holes
- 5.0 mm self-drilling, self-tapping locking head screws (LHS)
- 2.0 mm K-wires
- 6.5 mm cancellous bone screws

(Size of system, instruments, and implants can vary according to anatomy.)

Patient preparation and positioning
Antibiotics: single dose 2nd generation cephalosporin
Thrombosis prophylaxis: low-molecular heparin

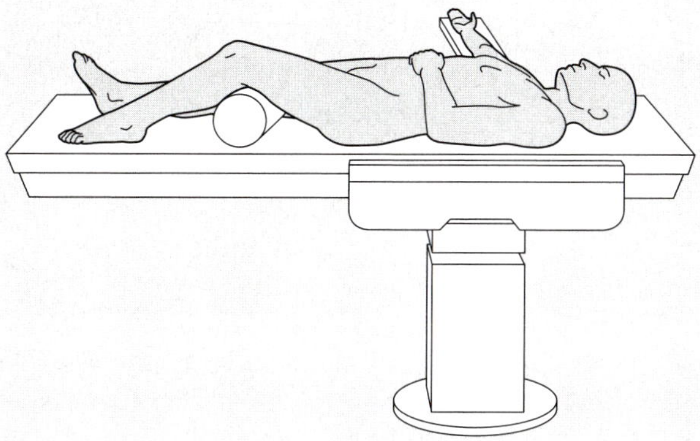

Fig 10.1.9-2 Supine position with elevation of the injured leg and flexion of the knee joint at approximately 30°, lowering of the contralateral leg for better intraoperative x-ray assessment, cushioning of the distal femur of the leg to be operated on, eg, with a towel roll.

2 Surgical approach

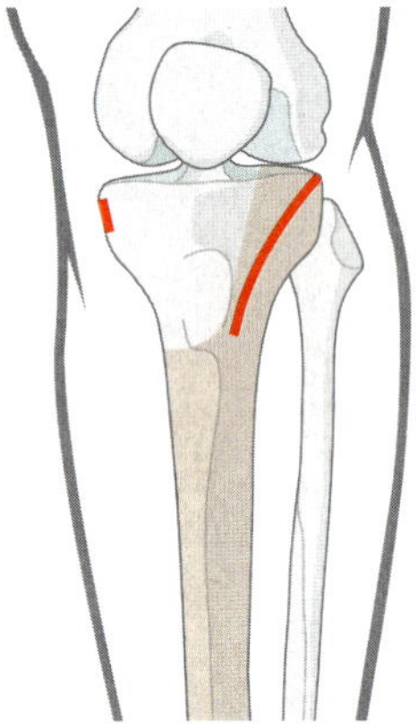

Fig 10.1.9-3 Hockey-stick incision approximately 5 cm long from Gerdy's tubercle extending in a distal direction, and dissection to the periosteum.

3 Reduction and fixation

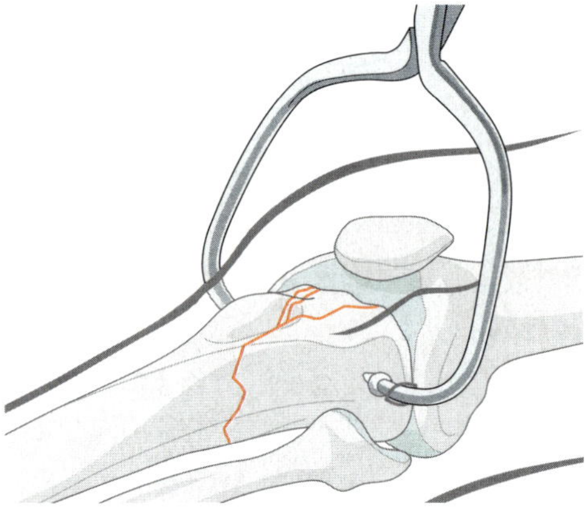

Fig 10.1.9-4 Approximate reduction of the joint surfaces by axial tension and tap out the collapsed joint surface components from the distal side with the help of pelvic reduction forceps.

3 Reduction and fixation (cont)

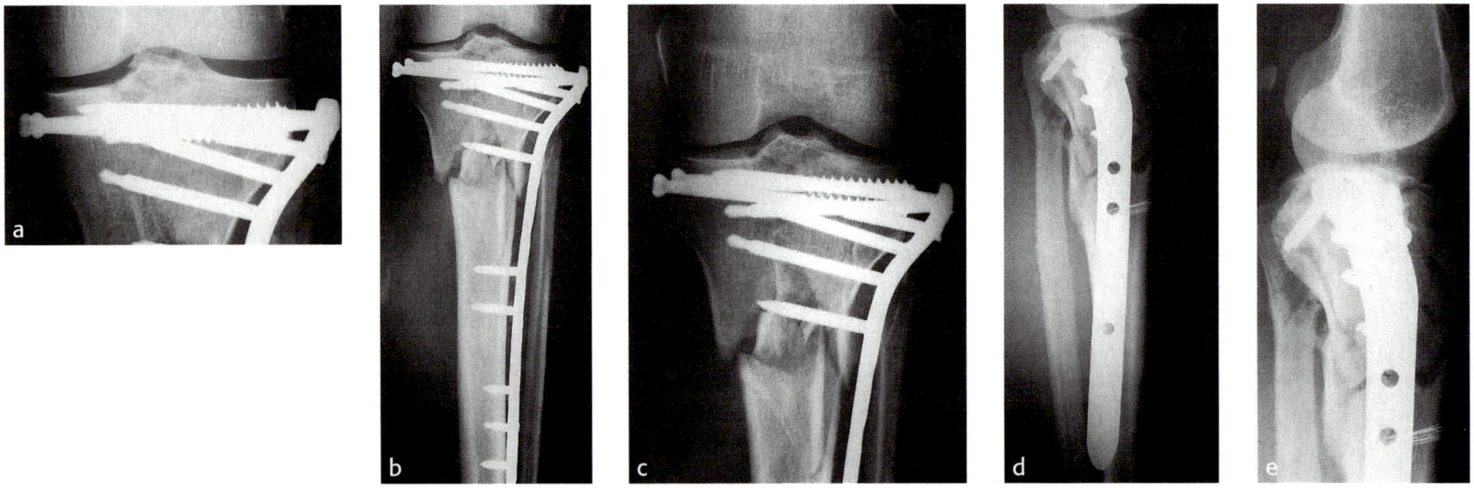

Fig 10.1.9-5a–e Secure reduction by inserting cancellous bone screws from the medial side and parallel to the joint surface through a stab incision.
Prepare the plate bed from proximal to distal epiperiosteally in the compartment of the anterior tibialis muscle with a long bone rasp.
Determine correct plate length under image intensification and slide the implant into the plate bed.
Stabilize the implant temporarily with K-wires and check plate position in two planes.
Precise reduction of the fragments with the pulling device.
Insert the screws alternately into the distal and proximal holes starting proximally, determine screw length according to Tab 3-2.

4 Rehabilitation

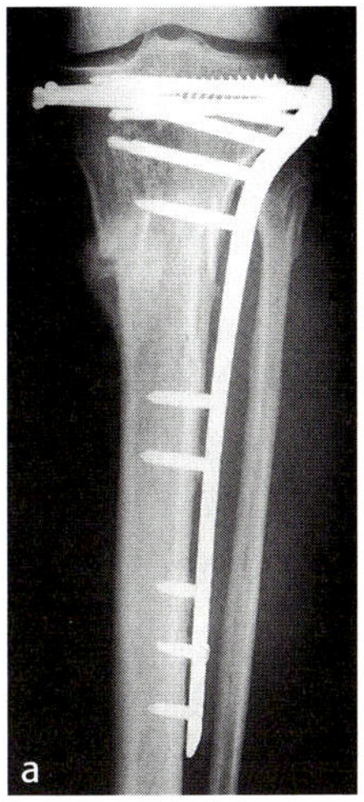

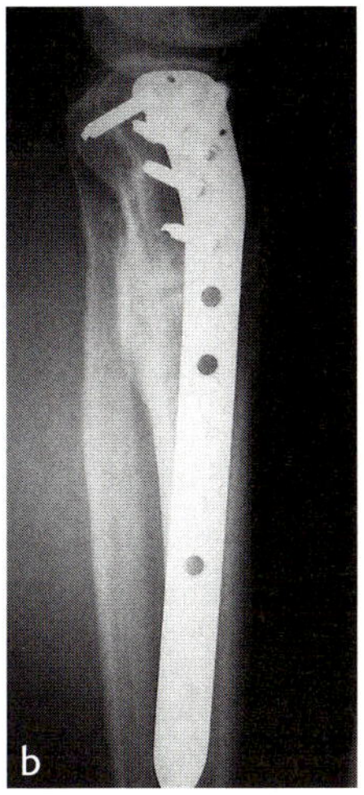

Weight bearing: half body weight after 2 weeks, full weight bearing after 10 weeks.
Physiotherapy: from the second postoperative day.
Pharmaceutical treatment: pain treatment and nonsteroid antiinflammatory drugs.

Fig 10.1.9-6a–b Bone healing after 12 weeks.
a AP view.
b Lateral view.

Implant removal

After approximately 12–18 months.
Reason for implant removal: mechanical irritation at the lateral tibial head caused by the implant.
Technique for implant removal: removal of screws through stab incision and removal of the LISS via the original proximal approach.

5 Pitfalls –

Equipment
Length of plate too short.

Approach
Inadequate preparation of the tibial head leads to incorrect plate positioning (too far posterior or too far anterior). Be aware of the peroneal nerve.

Reduction and fixation
Pull-out of the pulling device due to osteoporosis or too long a reduction distance.

Rehabilitation
Premature full weight bearing with joint involvement.

6 Pearls +

Equipment

Approach
Preservation of blood vessels due to a minimally invasive approach.

Reduction and fixation
Intraoperative x-ray controls to ensure that the plate is correctly positioned in the lateral plane.

Rehabilitation
Early mobilization with partial/full weight bearing.

Author **Michael Wagner**

10.1.10 Complete articular multifragmentary proximal tibial fracture—41-C3 and avulsion fracture of the fibular head

1 Case description

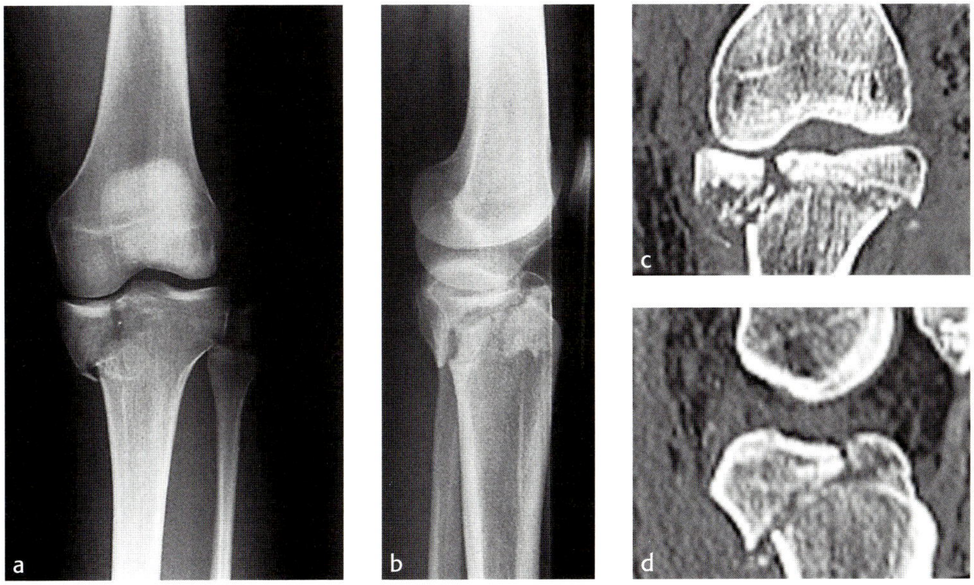

19-year-old woman fell from a horse. Multifragmentary articular fracture of the left tibial head with bone avulsion of the lateral ligament of the fibular head and contusion of the soft tissues.

Fig 10.1.10-1a–d
- a AP view.
- b Lateral view.
- c CT scan in the frontal plane shows the multifragmentary articular fracture with small fragments.
- d CT scan in the sagittal plane.

Indication

Displaced articular fracture with ligamentary instability is a clear indication for anatomical reduction and stable fixation in order to restore good function. The operation was performed on the third day after the accident after CT examination had been completed.

Preoperative planning

Equipment
- LCP T-plate 4.5/5.0, 5 holes
- 4.5 mm and 5.0 mm locking head screws (LHS)
- 4.0 mm cannulated cancellous bone screws, partially threaded
- 2.0 mm K-wires

(Size of system, instruments, and implants can vary according to anatomy.)

Patient preparation and positioning

Antibiotics: 3rd generation cephalosporin

Thrombosis prophylaxis: low-molecular heparin

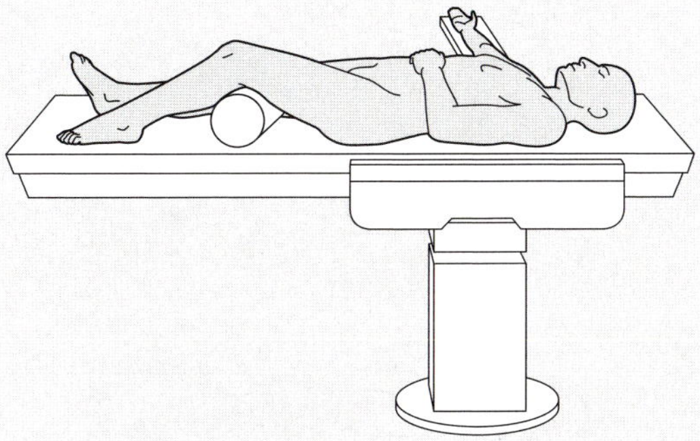

Fig 10.1.10-2 Supine position on radiolucent operating table with the leg freely moveable.

2 Surgical approach

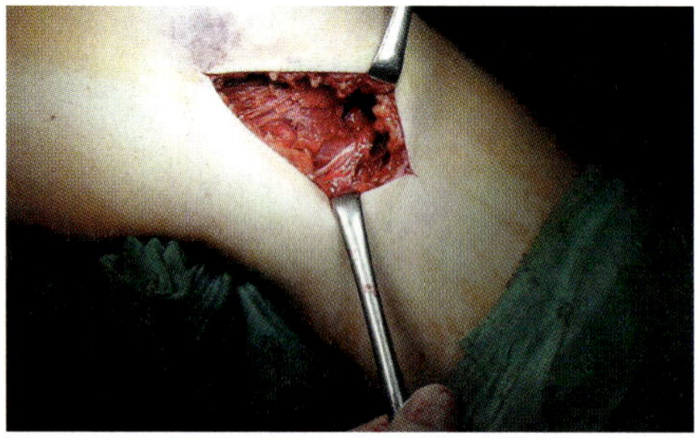

Fig 10.1.10-3 Medial approach for submeniscal medial arthrotomy, an additional medial distal approach for plate fixation in MIPO technique, and a third small lateral approach for reduction and fixation of the avulsion fracture of the fibular head.

3 Reduction and fixation

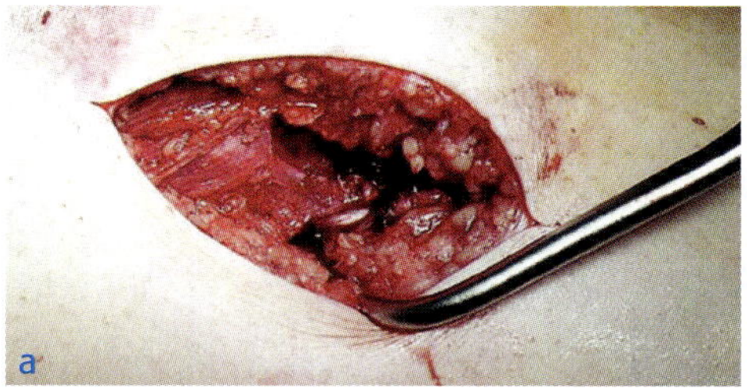

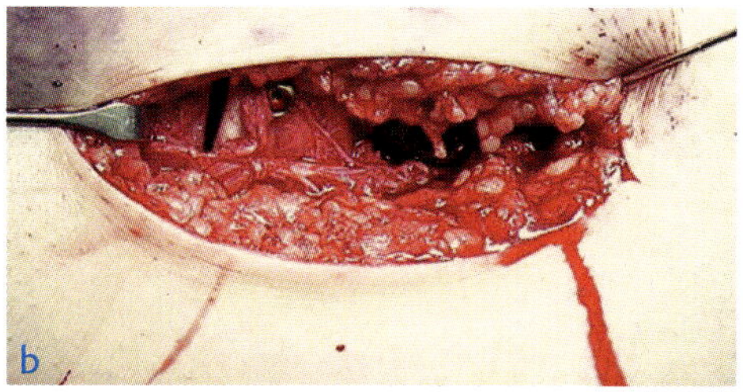

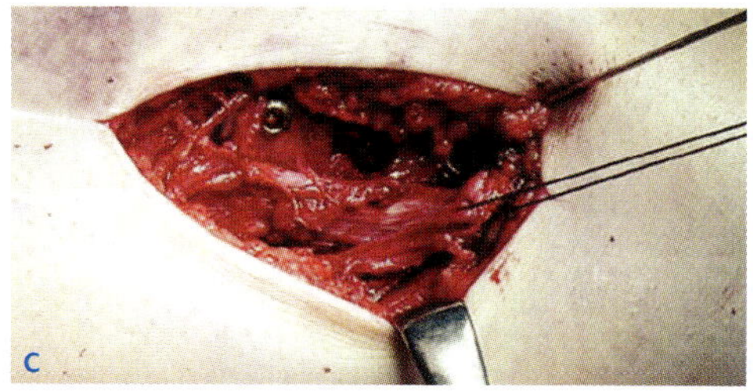

Fig 10.1.10-4a–h

a Reduction of the joint fragments and temporary fixation with pelvic reduction forceps and a ball spike.

b Shows the screw head of the 4.0 mm lag screw situated as far proximally as possible under the articular surface and the submeniscal arthrotomy through which the reduction was assessed.

c The partial rupture of the medial collateral ligament and the pes anserinus tendon can be seen.

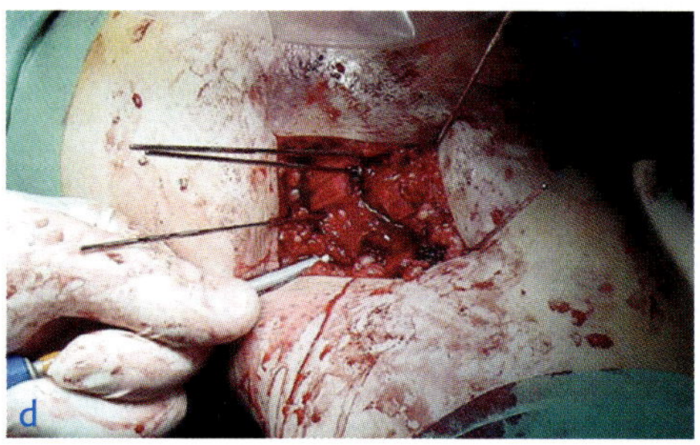

d The joint block that has been stabilized with two lag screws inserted from medial to lateral is then reduced in relation to the diaphyseal fragment by manual tension and ball spike. The reduction is stabilized by insertion of a guide wire in an anteroposterior orientation. The third lag screw is then inserted.

3 Reduction and fixation (cont)

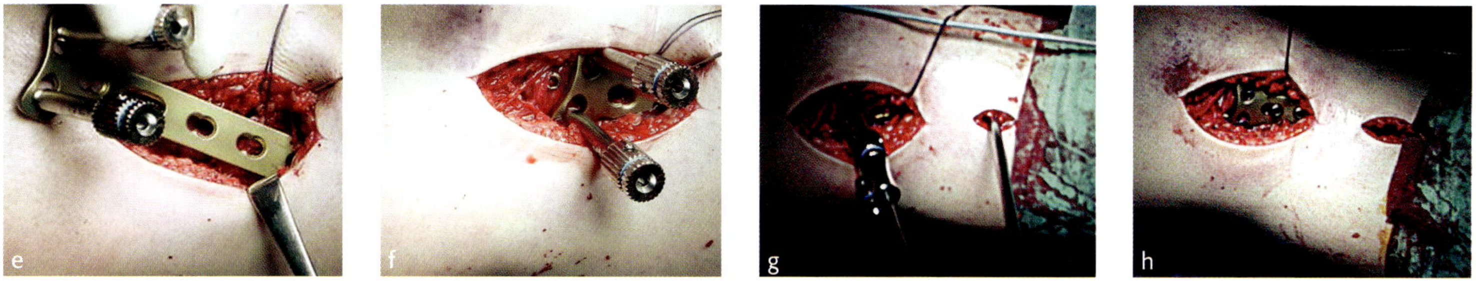

Fig 10.1.10-4a–h (cont)

e–f After securing the drill guides, insertion of the plate from proximal to distal. The plate comes to rest above the pes anserinus ligament and the insertion of the distal ligament.

g–h Additional incisions are made at the distal plate end. Temporary fixation with K-wires and assessment of implant position by image intensification; fixation with locking head screws.

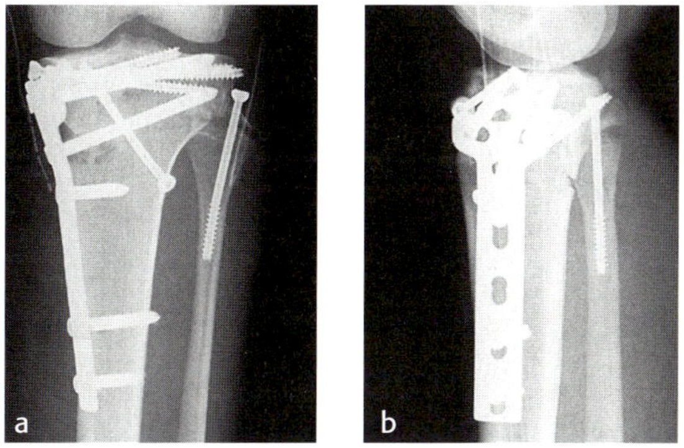

The last step is the fixation of the fibular head fracture with a cannulated 4.0 mm cancellous bone screw through an additional small lateral incision. The screw thread is anchored in the narrow intramedullary cavity of the fibular shaft.

Fig 10.1.10-5a–b Postoperative x-rays.

a AP view.

b Lateral view.

4 Rehabilitation

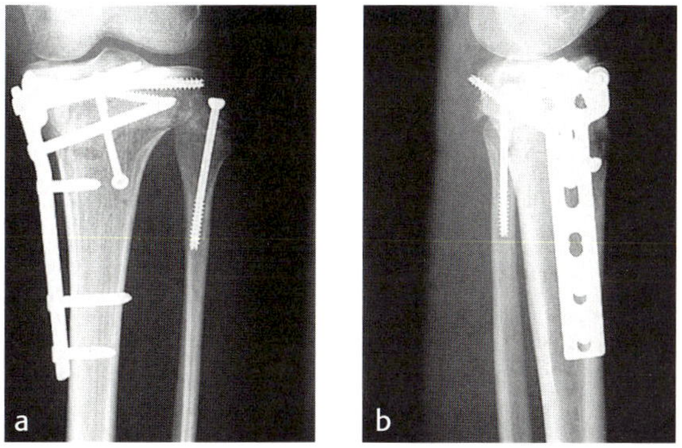

Mobilization began after removal of the drains in a removable knee brace to relieve the damaged ligaments of the knee. Initially 10–15 kg weight bearing and after 6 weeks half body weight.

Fig 10.1.10-6a–b Postoperative x-rays after 2 months show bone consolidation of all fractures and all implants in situ.

a AP view.

b Lateral view.

4 Rehabilitation (cont)

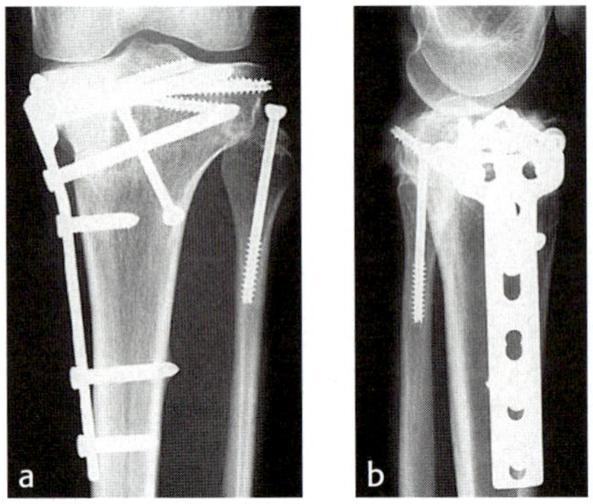

Fig 10.1.10-7a–b Postoperative x-rays after 1 year. All fractures have healed, function is unrestricted and the knee is stable and painfree.

a AP view shows the gap between the angular stable noncontact plate and the bone. The tendons of the pes anserinus and the distal insertion of the medial collateral ligament are placed in this space.

b Lateral view.

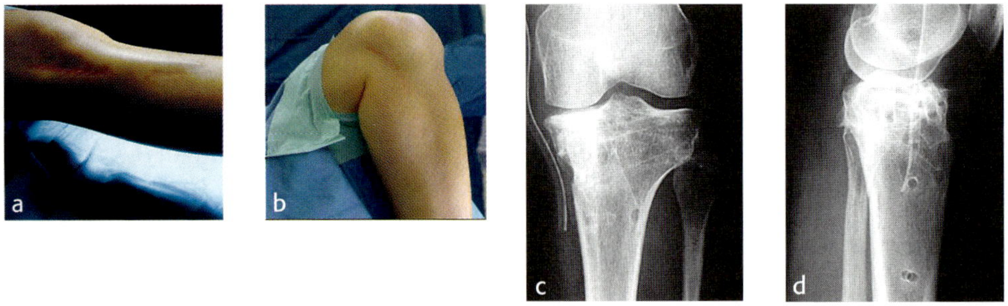

Implant removal

Fig 10.1.10-8a–d

a–b Functional result, full range of motion before implant removal.

c–d The implant was removed because it could be felt under the skin at the medial aspect.

5 Pitfalls –

Approach

The peroneal nerve may be damaged in a medial approach.

Reduction and fixation

Difficult to reduce an articular fracture in a less invasive technique.

6 Pearls +

Equipment

The submuscular arthrotomy permitted direct visualization of the reduced articular surface.

Reduction and fixation

Pelvic reduction forceps and the large pointed reduction forceps permit direct, percutaneous reduction of articular fragments. The fixation of cannulated screws inserted over a guide wire permits the optimal placement of the lag screws.

The LCP T-plate with LHS allows the stable fixation of very small joint blocks to the shaft and does not exert pressure on the tendons and ligaments beneath it. This stable fixation permits early functional rehabilitation.

Author Christoph Sommer

10.1.11 Inversed Y-fracture of the tibial head with impression of the anterolateral joint surface—41-C3

1 Case description

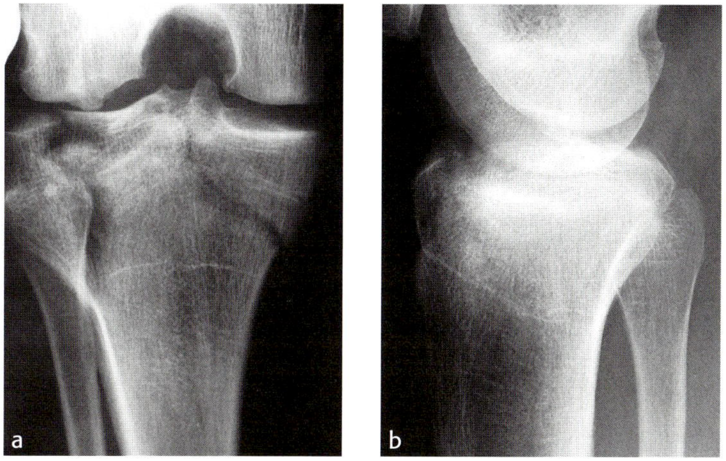

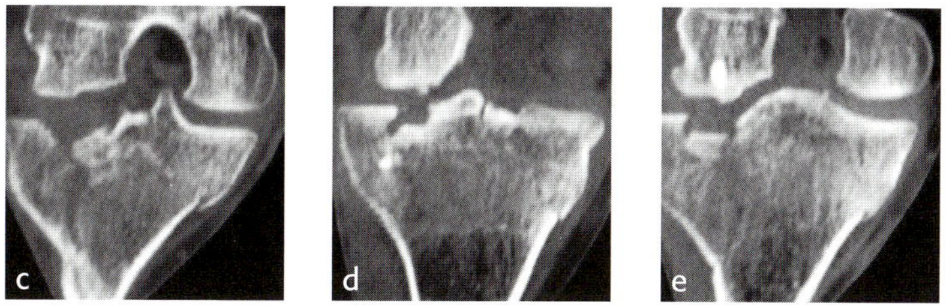

Fig 10.1.11-1a–e
a AP view.
b Lateral view.
c–e A preoperative CT scan was performed for more specific diagnosis. An anterolateral impression of 5–10 mm of the joint could be identified with only a slight displacement of the medial condyle.

30-year-old man sustained a valgization trauma while skiing. No soft-tissue damage. Status after operation of osteochondrosis dissecans of the lateral femoral condyle. An inversed Y-fracture of the tibial head can be seen on the x-ray with impression of the anterolateral joint surface (41-C3.1, complete articular fracture, lateral articular multifragmentary fracture). The medial tibial condyle is only minimally displaced.

Indication

This fracture is a clear indication for reduction and stabilization. Since the injury to the lateral tibial plateau is a multifragmentary fracture, there is the indication for a submeniscal arthrotomy and reduction under vision. The medial plateau is not displaced so a single anterolateral approach with an angular stable T-plate should be sufficient. Alternatively, a LISS-PLT could be used. If the medial plateau was displaced, a second posteromedial approach and a small posteromedial plate would be applied in a first step.

Preoperative planning

Equipment
- LCP L-plate 4.5/5.0, 6 holes
- 5.0 mm locking head screws (LHS)
- 4.5 mm cortex screws
- K-wires
- Pelvic reduction forceps

(Size of system, instruments, and implants can vary according to anatomy.)

Preoperative planning (cont)

Patient preparation and positioning

Antibiotics: single dose 2nd generation cephalosporin
Thrombosis prophylaxis: low-molecular heparin

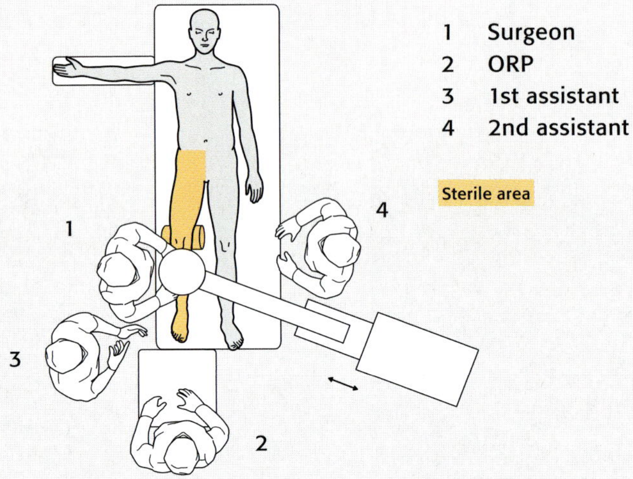

Fig 10.1.11-2 The entire leg is prepped and draped under sterile conditions, including the iliac crest so that cancellous bone can be harvested. The injured leg is extended but is supported below the knee with a metal triangular block or large towel roll, which can be removed as the situation requires.

2 Surgical approach

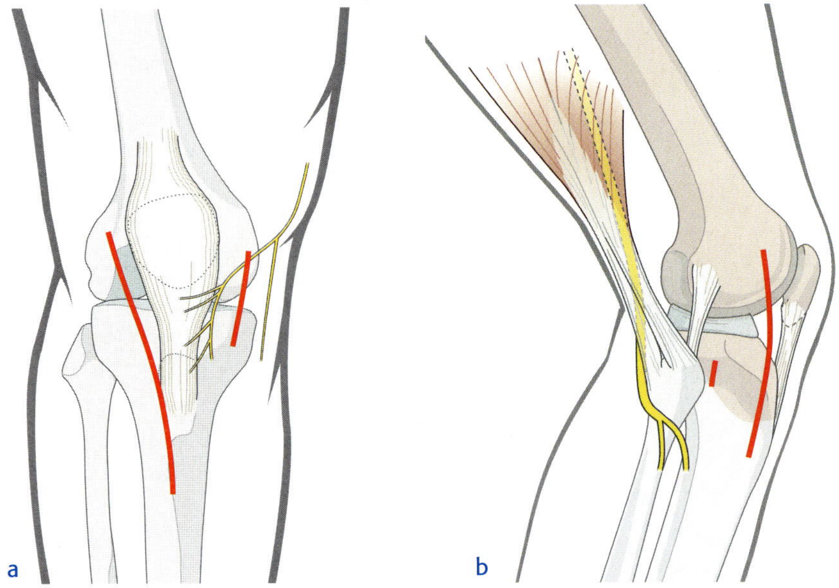

Fig 10.1.11-3a–b Anterolateral standard approach with two additional incisions for the percutaneous insertion of the pelvic reduction forceps.

3 Reduction and fixation

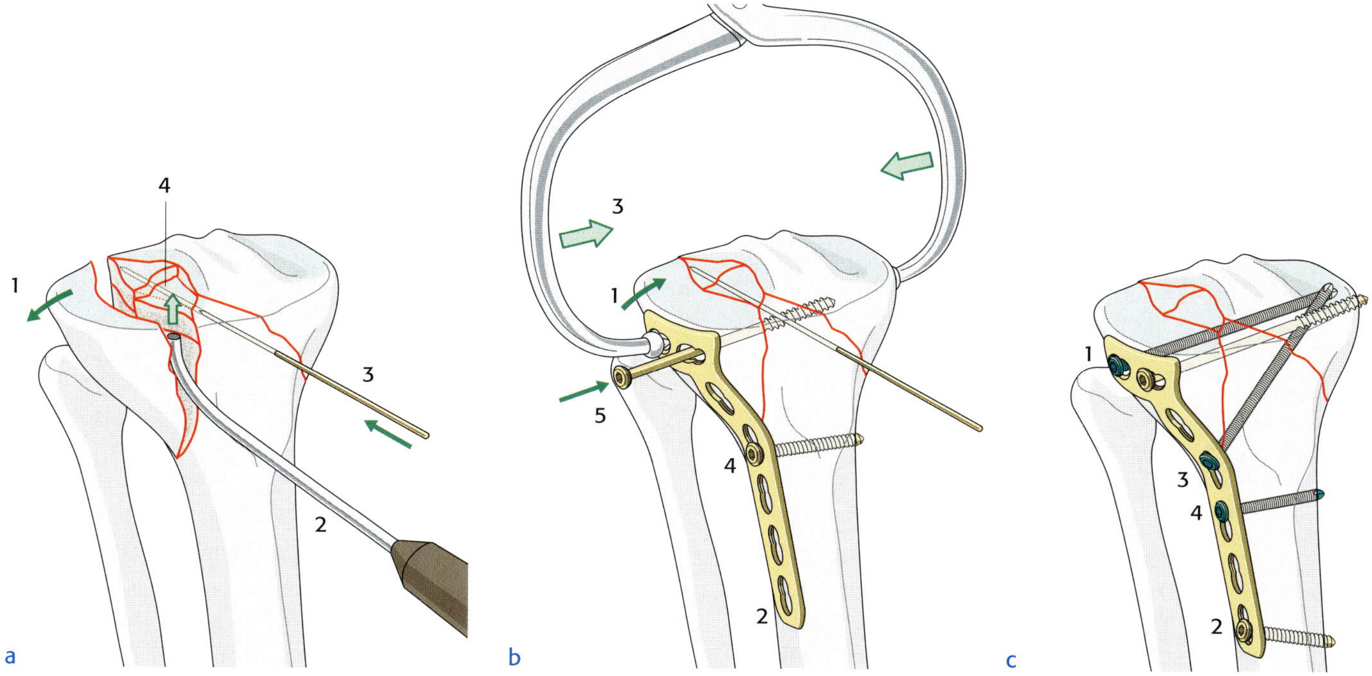

Fig 10.1.11-4a–c

a With the help of an anterolateral standard approach and release of the iliotibial tract from the lateral tibial head, a horizontal arthrotomy is performed and the fracture is stabilized in open reduction technique. The sagittal fracture line is presented and the lateral fragment is folded outwards with the help of a bone spreader (1). After removing the hematoma, the two joint fragments can be lifted into the correct position under vision (2). The reduced joint fragment can be held in place with a temporary K-wire inserted in an anteroposterior direction (3). If the bone fragment were narrow or the defect very large, the defect could be filled with cancellous bone and bicortical iliac bone graft (4).

b Replace the manually extracted joint fragment and apply the preshaped LCP 4.5 to the anterolateral aspect of the tibia (1, 2). With the help of the pelvic reduction forceps, (inserted medially and laterally via small incisions) and with the lateral fragment correctly positioned, the fracture can now be compressed. The forceps can be applied cranially or ideally through the posterior plate hole (3). The first screw to be used is a 4.5 mm cortex screw inserted into the metaphyseal combination hole (4). After verifying the reduction and the correct placement of the plate under image intensification, the fracture zone can be compressed with a 6.5 mm cancellous bone screw through the upper anterior hole (5).

c After removal of the pelvic reduction forceps and the K-wire, the other screws can be inserted (1). 5.0 mm LHS in the tibial head are ideal. Pay attention to the correct angle of the screws in relation to the plate. In the case described here, an LHS was inserted into the metaphyseal aspect of the plate to hold the medial condyle (3). The fixation of the plate onto the shaft can be accomplished with bicortical 4.5 mm cortex screws or in poor bone quality with bicortical LHS (2). In this case, the first 4.5 mm cortex screw was replaced with a LHS for a better hold (4).

3 Reduction and fixation (cont)

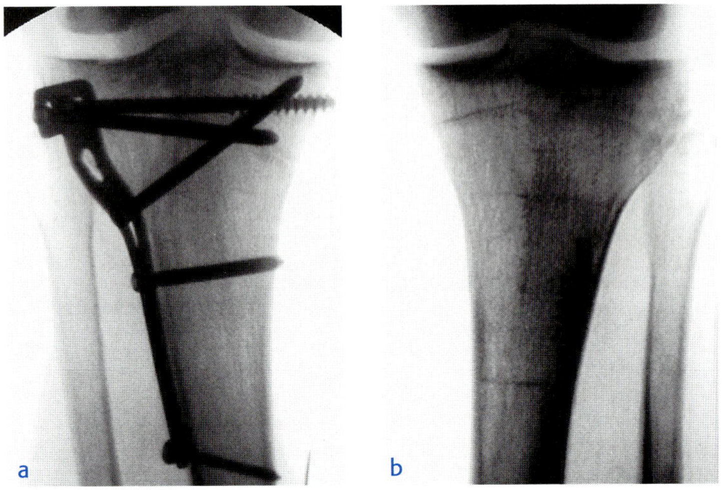

Fig 10.1.11-5a–b The x-rays at the end of the operation showed an anatomical reconstruction of all fracture components. The slight varus position on the AP projection (a) is symmetrical to the uninjured leg (b).

4 Rehabilitation

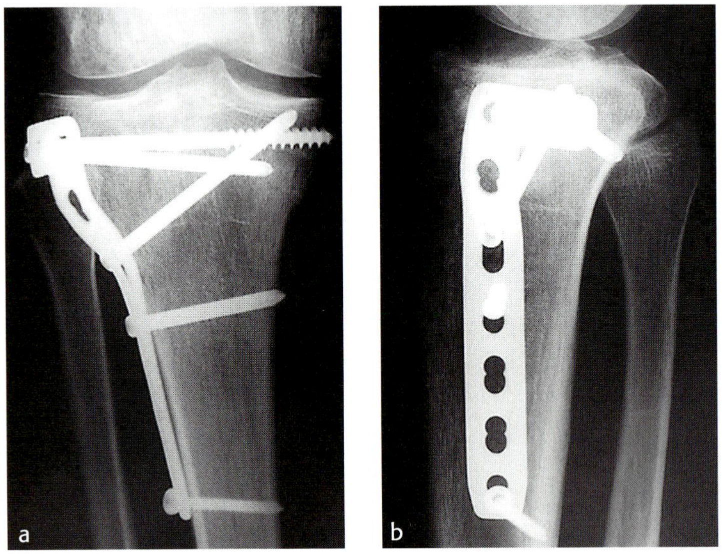

Given good stability of the knee joint (tested at the end of the operation), the joint could be treated functionally with a range of motion up to the first indication of pain. Mobilization started on the third day with 10–15 kg weight bearing for 6 weeks.

Fig 10.1.11-6a–h

a–b The first x-ray check-up after 7 weeks showed a good anatomical axis and a level joint surface with a stable fit for the plate.

4 Rehabilitation (cont)

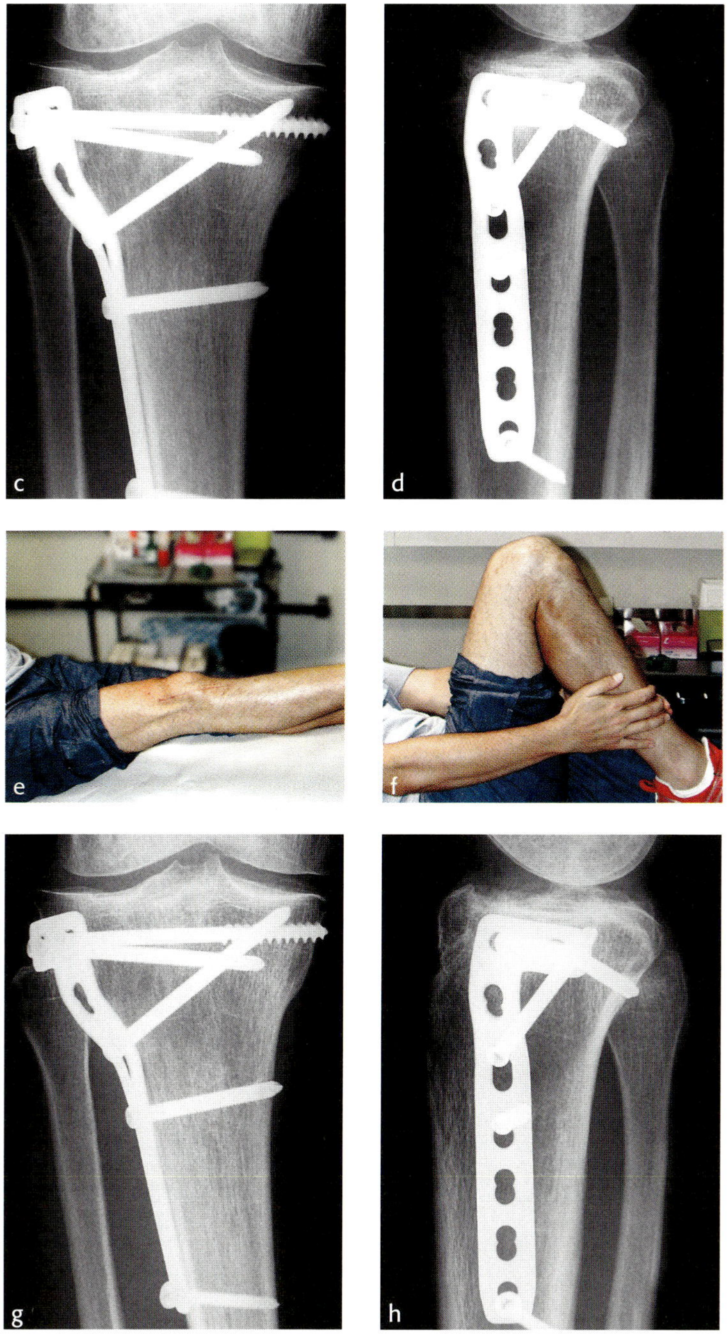

Fig 10.1.11-6a–h (cont)

c–d When the fracture line had nearly disappeared, weight bearing was increased to full weight after 3 months. The fracture was consolidated after this time.

e–f The range of motion was practically identical for both knees and the patient was able to go on a 7 hour cycling tour with 2700 m ascent.

g–h After 8 months the patient wished to have the plate removed because of a slight irritation of the iliotibial tract caused by the proximal plate end. At this time, there was complete radiological consolidation and remodeling of the fracture.

5 Pitfalls –

Equipment
During preshaping of the LCP 4.5/5.0 the holes may become bent and the locking head screws will not hold properly. Therefore, the plate should always be bent and twisted between the holes.

Approach
The standard approach has few risks. But the saphenous nerve and vein and the infragenicular nerve may be endangered by a medial approach (not performed in this case).

Reduction and fixation
Under early full weight bearing, the LCP 4.5/5.0 may twist, resulting in a varus malalignment.

Rehabilitation
Good compliance is required. Early full weight bearing can cause dislocation with change of joint surface level and/or varus malalignment.

6 Pearls +

Equipment
Ideal implant for treatment of a fracture in combination technique (compression of the joint surface with cortex screws and cancellous bone screws and buttressing of the metaphyseal zone with locking head screws).

Approach
An anterolateral approach allows the stabilization of a C-type fracture (in contrast to the double plate technique with medial and lateral approach).

Reduction and fixation
LCP 4.5 plates are ideal for medial and lateral partial joint fractures (41-B-type fractures). With a simple medial fragment and good bone quality, the LCP 4.5/5.0 with LHS can also be used for 41-C-type fractures (in contrast to the double plate technique). The less flexible LISS-PLT should be preferred in more complex fractures.

Rehabilitation

10.2 Tibia and fibula, shaft

Cases

Cases (cont)

Case	Classification	Method	Implant used	Implant function	Page
10.2.12 Open complex segmental tibial shaft fracture	42-C2	compression and locked splinting	LCP 4.5/5.0	lag screws and protection plate and locked internal fixator	755
10.2.13 Open complex irregular tibial and fibular shaft fracture	42-C3	locked splinting	LISS-PLT	lag screws and locked internal fixator	759
10.2.14 Open complex irregular tibial shaft fracture	42-C3	compression and locked splinting	LCP 4.5/5.0	lag screws and locked internal fixator	763
10.2.15 Spiral tibial shaft fracture in a child	42-A1	locked splinting	LCP metaphyseal plate 3.5/4.5/5.0	locked internal fixator	767
10.2.16 Periprosthetic fracture of the tibial shaft	42-B1	compression and locked splinting	LCP metaphyseal plate 3.5/4.5/5.0; LCP 3.5	locked internal fixator and compression plate	771
10.2.17 Pseudarthrosis of the tibia	42-B1	locked splinting	LCP 4.5/5.0, narrow	locked internal fixator	775

10 Tibia and fibula

Author Michael Wagner

10.2 Tibia and fibula, shaft

1 Incidence

Tibial shaft fractures are frequent in sports injuries and in road traffic accidents. Pedestrians are endangered when hit or jammed by bumper bars. For specific anatomical reasons the soft-tissue involvement is of path-breaking importance regarding fracture evaluation and treatment planning.

Any hint or evident sign of decreased local vascularization has to be taken into consideration as well as extensive soft-tissue deficiency and has to remain a warning component for a safe surgical schedule. In some cases, it may be advisable to await decreased soft tissue swelling before carrying out temporary bridging external fixation.

In tibial fractures, arterial injuries are more common than nerve involvements. Later on, the danger of a compartment syndrome is obvious, favoring the anterior compartment.

2 Classification

In the diaphysis, the Müller AO Classification distinguishes between simple (A), wedge (B), and complex (C) fractures.

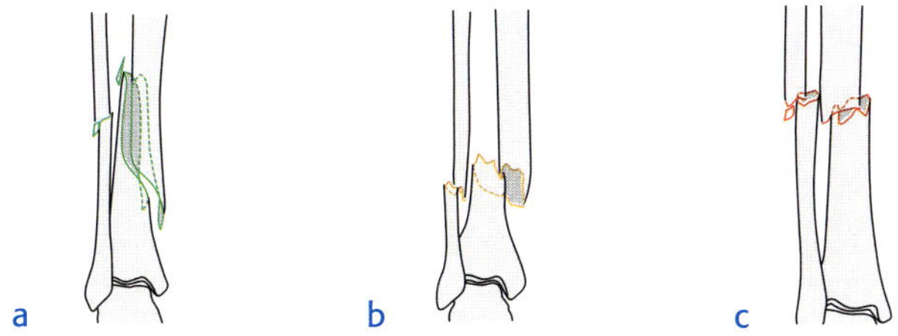

Fig 10.2-1a–c 42-A simple fracture.
a 42-A1 spiral
b 42-A2 oblique (≥ 30°)
c 42-A3 transverse (> 30°)

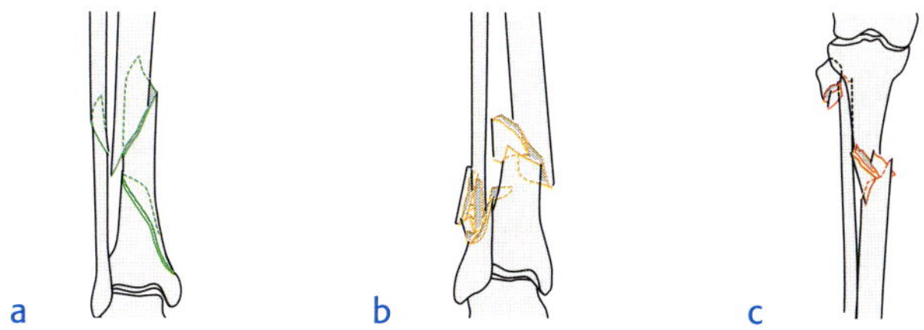

Fig 10.2-2a–c 42-B wedge fracture.
a 42-B1 spiral wedge
b 42-B2 bending wedge
c 42-B3 fragmented wedge

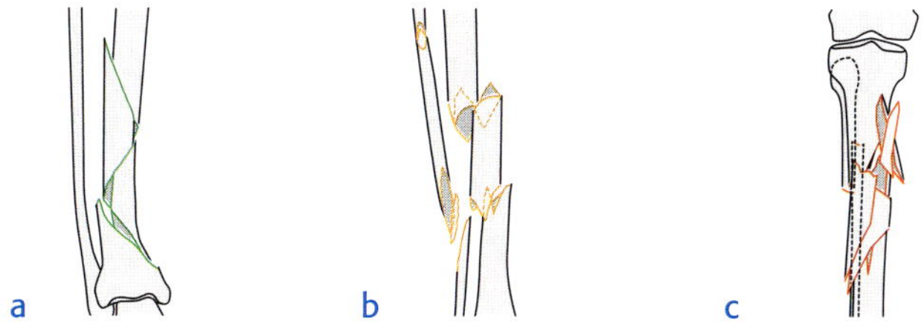

Fig 10.2-3a–c 42-C complete articular fractures.
a 43-C1 spiral
b 43-C2 segmental
c 43-C3 irregular

3 Treatment methods

Nonoperative treatment may be planned in exceptional cases if there are stable and minimally displaced fracture conditions. Good functional results are to be expected by initial immobilization in an appropriate cast followed by early weight bearing. In most cases, however, fractures of the tibial shaft reveal instability and displacement and need operative fixation.

For the majority of closed midshaft fractures as well as for open fractures with a sufficient soft-tissue cover intramedullary nailing is the key to success. In metaphyseal fractures the short fragment may be difficult to handle so that plating possibly seems more appropriate. In closed fractures reamed intramedullary nails are advantageous allowing the use of stronger implants and thus enhancing healing conditions. In most open tibial fractures, the solid "unreamed" nail is the implant of choice.

As a rule and to ensure indispensable stability, locking is recommended in all situations unless the nail has achieved excellent endosteal contact above and below a stable mid-diaphyseal fracture.

Locking results in a static bone–implant unit that impedes beneficial fracture loading. Consequently, and depending on the fracture type, only dynamic locking is recommended. Dynamization is required in delayed unions of the hypertrophic type at 4–6 months. In combined distal fractures it is advisable to fix the fibular component with a one-third tubular plate, thus assuring reduction and enhancing stability.

Inappropriate incision, nail entry point and nail positioning may cause considerable irritation of the patellar ligament. Therefore, any incision about the anterior aspect of the knee is to be avoided.

A further complication may be the breakage of locking screws due to the use of smaller nails or to prolonged bone healing time. On the other hand, a high rate of union and a low incidence of infection are to be stressed.

Displaced, unstable fractures of the proximal and distal thirds of the tibia shaft—with or without articular involvement—are best fixed with plates (because it is difficult to obtain an anatomical reduction and maintain it with an IM nail). In these areas the nail does not reduce the fracture nor does it maintain the reduction adequately. Plate fixation is also indicated in cases that require anatomically accurate reduction (more accurate than nailing will normally allow), for example, in high performance athletes.

Plating is contraindicated in unreliable patients or when the soft tissues are damaged or deficient. If the possibility of early weight bearing is more important than perfect alignment, intramedullary nailing is preferred.

The locking plates, ie, the LCP 4.5 and the Tibia LISS lend themselves to minimally invasive insertion and extraperiosteal positioning, especially in complex type C fractures.

Selection of the correct reduction technique is probably the most important part of internal fixation. When using direct or indirect methods, the goal is to restore the correct length, axial alignment, and rotation. Length is the key to the correct reduction and should be restored as the first step in most reductions. Manipulations to obtain reduction must be gentle and atraumatic in order not to compromise the essential blood supply to the fracture fragments.

With a simple type A or type B fracture pattern or bending and spiral wedges with a single fragment, direct anatomical reduction should be maintained by interfragmentary lag screw fixation and a protection or compression plate to provide absolute stability. Bridge plating, even with locking plates, should not be used for these fracture patterns. In complex type C fractures, exact reduction is not required and the plate should only have bridging function. Minimally invasive techniques with indirect reduction and extra long implants, preferably with locking head screws, provide relative stability with a low strain environment and allow healing by callus formation.

The LCP 4.5 can be used for diaphyseal fractures of the tibia. Conventional plating requires screw fixation in at least six cortices on either side of the fracture. Broad plates should not be used in the tibia; they are too stiff and too bulky. Smaller plates (eg, LCP 3.5) are occasionally indicated in the distal tibia in very small patients. In the LCP family there are metaphyseal plates with one end slightly precontoured and tapered as well as special form plates for both the proximal and the distal end of the tibia. For the proximal lateral tibia, a low profile L-shaped plate as well as the somewhat heavier LISS-PLT with combination holes are available and suitable for complex plateau fractures extending into the diaphysis. For the distal end of the bone there is the distal tibia LCP.

The current trend for both bridge plating and the conventional techniques is to use longer plates (8-hole to 10-hole) and not to fill every hole. Two or three bicortical screws above and two or three below the fracture focus are considered sufficient, provided they are spaced apart and anchored in good quality bone. More screws are probably unnecessary. In complex type C fractures a bridging plate should be about 3 times the length of the fracture zone.

Minimally invasive percutaneous plate application is a technique which can be used as an alternative to classical ORIF. It requires experience in indirect reduction techniques (with either a large distractor or external fixator), as correct length and axial alignment are mandatory before the plate is applied. In distal tibial fractures, indirect partial reduction and further stability may be achieved by plating the fibula. The length and rotation of the fibula must be exact or the tibia will be malaligned. Once the fracture is reduced and the plate contoured, the skin incision to introduce the plate is placed either proximally or distally to the fracture. With an elevator, an extraperiosteal tunnel is prepared to insert the plate. The LCP has a tapered end to facilitate the subcutaneous passage. The correct position is checked under fluoroscopy and subsequently the screws are inserted through stab incisions. As percutaneous plate application does not allow precise contouring of the implant, the LCP—used as an internal fixator—is the ideal implant for this technique. Thanks to the locking head screws the plate is not pressed against the bone, thereby preventing secondary malalignment.

Indications for external fixation may be in a way far-reaching. With rare exceptions however, external fixation will be intended to provide temporary fixation and to be supplemented by secondary internal fixation.

Therefore, its relevance is to be carefully considered in compromised soft tissue vascularization, in severe open fractures, in open fractures involving bone loss and/or soft tissue deficiency, in life-threatening polytrauma and in primary combination with an internal fixation.

The frame design should be as simple as possible, easy to handle and should allow access to the wound for secondary soft-tissue procedures and definitive internal fixation. In diaphyseal fractures the unilateral half pin frame might be favored in most situations whereas in proximal and distal fractures the use of a circular frame helps to avoid joint impairment. Finally, the use of a pinless fixator is advisable in view of secondary intramedullary nailing. To prevent plantar flexion contracture it may be helpful to add a pin in the first metatarsal to hold the foot in a neutral 90° position.

Summarizing, different and well-established treatment modalities are optional in the treatment of diaphyseal fractures of the tibia. The new angular stable plate with more "biological" approaches, especially in the proximal and distal third of the tibia, is opening up new dimensions in saving sufficient vascularization. However, the state of the soft-tissue cover is decisive for the choice of fixation device.

4 Implant overview

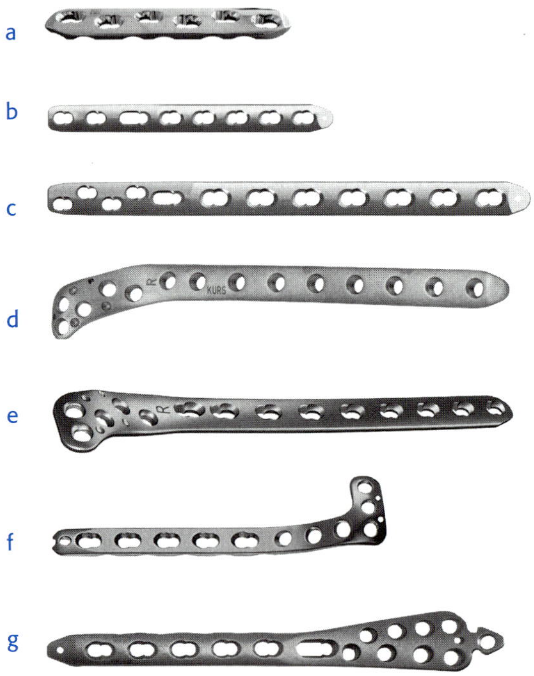

Fig 10.2-4a–g
- a LCP 4.5/5.0, broad
- b LCP metaphyseal plate 3.5
- c LCP metaphyseal plate 3.5/4.5/5.0
- d LISS-PLT 5.0 (left and right version)
- e LCP-PLT 4.5/5.0 (left and right version)
- f LCP proximal tibia plate 4.5/5.0, (lateral left and lateral right version)
- g LCP distal tibial plate 2.7/3.5, medial (left and right version)

5 Suggestions for further reading

Behrens F, Searls K (1986) External fixation of the tibia. Basic concepts and prospective evaluation. *J Bone Joint Surg [Br]*; 68 (2):246–254.

Bhandari M, Audige L, Ellis T, et al (2003) Operative Treatment of Extra-articular Proximal Tibial Fractures. *J. Orthop Trauma*; 17:591–595.

Bone LB, Sucato D, Stegemann PM, et al (1997) Displaced isolated fractures of the tibial shaft treated with either a cast or intramedullary nailing. An outcome analysis of matched pairs of patients. *J Bone Joint Surg [Am]*; 79 (9):1336–1341.

Gautier E, Sommer C (2003) Guidelines for the clinical application of the LCP. *Injury*; 34 (5-B63 – 5-B76).

Karladoni A, Granhad H, Edshage B, et al (2000) Displaced tibial shaft fractures. *Acta Orthop Scand*; 71:160–167.

Lang GJ, Cohen BE, Bosse MJ, et al (1995) Proximal third tibial shaft fractures. Should they be nailed? *Clin Orthop*; (315):64–74.

White RR, Babikian GM (2001) Tibia: shaft. In: Rüedi TP, Murphy WM, editors. AO Principles of Fracture Management. Stuttgart, New York: Thieme.

Author **Michael Wagner**

10.2.1 Simple spiral tibial shaft fracture—42-A1

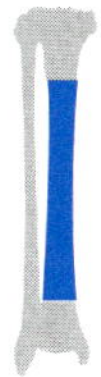

1 Case description

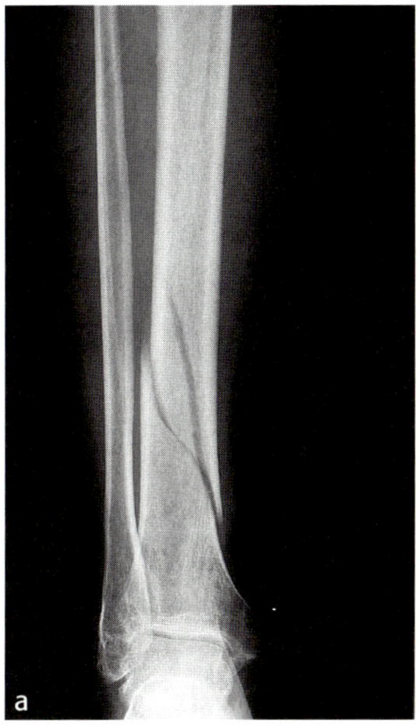

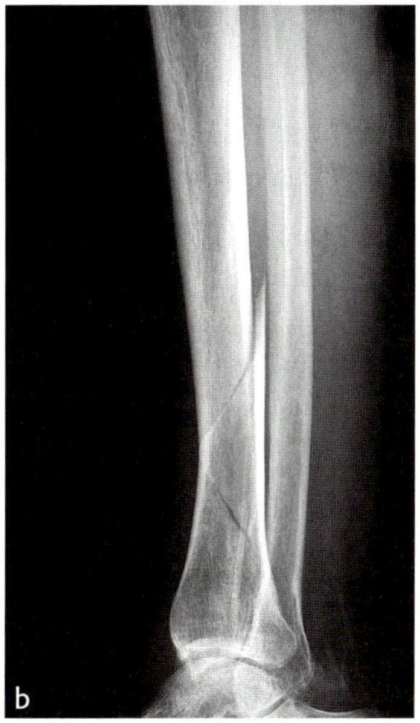

41-year-old patient slipped on the ice and sustained a spiral fracture of the right distal tibia. Monotrauma, closed fracture.

Fig 10.2.1-1a–b
a AP view.
b Lateral view.

Indication

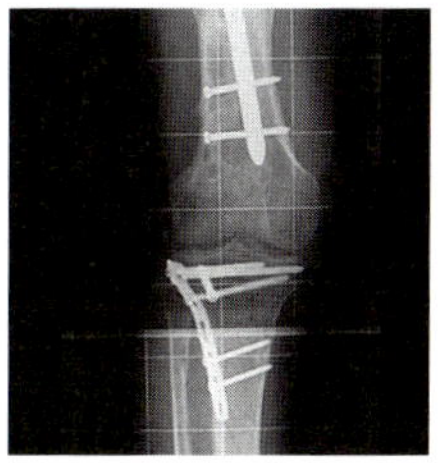

Fig 10.2.1-2 Intramedullary nailing is impossible because there is an implant in situ after a correction operation in the region of the lateral tibial head and, in addition, there is limited range of motion at the knee joint; flexion is only possible to 90°.

Preoperative planning

Equipment

- LCP 4.5/5.0, narrow, 14 holes
- Self-tapping locking head screws (LHS)
- 2.0 mm K-wires

(Size of system, instruments, and implants can vary according to anatomy.)

Patient preparation and positioning

Antibiotics: none
Thrombosis prophylaxis: low-molecular heparin

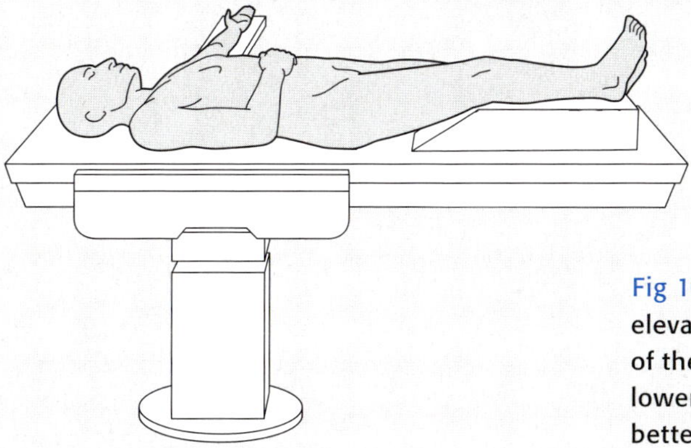

Fig 10.2.1-3 Supine position with elevation of the injured leg and flexion of the knee joint at approximately 30°, lowering of the contralateral leg for better intraoperative x-ray assessment.

2 Surgical approach

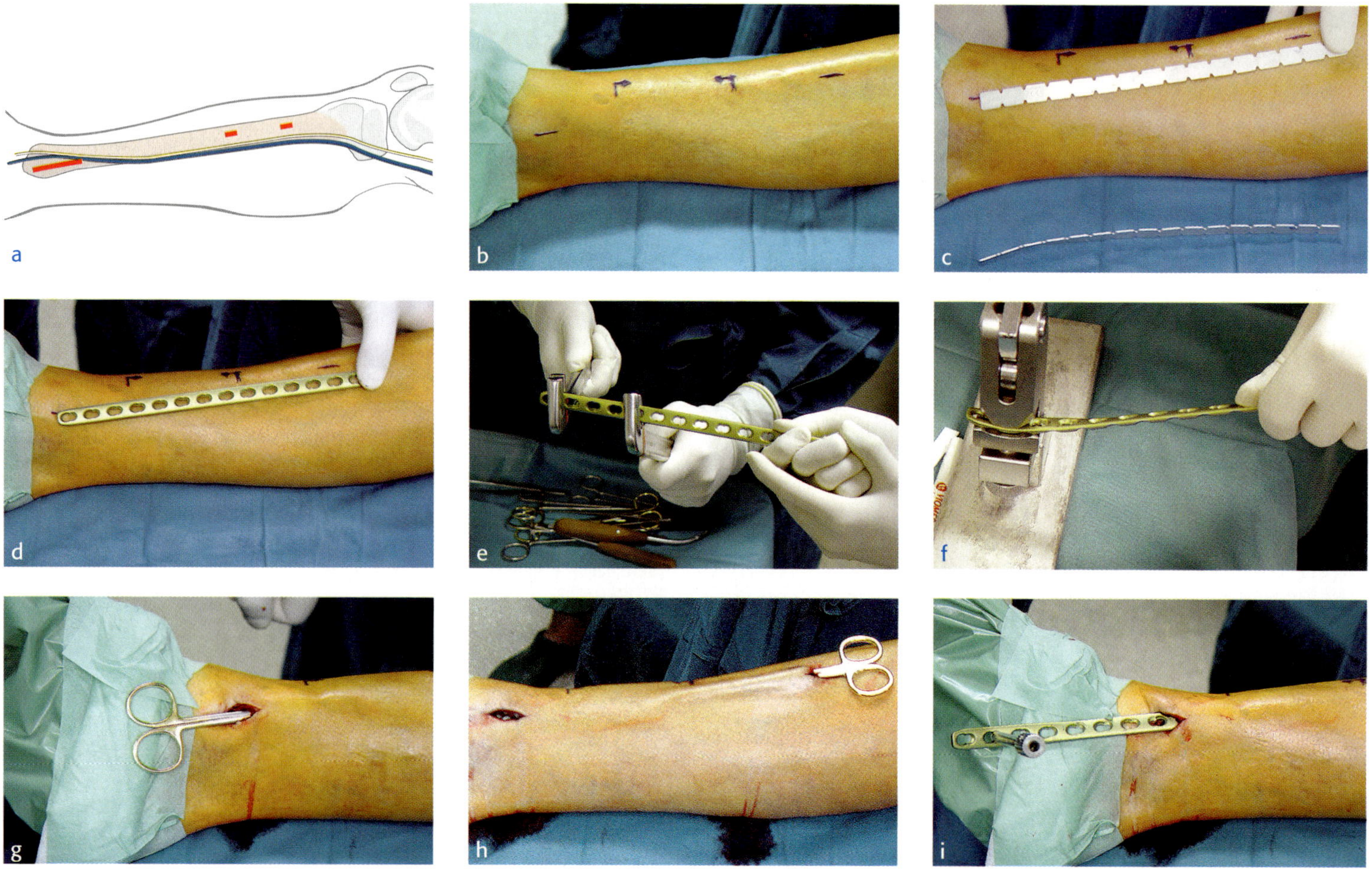

Fig 10.2.1-4a–i

- a Short incision over the medial malleolus taking care not to damage the great saphenous vein. Incision at the planned site for the proximal end of the plate and screw insertion.
- b Mark the planned incisions around the full extent of the fracture zone.
- c Measure for plate length using a template. Obtain the approximate surface contours of the distal tibia by applying the bending template.
- d Check the chosen plate length.
- e–f Preshape the plate with the bending press and bending irons. Prebend the plate to match the surface of the distal tibia.
- g Incision of the proximal side of the medial malleolus and preparation of the epiperiosteal space with surgical scissors.
- h Incision at the planned site for the proximal end of the plate. Preparation of the epiperiosteal space with surgical scissors.
- i After preparation of the epiperiosteal space, slip in the plate. A drill sleeve firmly anchored in the distal part of the plate acts as a handle. Slide-insertion of the plate from distal to proximal.

3 Reduction and fixation

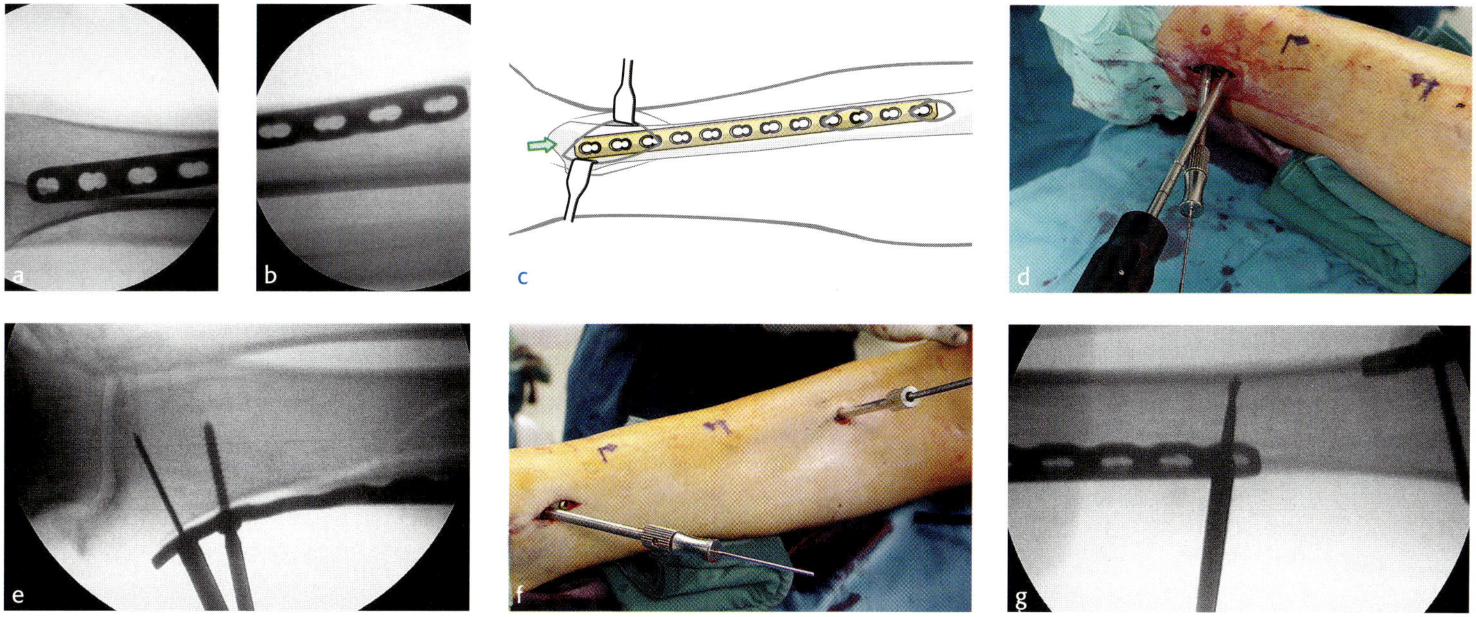

Fig 10.2.1-5a–j

a–b Check the necessary closed reduction maneuver under the image intensifier. Tension is applied at the heel to achieve closed reduction of the distal fragment. Assessment of plate position and fracture reduction by x-ray; align the plate on the longitudinal axis of the tibial shaft.

c One distal skin incision for plate insertion and two stab incisions for the proximal fixation.

d–e Insert a centering sleeve and a 2.0 mm K-wire into the most distal plate hole and use the K-wire to measure the required length of distal screw (protect the joint cavity!). The distal fragment is approximated to the plate with the aid of a cortex screw (reduction screw) and then finely adjusted.

f–g Preliminary proximal fixation of the plate with a drill bit. Radiological assessment of plate position.

3 Reduction and fixation (cont)

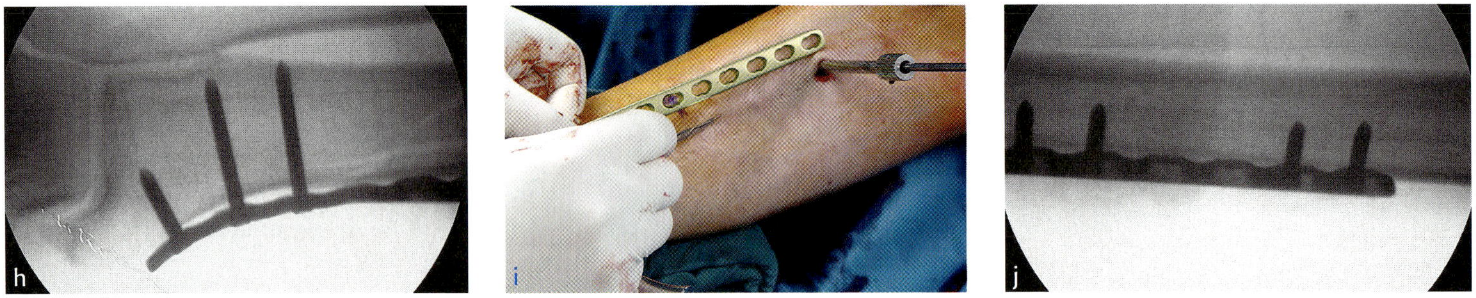

Fig 10.2.1-5a–j (cont)

- h Insertion of self-tapping locking head screws into the three most distal plate holes (the cortex screw that was used for reduction purposes is replaced by an LHS).
- i In order to locate the plate holes correctly, ie, in minimally invasive technique, a second plate with the same pattern of holes is used as an aid.
- j Proximal plate fixation with four monocortical LHS (good bone quality). Attention is paid to leaving the longest distance possible between screws one and four.

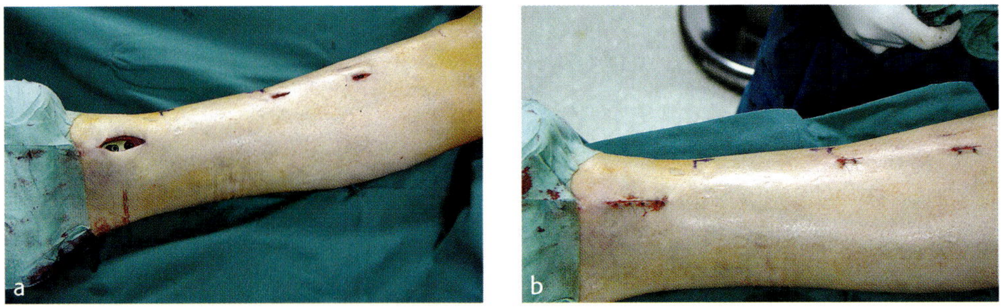

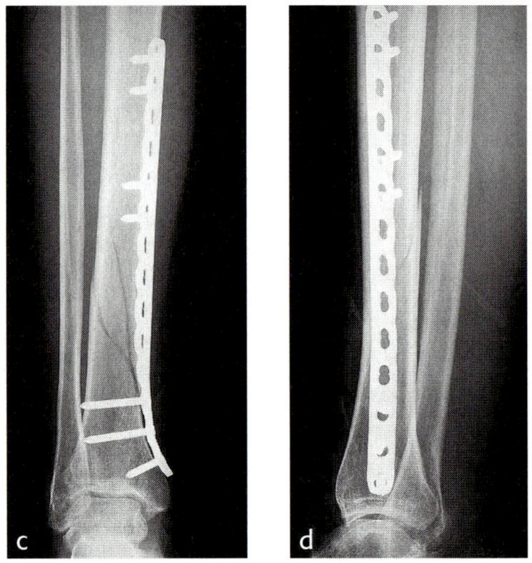

Fig 10.2.1-6a–d

- a Skin incisions before wound closure.
- b Skin suture, closing the incisions.
- c–d Postoperative x-rays, AP and lateral. The postoperative x-rays confirm correct axial alignment. It is deliberate that no attempt was made to achieve anatomical reduction of this simple spiral fracture.

4 Rehabilitation

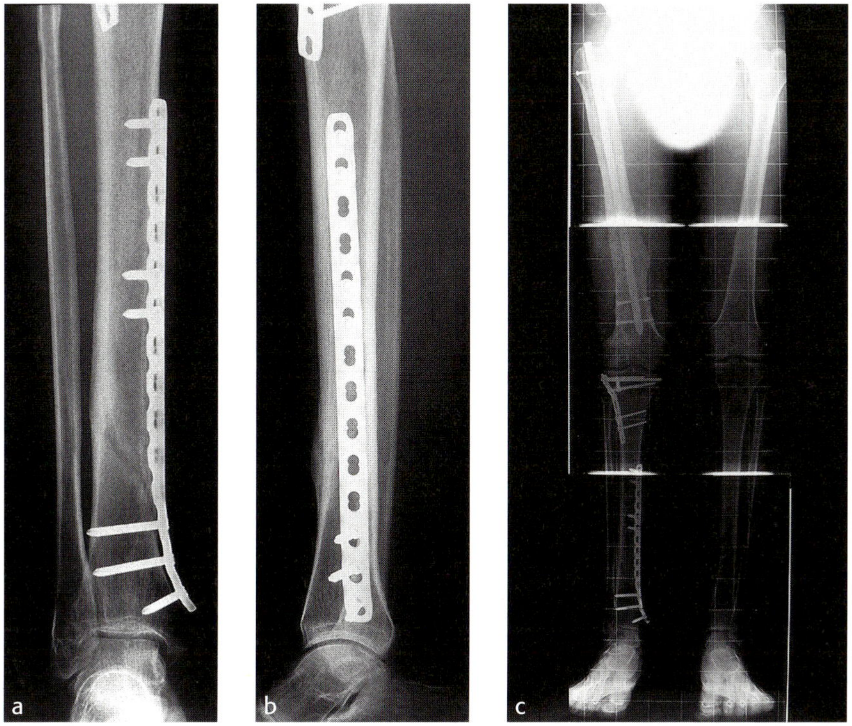

After 4 weeks, painless full weight bearing.
The 12 month follow-up confirmed complete radiological consolidation of the fracture with a very good clinical outcome.

Fig 10.2.1-7a–c
a–b AP and lateral at the one year follow-up. Bone consolidation of this healed fracture.
c X-ray view of the longitudinal leg axes.

5 Pitfalls –

Reduction and fixation
Varus/valgus tilting of the distal fragment.

Incorrect alignment of the plate on the longitudinal axis of the bone may lead to incorrect positioning of the LHS, a tangential screw position and, therefore, reduced anchorage in the bone. This will not be noticed when inserting and locking the screw because the screw head locks in the plate in any case.

Intraoperative evaluation of plate orientation in relation to the longitudinal axis.

The correct length of the distal LHS is important to avoid penetration of the articular surface

The thickness of the narrow LCP 4.5/5.0 may cause soft-tissue problems in the malleolar region. Alternatively a thinner metaphyseal plate can be used.

6 Pearls +

Reduction and fixation
Intraoperative correction is possible with the aid of a cortex screw (reduction screw) that pulls the fragment towards the plate.

The LCP metaphyseal plates 3.5/4.5/5.0, for distal tibia and the LCP distal medial tibial plate are anatomically preshaped and fit the distal end of the tibia.

Author Michael Wagner

10.2.2 Simple oblique tibial and fibular shaft fracture—42-A2

1 Case description

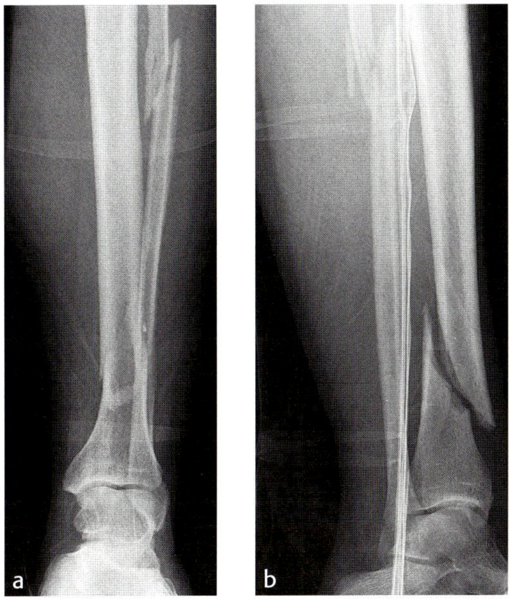

55-year-old man slipped in a field and fell on his left leg. There were no injuries other than the simple oblique tibial fracture.

Fig 10.2.2-1a–b
a AP view.
b Lateral view.

Indication

The diagnosis of an unstable fracture of the tibia at this age is an indication to operate. Insertion of an intramedullary nail would be possible. An alternative would be a slide-insertion plate in MIPO technique.

Preoperative planning

Equipment

- LCP metaphyseal plate 3.5/4.5/5.0, for distal tibia, 4 + 12 holes
- 3.5 mm locking head screws (LHS)
- 5.0 mm LHS
- 2.0 mm K-wires
- Small reduction table

(Size of system, instruments, and implants can vary according to anatomy.)

Patient preparation and positioning

Antibiotics: none
Thrombosis prophylaxis: low-molecular heparin

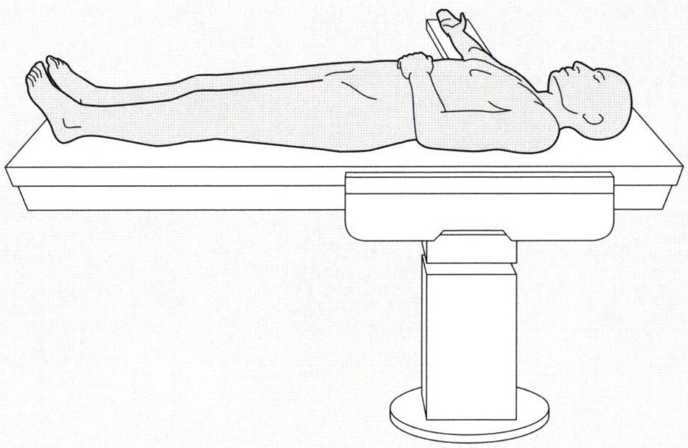

Fig 10.2.2-2 Supine position.

2 Surgical approach

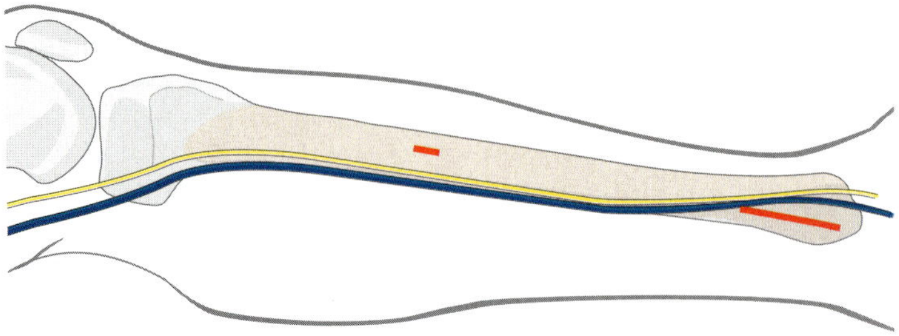

Fig 10.2.2-3 Medial incisions for plate insertion and fixation, and additional stab incisions are required for insertion of the Schanz screws.

3 Reduction and fixation

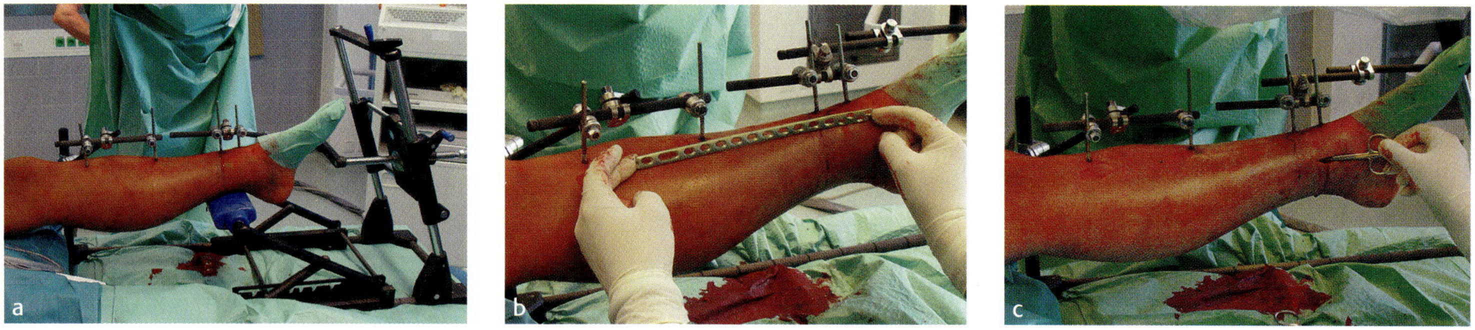

Fig 10.2.2-4a–i

a Indirect closed reduction by means of a small reduction table.

b The most appropriate plate length is determined.

c Preparation of the epiperiosteal space from distal to proximal.

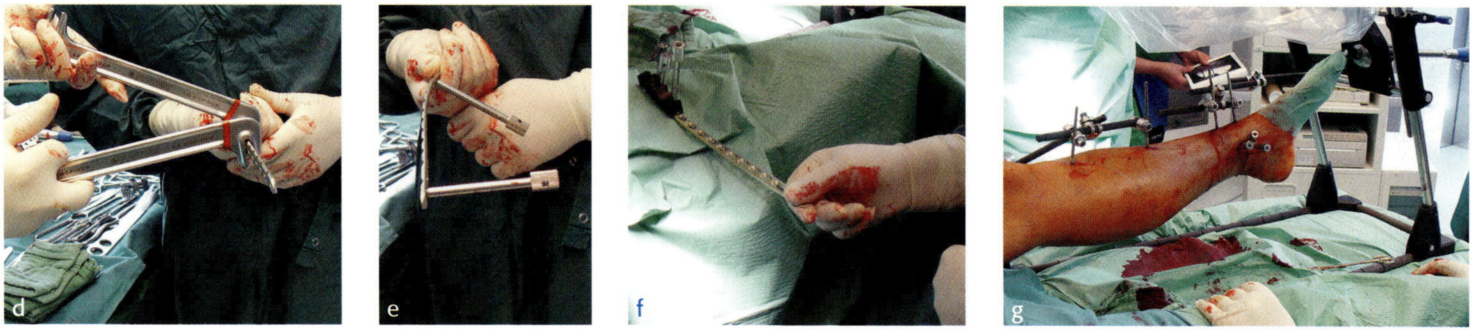

d–e Bending and twisting of the plate at the junction of the diaphysis and metaphysis.

f The drill sleeves are screwed into the distal end of the plate with the help of the guiding block.

g Insertion of the plate from distal to proximal.

3 Reduction and fixation (cont)

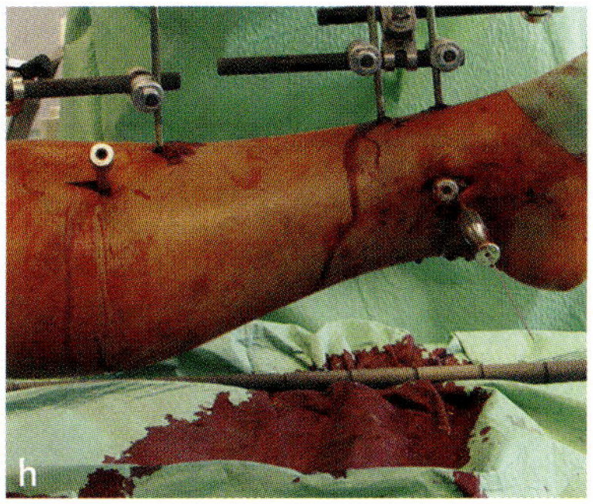

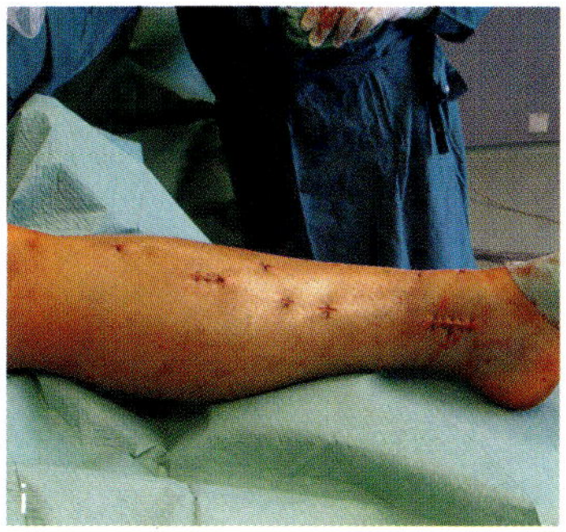

Fig 10.2.2-4a–i (cont)

h Temporary fixation with K-wires after assessment of plate position.

i Fixation of the plate with locking head screws through a total of four small incisions. Wound closure.

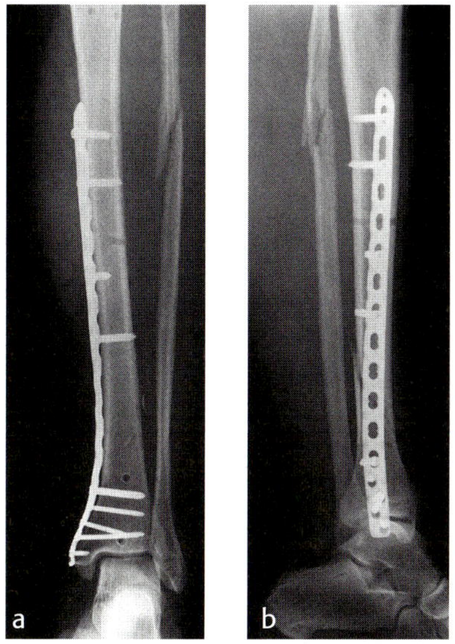

Fig 10.2.2-5a–b
Postoperative x-rays.

a AP view.

b Lateral view.

4 Rehabilitation

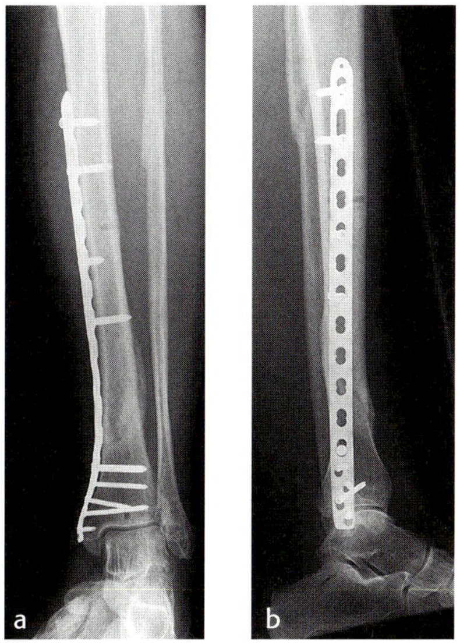

Partial weight bearing for 8 weeks.

Fig 10.2.2-6a–b Postoperative x-rays after 6 weeks. Only minimal callus formation was visible at this time, but weight bearing was increased because the patient did not feel any pain.

a AP view.

b Lateral view.

4 Rehabilitation (cont)

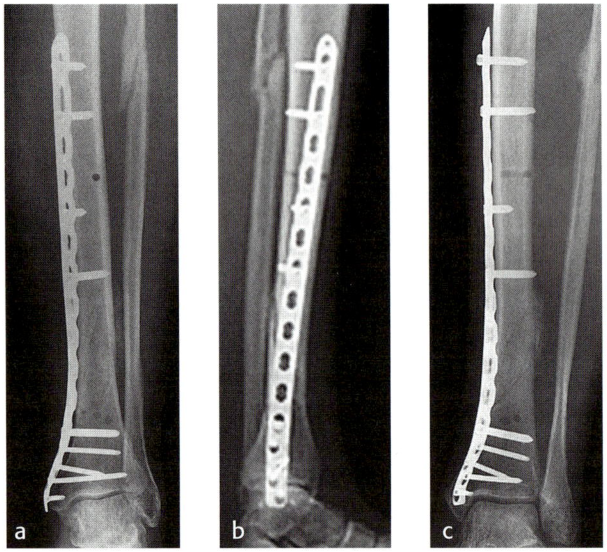

Fig 10.2.2-7a–c Postoperative x-rays after 3 months showing good callus healing.
a AP view.
b Lateral view.
c Lateral rotation.

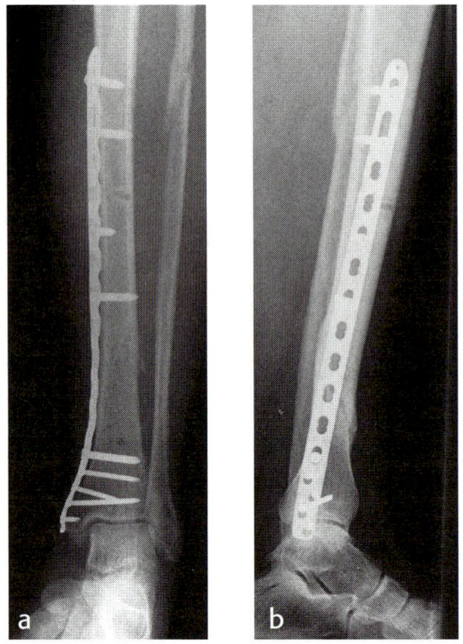

Fig 10.2.2-8a–b Postoperative x-rays after 6 months showing endosteal and callus healing of the fracture.
a AP view.
b Lateral view.

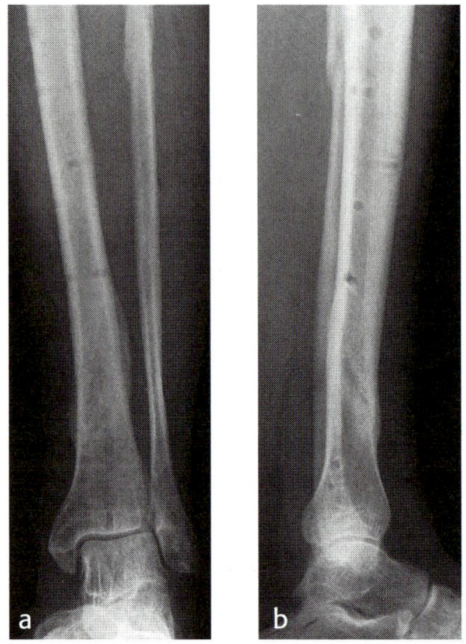

Implant removal
The implant was removed on the request of the patient. Difficulties relating to the implant did not occur.

Fig 10.2.2-9a–b
a AP view.
b Lateral view.

5 Pitfalls –

Fixation
The standard LCP may be too thick. The preferred implant is the LCP metaphyseal plate 3.5/4.5/5.0, for distal tibia.

6 Pearls +

Fixation
Angular stable screw-plate systems permit both stable fixation and a minimally invasive surgical technique. The operative time can be shortened and insertion of the plate eased if the fracture is reduced in advance. A large distractor, the external fixator, or a small reduction table can be used for these procedures.

Author Michael Wagner

10.2.3 Spiral wedge tibial shaft fracture—42-B1

1 Case description

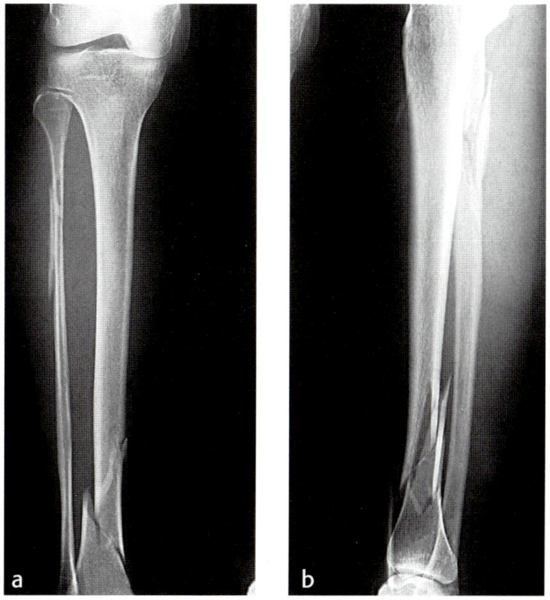

58-year-old woman fell on the street causing an isolated fracture of the tibial shaft of her right leg.

Fig 10.2.3-1a–b
a AP view.
b Lateral view.

Indication

An unstable fracture of the tibia is a good indication for operative stabilization. Nailing of this type of fracture is possible but would only be feasible with new generation nails that have a very distal locking option. Nonoperative treatment with extension and plaster cast requires a long hospital stay and a long period of immobility. MIPO using an LCP as a locked internal fixator is a good option.

Preoperative planning

Equipment

- LCP 4.5/5.0, narrow, 11 holes
- 5.0 mm self-drilling, self-tapping locking head screws (LHS)
- 5.0 mm self-tapping LHS
- 3.5 mm cortex screw
- 2.0 mm K-wires

(Size of system, instruments, and implants can vary according to anatomy.)

Patient preparation and positioning

Antibiotics: none

Thrombosis prophylaxis: low-molecular heparin

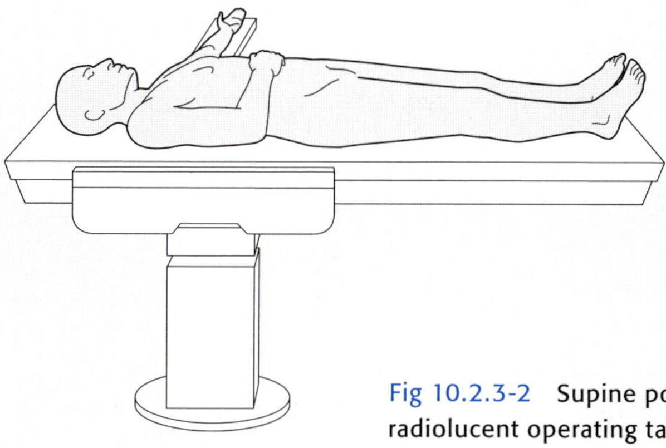

Fig 10.2.3-2 Supine position on radiolucent operating table.

2 Surgical approach

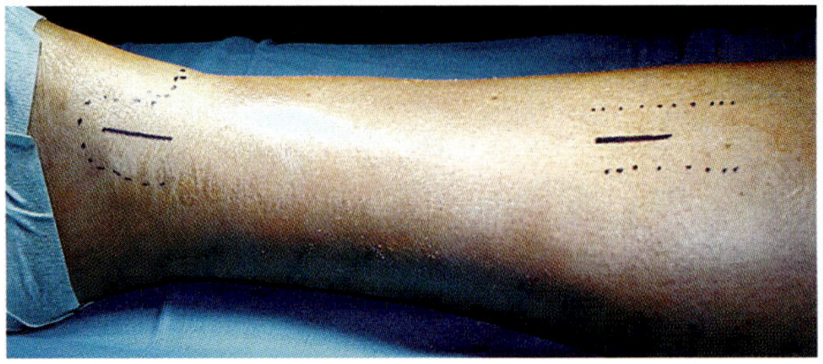

Fig 10.2.3-3 Preoperative marking of landmarks for the short medial incisions of the MIPO technique.

3 Reduction and fixation

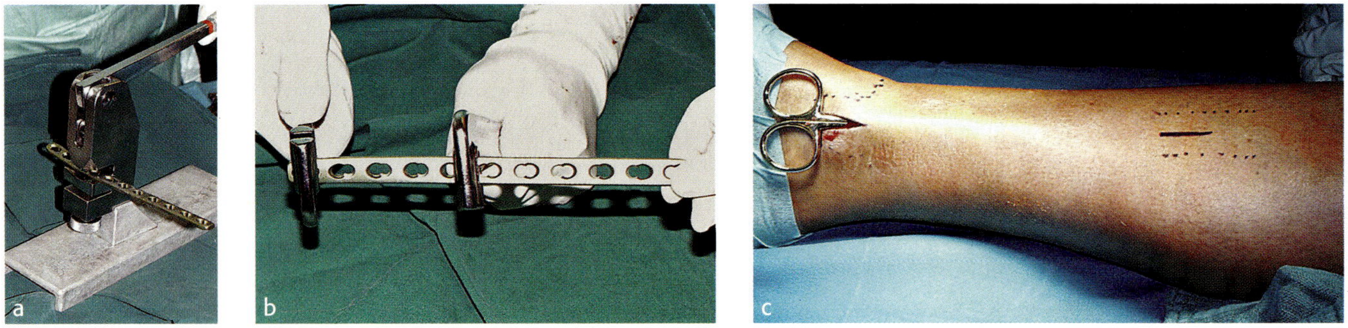

Fig 10.2.3-4a–i Closed indirect reduction with manual traction.

a–b The next step is to select the proper length of the plate and to bend and twist the distal part of the plate so that it approximates to the anatomical shape of the tibia.

c Preparation of the epiperiosteal space with the scissors from distal to proximal.

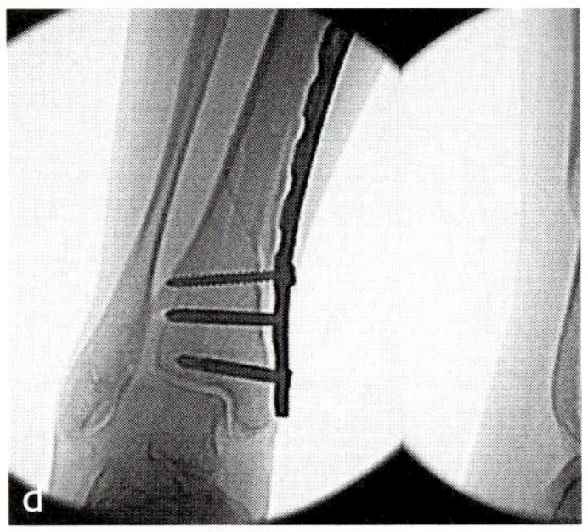

d A cortex screw is inserted in the third hole from the distal end as part of the definitive reduction. It functions as a reduction screw and pulls the fragment towards the plate. The distal fragment is then stabilized by insertion of two locking head screws in the distal fragment.

3 Reduction and fixation (cont)

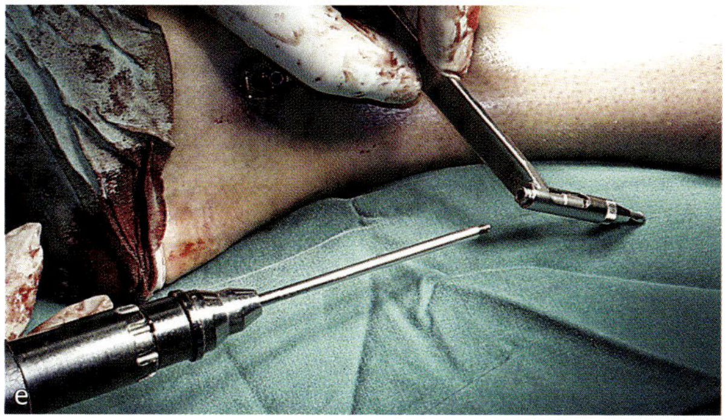

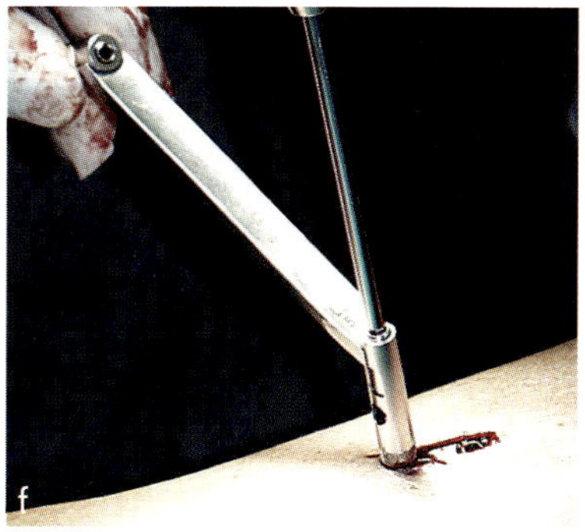

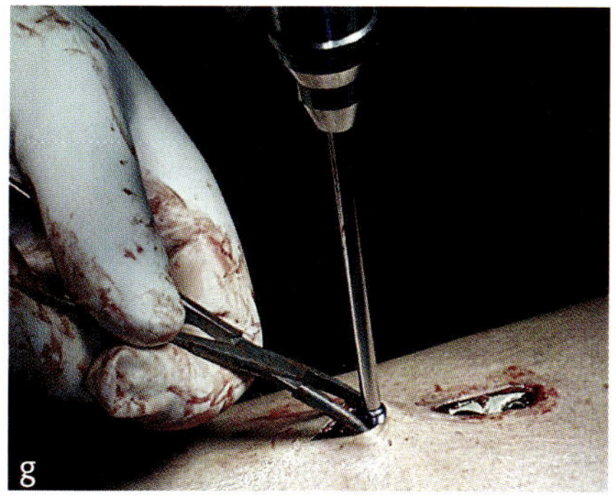

Fig 10.2.3-4a–i (cont)

e–g Definitive fixation of the proximal fragment by insertion of a total of four monocortical locking head screws, one of which is a self-drilling, self-tapping screw. It will be necessary to predrill with the help of the universal drill sleeve before inserting the self-drilling LHS if the diaphyseal cortex is thick and hard. This ensures optimal centering of the screw in the threaded part of the combination hole.

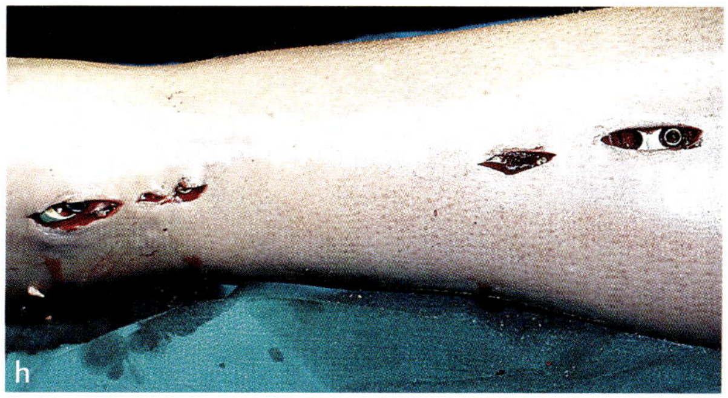

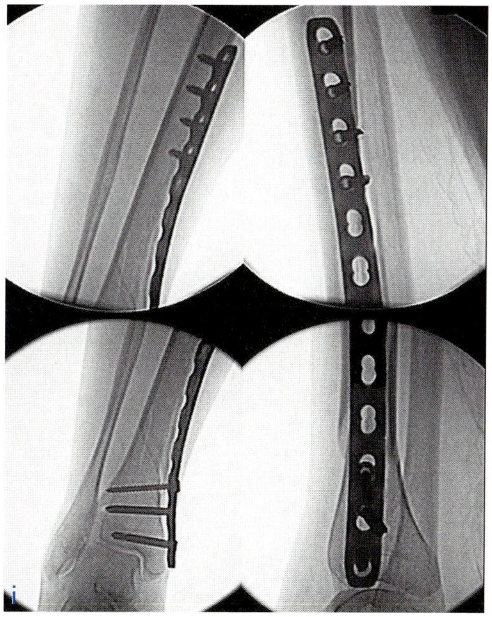

h All four incisions at completion of the osteosynthesis.

i Intraoperative x-ray evaluation.

4 Rehabilitation

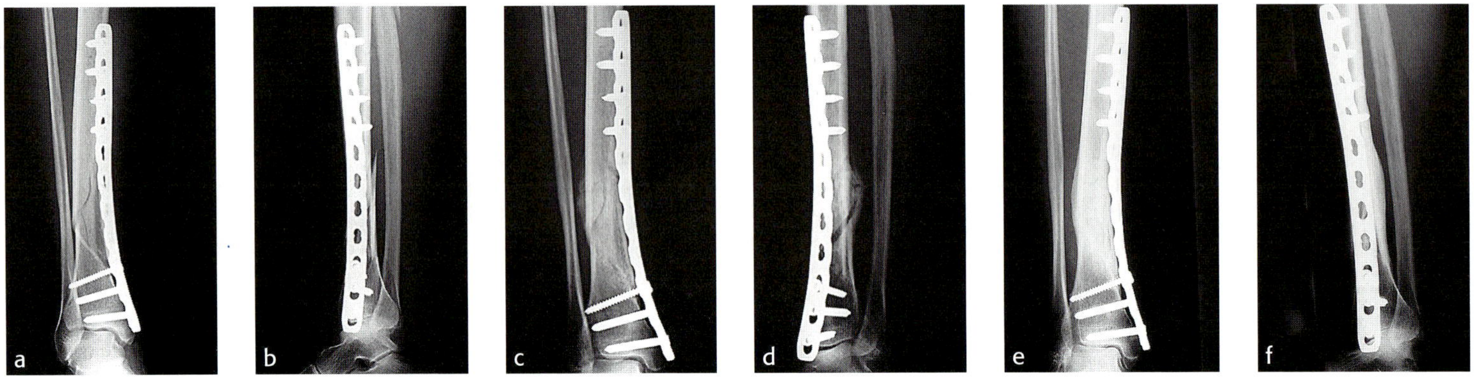

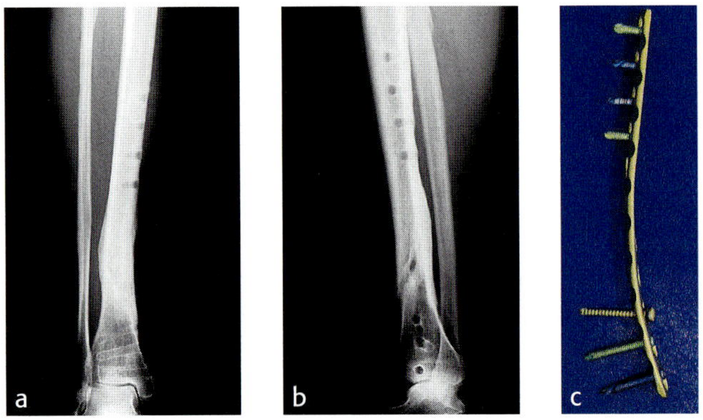

Mobilization with partial weight bearing and underarm crutches; increased weight bearing from the 4th week; full weight bearing after 8 weeks.

Fig 10.2.3-5a–f
a–b Postoperative x-rays after 1 week.
c–d The postoperative x-rays after 5 months show that endosteal and periosteal healing is not yet completed.
e–f The postoperative x-rays after 10 months show complete bone consolidation.

Fig 10.2.3-6a–c
a AP view.
b Lateral view.
c Implant after implant removal.

Implant removal

The standard narrow LCP 4.5/5.0 was palpable and caused visible thickening at the medial malleolus. This was uncomfortable for the patient and the implant was therefore removed.

5 Pitfalls –

Approach
The saphenous vein and nerve may be injured during the course of distal medial incision. The superficial peroneal nerve is endangered by lateral incision.

Fixation
The standard plate may be too thick. The preferred implant is the LCP metaphyseal plate 3.5/4.0/5.0, for distal tibia.

6 Pearls +

Approach

Fixation
The LCP metaphyseal plate 3.5/4.5/5.0, for distal tibia is anatomically preshaped and fits the distal end of the tibia.

Author Frankie Leung

10.2.4 Spiral wedge tibial shaft fracture—42-B1

1 Case description

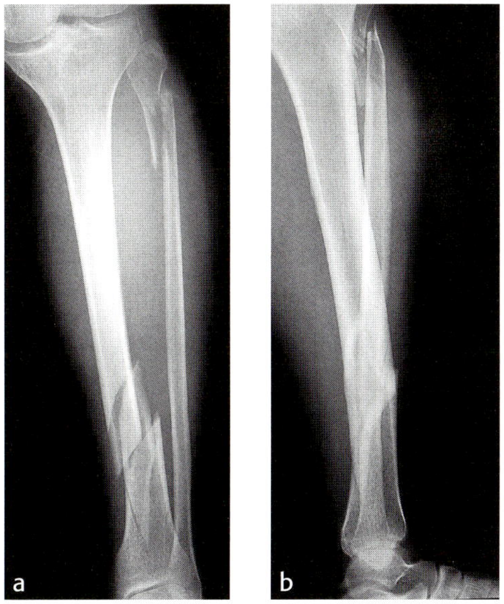

39-year-old man fell down the stairs. Low-energy, monotrauma, closed fracture.

Fig 10.2.4-1a–b Preoperative x-rays.
a AP view.
b Lateral view.

Indication

This is a distal diaphyseal extraarticular fracture of the tibia with displacement (42-B1.2). There is also a fracture of the fibula just below the fibular neck. Nonoperative treatment, ie, closed reduction and casting, is not recommended as the fracture is very unstable and will tend to heal with shortening and varus malalignment. Moreover, a long leg cast is needed for 6–8 weeks, which may cause joint stiffness and delay weight bearing.
Operative fixation of the tibia reduces the acute pain, achieves a better reduction of the fracture, and allows early mobilization of the adjacent joints.

The tibial fracture can be fixed with a bridging LCP inserted in minimally invasive technique. There is little disturbance of the vascularity of the fracture fragments and bone healing will be indirect with callus formation. The length and axis of the leg can also be maintained. An alternative fixation method is intramedullary nailing. However, it is difficult to obtain adequate stabilization of the short distal tibial fragment and the risk of malunion is higher. Another alternative fixation method is a hybrid external fixator. Ankle joint motion can be preserved as compared with bridging external fixation across the ankle joint. There is a certain risk of pin track infection and the duration of external fixation is usually up to 10–12 weeks.

Preoperative planning

Equipment

- LCP metaphyseal plate 3.5/4.5/5.0, 5 + 11 holes
- 3.5 mm self-tapping locking head screws (LHS)
- 3.5 mm cancellous bone screws
- 2.0 mm K-wires
- 3.0 mm Steinman pin for distraction at the heel
- (Optional) large distractor

(Size of system, instruments, and implants can vary according to anatomy.)

Patient preparation and positioning

Antibiotics: cephalosporin
Thrombosis prophylaxis: none

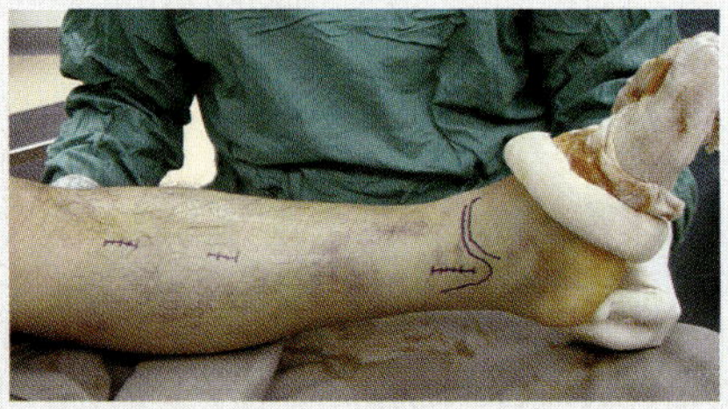

Fig 10.2.4-2 Supine position on radiolucent operating table.

2 Surgical approach

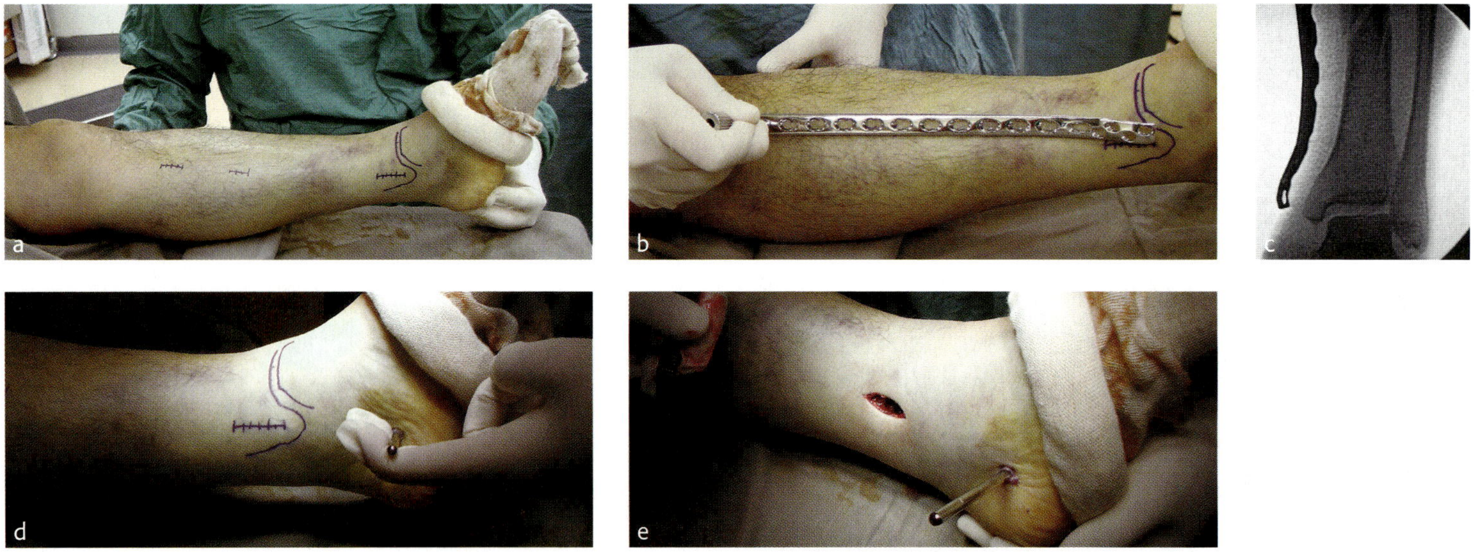

Fig 10.2.4-3a–e

a Identify the fracture site and mark the ankle joint and the medial malleolus. A minimally invasive approach with three small incisions is sufficient. There is no need to expose the fracture site. Restore the length and axial alignment. Remember that rotation is important but there is no need for anatomical reduction of the fracture itself.

b–c A straight 5 + 11 hole LCP metaphyseal plate 3.5/4.5/5.0 is contoured approximately to fit the medial aspect of the distal tibia.

d Insertion of a Steinman pin through the calcaneus for distraction, and reduction of the fracture by the surgical assistant. Alternatively, insert a large distractor for the same purpose.

e Make a small incision (3–4 cm long) just proximal to the medial malleolus for the insertion of the LCP.

3 Reduction

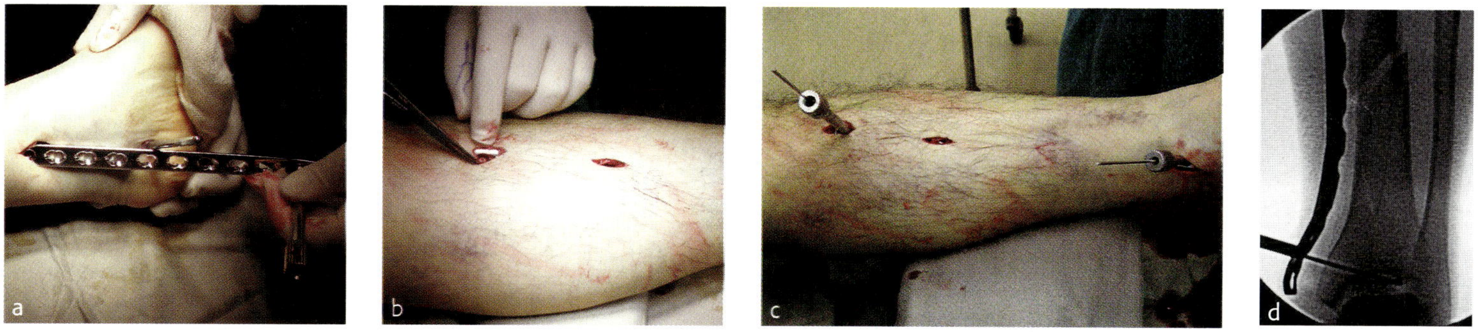

Fig 10.2.4-4a–d

a Insert the plate gently along the medial aspect of the tibia. Attach a locking drill sleeve to the plate and use it as a handle.

b Palpate the plate along the medial subcutaneous plane of the calf. Make small stab incisions (2–3 cm long) and expose the proximal end of the plate. Attach another locking drill sleeve to the proximal end of the plate.

c–d Fix the plate onto the tibia with K-wires after reduction of the fracture. Perform and check the reduction on the image intensifier.

4 Fixation

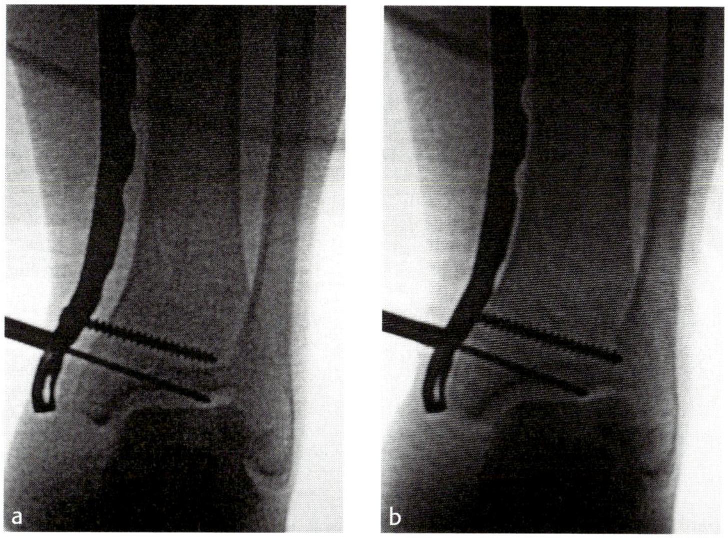

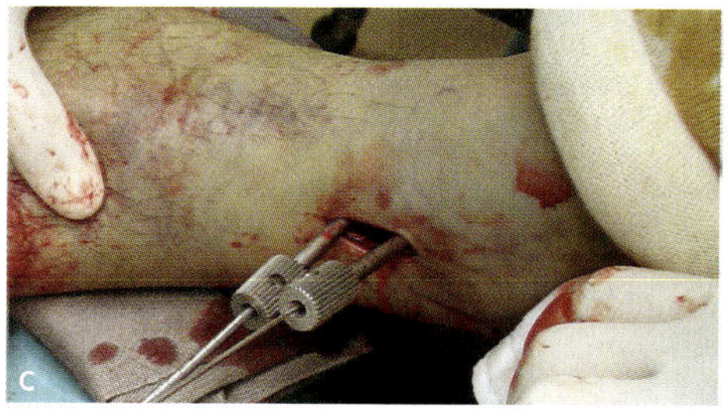

Fig 10.2.4-5a–c

a–b Insert a fully threaded 3.5 mm cancellous bone screw into the distal tibial fragment. This will help to fix the plate onto the bone and will greatly facilitate subsequent fixation.

c Insert a 3.5 mm self-tapping locking head screw into the distal fragment. Check the fracture reduction and axial alignment again.

4 Fixation (cont)

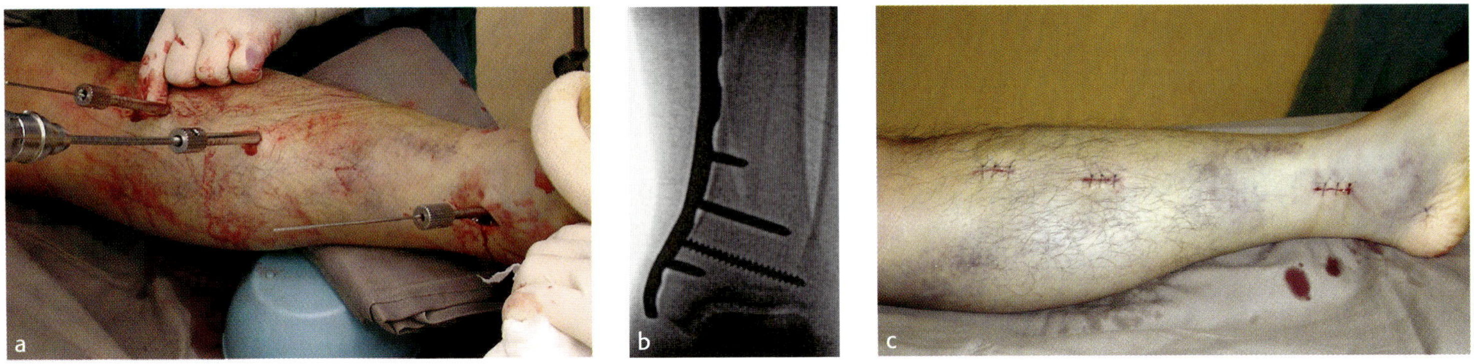

Fig 10.2.4-6a–c

a Insert a bicortical self-tapping 5.0 mm locking head screw into the proximal segment through one of the stab incisions.

b Complete the fixation by inserting two more 3.5 mm LHS distally, and one more bicortical 5.0 mm LHS proximally.

c Suture the skin incisions.

5 Rehabilitation

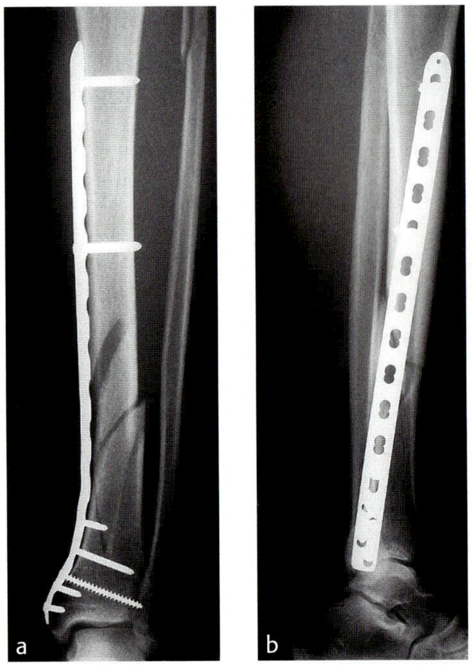

Weight bearing: 15 kg for 2 weeks, half body weight after 4 weeks; full weight bearing after 6 weeks.
Physiotherapy: Range of motion exercise of the ankle and knee joints to be started on day one postoperatively.

Fig 10.2.4-7a–b Postoperative x-rays after 6 weeks.

a AP view.

b Lateral view.

6 Pitfalls –

Equipment
A poorly contoured plate will lead to skin impingement and affect patient acceptance.

Approach
Open reduction of a displaced fracture with additional stripping of the periosteum.

Reduction and fixation
Overzealous effort to compress the plate onto the bone with a cortex screw will displace a reduced fracture.
Poor fixation of the distal fragment due to an inadequate number of screws.

Rehabilitation
In multifragmentary fractures, premature weight bearing may lead to valgus malalignment of the fracture.

7 Pearls +

Equipment
Precontouring the plate on a plastic bone will facilitate the application.

Approach
A minimally invasive approach will preserve vascularity. The emphasis is on restoration of length, axis, and rotation instead of fracture reduction.

Reduction and fixation
When the first conventional screw is inserted, check the reduction on the image intensifier.
Careful preoperative planning of the number and sites of the screws to be inserted.

Rehabilitation
If possible, perform fibular plating in order to increase the stability of the fixation. Moreover, weight bearing in multifragmentary fractures should be delayed to 4–6 weeks.

Author Michael Wagner

10.2.5 Spiral wedge tibial shaft fracture with extension into the joint—42-B1

1 Case description

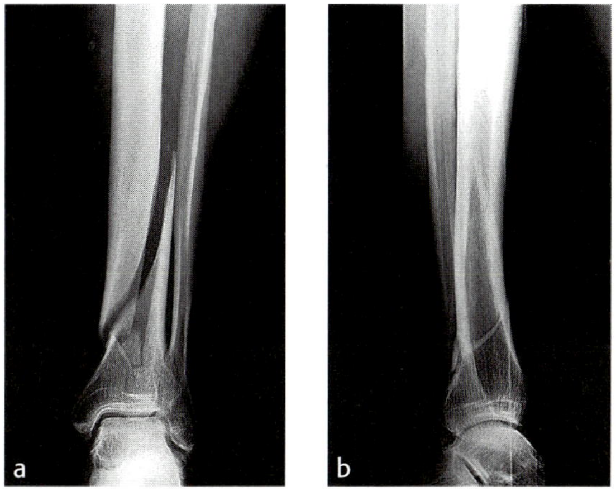

61-year-old man fell while skiing and sustained an unstable fracture of the left tibia.

Fig 10.2-5-1a–b
a AP view.
b Lateral view.

Indication

Unstable fracture with fissures extending into the joint. Good indication for MIPO.

Preoperative planning

Equipment

- LCP 4.5/5.0, narrow, 14 holes
- LCP 4.5/5.0, narrow, 20 holes
- 5.0 mm self-tapping locking head screws (LHS)
- 6.5 mm cancellous bone screw
- 2.0 mm K-wires
- Pointed reduction forceps

(Size of system, instruments, and implants can vary according to anatomy.)

Patient preparation and positioning

Antibiotics: none
Thrombosis prophylaxis: low-molecular heparin

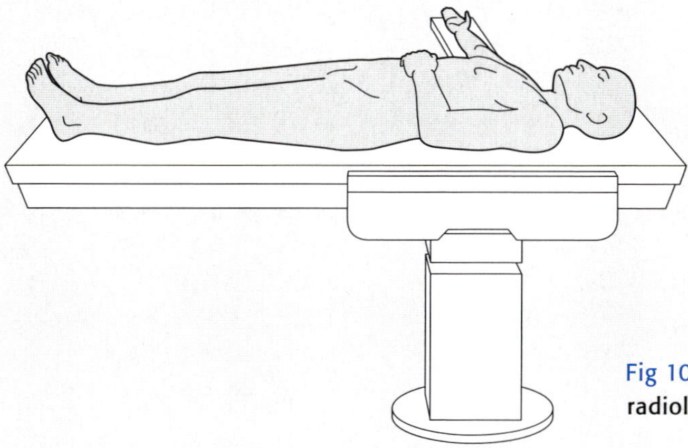

Fig 10.2.5-2 Supine position on radiolucent operating table.

2 Surgical approach

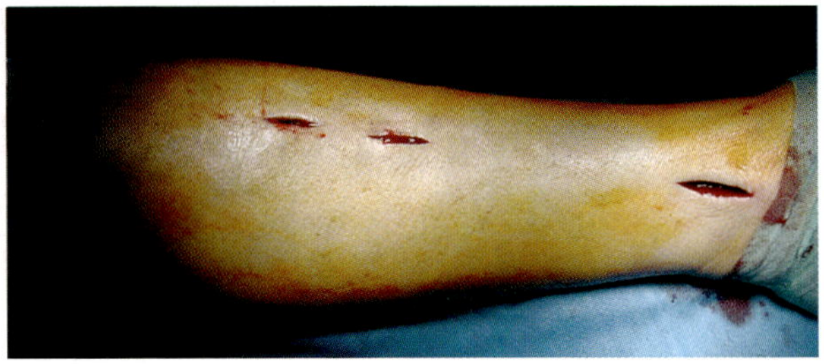

Fig 10.2.5-3 Medial incision proximal of the malleolus and two additional incisions in the region of the planned position of the proximal half of the plate.

3 Reduction and fixation

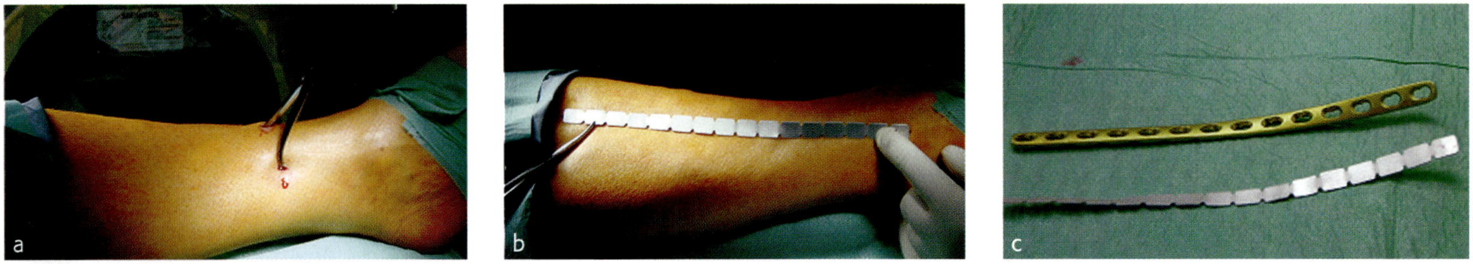

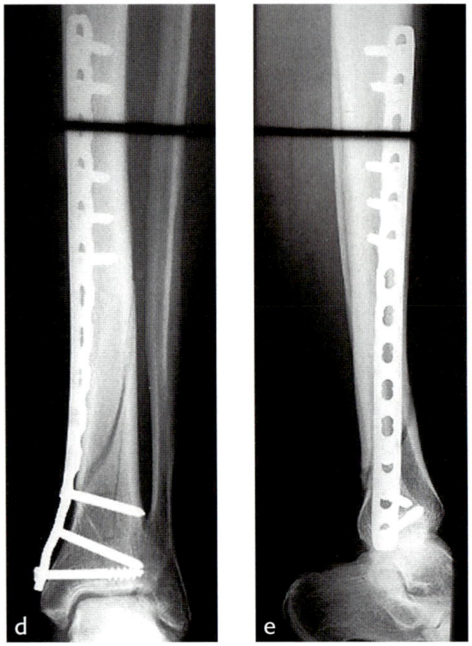

Fig 10.2.5-4a–e

- a Closed indirect reduction with manual traction and rotation of the foot, and direct reduction with percutaneously inserted, pointed reduction forceps. The forceps not only works as a reduction tool, but also makes temporary fixation possible.
- b–c Prebending of a 14-hole narrow LCP, 4.5/5.0 whereby a bending template is first applied to the skin on the medial aspect and contoured to determine the curvature and rotation of the distal tibia; also determination of the length of the plate. The plate is bent and twisted into shape with the bending press and bending irons.
- d–e Insertion of the plate from distal to proximal and distal fixation with a 6.5 mm cancellous bone screw parallel to the upper ankle joint and two additional locking head screws proximally. A total of five monocortical LHS are inserted to attach the plate to the tibial shaft.

4 Rehabilitation

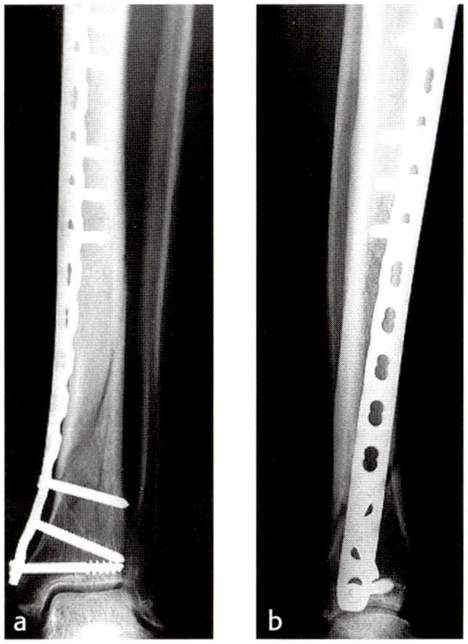

Mobilization with partial weight bearing and active exercise of the knee and ankle joint. Full weight bearing after 6 weeks.

Fig 10.2.5-5a–b
Postoperative x-rays after 6 weeks. Callus formation was not visible at this time.
a AP view.
b Lateral view.

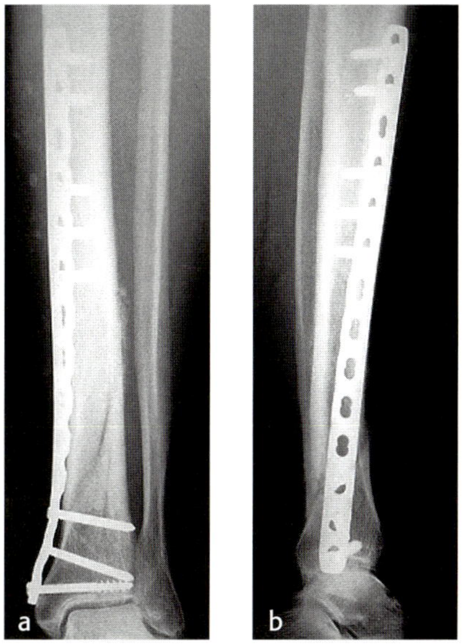

Fig 10.2.5-6a–b
The postoperative x-rays after 9 weeks show the beginnings of callus formation.
a AP view.
b Lateral view.

5 Refracture—Case description

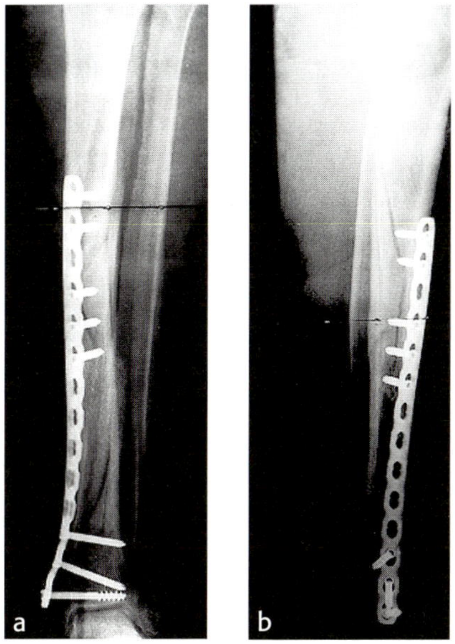

Fig 10.2.5-7a–b
11 weeks after the first operation, the patient fell off his motorbike and sustained an additional fracture at the proximal end of the plate.
a AP view.
b Lateral view.

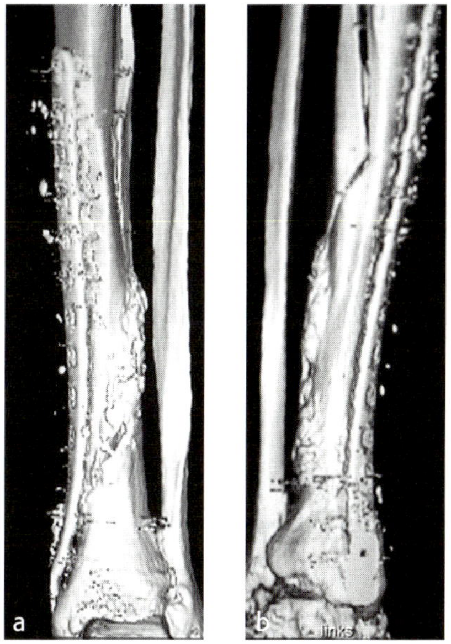

Fig 10.2.5-8a–b
CT scans show the most recent fracture at the proximal end of the plate, the first fracture with callus bridging and the LCP secured by the locking head screws, which had not loosened.
a 3D CT scan frontal plane.
b 3D CT scan sagittal plane.

6 Refracture—Indication

A revision osteosynthesis was required to treat the unstable spiral fracture with the plate in situ.

7 Refracture—Surgical approach

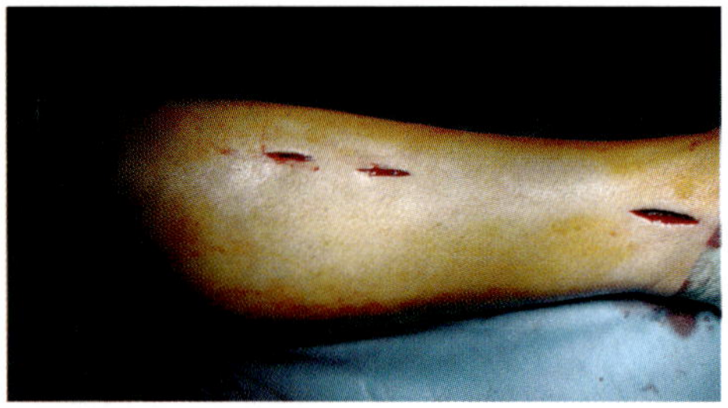

Same incisions as for the first operation. Additional proximal incisions were necessary because a longer plate was selected for the revision procedure.

Fig 10.2.5-9 Illustrates the requisite incisions for the revision operation and for implant removal.

8 Refracture—Reduction and fixation

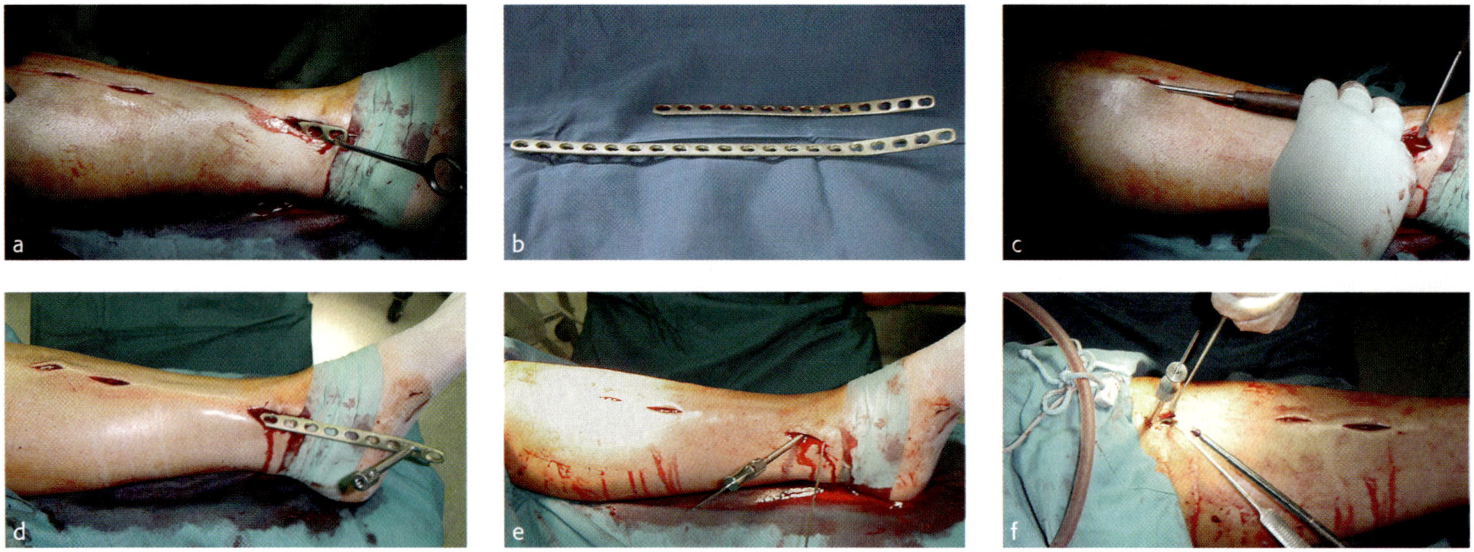

Fig 10.2.5-10a–f
- a Removal of the 14-hole LCP.
- b The explanted plate served as a template for the longer 20-hole LCP.
- c Tunneling through the epiperiosteal space from distal to proximal through the proximal incision.
- d Insertion of the longer plate from distal to proximal with the help of a threaded LCP drill sleeve used as a handle.
- e–f Temporary fixation distally and proximally with a K-wire.

8 Refracture—Reduction and fixation (cont)

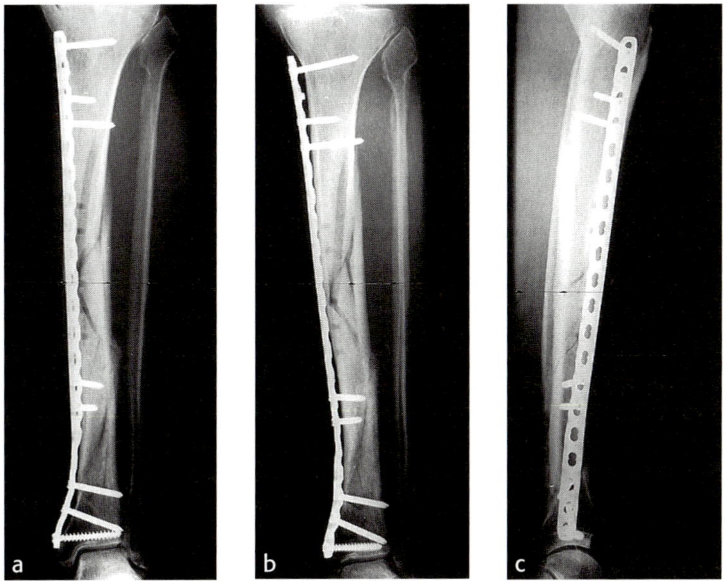

Fig 10.2.5-11a–c Definitive fixation of the 20 hole LCP distally with a fully threaded cancellous bone screw and two locking head screws, whereby care was taken to utilize the existing screw holes in the bone. Additional distal fixation at the level of the first and now consolidated fracture by insertion of two monocortical LHS, proximal plate fixation with three LHS, of which one should have bicortical anchorage. To ensure only limited plate-to-bone contact, a spacer was inserted in the second proximal hole.
The image of 20° outer rotation shows the gap between the plate and the bone. Fixation of the proximal fracture in 8° valgus.

a AP view.
b 20° outer rotation.
c Lateral view.

9 Refracture—Rehabilitation

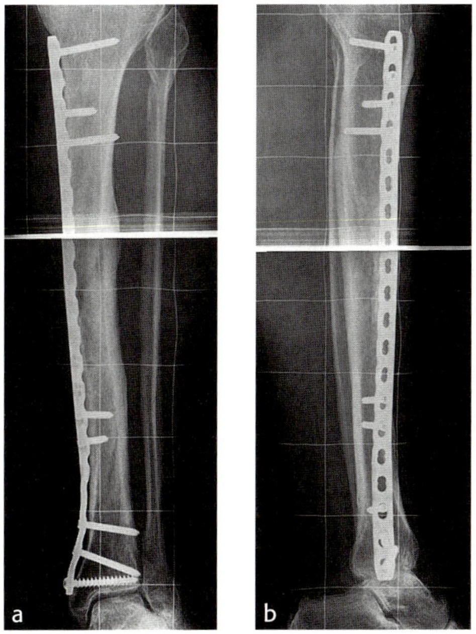

Partial weight bearing for 6 weeks; full weight bearing after 8 weeks.

Fig 10.2.5-12a–b Postoperative x-rays after 14 months. Both fractures show solid healing.

a AP view.
b Lateral view.

9 Refracture—Rehabilitation (cont)

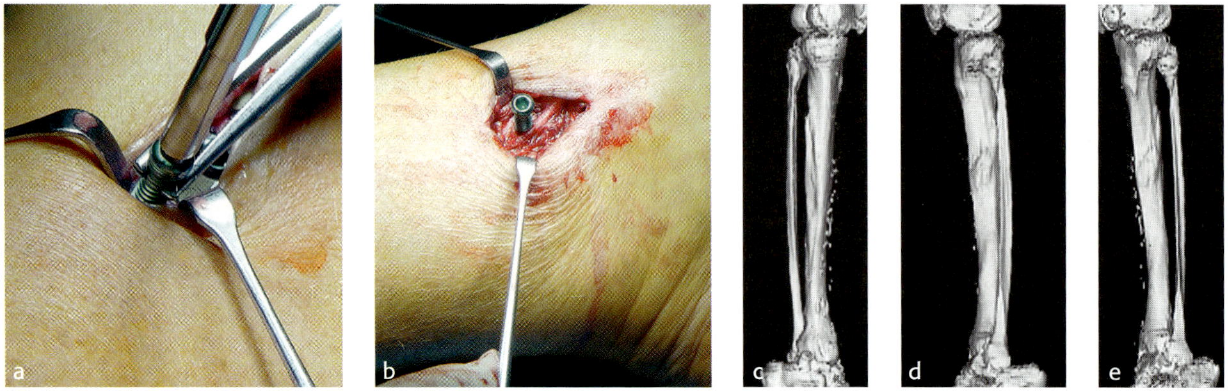

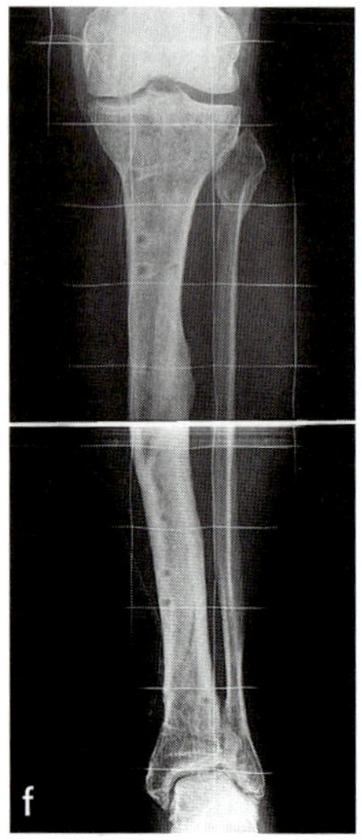

Implant removal

Implant removal after 15 months through stab incisions because of dysesthesia in the region of the saphenous nerve.

Fig 10.2.5-13a–f

a Removal of the LHS at the distal end of the plate.
b The nerve is seen here in direct contact with the screw.
c–e 3D CT scans in the anterior, posterior and lateral views reveal callus bridging of both fractures. There is incorrect axial alignment in the region of the proximal fracture.
f X-ray after implant removal, AP view.

10 Pitfalls –

Reduction and fixation

Problem of closed reduction and intraoperative axial assessment for the MIPO procedure.
Postoperative axial malalignment (8° valgus at reoperation).
Nerve lesions due to small incisions or MIPO technique.

11 Pearls +

Reduction and fixation

Internal fixator systems with locking head screws are complementary to MIPO technique and permit the stable fixation of complex fractures and situations that could not be treated by intramedullary nail fixation.

Author Christoph Sommer

10.2.6 Spiral wedge tibial and fibular shaft fracture—42-B1

1 Case description

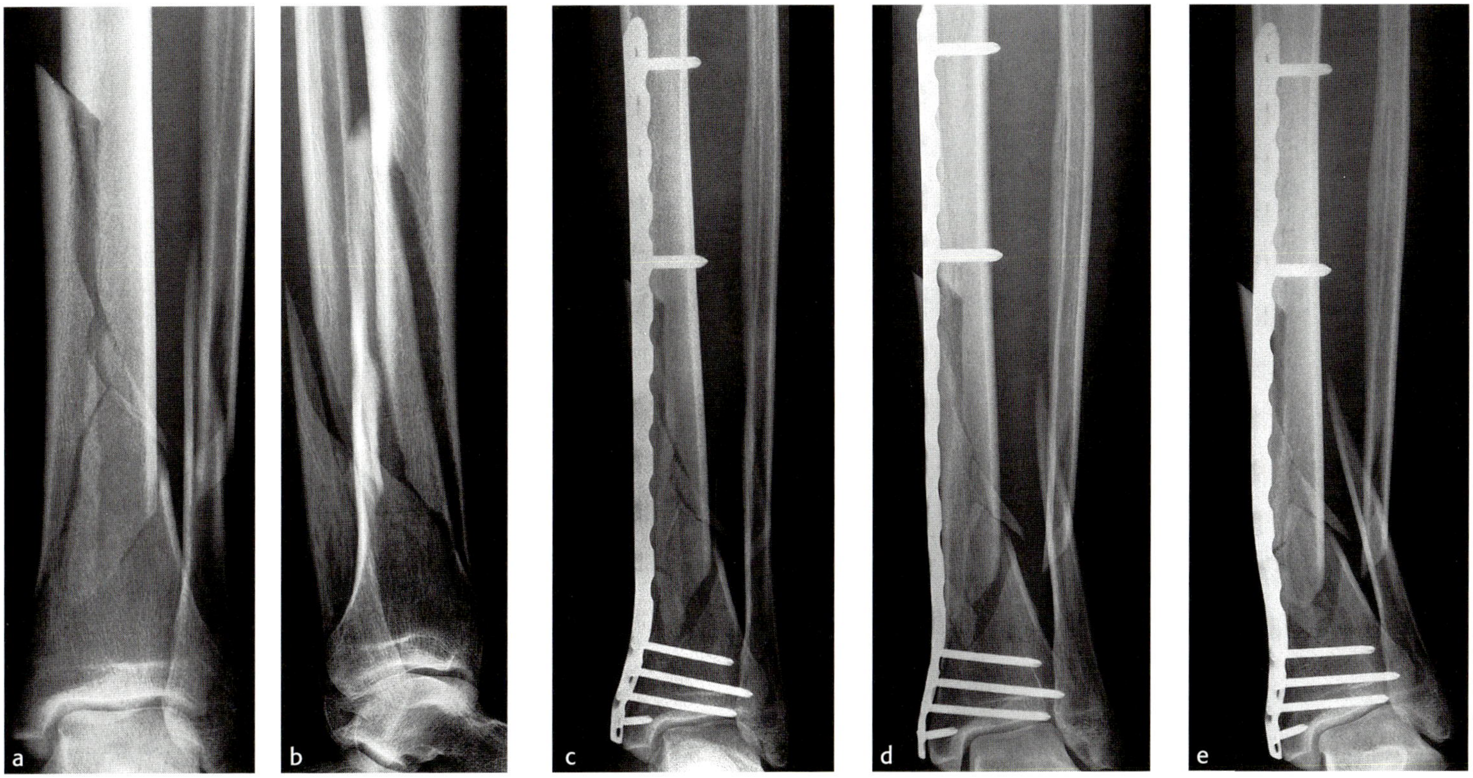

Fig 10.2.6-1a–e 41-year-old man under the influence of alcohol fell on an icy surface. 42-B1.3 extra-articular lower leg spiral fracture.

- a–b Preoperative x-rays.
- c The fracture was stabilized with a metaphyseal LCP (MIPO technique) immediately after trauma. The long fracture zone was bridged with a locked internal fixator.
- d On the first postoperative night, the patient mobilized himself with full weight bearing while in an alcoholic delirium. The plate became bent by 10° resulting in valgus malalignment of the fracture.
- e Even with all precautions taken, the patient mobilized himself again the next night and the plate bent even more, now with a valgus malalignment of 25°.

Indication

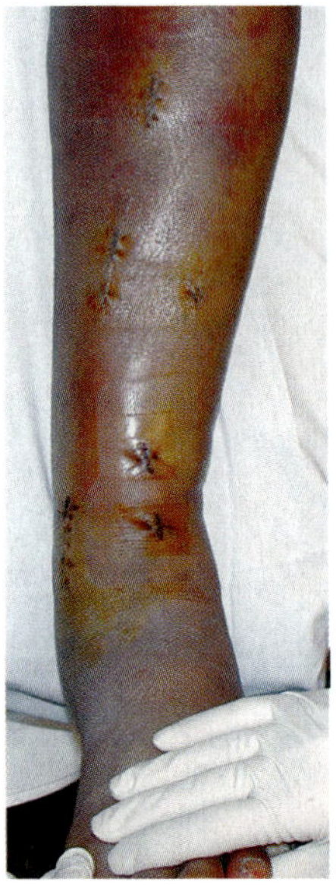

Fig 10.2.6-2 This malalignment cannot be tolerated and must be corrected. There are two possibilities:

- leave the plate in situ and bend it back as shown here.
- redo the osteosynthesis of the tibia, ie, remove the old plate and stabilize the tibia with a new plate.

If the plate bends shortly after the operation and all screws are still anchored tightly in the bone, the first possibility can be tried.
Stabilization of the fibula to support the long tibia bridging plate should also be considered. This additional stabilization of the fibula is recommended in patients with poor compliance. The clinical picture shows the valgus malalignment before the second operation.

Preoperative planning

Equipment

- LCP metaphyseal plate 3.5/4.5/5.0, 4 + 12 holes
- LCP 3.5, 10 holes
- Self-tapping locking head screws (LHS)
- 2.0 mm K-wires

(Size of system, instruments, and implants can vary according to anatomy.)

Patient preparation

Antibiotics: single dose 2nd generation cephalosporin
Thrombosis prophylaxis: low-molecular heparin

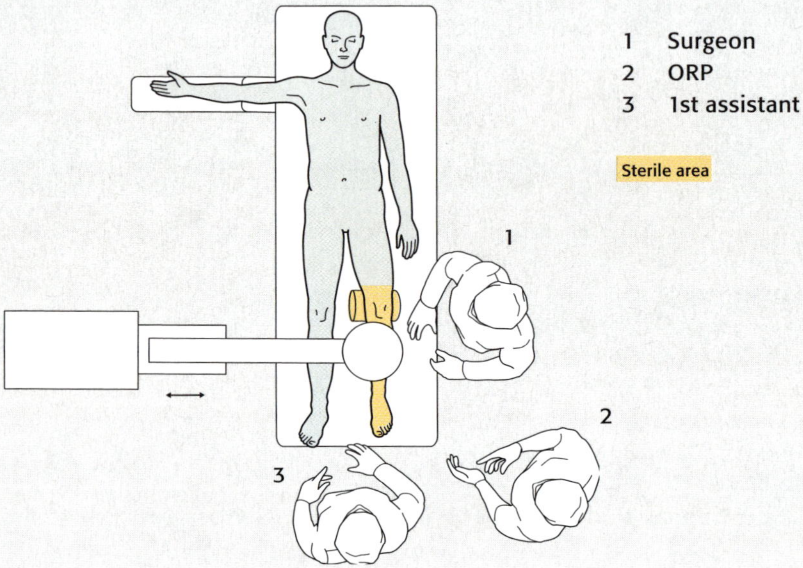

Fig 10.2.6-3 Positioning of OR team.

2 Surgical approach

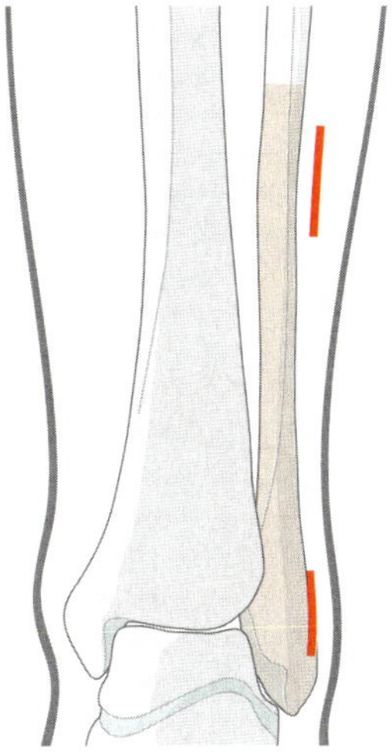

Fig 10.2.6-4 Two short incisions at the proximal and distal ends of the plate across the fibula are needed.

3 Reduction and fixation

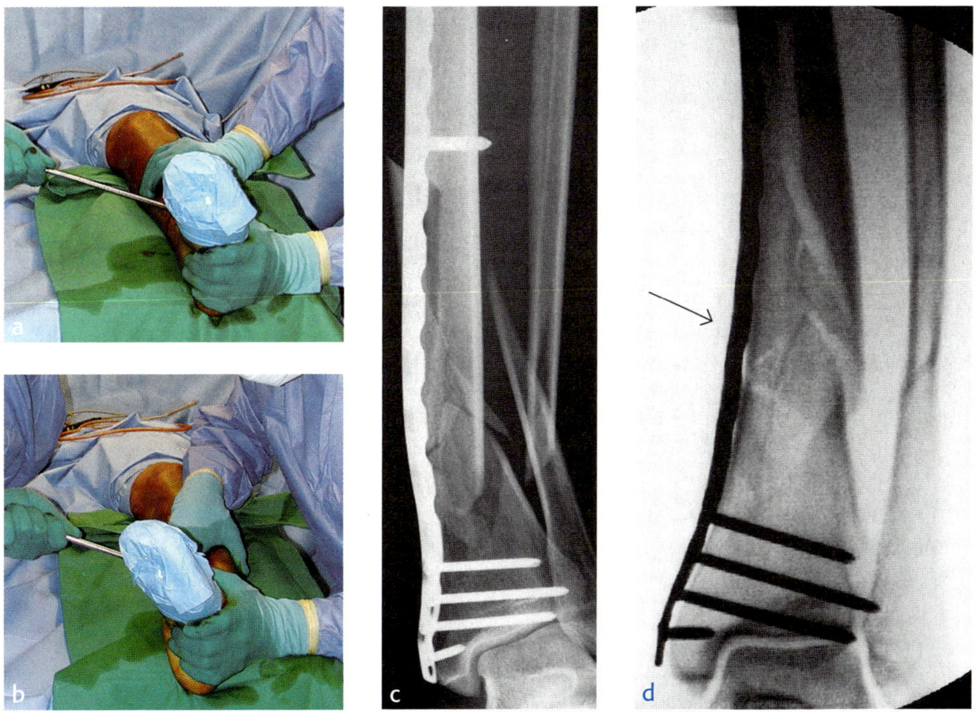

Fig 10.2.6-5a–d

a–b A short incision is made at the level of the bent tibia plate directly over a palpable plate hole. A ball spike with pointed ball tip is inserted into this hole and held by the assistant. The surgeon can bend the plate into the correct position by applying strong counterpressure on the foot and lower leg.

c–d Intraoperative x-ray shows successful bending of the tibial plate in contrast to the pre-operative images. The localization of the spike is marked on the image. The malalignment of the fibula is also corrected indirectly during this procedure.

3 Reduction and fixation (cont)

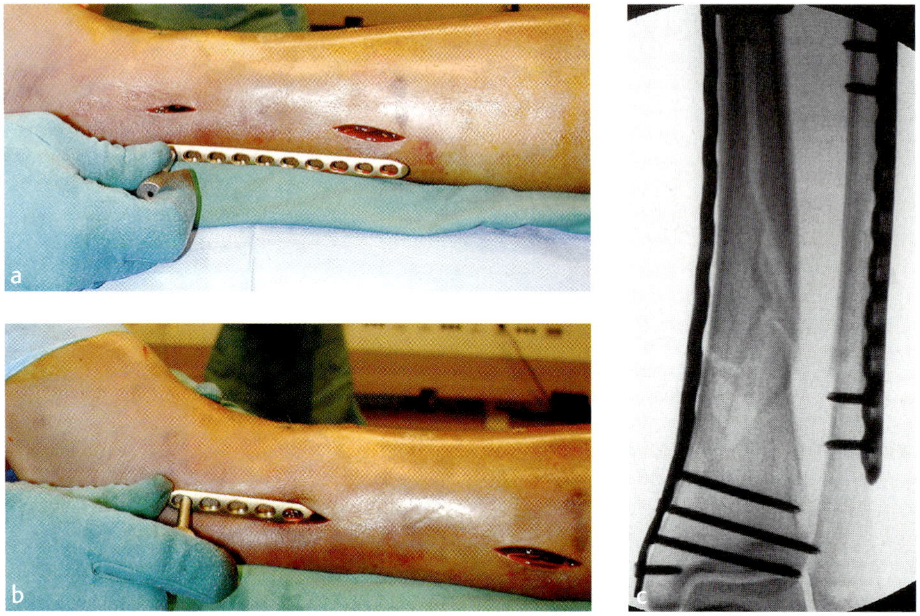

Fig 10.2.6-6a–c

a–b The simple fibular fracture can now be fixed in a routine way. Because of the marked soft-tissue swelling, a minimally invasive procedure is preferred. The straight 10-hole LCP 3.5 indicates the skin incisions proximally and distally. The plate bed is formed directly with the rounded and flattened end of the plate. A drill sleeve helps to hold and insert the plate in a distal to proximal direction.

c The plate is held in position proximally and distally with two bicortical self-tapping locking head screws to form a bridging plate on the fibula.

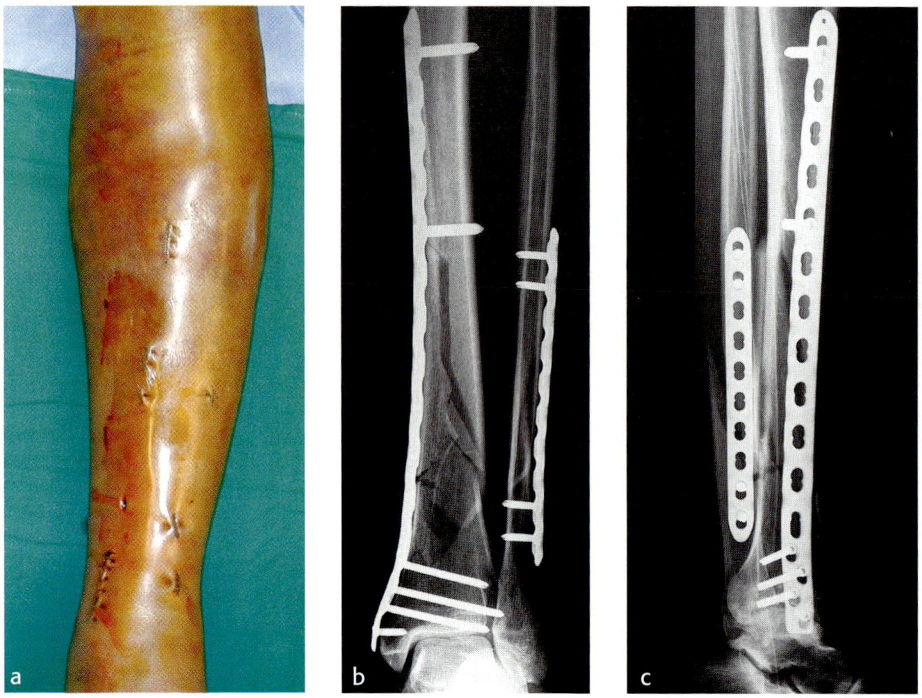

Fig 10.2.6-7a–c The postoperative images confirm the correct axis of the lower leg as well as a correct and congruent ankle joint.

4 Rehabilitation

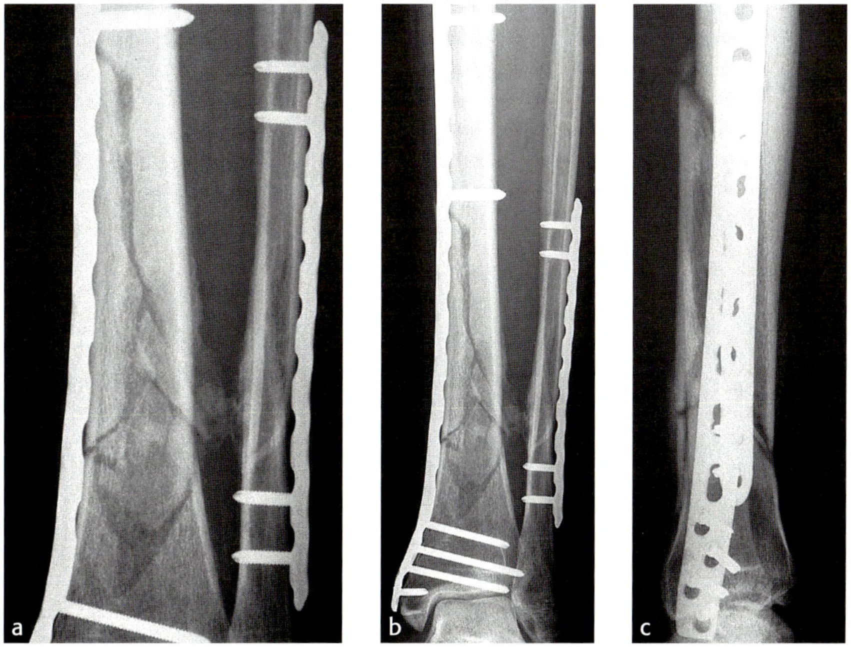

Fig 10.2.6-8a–g

a–c Functional rehabilitation began with 10–15 kg weight bearing for 6 weeks. The actual weight bearing was greater than stipulated in this patient with poor compliance. The patient bore full weight after the second operation almost all the time. Callus formation is seen 6 weeks after the operation at both the tibia and fibula without loosening of the screws.

d–g After 3 months clearly advanced callus and endosteal consolidation of both fractures is seen. Beginnings of synostosis between the distal fibula and tibia. The patient had no complaints at this time and was mobile with full weight bearing.

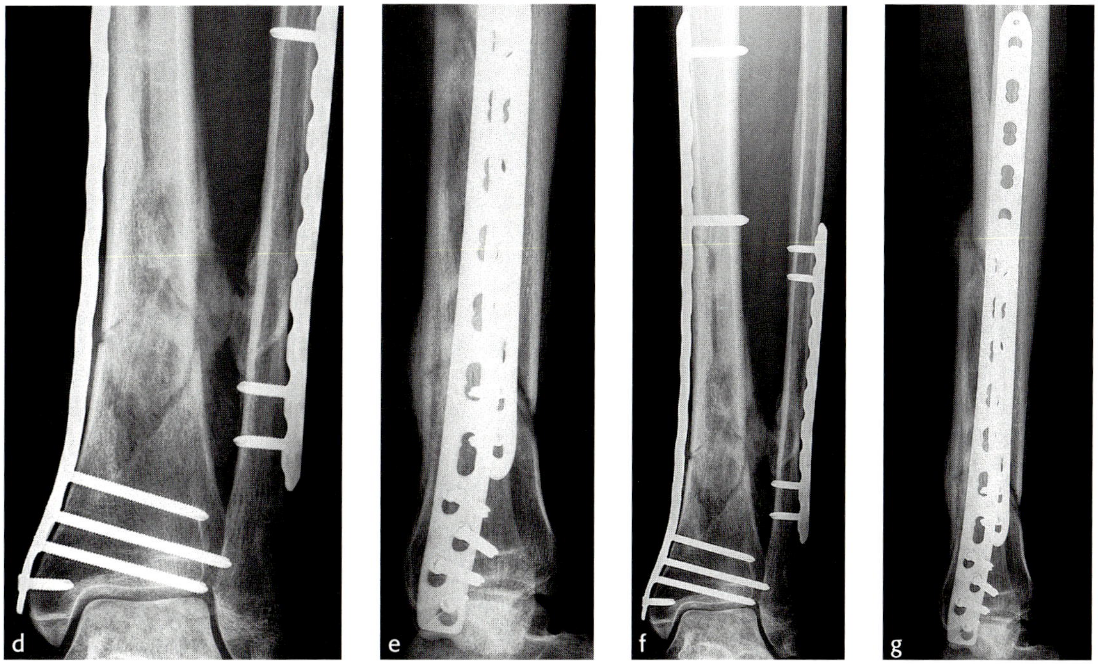

5 Pitfalls –

Equipment

Approach
The cranial incision on the lateral aspect of the fibula may endanger the superficial peroneal nerve.

Reduction and fixation

Rehabilitation
A long bridging LCP 4.5/5.0 on the tibia alone can bend in a patient with poor compliance who exercises full weight bearing. In these cases, fixation of the fibula is recommended, particularly in distal fibular fractures.

6 Pearls +

Equipment
The use of locking head screws simplifies minimally invasive procedures because the plate does not have to be anatomically bent. 3.5/4.5/5.0 metaphyseal LCPs are ideal for osteosynthesis of the distal tibia, particularly if the joint block is small.

Approach
Minimally invasive plate osteosynthesis (MIPO) spares the soft tissue and reduces the risk of iatrogenic vascular damage at the fracture level.

Reduction and fixation
Locking head screws enable good fixation of the plate, particularly in the metaphyseal part.

Rehabilitation
The additional fixation of the fibular fracture increases the stability of a lower leg fracture. Full weight bearing due to poor compliance often has no consequences.

Author Christoph Sommer

10.2.7 Fragmented wedge tibial and fibular shaft fracture—42-B3

1 Case description

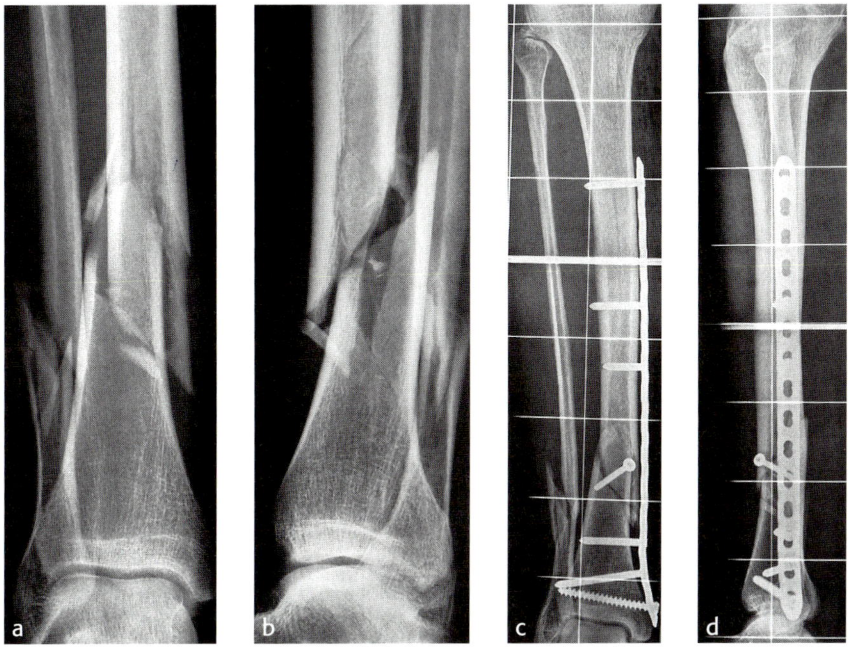

58-year-old man hit a post with his right lower leg while landing with his parachute; no relevant soft-tissue injury but a 42-B3.3 wedge fracture of his lower leg. The fracture was stabilized immediately after trauma with a 15-hole LCP 4.5/5.0 in MIPO technique and a percutaneous interfragmentary lag screw.

Fig 10.2.7-1a–g
- a–b AP and lateral view of preoperative x-rays.
- c–d The postoperative x-rays showed a valgus malalignment in a not perfectly reduced fracture.
- e–g An orthoradiogram and x-rays centered on the lower leg were obtained for precise documentation. The valgus malalignment measured about 15–20° compared with the uninjured leg. Malalignment represents one of the main problems of minimally invasive plate procedures because the position of the fragments can only be assessed by image intensification (>10° is unacceptable and must be corrected).

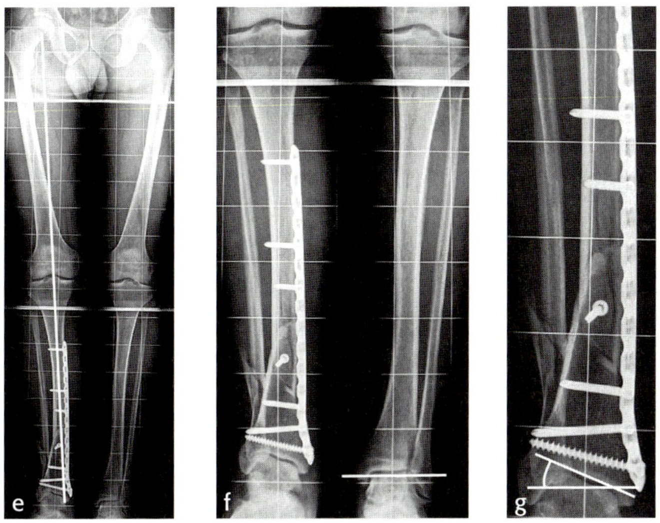

Indication

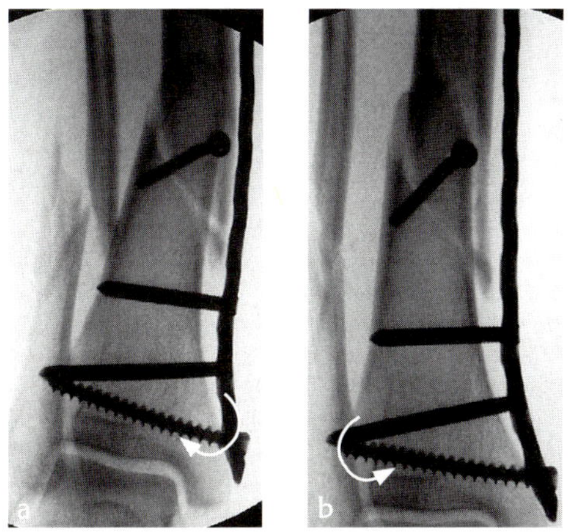

Fig 10.2.7-2a–b Functional testing under a second anesthetic showed the valgus (a) and varus (b) position by manual pushing-pulling. Because of the high flexibility of the LCP, it is possible to bend the plate into the correct position. In this situation, given that the syndesmosis is intact, plate stabilization of the fibula can result in a very stable fixation of this lower leg fracture.

Preoperative planning

Equipment

- LCP 3.5, 10 holes
- 3.5 mm self-tapping locking head screws (LHS)
- Small or large distractor

(Size of system, instruments, and implants can vary according to anatomy.)

Patient preparation and positioning

Antibiotics: single dose 2nd generation cephalosporin
Thrombosis prophylaxis: low-molecular heparin

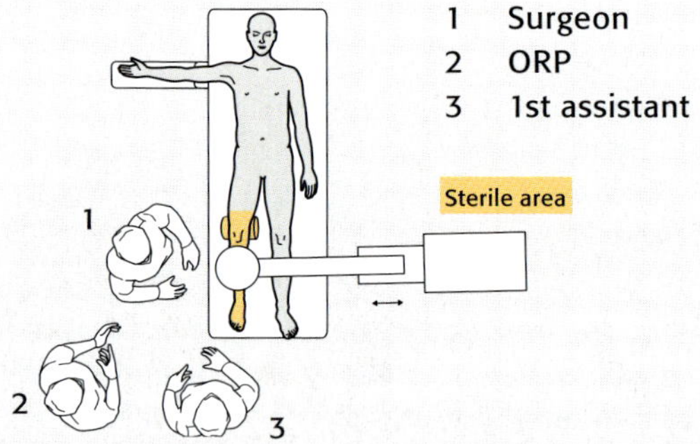

Fig 10.2.7-3 Lower leg elevated on a pad.

2 Surgical approach

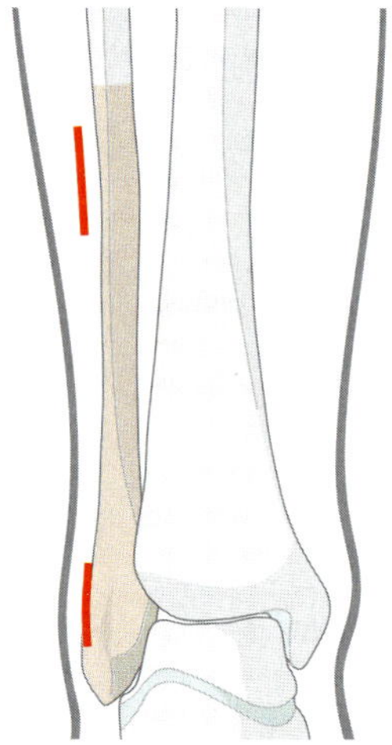

Fig 10.2.7-4 A 10-hole LCP 3.5 is chosen to bridge the multifragmentary fracture of the fibula. The ideal length of the plate is determined by image intensification and at both ends of the plate about 4 cm long incisions are made laterally over the fibula. The fracture zone is not exposed. At the cranial approach, the possible course of the superficial peroneal nerve across the fibula has to be taken into consideration.

3 Reduction and fixation

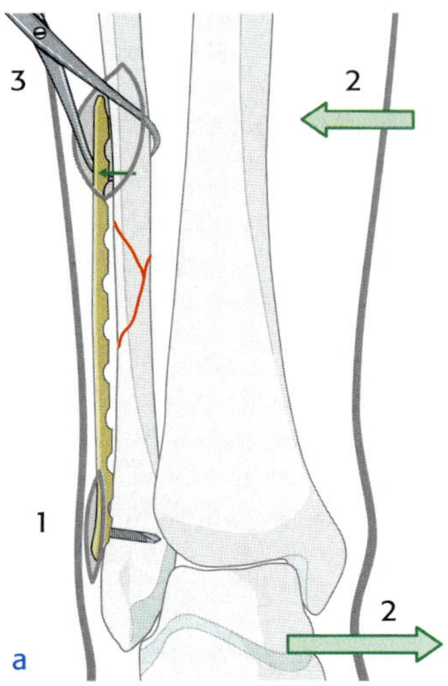

Reduction of the valgus malalignment is performed manually by the first assistant (or by the use of a distractor attached from proximal to distal tibia or to talus). The prebent LCP 3.5 is inserted epiperiosteally in a distal to proximal direction. A drill sleeve can be used as a handle. The plate is positioned under image intensification and is fixed distally at the center of the fibula with a 3.5 mm self-tapping, locking head screw. The plate has to fit tightly to the bone to avoid soft-tissue irritation. The plate is then fixed temporarily through the cranial incision with reduction forceps after correction of the axis and length.

Fig 10.2.7-5a–b

a Minimally invasive plate osteosynthesis of a distal fibular fracture. Fixation of the plate by insertion of a self-tapping locking head screw into the most distal plate hole (1). The valgus malalignment is corrected bimanually or with the help of a distractor (2). Reduction of the fibula and temporary plate fixation with the reduction forceps (3).

3 Reduction and fixation (cont)

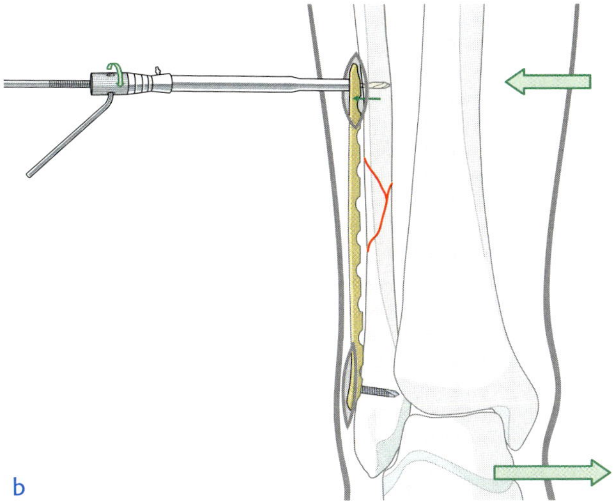

b

Fig 10.2.7-5a–b (cont)

b Alternatively, the reduction can be managed by insertion of a 2.8 mm drill bit into the cranial plate hole through a drill sleeve or by the use of the compression device.

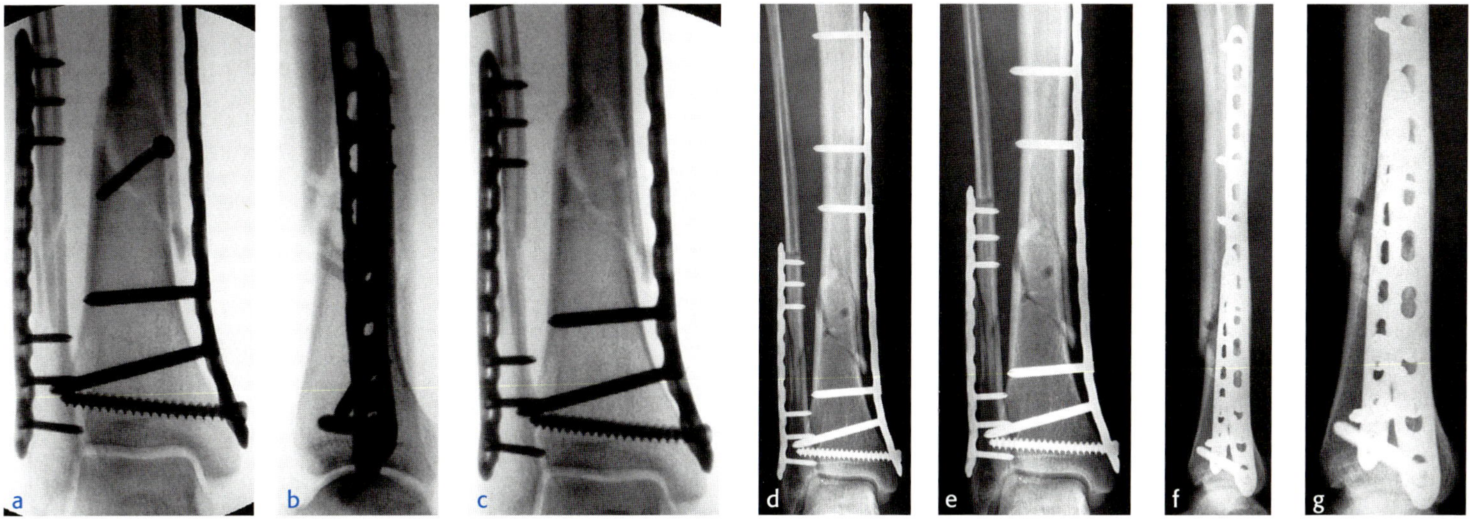

Fig 10.2.7-6a–g The fixed fibular length is definitively held by insertion of further self-tapping locking head screws. It is recommended that bicortical screws are used in the shaft area (two to three, depending on the bone quality). Self-tapping locking head screws are also used in the distal part. The screws should penetrate the metaphysis, but should not penetrate the far cortex as protrusion could irritate the syndesmosis.

In this case, three screws were used proximally and distally. The fibular fracture is reduced and bridged correctly. The interfragmentary lag screw from the first operation is removed. The screw is not needed with this bridging technique and can delay bone healing. The postoperative x-rays after the second operation show correct alignment of the tibia and fibula.

4 Rehabilitation

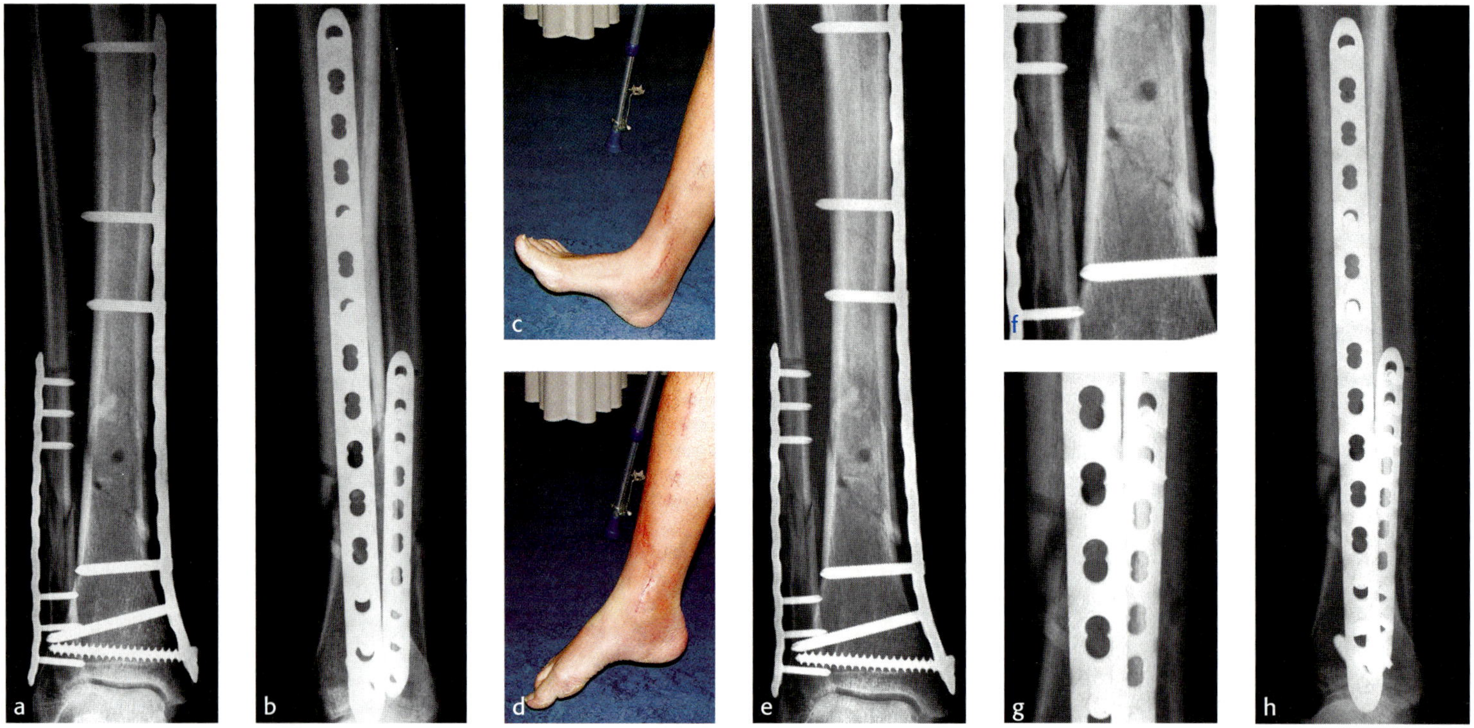

Fig 10.2.7-7a–h

a–d Mobilization began on the second postoperative day with 10–15 kg weight bearing for 6 weeks. After 6 weeks the fibula showed normal healing and callus. In contrast, the tibia showed no signs of healing at this time. The soft-tissue situation was normal.

e–h Full weight bearing was commenced after 9–10 weeks. There was still no sign of consolidation of the tibia after 10 weeks but there was normal healing of the fibula. None of the screws showed any signs of loosening. At this time, the patient was walking normally without a cane.

4 Rehabilitation (cont)

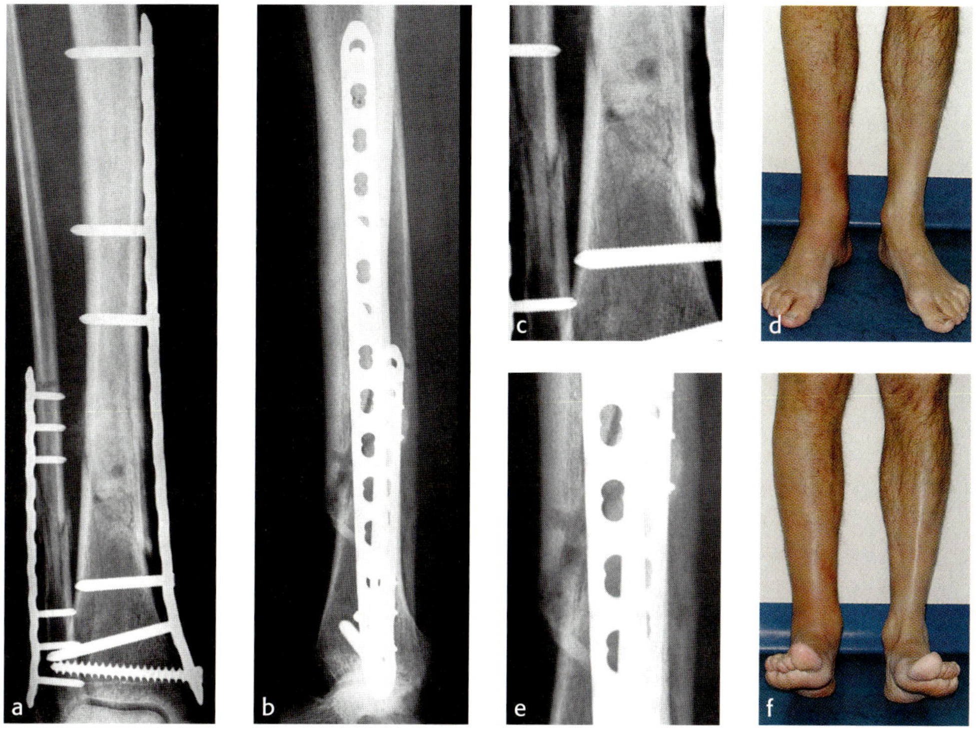

Fig 10.2.7-8a–f After 4 months callus formation had started at the tibia on the lateral side. Clinically, the fracture zone was slightly warm and slightly swollen but the patient had no complaints with regard to normal walking.

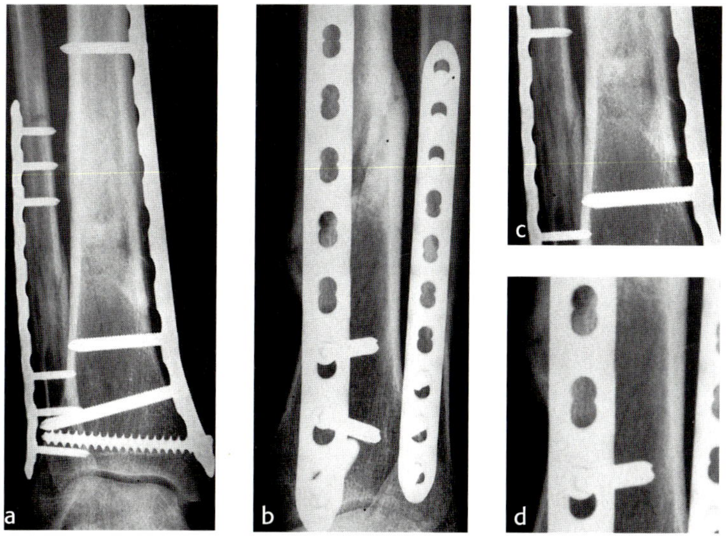

Fig 10.2.7-9a–d Both fractures had consolidated after 8 months and showed considerable endosteal remodeling.

5 Pitfalls –

Equipment

Approach
Lesion of the superficial peroneal nerve in the approach to the fibula.

Reduction and fixation
Axial deformity due to MIPO technique.
Bridging the fracture zone with a LIF in the splinting method is an elastic fracture fixation. Sometimes it is better to reduce the amount of elastic deformation by additional stabilization of the fibular fracture.

Rehabilitation

6 Pearls +

Equipment
The LCP is ideal for the MIPO technique (the plate must be contoured absolutely correctly).

Approach
Percutaneous approach to the fibula prevents iatrogenic damage to the vascularity of the numerous fragments of the fibular fracture.

Reduction and fixation
The drill inserted into the threaded drill sleeve is ideal for preliminary retention of corrected length.

Rehabilitation
Full weight bearing can be permitted early if both the tibia and fibula are stabilized.

Author Christoph Sommer

10.2.8 Fragmented wedge tibial shaft—42-B3 and multifragmentary suprasyndesmotic fibular shaft fracture—44-C2

1 Case description

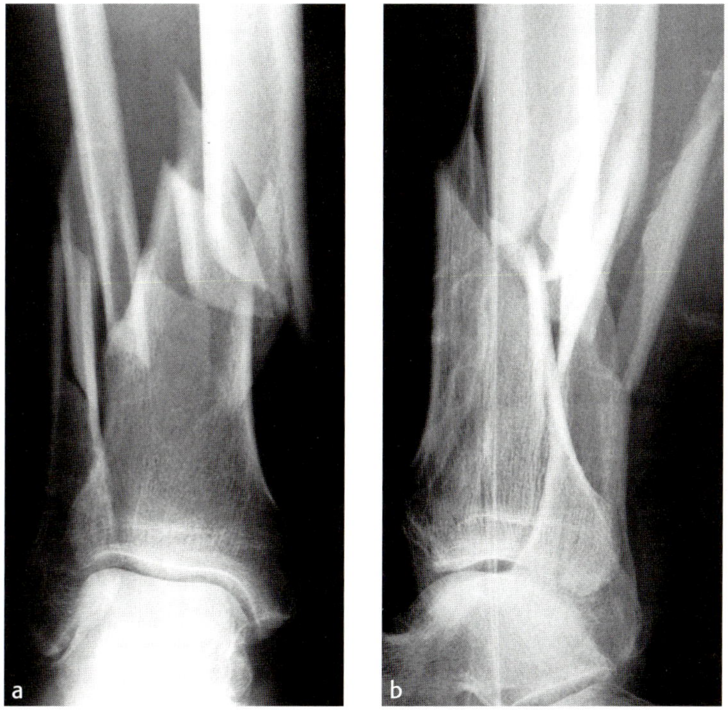

48-year-old man fell 1.5 m from a ladder and sustained a torsional injury of his lower leg and ankle. No obvious soft-tissue injuries.

Fig 10.2.8-1a–b Preoperative x-rays. Diaphyseal fracture of the distal third of the tibia with fracture line down to the metaphysis. The fibula fracture shows a long spiral wedge above the syndesmosis which does not appear to be disrupted. Taking the Volkmann triangle into account, this injury could be regarded as a combination type fracture of distal tibial and malleolar fracture.

a AP view.

b Lateral view. There are two intermediate fracture fragments and an additional isolated fracture of the Volkmann triangle.

Indication

This fracture is a clear indication for operative treatment. Because the fissure line extends close to the ankle joint, an intramedullary nail might not be suitable. Internal fixation with plates seems to be the optimal treatment in this case with only minor soft-tissue problems.

There are two reasons for additional fixation of the fibula:

1. Combination type injury
2. The relatively short distal tibia block with critical fixation to the plate

If both bones are stabilized as in this case the simpler fracture should be treated first. In our case the fibular fracture is simpler and can be reduced anatomically and stabilized absolutely using an open approach, anatomical reduction, and compression method and the conventional lag screw and protection plate technique.

The tibial fracture is not ideally suited to anatomical reduction of the different fracture fragments and therefore a minimally invasive plate osteosynthesis in a splinting method (bridge plate, internal fixator) is preferred.

Preoperative planning

Equipment

- LCP 4.5/5.0, 12 holes
- 5.0 mm locking head screws (LHS)
- 4.5 mm cortex screws
- LCP 3.5, 10 holes
- 3.5 mm LHS
- 2.7 mm cortex screws

(Size of system, instruments, and implants can vary according to anatomy.)

Patient preparation and positioning

Antibiotics: 2nd generation cephalosporin
Thrombosis prophylaxis: low-molecular heparin

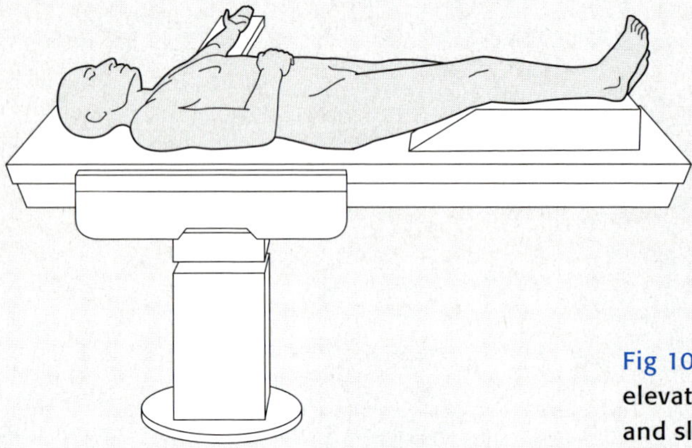

Fig 10.2.8-2 Supine position with elevation of the leg to be operated on and slight bending of the knee joint.

2 Surgical approach

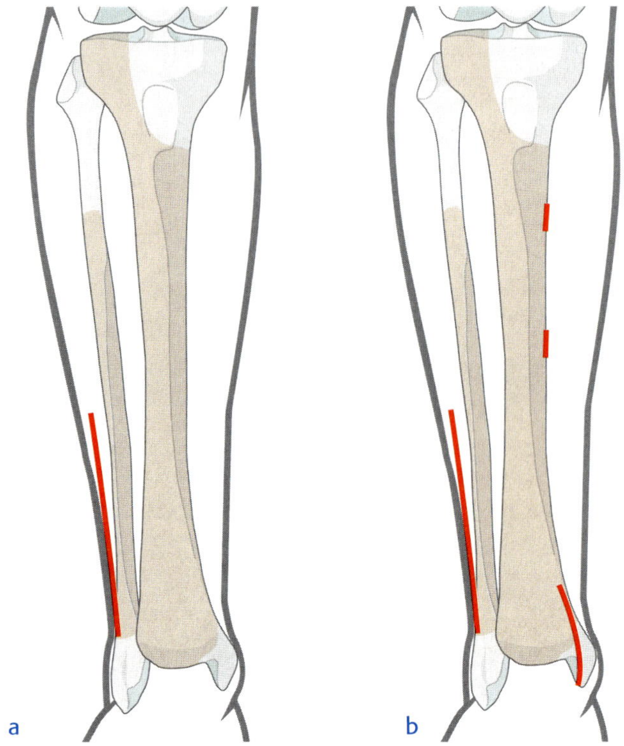

Fig 10.2.8-3a–b
a Fibula: lateral incision of 12 cm length for the fibula. The level of fracture access to the bone is in front of the peroneal muscles/tendons. Only minimal periosteal stripping of the butterfly fragment.
b Tibia: 3 cm slightly curved incision above the medial malleolus, preserving the saphenous vein and nerve, the approach goes straight down to the periosteum. Only stab incisions are used for insertion of the proximal screws.

3 Reduction and fixation

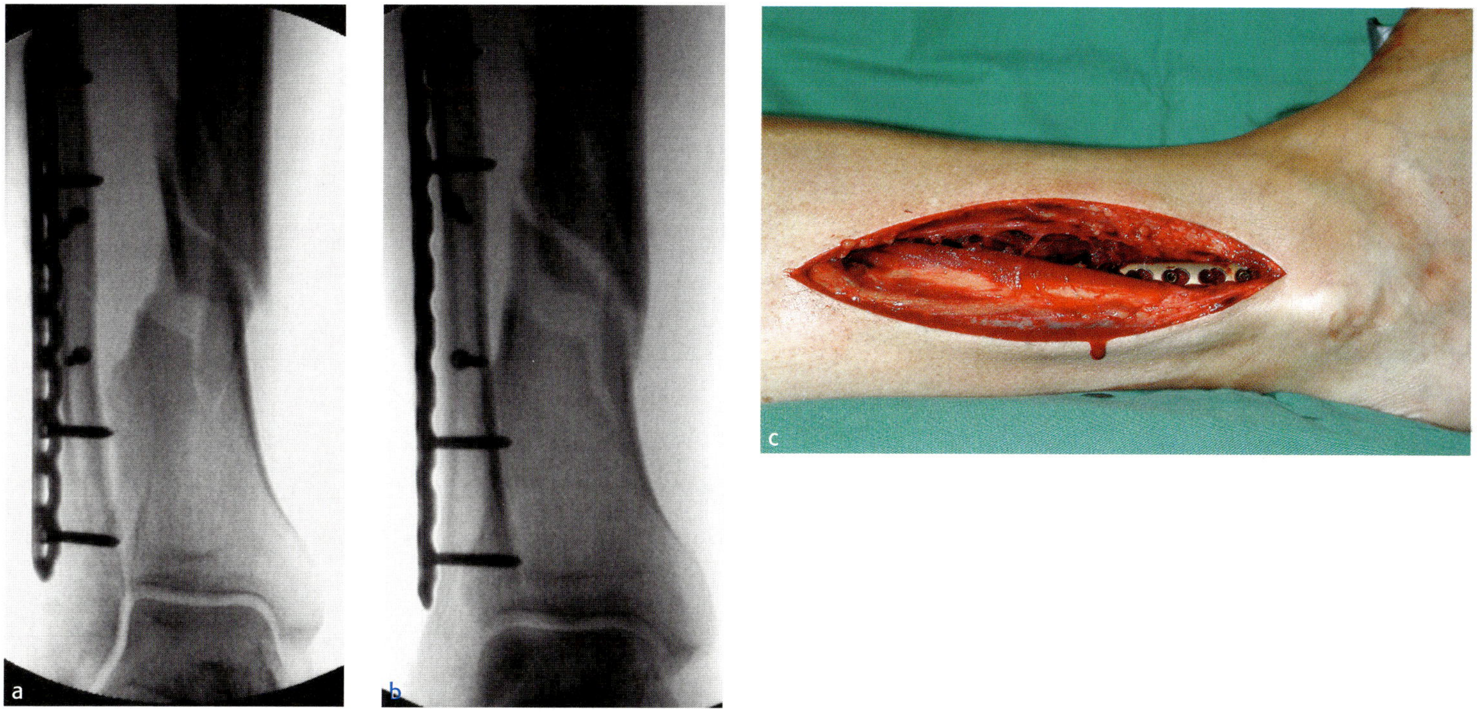

Fig 10.2.8-4a–c Reduction of the fibula. The fibula was reduced in a conventional open technique with direct reduction maneuvers using two small pointed reduction forceps. After absolutely precise, anatomical reduction, two 2.7 mm cortex screws were applied for interfragmentary compression. These two screws were protected in this case by a LCP 3.5 in an internal fixator method using two bicortical LHS on each side of the fracture. The advantage of this method is that the protection plate does not have to be bent and twisted precisely.

- a AP view.
- b Lateral view.
- c Clinical view of the lateral incision for the fibula and the internal fixator (LCP 3.5).

3 Reduction and fixation (cont)

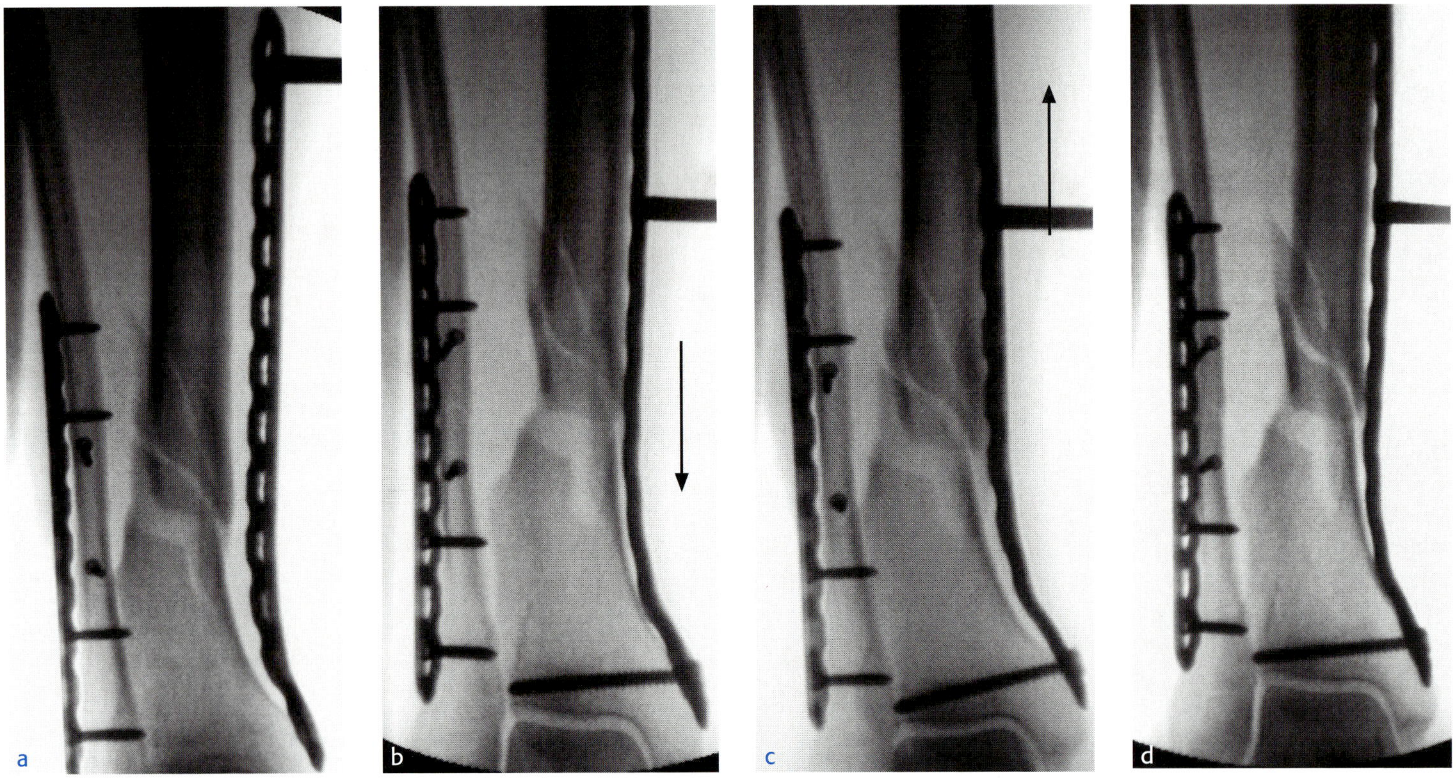

Fig 10.2.8-5a–i

- a Reduction of the tibia. The preshaped and slightly twisted LCP 4.5/5.0 is, prior to insertion, checked under image intensification. Care has to be taken not to overbend the plate, which would lead to a soft-tissue irritation at the distal end of the plate.
- b The plate is then inserted through the small supramalleolar incision and pushed cranially feeling and bypassing the fracture zone. In this case the most distal hole is first occupied using a 4.5 mm cortex screw which is not yet fully tightened. Through a small stab incision above the fracture, a drill sleeve is inserted in the threaded part of the combination hole. Using this drill sleeve as a handle, the alignment of the fracture in the coronal plane could be indirectly achieved: pushing the drill sleeve distally (arrow), the distal fragment angulated towards a valgus position.
- c While pushing the drill sleeve (and the plate) proximally (arrow), the fracture went into varus position. This is only possible if the screw already inserted is not a LHS and not fully tightened.
- d After correct alignment had been achieved, including correct rotation, which has to be checked clinically, a bicortical LHS was inserted through a stab incision in the most proximal hole of the plate and the distal screw was tightened.

3 Reduction and fixation (cont)

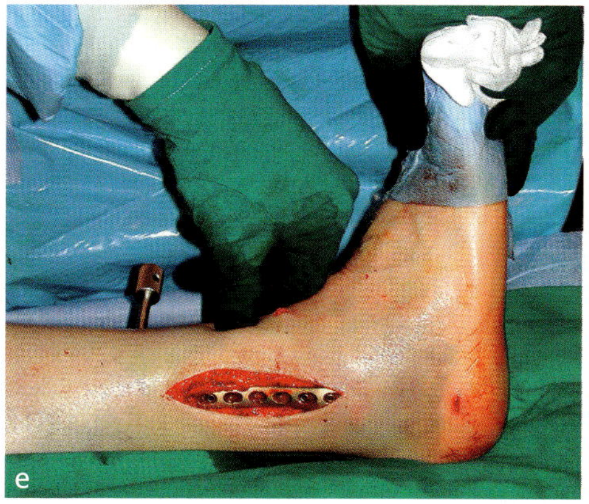

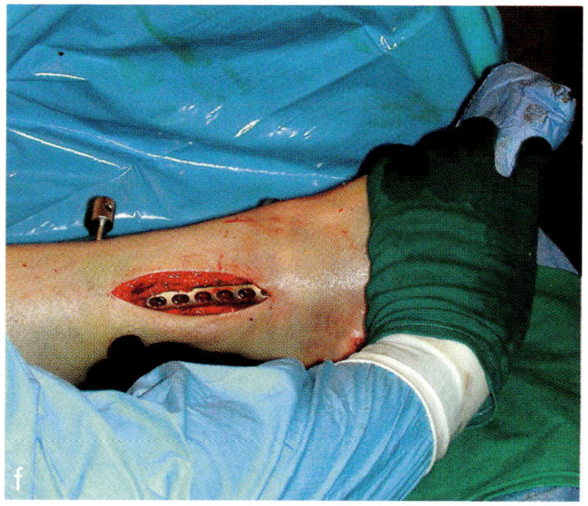

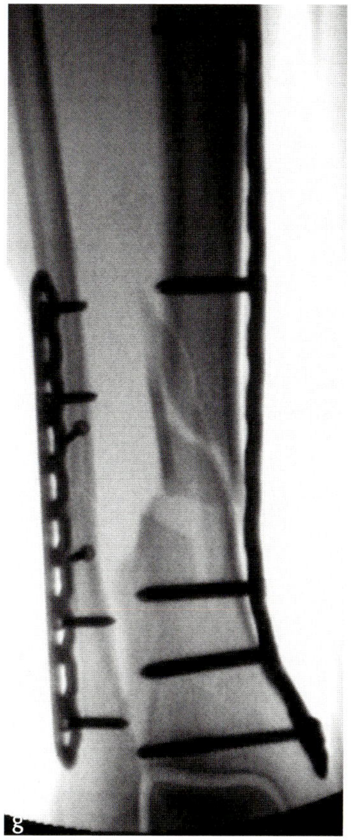

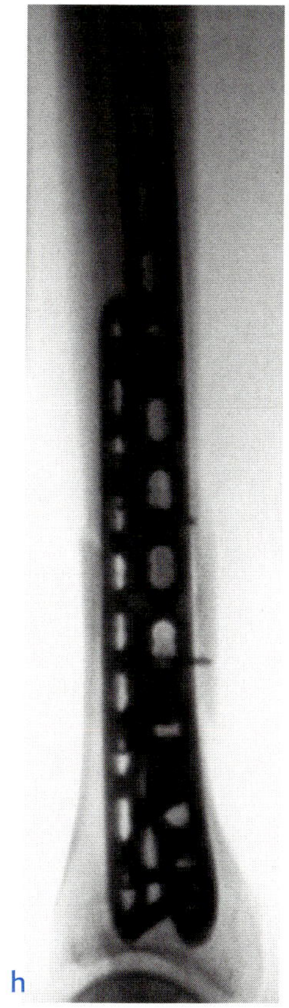

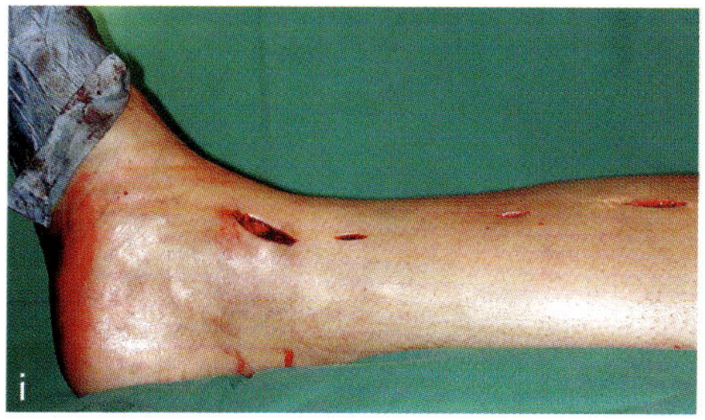

Fig 10.2.8-5a–i (cont)

e–f At this stage, the axis in the lateral view has to be controlled under image intensification. Residual axial deviation can then be finally adjusted using manipulation by hand. Both main fragments were able to rotate slightly around the single screws inserted in the most proximal and most distal plate holes.

g–h After this final alignment, further LHS are inserted. The second screw in each fragment is placed close to the fracture zone in a multifragmentary fracture situation. In good bone quality, two bicortical LHS (four cortices) are sufficient in the diaphysis. At least three screws should be used in the metaphysis.

i Final view after MIPO of the tibia.

4 Rehabilitation

Early movement is practised immediately following surgery. Mobilization is allowed 2–3 days after the operation, depending on the soft-tissue situation under toe-touch weight bearing (10–15 kg).

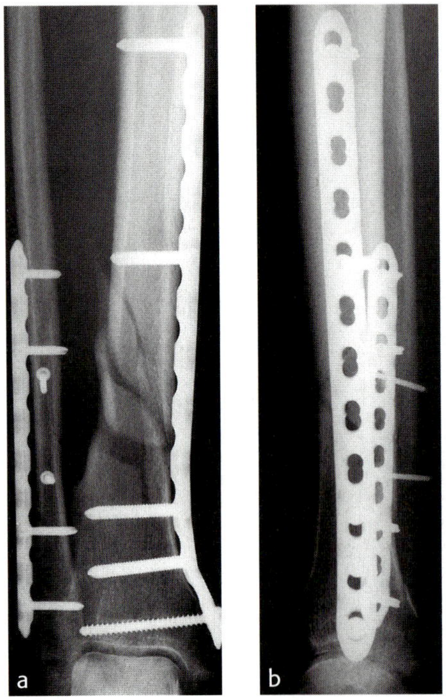

Fig 10.2.8-6a–b Follow-up x-rays after 6 weeks showed a stable situation and correct alignment and the beginnings of direct bone healing on the fibula (slight bone resorption at the fracture line). Loading was gradually increased depending on the clinical situation (swelling and pain at the fracture zone). Full weight bearing was allowed after 3 months.

a AP view.

b Lateral view.

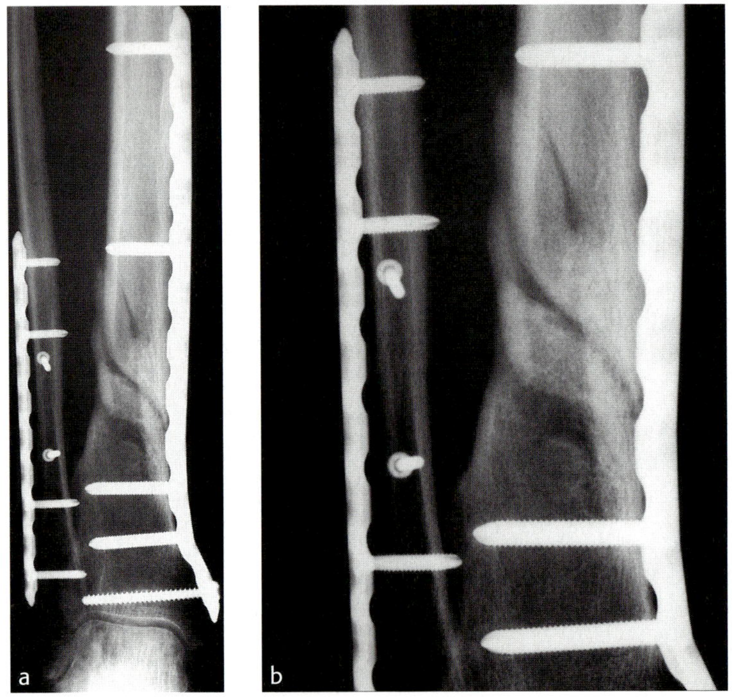

Fig 10.2.8-7a–b Follow-up x-rays after 6 months. Complete direct bone healing of the fibula and ongoing indirect healing of the tibia, mainly by endosteal callus formation.

4 Rehabilitation (cont)

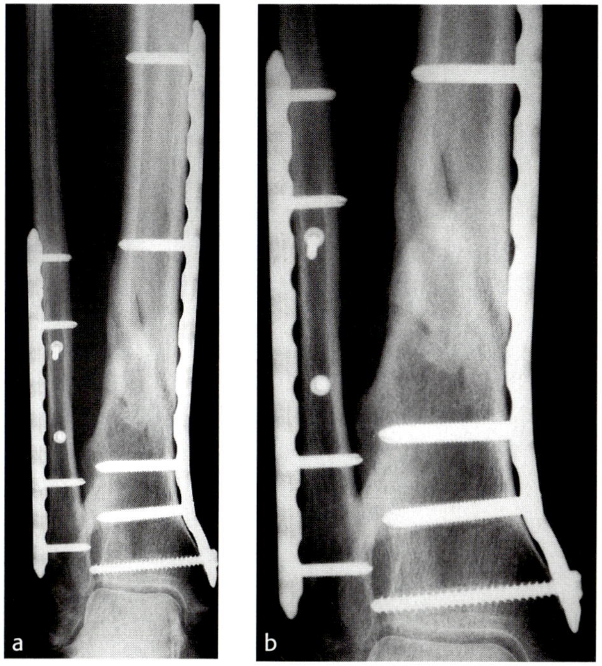

Fig 10.2.8-8a–b After 14 months the fracture was completely healed whereby the remodeling process on the tibia was still going.

5 Pitfalls –

Approach

Reduction and fixation

Omitting anatomical reduction of the fibula will lead to incorrect alignment of the tibia.

In complex fibular fractures, the tibia must be addressed first.

6 Pearls +

Approach

The percutaneous approach to the tibia is safe and can be performed on the day of the injury. A double open approach to the fibula and the tibia can be dangerous and can lead to wound necrosis.

Reduction and fixation

LCP with different screw types allows for indirect reduction in a minimally invasive approach using the drill sleeves as reduction tools (handles).

Author Michael Wagner

10.2.9 Complex spiral tibial shaft fracture—42-C1

1 Case description

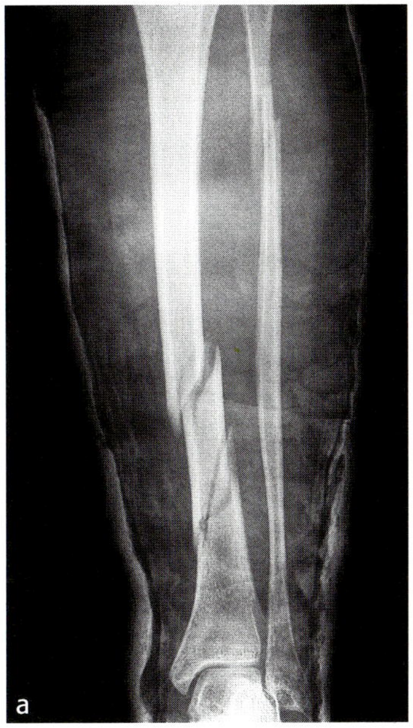

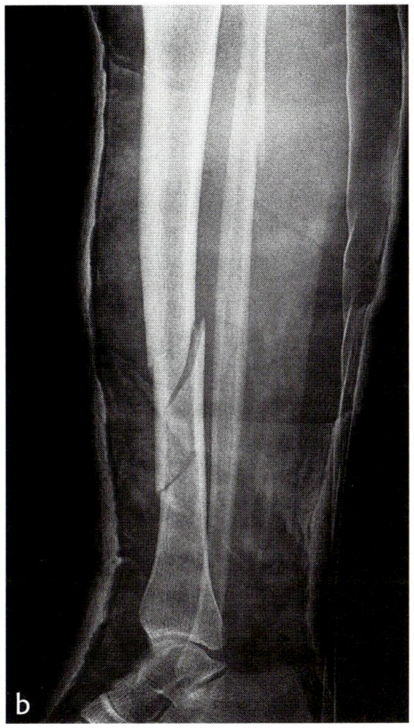

28-year-old man fell on ice.

Fig 10.2.9-1a–b Emergency care in another hospital with long-leg cast.
a AP view.
b Lateral view.

Indication

Unstable tibial shaft fracture.

Preoperative planning

Equipment

- LCP metaphyseal plate 3.5/4.5/5.0, for distal tibia, 4 + 12 holes
- 3.5 mm locking head screws (LHS)
- 5.0 mm LHS
- 2.0 mm K-wires

(Size of system, instruments, and implants can vary according to anatomy.)

Patient preparation and positioning

Antibiotics: none
Thrombosis prophylaxis: low-molecular heparin

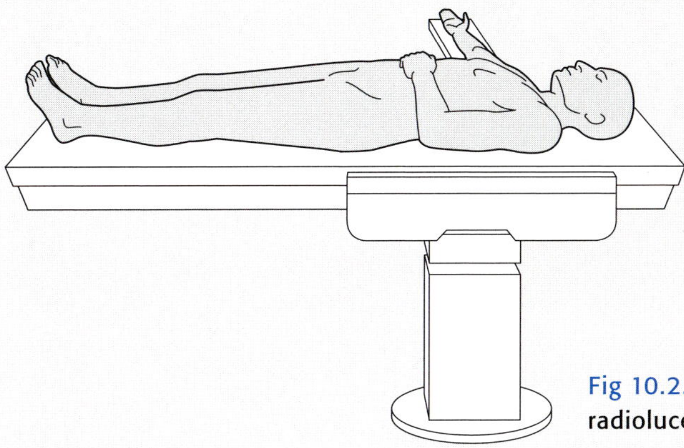

Fig 10.2.9-2 Supine position on radiolucent operating table.

2 Surgical approach

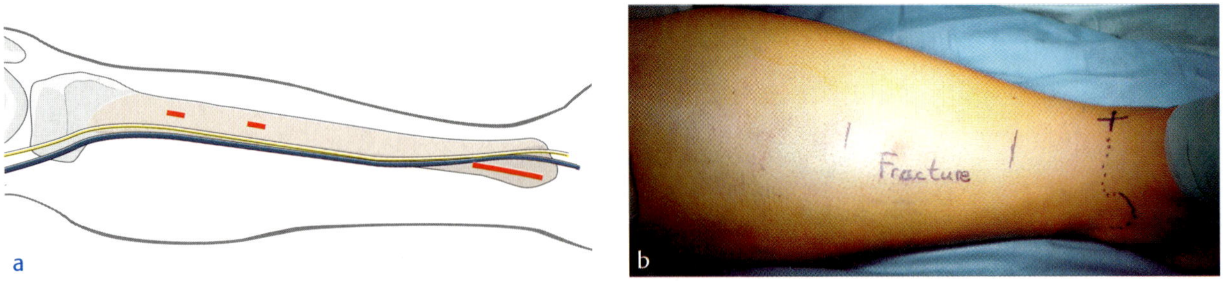

Fig 10.2.9-3a–b MIPO; three incisions on the medial side of the tibia.

a Short incision over the medial malleolus taking care not to damage the great saphenous vein. Incision at the planned site for the proximal end of the plate.

b Preoperative marking of landmarks.

3 Reduction and fixation

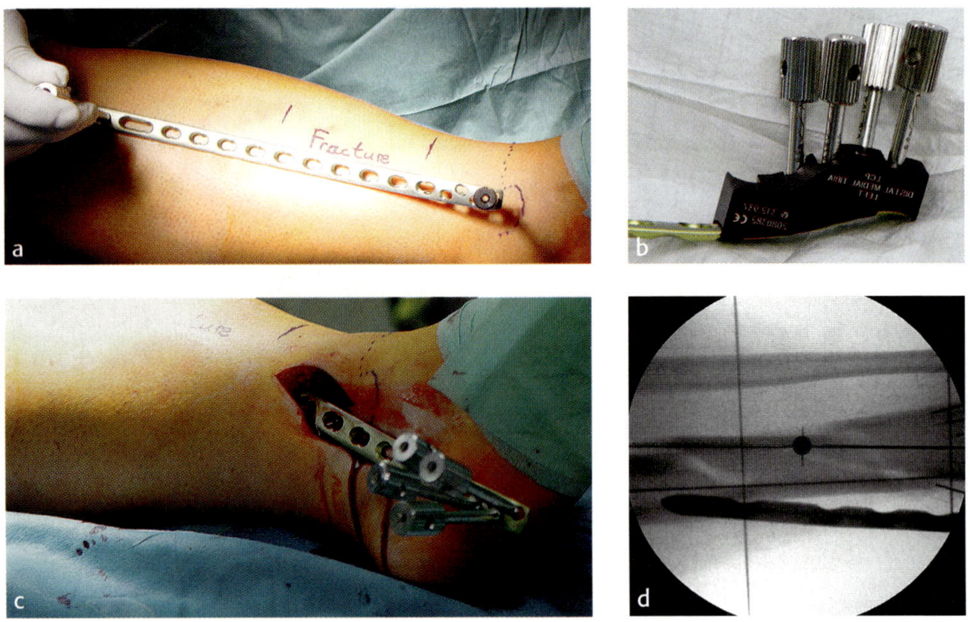

Fig 10.2.9-4a–m

a LCP metaphyseal plate 3.5/4.5/5.0, for distal tibia is chosen according to length.

b With the aid of the guiding block the threaded drill sleeves are inserted in the predefined direction.

c–d After preparing the epiperiosteal space with a long bone rasp the plate is inserted from a distal to proximal direction; control using image intensifier.

3 Reduction and fixation (cont)

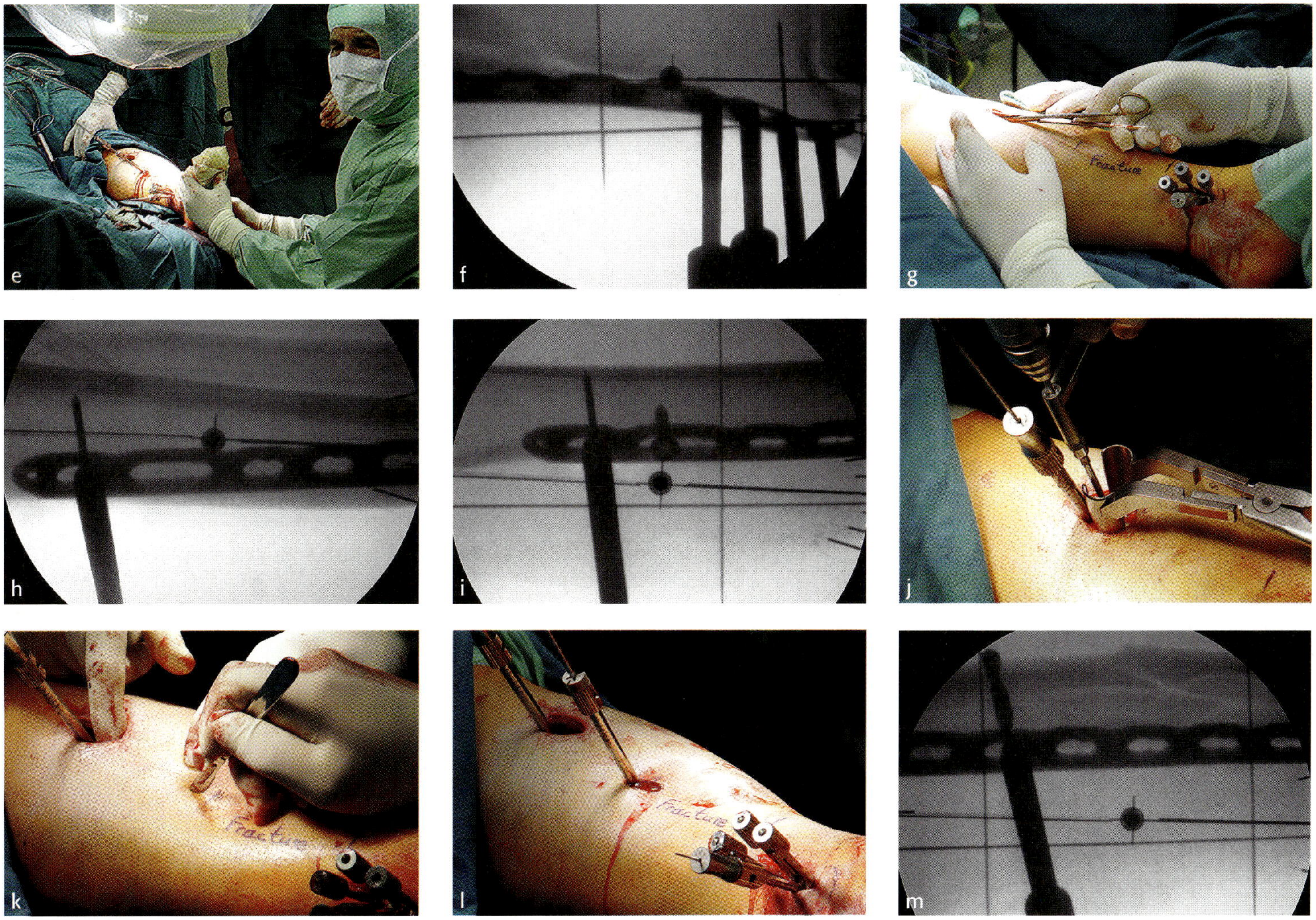

Fig 10.2.9-4a–m (cont)

- e Closed reduction by manual traction; control using image intensifier.
- f Control of plate position with regard to the lateral aspect of the bone. Then temporary fixation with a K-wire distally.
- g–h At the proximal end of the plate an incision is made and the plate is secured with a K-wire.
- i–j In order to prevent the plate from protruding beyond the bone, the plate is pulled close to the bone with the aid of a cortex screw. In this case the cortex screw was only placed monocortically through the oval long hole.
- k–m Additional incision and fixation of the proximal main fragment close to the fracture site, temporarily with the drill bit inserted through the drill sleeve in order to increase stability for definitive reduction.

3 Reduction and fixation (cont)

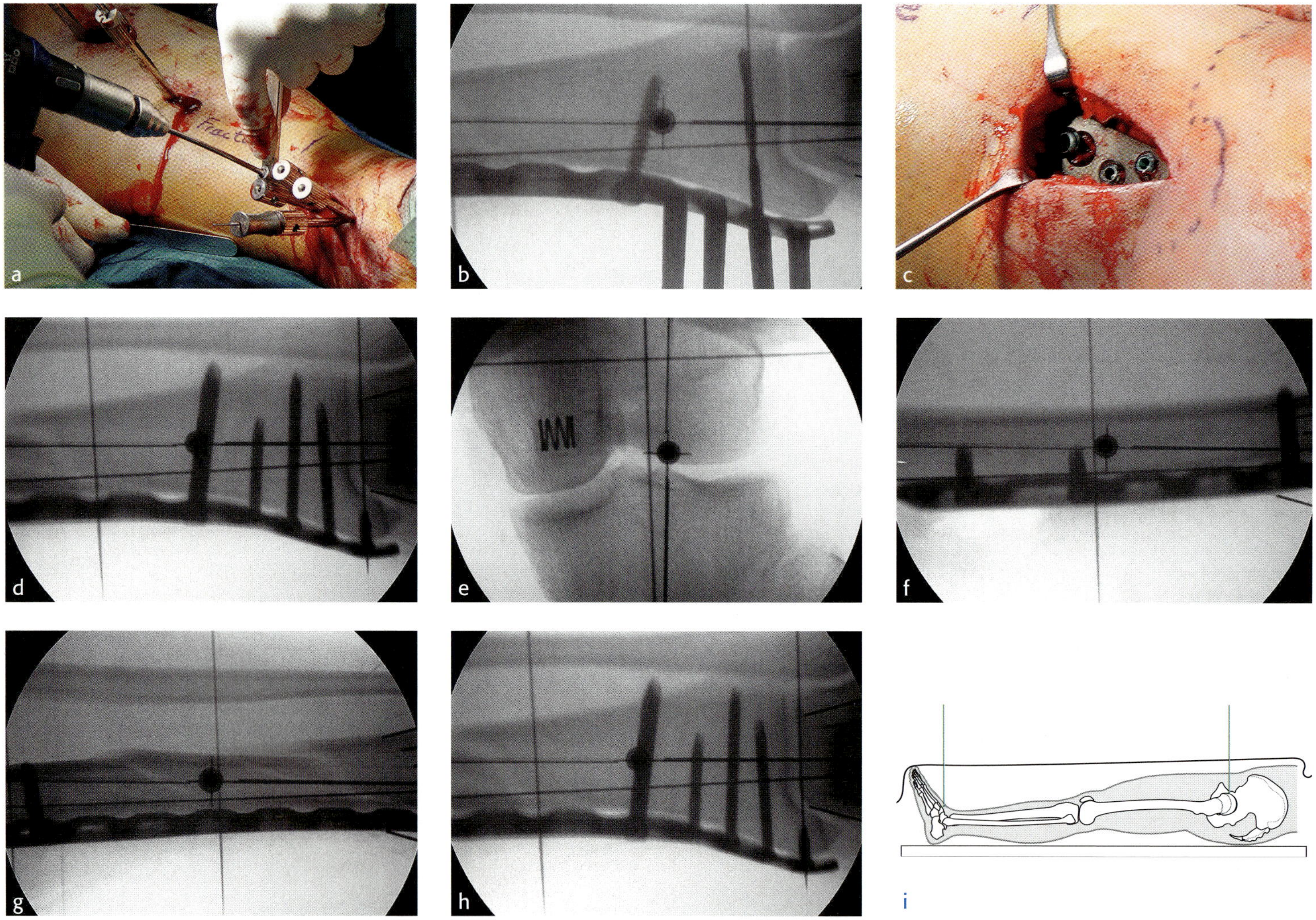

Fig 10.2.9-5a–i

a Place LHS in the distal main fragment.

b In order to avoid tilting of the distal fragment and to retain the reduction while inserting the distal LHS, a cortex screw is placed as a reduction screw. Then the drill bit is used through the drill sleeve to predrill parallel to the upper ankle joint. Subsequently, a 3.5 mm LHS is inserted.

c–d After a total of four 3.5 mm LHS have been inserted into the distal fragment, the reduction screw (cortex screw) is replaced by a bicortical 5.0 mm LHS.

e–i The correction of the axis is checked using the cable method.

3 Reduction and fixation (cont)

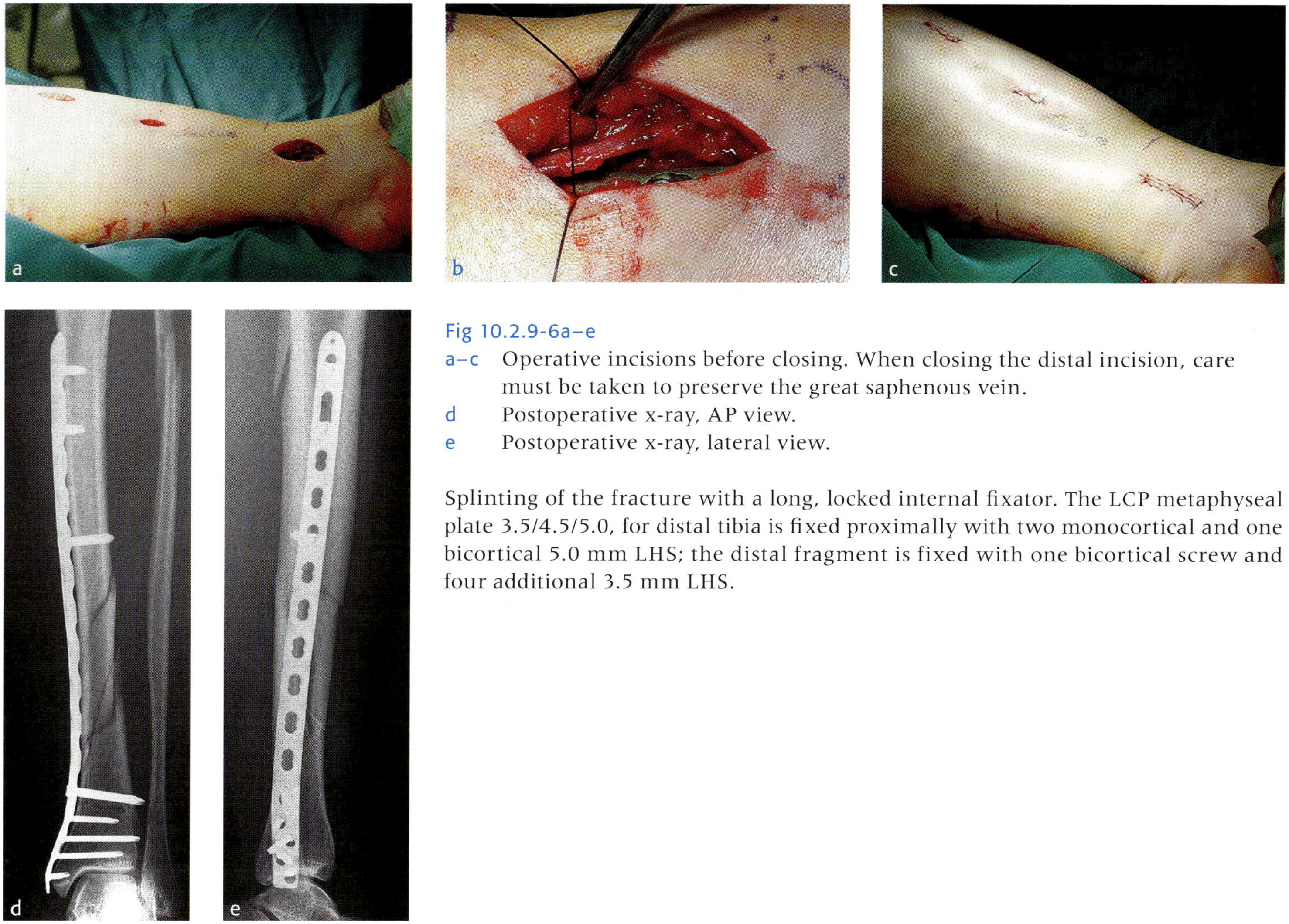

Fig 10.2.9-6a–e
a–c Operative incisions before closing. When closing the distal incision, care must be taken to preserve the great saphenous vein.
d Postoperative x-ray, AP view.
e Postoperative x-ray, lateral view.

Splinting of the fracture with a long, locked internal fixator. The LCP metaphyseal plate 3.5/4.5/5.0, for distal tibia is fixed proximally with two monocortical and one bicortical 5.0 mm LHS; the distal fragment is fixed with one bicortical screw and four additional 3.5 mm LHS.

4 Rehabilitation

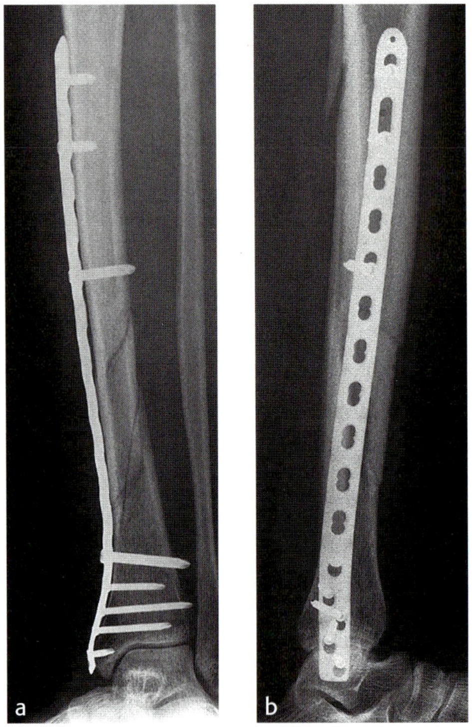

Fig 10.2.9-7a–b Partial weight bearing for 8 weeks. Postoperative x-rays after 2 months.

a AP view.

b Lateral view.

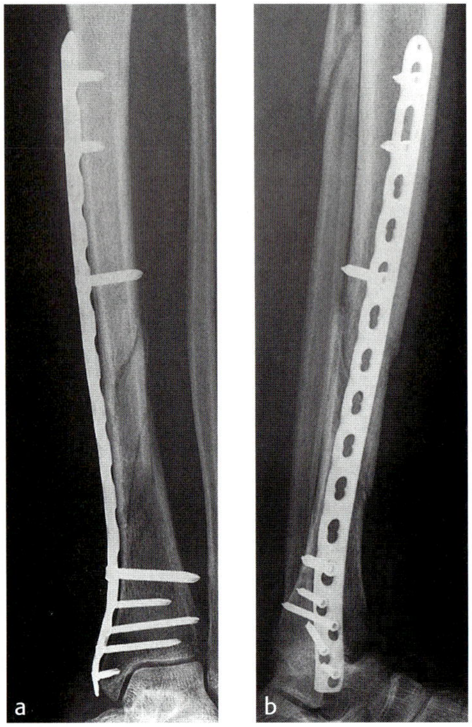

Fig 10.2.9-8a–b Radiological procedure. No radiological signs of callus formation after 3 months. The patient was pain free when totally mobilized with full weight bearing.

a AP view.

b Lateral view.

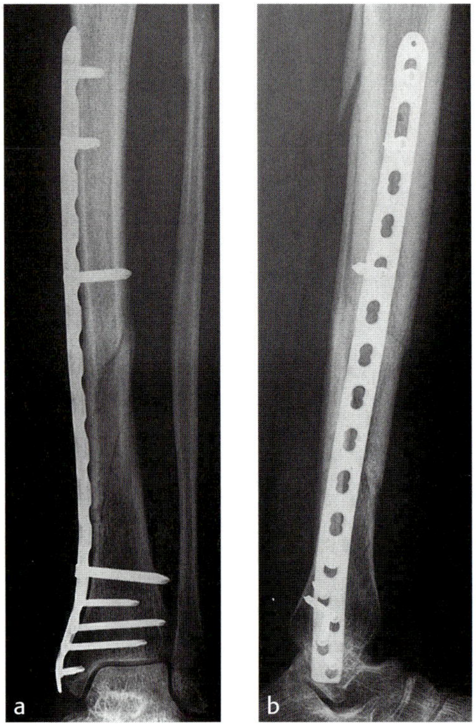

Fig 10.2.9-9a–b Callus formation visible on x-ray after 4 months.

a AP view.

b Lateral view.

4 Rehabilitation (cont)

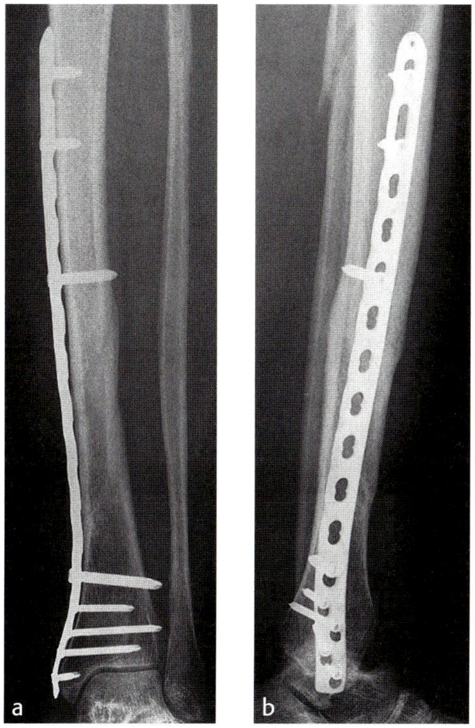

Fig 10.2.9-10a–b Fracture consolidation after 7 months.

- a AP view.
- b Lateral view.

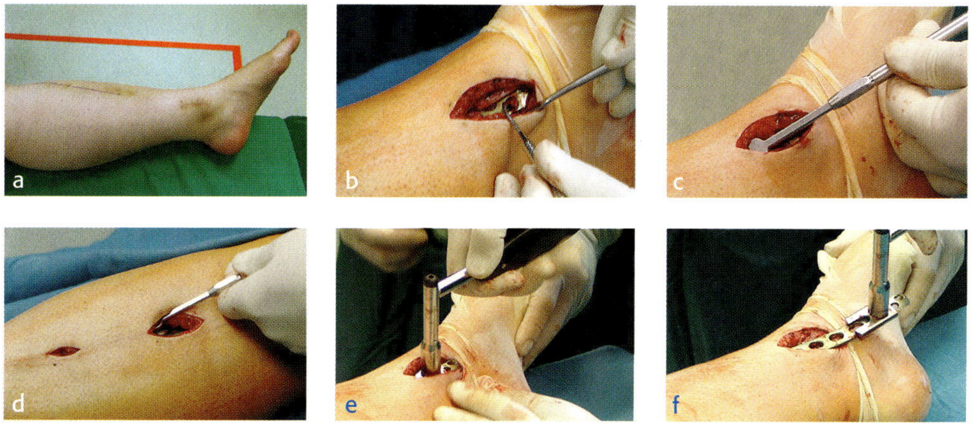

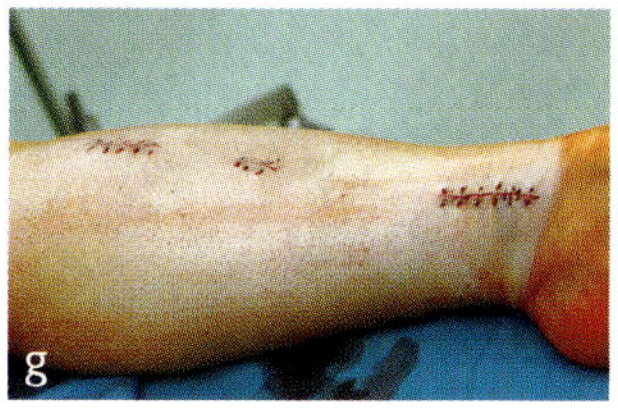

Implant removal

Due to slight pain at the distal end of the plate the patient requested implant removal after 14 months.

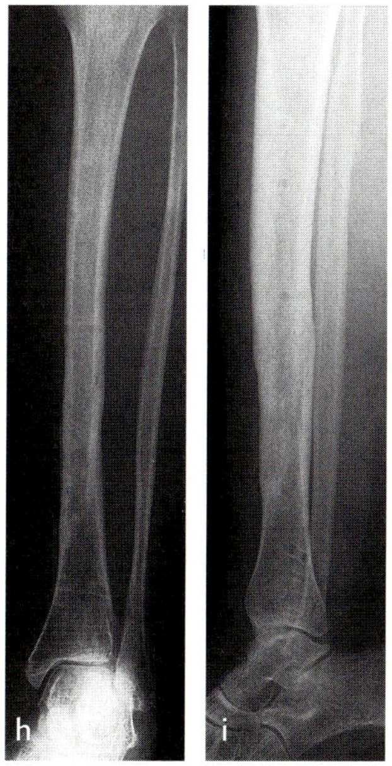

Fig 10.2.9-11a–i

- a–b Use of the existing scars. After cleaning the socket of the screw head with the fine dentist's hook and the small bone rasp, first the distal, then the proximal LHS are removed.
- c–d Subsequently, using the soft-tissue retractor in a proximal direction, the plate is freed of soft-tissue adhesiolysis.
- e–f With the aid of the plate holder fixed to the distal end of the plate, tilting movements can be performed with the plate so that the last soft-tissue remnants are released. Then the plate is pulled out in a distal direction.
- g Closure of the incisions after implant removal, which was performed via the scars from the initial operation.
- h X-ray after implant removal, AP view.
- i X-ray after implant removal, lateral view.

5 Pitfalls –

Equipment

Approach

Reduction and fixation
Varus/valgus tilting of the distal fragment

Rehabilitation
If mobilized too early with too much weight bearing or in a noncompliant patient, the plate may bend.

6 Pearls +

Equipment
The LCP metaphyseal plate 3.5/4.5/5.0, for distal tibia is anatomically preshaped and fits the distal end of the tibia.

The use of locking head screws simplifies minimally invasive procedures because the plate does not have to be anatomically bent. The distal metaphyseal LCPs are ideal for osteosynthesis of the distal tibia, particularly if the joint block is small.

Approach
Minimally invasive plate osteosynthesis (MIPO) preserves soft tissues and reduces the risk of iatrogenic vascular damage at fracture level.

Reduction and fixation
Intraoperative correction is possible with the aid of a cortex screw = "reduction screw" that pulls the fragment towards the plate.

Locking head screws enable good fixation of the plate, particularly in the metaphyseal part.

Rehabilitation
Early functional postoperative treatment is possible even in complex fractures if the fracture is well stabilized.

Authors Michael Wagner, Thomas Neubauer

10.2.10 Open complex segmental tibial shaft fracture—42-C1

1 Case description

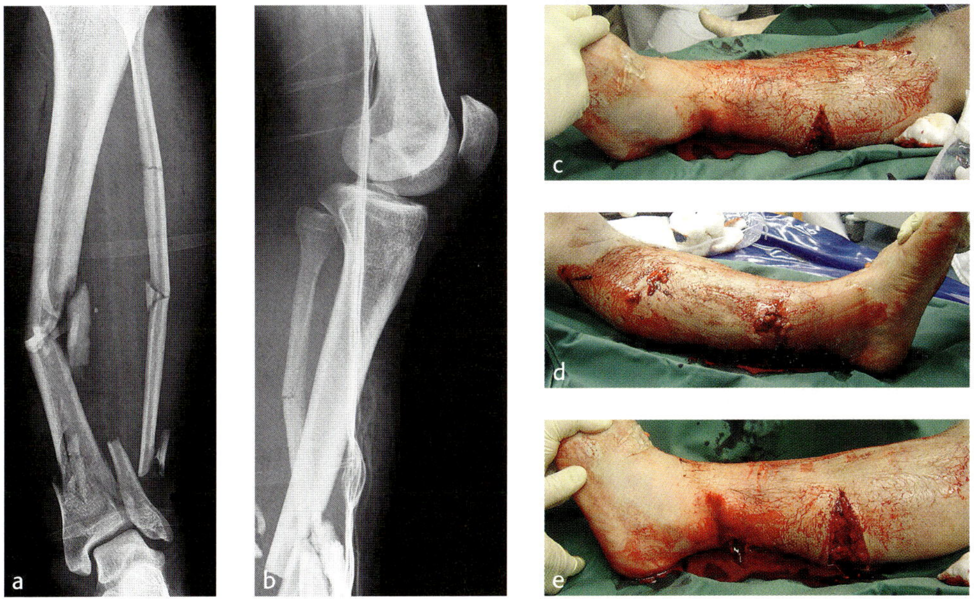

36-year-old man fell off his motorbike and the motorbike fell on his left leg. This caused a Gustilo type III open tibial fracture with a semicircular wound on the posterior aspect of the lower leg and traumatic severage of the posterior tibial artery.

Fig 10.2.10-1a–e
a AP view.
b Lateral view.
c–e Semicircular wound.

Indication

Gustilo type III open segmental fracture of the lower leg with traumatic severance of the posterior tibial artery is an absolute indication for surgical treatment. Wound decontamination, vessel suture, and stabilization of the fracture must be performed immediately. Revision operations and plastic surgery must be incorporated into plans for subsequent treatment.

Preoperative planning

Equipment

- LCP metaphyseal plate 3.5/4.5/5.0, for distal tibia, 4 + 16 holes
- 3.5 mm locking head screws (LHS)
- 5.0 mm LHS
- 2.0 mm K-wires
- 2.0 mm titanium elastic nail

(Size of system, instruments, and implants can vary according to anatomy.)

Patient preparation and positioning

Antibiotics: 3rd generation cephalosporin
Thrombosis prophylaxis: low-molecular heparin

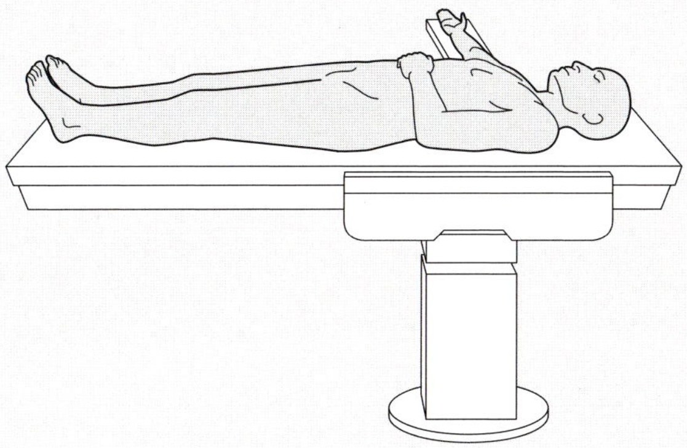

Fig 10.2.10-2 Supine position.

2 Surgical approach

The approach is partly given because the injury is an open fracture. Additionally, distal medial and proximal medial incisions are made.

3 Reduction and fixation

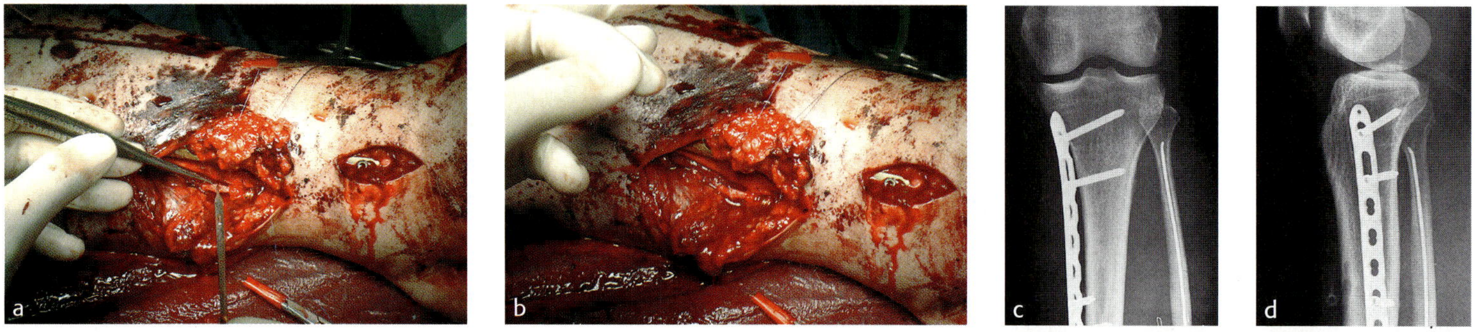

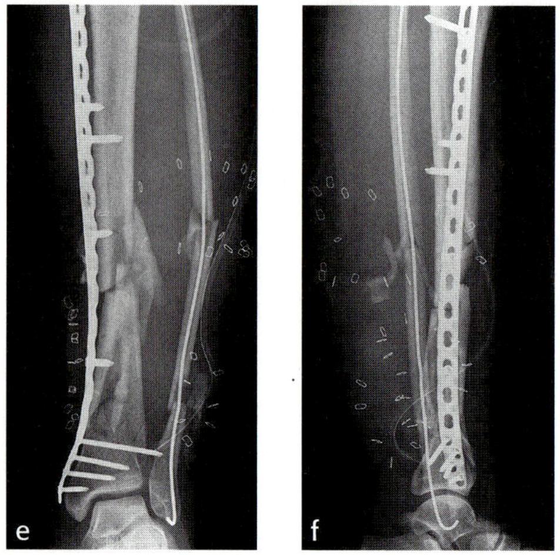

Fig 10.2.10-3a–f After wound debridement and manual traction, the plate is inserted from distal to proximal through the distal medial surgical incision. It is positioned over the distal and proximal main fragments and stabilized. Four 3.5 mm locking head screws are inserted distally and four 5.0 mm LHS proximally. The intermediary segment is stabilized with a monocortical LHS. Intramedullary osteo-synthesis of the segmental fracture of the fibula is achieved with a 2.0 mm titanium elastic nail. The wound is closed with artificial skin.

4 Rehabilitation

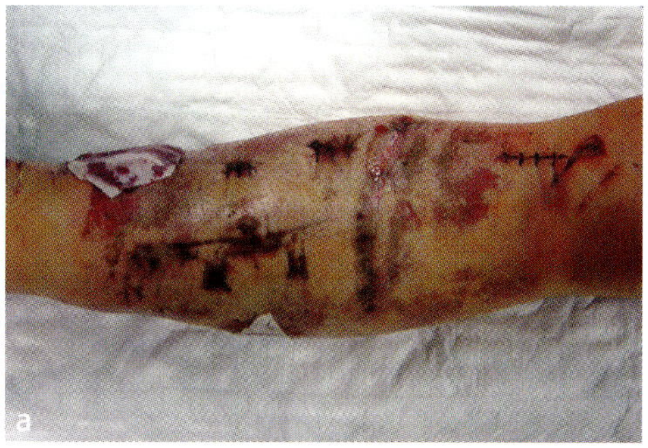

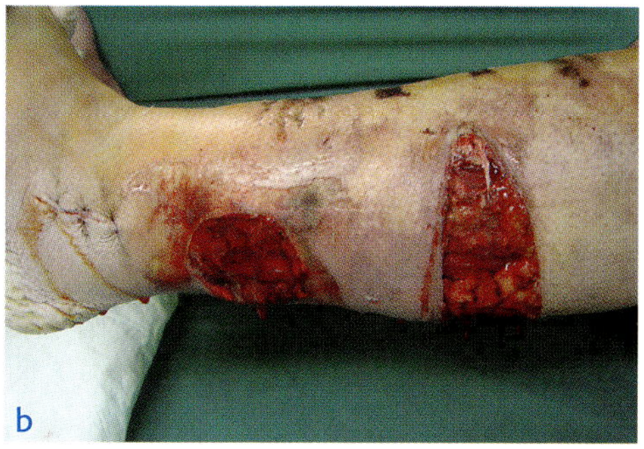

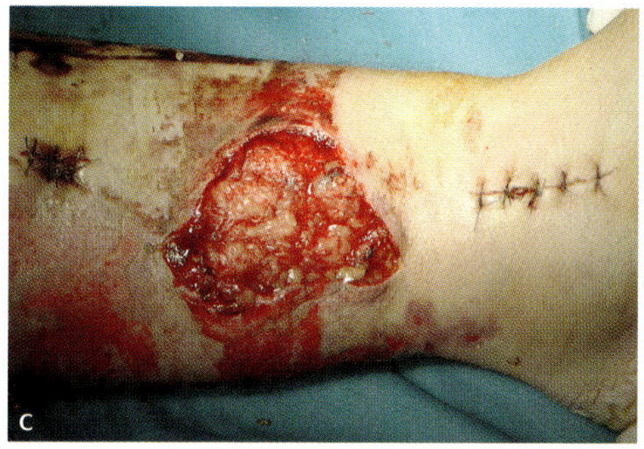

Further course of treatment: several second look operations planned to treat the severe soft-tissue damage.

Fig 10.2.10-4a–h
a–c Clinical picture of the soft-tissue situation at the second look operation on the 4th day after the operation. Severe skin contusions and skin defects are visible.

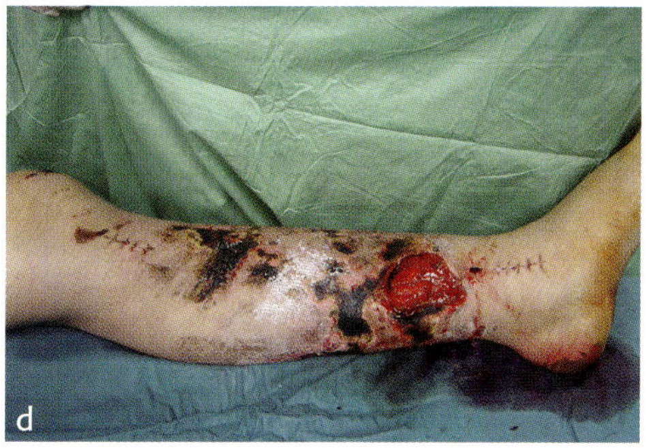

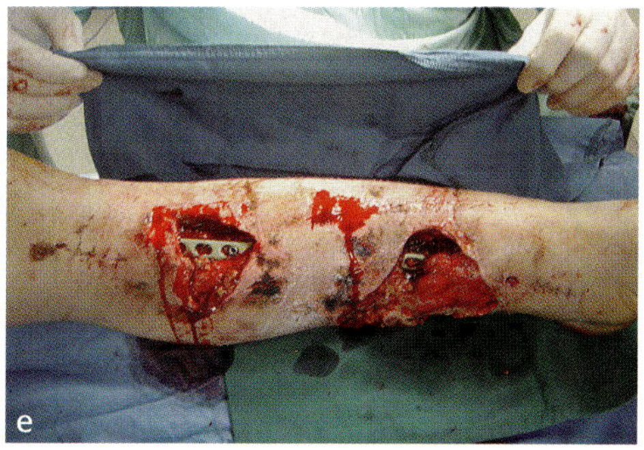

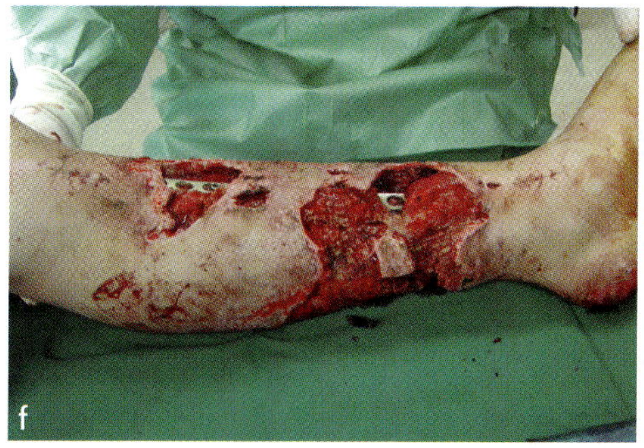

d Extent of skin necrosis and defects.

e Extent of skin defects after excision of the necrotic skin. The internal fixator is partially exposed.

f Definitive size of the skin defect after several necrosectomies.

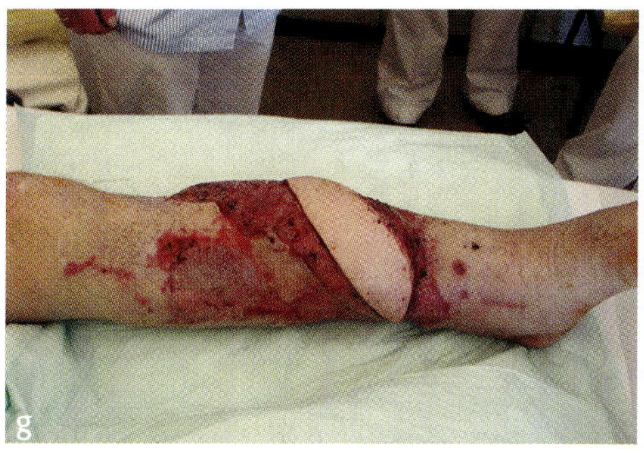

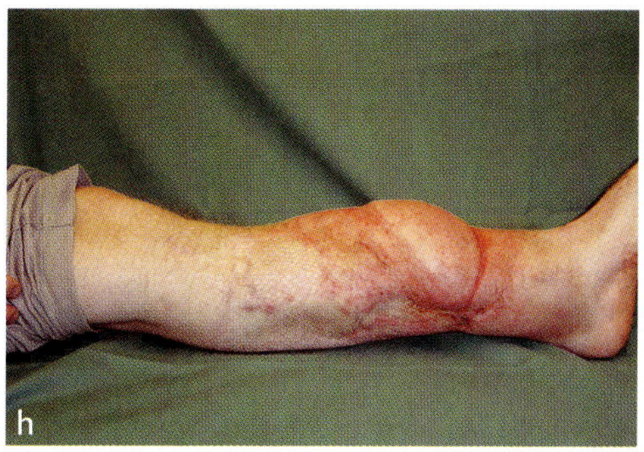

g The soft-tissue defects are covered with gastrocnemius flaps proximally and latissimus flaps distally.
h Soft-tissue situation after consolidation.

4 Rehabilitation (cont)

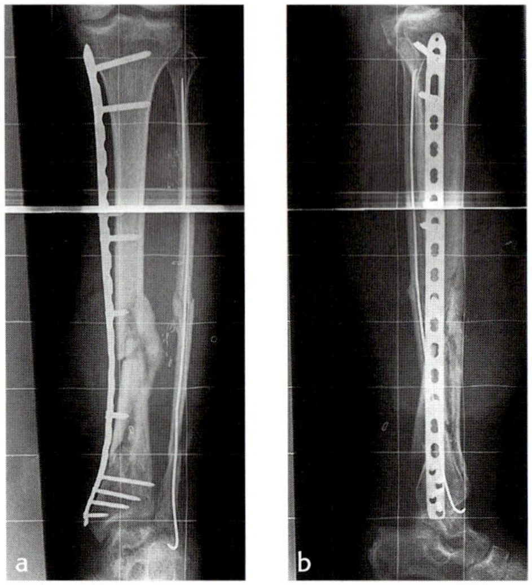

Fig 10.2.10-5a–b
Postoperative x-rays after 6 months show the start of fracture consolidation.
a AP view.
b Lateral view.

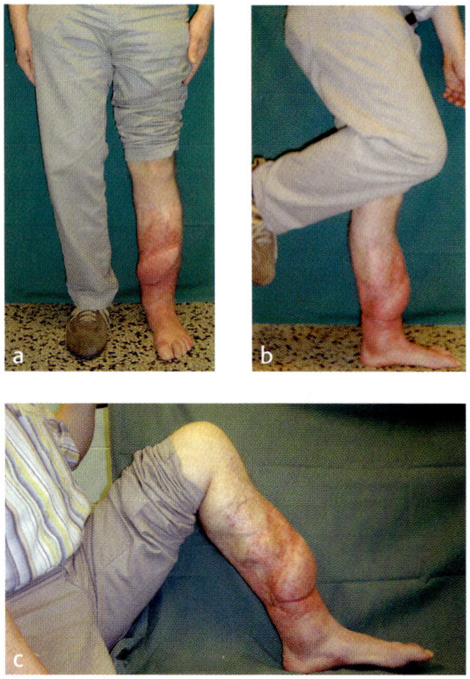

Fig 10.2.10-6a–c Clinical situation 6 months after soft-tissue consolidation. Full weight bearing.

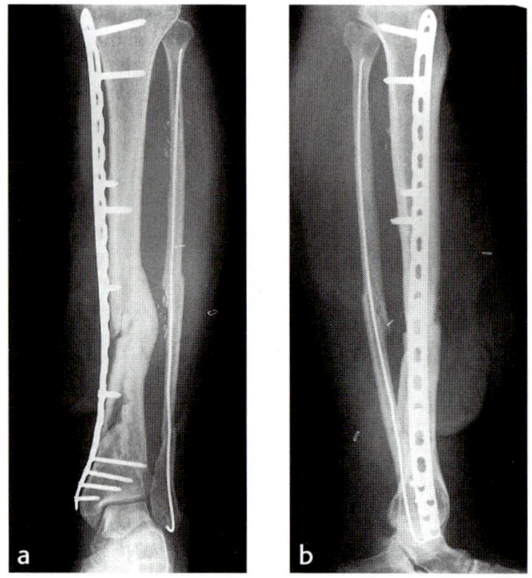

Fig 10.2.10-7a–b
Postoperative x-rays after 20 months show that the fracture has been bridged at the posterior and lateral aspects. The fibular fractures have healed.
a AP view.
b Lateral view.

5 Pitfalls –

Fixation

6 Pearls +

Fixation
Locked internal fixators are a good alternative to the external fixator in the treatment of fractures with severe soft-tissue involvement. They are less distressing for the patient.

Author Christoph Sommer

10.2.11 Complex segmental tibial shaft fracture with one intermediate segment and additional wedge fragment—42-C2

1 Case description

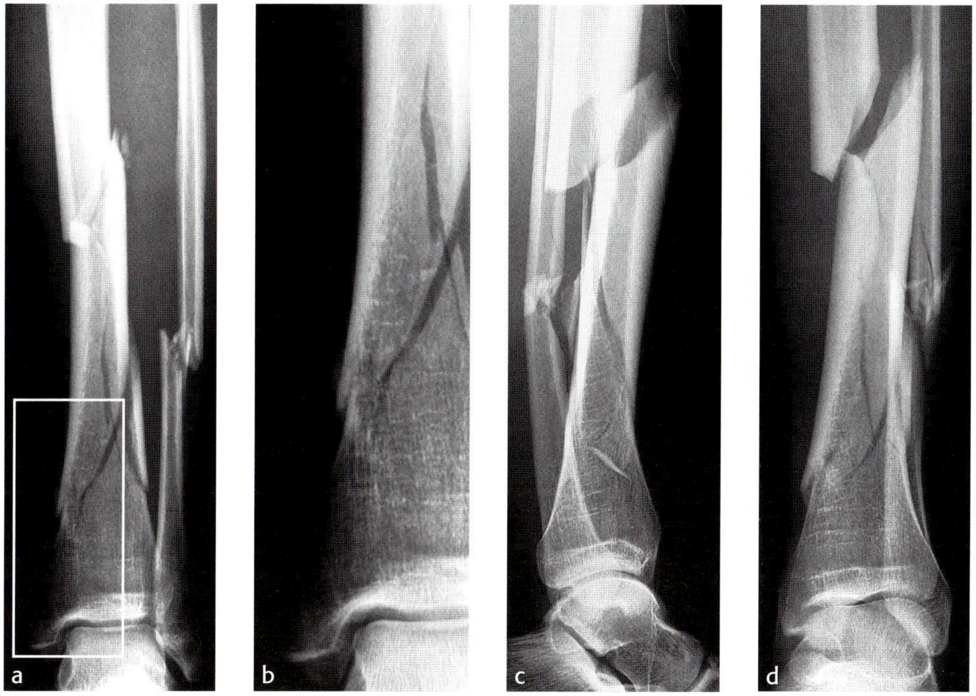

31-year-old woman fell while skiing at high velocity and fractured her left lower leg at two levels (closed fracture).

Fig 10.2.11-1a–d
- a AP view.
- b Detail AP view of the fissure into the upper ankle joint.
- c Lateral view.
- d Oblique view.

Indication

Complex fracture, segmental with one intermediate segment and additional wedge fragment. Fissure in the direction of the upper ankle joint. Because the tibial fracture had a fissure into the upper ankle joint, a nail osteosynthesis was not suitable. This fracture is a good indication for stabilization with a metaphyseal LCP 3.5/4.5/5.0. In addition, an intramedullary fixation of the long fibular fracture was performed (elastic nail).

Preoperative planning

Equipment
- LCP metaphyseal plate 3.5/4.5/5.0, 5 + 11 holes
- 3.5 mm self-tapping locking head screws (LHS)
- 5.0 mm self-tapping LHS
- Titanium elastic nail

(Size of system, instruments, and implants can vary according to anatomy.)

Patient preparation and positioning

Antibiotics: single dose 2nd generation cephalosporin

Thrombosis prophylaxis: low-molecular heparin

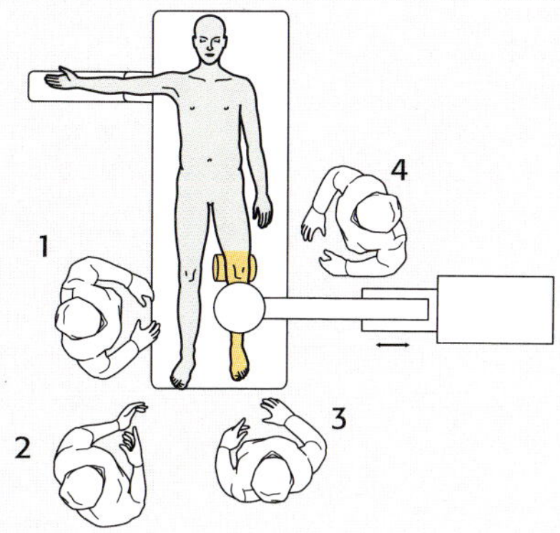

1 Surgeon
2 ORP
3 1st assistant
4 2nd assistant

Sterile area

Fig 10.2.11-2 Lower leg elevated on a pad.

2 Surgical approach

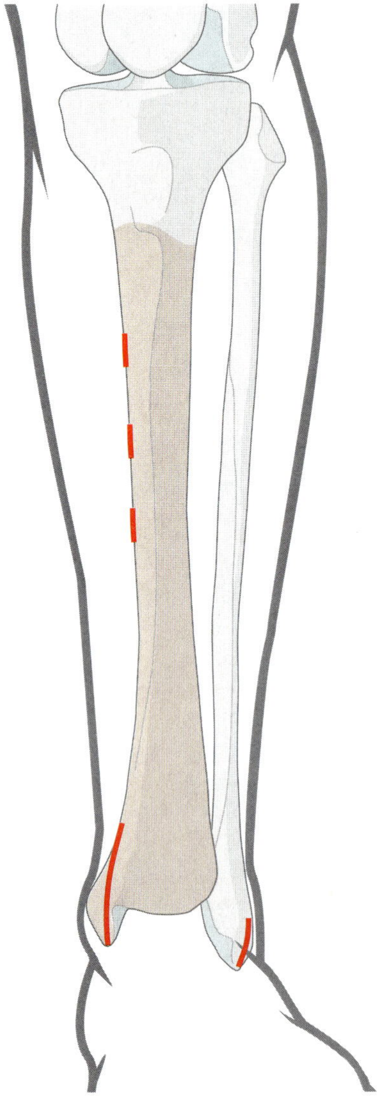

Fig 10.2.11-3 Short 4 cm approach on the anteromedial aspect of the distal and proximal tibia. Additional incisions on the lateral tibial shaft and over the tip of the lateral malleolus.

3 Reduction and fixation

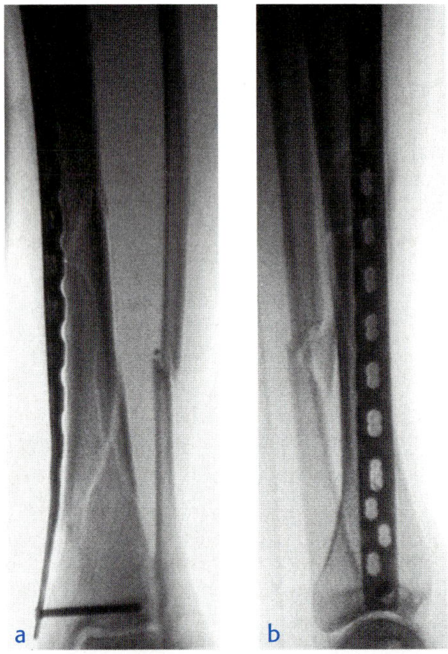

Fig 10.2.11-4a–b Epiperiosteal and subfascial tunneling with the bent 5 + 11-hole metaphyseal LCP to prepare the intended plate bed. The plate position is close to the ankle joint since the joint block is quite short. A 3.5 mm self-tapping LHS is inserted under image intensification into the most distal hole. The screw should penetrate the whole metaphysis but should not go beyond the far cortex so as not to irritate the syndesmosis.

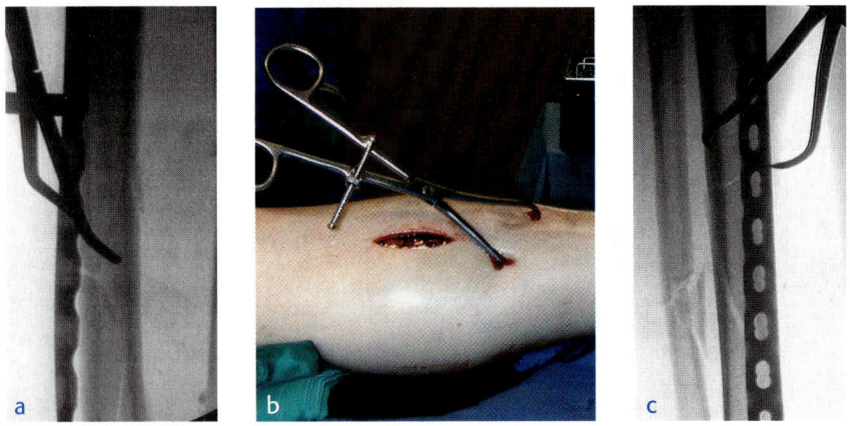

Fig 10.2.11-5a–c The fracture is reduced manually with slight traction on the foot and is supported by a plate. A drill sleeve is inserted into the proximal hole. With the help of this drill sleeve, the fracture can be indirectly reduced (length, rotation). Simple fracture components should be accurately reduced, either with a percutaneously applied Weber forceps or collinear reduction clamp.

3 Reduction and fixation (cont)

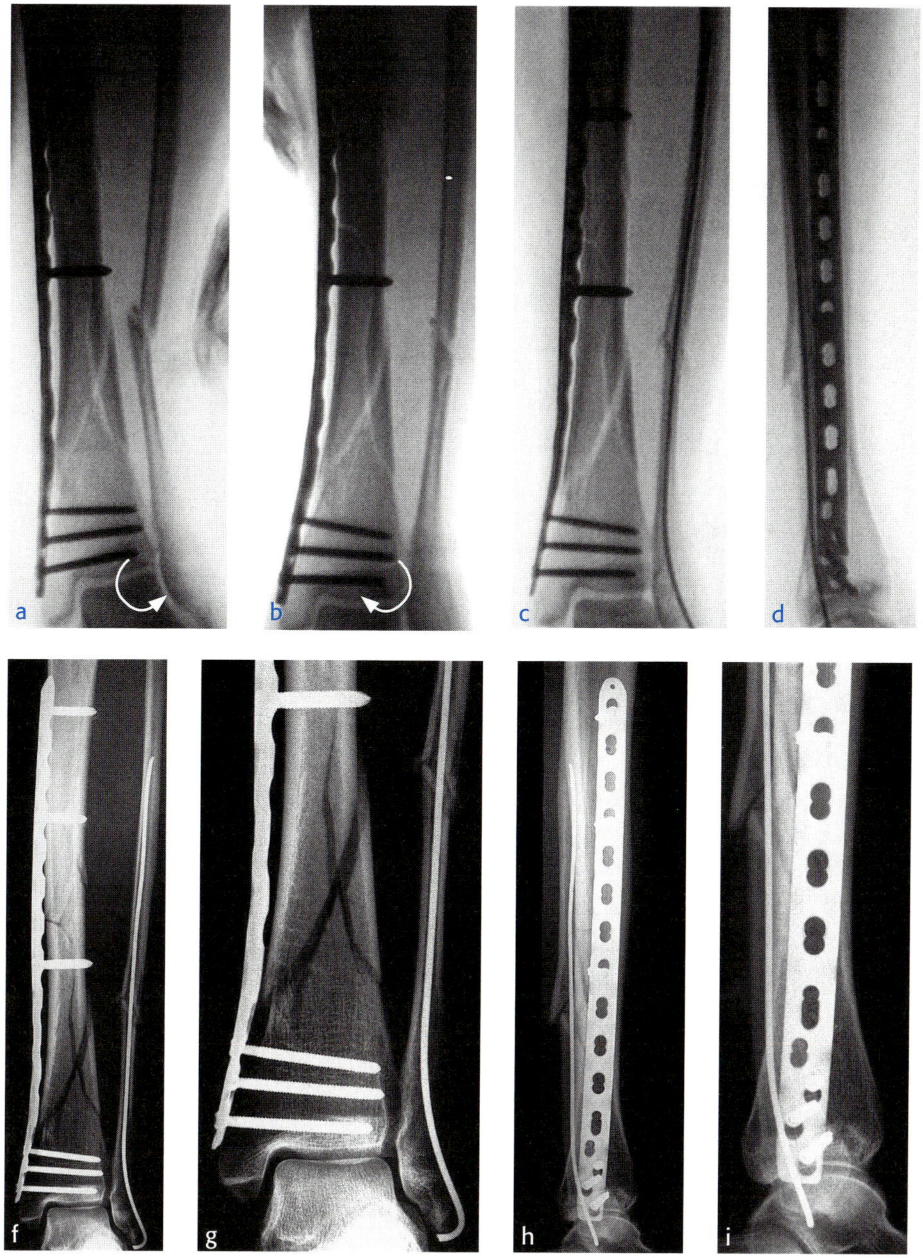

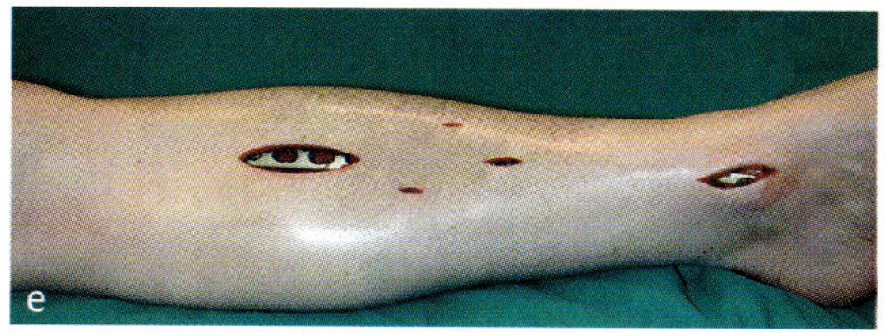

Fig 10.2.11-6a–i

a–b After careful reduction and image intensifier control, further LHS are inserted. 3.5 mm self-tapping LHS are used in the distal metaphyseal part. Two 5.0 mm self-tapping bicortical LHS in the proximal part are sufficient (four cortices in the shaft area are sufficient). In addition, the intermediate fragment was stabilized with a 5.0 mm bicortical self-tapping LHS. Under intraoperative valgus and varus stress, the lower leg showed malalignment due to the high flexibility of the internal fixator.

c–e Because of this circumstance, the fibula was additionally stabilized with an intramedullary titanium elastic nail. Postoperative x-rays are shown and the soft-tissue situation before wound closure.

f–i The postoperative x-rays in two planes reveal good reduction of the fracture.

4 Rehabilitation

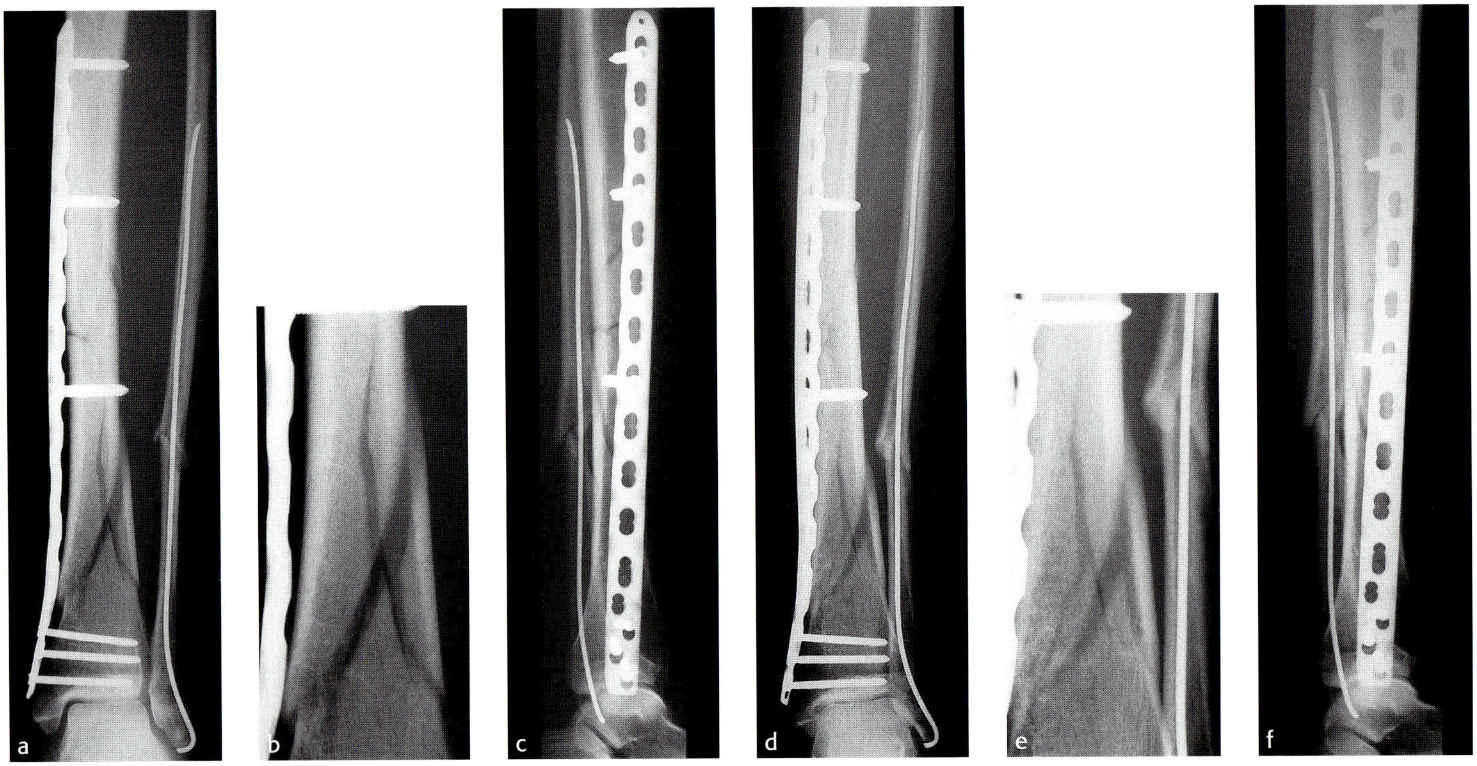

Mobilization began on the first postoperative day with 10–15 kg weight bearing. Functional treatment of the upper ankle joint was added.

Fig 10.2.11-7a–f

a–c The beginning of callus formation was seen 6 weeks after the operation on the proximal tibia and fibula.

d–f Weight bearing was increased to 20–30 kg for another 6 weeks. Callus formation increased on the upper tibia and fibula. The distal fracture segment had healed endosteally from the medial to the lateral side.

4 Rehabilitation (cont)

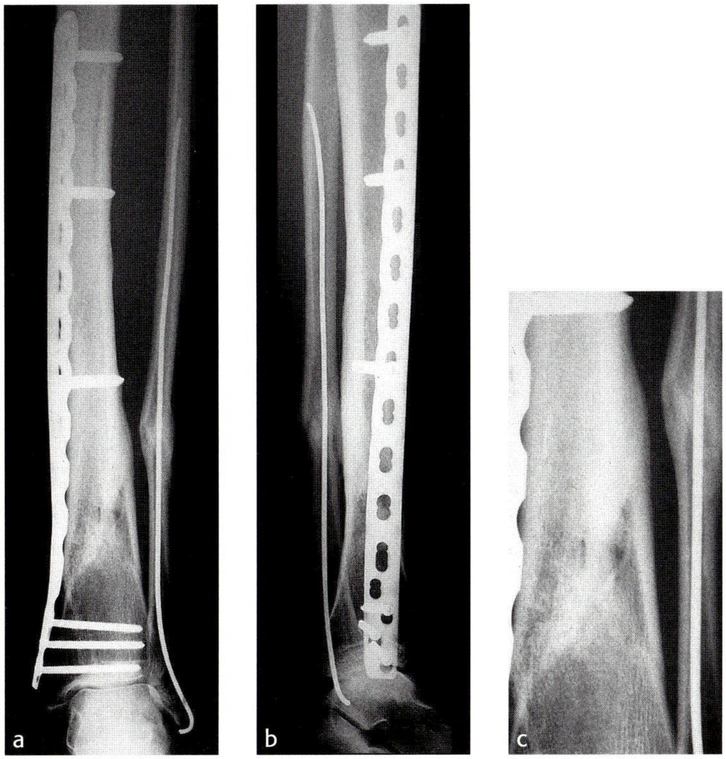

Fig 10.2.11-8a–c After one year the fracture was entirely consolidated and the callus remodeled. The implant position was unchanged.

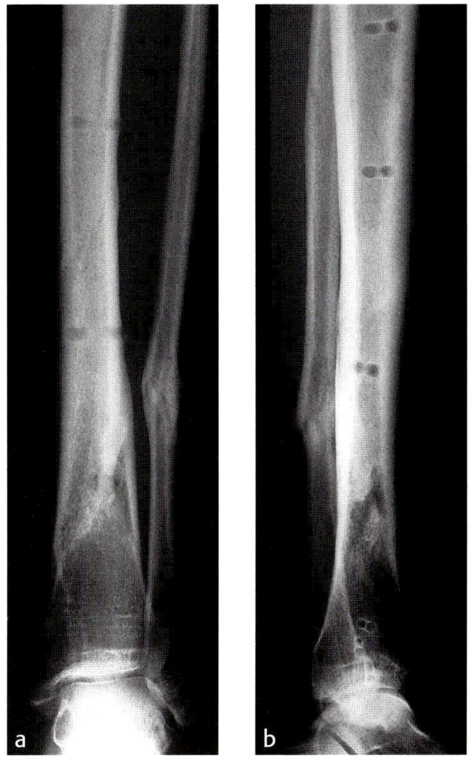

Implant removal

Fig 10.2.11-9a–b Implant removal after 14 months.

5 Pitfalls –

Equipment

Approach
The great saphenous vein and the saphenous nerve can be endangered by the distal approach.

Reduction and fixation
Malalignment because of the minimally invasive approach. Assessment x-rays must be obtained.

Rehabilitation
If mobilized too early with too much weight or in a noncompliant patient, the plate may bend.

6 Pearls +

Equipment
The LCP metaphyseal plates 3.5/4.5/5.0 are ideal for proximal or distal fractures close to a joint (the distances between the holes are shorter in the 3.5 plate part compared with the 4.5/0.5 plate part).

Approach

Reduction and fixation
Locking head screws also stabilize small joint fragments. Splinting a long fracture zone with a locked internal fixator results in an elastic stabilization. In this cirum-stance, an additional osteosynthesis of the fibular fracture is recommended.

Rehabilitation
Early functional postoperative treatment is possible even in complex fractures if the fracture is well stabilized and if the soft tissue allows.

Author Christian Ryf

10.2.12 Open complex segmental tibial shaft fracture—42-C2

1 Case description

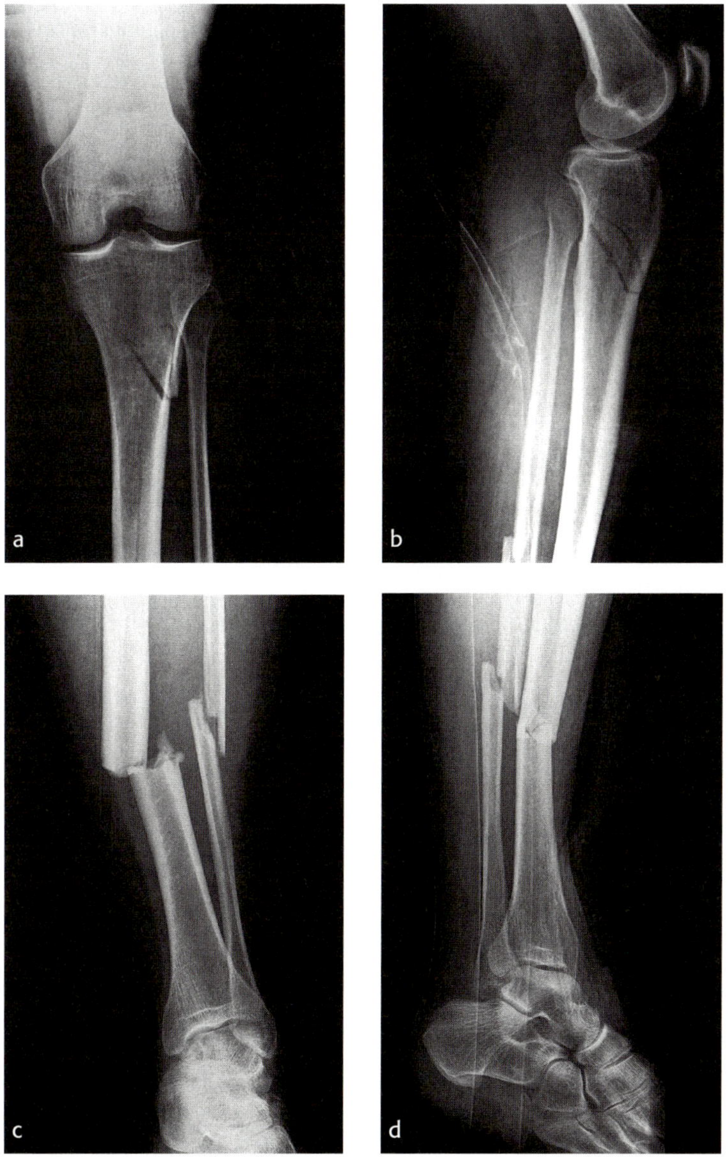

50-year-old man with ski injury; open tibial shaft fracture Gustilo type II.

Fig 10.2.12-1a–d
a AP view, proximal fracture.
b Lateral view, proximal fracture.
c AP view, shaft fracture.
d Lateral view, shaft fracture.

Indication

The patient suffered an open segment fracture while skiing. The compartment pressures and neurology were normal.

Preoperative planning

Equipment

- LCP 4.5/5.0, narrow, 20 holes
- 5.0 mm locking head screws (LHS)
- 4.5 mm cortex screws

(Size of system, instruments, and implants can vary according to anatomy.)

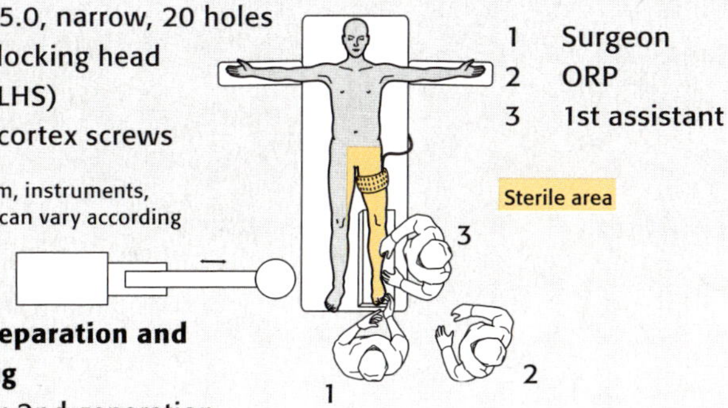

Fig 10.2.12-2 Patient in supine position. Tourniquet on the femur.

Patient preparation and positioning

Antibiotics: 2nd generation cephalosporin for 48 hours

Thrombosis prophylaxis: low-molecular heparin

2 Surgical approach

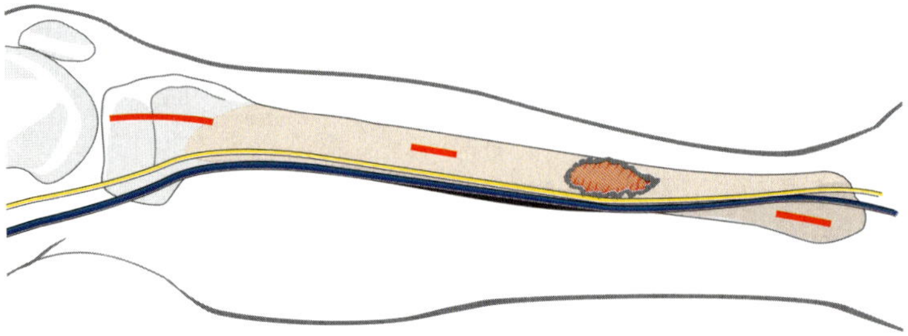

Fig 10.2.12-3 The wound is debrided and jet-lavaged. The preexisting wound is extended some 2 cm.

3 Reduction and fixation

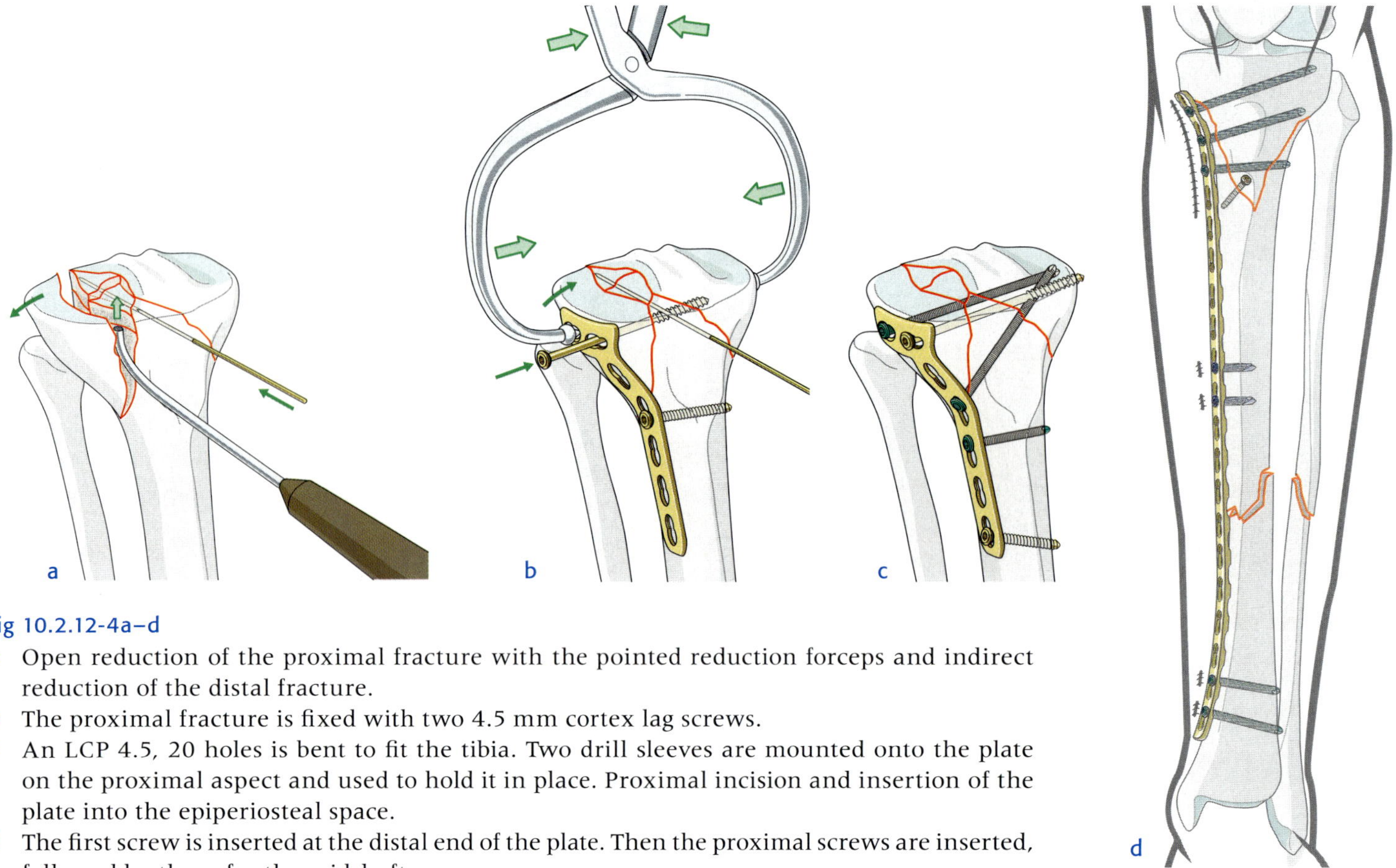

Fig 10.2.12-4a–d

a Open reduction of the proximal fracture with the pointed reduction forceps and indirect reduction of the distal fracture.

b The proximal fracture is fixed with two 4.5 mm cortex lag screws.

c An LCP 4.5, 20 holes is bent to fit the tibia. Two drill sleeves are mounted onto the plate on the proximal aspect and used to hold it in place. Proximal incision and insertion of the plate into the epiperiosteal space.

d The first screw is inserted at the distal end of the plate. Then the proximal screws are inserted, followed by those for the midshaft.

3 Reduction and fixation (cont)

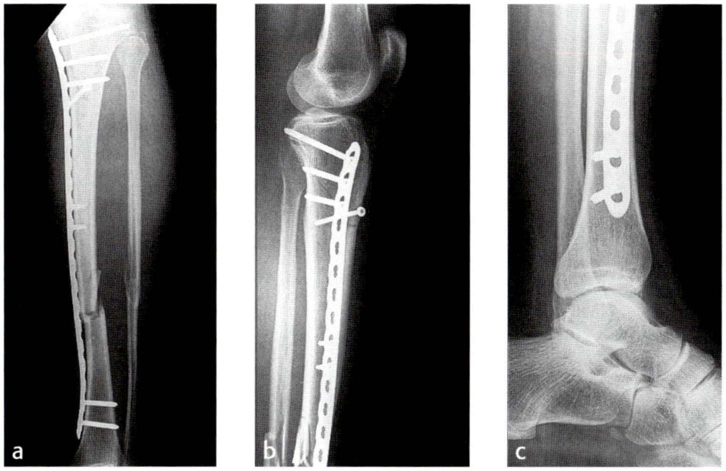

Fig 10.2.12-5a–c Postoperative x-rays.
a AP view.
b Lateral view, proximal part.
c Lateral view, distal part.

After open, direct precise reduction of this proximal simple fracture, the fracture was compressed by a lag screw. The LCP acts here as a noncontact plate with the function of a protection plate. Indirect, closed reduction of the multifragmentary, open shaft fracture and fixation by the locked splinting method.

4 Rehabilitation

Weight bearing: 15 kg for 6 weeks; half body weight after 12 weeks; full weight bearing after 16 weeks.

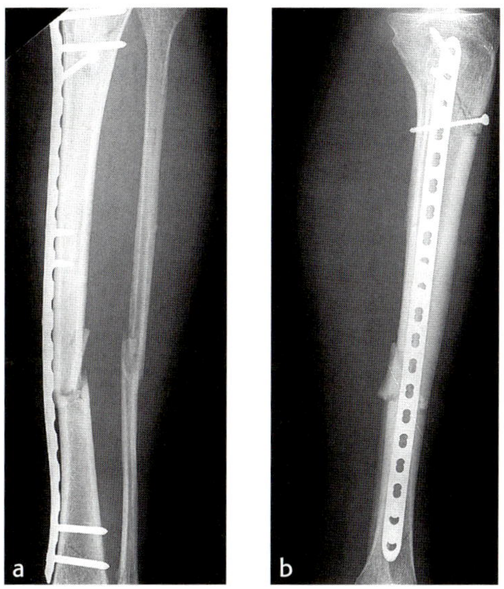

Fig 10.2.12-6a–b Postoperative x-ray after 6 weeks
a AP view.
b Lateral view.

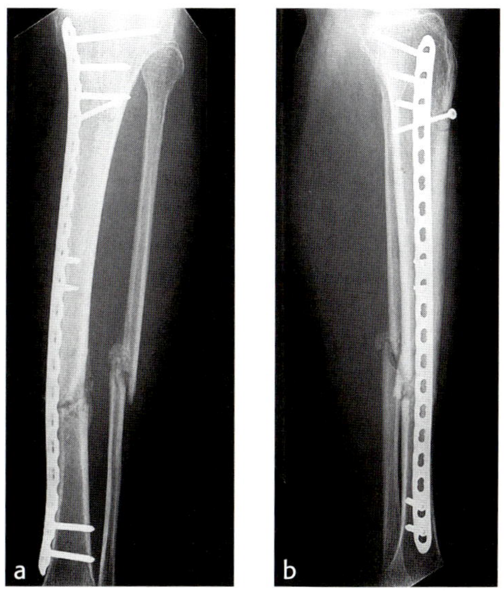

Fig 10.2.12-7a–b Postoperative x-ray after 6 months
a AP view.
b Lateral view.

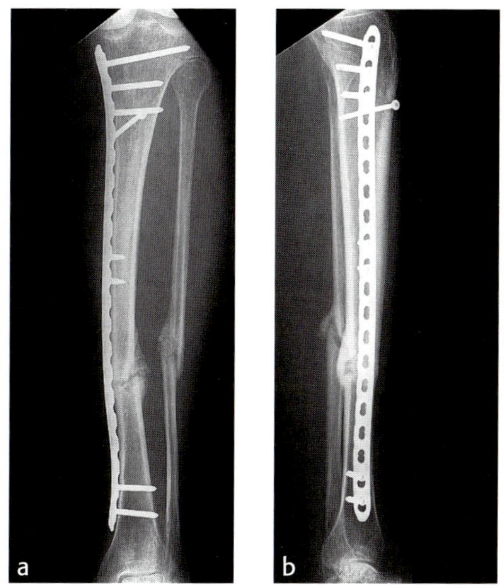

Fig 10.2.12-8a–b Postoperative x-ray after 8 months
a AP view.
b Lateral view.

5 Pitfalls –

Equipment

6 Pearls +

Equipment

The LCP supports the MIPO technique.
The percutaneous approach to the tibia is safe.

The LCP with combination holes allows a fracture specific fixation method—compression for simple fractures and locked splinting for mulifragmentary fractures.

Authors Gabriele Streicher, Andreas Gruner, Thomas Hockertz, Heinrich Reilmann

10.2.13 Open complex irregular tibial and fibular shaft fracture—42-C3

1 Case description

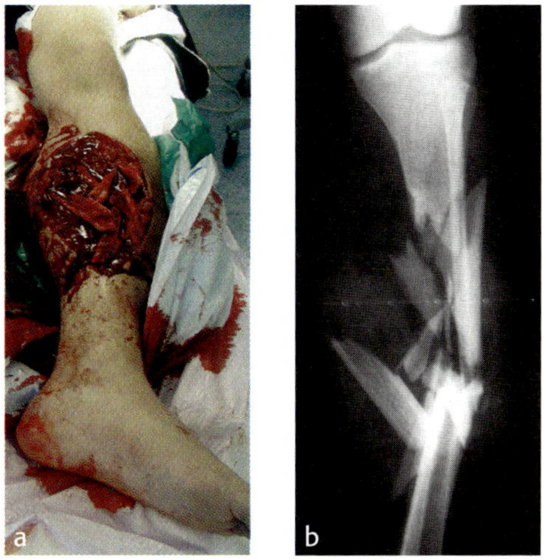

17-year-old patient who was run into by a car and suffered an injury to the left leg.

Fig 10.2.13-1a–b
a Preoperative clinical picture.
b Preoperative x-ray AP view.

Indication

As the result of a high-energy incident the patient sustained an open fracture with soft-tissue involvement (Gustilo type IIIB). This open fracture is an absolute indication to operate.

Preoperative planning

Equipment
- LISS-PLT, 13 holes
- 5.0 mm self-drilling, self-tapping locking head screws (LHS)
- 3.5 mm cortex screw
- 2.0 mm K-wires

(Size of system, instruments, and implants can vary according to anatomy.)

Patient preparation and positioning
Antibiotics: single dose 2nd generation cephalosporin.
Thrombosis prophylaxis: low-molecular heparin.

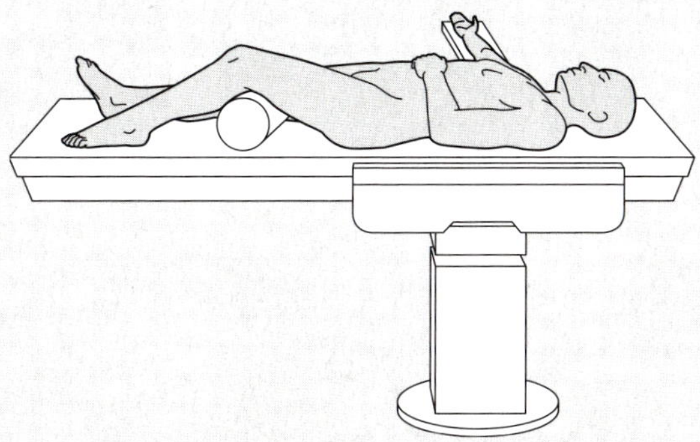

Fig 10.2.13-2 Supine position with elevation of the leg to be operated on and flexion of the knee joint to approximately 30°, lowering of the other leg to improve intraoperative radiographic diagnosis, cushioning of the distal femur of the injured leg, eg, with a towel roll.

2 Surgical approach

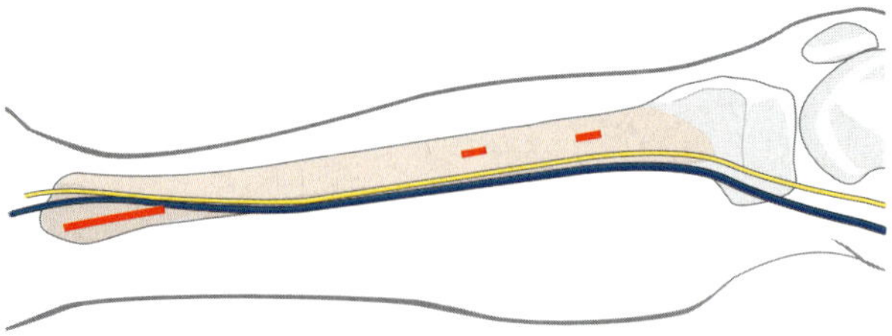

Fig 10.2.13-3 Anterolateral approach to the tibial head through a 5 cm incision into the proximal region of the compartment of the tibialis anterior muscle.

Preparation to the periosteum and the implant bed with the long bone rasp.

3 Reduction and fixation

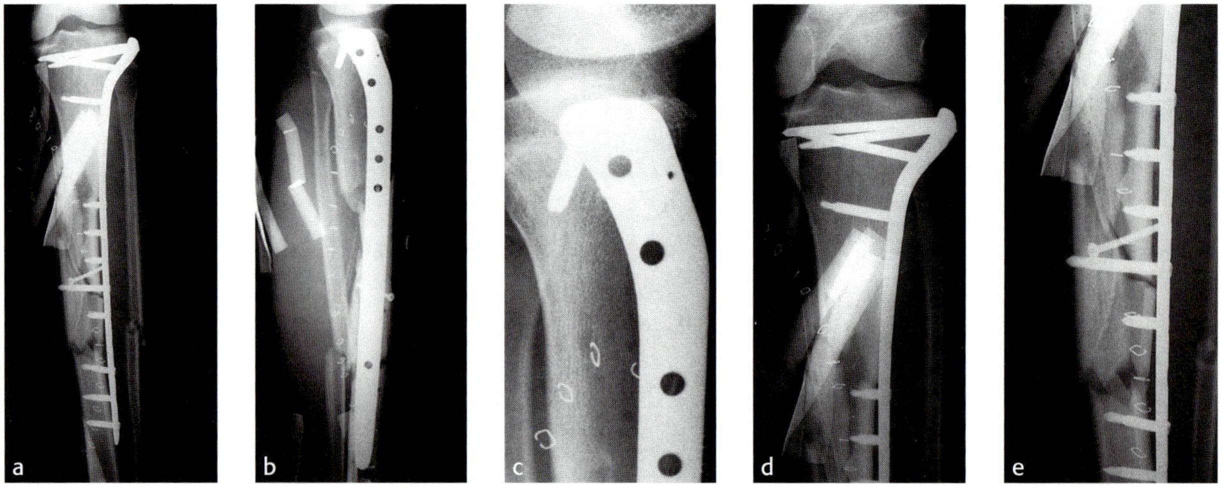

After determining plate length under image intensification, insertion of the implant into the plate bed from the proximal aspect and bridging of the approximately reduced fracture zone.

Second incision at the distal end of the plate, completion of the LISS frame and temporary fixation of the proximal and distal ends of the plate with K-wires.

Proximal and distal fixation of LISS to the bone by insertion of locking head screws.

Interpolation of the multiple intermediary fragments and fixation of the two large fragments with LHS and cortex screws.

Fig 10.2.13-4a–j

a Postoperative x-ray, AP view.
b Postoperative x-ray, lateral view.
c Postoperative x-ray, lateral view knee.
d Postoperative x-ray, AP view detail.
e Postoperative x-ray, AP view fragment fixation.

3 Reduction and fixation (cont)

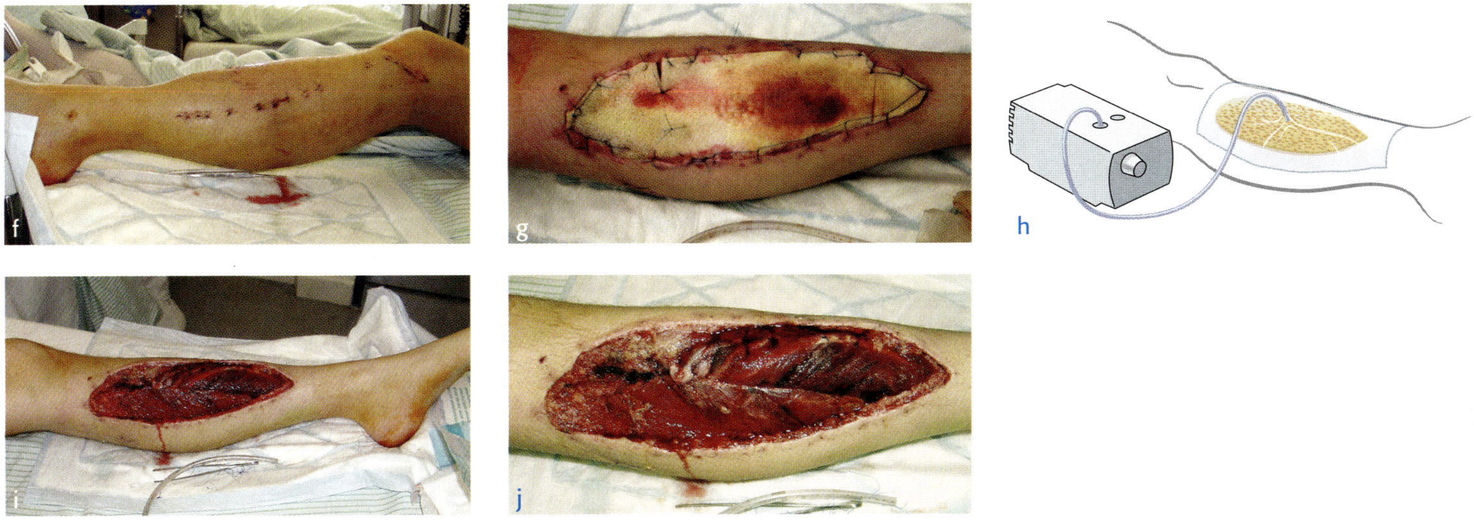

Fig 10.2.13-4a–j (cont)
f Postoperative picture of the lateral approach.
g Postoperative picture of the vacuum dressing.
h Vacuum dressing.
i Clinical status after vacuum dressing.
j Granulation after vacuum dressing.

4 Rehabilitation

Weight bearing: 15 kg for 6 weeks; half body weight after 6 weeks; full weight bearing after 12 weeks.
Physiotherapy: from the 2nd postoperative day
Pharmaceutical treatment: Non-steroidal antiinflammatory drugs

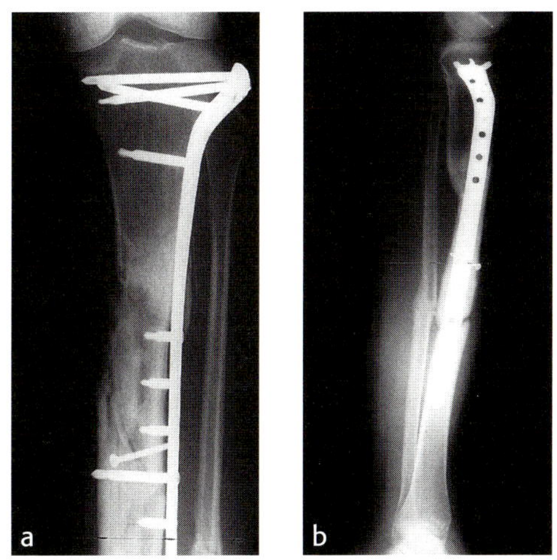

Fig 10.2.13-5a–e
a Postoperative x-ray after 2 weeks, AP view.
b Postoperative x-ray after 2 weeks, lateral view.

4 Rehabilitation (cont)

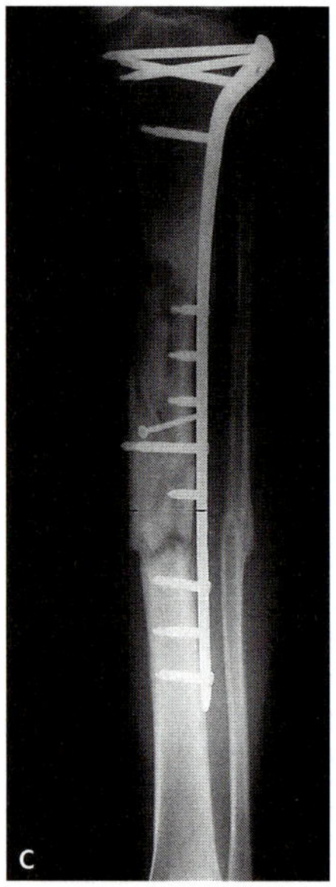

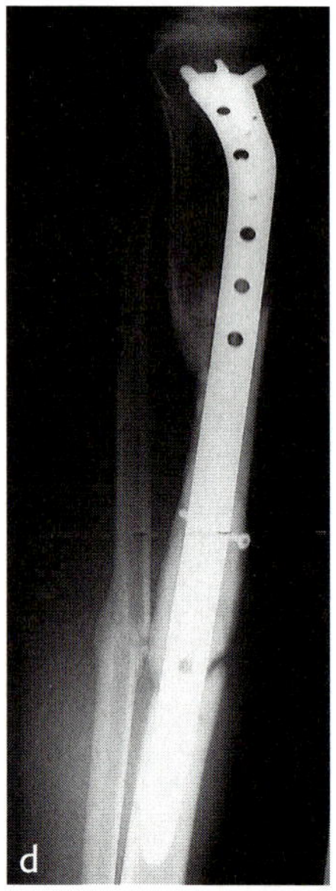

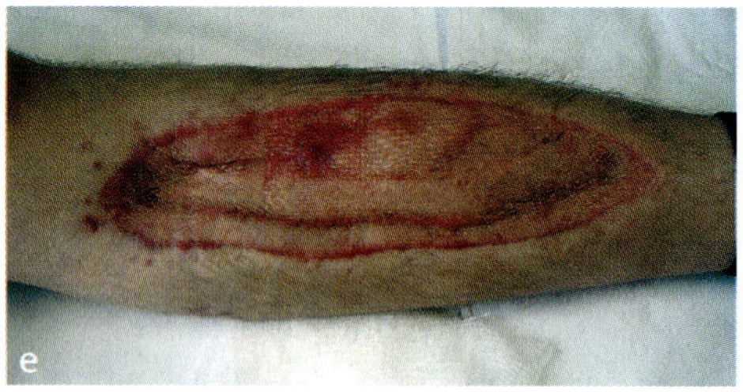

Fig 10.2.13-5a–e (cont)
c Postoperative x-ray after 5 weeks, AP view
d Postoperative x-ray after 5 weeks, lateral view
e Clinical picture.

Implant removal
Reason for implant removal: mechanical irritation of the lateral tibial head by the implant.
Technique for implant removal: Removal of the screws through stab incisions and removal of the LISS through the previous proximal incision.

5 Pitfalls –

Equipment
An implant that is almost too short so that adequate distal fixation is only just possible.

Approach
Inadequate preparation of the tibial head leads to incorrect plate positioning (too far on the anterior or posterior side).

Reduction and fixation
Rotational errors if the fracture zone is too lengthy.

Rehabilitation
In open fractures, a procedure only for specialists.

6 Pearls +

Equipment

Approach

Reduction and fixation

Rehabilitation
Primary definitive fracture treatment is possible despite exposed bone and massive soft-tissue injury.

Author Christian Ryf

10.2.14 Open complex irregular tibial shaft fracture—42-C3

1 Case description

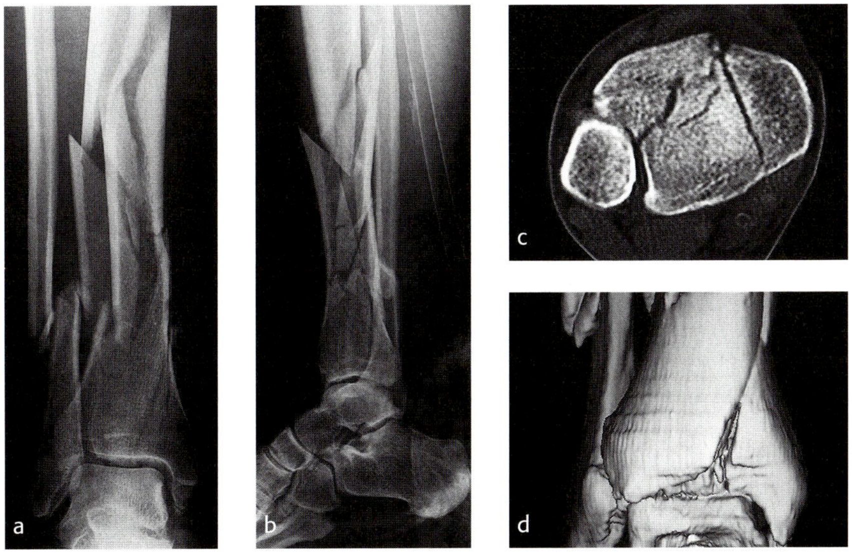

52-year-old man fell from a ladder and fractured his right lower leg. Open fracture Gustilo type II.

Fig 10.2.14-1a–d
a AP view.
b Lateral view.
c–d CT scans.

Indication

The patient suffered a massive soft-tissue swelling of the whole lower leg. The fractured distal fibula perforated the skin. Even with this extended swelling, no compartment syndrome was observed. The distal blood supply and nerves were not damaged. So an operative treatment seemed possible. A percutaneous screw osteosynthesis and a bridging plate for the shaft fracture (MIPO), ie, a long LCP 4.5/5.0, were planned.

Preoperative planning

Equipment

- LCP 4.5/5.0, narrow, 16 holes
- Locking head screws (LHS)
- 4.5 mm cortex screws
- 2.4 mm cancellous bone screws
- External fixator used as a reduction tool

(Size of system, instruments, and implants can vary according to anatomy.)

Patient preparation and positioning

Antibiotics: 2nd generation cephalosporin for 48 hours
Thrombosis prophylaxis: low-molecular heparin

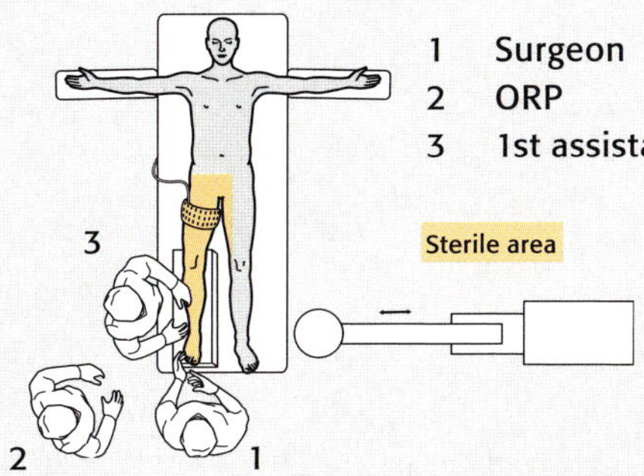

1 Surgeon
2 ORP
3 1st assistant

Fig 10.2.14-2 Supine position of the patient with a tourniquet on the thigh. The lower leg is positioned on a pillow on a radiolucent operating table.

2 Surgical approach

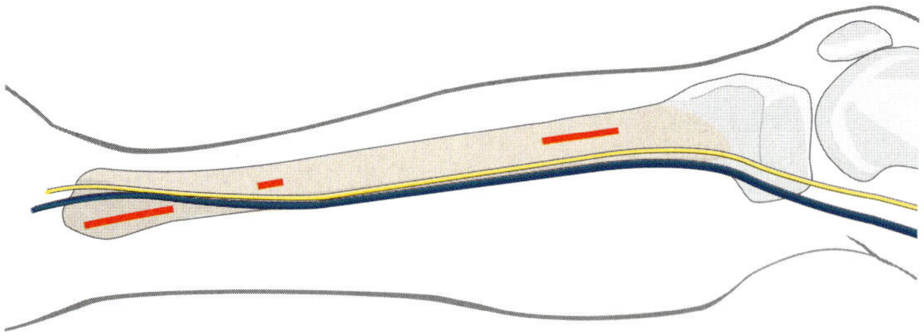

Fig 10.2.14-3 Debridement of the lateral wound. Jet lavage of the lateral wound with polihexanid. Plate position and length are marked. Stab incisions for the two articular screws under image intensifier and length incision distal medial and anterior to the medial malleolus. The great saphenous vein and the saphenous nerve must be identified and spared to prevent irritation. The proximal incision is performed proximally over the tibial edge at the previously marked position.

3 Reduction and fixation

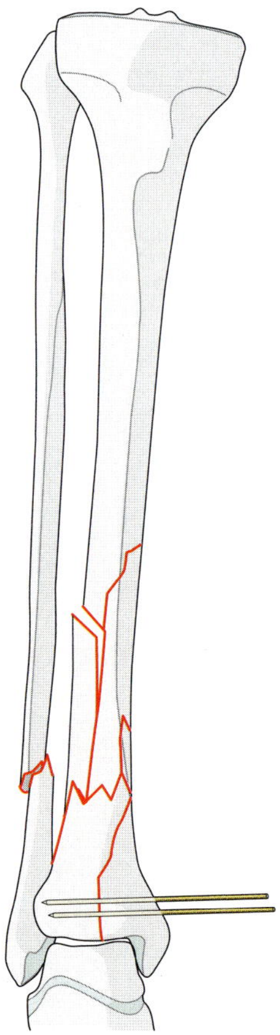

a

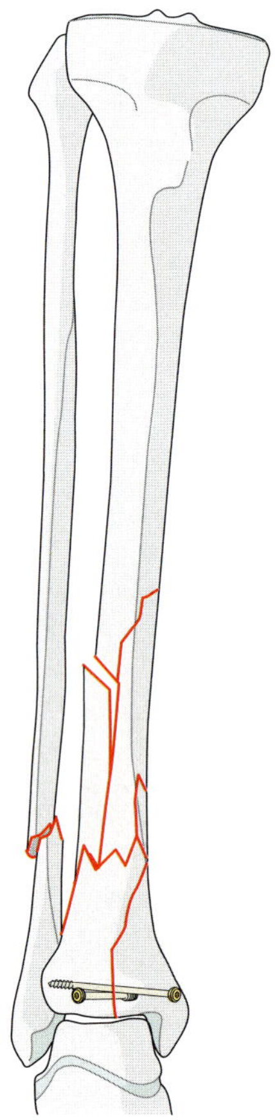

b

Fig 10.2.14-4a–c

a The articular fracture is reduced by external pressure under image intensifier control and manipulated with K-wires. The joint fracture is temporarily fixed with percutaneous K-wires.

b Definitive stabilization of the articular fragments with 2.4 mm cancellous bone screws as lag screws. The two Schanz screws are inserted. The proximal screw is placed directly distal to the tibial tuberosity in an anteroposterior direction and the distal screw transverses the calcaneus.

c The external fixator is mounted anterolaterally so as not to disturb the plate position.
The fracture can now be reduced under image intensifier control and held in this position with the external fixator.

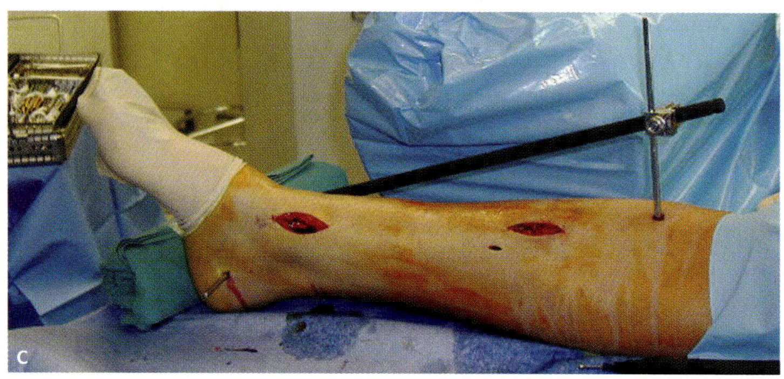

c

4 Fixation

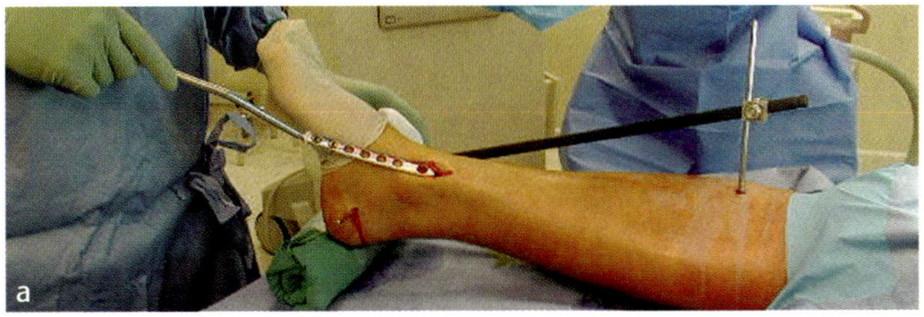

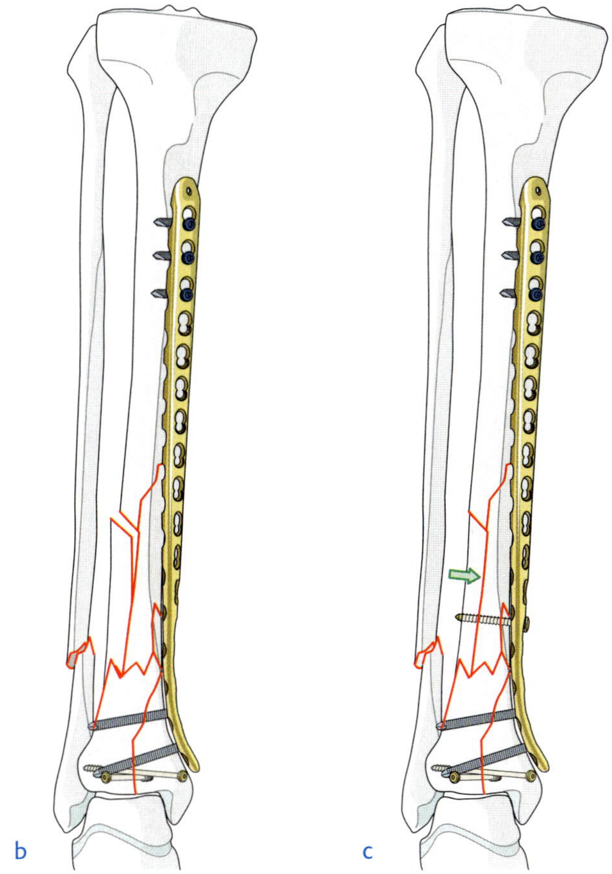

Fig 10.2.14-5a–c

a Two drill sleeves are used as handles to insert the plate into the preformed subfascial space. The plate is inserted under image intensifier control to prevent misplacement of the fragments. Attention has to be paid to not harming the saphenous vein or nerve and to preventing posterior misplacement.

b A first distal locking head screw is inserted. Lock the screw after insertion of a proximal screw. In this manner, correction is still possible.
After correct reduction was confirmed, a total of three proximal monocortical locking head screws and two distal bicortical locking head screws were inserted.

c The dislocated intermediate fragment is approached with a 4.5 mm cortex screw (reduction screw). Care must be taken not to push the fragment while drilling. A formal interfragmentary compression is not possible because of a lack of anatomical reduction. An elastic bridging osteosynthesis is achieved.

5 Rehabilitation

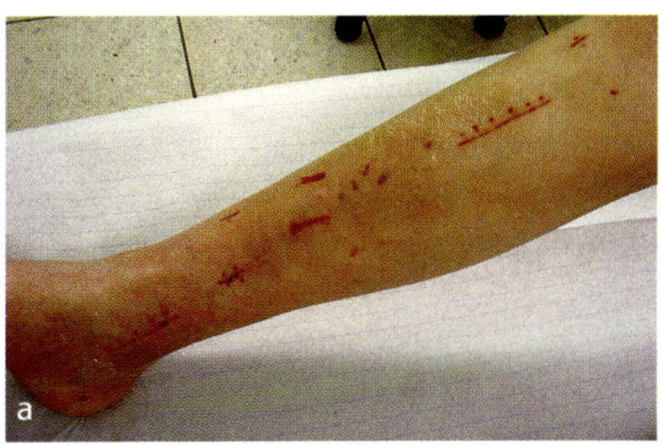

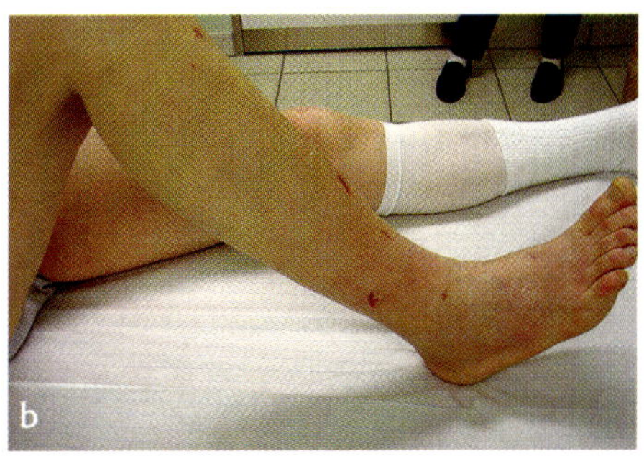

Fig 10.2.14-6a–b Functional results after 6 weeks.

Weight bearing: 15 kg for 12 weeks; half body weight after 12 weeks; full weight bearing after 18 weeks.

Physiotherapy: active therapy of the neighboring joints postoperatively. Lymphatic drainage and compression therapy is applied because of a tendency towards swelling.

5 Rehabilitation (cont)

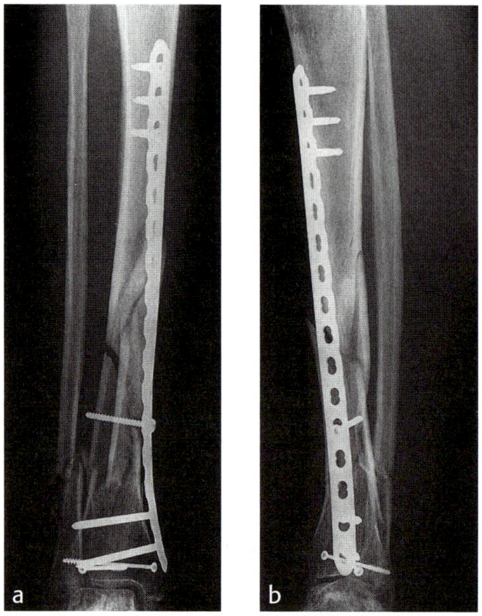

Fig 10.2.14-7a–b Postoperative x-rays after 18 weeks.
a AP view.
b Lateral view.

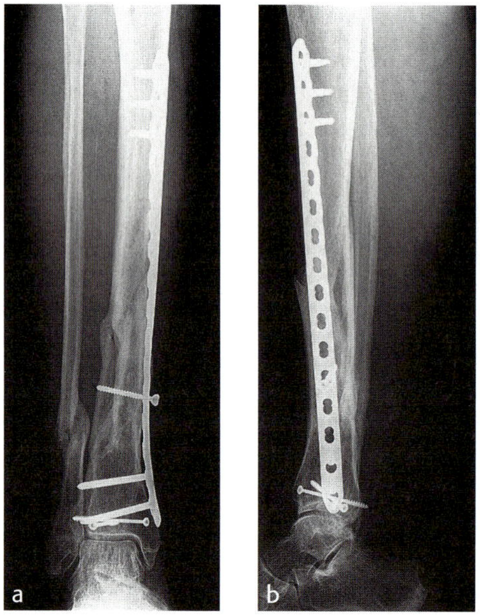

Fig 10.2.14-8a–b Postoperative x-rays after 36 months.
a AP view.
b Lateral view.

Author Michael Wagner

10.2.15 Spiral tibial shaft fracture in a child—42-A1

1 Case description

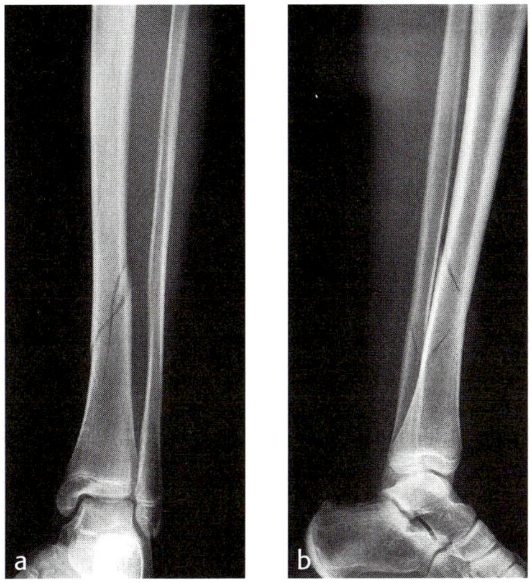

15-year-old boy fell off his bicycle and sustained an isolated tibial shaft fracture.

Fig 10.2.15-1a–b
a AP view.
b Lateral view.

Indication

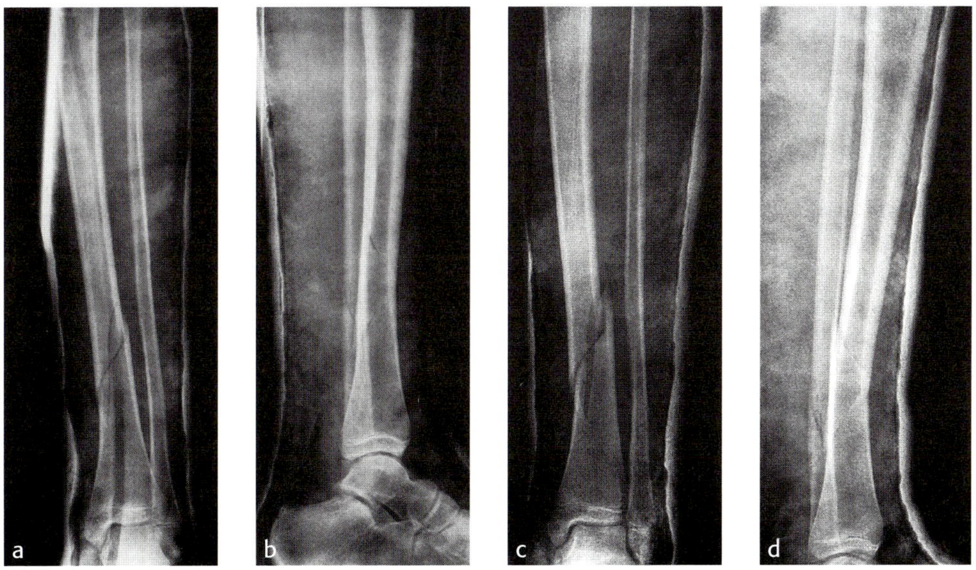

Primary undisplaced fracture of the tibia at this age is a good indication for non-operative treatment. If this is performed inconsequentially, varus malalignment will occur in the plaster cast and this then provides the indication for surgical treatment. An alternative to MIPO would be the application of independent screws, an external fixation, or elastic nailing in patients in this age group.

Fig 10.2.15-2a–d
a–b Fracture treated with plaster cast.
c–d Varus malalignment.

Preoperative planning

Equipment

- LCP metaphyseal plate 3.5/4.5./5.0, 5 + 14 holes
- 3.5 mm locking head screws (LHS)
- 5.0 mm LHS
- 2.0 mm K-wires

(Size of system, instruments, and implants can vary according to anatomy.)

Patient preparation and positioning

Antibiotics: none
Thrombosis prophylaxis: low-molecular heparin

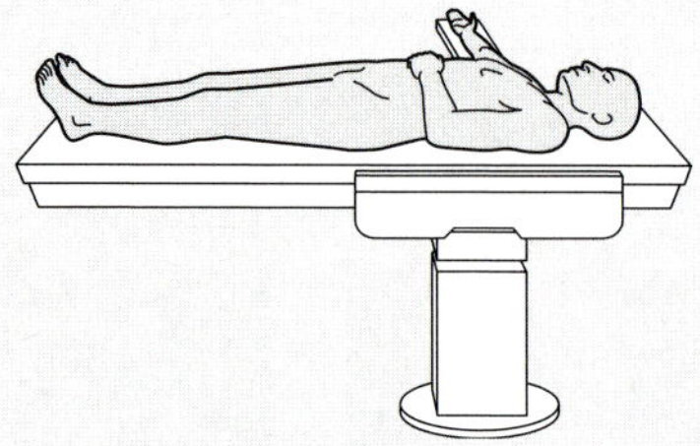

Fig 10.2.15-3 Supine position.

2 Surgical approach

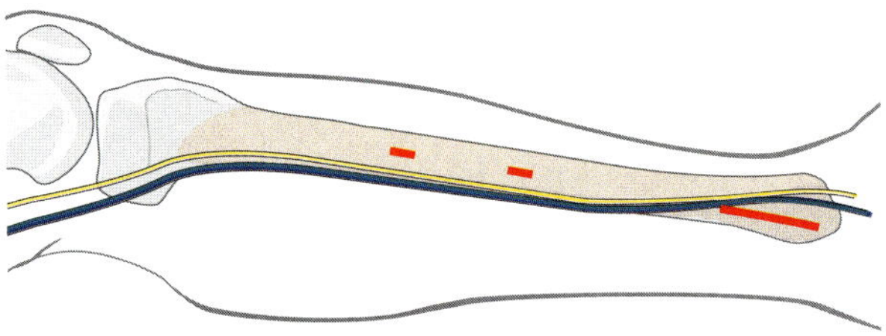

Fig 10.2.15-4 Three medial incisions.

3 Reduction and fixation

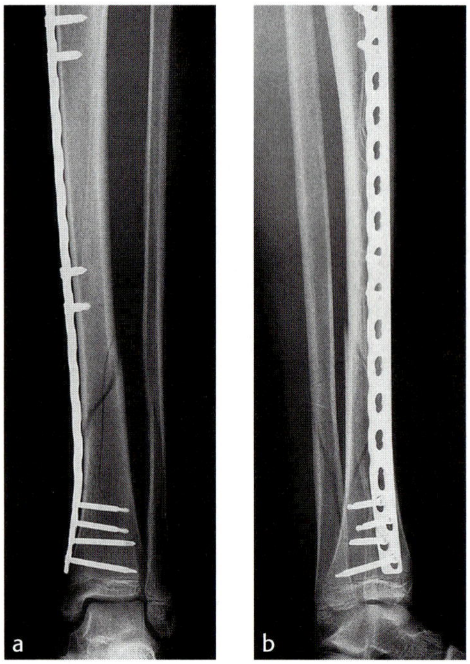

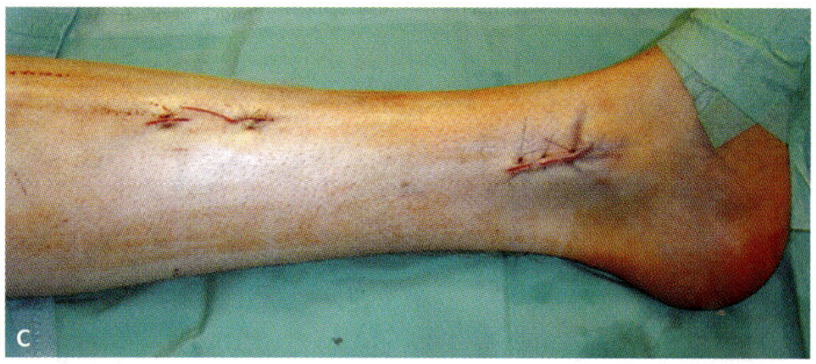

Fig 10.2.15-5a–c
a AP view.
b Lateral view.
c Skin closure.

Closed reduction with manual traction; control using the image intensifier.
Preparation of the epiperiosteal space with the scissors from distal to proximal and proximal to distal.
Plate insertion from distal to proximal and temporary fixation with K-wires at the distal and proximal fragments.
Distal fixation with four 3.5 mm LHS and proximal fixation with four 4.5/5.0 mm monocortical LHS.

4 Rehabilitation

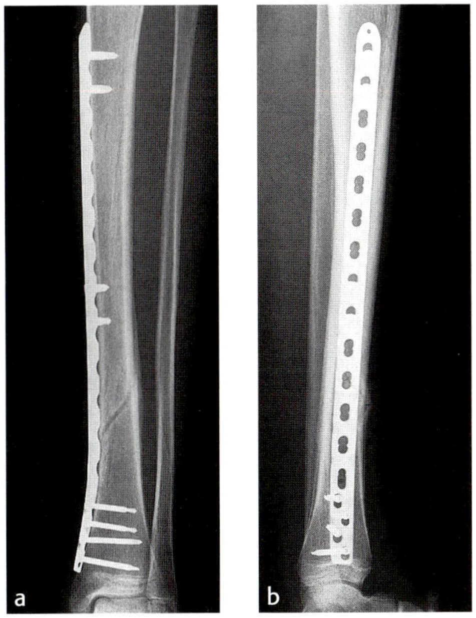

Fig 10.2.15-6a–b Postoperative x-rays after 2 months show callus bridging of the fracture.

a AP view.

b Lateral view.

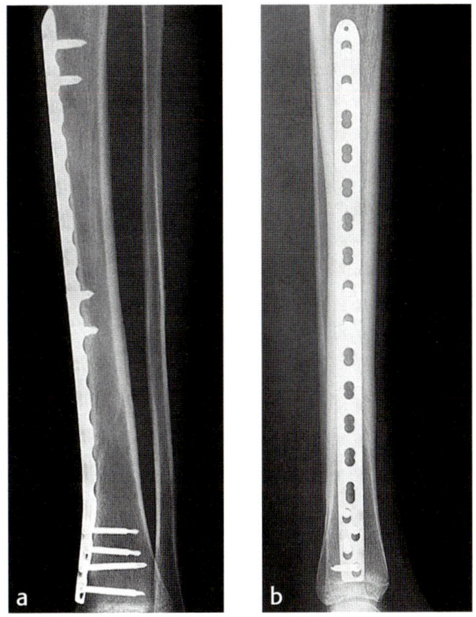

Fig 10.2.15-7a–b Postoperative x-rays after 8 months show endosteal and callus bridging of the fracture.

a AP view.

b Lateral view.

Full weight bearing after 2 weeks.

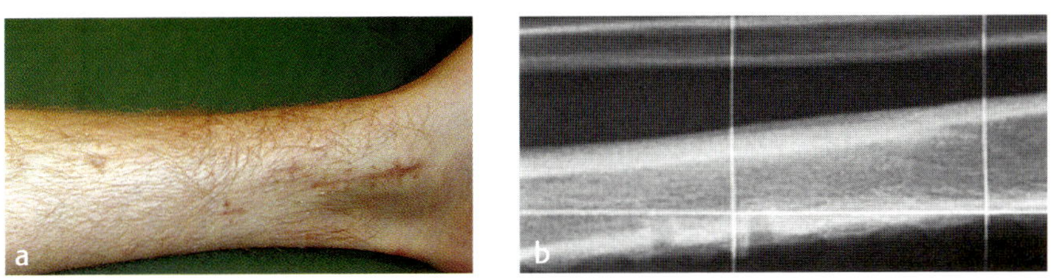

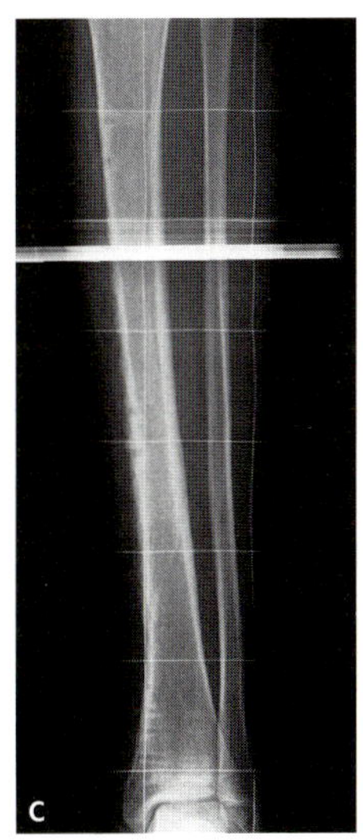

Fig 10.2.15-8a–c

a The contour of the plate is seen beneath the skin at the medial tibia. Good cosmetic result.

b X-ray examination after implant removal. Periosteal callus is formed on the side opposite to the plate; in the case of a noncontact plate there is also callus formation beneath the plate and in the region of the plate undercuts.

c AP view after implant removal. Osseous healing of the fracture. Correct axial alignment.

Implant removal

Implants should be removed from children. Furthermore, the plate was situated directly under the skin.

5 Pitfalls –

Fixation

Isolated tibial fractures in children tend to consolidate in varus malalignment if treated in a plaster cast and need to be corrected surgically later.

6 Pearls +

Fixation

MIPO using a LIF is a good alternative in fractures in children of this age and allows full weight bearing after 2 weeks.

Bridging a fracture with a locked internal fixator induce indirect bone healing.

In the case of a noncontact plate, there is also callus formation beneath the plate.

Author Michael Wagner

10.2.16 Periprosthetic fracture of the tibial shaft—42-B1

1 Case description

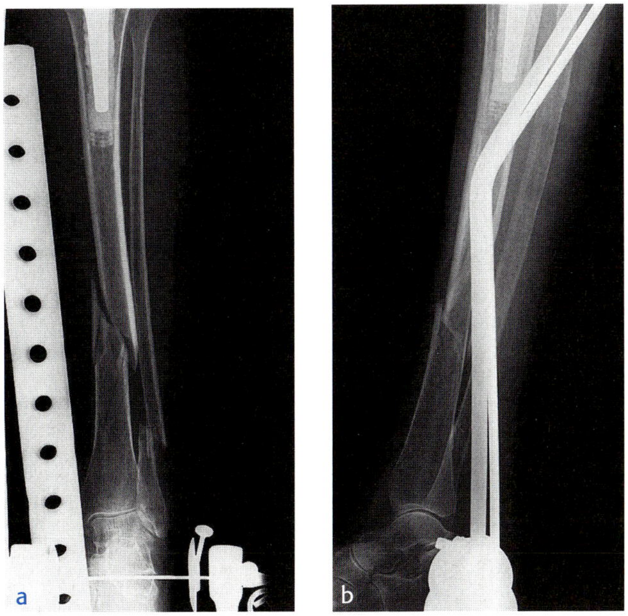

76-year-old woman fell while out walking.

Fig 10.2.16-1a–b
a AP view.
b Lateral view.

Indication

Intramedullary treatment was not possible because there was a total endoprosthesis of the knee in situ. The best solution in terms of surgical treatment is bridging the fracture with a locked internal fixator in MIPO technique.
Emergency treatment: Traction by insertion of a K-wire through the calcaneus and positioning on a traction bed.

Preoperative planning

Equipment

- LCP metaphyseal plate 3.5/4.5./5.0, 4 + 16 holes
- LCP 3.5, 7 holes
- 3.5 mm locking head screws (LHS)
- 5.0 mm LHS
- 2.0 mm K-wires

(Size of system, instruments, and implants can vary according to anatomy.)

Patient preparation and positioning

Antibiotics: 3rd generation cephalosporin
Thrombosis prophylaxis: low-molecular heparin

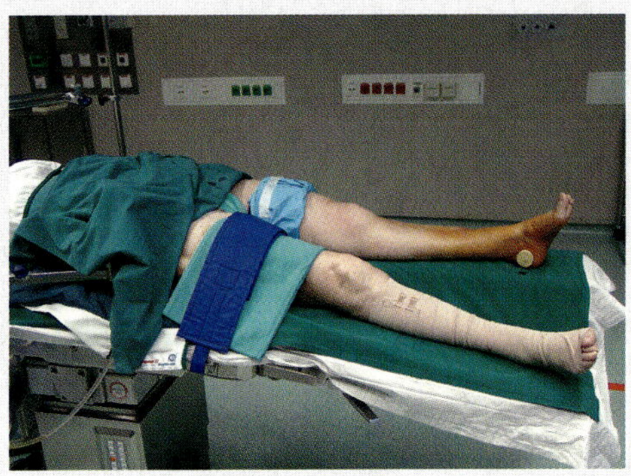

Fig 10.2.16-2 Supine position with the intact limb lowered to facilitate x-ray assessment in the lateral plane with the image intensifier.

2 Surgical approach

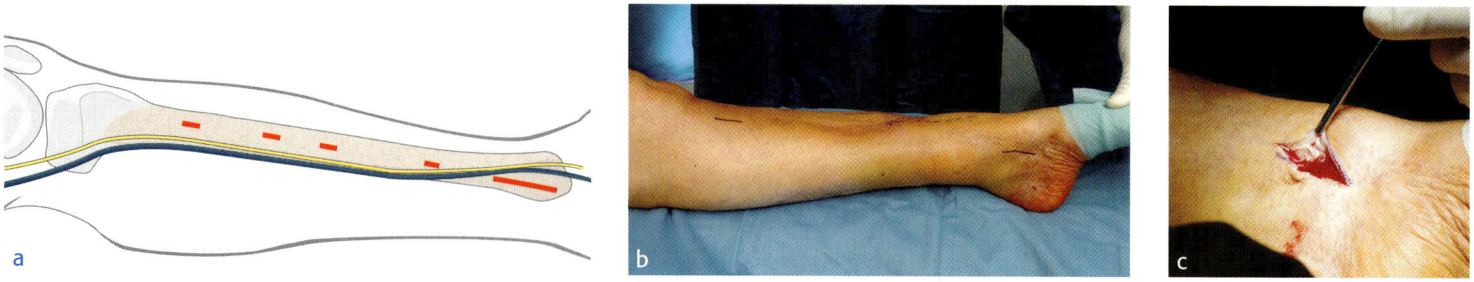

Fig 10.2.16-3a–c MIPO five incisions on the medial side of the tibia.

a Short incision over the medial malleolus taking care not to damage the great saphenous vein. Incision at the planned site for the proximal end of the plate and additional stab incisions for the LHS.

b Preoperative marking of landmarks.

c Care should be taken not to damage the saphenous nerve and vein during distal incision.

3 Reduction and fixation

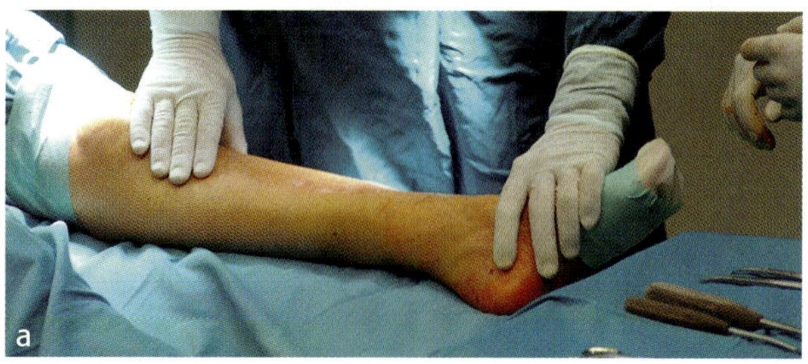

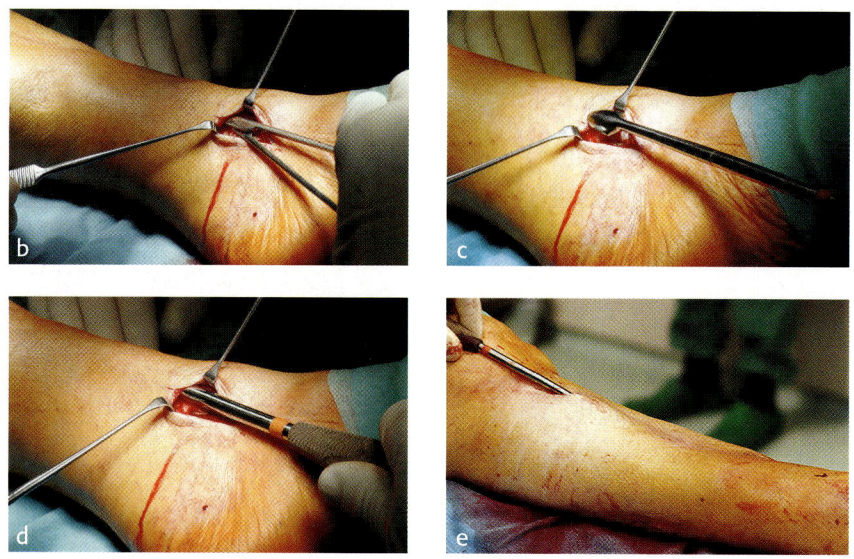

Fig 10.2.16-4a–l

a Closed reduction with manual traction; control using the image intensifier.

b–e Preparation of the epiperiosteal space with the scissors and long bone rasp from distal to proximal and proximal to distal.

3 Reduction and fixation (cont)

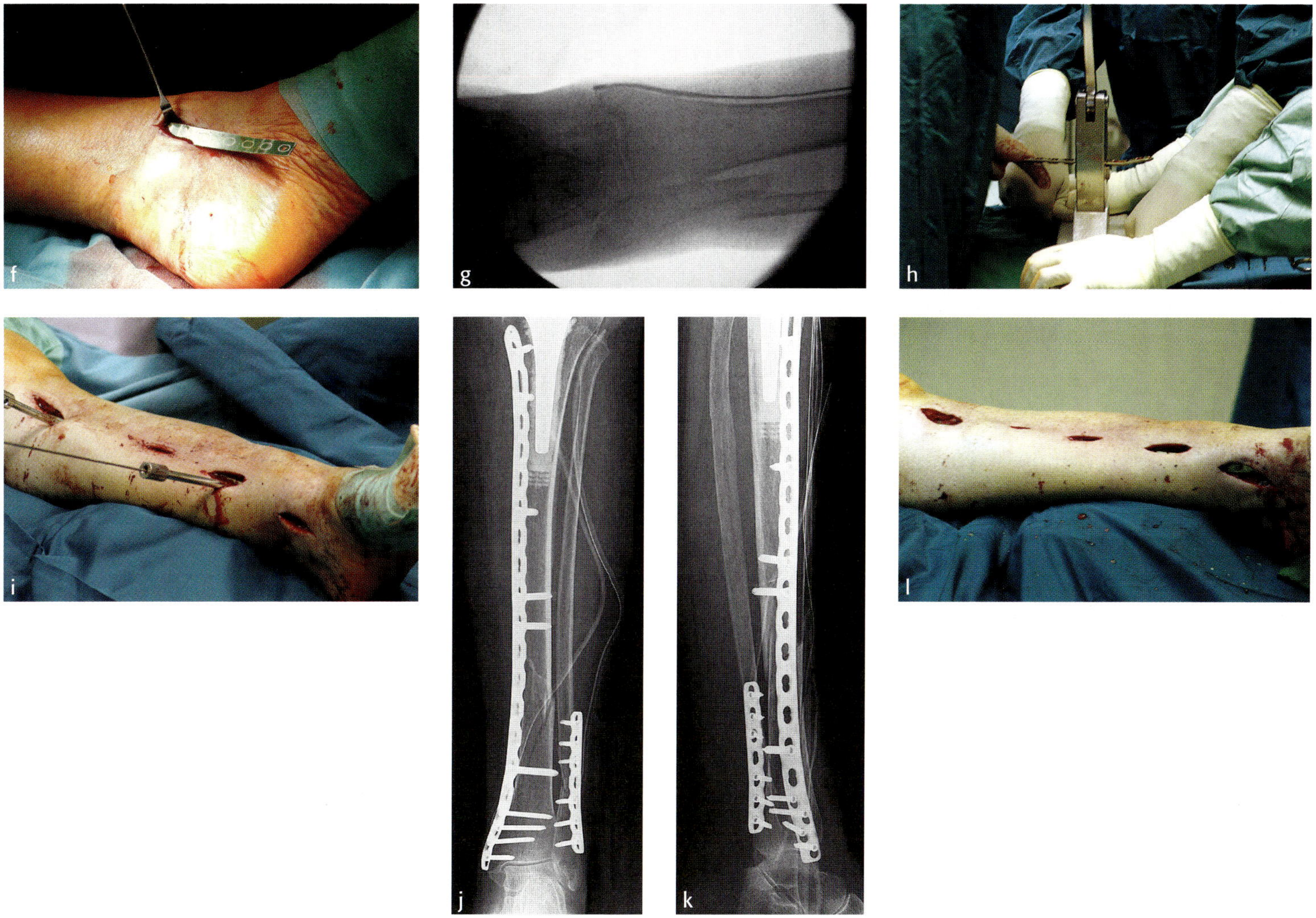

Fig 10.2.16-4a–l (cont)

f–g The anatomical shape of the tibia is determined with the help of a bending template.

h Preshaping of the plate.

i Plate insertion from distal to proximal and temporary fixation with K-wires at the distal and proximal fragments.

j–k This is followed by fixation of the two main fragments with five locking head screws in the distal fragment and five LHS in the proximal fragment. Short monocortical screws are inserted in the proximity of the knee prosthesis. The lateral malleolar fracture is stabilized by application of a 7-hole LCP 3.5 with locking head screws.

l Incisions after completion of the osteosynthesis.

4 Rehabilitation

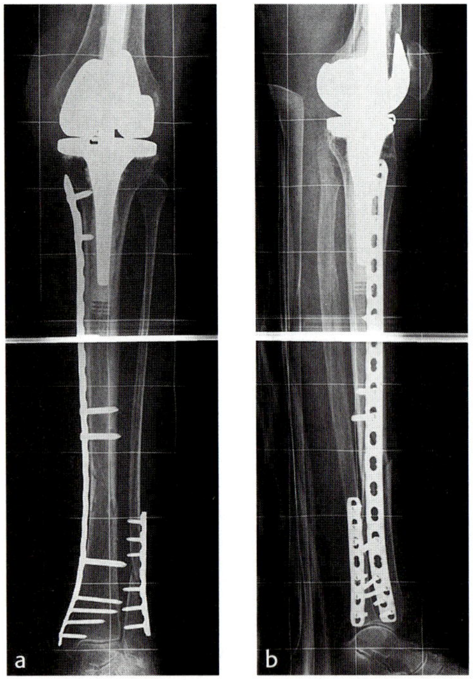

Fig 10.2.16-5a–b Partial weight bearing for 8 weeks. Postoperative x-rays after 8 weeks.

a AP view.

b Lateral view.

5 Pitfalls –

Approach

The saphenous vein and nerve may be injured during the course of distal, medial incision. The superficial peroneal nerve is endangered by lateral incision.

6 Pearls +

Equipment

The LCP metaphyseal plate 3.5/4.5/5.0, for distal tibia is anatomically preshaped and fits the distal end of the tibia. The use of locking head screws simplifies minimally invasive procedures because the plate does not have to be precisely contoured to anatomical shape. 3.5/4.5/5.0 metaphyseal LCPs are ideal for osteosynthesis of the distal tibia, particularly if the joint block is small.

In this case, the proximal end of the plate had to be adapted to the bone contours because the plate was extremely long.

The metaphyseal plate has 3.5 mm holes in the area of the joint so that it is possible to insert several locking head screws within a small space. These can be inserted divergently to each other and are angled away from the articular surface.

Author Michael Wagner

10.2.17 Pseudarthrosis of the tibia—42-B1

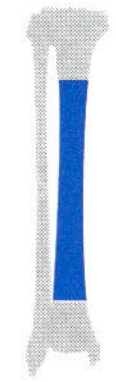

1 Case description

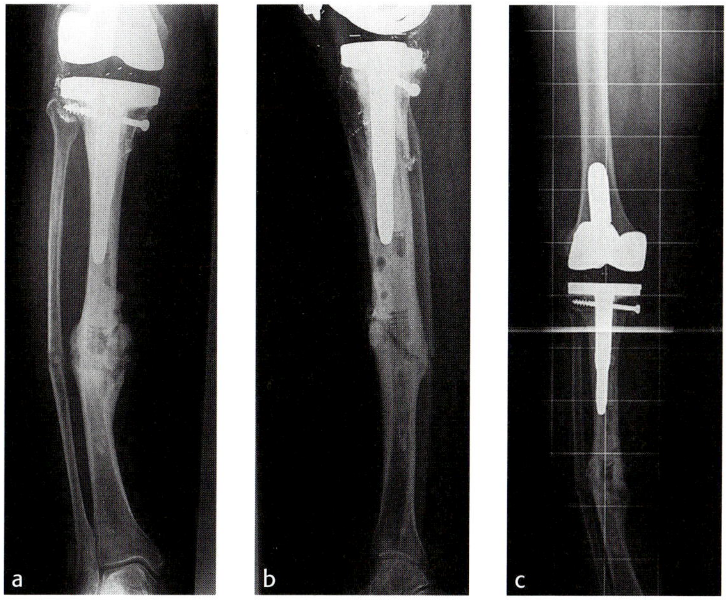

81-year-old woman suffered a spontaneous fracture of the tibial shaft at the end of the cemented stem of a revised knee prosthesis. The spontaneous fracture was treated nonoperatively and ended in a pseudarthrosis with varus malalignment.

Fig 10.2-17-1a–c
a AP view.
b Lateral view.
c Varus malalignment.

Indication

Stabilization of the nonunion and correction of the axial malalignment.

Preoperative planning

Equipment
- LCP 4.5/5.0, narrow, 15 holes
- 5.0 mm locking head screws (LHS)
- 3.5 mm cortex screws
- 2.0 mm K-wires

(Size of system, instruments, and implants can vary according to anatomy.)

Patient preparation and positioning
Antibiotics: 3rd generation cephalosporin
Thrombosis prophylaxis: low-molecular heparin

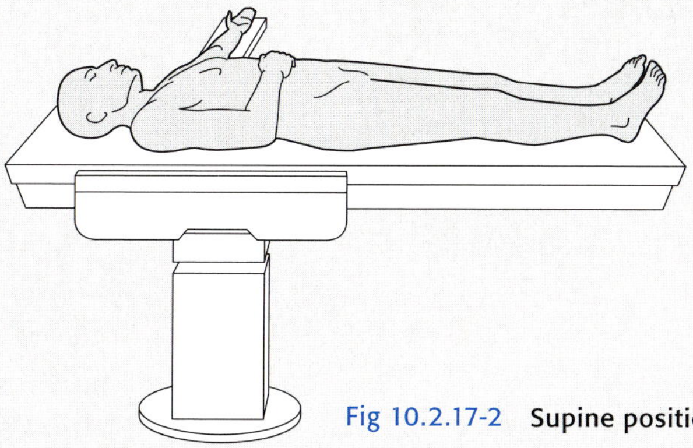

Fig 10.2.17-2 Supine position.

2 Surgical approach

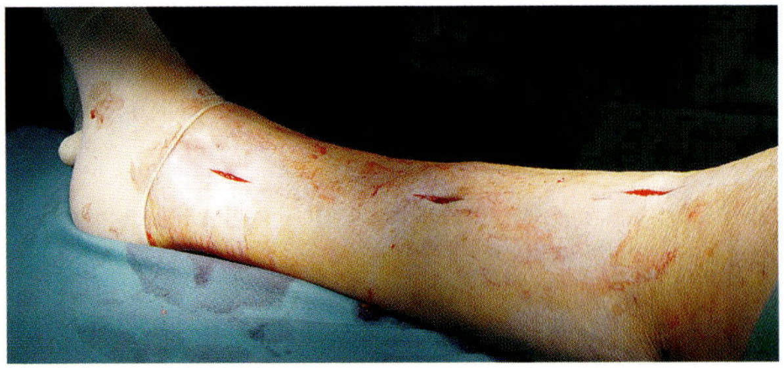

Fig 10.2.17-3 Medial incisions over the distal tibia and two additional stab incisions for the introduction of the screws.

3 Reduction and fixation

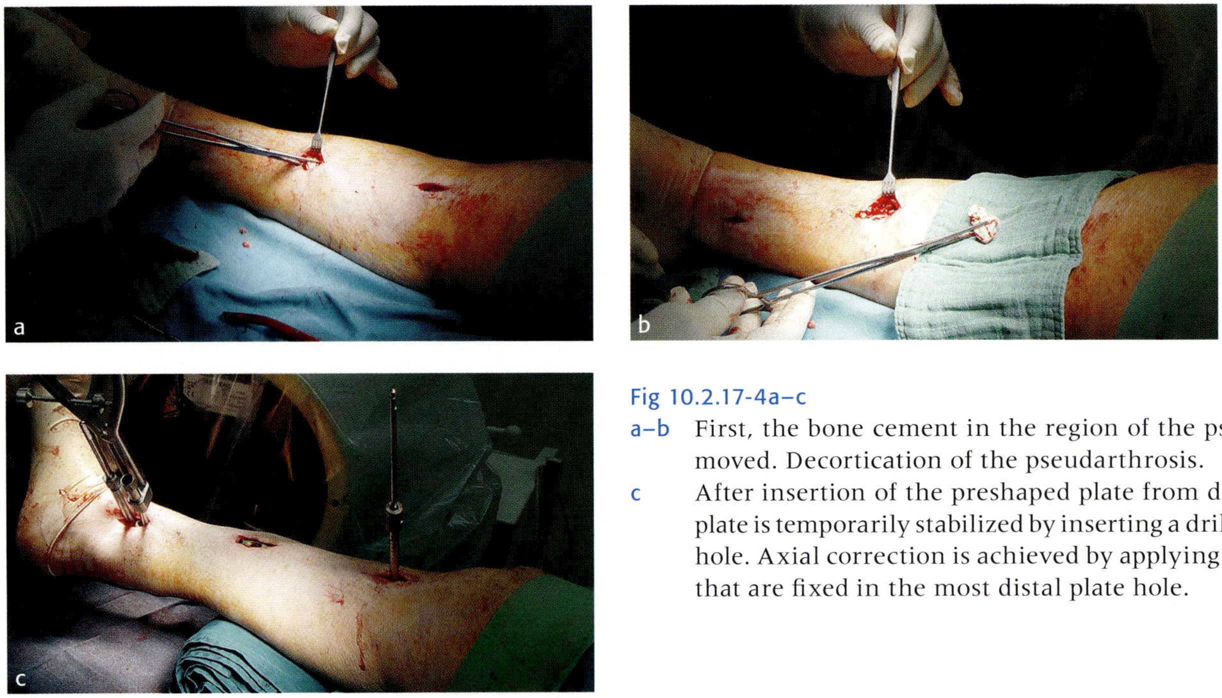

Fig 10.2.17-4a–c

a–b First, the bone cement in the region of the pseudarthrosis was removed. Decortication of the pseudarthrosis.

c After insertion of the preshaped plate from distal to proximal, the plate is temporarily stabilized by inserting a drill bit into the proximal hole. Axial correction is achieved by applying the push-pull forceps that are fixed in the most distal plate hole.

3 Reduction and fixation (cont)

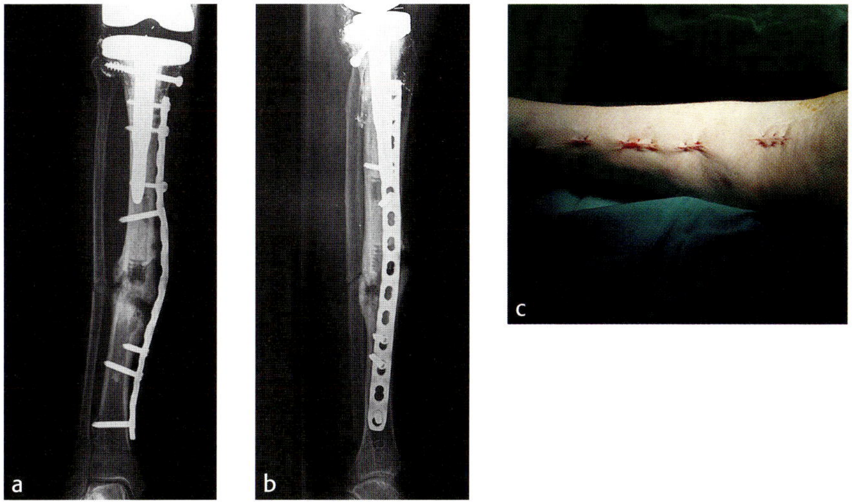

Fig 10.2.17-5a–c
a–b Three locking head screws are inserted into the distal fragment. One locking head screw and three cortex screws are inserted into the proximal fragment.
c Skin closure.

4 Rehabilitation

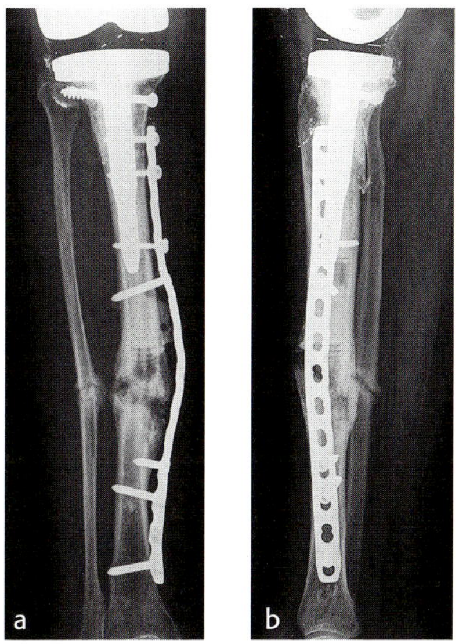

Immediate full weight bearing.

Fig 10.2.17-6a–b
Postoperative x-rays after 8 weeks.
a AP view.
b Lateral view.

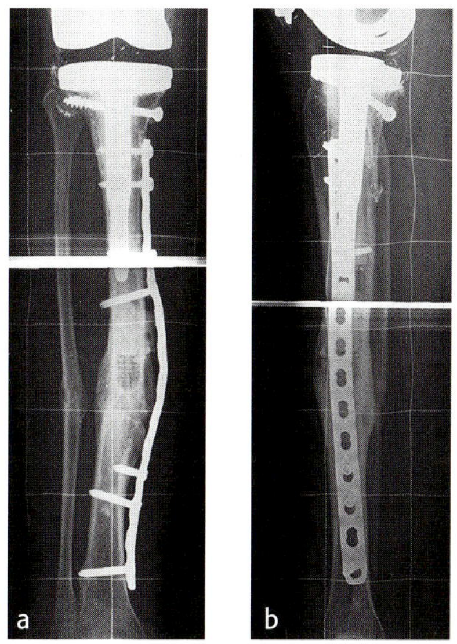

Fig 10.2.17-7a–b
Postoperative x-rays after 1 year show solid bone consolidation and good axial alignment.
a AP view.
b Lateral view.

4 Rehabilitation (cont)

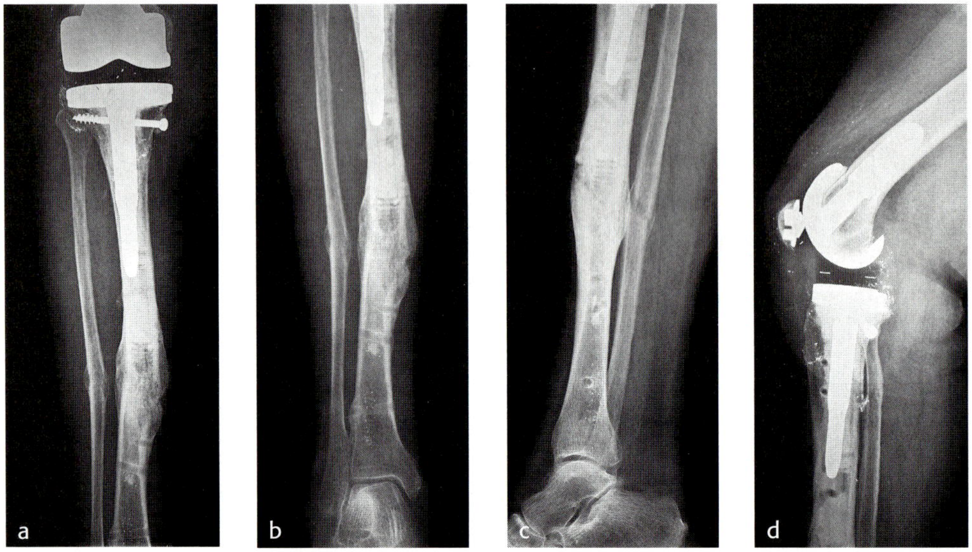

Implant removal

The distal end of the implant was the cause of slight pain and so the implant was removed 18 months after the operation.

Fig 10.2.17-8a–d Postoperative x-rays after implant removal. Bone healing in correct alignment. Note the callus formation (without bone grafting) also on the medial side beneath the non-contact plate.
a–b AP view.
c–d Lateral view.

5 Pitfalls –

Reduction and fixation

6 Pearls +

Reduction and fixation

The combination hole of the LCP permits the insertion of LHS and cortex screws. This facilitates application of the LCP in the treatment of periprosthetic fractures. The push-pull forceps provide a less invasive technique for the correction of axial malalignment by means of plating.

10.3 Tibia and fibula, distal

Cases

10 Tibia and fibula

Author Thomas P Rüedi

10.3 Tibia and fibula, distal

1 Incidence

Fractures of the distal end of the tibia AO type 43-A–C—so-called pilon fractures—have for a long time been considered not amenable to operative treatment. With the introduction of AO techniques and equipment, it became evident that only anatomical reconstruction of the articular surface and correct alignment of the axis, together with rigid fixation, would permit satisfactory results to be obtained in the long-term. Today, nonoperative treatment may be considered in minimally displaced fractures only.

Although the majority of low-energy injuries from sports accidents were originally treated by emergency ORIF, a similar approach to high-energy road traffic injuries associated with severe soft-tissue lesions often resulted in serious complications and disability. Today the majority of complex pilon fractures are therefore treated in two or more steps or stages, which permits not only the appropriate timing according to the soft-tissue recovery but also careful preoperative evaluation (including CT scan) and detailed planning.

2 Classification

The Müller AO Classification gives detailed consideration to the degree of involvement of the ankle joint.

3 Treatment methods

The most widely used techniques for the reconstruction of pilon fractures involve plates and screws, which are applied according to the four well established AO principles. Alternatively, external fixators as well as ring or hybrid fixators have been proposed and more recently even special intramedullary nails with very distal interlocking possibilities. The original

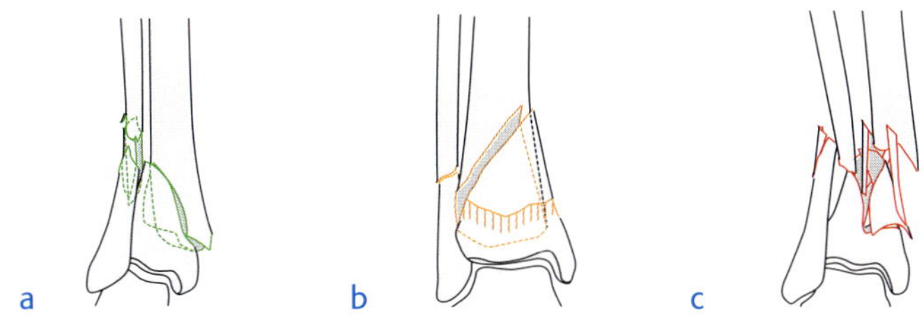

Fig 10.3-1a–c 43-A Extraarticular fractures.
a 43-A1 simple
b 43-A2 wedge
c 43-A3 complex

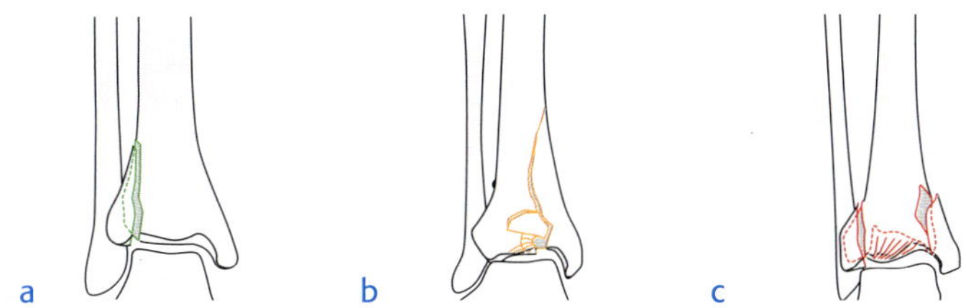

Fig 10.2-2a–c 43-B Partial articular fractures.
a 43-B1 pure split
b 43-B2 split-depression
c 43-B3 multifragmentary depression

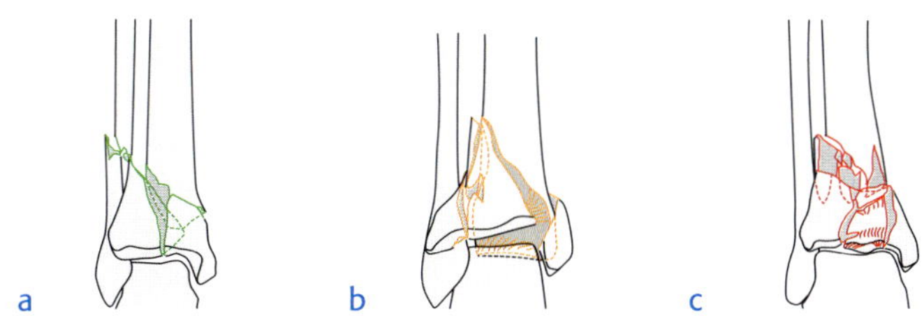

Fig 10.2-3a–c 43-C Complete articular fractures.
a 43-C1 articular simple, metaphyseal simple
b 43-C2 articular simple, metaphyseal multifragmentary
c 43-C3 articular multifragmentary

wide exposure of the entire fracture zone has been replaced by a more limited approach to the reconstruction of the articular components, combined with a sliding in of the implant for the bridging of the metaphysis according to the MIPO technique. The introduction of specially designed plates with combination holes (LCP) and locking head screws (LHS) that provide angular stability has considerably extended the possibilities of plating. Furthermore, the risk of secondary displacement has been minimized, while the need for cancellous autograft could be reduced. The actual choice of implant depends very much on the fracture pattern, the size of the distal fragments and the location of the major impaction. Nevertheless the correct timing of surgery and careful soft-tissue handling are the most important and decisive factors for success or failure of any surgical procedure in the distal tibia. Preoperative planning and skillful surgery are next in importance.

Videos 10.3-1, 10.3-2

4 Implant overview

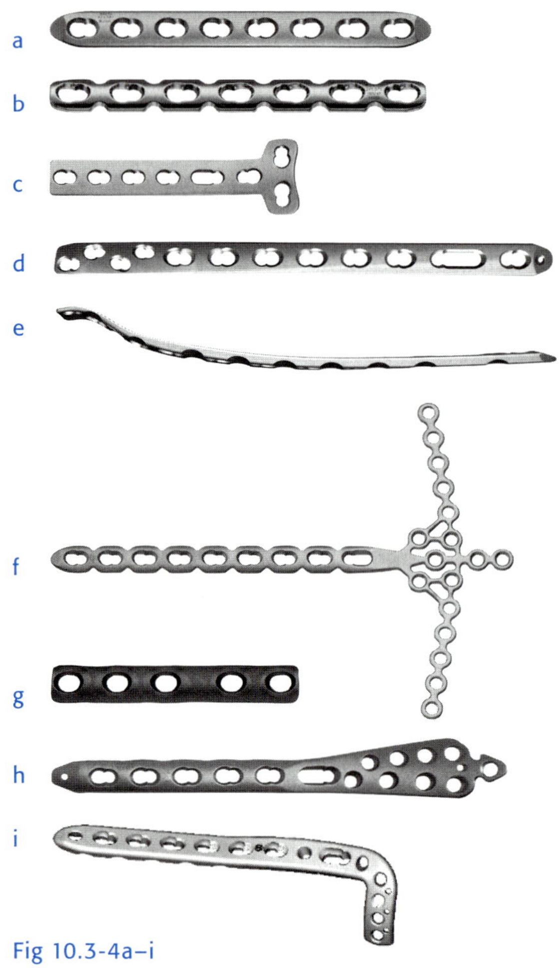

Fig 10.3-4a–i
a LCP 3.5
b LCP reconstruction plate 3.5
c LCP T-plate 3.5
d–e LCP metaphyseal plate 3.5/4.5/5.0 for distal tibia
f LCP pilon plate 2.7/3.5
g LCP one-third tubular plate 3.5
h LCP distal medial tibial plate 3.5
i LCP anterolateral distal tibial plate 3.5

5 Suggestions for further reading

Bastian L, Blauth M, Thermann H et al (1995) [Various therapy concepts in severe fractures of the tibial pilon (type C injuries). A comparative study]. *Unfallchirurg*; 98 (11):551-558

Beck E (1993) Results of operative treatment of pilon fractures. In:Tscherne H, Schatzker J, editors. Major Fractures of the Pilon, the Talus and the Calcaneus. Berlin Heidelberg New York: Springer-Verlag, 49-51.

Blauth M, Bastian L, Krettek C, et al (2001) Surgical options for the treatment of severe tibial pilon fractures: a study of three techniques. *J Orthop Trauma*; 15(3):153–160.

Crutchfield EH, Seligson D, Henry SL et al (1995) Tibial pilon fractures: a comparative clinical study of management techniques and results. *Orthopedics*; 18 (7):613-617

Trentz O, Friedl HP (1993) Critical soft- tissue conditions in pilon fractures. In: Tscherne H, Schatzker J, editors. Major Fractures of the Pilon, the Talus and the Calcaneus. Berlin Heidelberg New York: Springer- Verlag, 59-64.

Author Christian Ryf

10.3.1 Extraarticular simple distal tibial and fibular fracture—43-A1

1 Case description

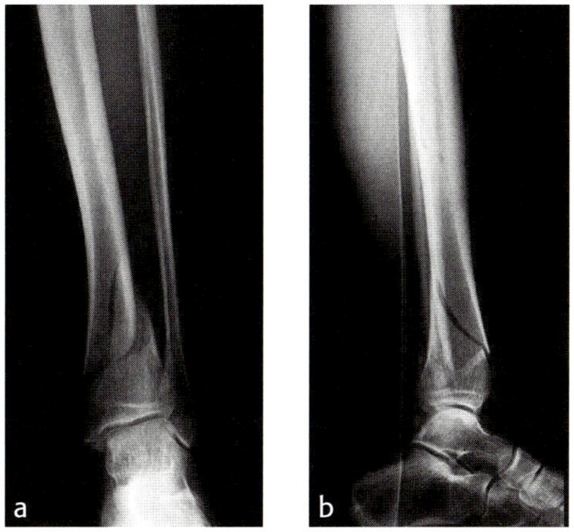

60-year-old man fell while skiing and sustained a distal tibial and fibular shaft fracture.

Fig 10.3.1-1a–b
a AP view.
b Lateral view.

Indication

The patient suffered a complete lower leg fracture. After decreased soft-tissue swelling, the fracture was operated on.

Preoperative planning

Equipment

- LCP metaphyseal plate 3.5/4.5/5.0, 5 + 13 holes
- One-third tubular plate, 5 holes
- Locking head screws (LHS)
- 3.5 mm cortex screws
- 4.0 mm cancellous bone screws

(Size of system, instruments, and implants can vary according to anatomy.)

Patient preparation and positioning

Antibiotics: single dose 2nd generation cephalosphorin
Thrombosis prophylaxis: low-molecular heparin

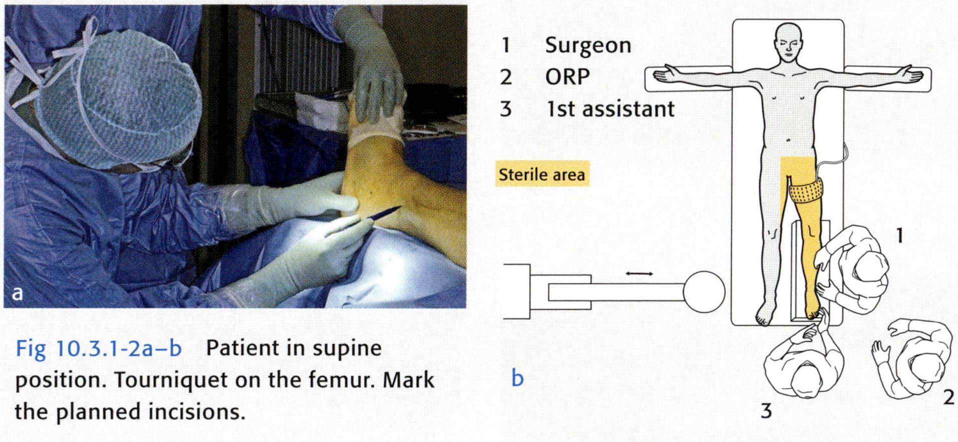

Fig 10.3.1-2a–b Patient in supine position. Tourniquet on the femur. Mark the planned incisions.

2 Surgical approach

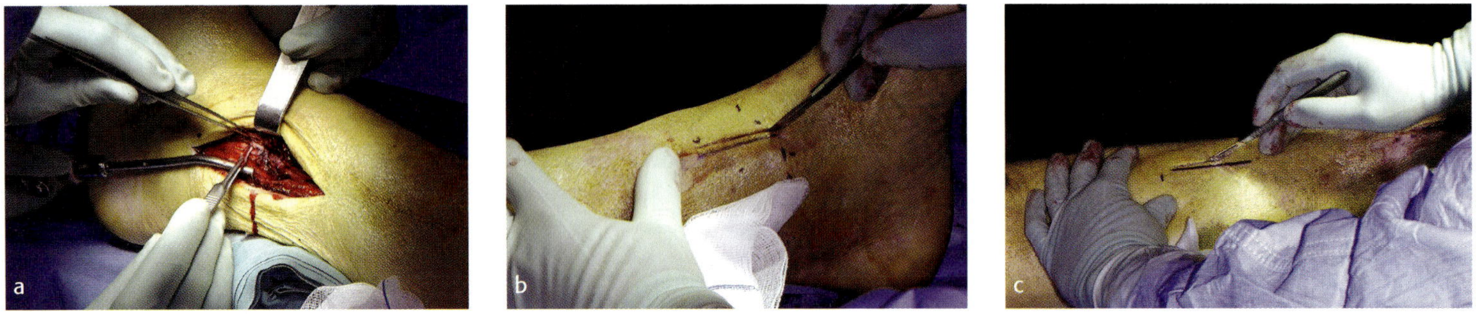

Fig 10.3.1-3a–c

a In a first step, the fibula is reduced and fixed to determine the correct lower leg length. The incision is made directly over the fracture zone.

b The distal incision is made over the medial malleolus to allow reduction and the insertion of the metaphyseal plate.

c The proximal incision is localized directly over the proximal part of the plate for fixation.

3 Reduction—fibula

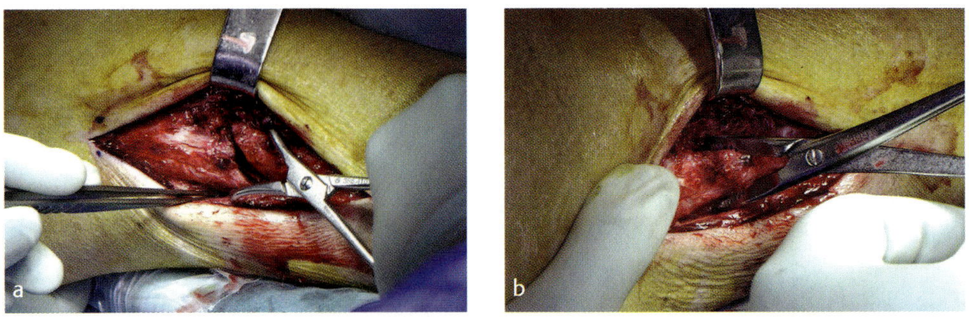

Fig 10.3.1-4a–b The distal fragment of the fibular fracture is lifted slightly. The fracture is then reduced anatomically and held in position with the pointed reduction forceps.

4 Reduction—tibia

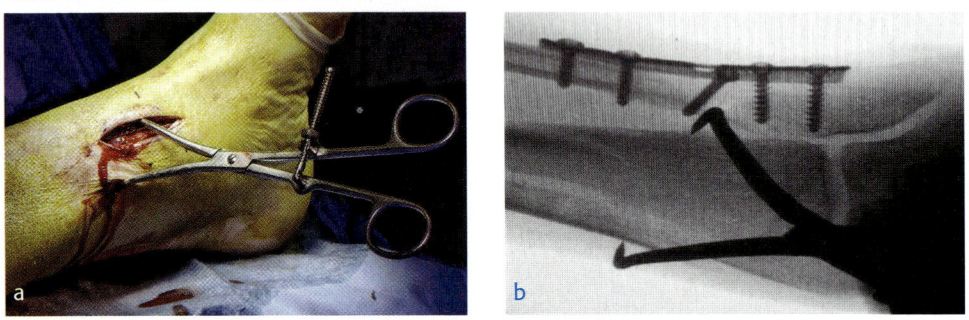

Fig 10.3.1-5a–b After complete reduction and plate fixation of the fibula, the tibia is reduced under image intensifier control with the pointed reduction forceps.

5 Fixation—fibula

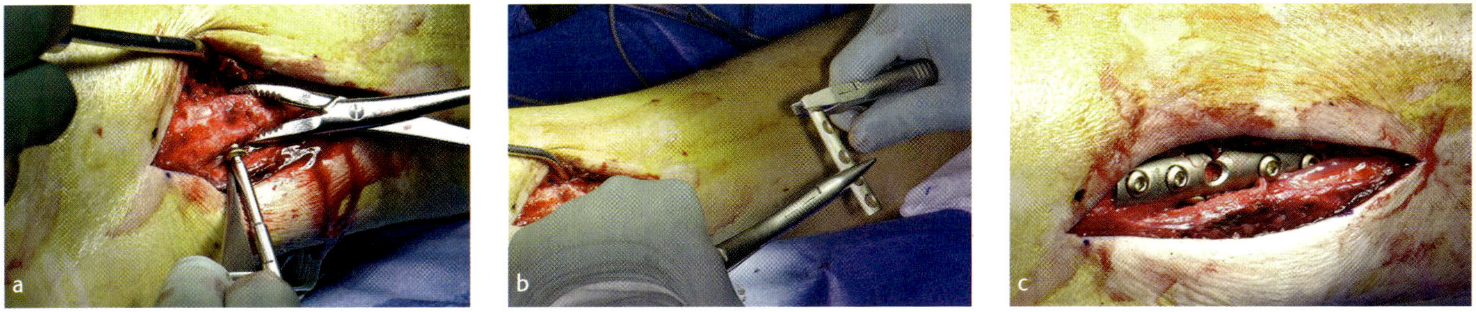

Fig 10.3.1-6a–c

a A first anteroposterior screw secures the reduced fibular fracture.

b–c For the definitive fixation a one-third tubular plate is anatomically prebent and screwed onto the bone, holding the fracture stable for the further tibial osteosynthesis.

6 Fixation—tibia

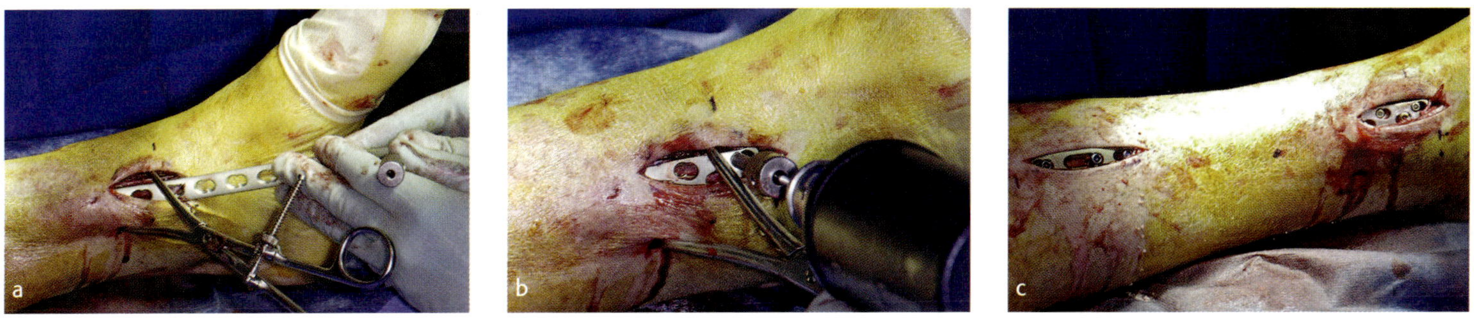

Fig 10.3.1-7a–c

a A 5 + 13-hole metaphyseal LCP is inserted from distal to proximal. The firmly attached drill sleeve in the most distal hole is used as a handle to guide the plate.

b Distal fixation of the plate with locking head screws and cortex screws.

c Proximal locking head screws are used to fix the plate onto the bone.

7 Rehabilitation

Additional immobilization: none.
Weight bearing: 15 kg for 6 weeks; half body weight after 8 weeks.

Implant removal
Implant removal not before 12–18 months.

8 Pitfalls –

Equipment

Approach

Reduction and fixation

9 Pearls +

Equipment
The LCP metaphyseal plate 3.5/4.5/5.0, for distal tibia is anatomically preshaped and fits the distal end of the tibia. The use of locking head screws simplifies the minimally invasive procedures because the plate does not have to be anatomically contoured. The distal metaphyseal LCPs are ideal for osteosynthesis of the distal tibia, particularly if the joint block is small.

Approach
Minimally invasive plate osteosynthesis (MIPO) preserves the soft tissues and reduces the risk of iatrogenic vascular damage at fracture level.

Reduction and fixation
Precise anatomical reduction and stable fixation (of the fibular fracture) with a lag screw and protection plate facilitates the direct percutaneous reduction of the tibia and its temporary retention with pointed reduction forceps. After reduction, locked splinting using the MIPO technique is easy.

Locking head screws enable good fixation of the plate, particularly in the metaphyseal area.

A long internal fixator is mandatory for locked splinting.

Authors Gabriele Streicher, Andreas Gruner, Thomas J Hockertz, Heinrich Reilmann

10.3.2 Extraarticular wedge distal tibial and fibular fracture—43-A2

1 Case description

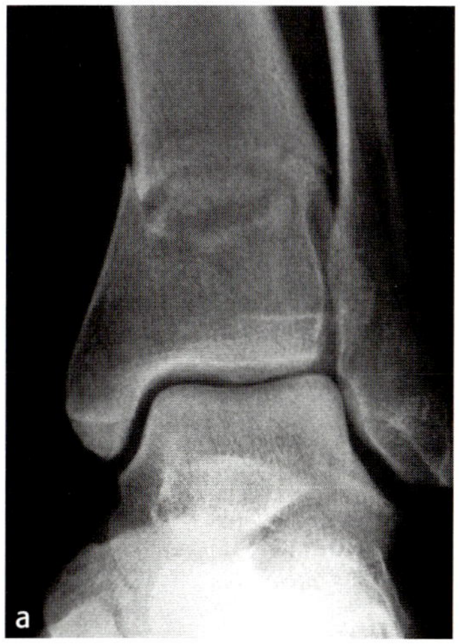

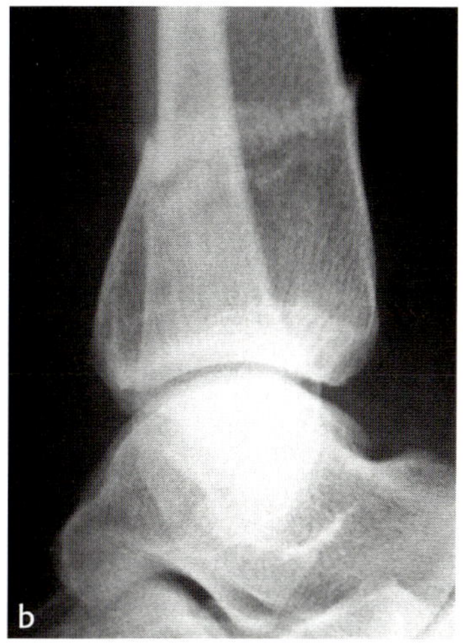

67-year-old woman with injury to the distal tibia.
Type of injury: low-energy trauma, monotrauma, closed fracture.

Fig 10.3.2-1a–b
a AP view.
b Lateral view.

Indication

Gross axial malalignment and instability of the fracture of the distal tibia, imminent risk of incorrect loading of the ankle joint.

Preoperative planning

Equipment

- LCP metaphyseal plate 3.5/4.5/5.0, 5 + 4 holes
- 5.0 mm locking head screws (LHS)
- 3.5 mm LHS
- 4.5 mm cortex screw (reduction tool)
- 2.0 mm K-wires

(Size of system, instruments, and implants can vary according to anatomy.)

Patient preparation and positioning

Antibiotics: single dose 2nd generation cephalosporin
Thrombosis prophylaxis: low-molecular heparin

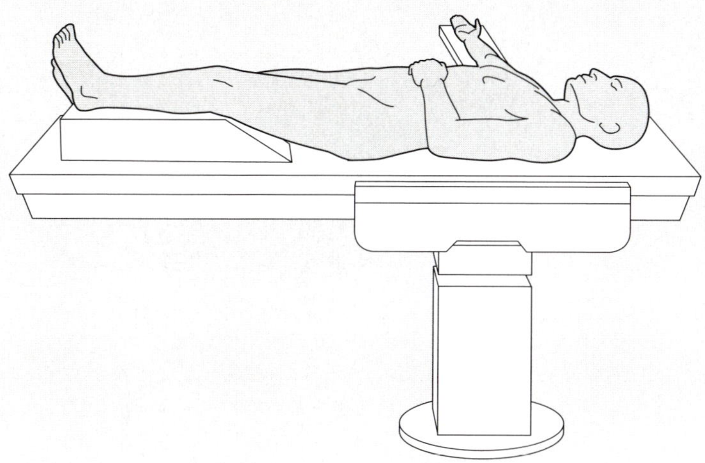

Fig 10.3.2-2 Supine position with elevation of the leg to be operated on and slight bending of the knee joint.

2 Surgical approach

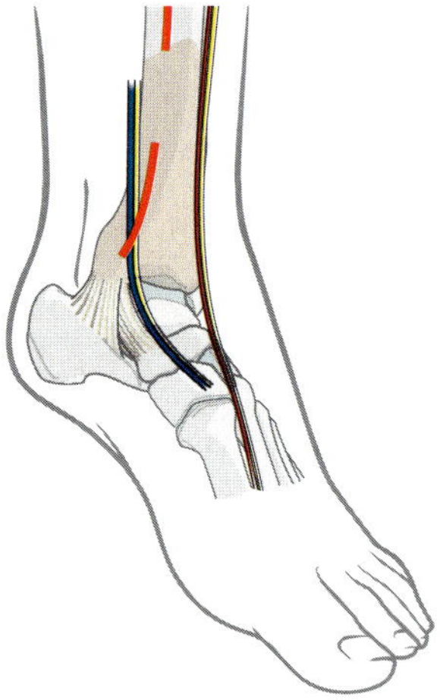

Fig 10.3.2-3 Make an incision approximately 4–5 cm long anteromedially at the inner malleolus and dissect to the periosteum. Prepare the plate bed along the medial tibial crest from distal to proximal with the bone rasp. Make a counter-incision over the proximal end of the plate through which to insert the screws.

3 Reduction

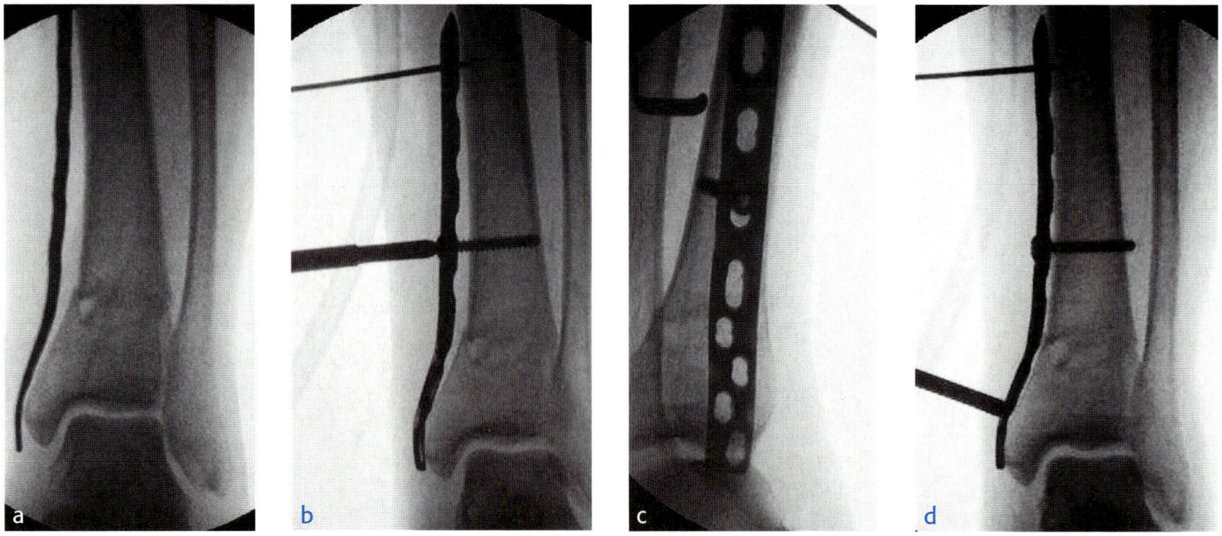

Fig 10.3.2-4a–d

a Prebend the plate and insert it from distal to proximal into the plate bed.

b–c After approximate reduction and temporary fixation of the plate with a K-wire, the fragment and plate can be aligned with a cortex screw (reduction screw).

d Situation after reduction: the bone is in correct axial alignment adjacent to the plate. Fixation can now start.

4 Fixation

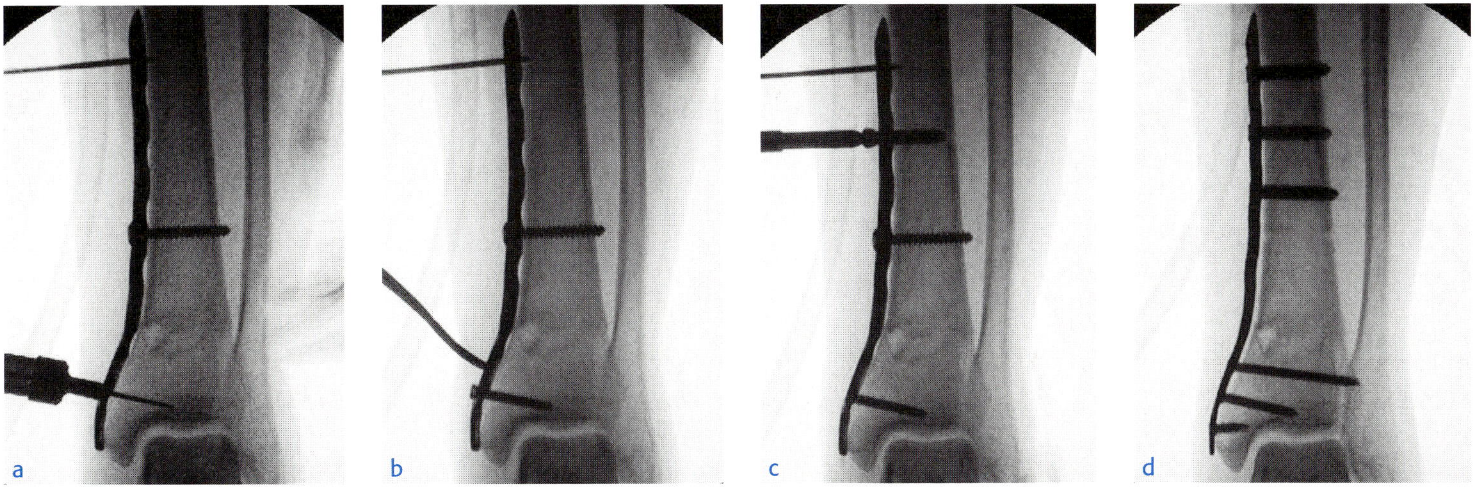

Fig 10.3.2-5a–d
a–c The LHS are inserted alternately into the distal and proximal plate holes.
d In this way, bridging of the fracture zone is achieved; the screw holes in the immediate vicinity of the fracture are left empty. The cortex reduction screw is removed.

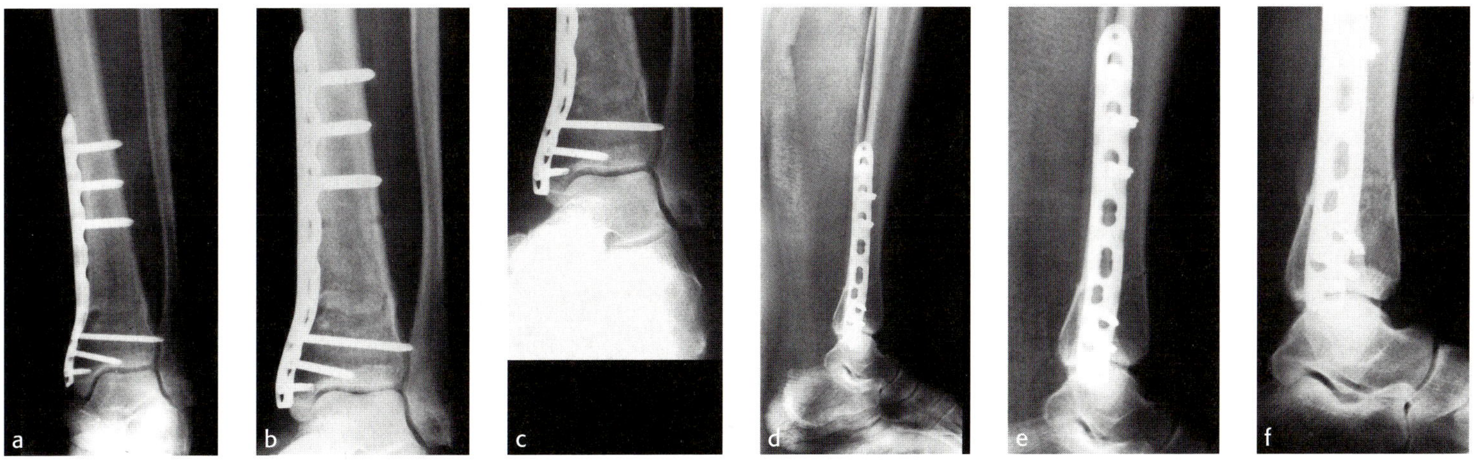

Fig 10.3.2-6a–f Postoperative x-rays.
a AP axis view.
b AP view.
c Ankle joint centered, AP view.
d Lateral axis view.
e Lateral view.
f Ankle joint centered, lateral view.

5 Rehabilitation

Additional immobilization: lower limb plaster cast until definitive healing.
Weight bearing: half body weight after 4 weeks, full weight bearing after 6 weeks.
Physiotherapy: from the second postoperative day.
Pharmaceutical treatment: nonsteroid antiinflammatory drugs.

Implant removal
Remove the plate through a small incision in the region of the previous approaches.
Reason for implant removal: the implant was causing mechanical irritation of the inner malleolus.

6 Pitfalls –

Equipment
Incorrect prebending of the plate.

Approach
Injury to the saphenous vein and nerve if the approach is too far on the ventral side of the inner malleolus.

Reduction and fixation
Incorrect positioning of the plate, especially in the lateral plane.

Rehabilitation

7 Pearls +

Equipment
Application of an LCP metaphyseal plate for the distal tibia (anatomically precontoured plate) or a metaphyseal LCP (easier to preshape than an LCP 4.5/5.0) facilitates better adaptation to the shape of the bone.

Approach
Preservation of soft tissue in the region of the fracture due to a minimally invasive approach.

Reduction and fixation
Intraoperative x-ray controls to ensure that the plate is correctly positioned in the lateral plane.
Final reduction in the frontal plane with a cortex screw—pulls the bone onto the plate (reduction screw).

Rehabilitation
Early mobilization with partial loading is possible.

Author Christoph Sommer

10.3.3 Partial articular multifragmentary distal tibial fracture (pilon)—43-B3

1 Case description

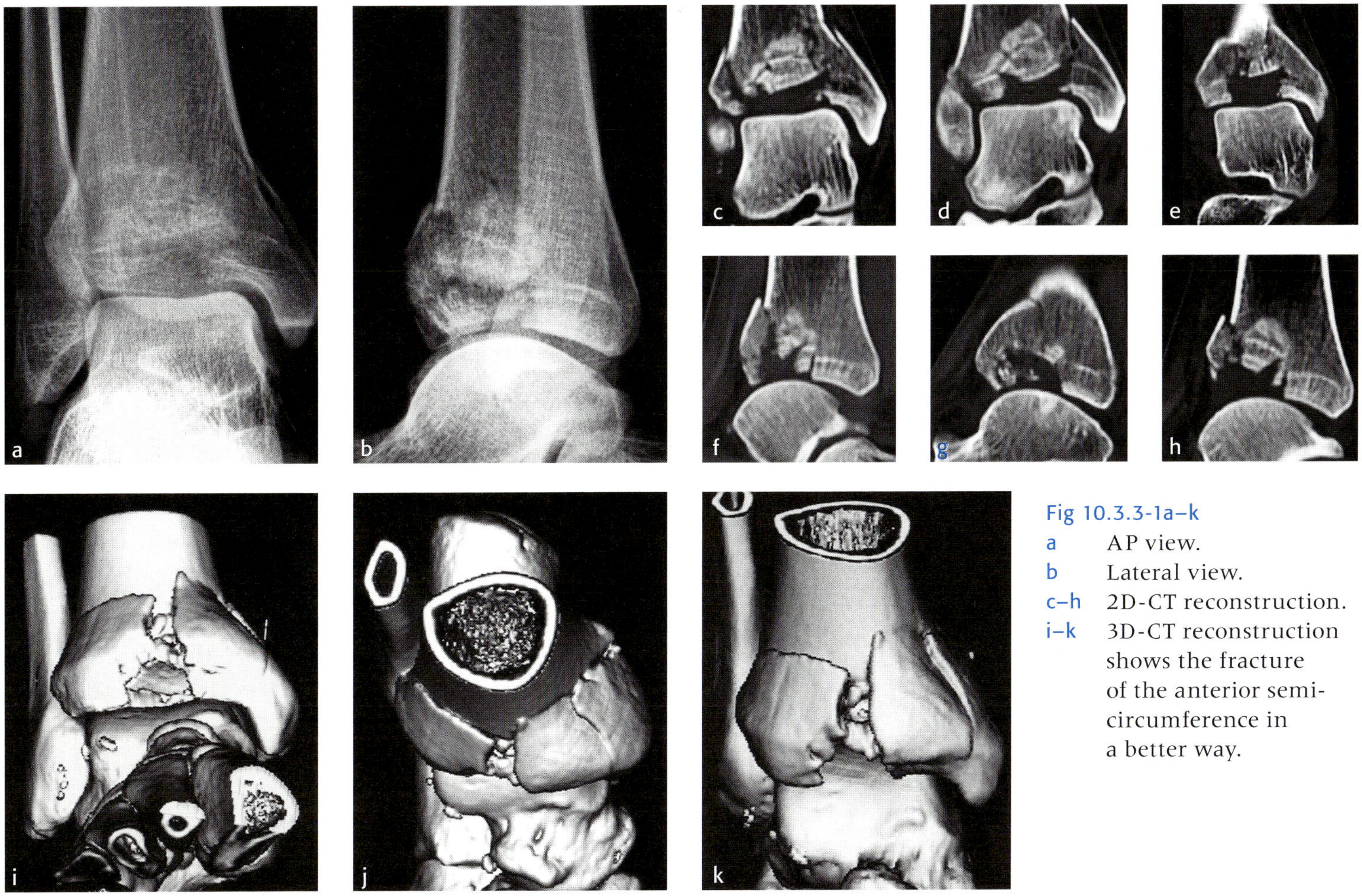

Fig 10.3.3-1a–k
a AP view.
b Lateral view.
c–h 2D-CT reconstruction.
i–k 3D-CT reconstruction shows the fracture of the anterior semi-circumference in a better way.

29-year-old woman slipped while icefall climbing. She fell approximately 5 m and suffered a hyperextension injury to the upper ankle joint. The x-ray showed an articular tibial fracture without a fracture of the fibula (43-B3.2). The anterior tibial joint surface was impacted and had fractured into multiple fragments, and both the anterolateral and the anterior parts of the medial malleolus were fractured.

Indication

Because of the incongruent joint, this fracture is an absolute indication for an operative procedure. With only slight malalignment and no subluxation or dislocation, a one-stage procedure can be performed. This operation is best done 5–10 days after injury. This multifragmentary fracture cannot be reduced closed (insufficient ligamentotaxis for impacted articular fragments), and requires an open procedure. Given this fracture pattern, an anterior implant is ideal to hold the anterior joint rim. The new pilon LCP 3.5 is ideal or, alternatively, a double plate osteosynthesis with conventional plates could be used (two one-third tubular plates 3.5). Cancellous bone grafting may be necessary depending on the size of the metaphyseal defect and the impacted fragments.

Preoperative planning

Equipment

- LCP pilon plate 2.7/3.5, 6 holes
- Locking head screws (LHS)
- 3.5 mm cortex screw
- 1.2 mm K-wires
- Large distractor

(Size of system, instruments, and implants can vary according to anatomy.)

Patient preparation and positioning

Antibiotics: single dose 2nd generation cephalosporin

Thrombosis prophylaxis: low-molecular heparin

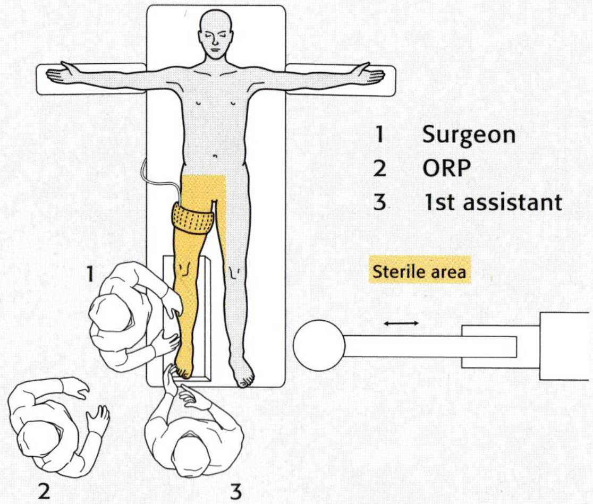

Fig 10.3.3-2 Positioning of OR team.

2 Surgical approach

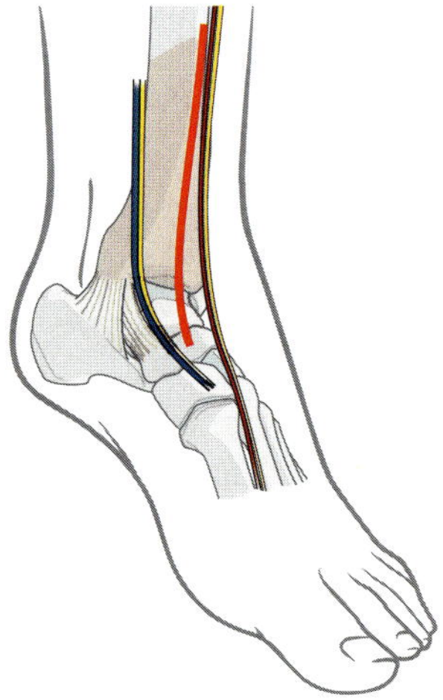

Fig 10.3.3-3 Only one anteromedial approach is necessary (fibula intact). This approach has to be long enough for adequate open joint reduction, but does not have to be extended to the full length of the plate, which can be inserted retrograde to the diaphysis.

3 Reduction and fixation

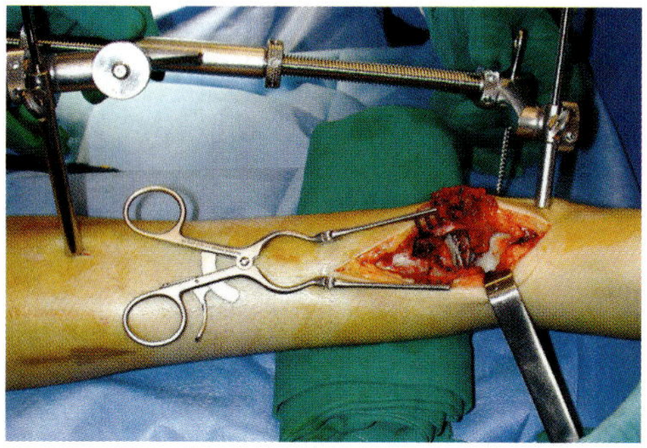

Fig 10.3.3-4 The optimal time for this operation was after seven days (skin wrinkles were visible). First the large distractor is positioned on the tibial shaft and the talus neck. The talus is pulled in a caudal and posterior direction under distraction to allow a good view into the ankle joint.

3 Reduction and fixation (cont)

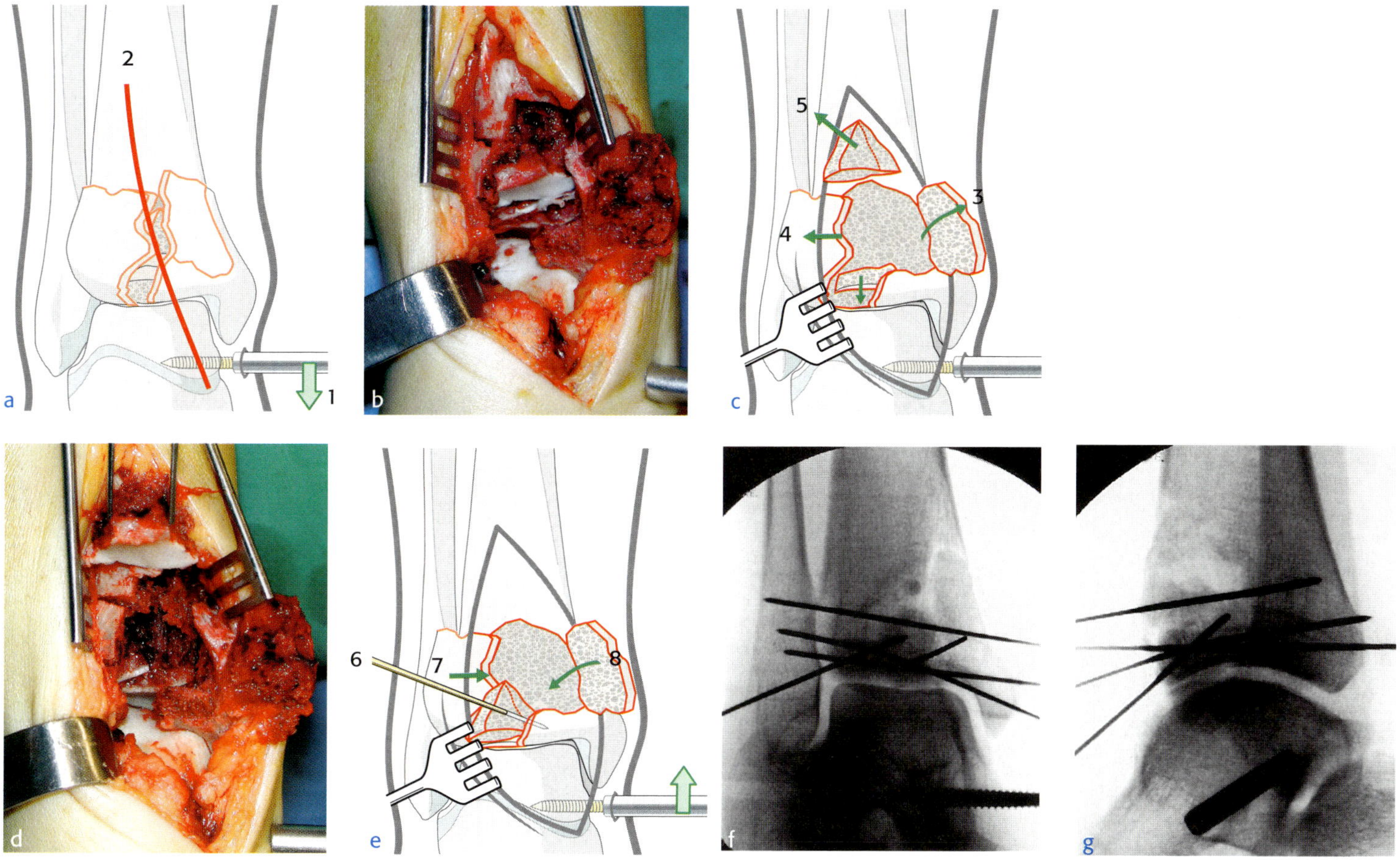

Fig 10.3.3-5a–o

a The approach (2) is straight and runs from the anterior tibial margin to the base of the navicular bone. The large distractor is still in place (1).

b–c The anteromedial fragment is held medially (3) and the anterolateral fragment (4) is held laterally. Now the large impacted main fragment can be seen. This fragment is removed and temporarily set aside (5).

d–e The small impacted central fragment is reduced anatomically under vision onto the posterior joint rim. Now the large impacted fragment, that had previously been removed, is reduced anatomically onto the central, posterior fragment and held by a K-wire inserted in an anterior to posterior direction (6). In the next step, the anteromedial and the anterolateral fragments are rotated back to their anatomical positions (7, 8). To do this, distraction with the large distractor must be interrupted because these two fragments are attached at the joint capsule. These two fragments are held in their anatomically correct positions with the help of the Weber forceps.

f–g K-wires are inserted for further stabilization. Image intensification images show the correct reduction of the joint surfaces. With this good quality of bone and the small metaphyseal defect zone, cancellous bone grafting is not necessary.

3 Reduction and fixation (cont)

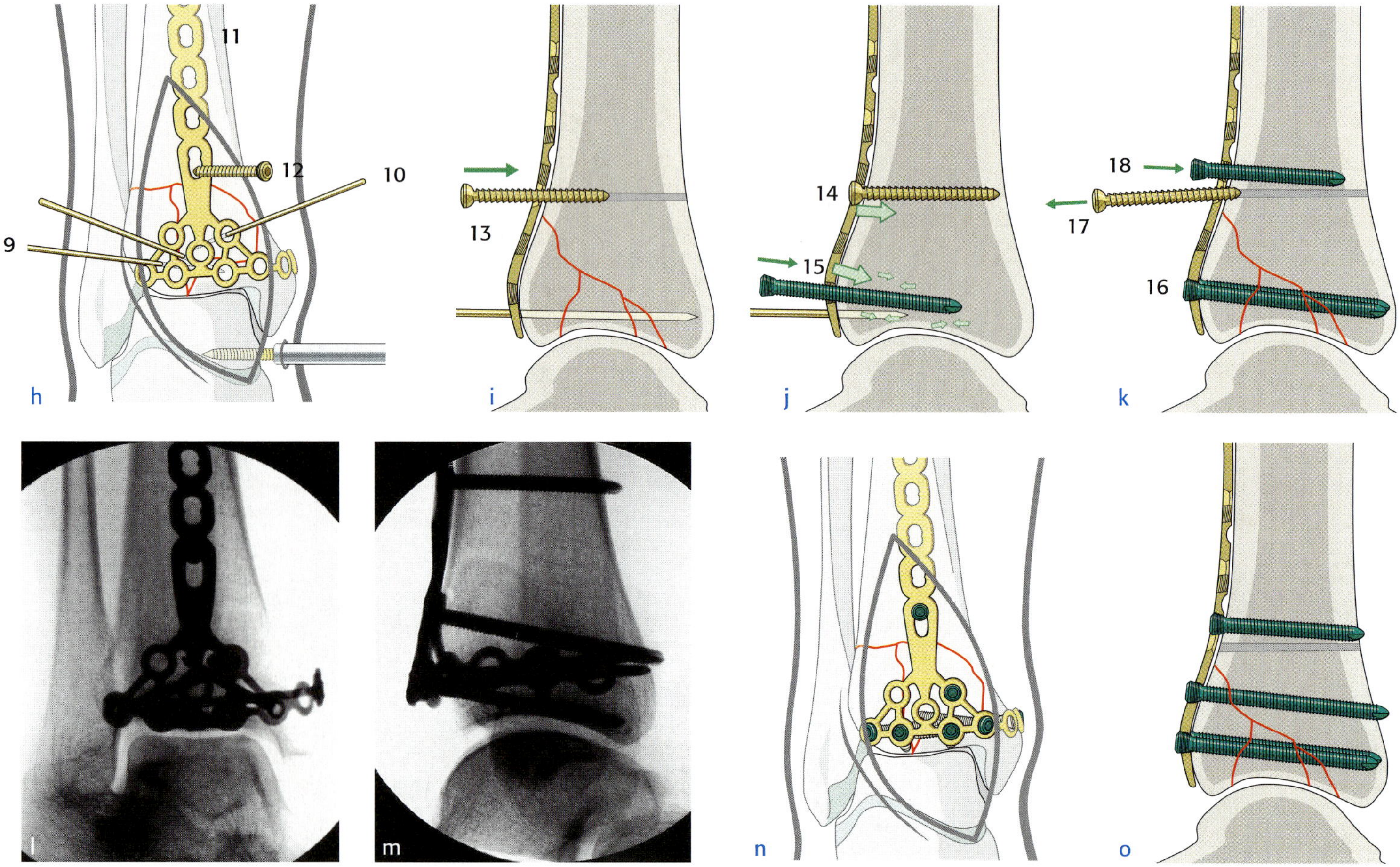

Fig 10.3.3-5a–o (cont)

h–i A 6-hole LCP pilon plate 2.7/3.0 is cut distally to fit the bone. The lateral sides of the plate will hold the anterolateral fragment and the medial malleolus. The plate is bent so that the middle part of the plate is not touching the bone (**9, 10, 11**). A 3.5 mm cortex screw is inserted proximal to the fracture, thus compressing the fragments with the inferior end of the plate (**12, 13, 14**).

j–k Locking head screws are now inserted into the joint block to hold the anatomical reduction in place (**15**). A screw is inserted into the most proximal hole (**16**) and the first screw is exchanged for a locking head screw to reduce the pressure on the periosteum (**17, 18**).

l–o The x-ray control at the end of the operation confirms the anatomical reduction and the correct position of the screws and plate. Two central locking head screws are very near to the joint surface. To exclude penetration of the joint surface, an x-ray in the direction of the screws can be obtained. This view will show screw position in relation to the joint.

3 Reduction and fixation (cont)

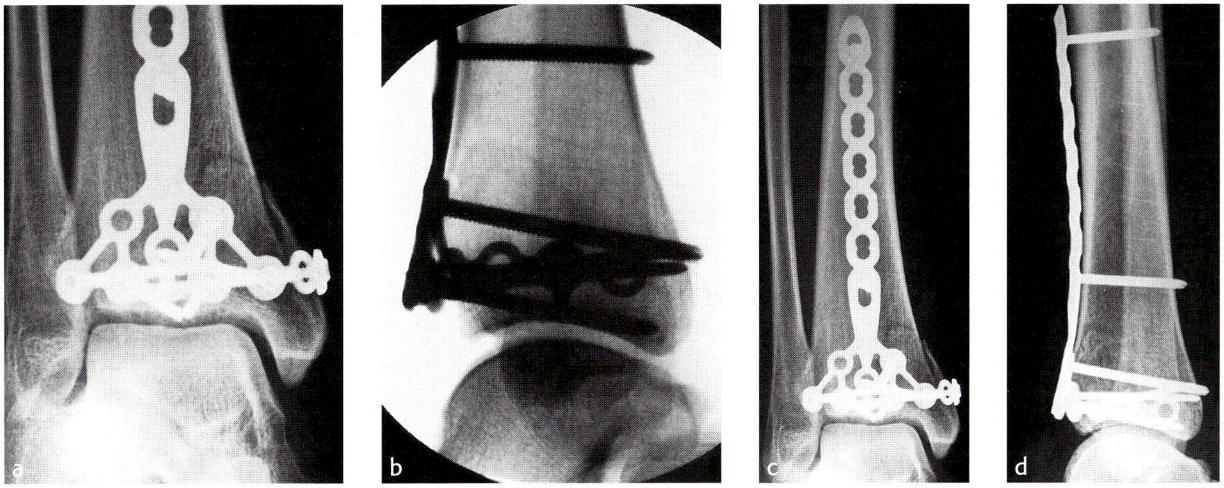

Fig 10.3.3-6a–d The postoperative x-rays show good anatomical reduction and stabilization of the pilon fracture.

4 Rehabilitation

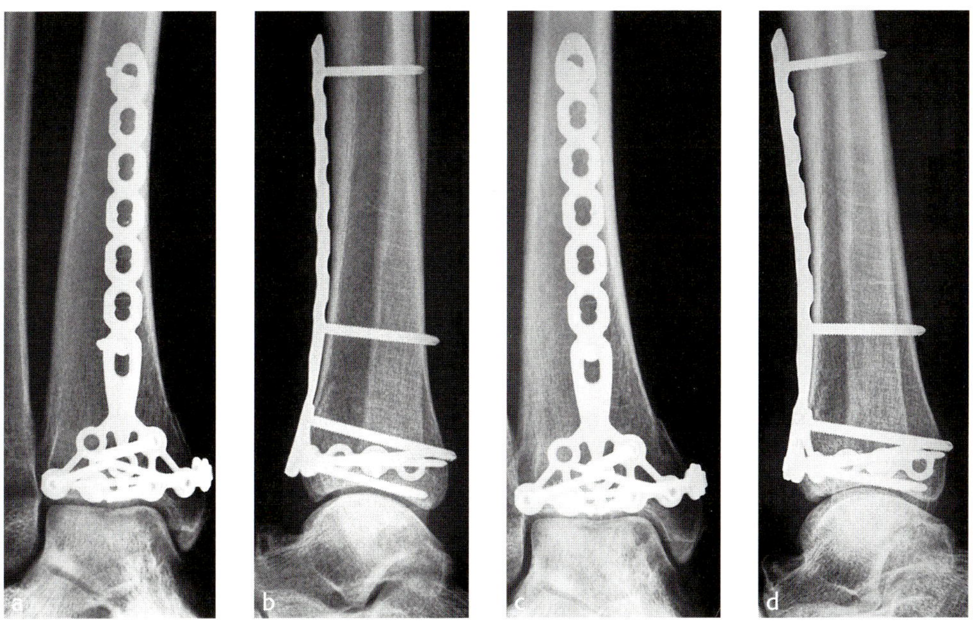

Mobilization begins after wound healing on the 1–5 postoperative day with toe-touch weight bearing (10–15 kg). Early functional and active movement must be started.

Fig 10.3.3-7a–d

a–b 6 weeks after surgery, the fracture is practically consolidated and the implant is in the correct position; weight bearing can be increased to 30 kg.

c–d After 11 weeks, the fracture is completely consolidated. Osteopenia due to partial weight bearing will diminish rapidly. There were no further problems and the plate could be removed after 11 months with good range of motion.

5 Pitfalls –

Equipment
If the plate is badly bent, irritation of the extensor tendons can occur.

Approach
An approach too far medially could complicate the reduction of the anterolateral fragment and the insertion of the plate.

Reduction and fixation
Insufficient reduction and fixation of the anterolateral fragment provokes instability of the ankle joint with post-traumatic osteoarthritis. The same can happen due to a badly reduced central fragment.

Rehabilitation
Full weight bearing too early can redisplace the fragments and/or lead to an implant failure. The screws may cut through the joint in osteoporotic bone.

6 Pearls +

Equipment
The LCP pilon plate is an ideal plate for the treatment of anterior semicircular multifragmentary fractures.

Approach
An anterior or anteromedial approach is ideal for the treatment of these fractures.

Reduction and fixation
The large distractor is a helpful instrument for the preliminary distraction of fractures and allows a good view of the tibial joint surface. The 2.7 mm locking head screws are ideal for multifragmentary and very distal pilon fractures.

Rehabilitation
Early functional movement is usually possible in all stabilized fractures where sufficient primary stability has been achieved.

Author Christopher W Geel

10.3.4 Complete articular simple distal tibial and fibular fracture—43-C1

1 Case description

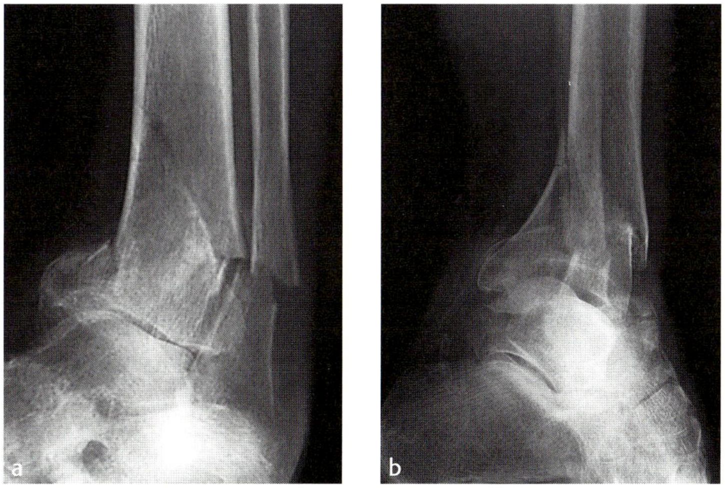

68-year-old-man has a left pilon fracture due to falling off a ladder. Type of injury: low-energy, monotrauma, closed fracture.

Fig 10.3.4-1a–b
a AP view.
b Lateral view.

Indication

Insulin dependent diabetic with articular fracture with proximal extension. Moderate osteoporotic bone. Very active lifestyle with daily walking.

Preoperative planning

Equipment
- LCP distal tibial plate 2.7/3.5, medial, 8 holes
- Locking head screws (LHS)
- 3.5 mm cortex screw

(Size of system, instruments, and implants can vary according to anatomy.)

Patient preparation and positioning
Antibiotics: cephalosporin
Thrombosis prophylaxis: low-molecular heparin

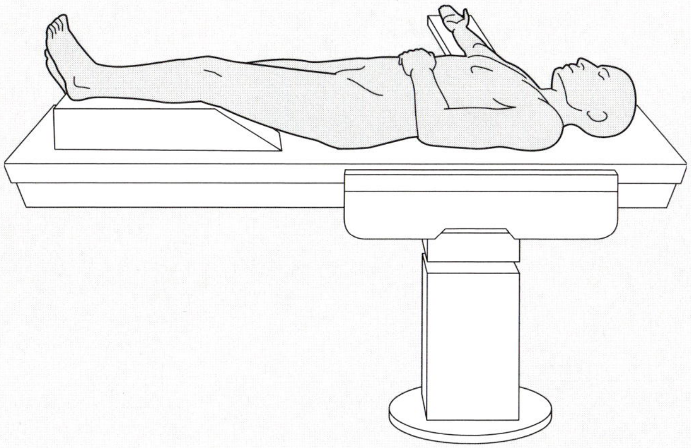

Fig 10.3.4-2 Supine on a radiolucent operating table. Image intensification, contralateral, perpendicular to table axis.

2 Surgical approach

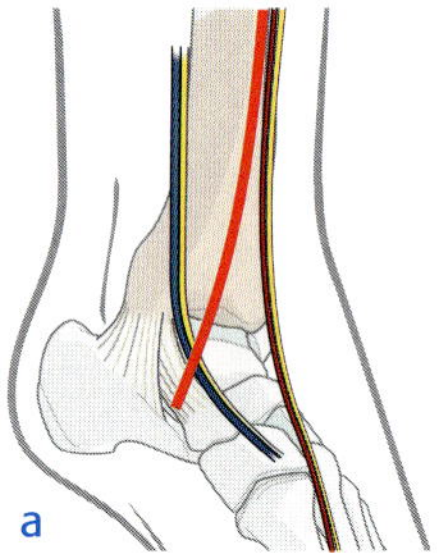

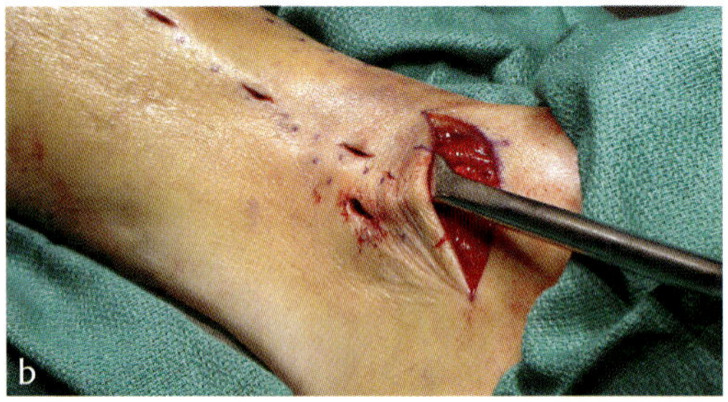

Fig 10.3.4-3a–b
a Curvylinear anteromedial malleolus incision with preservation of the greater saphenous vein.
b Preparation of the future plate position using a wide Cobb elevator to tunnel subcutaneously; preservation of the periosteum.

3 Reduction

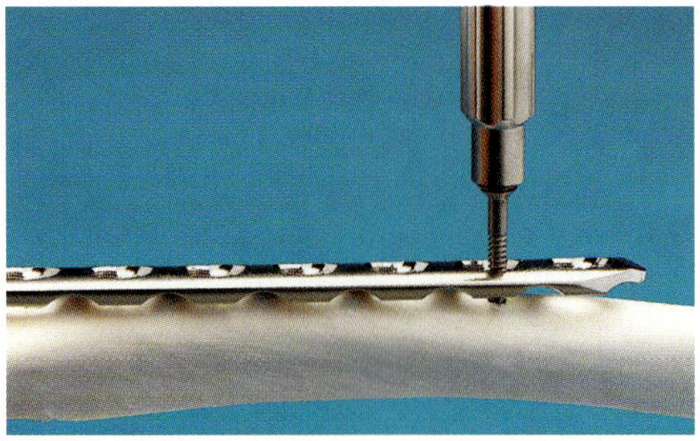

Closed reduction with traction under image intensification.

Fig 10.3.4-4 Place plate and verify its proper position by making on additional 2.5 cm long incision proximally.
First, fixation of the plate distally to have an anchor to aid reduction.
Finishing the reduction with the plate and push-pull screw proximally in the last locking screw hole.
Verify the reduction and the plate position under image intensifier in AP and lateral view.

4 Fixation

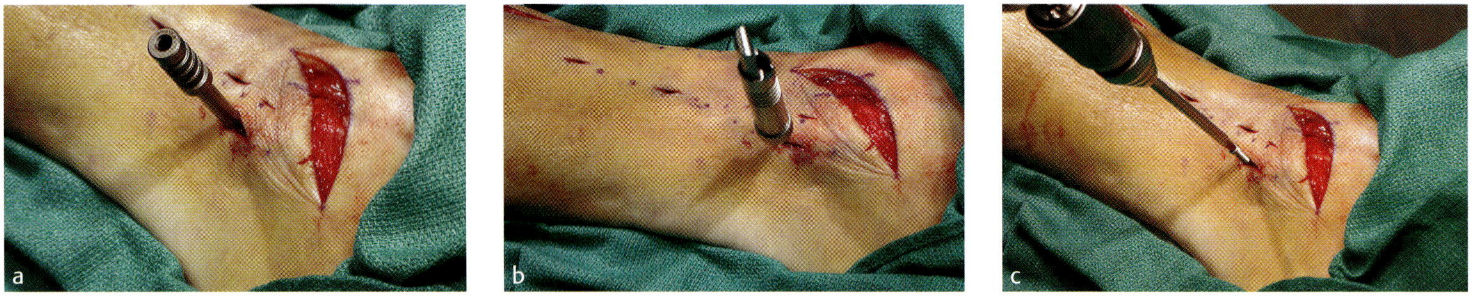

To ensure anatomical joint reconstruction, first fix the LCP distal tibial plate 2.7/3.5 medial, 8 holes distally.
Use a second plate as a template that is placed on the skin so that the insertion sites for both the locking and conventional screws can be marked with a marker pen.
Stab incision at desired locking or standard hole.

Fig 10.3.4-5a–c
a Insert drill guide and check its proper alignment in the locking hole.
b–c After drilling measure length using the depth gauge and insert the locking head screw with torque limiter.

4 Fixation (cont)

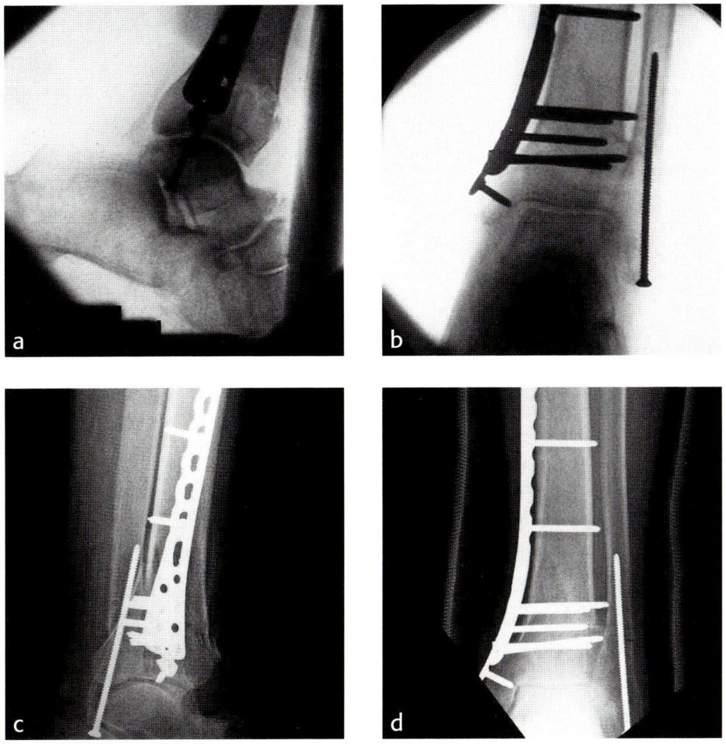

Fig 10.3.4-6a–d

a–b Final fixation and evaluation with image intensifier in AP and lateral views, including the mortise view. To improve stability, place screws as far and as near to the fracture site as possible.

c–d Percutaneously drill and insert an 3.5 mm cortex screw (length 85 mm) under image intensifier guidance to stabilize the transverse distal fibular fracture.

5 Rehabilitation

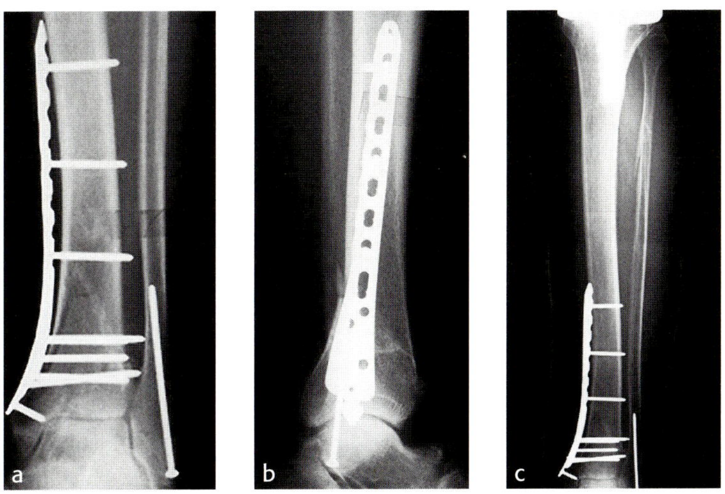

Additional immobilization: u-splint.
Weight bearing: 15 kg for 4 weeks; half body weight after 8 weeks; full weight bearing after 12 weeks.
Physiotherapy: starting one day postoperatively.
Pharmaceutical treatment: codeine.

Fig 10.3.4-7a–c Postoperative x-rays after 8 weeks.

a AP view.

b Lateral view.

c Overview.

5 Rehabilitation (cont)

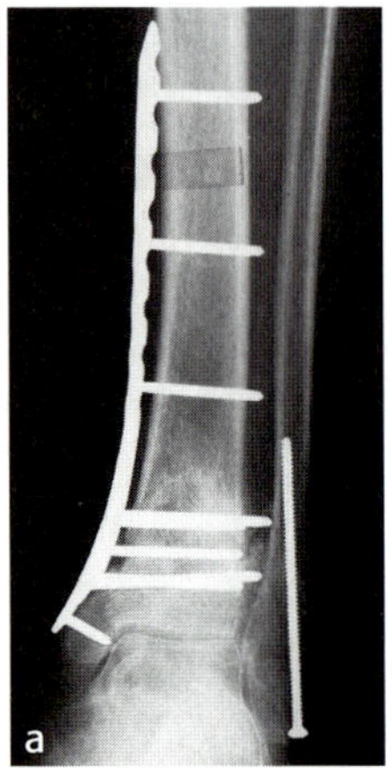

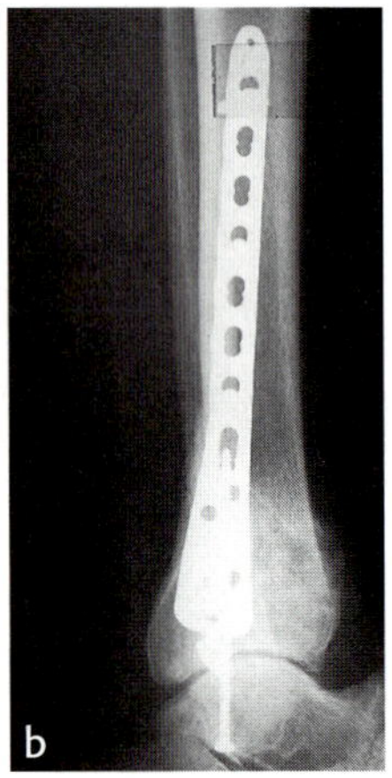

Fig 10.3.4-8a–b Postoperative x-rays after 12 months.
a AP view.
b Lateral view.

6 Pitfalls –

Equipment

Reduction and fixation

Rehabilitation

7 Pearls +

Equipment

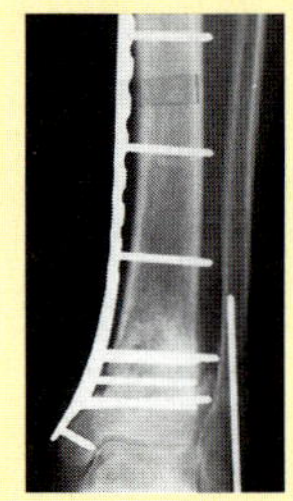

Fig 10.3.4-9 Osteoporotic and osteopenic bone requires long plates and bicortical locking head screws.

Reduction and fixation

Placement of screws: as close and as far away from the fracture site provides adequate stability.

Rehabilitation

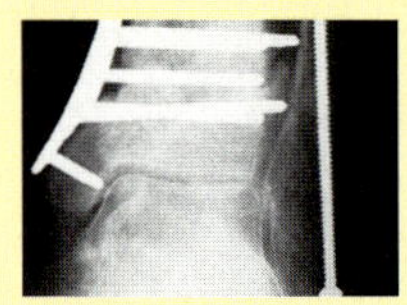

Fig 10.3.4-10 Percutaneous fixation requires no compromise in the reduction of articular fractures.

Authors Michael J Gardner, Dean G Lorich, David L Helfet

10.3.5 Articular multifragmentary distal tibial and fibular fracture—43-C3

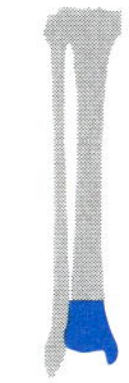

1 Case description

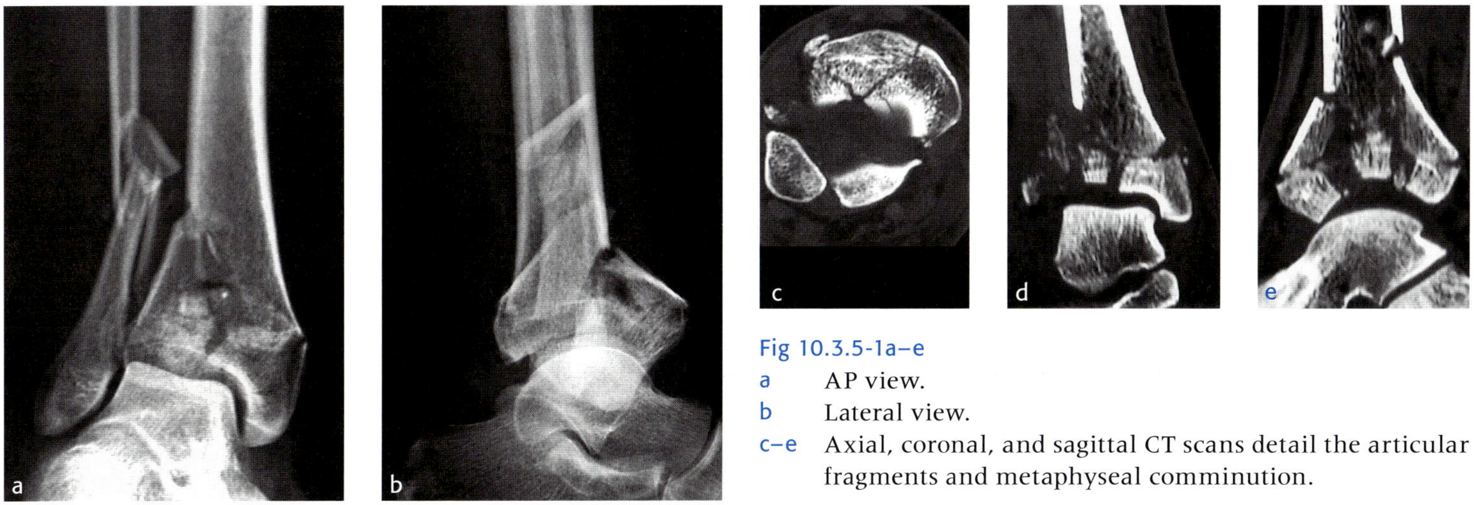

Fig 10.3.5-1a–e
a AP view.
b Lateral view.
c–e Axial, coronal, and sagittal CT scans detail the articular fragments and metaphyseal comminution.

55-year-old man riding a slow moving motorcycle, when it slipped out from underneath him and landed on his right ankle. He came to the emergency department complaining of significant pain and deformity. X-rays revealed a right articular pilon fracture, and an ankle-bridging external fixator was placed immediately. There were no associated injuries.
Moderate soft-tissue swelling was present with fracture blisters anteriorly and medially which persisted for 15 days before the soft tissues were suitable for surgery. There was no evidence of neurovascular compromise.

Indication

The intraarticular displacement and impaction warrants anatomical reduction and fixation to minimize the risk of the development of osteoarthrosis.
In addition, the metaphyseal comminution makes this fracture highly unstable, and warrants internal stabilization to ensure anatomical alignment.

Preoperative planning

Equipment
- LCP 3.5, 9 holes
- LCP reconstruction plate 3.5, 6 holes
- LCP buttress plate 3.5, 8 holes
- Locking head screws (LHS)
- 2.0 mm K-wires
- Large pelvic reduction forceps
- Large distractor
- Synthetic bone substitute

(Size of system, instruments, and implants can vary according to anatomy.)

Preoperative planning (cont)

Immediate treatment

Antibiotics: single dose 2nd generation cephalosporin
Place an external fixator immediately using a transverse Schanz screw through the proximal tibia and the calcaneus. This allows gross alignment of the fracture fragments by ligamentotaxis.
Elevate the patient's leg for 10–14 days until the soft tissues permit a surgical incision, as judged by wrinkling of the skin upon palpation.

Patient preparation and positioning

Fig 10.3.5-2 Position the patient supine on the operating table, place a tourniquet on the upper thigh, prepare and drape the leg free, and position the image intensifier to ensure adequate AP and lateral views.

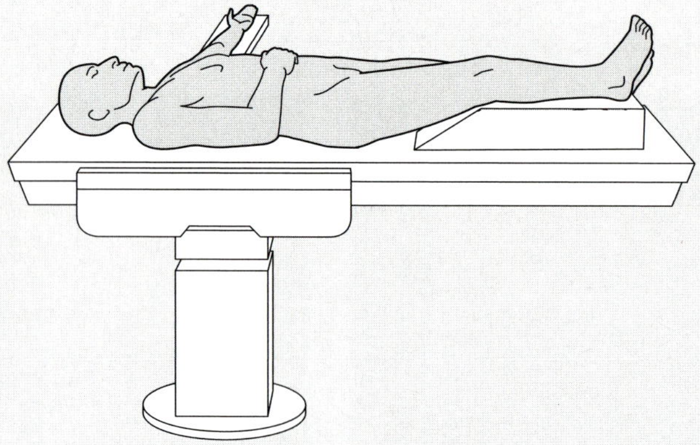

2 Surgical approach

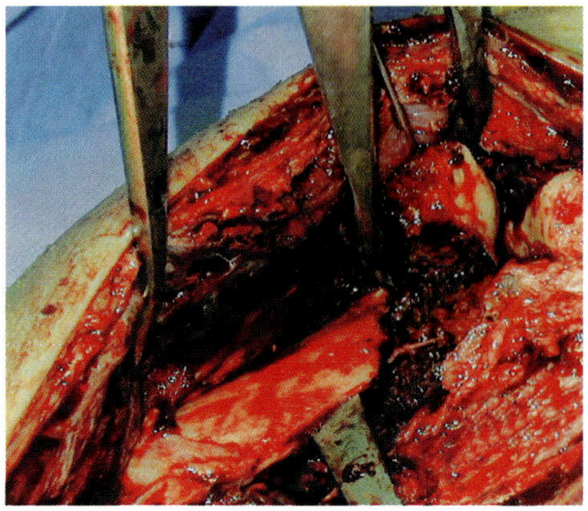

Fig 10.3.5-3 Make an incision directly over the fibula laterally, from the lateral malleolus and extending approximately 20 cm proximally.
Dissect to the level of the fascia of the peroneal muscles. Identify and protect the superficial peroneal nerve as the incision extends proximally.
Continue anterior to the peroneal muscles to expose the fibula, and then follow the interosseous membrane and anterior inferior tibiofibular ligament (AITFL) medially to the lateral border of the tibia. Take care to preserve the soft-tissue attachments, to the Chaput fragment, including the AITFL.
Elevate the anterior compartment muscles subperiosteally. Take care not to stray into the anterior compartment to avoid damage to the anterior tibial neurovascular bundle. The fibula and anterior and lateral tibia are now exposed.
For percutaneous application of the LCP buttress plate, make a 3 cm incision over the medial malleolus extending distally past the tip. Make a second 3 cm incision proximally, centered on the tibia in the lateral view, over where the planned site for the proximal end of the plate. Place the plate over the skin as a rough guide for placement. Gently slide tonsil clamps from each incision towards the other to bluntly develop the epiperiosteal space. Attach a threaded drill guide to the distal end of the plate for use as an insertion handle, and slide the plate subcutaneously up the medial tibia.

3 Reduction and fixation

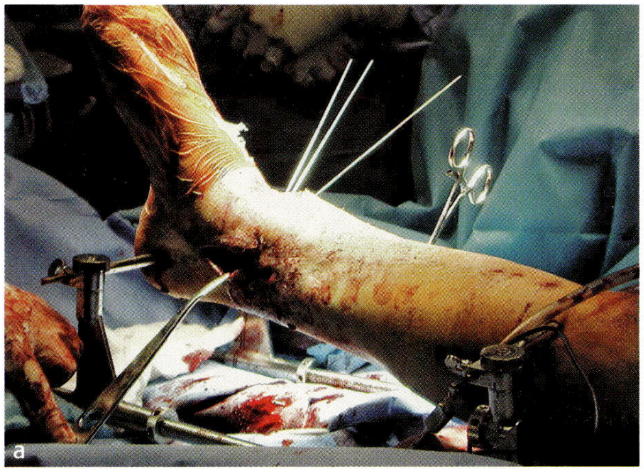

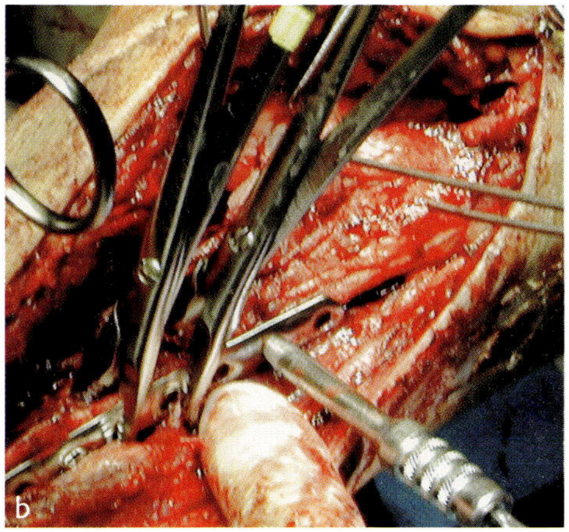

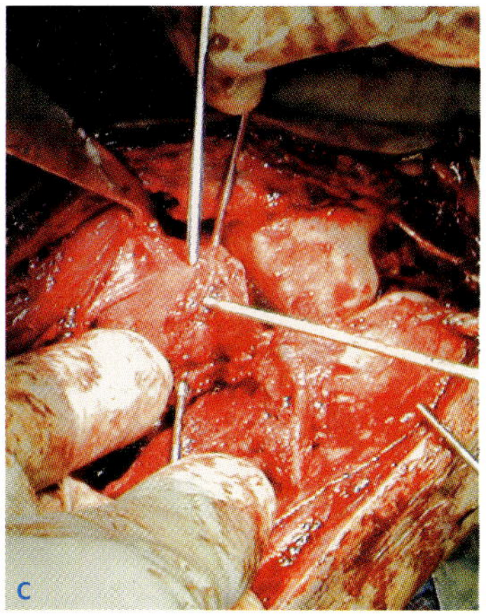

Fig 10.3.5-4a–f

a Remove the external fixator and place the large distractor on the same Schanz screws, both medially and laterally. Position the threaded bars posteriorly to elevate the leg off the table.

b First, reduce and stabilize the fibula using a straight LCP. If comminution exists and the fibula is shortened, a push-pull technique may be used with a laminar spreader and a screw outside the plate to aid reduction. Extreme care must be taken to achieve anatomical reduction of the fibula, as this will ultimately affect reduction of the tibia.
Next, identify the anterolateral key tibial fragment. This Chaput tubercle fragment is frequently large and attached to an intact anterior tibiofibular ligament. Following reduction of the fibula, this may be roughly reduced to the tibia.
Hinge the Chaput fragment anteriorly to identify the posterior Volkmann fragments. These may be visualized directly and reduced and stabilized. This step is critical in achieving anatomical articular reduction.

c Next, insert threaded K-wires into the Chaput tubercle to use as joysticks. Reduce the tubercle directly using the talus as a mold, and stabilize it provisionally with K-wires. Assess reduction under image intensification.
Disimpact any additional articular fragments from the metaphyseal defect.

3 Reduction and fixation (cont)

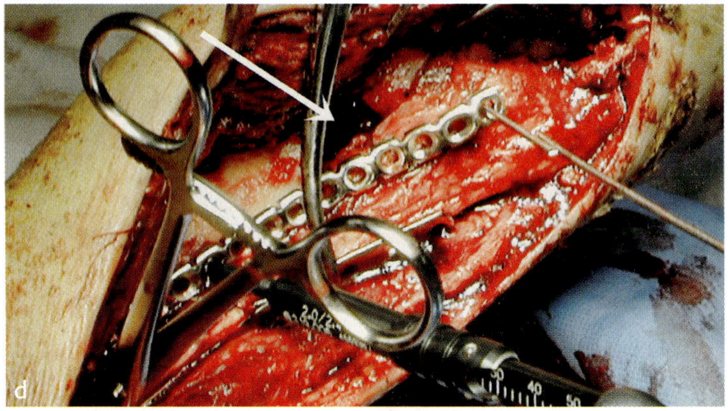

d

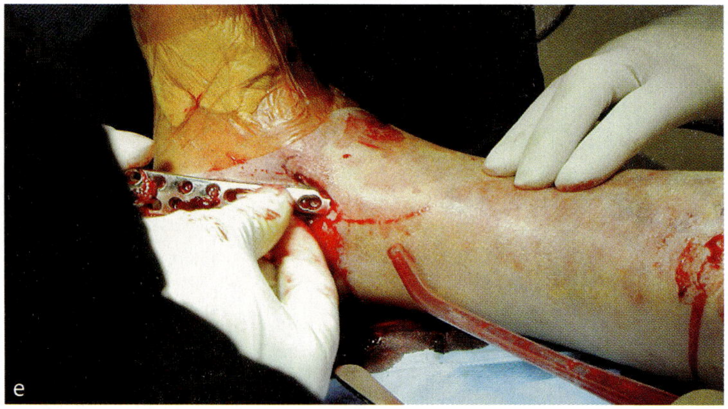

e

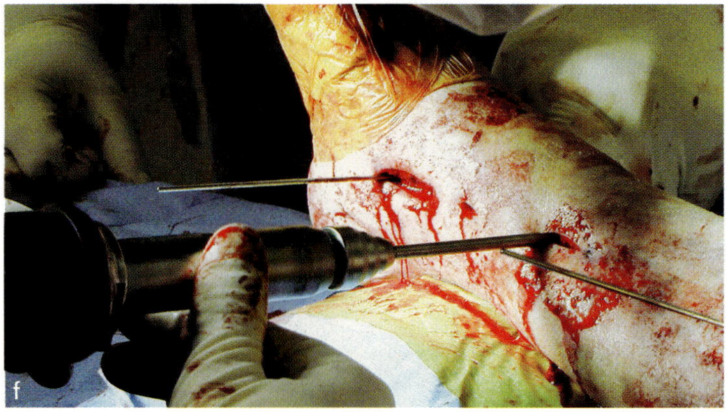

f

Fig 10.3.5-4a–f (cont)

d Contour a locking reconstruction plate 3.5, and secure it to the anterolateral surface of the tibia.
Most high-energy pilon fractures will have some element of metaphyseal impaction. Confirm under image intensification that the length of the articular block has been restored. Adjusting the femoral distractors can improve length. Place a locking head screw proximally to secure the anterior plate.

e Next, place a LCP buttress plate subcutaneously through a small distal incision. A lag screw may be placed if an oblique or spiral fracture line exists. Compression screws may be directed through the plate anteriorly or posteriorly to capture the Chaput or Volkmann fragments, respectively.

f Use the image intensifier to determine the location of the plate holes, and place proximal locking head screws percutaneously through stab incisions.
Having achieved overall stability of the metaphyseal and articular fragments with the previously placed anterolateral and medial plates, fine tune the articular reduction under direct and image intensifier visualization, and provisionally secure with K-wires. Strategically direct subchondral lag screws across the articular fragments to achieve ultimate fixation.
Fill the metaphyseal defect with iliac crest bone graft or synthetic bone substitute.
Close the wound over medium suction drains. Apply a short leg plaster splint in the operating room.

4 Rehabilitation

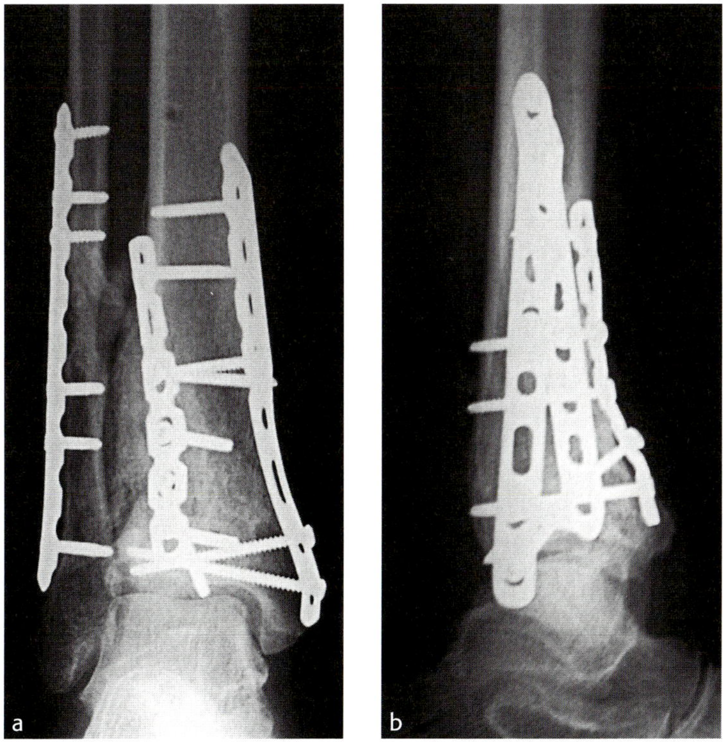

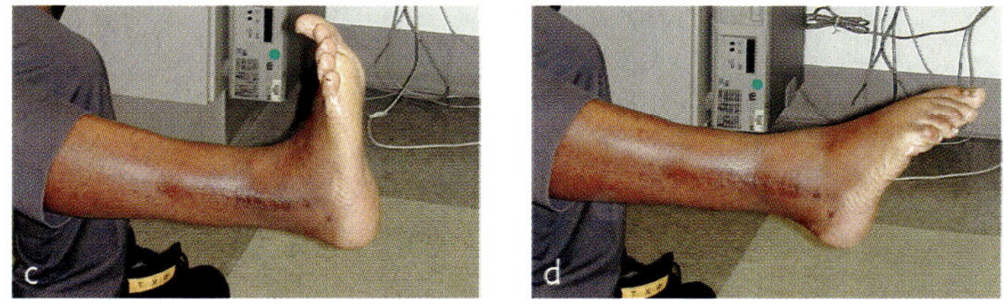

Continue prophylactic antibiotics for 24 hours.
Initiate deep venous thrombosis prophylaxis with low-molecular heparin.
On postoperative day 2, remove the splint, check the wound, and apply a rigid walking boot.

Fig 10.3.5-5a–d Postoperative x-rays.
a AP view.
b Lateral view.
c–d Physiotherapy should commence early, and include crutch or walker training, 9 kg touchdown weight bearing, and aggressive active and passive ankle range of motion exercises.

5 Pitfalls –

Equipment

If a locking plate is bent through a hole, the locking hole threads become distorted and will no longer fit a threaded guide or locking head screw.

Approach

The superficial peroneal nerve is at risk during the fibular approach.
The anterior tibial neurovascular bundle may be damaged while dissecting across the interosseous membrane. The fascial envelope is often disrupted by the fracture and the anatomy is distorted.
Several large veins are located subcutaneously along the medial side of the leg and are at risk when making stab incisions.

Reduction and fixation

Visualizing and reducing the articular fragments may be difficult.
Significant metaphyseal impaction often exists.

Rehabilitation

Some degree of ankle stiffness frequently occurs following multifragmentary intraarticular pilon fractures.

6 Pearls +

Equipment

Use standard plate benders to contour the plate. Plan which holes will be used for locking head screws, and be certain not to bend the plate through these holes. Only bend locking reconstruction plates through the notches.

Approach

The superficial peroneal nerve pierces the fascia in the line of the lateral incision as it extends proximally. Be aware of its position and protect it.
As dissection progresses medially, raise the anterior compartment musculature subperiosteally from the fibula and tibia, and directly from the interosseous membrane. Do not stray anteriorly into the muscle bellies to avoid the anterior tibial vessels and nerve.
Be aware of these large veins, they can often be visualized or palpated through the skin. Make incisions through the subcutaneous layer, and spread it gently to avoid incising the veins.

Reduction and fixation

In order to adequately reduce the articular surface, begin posteriorly with the Volkmann fragment. Visualize this by retracting the Chaput tubercle. Progress sequentially in an anterior direction. Stabilize provisionally with K-wires.
Reducing the fibula anatomically at first will help estimate the appropriate length of the distal tibia. Use the large distractor, and assess joint line obliquity to finalize length determination.

Rehabilitation

Prior to discharge, replace the plaster splint with a removable rigid cast boot. Initiate early physiotherapy to assist in aggressive active and passive range of motion.

Author Christoph Sommer

10.3.6 Complete articular multifragmentary distal tibial fracture (pilon)—43-C3

1 Case description

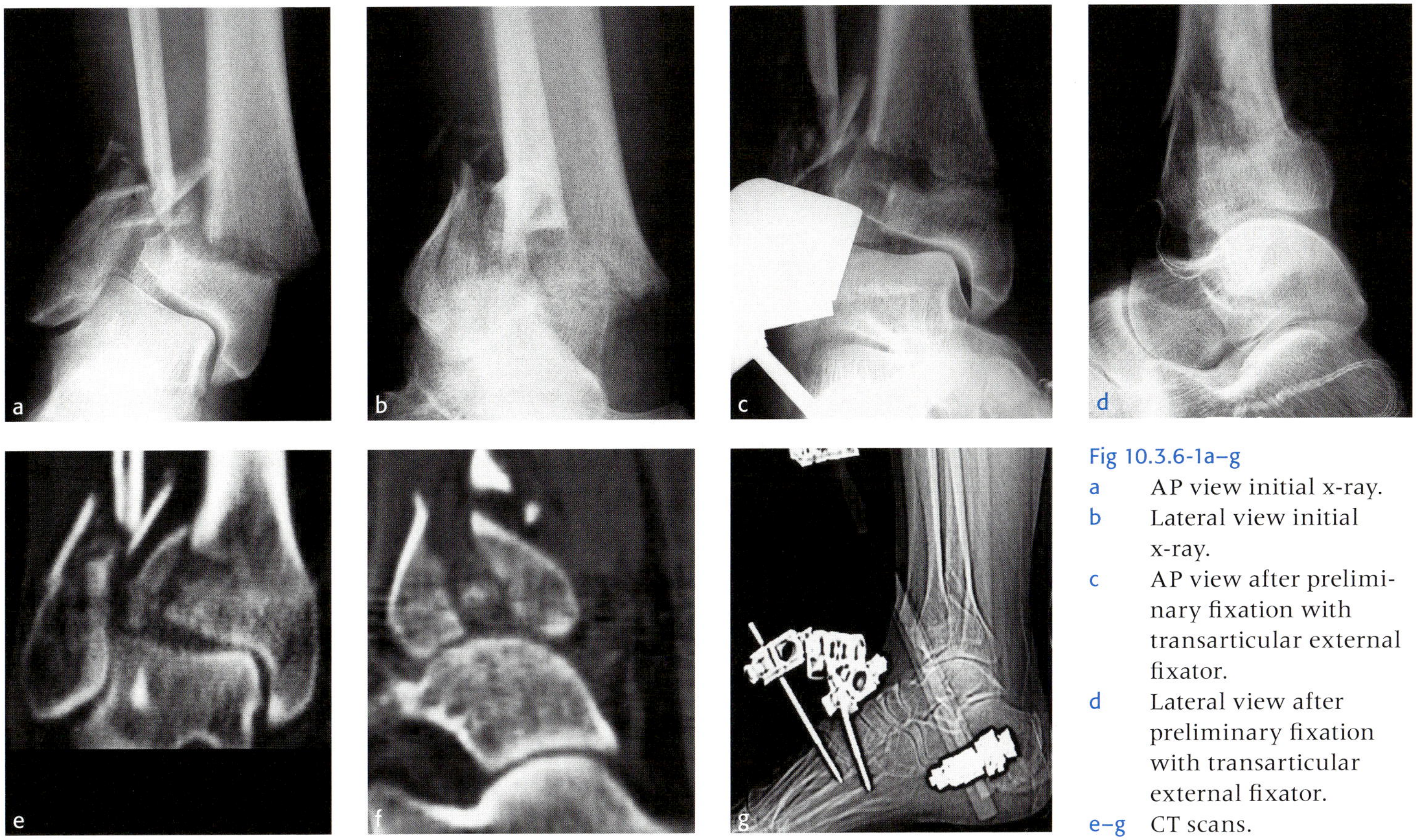

Fig 10.3.6-1a–g

- a AP view initial x-ray.
- b Lateral view initial x-ray.
- c AP view after preliminary fixation with transarticular external fixator.
- d Lateral view after preliminary fixation with transarticular external fixator.
- e–g CT scans.

62-year-old woman slipped on a ladder and fell approximately 1 m to the ground. She suffered a distal articular lower leg fracture. There was a severe displacement in the metaphyseal zone with major soft-tissue injury above the medial malleolus (Tscherne grade II). The articular surface of the tibia as well as the supramalleolar fibula had fractured into several fragments. The valgus malalignment was reduced with an external fixator bridging the ankle joint. CT imaging showed a multifragmentary joint fracture of the tibia (43-C3) with at least one large impacted central fragment. The anterolateral fragment appeared to be still attached to the distal fibula by the intact anterior syndesmotic ligament.

Indication

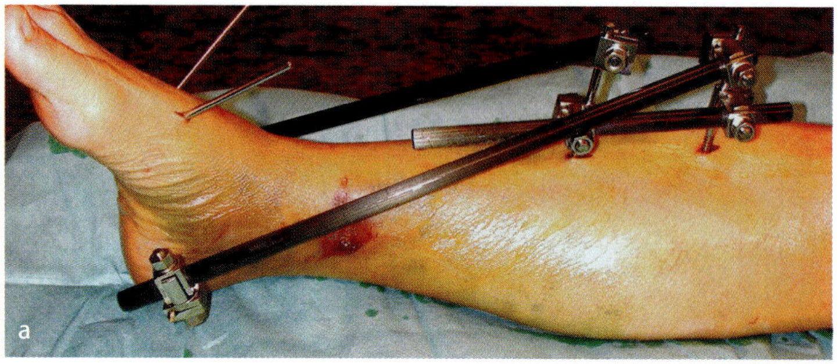

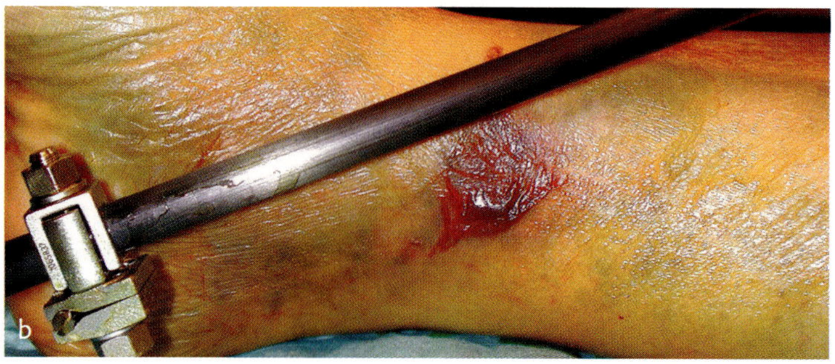

Fig 10.3.6-2a–b This displaced pilon fracture is an absolute indication for reduction and fixation of the tibia and the fibula. Due to the soft-tissue injury and the complexity of the fracture, a staged procedure is advised. First the fracture is bridged with a transarticular external fixator until the swelling has diminished.

Conventional definitive reconstruction according to the AO Principles of Fracture Management consists of four steps:
1. the reconstruction of the fibula,
2. the reconstruction of the tibial joint surface,
3. cancellous bone grafting at the metaphyseal defect, and
4. anteromedial plate osteosynthesis of the tibia.

Alternatively, a percutaneous screw osteosynthesis and a hybrid fixator could be used. Nevertheless, a minimal open joint approach is required to reduce the central impacted fragment.
In this case, prior fixation of the tibia and subsequent fixation of the fibula is preferable because, given the multifragmentary fracture of the fibula, correct reduction in length and rotation of the fibula would be very difficult.

Preoperative planning

Equipment
- One-third tubular plate, 4 holes
- LCP T-plate 3.5, 6 hole
- LCP 3.5, 10 holes
- 3.5 mm self-tapping locking head screws (LHS)
- 3.5 mm cortex screw
- 1.2 mm and 1.6 mm K-wires
- Large Weber forceps
- Large distractor

(Size of system, instruments, and implants can vary according to anatomy.)

Patient preparation and positioning
Antibiotics: single dose 2nd generation cephalosporin
Thrombosis prophylaxis: low-molecular heparin

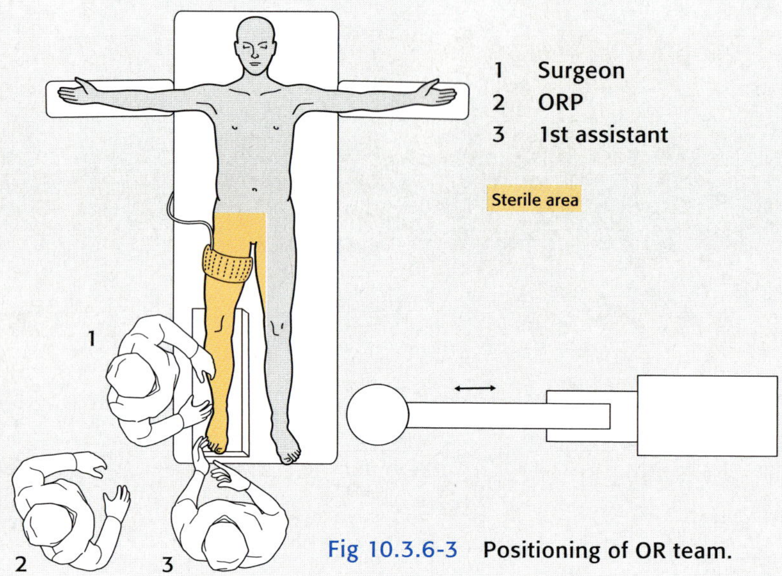

Fig 10.3.6-3 Positioning of OR team.

2 Surgical approach

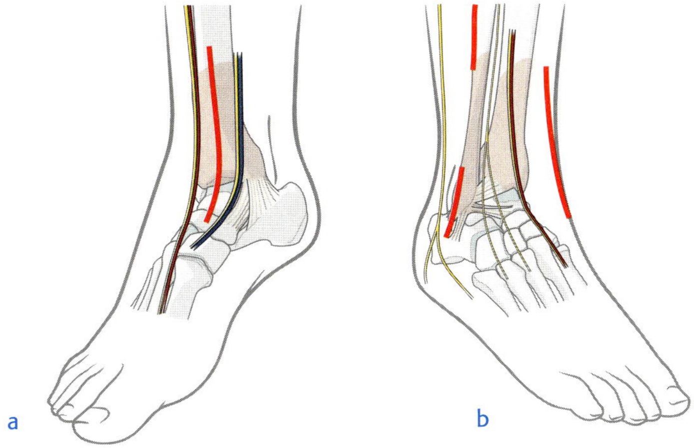

Fig 10.3.6-4a–b A small anteromedial straight approach of limited length is made in the direction of the ankle joint. The incision begins about 5 cm cranial to the ankle joint over the anterior tibial edge in the direction of the talonavicular joint. The bridging (MIPO) of the fibula is carried out in minimally invasive technique. The approach is limited to the proximal and distal ends of the plate at the posterolateral margin of the fibula.

3 Reduction and fixation

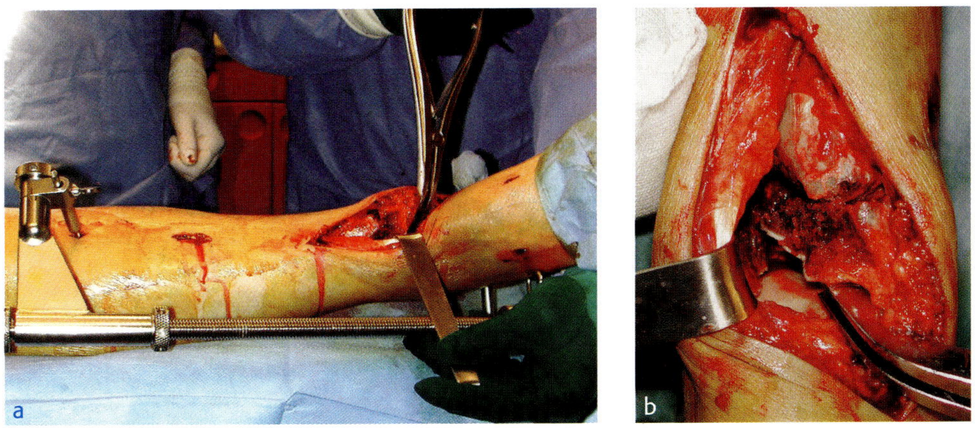

Fig 10.3.6-5a–b

a The definitive stabilization of the pilon fracture is performed on the seventh day after injury. The external fixator is removed except for the Schanz screws in the calcaneus and in the proximal tibial shaft. The large distractor is now mounted on these two screws. The ankle joint is reduced and distracted. The distraction permits excellent direct vision of the tibial joint surface.

b The anteromedial approach is made onto the periosteum. A limited horizontal capsulotomy is performed in a caudal direction. The anterolateral fragment is held aside. The periosteum is handled carefully and detached minimally at the fracture lines (1–2 mm).

3 Reduction and fixation (cont)

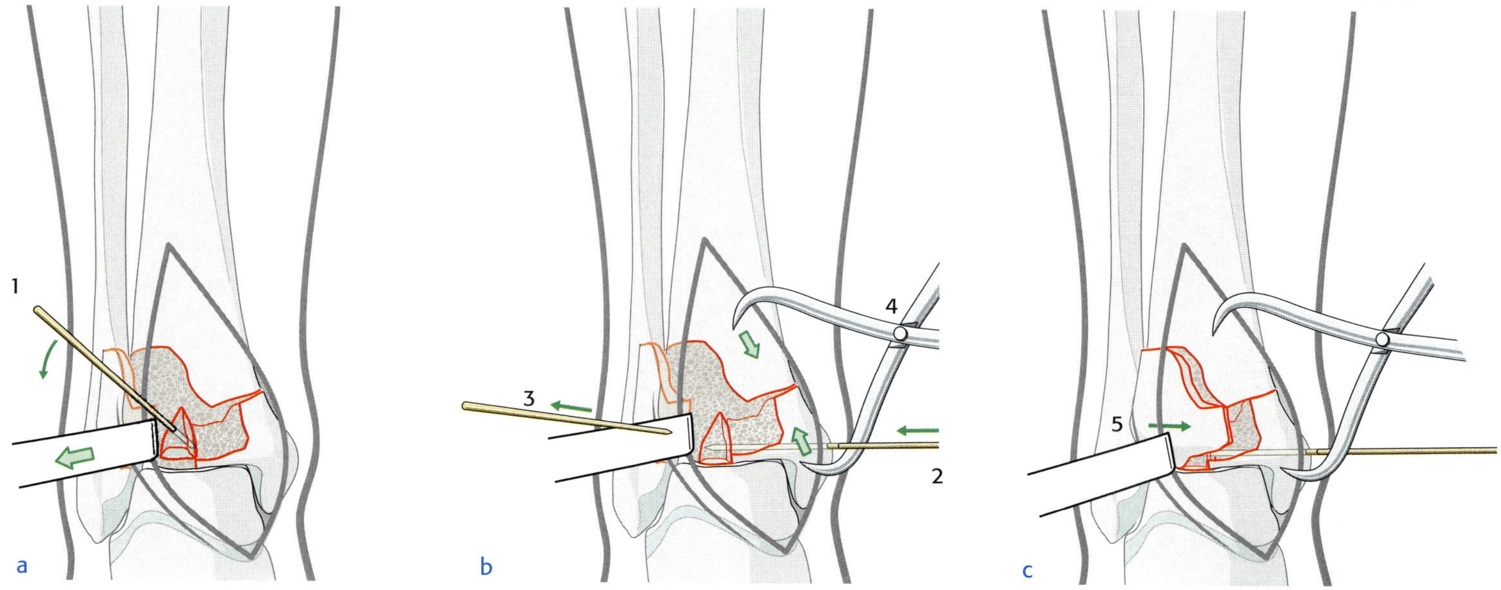

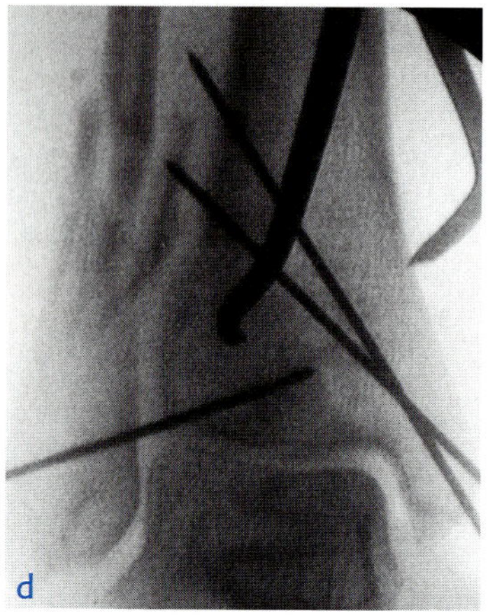

Fig 10.3.6-6a–n

a The impacted central fragment is now visible. A 1.2 mm K-wire is inserted as a joystick into the central fragment (**1**). With the help of this joystick, the fragment can be rotated and reduced to its anatomical position. After correct reduction, the K-wire is drilled into the posterior articular fragment (**2**).

b–c As this K-wire prevents the reduction of the anterolateral fragment, it will be replaced by a second K-wire inserted percutaneously over the medial malleolus (**3**). The reconstructed joint block is now finally reduced to the metaphysis by a large Weber forceps (**4**). To achieve this, the distraction over the large distractor has to be released.

d Preliminary fixation is achieved by two 1.6 mm K-wires inserted from the medial malleolus. The anterolateral fragment can be reduced and temporarily fixed with another K-wire (**5**).

3 Reduction and fixation (cont)

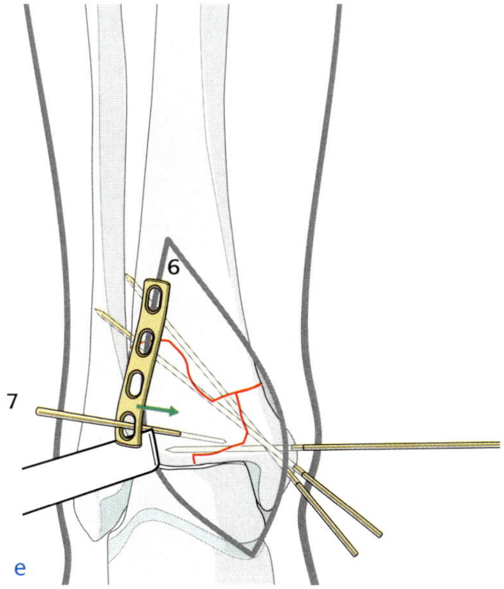

e

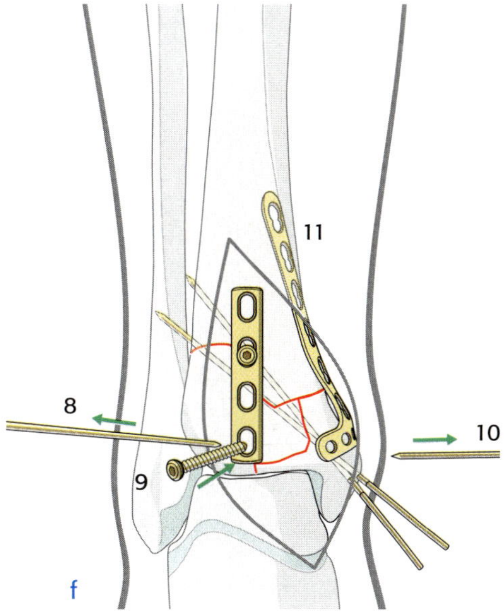

f

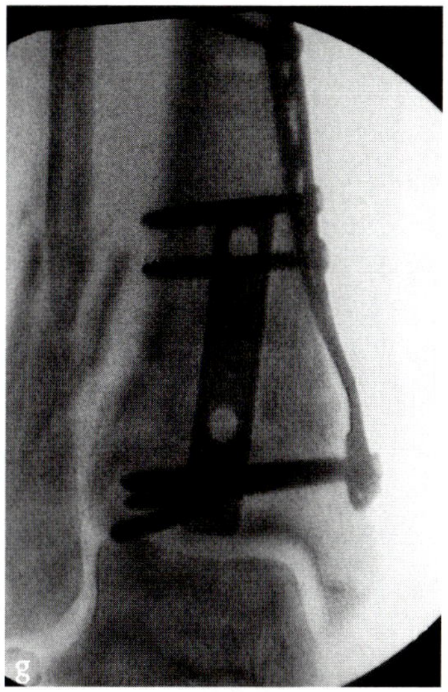

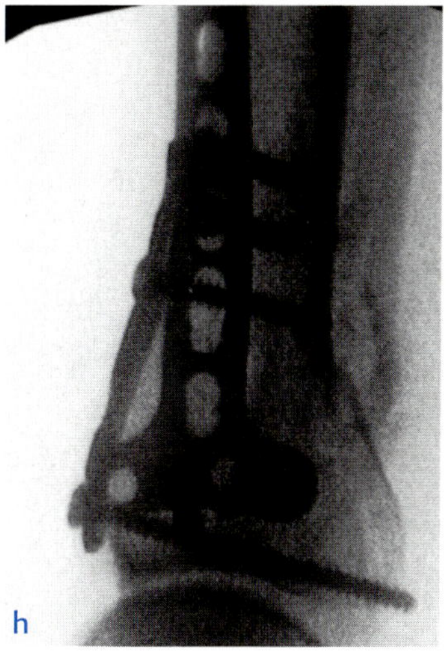

h

Fig 10.3.6-7a–n (cont)

e A bent 4-hole one-third tubular plate (**6**) is placed over the anterolateral K-wire (**7**) and onto the anterolateral tibia. The plate is fixed first by insertion of a 3.5 mm cortex screw into the second proximal hole. The plate pushes the fragment against the bone (antiglide plate). Now the anterolateral K-wire can be removed (**8**). A 3.5 mm cortex lag screw is inserted through the distal hole, compressing the anterolateral syndesmotic fragment to the central and posterior joint fragments (**9**).

f The K-wire holding the central fragment is now removed (**10**). An LCP T-plate 3.5 is bent and inserted medially close to the level of the joint space (**11**). This plate is first fixed with a 3.5 mm cortex screw proximal to the fracture. 3.5 mm self-tapping LHS are chosen for the most distal holes; the screws should be as long as possible without penetrating the opposite cortex (syndesmosis). The holes are drilled over the drill sleeves allowing correct measurement of ideal screw length. Finally, the plate is fixed proximally by two further screws.

g–h Intraoperative x-rays confirm the anatomical reduction and stable fixation of the tibia. They also show the epiperiosteal position of the two plates.

3 Reduction and fixation (cont)

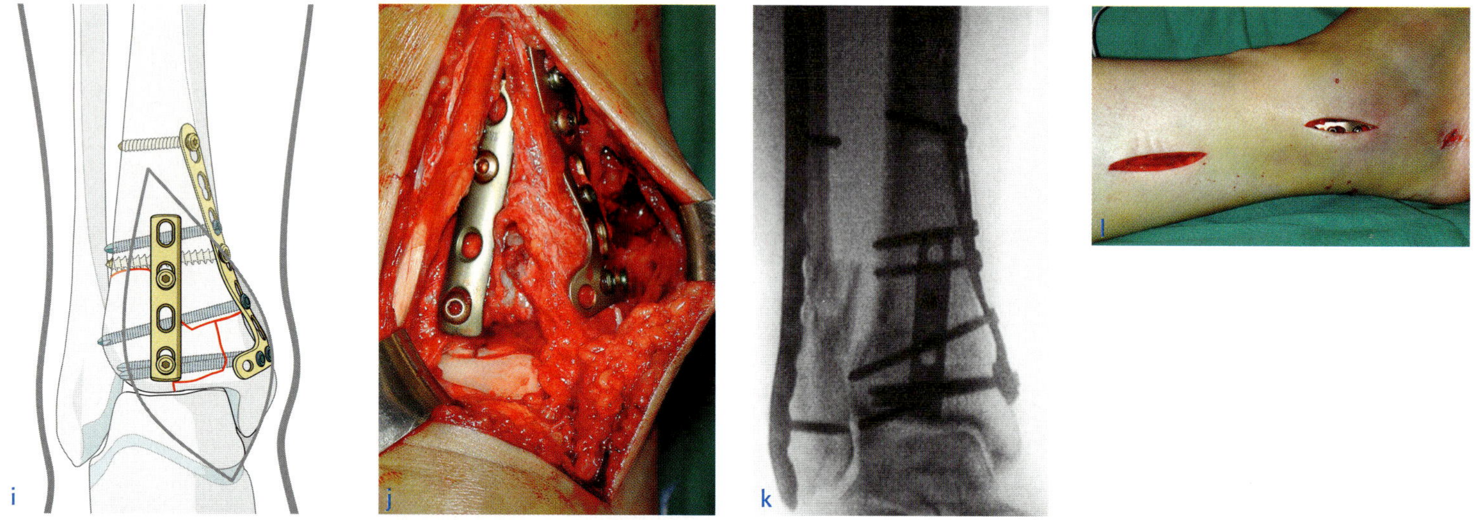

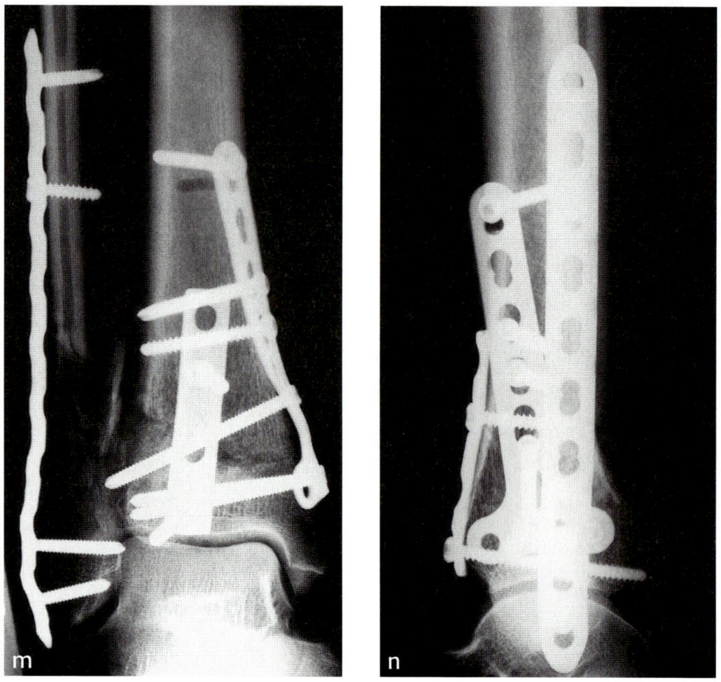

Fig 10.3.6-6a–n (cont)

i–j The small periosteal "window" can be seen between the two plates. Also, the limited horizontal arthrotomy at the joint rim level is visible.

k Minimally invasive osteosynthesis (MIPO) of the fibula is the final step. A slightly contoured 10-hole LCP 3.5 is inserted from distal to proximal through the small incisions mentioned earlier. First the plate is fixed with an LHS in the distal fragment. The correct length of the fibula is assessed under image intensification. Subsequently, a 3.5 mm cortex screw fixes the plate tightly to the proximal shaft fragment.

l After correct axial alignment has been achieved and confirmed in the lateral view, definitive fixation with LHS proximally and distally is performed. The clinical appearance before skin closure is shown.

m–n The postoperative x-rays two days after surgery show anatomical reduction and stable fixation of the tibia with a congruent ankle and correct axial alignment. The fibula is also correct in length.

4 Rehabilitation

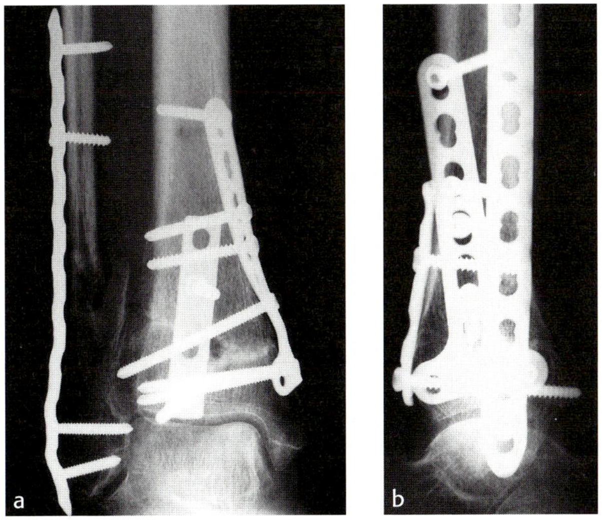

The skin lesion above the medial malleolus developed into a dry necrosis of about 2 cm and had to be treated with a fasciocutaneous flap. For this reason, the ankle was stabilized with a removable hinged splint for 6 weeks. Mobilization started two weeks after the operation with 0–15 kg weight bearing, changed to full loading after 3 months. The tibia was fully consolidated after 4 months with still ongoing bone healing of the fibula.

Fig 10.3.6-7a–b Postoperative x-rays after 4 months.
a AP view.
b Lateral view.

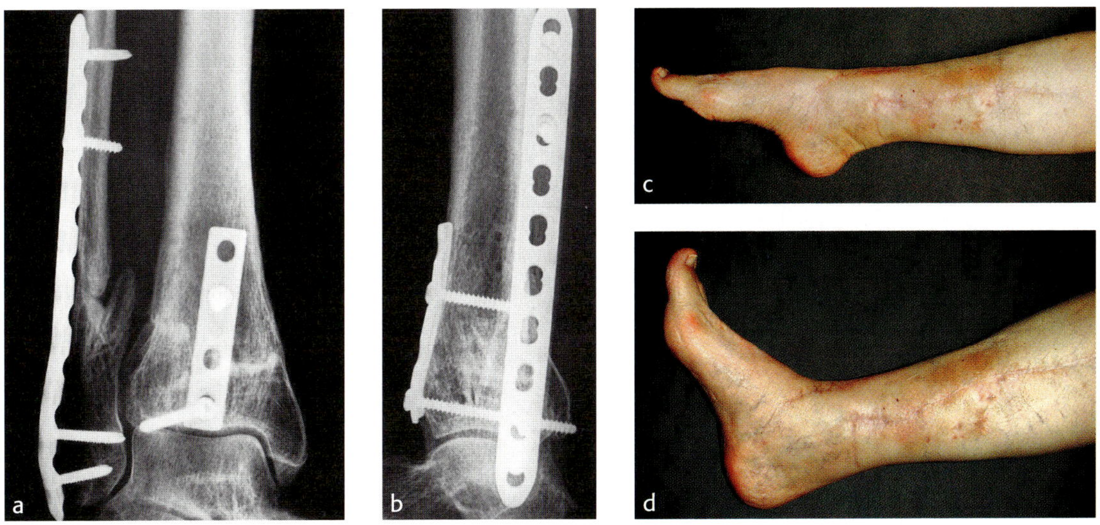

Fig 10.3.6-8a–d The medial plate was removed 1 year after surgery on the request of the patient. Scar correction was performed at the same time. The x-rays at this point show a fully consolidated tibia and fibula and no signs of posttraumatic osteoarthritis. Full range of motion was present at that time and the skin lesion had healed.

5 Pitfalls –

Equipment

Approach
A too small incision for the tibia could complicate or even prevent an anatomical joint reduction. A too wide exposure could provoke skin necrosis.

Reduction and fixation
Double plate osteosynthesis is only recommended with low profile plates. In the presence of joint incongruence, posttraumatic arthrosis may occur. The fixation of the articular part has to be absolutely stable—using the compression method with lag screws and buttress plating. If not, osteonecrosis, mainly of the central fragment, may become manifest.

Timing is crucial: if the ORIF is performed too early, wound healing problems may occur.

Rehabilitation
If mobilized too early or with too much weight, secondary collapse and/or implant failure can occur.

6 Pearls +

Equipment
Angular stable screw-plate systems such as the LCP are ideal for complex pilon fractures. MIPO technique is facilitated by these implants.

Approach
A limited open approach to the tibia offers the possibility of correct anatomical reduction with a limited risk of wound healing problems. A minimally invasive approach decreases the risk of perfusion damage to an already endangered multifragmentary zone (fibula).

Reduction and fixation
Locking head screws also stabilize the small joint block.

Rehabilitation
Early functional postoperative treatment is possible even in complex fractures provided that the fracture is well stabilized.

Authors Michael D Stover, Hobie D Summers

10.3.7 Open complete articular multifragmentary distal tibial and fibular fracture—43-C2

1 Case description

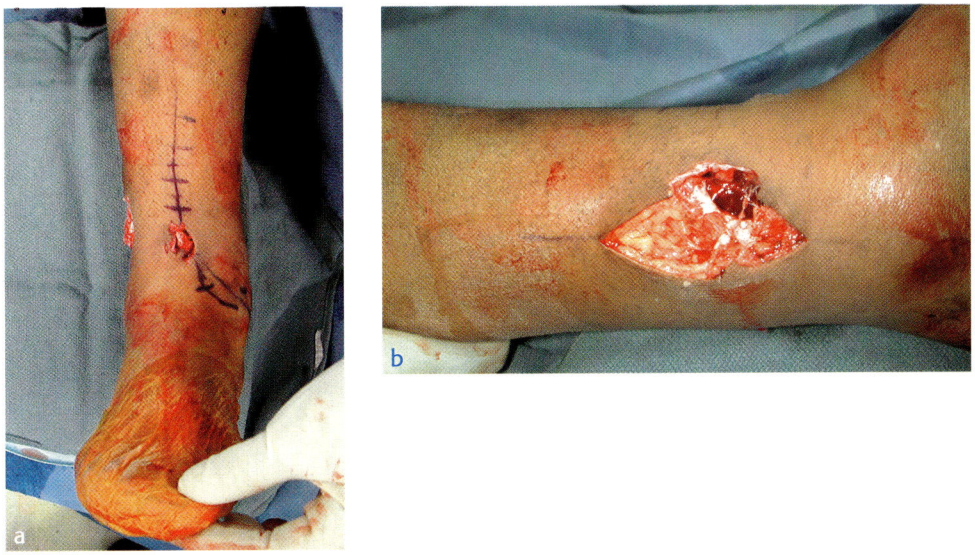

27-year-old man suffered a high velocity ballistic injury on the right distal tibia; high energy trauma with open fracture (Gustilo type IIIB).

Fig 10.3.7-1a–f
a–b Clinical pictures of extremity: Planned incision incoporates anterior entrance wound, the lateral exit wound is also shown.
c–d Initial AP and lateral x-rays.
e–f Traction views can be helpful in identifying fracture fragments.

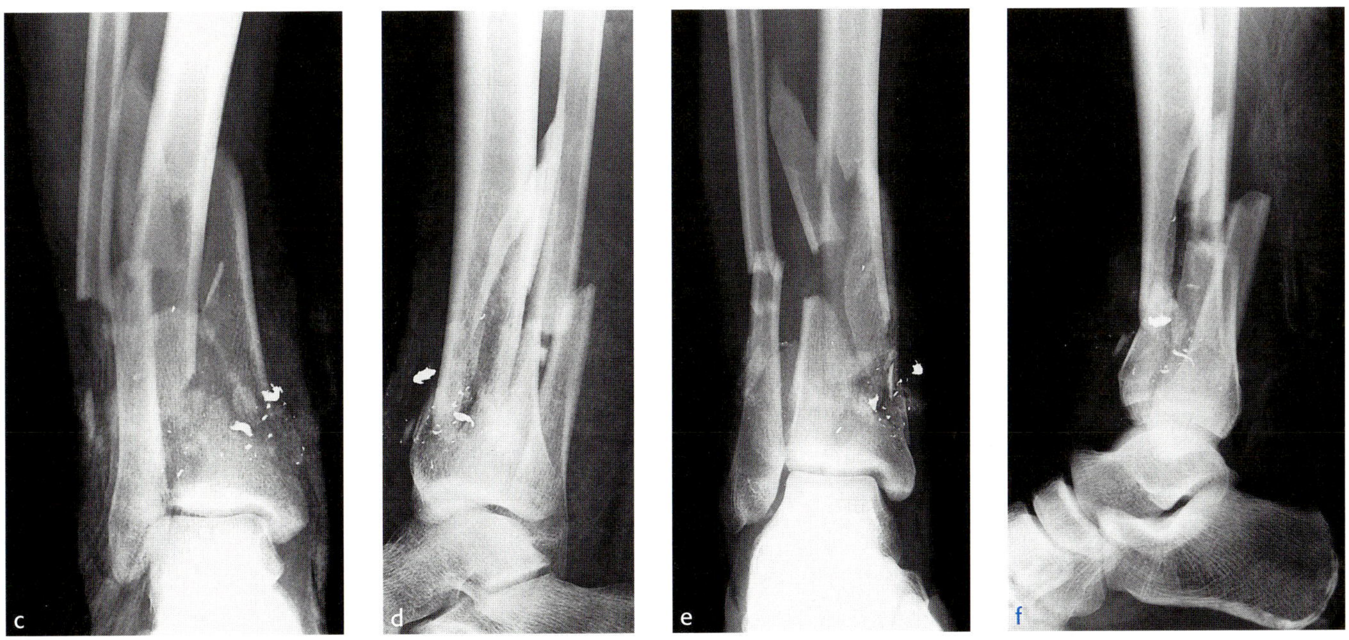

Indication

Complete articular fracture of the distal tibia with metaphyseal fragmentation and associated fracture of the fibula. Operative indications include articular displacement greater than 2 mm, ankle joint instability, and unacceptable axial alignment of the limb. Operative treatment will restore joint congruity, skeletal stability, overall limb alignment, and allows for early functional rehabilitation and joint motion to improve cartilage nutrition and healing. The primary risk of surgical intervention concernes the soft-tissue envelope. Careful handling of the skin and surrounding soft tissues is crucial for a successful outcome. In this case, nonoperative treatment is likely to lead to a poor result with possible malunion, nonunion, stiffness from immobilization, and arthrosis of the ankle joint. Operative treatment also provides skeletal stability for appropriate care of the soft-tissue injury associated with open fractures.

Preoperative planning

Equipment

- LCP distal tibial plate 2.7/3.0, medial, 12 holes
- 3.5 mm locking head screws (LHS)
- 3.5 mm cortex screws
- 2.0 mm K-wires
- Large distractor
- Pulsatile irrigator (open fracture)
- Intramedullary device, small fragment for fibular stabilization

(Size of system, instruments, and implants can vary according to anatomy.)

Patient preparation and positioning

Antibiotics: cephalosporin

Thrombosis prophylaxis: low-molecular heparin

Lateral column (fibular) fixation may not be necessary with the use of an angular stable device. This may be used as a tool for indirect reduction of the tibia or in the case of an open fracture with residual displacement (as in this case).

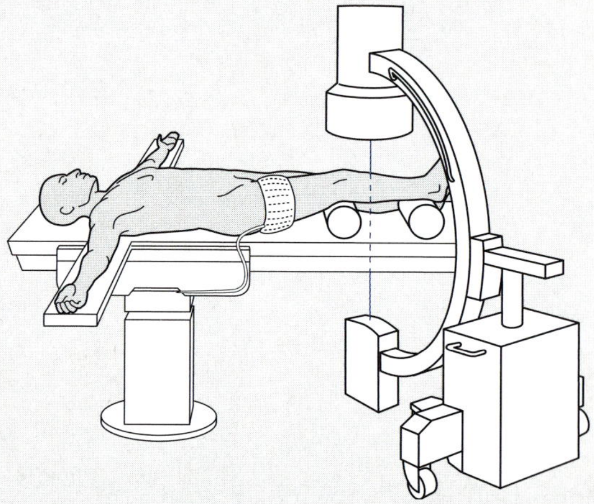

Fig 10.3.7-2 Supine on radiolucent table. Nonsterile pneumatic tourniquet around thigh. Bump under affected hip to internally rotate the limb.

2 Surgical approach

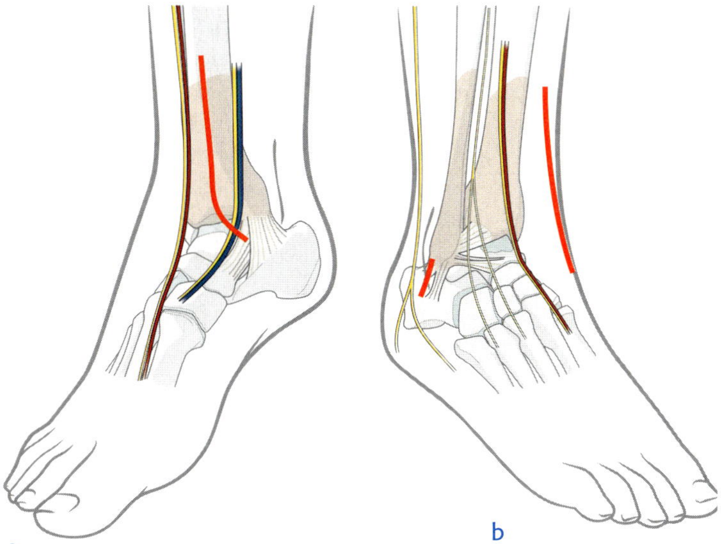

a

b

Fig 10.3.7-3a–b Make a 3–5 cm curvilinear skin incision over the anterior portion of the medial malleolus and anterior medial joint to allow for adequate joint visualization in the presence of articular involvement. Alternatively for extraarticular (A-type) fractures, a 2–3 cm longitudinal incision can be made over the medial malleolus to expose the distal tip without entering the ankle joint, preserving the periosteum when possible.

Preserve the saphenous vein and nerve as they pass anterior to the medial malleolus. Anterior horizontal arthrotomy can be performed to evaluate joint reduction or anterolateral fragments can be hinged open on their distal lateral ligaments. Talar access for placement of a Schanz screw and medium distractor for indirect reduction is anterior to the deep deltoid ligament in the nonarticular anterior talar body.

3 Reduction

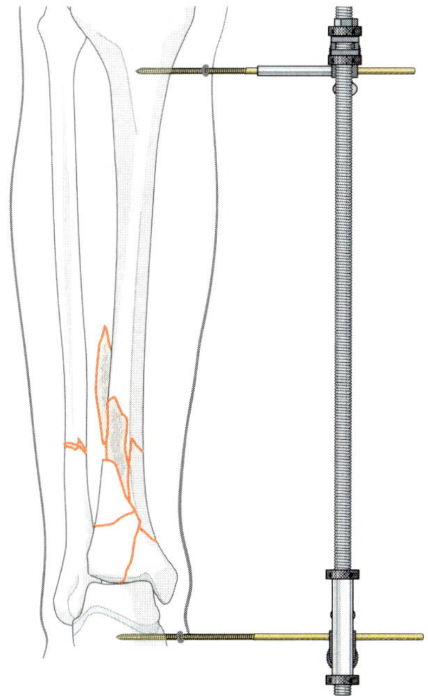

Articular reconstruction should precede placement of the plate. Reduce the articular fragments under direct visualization and/or with the assistance of an image intensifier using periarticular clamps or K-wires as joysticks. The fragments may be provisionally fixed with 2.0 mm K-wires.

Obtain indirect reduction of axial and rotational alignment. This can be performed with a medium distractor. Manual indirect reduction through the foot can be facilitated with the use of small towel bumps, slightly larger just below the knee than at the metaphyseal fracture site to allow for posterior proximal tibial slope.

Fig 10.3.7-4 Indirect reduction of axial and rotational alignment can be performed with a medium distractor.

4 Fixation

Obtain interfragmentary fixation of the articular fragments with small or mini fragment screws. Fixation immediately cephalad to the joint surface, if possible, will allow for subsequent placement of angular stable locking head screws without interference. Fixation of articular fragments must precede fixation of the articular block to the metaphyseal/diaphyseal segment.

Assemble the LCP distal tibial plate with 2–3 screw guides threaded into the plate along with a threaded plate holder to assist with insertion and subsequent distal screw placement. Insert the LCP distal medial tibial plate in the incision and slide it subcutaneously and extraperiosteally along the posteromedial border of the bone. Due to the subcutaneous nature of the medial surface of the tibia, direct palpation and guidance of the plate placement is possible. Verify plate position on AP and lateral x-rays. When the plate is correctly positioned over the distal block, temporary fixation may be accomplished with a 2.0 mm K-wire through the hole provided in the plate.

Once length, rotation, and axial alignment have been corrected, secure the plate to the proximal fragment. A small incision (5 mm) is made over a plate hole proximally. Drill 2.5 mm monocortical holes through the plate proximally and distally, placing 3.5 mm cortex screws into each fragment to secure the plate to the bone.

Full length biplanar x-rays may be indicated prior to final fixation to confirm alignment. Begin locking head screw insertion distally using the 2.8 mm threaded drill guide and drill bit for 3.5 mm locking head screws. It is important to note that all lag/compression screws must be placed prior to the placement of locking head screws. The distal screw holes are designed to be parallel to the joint surface. Monocortical fixation is generally adequate but bicortical fixation may be considered in osteoporotic bone. The number of fixation points will be determined based on bone quality and fracture reduction.

Place proximal screws by making small incisions over plate holes and securing 2.8 mm guide into plate. The screw length can be determined by direct measurement. Working screws can be removed once locked fixation is obtained in each fragment, since these were placed in a monocortical fashion and have now been replaced with a bicortical locking head screw.

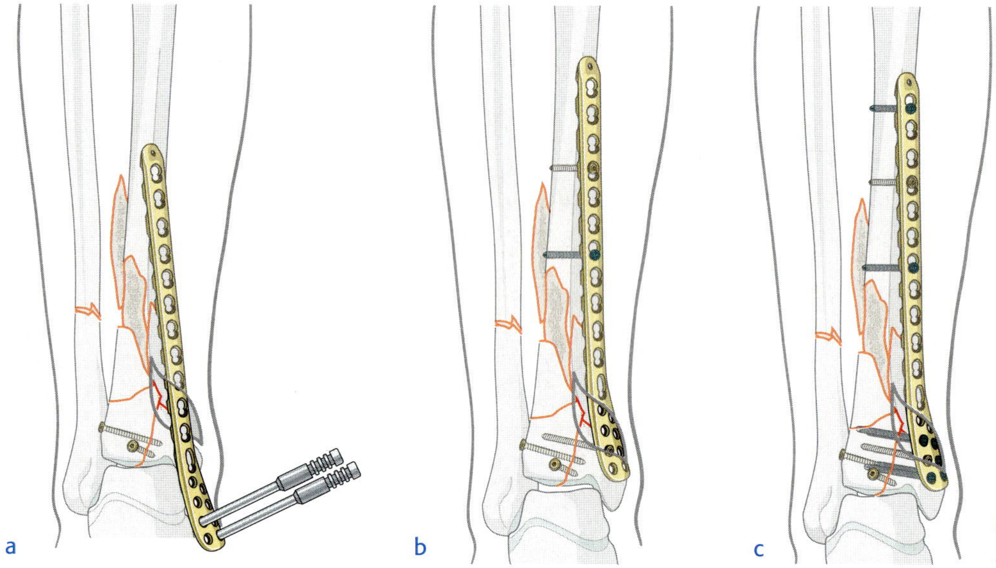

Fig 10.3.7-5a–c Insertion and fixation of the LCP distal tibial plate.

4 Fixation (cont)

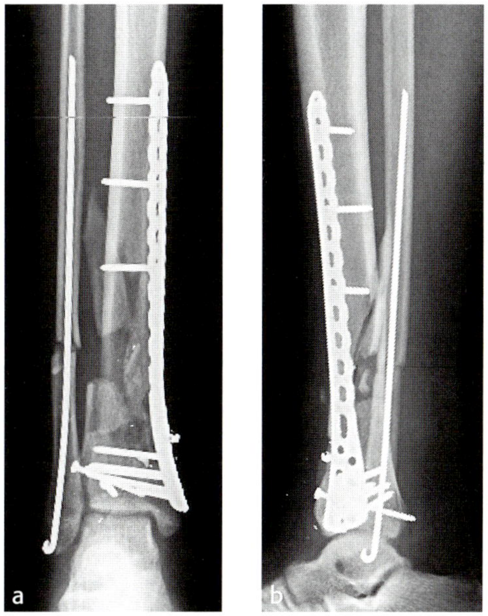

Fig 10.3.7-6a–b Obtain plain x-rays prior to the end of the operation.

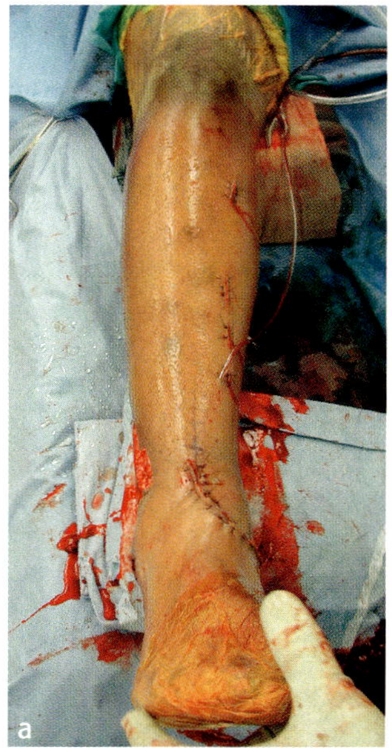

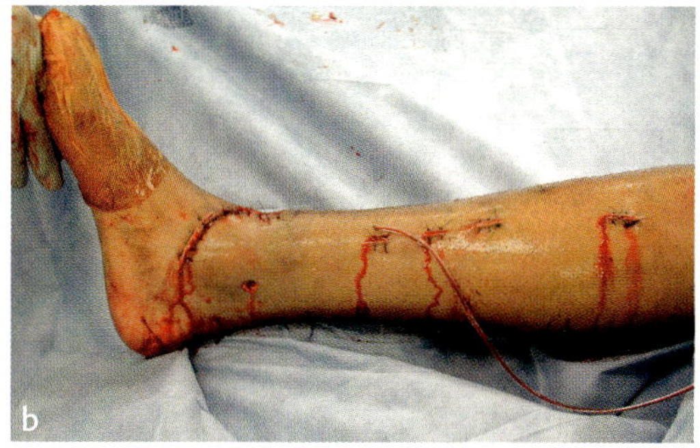

Fig 10.3.7-7a–b Postoperative images of the extremity showing the closed incision anteriorly with the small stab incisions medially for screw placement.

5 Rehabilitation

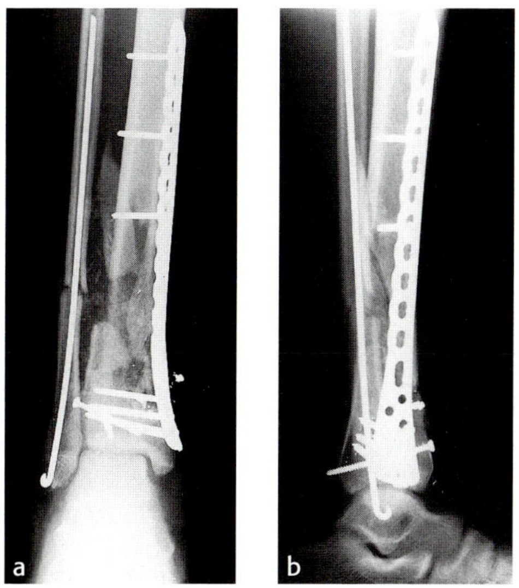

Additional immobilization: A short leg splint is used for 3–7 days to allow soft-tissue swelling to subside and the wound edges to seal.
Weight bearing: 15 kg for 6 weeks; half body weight after 6 weeks; full weight bearing after 10 weeks.
Mobilization: active mobilization after 7 days
Physiotherapy: Active and active-assisted range of motion is started as soon as the patient is comfortable. Passive dorsiflexion stretching is allowed with foot flat. No strengthening is permitted until the fracture has healed.
Pharmaceutical treatment: Pain management as needed.

Fig 10.3.7-8a–b Postoperative x-ray after 12 weeks. Bone graft was performed.
a AP view.
b Lateral view.

5 Rehabilitation (cont)

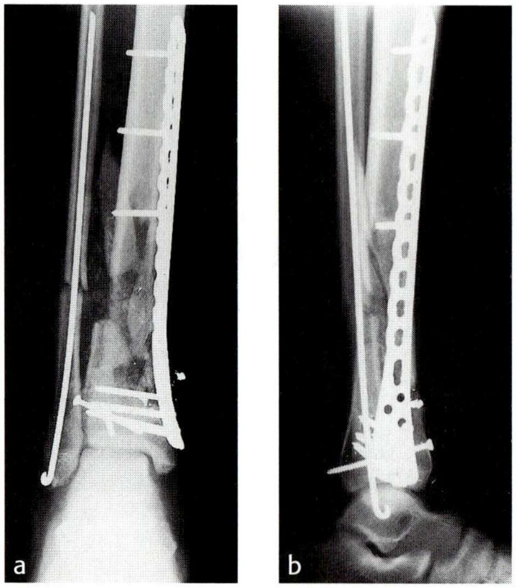

Fig 10.3.7-9a–b Postoperative x-rays after union.
a AP view.
b Lateral view.

6 Pitfalls –

Equipment

Reduction can be difficult with manual distraction alone.

Approach

Be aware of soft-tissue complications.

Reduction and fixation

Relying on image intensification to determine axial alignment. Poor attention to rotational reduction.

7 Pearls +

Equipment

The use of an external fixator or a large distractor is key to maintaining length and alignment.
Insert two to three 2.8 mm threaded drill guides into distal plate to ease initial locking head screw insertion.

Approach

Avoid raising flaps and perform extraperiosteal dissection to maintain vascularity of fracture fragments.

Reduction and fixation

Full length x-rays following provisional reduction.

Authors Hermann Josef Bail, Klaus-Dieter Schaser, Norbert P Haas

10.3.8 Bilateral complete articular multifragmentary distal tibial fracture—43-C3

1 Case description

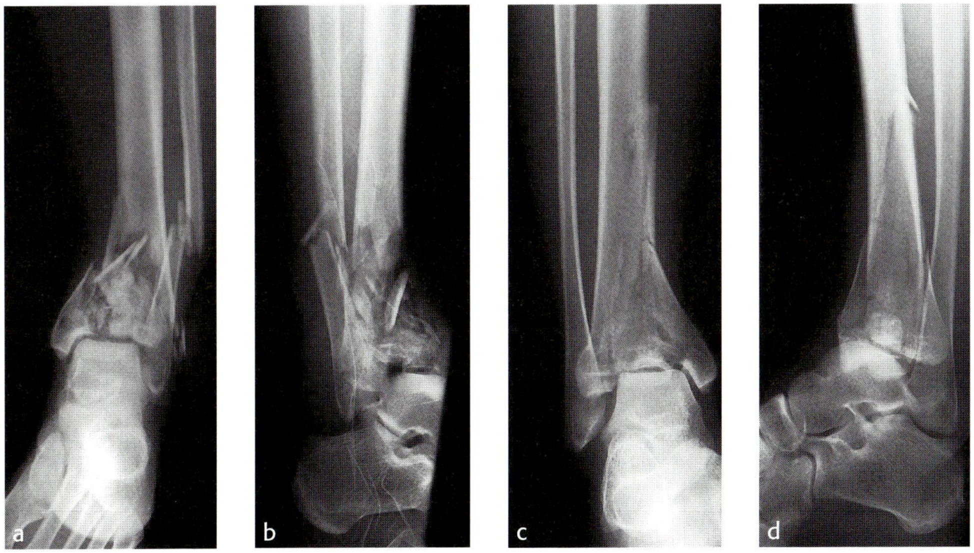

28-year-old woman, jumped off a building (6–8 m height) in suicidal intent, which resulted in polytrauma with pelvic ring injury (type B-fracture), moderate chest trauma, distal radial (type A-fracture) and bilateral closed pilon fractures (type C3).

Fig 10.3.8-1a–d Lateral and AP x-rays show the multifragmentary pilon fractures on both distal tibiae. On the left side severe metaphyseal comminution is present.

- a AP view of left pilon fracture.
- b Lateral view of left pilon fracture.
- c AP view of right pilon fracture.
- d Lateral view of right pilon fracture.

Indication

These impacted, intraarticular, and also metaphyseal multi-fragmentary fractures with multifragmentary joint incongruence are an absolute indication for surgical intervention, ie, anatomical reconstruction. Due to the severe closed soft-tissue damage on both sides and in the face of the patient's overall condition (polytrauma) a preliminary closed reduction and external fixation was performed (orthopedic damage control surgery).

In a second step and after soft-tissue consolidation, sequential open reduction and internal fixation was performed on both sides via an anteromedial approach using several lag screws and a LCP metaphyseal plate 3.5/4.5/5.0 on the right, and an LCP distal tibial plate 2.7/3.5 on the left. The right fibular fracture was stabilized by an LCP 3.5. Primary cancellous bone grafting was necessary because of the severely impacted fragments and the extensive metaphyseal defect situation.

Indication (cont)

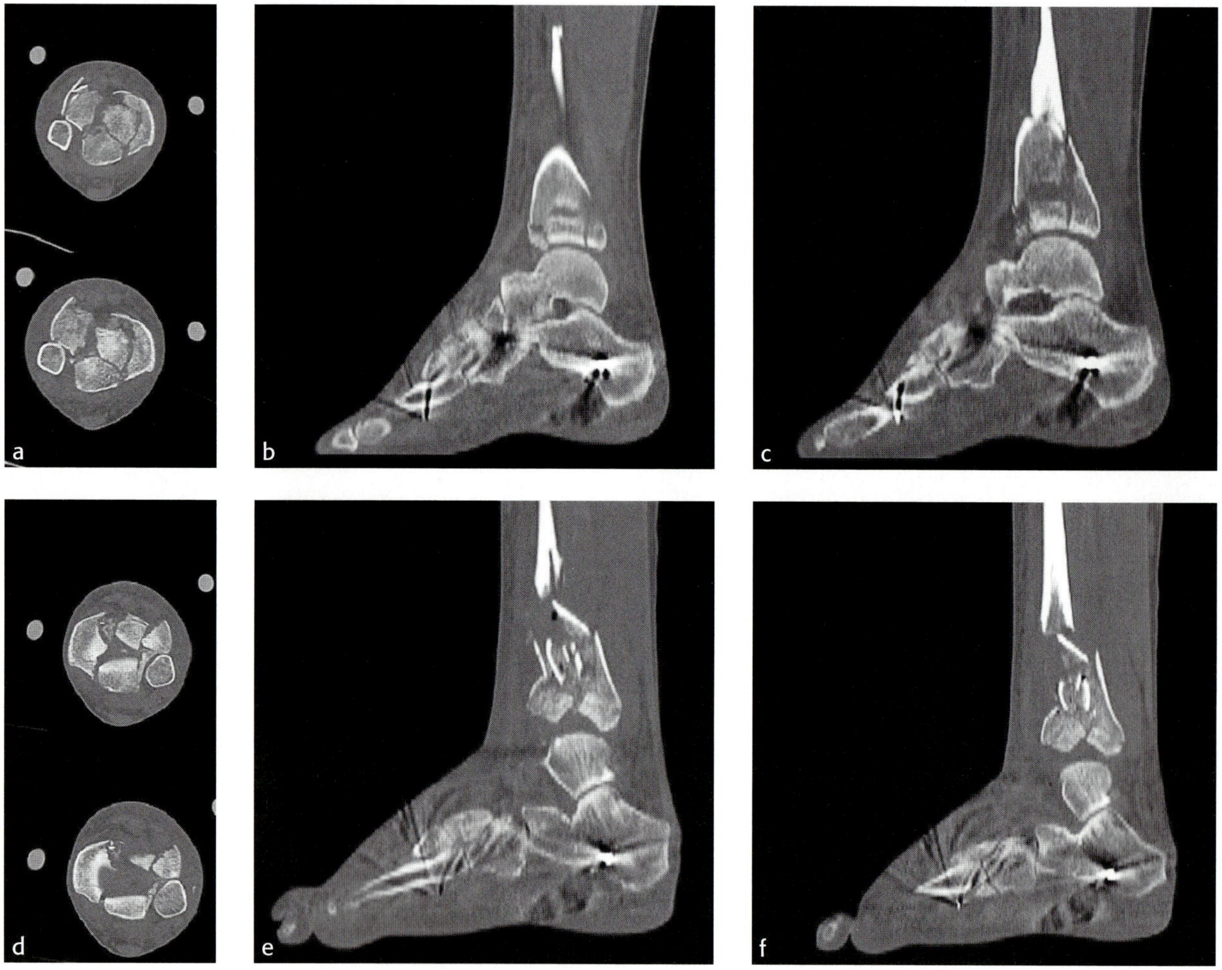

Fig 10.3.8-2a–f After primary external fixation, preoperative CT scans of both sides show a displaced anterolateral fragment, a centrally impacted fragment, a medial malleolar fragment, and a Volkmann fragment. The sagittal reconstructions reveal that on the right side the closed reduction produced a better alignment compared with the left side.

a–c Left side.

d–f Right side.

Preoperative planning

Equipment

- LCP distal tibial plate 2.7/3.5, medial, 5 holes
- LCP metaphyseal plate 3.5/4.5/5.0, 10 holes
- 3.5 mm cortex screws
- 3.5 mm locking head screw (LHS)
- 5.0 mm LHS
- 1.6/2.0 mm K-wires
- Pelvic reduction forceps
- Large external fixator

(Size of system, instruments, and implants can vary according to anatomy.)

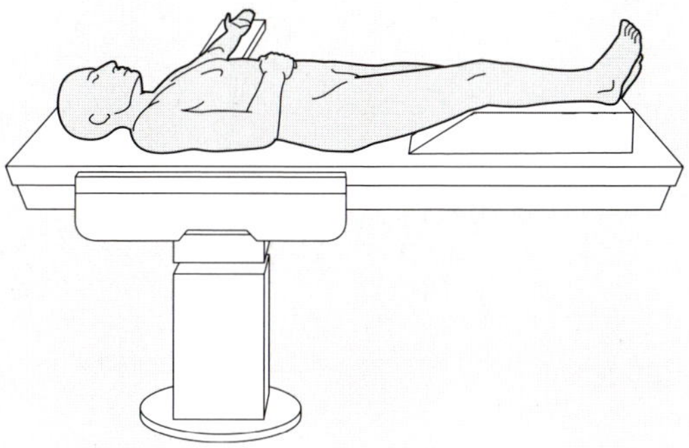

Fig 10.3.8-3 Supine position with elevation of the injured limb or contralateral leg lowered below the table level (allowing lateral intraoperative x-ray).

Patient preparation and positioning

Antibiotics: cephalosporin

Thrombosis prophylaxis: low-molecular heparin

2 Surgical approach

Fig 10.3.8-4a–b An anteromedial approach (extending sigmoidally from the medial malleolus to the anterior rim of the tibial shaft) was chosen for sufficient visualization and reconstruction of the joint surface at the joint level. Fixation of the plate at the dia/-metaphysis may be performed percutaneously.

a Anteromedial approach to the right distal tibia.

b Anteromedial approach to the left distal tibia. Additional lateral approach to the left fibula is not shown.

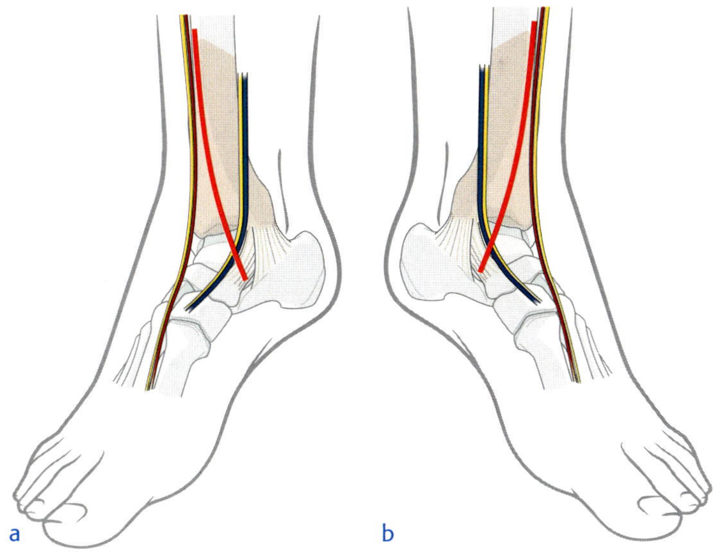

3 Reduction—left distal tibia

The external fixator was left in place, thereby maintaining length and axis as well as slight distraction of the ankle joint. The operation started with a lateral approach to the distal fibular fracture. The fibula was reduced and fixed with an LCP 3.5. During the complete surgical procedure, the calcaneal Schanz' screw was used for distraction of the ankle joint and maintenance of the ligamentotaxis. While the lateral approach to the fibula was left open, the anteromedial approach was performed. After gently retracting the anteromedial fragment, the impacted central pilon fragment became visible. Before this key fragment was reduced, the posterolateral fragment, which was additionally impacted and dislocated, was reduced to the posterior aspect of the talus and temporarily fixed with a K-wire. Subsequently, the central, impacted pilon fragment was anatomically reduced and pinned with a K-wire to the posterolateral already reduced and fixed fragment. Finally, the anteromedial and anterolateral fragments were reduced and held in position by reduction forceps and K-wires in the sagittal plane. Subsequently, two cortex lag screws were inserted perpendicular to the central fragment and fracture lines and parallel to the joint line for interfragmentary compression. Anatomical reduction and absolute stability was achieved for the joint block. The defect at the metaphyseal level was filled by cancellous bone graft harvested from the ipsilateral iliac crest. The fragment involving the medial malleolus was relatively large in the horizontal plane but only thin in a vertical direction making fixation to the other joint fragments insecure. Therefore, a long cortex screw was placed from the medial malleolus to the adjacent intact lateral cortex of the proximal meta-/diaphysis. Finally a LCP distal tibial plate 2.7/3.5, medial was introduced and a cortex screw was inserted through the plate and fixed to the diaphysis followed by three locking head screws to the shaft. Thus, the metaphyseal defect zone was bridged by using the LCP as a pure internal fixator. The long lag screw only engages the medial malleolus and has no mechanical effect in the metaphyseal area.

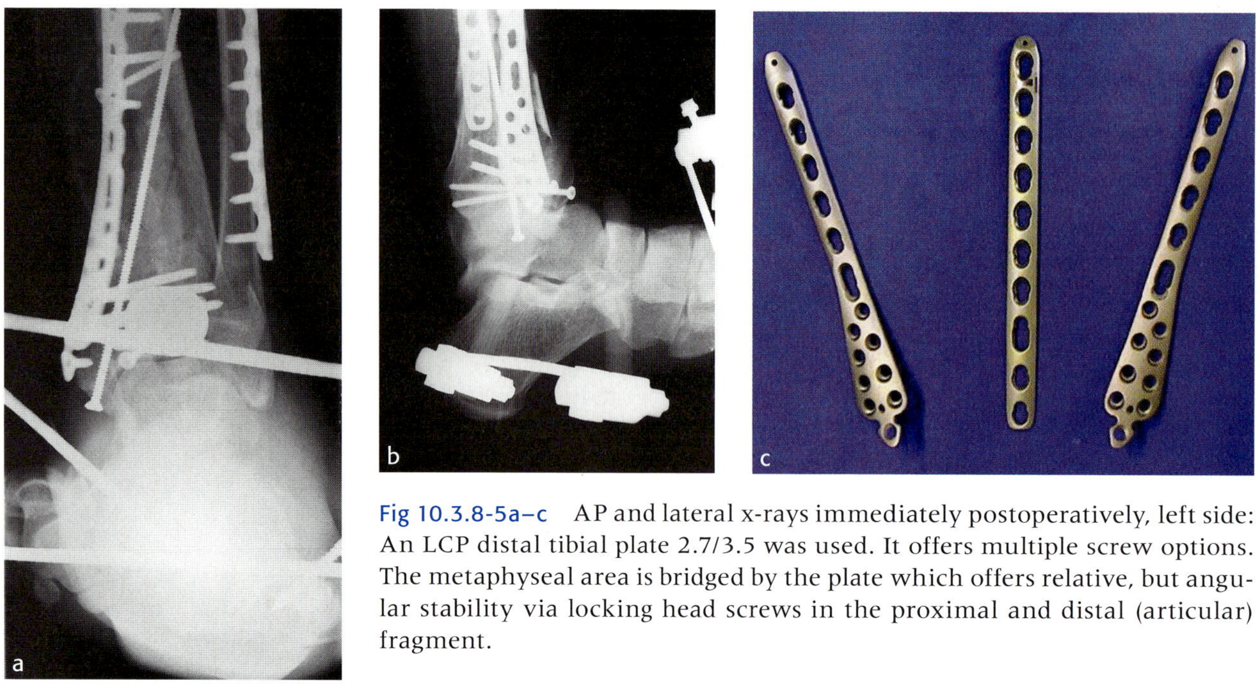

Fig 10.3.8-5a–c AP and lateral x-rays immediately postoperatively, left side: An LCP distal tibial plate 2.7/3.5 was used. It offers multiple screw options. The metaphyseal area is bridged by the plate which offers relative, but angular stability via locking head screws in the proximal and distal (articular) fragment.

4 Reduction—right distal tibia

Neither a lateral approach nor cancellous bone grafting were necessary in the metaphyseal area as there were fewer fragments and the fibula was not fractured.

The reduction technique was similar to that for the left side with temporary reduction forceps and K-wire fixation. One lag screw was inserted percutaneously for fixation of the previously reduced anterolateral fragment. Another lag screw compressed the joint block for absolute stability. Two more lag screws were placed in the sagittal plane for fixation/interfragmentary compression of metaphyseal split fragments. However, as a consequence of the large split fragment extending to the medial aspect of the meta-/diaphysis, a distal tibial LCP was not considered to provide enough fixation in the diaphysis. Thus, a LCP metaphyseal plate 3.5/4.5/5.0 was used and inserted subcutaneously at the diaphysis where the 5.0 mm locking head screws were inserted percutaneously. All angular stable options adjacent to the joint level were used with 3.5 mm locking head screws. The angular stable LCP neutralizes incoming shear forces. Principally, one can discuss whether the fifth 5.0 mm screw from proximal is needed. This LHS crosses the fracture gap in the meta-/diaphyseal transition zone and results in a mixture of principles. If the LCP is used as a protection plate, another lag screw would follow the principle of absolute stability, which can be applied in the treatment of simple metaphyseal fractures. If the LCP were being used as a bridging internal fixator, the fifth and the fourth LHS (counted from proximal) should be omitted. An angular stable screw which crosses the fracture zone may bother slight interfragmentary movement which is helpful for healing.

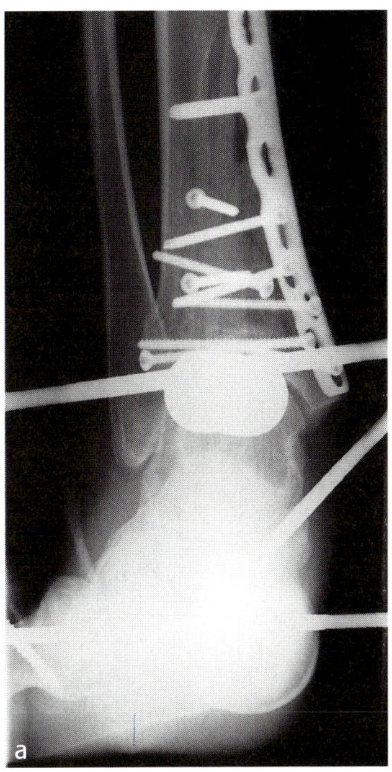

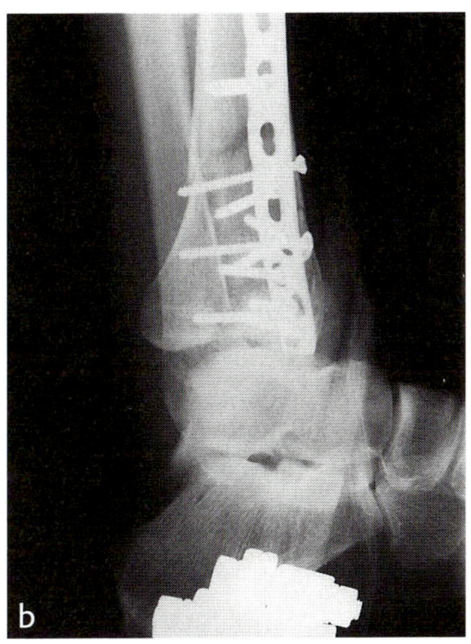

Fig 10.3.8-6a–b AP and lateral x-rays directly postoperatively, right side: An LCP metaphyseal plate 3.5/4.5/5.0 is used as a neutralization plate to protect the absolute stability achieved with the lag screws in the distal metaphyseal fracture area. For protection of the soft tissues on both sides, the external fixator was maintained until the tenth postoperative day.

5 Rehabilitation

After 12 weeks of partial weight bearing on both sides the patient started full weight bearing first on the right side followed by the left side at 15 weeks.
5 months after surgery the patient was able to walk without crutches and stand on tiptoe.

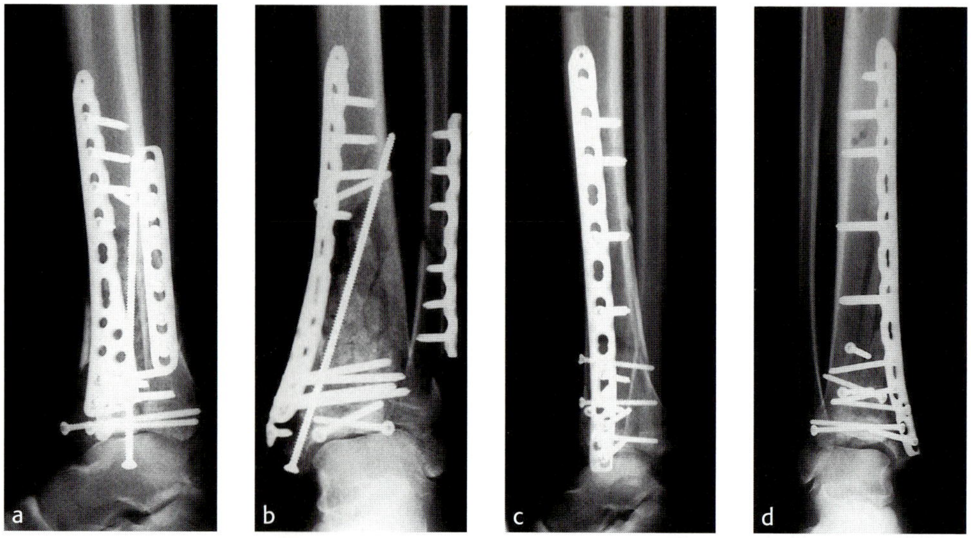

Fig 10.3.8-7a–d 6 weeks postoperative: On the left side, good callus formation in the metaphyseal defect area is visible. On the right side, no loss of reduction could be identified. As discussed in the text, in the meta-/diaphyseal transition area, no lag screw was inserted but a locking head screw crosses the fracture gap.

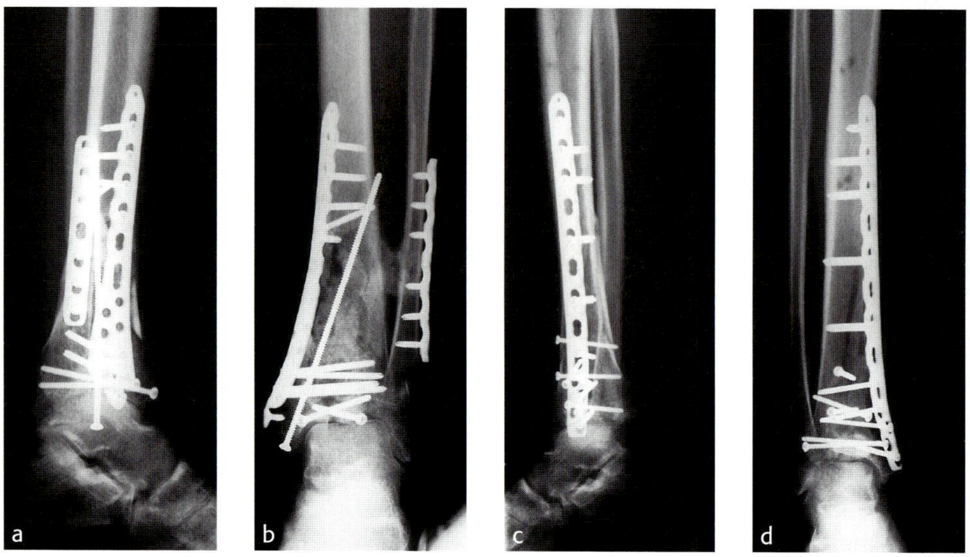

Fig 10.3.8-8a–d 12 weeks postoperative: No implant loosening or breakage is visible. The metaphyseal zone and joint area is healed on both sides. At this time, full weight bearing was allowed starting with the right side.

5 Rehabilitation (cont)

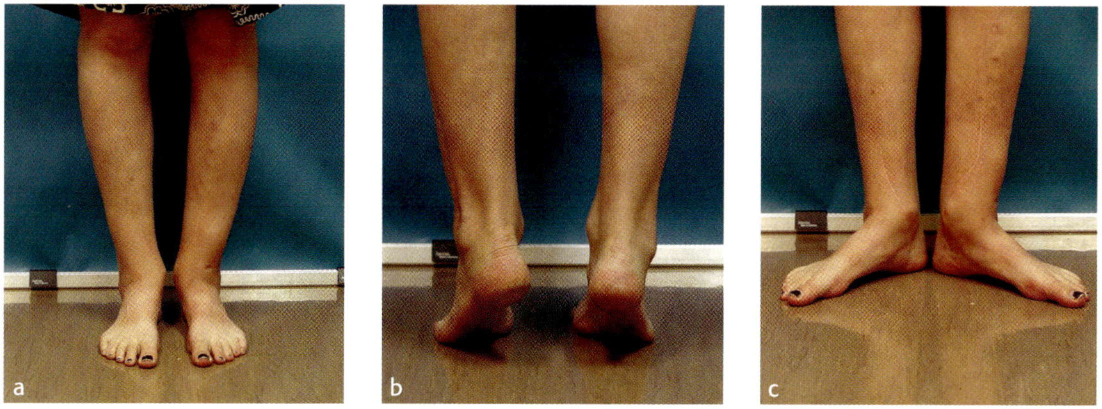

Fig 10.3.8-9a–c The clinical images show uneventful soft-tissue healing and good motor function on both sides.

6 Pitfalls –

Equipment
The distal tibial LCP may be too short for fractures which extend into the diaphyseal area.

The metaphyseal LCP may offer too few fixation options in the distal part to fix complete multifragmentary articular fractures.

Approach
With the anteromedial approach the control of the Volkmann fragment may be difficult.

7 Pearls +

Equipment
The distal tibial LCP is an ideal plate for multifragmentary complete articular fractures.

The LCP metaphyseal plate 3.5/4.5/5.0 is an ideal implant for fractures which extend into the diaphyseal area.

Approach
The anteromedial approach allows optimal control of the anterior and the medial fragments. For control of the anterolateral fragment, the approach can be extended proximally and distally as needed.

6 Pitfalls – (cont)

Reduction and fixation

In complete multifragmentary pilon fractures, reference contours for reduction of key fragments are generally hard to find.

In complete articular distal tibial fractures with a multifragmentary metaphyseal zone, no proximal reference fragments for reconstruction of the joint segment are available.

Exposure of the multifragmentary metaphyseal area in order to find a reference fragment leads to periosteal stripping and soft-tissue stress.

Rehabilitation

Too early full weight bearing in cases with metaphyseal defect areas may lead to implant failure.

Mixture of principles (here a locking head screw crossing the fracture line) may lead to prolonged fracture consolidation.

7 Pearls + (cont)

Reduction and fixation

If the posterolateral fragment (Volkmann fragment) can be reduced to the metaphyseal fragment, the joint can be reconstructed based on the correct position of that fragment.

If no direct reduction of an articular fragment to a metaphyseal fragment is possible, the reconstructed fibula provides the reference for the orientation of the joint segment.

For reconstruction of the articular surface, the surface of the joint partner (here: talus) can serve as a reference.

Rehabilitation

In multifragmentary metaphyseal fractures angular stability allows early functional postoperative treatment with continuous passive motion of the joint.

In multifragmentary articular fractures (with absolute stability), angular stable fixation of the reconstructed joint segment in many cases allows partial weight bearing.

Authors Andreas Gruner, Thomas J Hockertz, Gabriele Streicher, Heinrich Reilmann

10.3.9 Adolescent bone cyst—with imminent fracture of the distal tibia

1 Case description

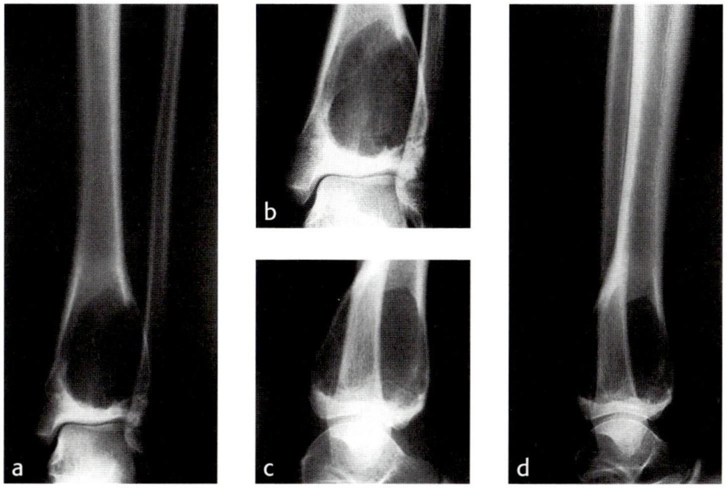

14-year-old female patient with an abnormal condition.
Type of disorder: tumor of the distal tibia—adolescent bone cyst—with imminent fracture of the distal tibia

Fig 10.3.9-1a–d
a AP view.
b AP view detail.
c Lateral view detail.
d Lateral view.

Indication

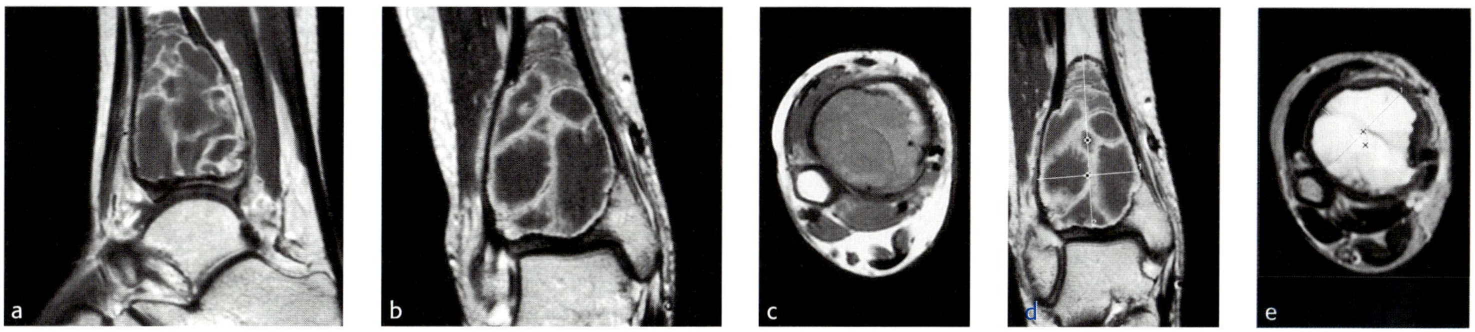

Bone cyst of the distal tibia, left, in a 14-year-old girl. The position of the cyst at the distal tibial metaphysis immediately adjacent to the epiphysis is associated with the risk of fracture. The cyst was filled with serous fluid, unicameral, contained pseudosepta, and affected the entire distal tibia (see CT scan).

Fig 10.3.9-2a–e CT scans of the adolescent bone cyst.

Preoperative planning

Equipment
- LCP metaphyseal plate 3.5/4.5/5.0, 5 + 9 holes
- 5.0 mm locking head screws (LHS)
- 3.5 mm LHS
- K-wires

(Size of system, instruments, and implants can vary according to anatomy.)

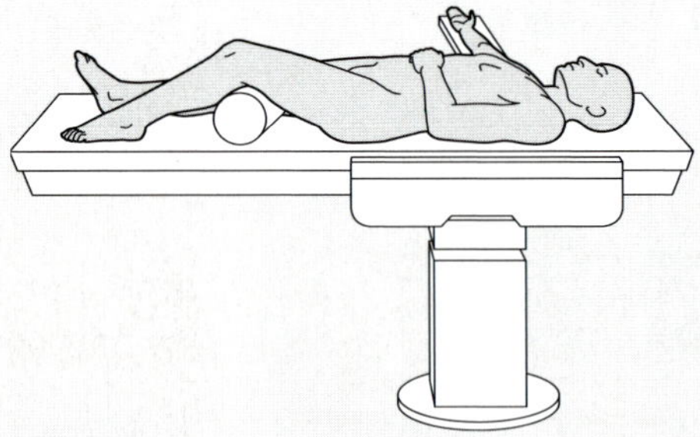

Fig 10.3.9-3 Supine position, the left leg is free-draped for intraoperative mobility, thigh tourniquet, right leg lowered by approximately 20°, image intensifier from the right.

Patient preparation and positioning
Antibiotics: single dose 2nd generation cephalosporin
Thrombosis prophylaxis: low-molecular heparin

2 Surgical approach

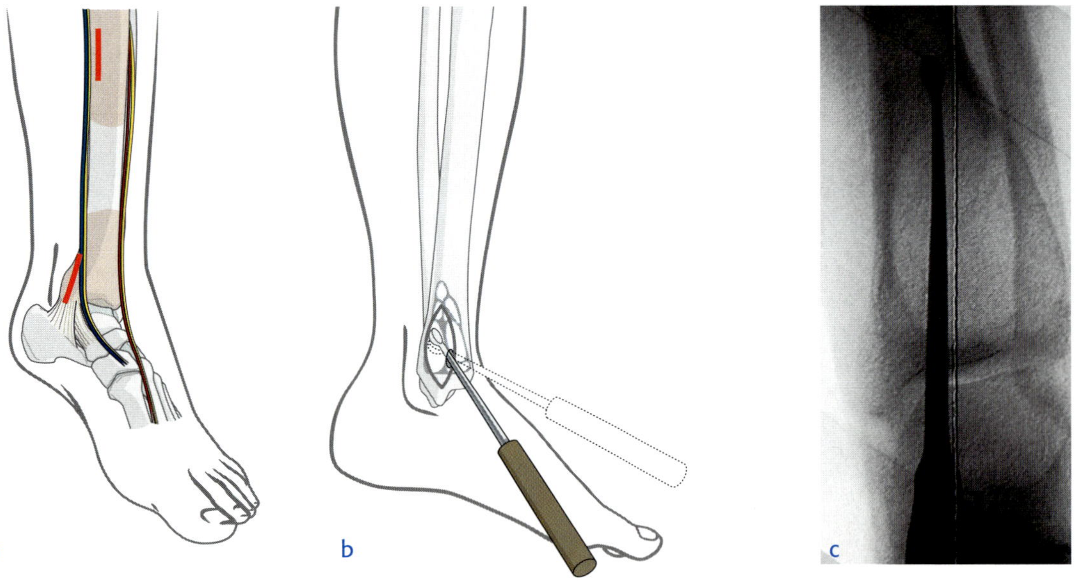

a b c

Fig 10.3.9-4a–c Anterior incision over the distal tibia, dissection to the periosteum, create a bone aperture, mobilize the cystic content down to the cyst-shaft interface.
Approximately 5 cm long, central skin incision longitudinally over the inner malleolus, dissect to the periosteum, prepare the plate bed by epiperiosteal tunneling from distal to proximal with a long bone rasp.

Prebending of the metaphyseal LCP with the plate bending press and adaptation under image intensification.
Skin incision parallel to the tibial axis at the proximal end of the implant bed.

3 Reduction and fixation

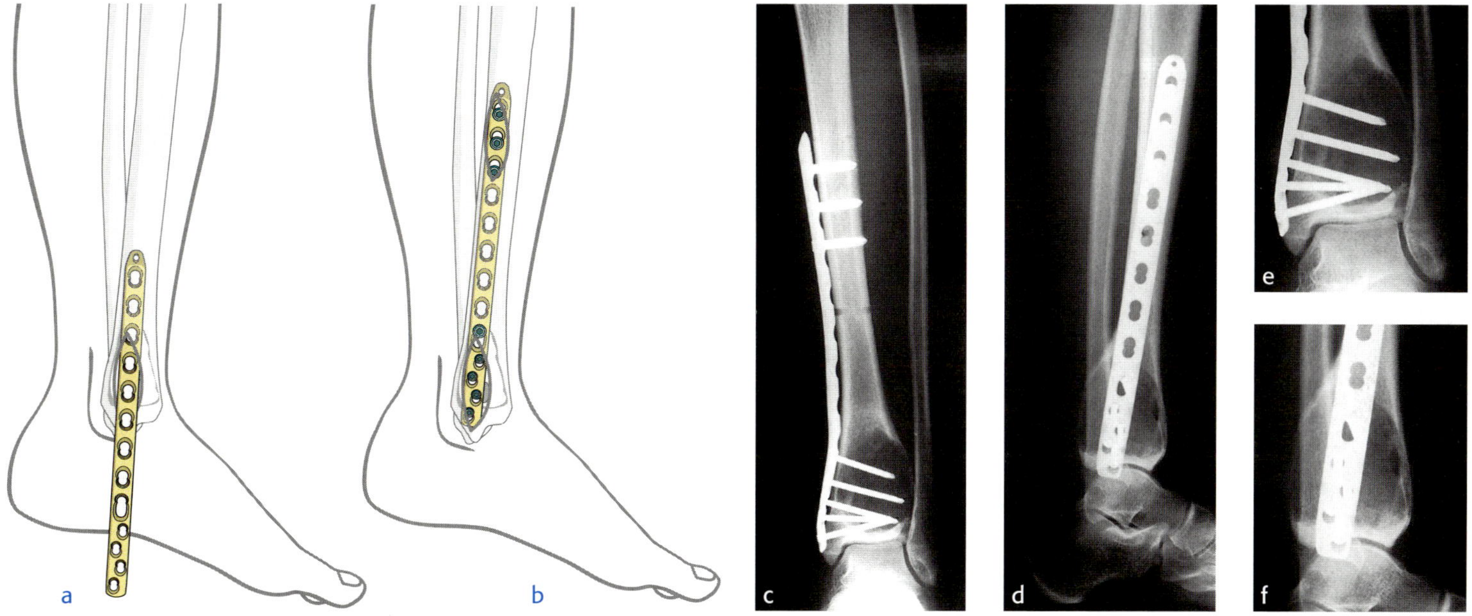

Fig 10.3.9-5a–f

a No reduction is required since this is not a case of fracture. Plate insertion, temporary fixation using K-wires proximally, image intensification in two planes, possibly adaptation of the LCP to the tibial shaft with the pulling device.

b–f Fixation with three 5.0 mm locking head screws proximally and five 3.5 mm monocortical locking head screws distally. Ensure that the screws have secure anchorage in the distal epimetaphysis and protrude into the cystic structure, skin incision is always a stab incision over the plate bed.

4 Rehabilitation

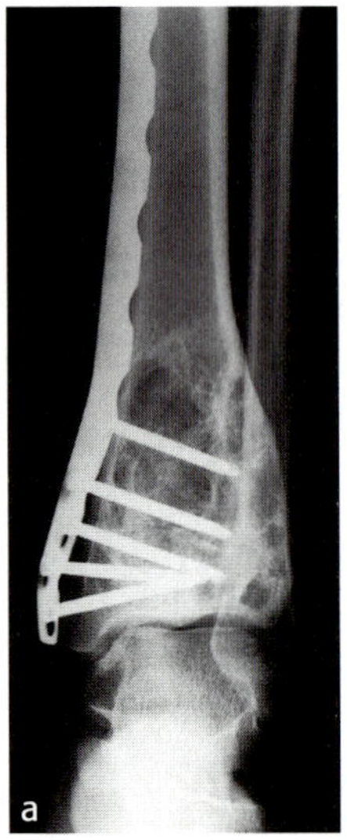

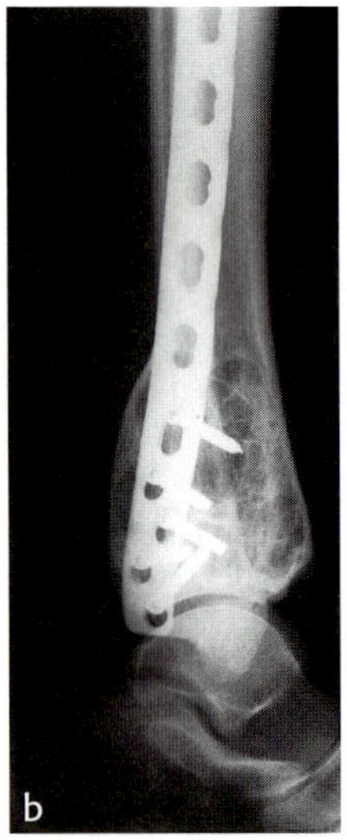

Fig 10.3.9-6a–b Postoperative x-rays after 18 months.
a AP view.
b Lateral view.

Additional immobilization: functional postoperative treatment.
Weight bearing: full weight bearing after 4 weeks.
Passive mobilization after 1 day.
Active mobilization after 2 days.
Physiotherapy: from the first postoperative day.
Pharmaceutical treatment: perioperative pain medication.

Implant removal
Implant removal after definitive healing of the bone cyst.

5 Pitfalls –

Equipment
Incorrect prebending of the LCP.

Approach
Injury to the saphenous vein and nerve if the approach is too far on the anterior side of the inner malleolus.

Reduction and fixation
Correct positioning of the implant, whereby the curvature of the plate should be slightly less than the curvature of the bone.
Incorrect positioning of the plate, especially in the lateral plane.

Rehabilitation

6 Pearls +

Equipment
LCP metaphyeal plate does not rest on the inner malleolus in the distal region.

Approach

Reduction and fixation

Rehabilitation
Early mobilization with partial loading is possible.

Author **Michael Wagner**

10.3.10 Fibular fracture with medial ligamentous lesion—44-B2

1 Case description

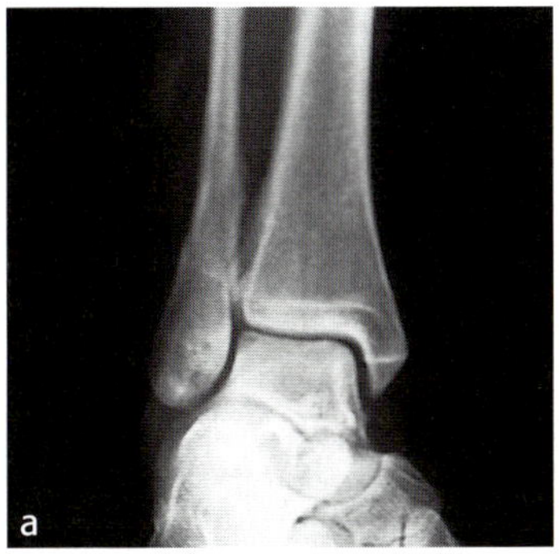

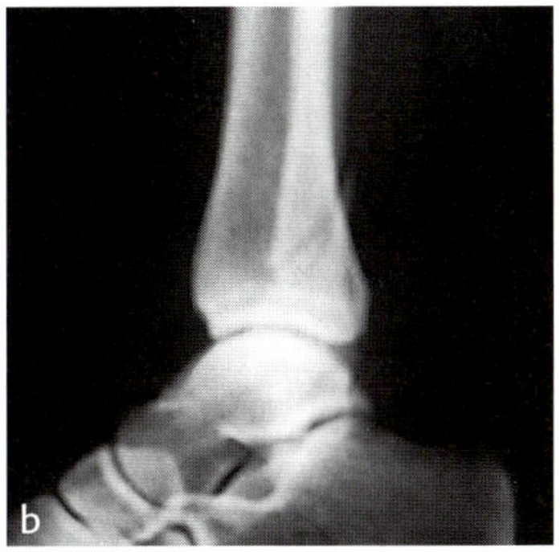

50-year-old woman fell while out walking and sustained an isolated fracture of the right ankle joint.

Fig 10.3.10-1a–b
a AP view.
b Lateral view.

Indication

Displaced malleolar fracture with ligament on the medial side.

Preoperative planning

Equipment

- LCP one-third tubular plate 3.5, 6 holes
- 3.5 mm cortex screw
- 3.5 mm locking head screws (LHS)

(Size of system, instruments, and implants can vary according to anatomy.)

Patient preparation and positioning

Antibiotics: none
Thrombosis prophylaxis: low-molecular heparin

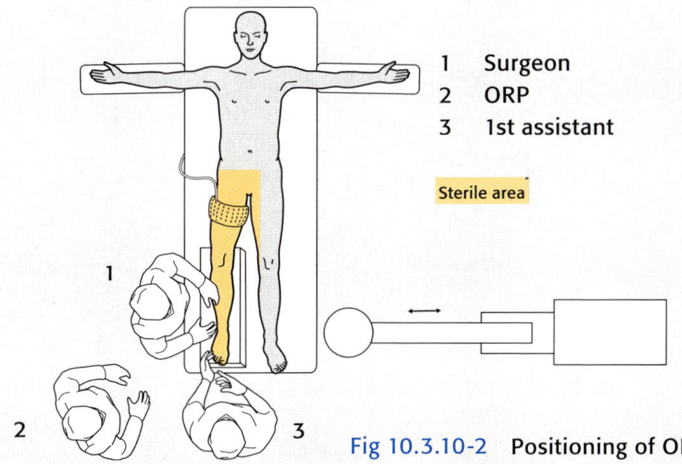

Fig 10.3.10-2 Positioning of OR team.

2 Surgical approach

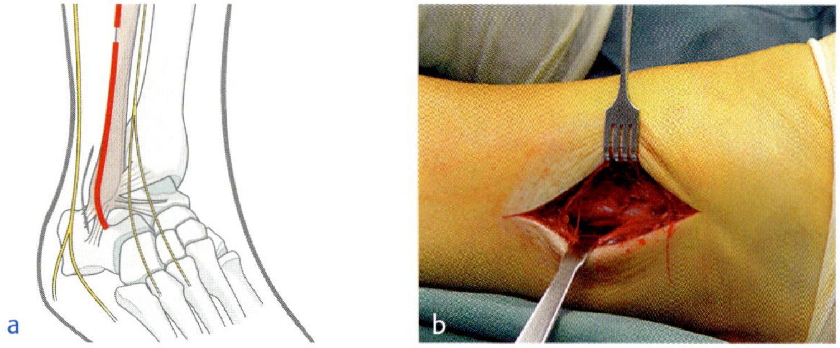

Fig 10.3.10-3a–b Lateral approach to the lateral malleolar fracture.

3 Reduction and fixation

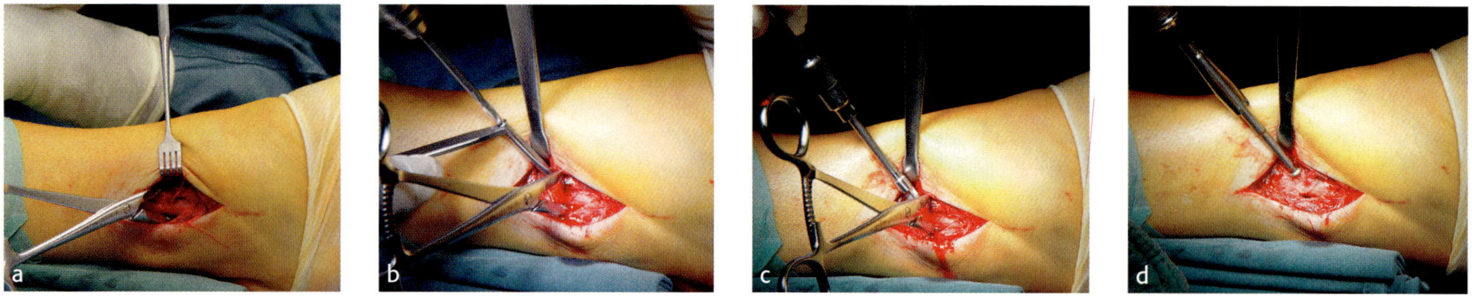

Fig 10.3.10-4a–d

a Open reduction of the lateral malleolus fracture with reduction forceps with serrated jaws.

b After anatomical reduction, fixation with a lag screw (3.5 mm cortex screw). A gliding hole and a threaded hole are drilled.

c The thread is tapped.

d The lag screw (cortex shaft screw) is inserted.

3 Reduction and fixation (cont)

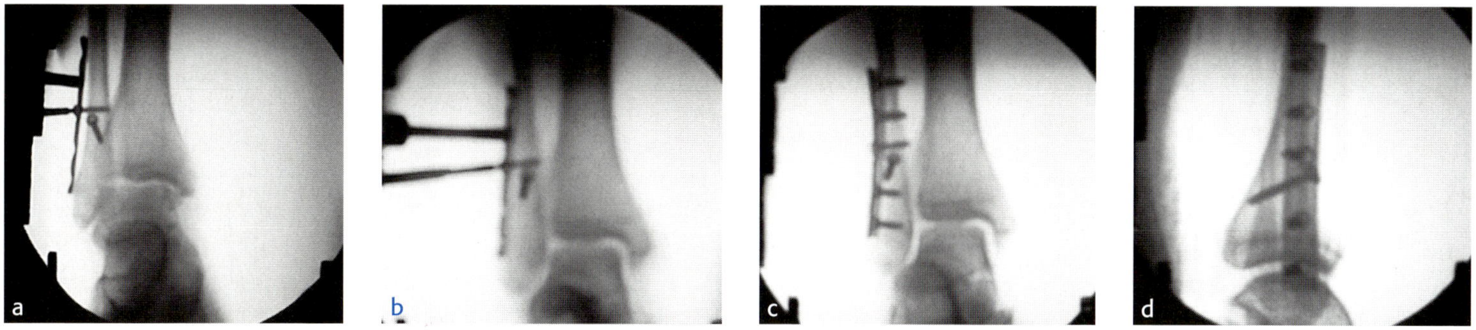

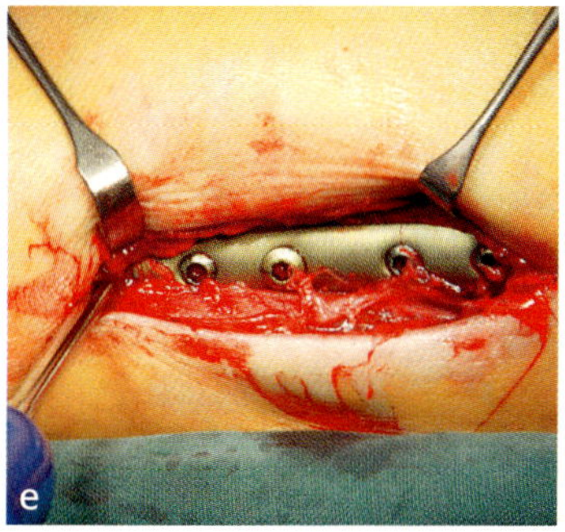

Fig 10.3.10-5a–e
a–b A straight LCP one-third tubular plate is fixed by insertion of a cortex screw to the slightly curved lateral aspect of the fibular malleolus and takes on the additional function of a buttress plate to counteract lateral fragment displacement.
c–d Additional stabilization with a 6-hole LCP one-third tubular plate stabilized by LHS — two in the proximal and two in the distal fragment.
e The plate in situ after completion of the operation shows the different types of screws inthe LCP coaxial combination holes of the one-third tubular plate.

4 Rehabilitation

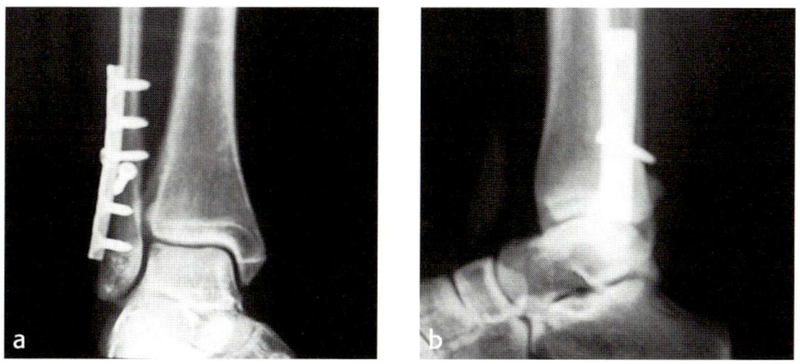

Fig 10.3.10-6a–b Postoperative x-rays after 6 months. No pain, full function, no need for implant removal.
a AP view.
b Lateral view.

Additional immobilization postoperatively in a split plaster cast. As soon as the redon drains have been taken out, the cast can be removed to permit immediate early functional treatment. After removal of stitches 12 days postoperatively, mobilization of the patient with full weight bearing in a short-leg walking cast for 6 weeks following surgery.

5 Pitfalls –

Approach
A lateral incision can place the superficial peroneal nerve at risk. During the operation care should be taken to traumatize the soft tissue as little as possible by careful division of structures.

Reduction and fixation
Standard screws may become loose if the bone is osteoporotic.

6 Pearls +

Approach

Reduction and fixation
Anatomical reduction of a malleolar fracture is imperative. Revision and treatment of the medial ligamentous injury may not be necessary if precise anatomical reduction and positioning of the trochlear of the talus in the mortise can be achieved. The insertion of LHS into the distal fragment permits stable fragment fixation.

The LCP reduces the risk of screw loosening in osteoporotic bone.

Author Michael Wagner

10.3.11 Bimalleolar fracture with medial lesion—44-B2

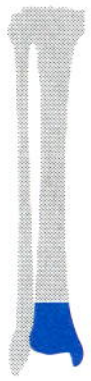

1 Case description

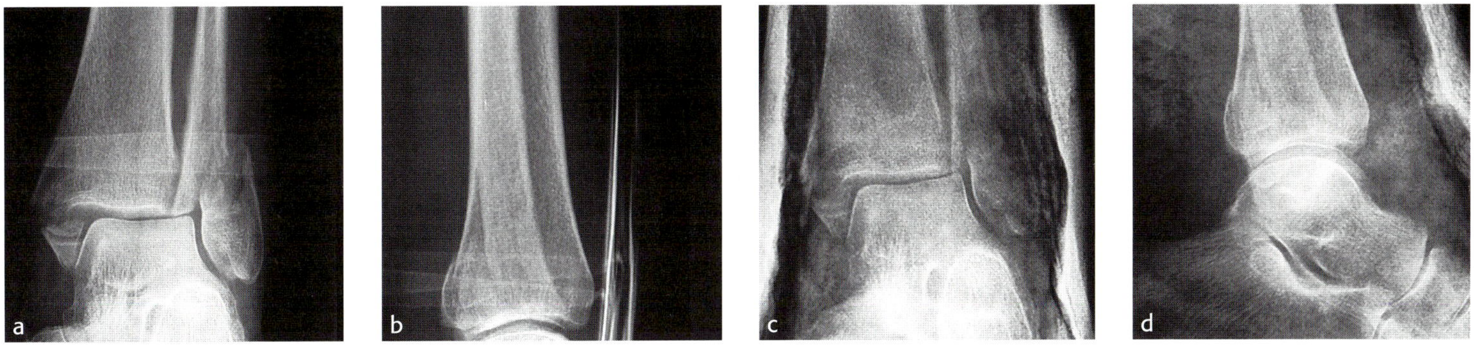

61-year-old woman fell while out walking, dislocated fracture of the left ankle joint.

Fig 10.3.11-1a–d
a AP view.
b Lateral view.
c–d AP view and lateral view after closed reduction and fixation in split plaster cast.

Indication

Displaced bimalleolar fracture. As this is an unstable fracture of the ankle joint, this is a clear indication for stable fixation.

Preoperative planning

Equipment

- LCP one-third tubular plate 3.5, 6 holes
- 4.0 mm cannulated screws with metal washers
- 3.5 mm cortex screw
- 3.5 mm locking head screws (LHS)

(Size of system, instruments, and implants can vary according to anatomy.)

Patient preparation and positioning

Antibiotics: none

Thrombosis prophylaxis: low-molecular heparin

Lateral malleolus
1 Surgeon
2 ORP
3 1st assistant

Sterile area

Medial malleolus
1 1st assistant
2 ORP
3 Surgeon

Sterile area

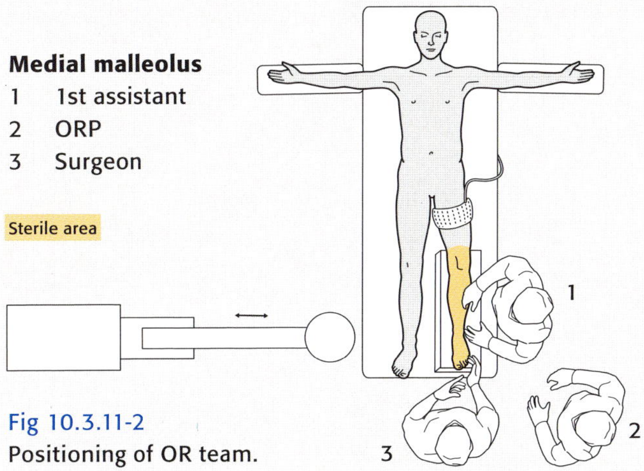

Fig 10.3.11-2
Positioning of OR team.

2 Surgical approach

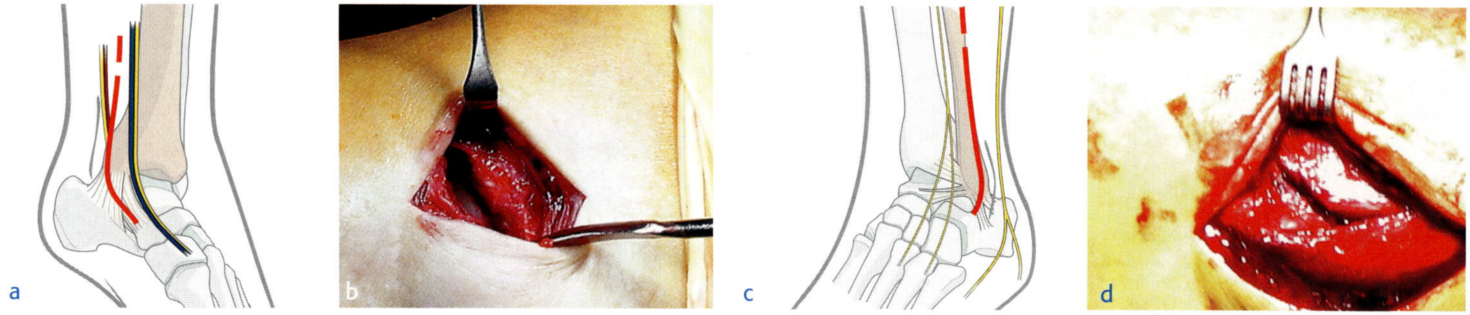

Fig 10.3.11-3a–d

a–b Medial approach. The articular surface of the talus dome is seen through the fracture of the inner malleolus.

c–d Lateral approach. The fracture of the lateral malleolus is visible.

3 Reduction and fixation

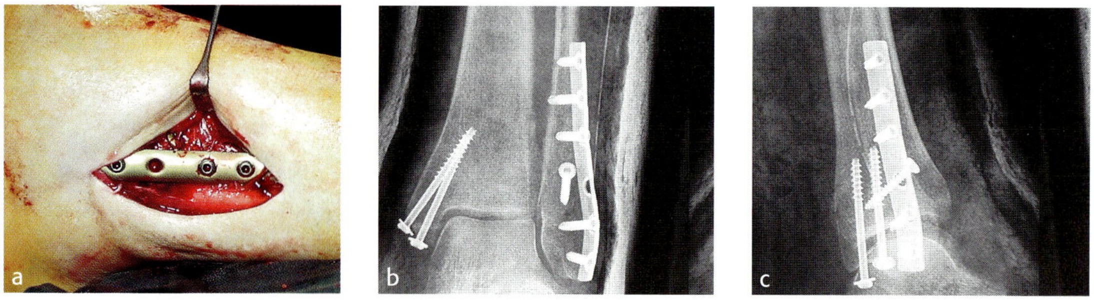

Open reduction of the lateral malleolus fracture and fixation with a lag screw (3.5 mm cortex screw). Additional stabilization with a 6-hole LCP one-third tubular plate, fixed with 5 LHS. Despite osteoporosis, the distal LHS find purchase in the small distal malleolar fragment and the plate acts as an "individual" blade plate.
After exact reduction the medial malleolus is stabilized with two 4.0 mm cannulated screws with washers. The screws are only partially threaded and act as lag screws.

Fig 10.3.11-4a–c

a The LCP one-third tubular plate stabilizes the lateral malleolar fracture.

b AP view.

c Lateral view.

4 Rehabilitation

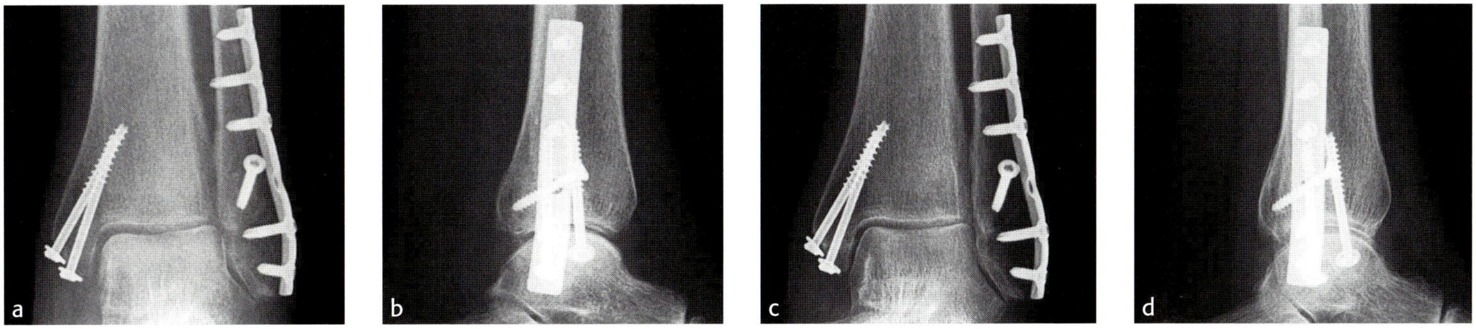

Additional immobilization postoperatively in a split plaster cast. After removal of the redon drains the cast is removed for intermediate early functional treatment. After removal of stitches 12 days postoperatively, mobilization of the patient with full weight bearing a in short-leg walking cast for 6 weeks following surgery.

Fig 10.3.11-5a–d
a Postoperative x-ray after 6 weeks, AP view.
b Postoperative x-ray after 6 weeks, lateral view.
c Postoperative x-ray after 5 months, AP view.
d Postoperative x-ray after 5 months, lateral view.

5 Pitfalls –

Equipment
In the event of severe osteoporosis loosening of the implants may sometimes occur (conventional screws and one-third tubular plate with secondary fracture displacement).

Reduction and fixation
Operative injury to the superficial peroneal nerve as a result of incision or intraoperative trauma.
Also inadequate technique can lead to skin necrosis.

6 Pearls +

Equipment
LCP reduces the risk of screw loosening in osteoporotic bone.

Reduction and fixation
After anatomical open direct reduction, fixation with a plate-independent lag screw to achieve interfragmentary compression. The plate acts as protection plate. Two monocortical LHS secure the small distal fragment, even in osteoporotic bone.

11 Calcaneus

Cases

11 Calcaneus

Author Hans Zwipp

11 Calcaneus

1 Incidence

Calcaneal fractures occur in 1–2% of all fractures of the human skeleton but represent 60–75% of all foot fractures. The mean age is 42 years. The male:female-ratio is recorded as 5:1. A high-velocity trauma is the basic cause in falls from a height (43–82%), in traffic accidents (13–53%), in sports (5%) and in polytrauma (35%). The fractures are open in 3–12%, with compartment syndrome in 4–5%, and bilateral in 10–20%.

2 Classification

A-type fractures are not often seen (13%).
B-type frctures are most common (82%).
C-type fractures are rare (5%).

3 Treatment methods

Extraarticular fractures of 1–3 segments are treated conservatively if they have only slightly displacement. In cases of severe displacement and varus/valgus malalignment they are most often treated with ORIF or in minimally invasive technique with screws.

Intraarticular fractures of 1–3 joints are treated by ORIF if the joint displacement is more than 1–2 mm as visualized on the CT scans and if contraindications for surgery are not given.

Fracture dislocations of 1–3 joints greatly need ORIF because late reconstructions are the most difficult ones. In cases of contraindications for ORIF, minimally invasive techniques with percutaneous screw fixation should be performed to restore the statics of the hindfoot.

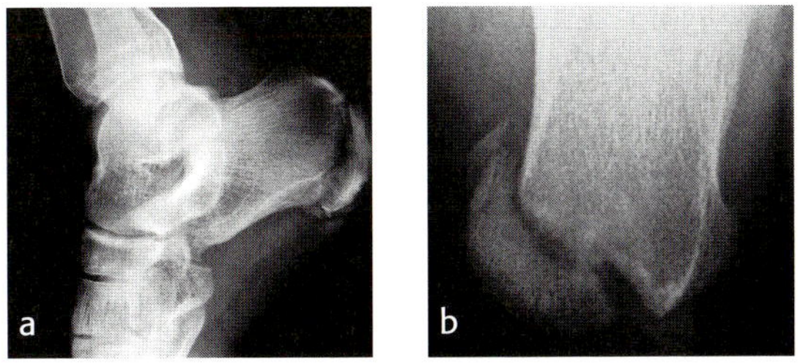

Fig 11-1a–b A-type fracture.

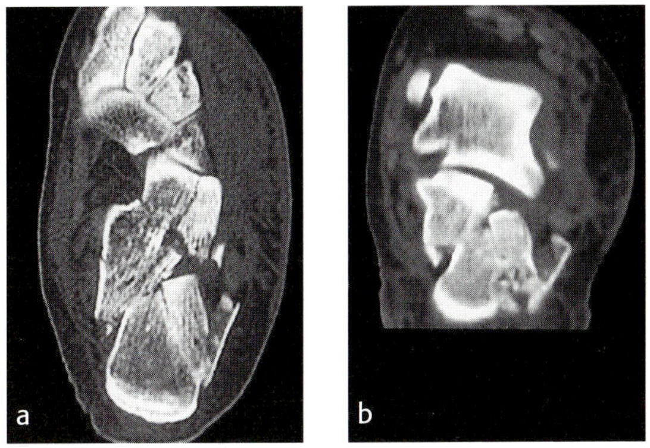

Fig 11-2a–b B-type fracture.

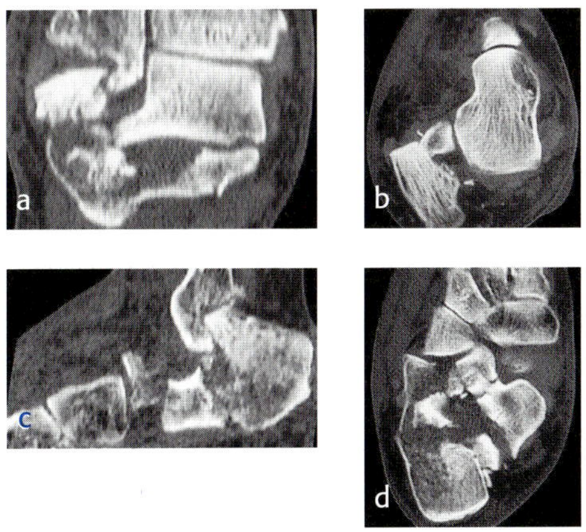

Fig 11-3a–d C-type fracture.

4 Implant overview

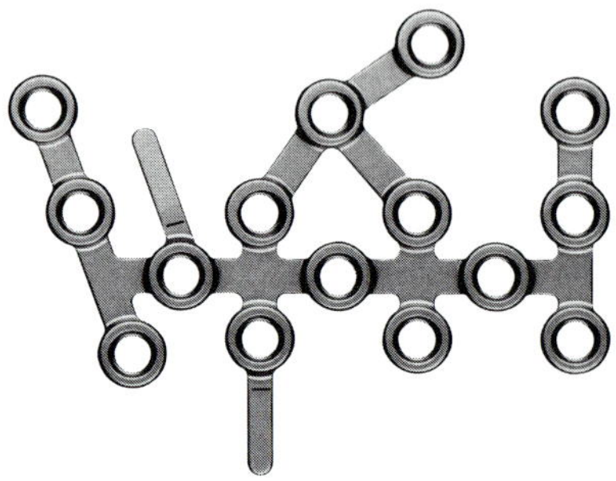

Fig 11-4 Calcaneal locking plate 3.5.

5 Suggestions for further reading

Zwipp H (1994) *Surgery on the foot.* Berlin: Springer Verlag.

Zwipp H, Rammelt S, Barthel S (2005) Fracture of the calcaneus. *Unfallchirurg;* 108(9):737–747.

Author Hans Zwipp

11.1 Intraarticular calcaneal fracture

1 Case description

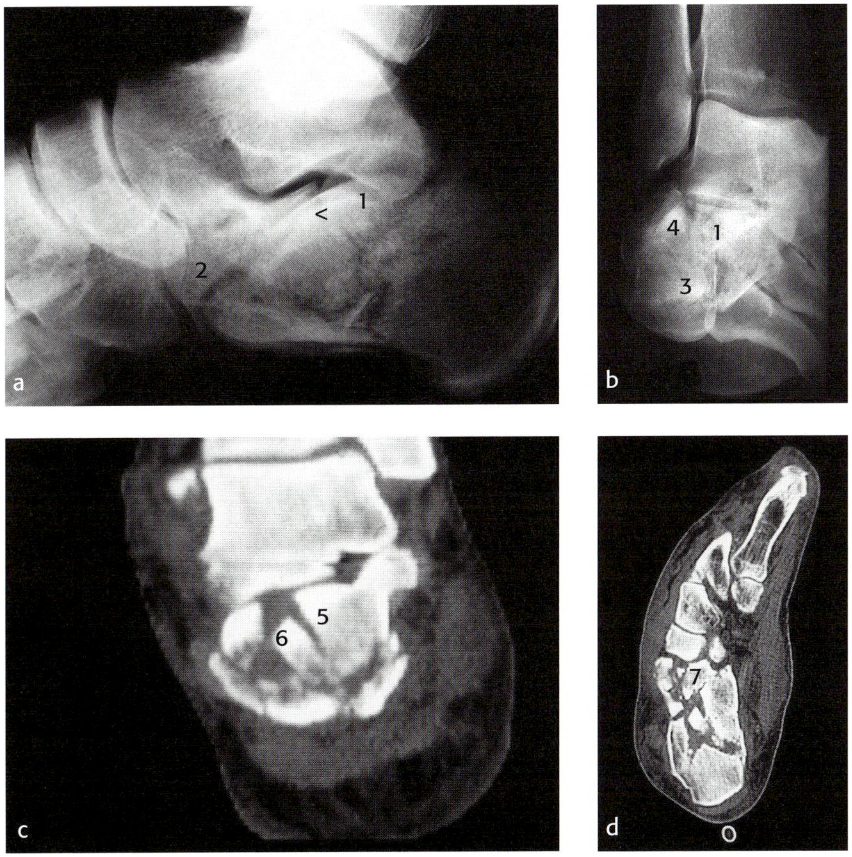

49-year-old man jumped during a psychotic attack from the second floor and fractured the right calcaneus.

Fig 11.1-1a–d

a–b Lateral view and Broden's view (20°) show the deep impaction of the posterior facet (1), the involvement of the cuboidal facet (2), the lateral translation of the tuberosity fragment (3), the tilting of the lateral part of the posterior facet (4), and a suspicious intermediate fragment of the posterior facet.

c–d Coronal CT scan and axial cut show precisely the shifting of the medial part of the posterior facet (5) with adjacent sustentaculum tali medially, the tilted and impacted intermediate fragment of the posterior facet (6), and the severely dislocated medial part of the cuboidal facet (7) medially.

Indication

Severe displacement of the subtalar and calcaneocuboid joint. There are no general or local contraindications for ORIF.

Preoperative planning

Equipment

- Calcaneal locking plate 3.5
- 3.5 mm locking head screws
- 3.5 mm cortex screws
- 2.0 mm cortex screws
- 2.0 mm K-wires
- Arthroscopy set

(Size of system, instruments, and implants can vary according to anatomy.)

Patient preparation and positioning

Soft-tissue recovery after 8 days with elevation, ice or lymph drainage. Tourniquet (200–300 mm mercury) for 30–45 minutes.

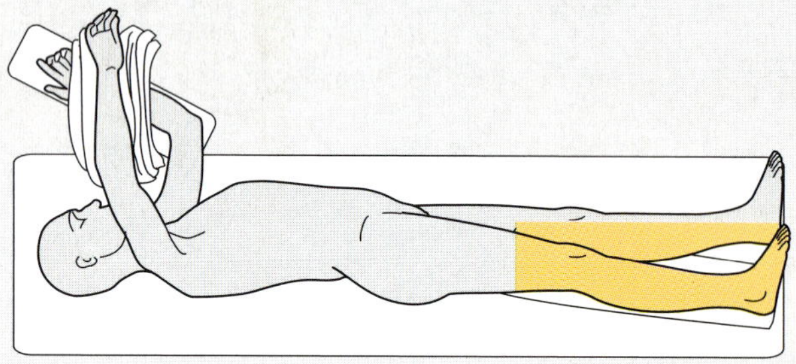

Fig 11.1-2 Lateral positioning of the patient on the operating table.

2 Surgical approach

Extended lateral approach (Seattle approach).

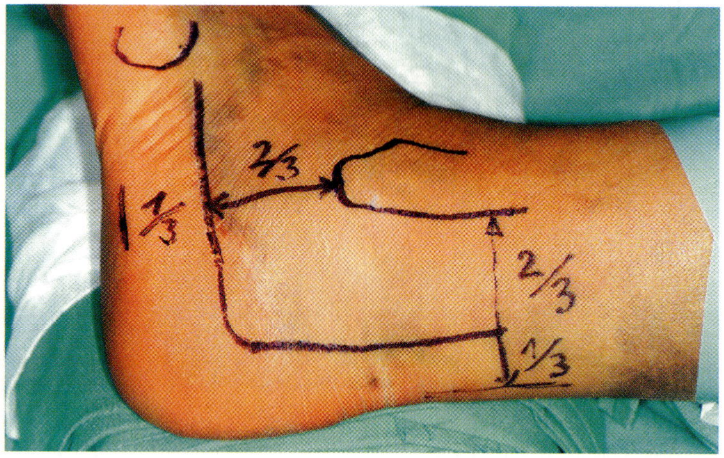

Fig 11.1-3 The L-shaped incision is performed as a full thickness flap including the sural nerve. The peroneal tendons should not be seen, except in the area of the peroneal tubercle where a medial sheath is missing. Distally the peroneal tendons have to be mobilized within their sheaths for exposure of the calcaneocuboid joint. The fibulo-calcaneal ligament is detached from the bone and all preparation is done epiperiosteally. Generally no sharp hooks are used. As soon as the subtalar joint is visualized, three 2.0 mm K-wires are introduced close to the joint into the talar body and neck, a fourth into the cuboid if exposure of the calcaneocuboid joint is needed.

3 Reduction and fixation

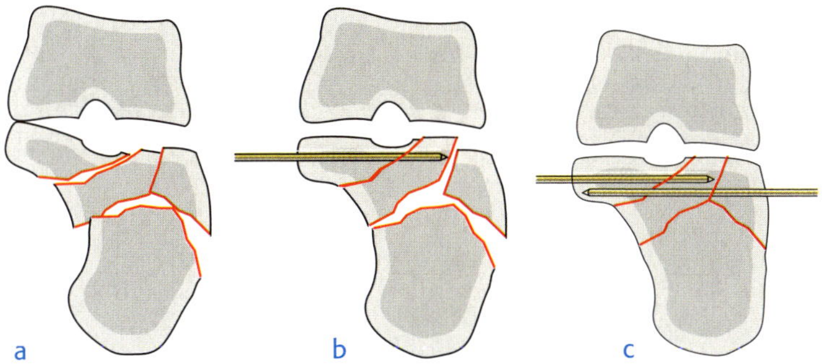

Fig 11.1-4a–c If the medial part of the posterior facet is not congruent to the talus one has to first reduce this sustentacular fragment congruent to the talus, keeping it temporarily reduced with a 2.0 mm K-wire coming from the plantar side and fixing it anatomically to the talus. After this the intermediate posterior facet fragment should be reduced and fixed temporarily with 1–2 K-wires which run from lateral through the skin medially. They are retracted so far medially that one can now reduce the larger lateral part of the posterior facet congruent to the intermediate and medial part of the posterior facet as well as to the talus by advancing the K-wires from medial to lateral to have the complete subtalar joint temporarily fixed in an anatomical position.

After this maneuver the tuberosity fragment and the anterior process fragments are reduced, keeping them in the correct position with K-wires. After this anatomical reduction the plate is roughly modeled and applied to the calcaneal wall.

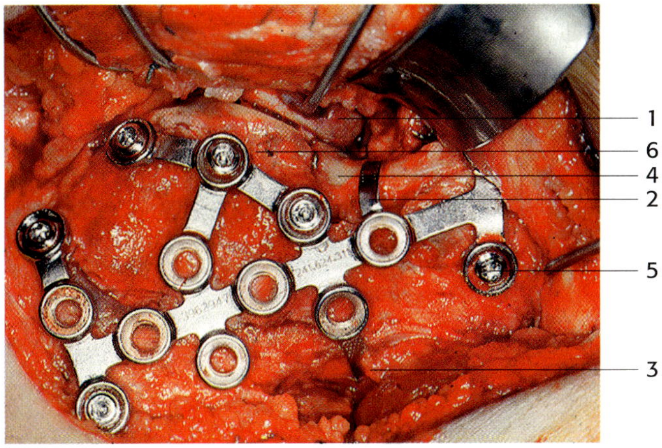

Fig 11.1-5 The tab in the critical angle of Gissane (CAG) is precisely bent into place with special forceps to keep the anterior process fragment in position. Usually 6–7 screws are inserted into the calcaneal bone: 2–3 from the subthalamic area into the sustentaculum, 2 into the tuberosity fragment far dorsally, and 2 screws into the anterior process fragment close to the calcaneocuboid joint. Fine-tuning adaptation of the plate before inserting the locking head screws is achieved by using the threaded tab benders especially in the subthalamic and calcaneocuboid joint area. Be aware that the very first subthalamic screw should not be a locking head screw but a 3.5 mm cortex screw (compression screw) so as not to leave a gap in the posterior facet.

The intraoperative picture (Fig 11.1-5) shows the situation after anatomical reduction and fixation with the locking plate. **1**) One of the four 2.0 mm K-wires which are inserted in the talus and cuboid is keeping the full thickness flap up for optimal exposure. **2**) Tab bent close to the bone in the calcaneal neck area to keep the anterior process fragment in anatomical position. **3**) Tab bent towards the bone, which optionally might keep a plantar triangular fragment in position. **4**) 2.0 mm cortex screw fixing the lateral part of the posterior facet which was additionally broken in itself. **5**) One of the locking head screws, here close to the calcaneocuboid joint. **6**) 3.5 mm cortex screw which has to be inserted as a compression screw at the very beginning so as not to leave a gap in the subtalar joint.

4 Rehabilitation

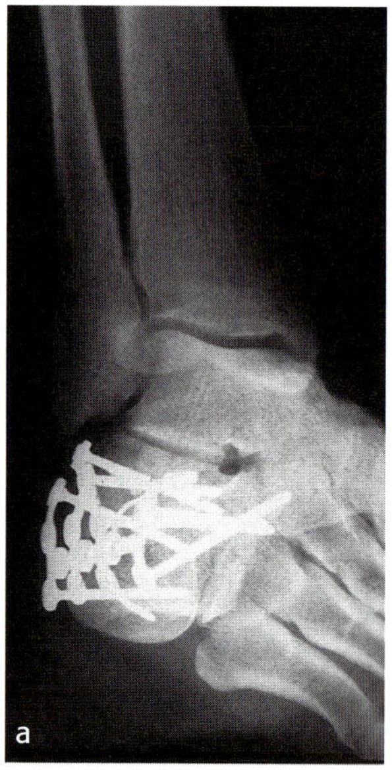

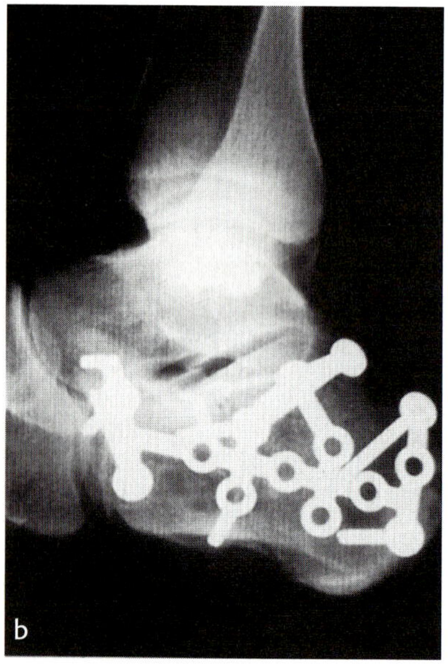

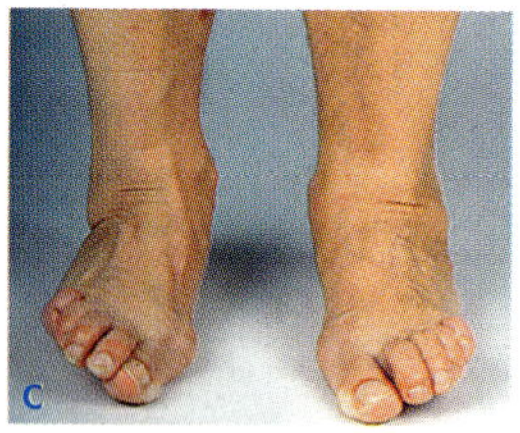

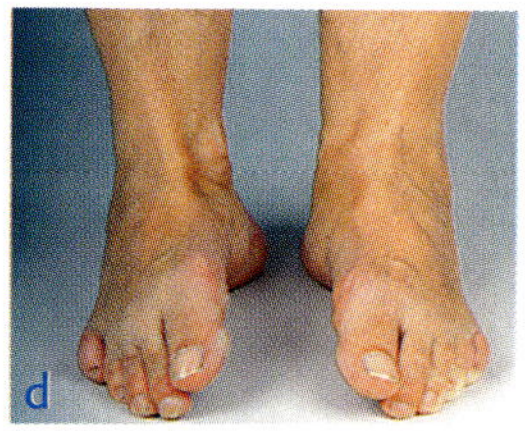

With split lower leg cast (8 days), continuous passive motion (starting 2nd day), active motion, partial weight bearing (20 kg) for 6 weeks in patient's own shoes, full weight bearing after 8–9 weeks.

Fig 11.1-6a–d
a–b Anatomical reduction and fixation with the locking calcaneal plate is achieved without the need for bone grafting.
c–d Extension, flexion, as well as pronation, supination of the foot after 3 months.

5 Pitfalls –

Approach

If the horizontal part of the extended lateral approach is positioned too far in the plantar direction, the overview of the subtalar might be limited; if the vertical part of the incision is not positioned dorsally enough, the sural nerve might be injured.

6 Pearls +

Approach

Fig 11.1-7a–b The limited sustentacular approach in addition to the extended lateral approach (patient in the supine position) is very helpful in cases where the medial facet is broken in itself (see Fig 11.1-9b–d). Reconstruction of the multifragmented subtalar joint (medial and posterior facet) always has to be started from medial to lateral. This approach is recommended also for isolated fractures of the sustentaculum tali.

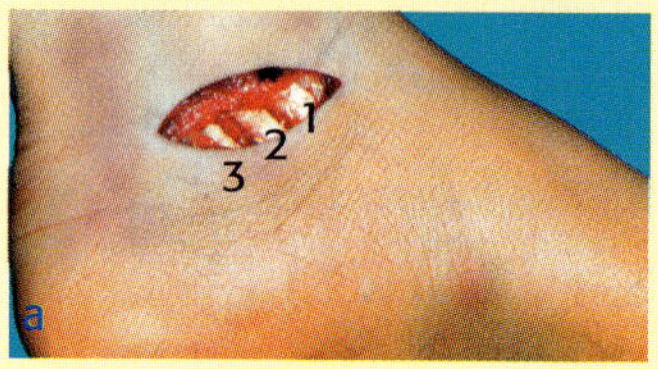

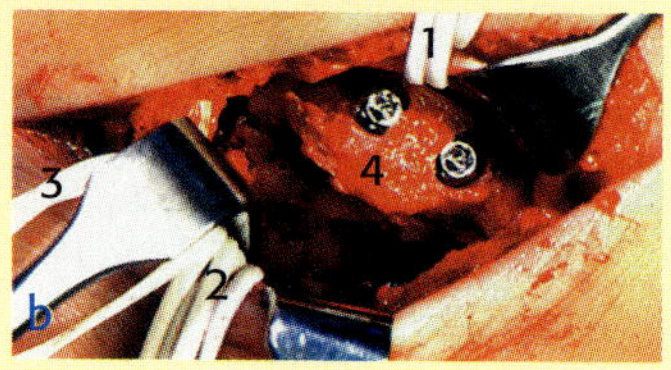

1 Posterior tibialis tendon.
2 Flexor digitorum longus tendon.
3 Flexor hallucis longus tendon held away with rutter bands.
4 Sustentaculum tali.

5 Pitfalls – (cont)

Reduction

Fig 11.1-8a–b Be aware of the tilted part of the medial portion of the posterior facet which must first be reduced congruent to the talus and temporarily fixed with a K-wire as shown in Fig 11.1-4a–c.

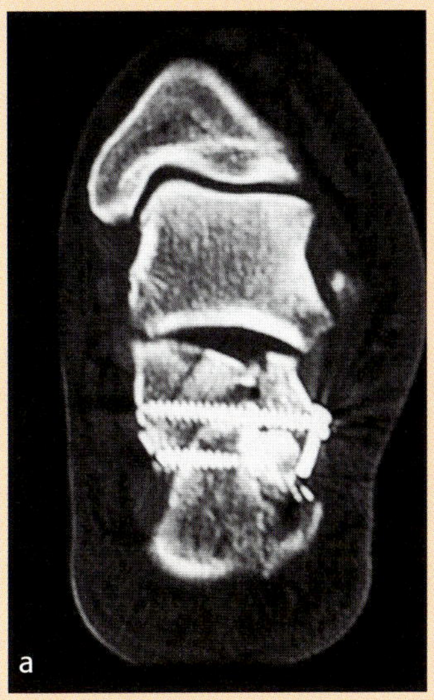

a

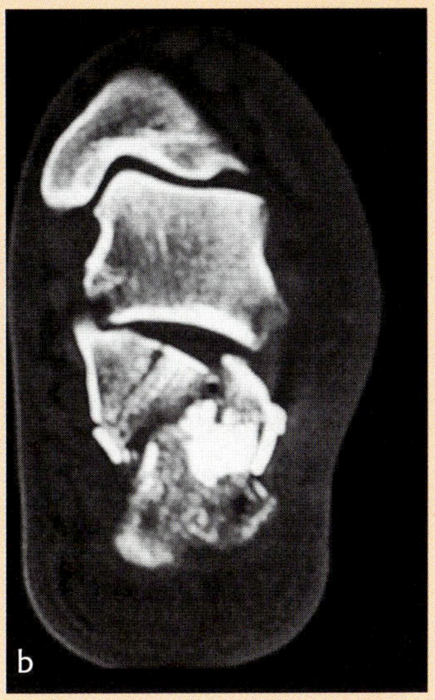

b

6 Pearls + (cont)

Reduction

Fig 11.1-9a–b After reducing the four parts of the subthalamic zone, using the extended lateral and the limited sustentacular approach simultaneously, one can screw and fix the subthalamic block with 4.0 mm cancellous lag screws.

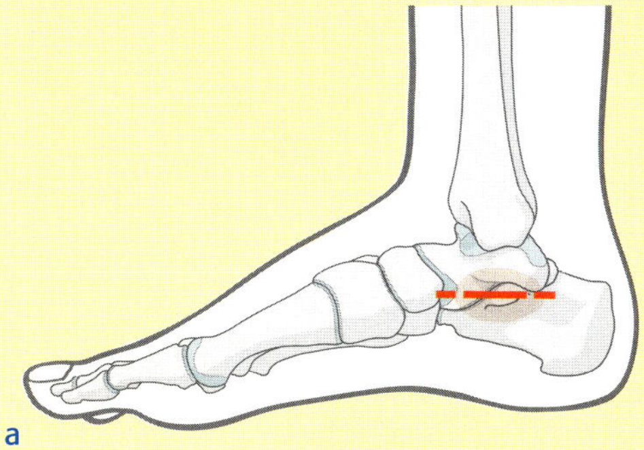

a

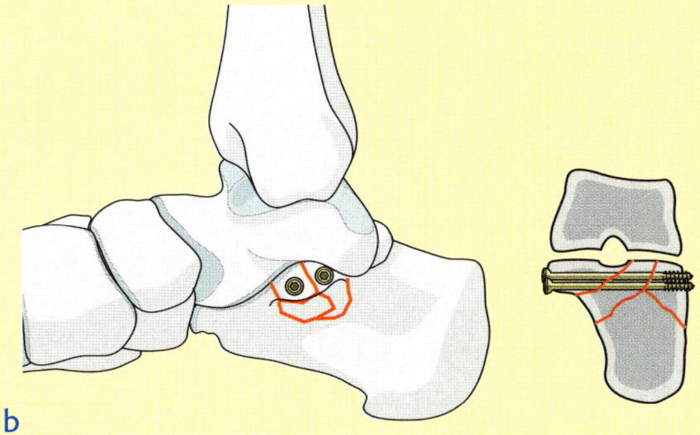

b

Author Hans Zwipp

11.2 Severe fracture dislocation of the calcaneus

1 Case description

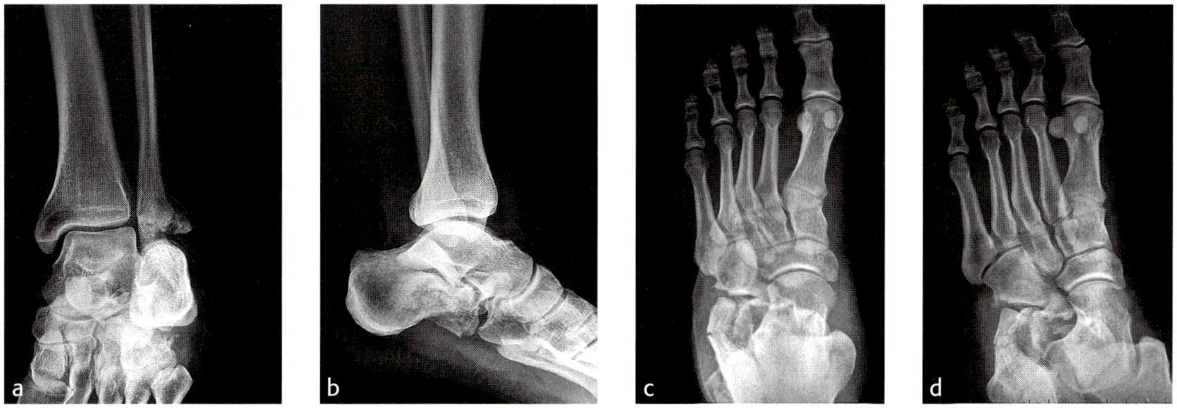

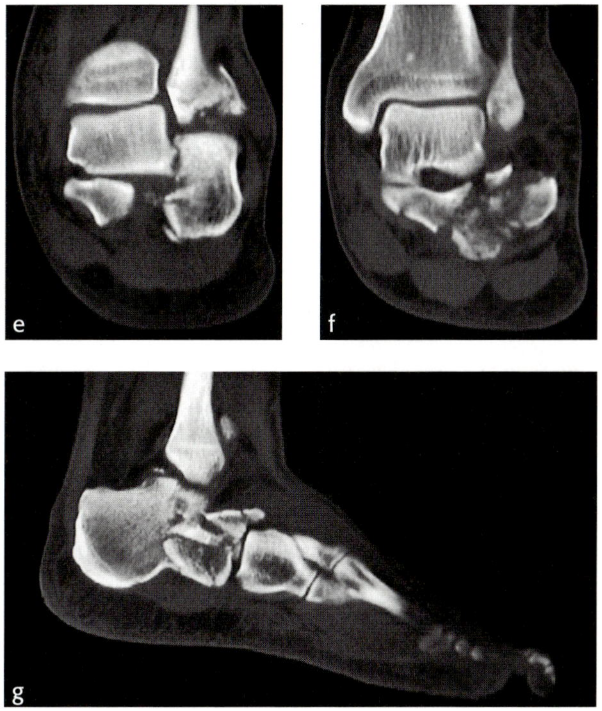

28-year-old man fell downstairs and sustained a severe fracture dislocation of the calcaneus.

Fig 11.2-1a–g

a–b AP ankle view and lateral x-ray show severe dislocation of the tuberosity and bursting of the lateral malleolus. Severe comminution of the anterior part of the calcaneus also affecting the calcaneocuboid joint.

c–g The dorso-plantar x-ray and the CT scans impressively show the dislocated tuberosity, including the main part of the posterior facet. Comminution of the distal fibula and the anterior half of the calcaneus involving the medial and cuboidal facets.

Indication

Severest fracture dislocation of the left calcaneus with complete dislocation at the subtalar level, intraarticular fracture of the posterior facet, medial/anterior facet and cuboidal facet, latter comminuted. Additional multifragmentary fracture of the distal fibula. Despite diabetes the indication for ORIF is given because of the severity of the dislocated hindfoot and youth of the patient.

Preoperative planning

Equipment

- Calcaneal locking plate 3.5
- 3.5 mm locking head screws
- 4.0 mm cancellous bone screw
- 2.0 mm cortex screws
- Cancellous 6.5 mm Schanz screw with handle to reduce the tuberosity fragment
- Large pelvic reduction forceps
- Arthroscopy set

(Size of system, instruments, and implants can vary according to anatomy.)

Patient preparation and positioning

Preoperative antibiotics.

Lifting the left pelvis with a 45° wedge.

Fixing the pelvis laterally on both sides to allow table tilting.

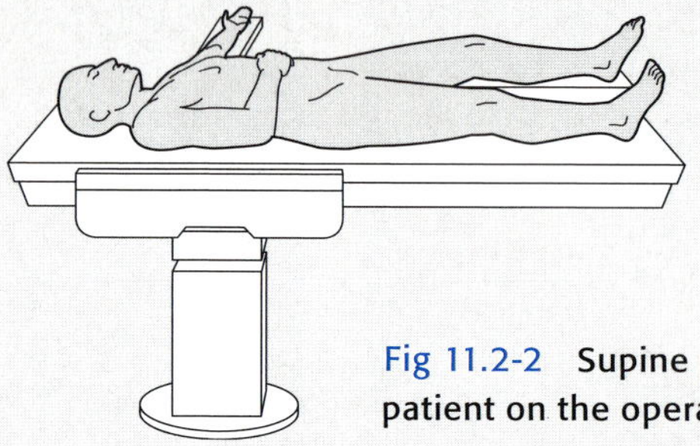

Fig 11.2-2 Supine position of the patient on the operating table.

2 Surgical approach

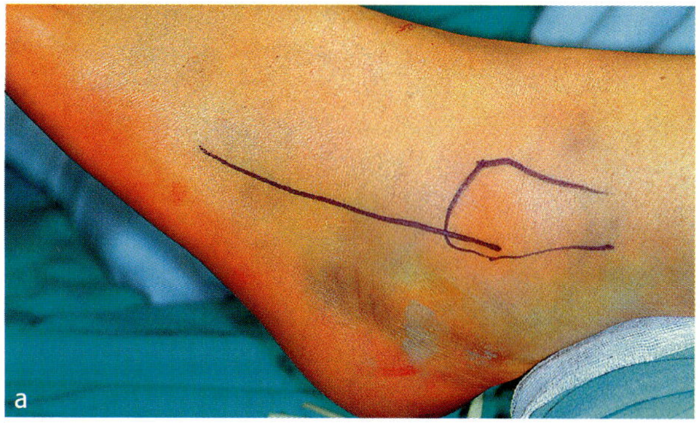

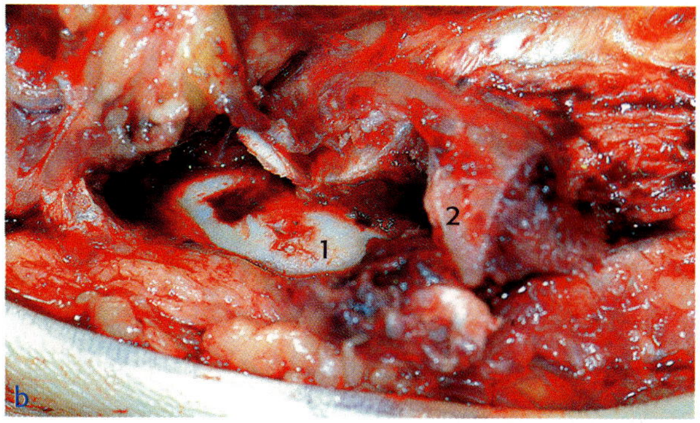

Fig 11.2-3a–b Modified palmar approach runs from the dorsal aspect of the fibula to the anterior aspect of the base of the fifth metatarsal, taking care of the peroneal tendons which, in these cases, unnon-anatomically because of their avulsion from the proximal retinaculum and consecutive dislocation. Severe cartilage damage (1) to the posterior facet which is dislocated far lateral just below the multifragmented distal fibula (2).

2 Surgical approach (cont)

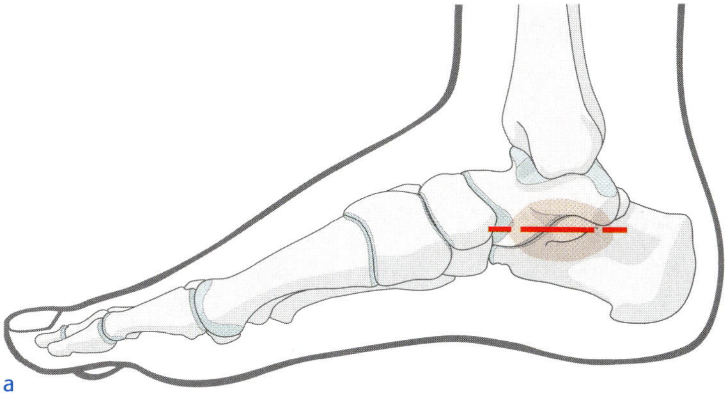

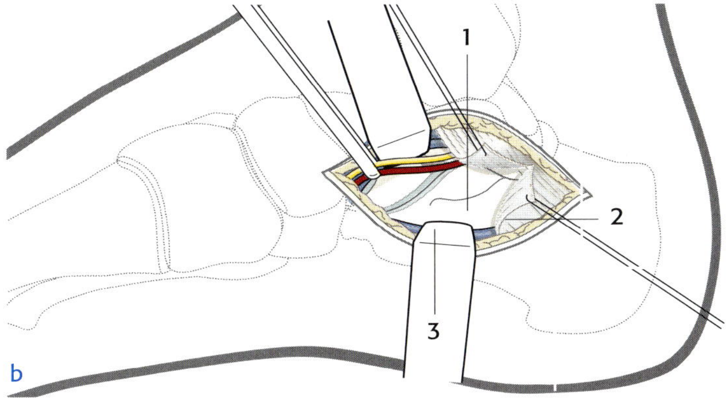

Fig. 11.2-4a–b Modified McReynolds approach. The incision is made horizontally or as a lazy S, about 8–10 cm, exactly halfway between the tip of the medial malleolus and the sole. The neurovascular bundle is identified and carefully held away with a penrose drain. The abductor hallucis muscle is retracted downwards, whereas the flexor hallucis longus tendon is only identified and left in place.

1 Sustentacular fragment
2 Anterior process fragment
3 Tuberosity fragment

3 Reduction and fixation

After approaching from laterally and medially and having cleaned the fracture sites in the **first step,** a 6.5 mm cancellous Schanz screw with handle is positioned into the large tuberosity fragment after stab incision and predrilling (3.2 mm).

By pulling the tuberosity fragment down and shifting it medially, the posterior facet can be reduced below the talus.

Controlling the position of the tuberosity fragment with the adjacent posterior facet from lateral, the reduction towards the sustentacular fragment is controlled from medial.

As soon as an anatomical reduction has been achieved, the large pelvic reduction forceps with ball and spike is brought into place, ie towards the medial sustentacular wall and the lateral subthalamic area, in this way completing medial shifting and safe anatomical reduction.

While compressing the tuberosity fragment towards the sustentacular fragment with the large pelvic reduction forceps, a 4.0 mm cancellous bone lag screw is inserted from the lateral subthalamic zone into the sustentacular fragment.

A two-hole part of the locking calcaneal plate is cut off with the special smooth-cutting forceps to fix the sustentacular and the large tuberosity fragment from the medial side using screws for locking, and rebuilding in this way a stable medial wall.

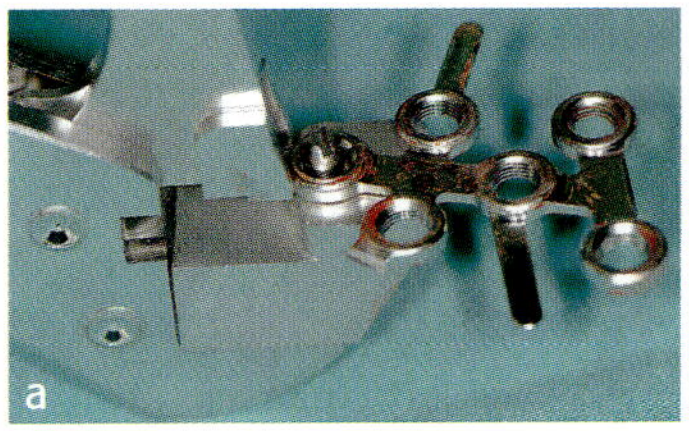

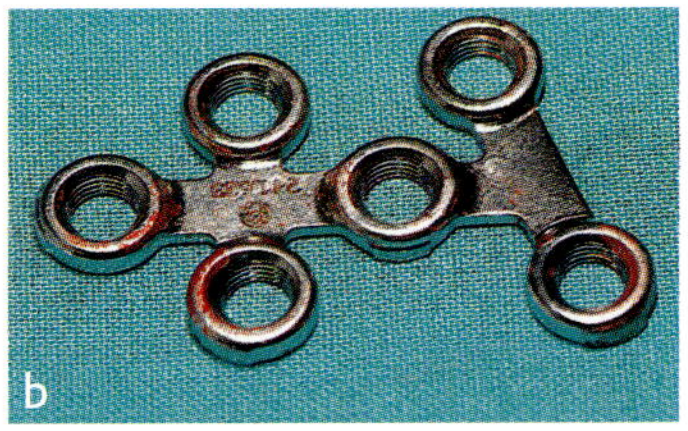

Fig 11.2-5a–d

a–b After anatomical reduction of the multifragmented anterior half of the calcaneus by remodeling the cuboidal facet towards the cuboid and fixing the fragments temporarily with K-wires, a 6-hole part of the locking calcaneal plate is cut off.

3 Reduction and fixation (cont)

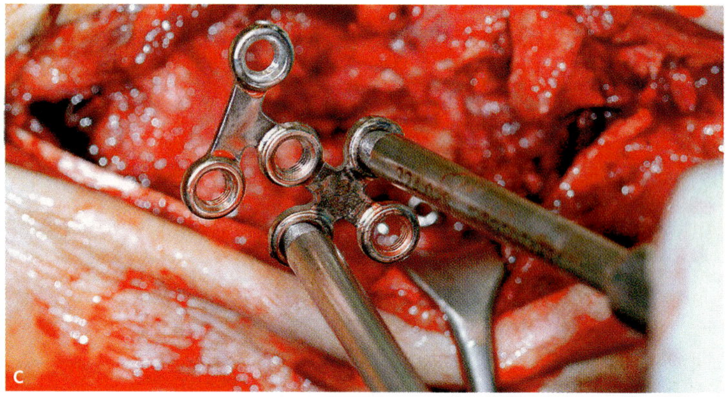

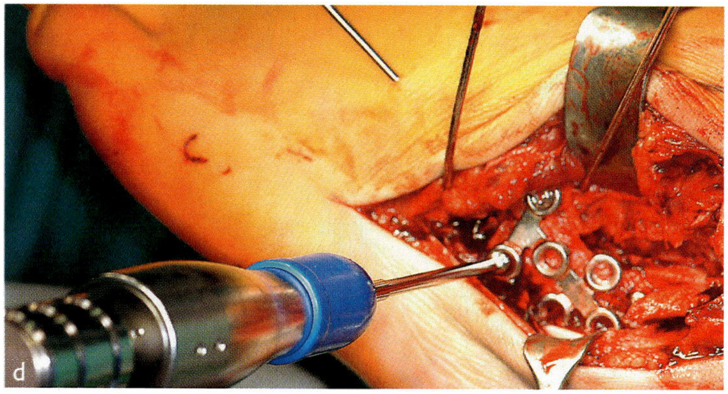

Fig 11.2-5a–d (cont)

c The plate is anatomically bent with the threaded tab benders and brought down to the calcaneal wall.

d Four locking head screws are inserted using the torque limiter.

After completely restoring the calcaneus, the multifragmented lateral distal malleolus is rebuilt with four 2.0 mm cortex screws. At the least, the dislocated peroneal tendons are reduced behind the lateral malleolus and the proximal retinaculum is sutured back to its origin in transosseus suture technique.

4 Rehabilitation

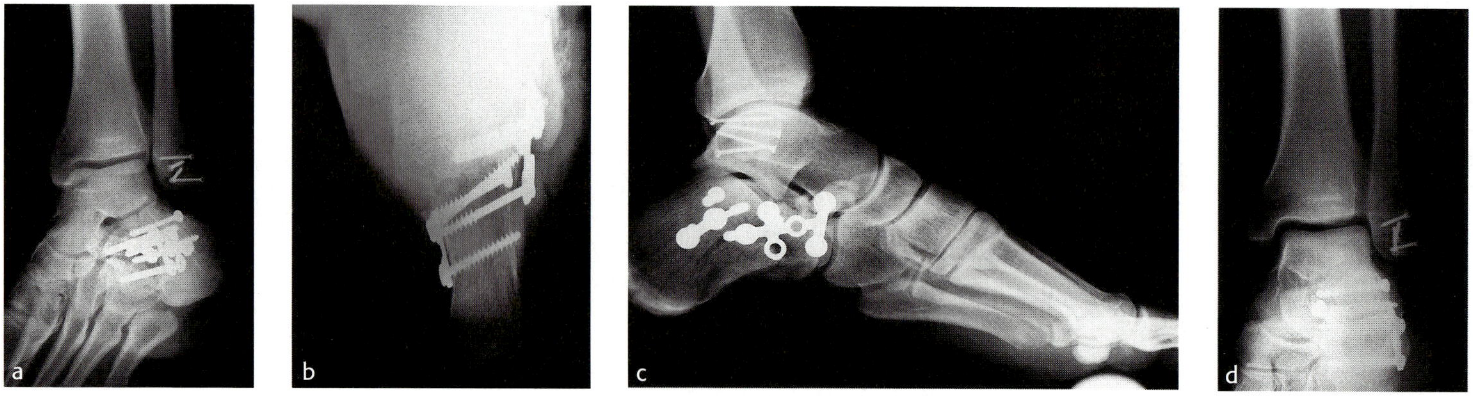

With split lower leg cast (8 days), continuous passive motion (starting second day), active motion, partial weight bearing (20 kg) for 6–8 weeks in patient's own shoes, full weight bearing is achieved after 8 weeks.

Fig 11.2-6a–k Anatomical reduction and fixation with the locking calcaneal plate is performed without use of any bone graft. Extension, flexion, as well as pronation/supination of the foot are close to normal. Fully active as a beer brewer.

4 Rehabilitation (cont)

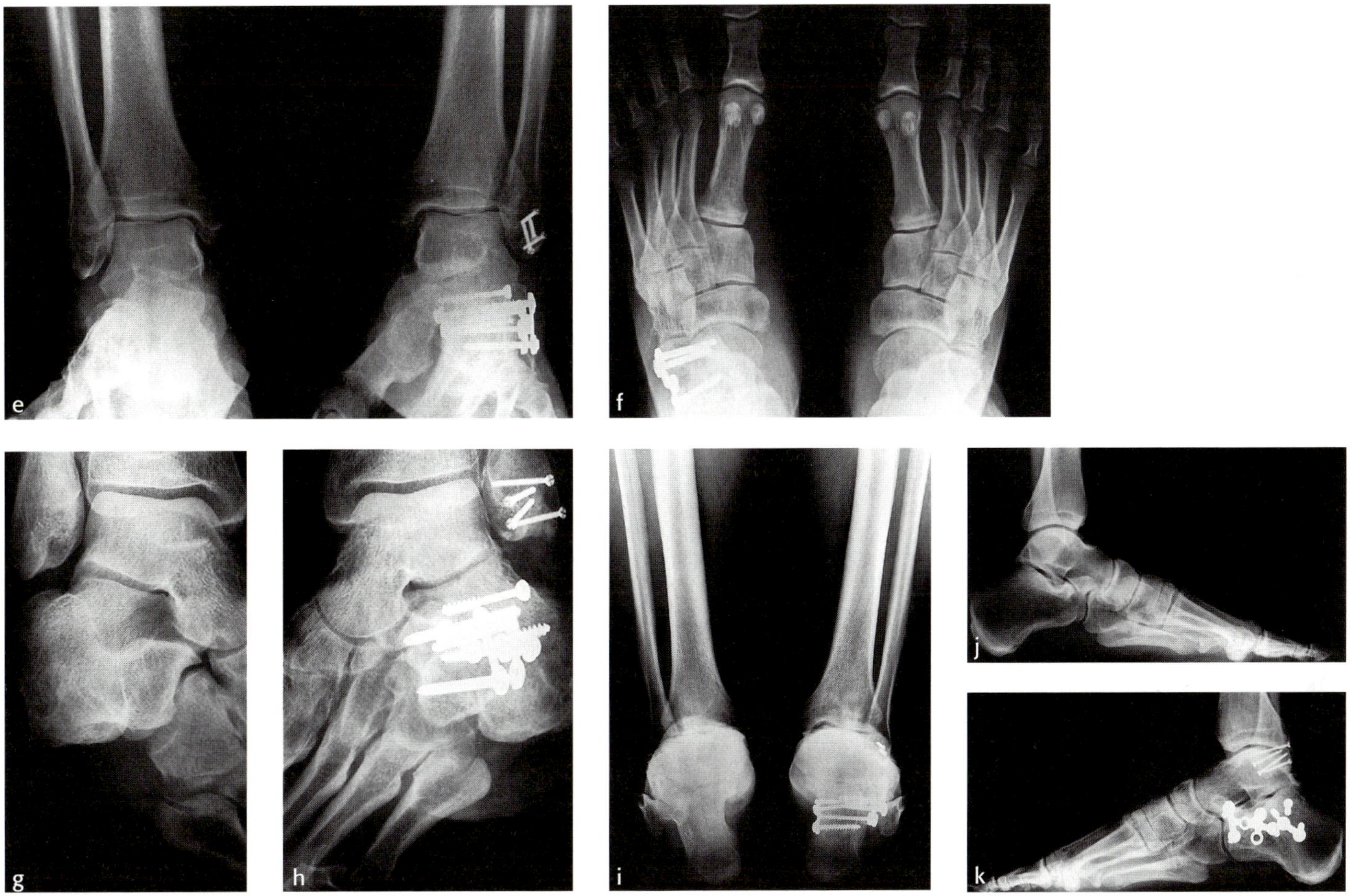

Fig 11.2-6a–k (cont) The fracture has healed anatomically without signs of posttraumatic arthritis at 15 months follow-up.

5 Pitfalls –

Exposure

Choosing the incorrect approach, like the extended lateral approach in these cases, means that the lateral malleolus and the dislocated peroneal tendons cannot be controlled and repaired.

Reduction

Not using a bilateral approach or the 6.5 mm cancellous Schanz screw with handle to manipulate the tuberosity fragment, or failing to use the big round pelvis clamp, one will probably not be able to achieve anatomical reduction of these severely dislocated fractures as demonstrated by the following malunited case.

Fig 11.2-7a–d By using a bilateral approach, mobilizing the malunited fragments, shifting the tuberosity fragment with the inserted Schanz screw (6.5 mm) with handle and using the large pelvic reduction forceps (a) the large laterally dislocated tuberosity fragment including the posterior facet can be reduced and fixed anatomically freeing up the lateral malleolus (compare to b and d).

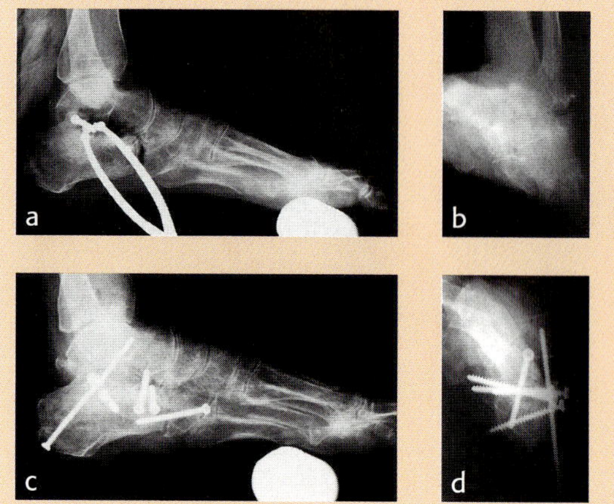

6 Pearls +

Exposure

In the case of a completely destroyed cuboidal facet, the skin incision should run beyond the cuboidal joint to achieve enough exposure of its calcaneal facet using the cuboid as a mold.

Reduction

Fig 11.2-8a–d By using a mini distractor after having placed one pin into the cuboid and one pin into the unbroken part of the calcaneus, reduction of the comminuted cuboidal facet becomes possible. Fixation with a locking plate offers stability, even in complex foot fractures like this one.

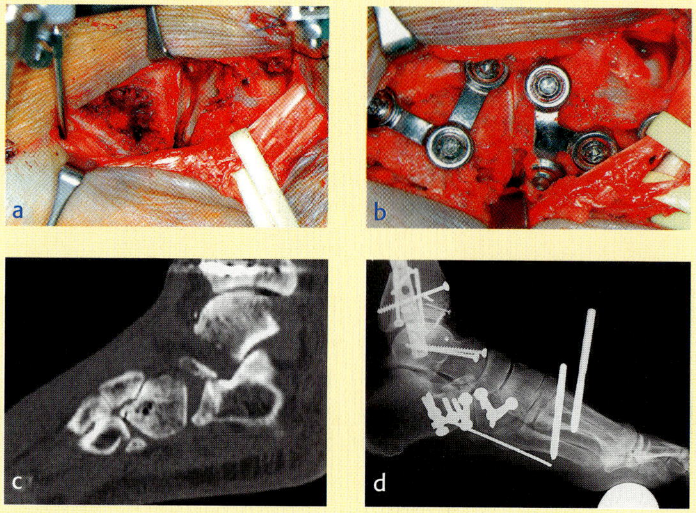

Glossary

With acknowledgements to Christopher L Colton, Christopher G Moran, and Stephan M Perren

The glossary provides the working definitions for terms that have been used by authors throughout the book. We hope the glossary will help readers understand the text.

abduction   Movement of a part away from the midline.

absolute stability   See stability, absolute.

adduction   Movement of a part towards the midline.

algodystrophy   Alternatively known as Reflex Sympathetic Dystrophy, Sudek's atrophy, or type II complex regional pain syndrome (CRPS)—see also fracture disease.

allograft   Bone or tissue transplanted from one individual to another.

anatomical position   The reference position of the body—standing facing the observer, with the palms of the hands facing forward.

anatomical reduction   Reinstatement of the exact pre-fracture shape of the bone.

angular stability   The property of an implant construct, which is designed so that the discreet parts of the implant, when assembled, are fixed in their angular relationship to each other, to stabilize the fracture. Usually applied to plates and screws, when the screw heads, once driven home in the plate hole, are interconnected with the plate—this is achieved by an external thread on the screw head which engages with an internal thread in the plate hole.

antibiotic   Any drug or naturally occurring substance, which can inhibit the growth of, or destroy, microorganisms.

antiglide plate   Prevents shear displacement of an oblique fracture fragment whereby the antiglide plate functions as a buttress.

arthritis   An inflammatory condition of a synovial joint. It may be septic or aseptic.

arthrodesis   Fusion of a joint by bone as a planned outcome of a surgical procedure.

articular fracture–partial   Only part of the joint is involved while the remainder remains attached to the diaphysis. There are several varieties:

- pure depression   An articular fracture in which there is depression alone of the articular surface without split. The depression may be central or peripheral—see impacted fracture.
- pure split   An articular fracture in which there is a longitudinal metaphyseal and articular split, without any additional osteochondral lesion.
- split-depression   A combination of a split and a depression, in which the joint fragments are usually separated.
- multifragmentary-depression   A fracture in which part of the joint is depressed and the fragments are completely separated.

articular fracture–complete   The entire articular surface is separated from the diaphysis.

autograft   Graft of tissue from one site to another within the same individual (homograft).

avascular necrosis (often abbreviated as AVN) Bone which has been deprived of its blood supply dies. In the absence of sepsis, this is called avascular necrosis. The dead bone retains its normal strength until the natural process of revascularization, by creeping substitution, starts to remove the dead bone, in preparation for the laying down of new bone.

avulsion Pulling off, eg, a bone fragment pulled off by a ligament or muscle attachment is an avulsion fracture.

bactericidal Capable of killing bacteria.

bicortical screw A screw that engages in both the near and the far cortex.

biocompatibility The ability to exist in harmony with, and not to injure, associated biological tissues or processes.

biological internal fixation A technique of surgical exposure, fracture reduction and fixation including the bone-implant interface which favors the preservation of the blood supply and thereby optimizes the healing potential of the bone and soft tissues.

bone graft Bone removed from one skeletal site and placed at another. Bone grafts are used to stimulate bone union and also to restore skeletal continuity where there has been bone loss—see allograft, autograft, and xenograft.

bone healing See healing.

butterfly fragment Where there is a fracture complex with a third fragment which does not comprise a full cross section of the bone (ie, after reduction there is some contact between the two main fragments), the small wedge-shaped fragment, which may be spiral, is occasionally referred to as a butterfly fragment—see wedge fracture.

buttress Construct that resists axial load by applying force at 90° to the axis of potential deformity.

callus A complex tissue of immature bone and cartilage that is formed at the site of bone repair.

cancellous bone Trabecular bone of spongy structure, found mostly at the proximal and distal bone ends.

chondrocytes The active cells of cartilage which produce type II collagen and proteoglycans that make up the chondral matrix.

compartment syndrome Raised pressure in a closed fascial compartment that results in local tissue ischaemia—see muscle compartment.

complex fracture Fracture with one or more intermediate fragments in which there is no contact between the main fragments after reduction.

compression screw See lag screw.

compression plate A plate applied under axial tension to compress fracture surfaces and oriented more or less perpendicularly to the long axis of the bone.

compression method The act of pressing together to increase or achieve stability. Compression stabilizes by preloading and/or producing friction.

contact healing Occurs between two fragments of bone maintained in motionless contact. The fracture is then repaired by direct internal remodeling.

conventional plate All plates without threaded screw holes. Compare: angular stable plate.

conventional screw Cortex screws or cancellous bone screws, ie, not locking head screw.

coronal This is a vertical plane of the body passing from side to side, so that a coronal bisection of the body would cut it into a front half and a back half. Also called the frontal plane.

cortical bone The dense bone forming the tubular element of the shaft, or diaphysis (middle part) of a long bone. The term is also applied to the dense, thin shell covering the cancellous bone of the metaphysis.

corticotomy A special osteotomy where the cortex is surgically divided but the medullary content and the periosteum are not injured.

continuous passive motion—CPM The use of apparatus to provide periods of passive movement of a joint through a controlled range of motion.

creeping substitution The slow replacement of dead bone with living, vascular bone.

debridement The surgical excision from a wound or pathological area, of foreign material and all avascular, contaminated and infected tissue.

deformability A material (bone, implant, etc.) placed under load is deformed. The larger the deformability, the larger the deformation under a given load. Deformability is inverse to stiffness. The implants are generally more deformable than bone. As an example: under an applied bending moment the nail may deform about 10 times more and a plate about 50 times more than the corresponding bone.

deformation Deformation may be elastic (reversible) or plastic (irreversible).

deformation-tissue For a given load the deformation of different repair tissues may differ by a factor of about 1:1,000,000 (granulation tissue:cortical bone).

deformity Any abnormality of the form of a body part.

delayed union Union is not taking place at what is accepted as the expected time course for a particular fracture (and the patient's age).

diaphysis The cylindrical or tubular part between the ends of a long bone, often referred to as the shaft.

dislocation A displacement of a joint such that no part of one articular surface remains in contact with the other. Sometimes used incorrectly to denote fracture displacement.

displacement The condition of being or moving out of place. A fracture is displaced if the fragments are not perfectly anatomically aligned. The fragments of a fracture displace in relation to each other. The displacement may be reversible or irreversible.

distal Away from the center of the body, more peripheral.

ductility The ability of a material to develop significant, permanent deformation before it breaks—see plastic deformation.

dynamization Increasing mechanical load across a fracture to enhance bone formation.

elastic deformation See plastic deformation.

endosteum A single layered membrane that lines the interior surface of the bone, ie, the wall of the medullary cavity. Its cells have osteogenic potential.

energy transfer When tissues are injured, the damage is due to energy that is transferred to the tissues. This is most commonly due to the transfer of kinetic energy from a moving object (car, missile, falling object, etc).

epiphysis The end of a long bone which lies upon the growth plate in a child's skeleton—see metaphysis.

external fixation Skeletal stabilization using pins, wires, or screws that protrude through the skin and are linked externally by bars or other devices.

extraarticular fracture Does not involve the articular surface but may be within the capsule of the joint.

far cortex The cortex more distant from the operator.

fasciocutaneous Soft-tissue flaps, based upon a perforating artery, which include the skin, the subcutaneous tissues and the deep fascia.

fasciotomy The surgical division of the wall of a muscle compartment, usually to release high intracompartmental pressure—see compartment syndrome and muscle compartment.

fibrocartilage Tissue consisting of elements of cartilage and of fibrous tissue. It is the normal constituent of the menisci and the triangular fibrocartilage at the wrist. It forms as the repair tissue after injury to articular cartilage.

fracture disease A condition characterized by disproportionate pain, soft-tissue swelling, patchy bone loss, and joint stiffnes. Linked terms are algodystrophy, reflex sympathetic dystrophy (RSD), Sudeck's atrophy and type II complex regional pain syndrome.

fracture fixation Application of a mechanical device to a broken bone to allow healing in a controlled position and (usually) early functional rehabilitation. The surgeon determines the degree of reduction required and the mechanical environment that influences the mode of healing.

fracture zone The area adjacent to the fracture

gliding hole The cortex under the screw head is drilled to the size of the outer thread diameter so that the thread gets no purchase. It is used for lag screw techniques.

gliding splint A splint (such as a nonlocked intramedullary nail) which allows some displacement of the fracture fragments, eg, axial shortening.

Haversian system The cortical bone is composed of a system of small channels (osteons) about 0.1 mm in diameter. These channels contain the blood vessels and are remodeled after a disturbance of the blood supply to bone. There is a natural turnover of the Haversian systems by continuous osteonal remodeling; this process is part of the dynamic and metabolic nature of bone. It is also involved in the adaptation of bone to an altered mechanical environment. Direct fracture healing may by a side effect of osteonal remodeling of necrotic bone.

healing Recovery of original integrity; clinical bone healing; regarded as complete when bone has regained adequate stiffness and strength to withstand functional loading.

healing—direct Observed following internal fixation with absolute stability. It is characterized by the absence of callus; there is no resorption at the fracture site. Bone forms by internal remodeling without intermediate repair tissue. Direct fracture healing was formerly called "primary" healing. Direct healing takes one to two years until safe functional loading after implant removal is possible.

healing—contact Direct bone healing due to internal remodeling when there is absolute stability and the bone ends are in contact.

healing—gap Direct bone healing when there is absolute stability but a small gap between the fracture fragments. Lamellar bone forms in the gap and is then remodeled by penetrating osteons.

healing—indirect Bone healing by callus formation in fractures treated either with relative stability, or left untreated. Indirect healing takes only a few months to regain adequate stiffnes and strength for functional loading—see callus.

impacted fracture A fracture in which the opposing bony surfaces are driven one into the other.

interfragmentary compression Bone fragments are pressed together, either with a lag screw or plate, to produce preloading and friction between the fragments according to the principle of absolute stability.

fixator A device attached to the fragments of a fracture using a splint and pins. The fixator bridges the fracture site and reduces load-dependent instability.

external fixator A fixator placed outside the body and connected to the bone using transcutaneous pins and clamps.

internal fixator A fixator placed inside the body. The internal fixator replaces the clamps by locking threaded pins (screws) within the plate hole. The fully implanted internal fixator resembles a plate but functions like a fixator, ie, its stiffness reduces load dependent deformation or displacement. Like the external fixator, when elevated from the bone surface, it does not require exact shaping to fit the bone surface. It can, therefore, be used without broad surgical exposure (MIPO).

ischemia Reduction in blood flow resulting in tissue hypoxia and metabolic standstill.

kinetic energy The energy stored by a body by virtue of the fact that it is in motion. Kinetic energy is calculated according to the formula $E = mv^2/2$, where m is the mass of the moving object and v its velocity.

lag screw A screw that passes through a gliding hole to grip the opposite fragment in a threaded hole, producing interfragmentary compression when it is tightened.

locking plate A plate with screw holes that allow tight mechanical coupling to a locking head screw. The less invasive stabilization system (LISS) will accept only this type of screw, while locking compression plates (LCP) have a combination hole that will accept conventional (nonlocking) screw heads or locking screw heads.

locking head screw (LHS) Screws with, for instance, threads cut into the head which provide a mechanical coupling to a threaded screw hole in a plate, thereby creating an angular and axial stable device, ie, after application the screw can not tilt or move along its long axis. The locking head screws of the internal fixator resemble and act more like threaded bolts than conventional screws. The LHS maintains the relative positions of the body of the fixator and the bone.

malunion The fracture has healed in a position of deformity.

metaphysis In the adult, this is the segment of a long bone located between the articular surface and the shaft (diaphysis). It consists mostly of cancellous bone within a thin cortical shell.

method of fracture fixation The two basic methods are compression and splinting.

minimally invasive surgery Any surgical procedure undertaken using small skin incisions. Examples include laparoscopic abdominal surgery, arthroscopy, and closed intramedullary nailing.

minimally invasive plate osteosynthesis (MIPO) Reduction and plate fixation without direct surgical exposure of the fracture site, using small skin incisions and subcutaneous, or submuscular, insertion of the plate. Preferably locked and slightly elevated implants are used. Instruments with small footprint are mandatory.

monocortical screw A screw that engages only in one (the near) cortex.

multifragmentary fracture A fracture with more than one fracture line so that there are three pieces or more—see also complex fracture.

muscle compartment An anatomical space, bounded on all sides either by bone or deep fascia which contains one or more muscle bellies.

near cortex The cortex near the operator and on the side of insertion of an implant.

neutralization A plate, or other implant, which reduces the load placed upon a lag screw fixation, thus protecting it from overload. This term has been replaced by protection (protection plate).

noncontact plate Plates elevated from the bone surface in order to avoid disturbance of blood supply to soft tissues and bone. The locking head screw (threaded bolt) of the locked internal fixator does not press the plate (body of the fixator) toward the bone—see also internal fixator, locking plate, locking head screw (LHS).

nonunion The fracture is still present and healing has come to a standstill. Under no circumstances will the fracture unite without surgical intervention. It is usually due to improper mechanical or biological conditions—see union, pseudarthrosis, and delayed union.

ORIF A widely used abbreviation for open reduction and internal fixation (osteosynthesis).

osteoarthritis A condition of synovial joints which is characterized by loss of articular cartilage, subchondral bone sclerosis, bone cysts, and the formation of osteophytes.

osteolysis Softening and absorption of bone tissue.

osteomyelitis An acute or chronic inflammatory condition affecting bone and its medullary cavity, usually the result of infection.

osteon The name given to the small channels which combine to make up the Haversian system in cortical bone.

osteopenia A reduction in bone mass between 1 and 2.5 standard deviations below the mean for a young adult (ie, a T score of -1 to -2.5)—see osteoporosis.

osteoporosis A reduction in bone mass more than 2.5 standard deviations below the mean for a young adult (ie, a T score of < -2.5)—see osteopenia and pathological fracture.

osteosynthesis A term coined by Albin Lambotte to describe the "synthesis" (derived from the Greek for putting together, or union) of a fractured bone by a surgical intervention using implanted material. It differs from "internal fixation" in that it also includes external fixation.

osteotomy Controlled surgical division of a bone.

overbending (of plate) An exactly contoured plate is slightly arched at the level of a transverse fracture, so that its central portion stands slightly off the underlying cortex. As compression is applied, the far cortex is compressed first, then the near cortex (without the arch, the plate will only compress the near cortex—this is not a stable situation).

pathological fracture A fracture through abnormal bone which occurs at normal physiological load or stress.

periosteum The fibrovascular membrane covering the exterior surface of a bone. The deep cell layer has osteogenic potential.

pilot hole A drill hole which has the same diameter as the core of the screw. This can then be used to guide the insertion channel for screws that cut their own thread (self-tapping) or a tap that will cut the threads and produce a threaded hole.

pin loosening Bone resorption at a fixator pin-bone interface usually the result of interface micromotion.

plastic deformation A permanent change in a material's length or angle, ie, it will not be reversed when the deforming force is released.

polytrauma Multiple injury to one or more body systems or cavities with sequential systemic reactions. An Injury Severity Score (ISS) of more than 15 is usually taken to indicate polytrauma.

prebending of plate (precontouring, preshaping) Preoperative or intraoperative bending of a plate to fit the shape of the plated bone exactly.

precise reduction See anatomical reduction.

protection plate A plate, or other implant, which shares load with bone and thus reduces the load placed upon a lag screw fixation, thus protecting it from destructive overload. This term has replaced neutralization.

pseudarthrosis literally means "false joint". When a nonunion is mobile and allowed to persist for a long period, the bone ends become sclerotic and the intervening soft tissues differentiate to form a type of synovial articulation—see delayed union, nonunion, union.

reduction The realignment of a displaced fracture.

reduction–direct Reduction achieved by direct manipulation using hands or instruments.

reduction–indirect Fragments are manipulated indirectly by applying corrective force at a distance from the fracture, or by distraction or other means.

reduction screw A screw that pulls a bone, or bone fragment towards the screw head or plate.

reflex sympathetic dystrophy (RSD) One of the names given to algodystrophy—see fracture disease.

refracture A further fracture occurring after a fracture has been solidly bridged by bone, at a load level otherwise tolerated by normal bone. The resulting fracture line may coincide with the original fracture line, or be within the area of bone that has undergone changes as a result of the fracture and its treatment.

relative stability See stability, relative.

remodeling (of bone) The process of transformation of external bone shape (external remodeling), or of internal bone structure (internal remodeling, or remodeling of the Haversian system).

rigidity The ability to resist deformation under an applied load.
Rigid fixation: This term is sometimes used to define a fixation using a rigid implant. The term is incorrect because most implants have a structural rigidity, which is less than that of bone. The implant materials rigidity is less important that the geometry or dimensions of the implant—see stability, absolute.

sagittal This is a vertical plane of the body passing from front to back, so that a sagittal bisection of the body would cut it into a right half and a left half.

second look Surgical inspection of a wound or injury zone, 24 to 72 hours after the initial management of a fracture or wound.

segmental If the shaft of a bone is broken at two levels, leaving a separate shaft segment between the two fracture sites, it is called a "segmental" fracture complex.

sequestrum A piece of dead bone lying alongside, but separated from, the bony bed from which it came. Infected sequestra are formed in chronic osteomyelitis.Intensification of necrosis-induced porosity may lead to confluence of the pores whereby the dead bone becomes separated and a sequestrum is formed—see osteomyelitis.

shear A shearing force is one which tends to cause one segment of a body to slide upon another, as opposed to tensile forces, which tend to elongate a body.

simple fracture There is a single fracture line producing two fracture fragments.

splinting method Splinting is a method of fracture fixation. Movement at the fracture site is reduced by attaching a rigid support to the main bone fragments. The splint may be external (plaster, external fixators) or internal (plate, internal fixator, intramedullary nail).

splint—locked There are fixed connections between the bone and splinting device, above and below the fracture zone, so that the working length between the main fragments cannot change (eg, static, locked nail).

splint—gliding The connection between the bone and the splinting device allows (controlled) axial movement, so that the distance between the main fragments can change (eg, dynamic, locked nail).

splint-nonlocking No axial connections between the bone and the splint (eg, nonlocking nail, TEN).

split depression An articular injury with a fracture line running into the metaphysis (split) and impaction of separate osteochondral joint fragments (depression).

spontaneous fracture A fracture that occurs at physiological load or stress, usually in abnormal bone—see pathological fracture.

stability of fixation This is characterized by the degree of residual motion at the fracture site after fixation.

stability, absolute One of the principles of fracture fixation. Fixation of fracture fragments so that there is virtually no displacement of the fracture surfaces under physiological load. This allows direct bone healing. The fracture is more or less repaired as a result of normal tissue renewal. The process of healing is mainly effected by the removal of necrotic bone during internal remodeling.

stability, relative Another principle of fracture fixation. A fixation construct that allows small amounts of motion in proportion to the load applied. This results in indirect healing by callus formation. The small degree of fracture instability allows the repair tissue to recognize the presence of the fracture whereby an early repair process is initiated.

stiffness The resistance of a structure to deformation. The stiffness of a structure is expressed for instance as its Young's modulus of elasticity, which is the ratio of stress to strain.

stiffness, bending bending stiffness of an implant is inversely proportional to the square of its working length.

stiffness, torsional Torsional stiffness of an implant is inversely proportional to its working length.

stiffness and geometrical properties The thickness of a structure affects deformability by its third power. Changes in geometry are, therefore, much more critical than changes in material properties.

strain Change in the length of a material when a given force is applied. Normal strain is the ratio of deformation (lengthening or shortening) to original length. It has no dimensions but is often expressed as a percentage.

strain induction Tissue deformation—among other things—may result in induction of callus. This is an example of a mechanically induced biological reaction.

strain tolerance This determines the tolerance of tissues to deformation. No tissue can remain intact and function properly when an increase in length (ie, strain) causes the tissue to disrupt. This is the critical strain level.

strain theory–Perren With a small fracture gap, any movement will result in a relatively large change in length (ie, high strain). If this exceeds the strain tolerance of the tissue, healing will not take place. If a larger fracture gap is subject to the same movement, the relative change in length will be smaller (ie, less strain) and, if the critical strain level is not exceeded, there will be normal tissue function and indirect healing by callus. If the distance between the fractured surfaces is excessive, healing will not occur.

strength The ability to withstand load without structural failure. The strength of a material can be expressed as ultimate tensile strength, bending strength, or torsional strength.

stress concentration In the vicinity of a small notch in the bone excessive stress may occur within the material under load. Refracture may result when a fracture gap is not adequately bridged due to an impaired blood supply at the bone-implant interface.

stress distribution The pattern of stress within a material—see stress concentration.

stress protection Using an implant to reduce peak loads applied to a screw fixation, for example. The theory of "stress protection", that is the explanation that early temporary porosis of bone in the vicinity of the implant contact is the result of unloading according to Wolff's law, is no longer acceptable.

stress riser A small surface defect (notch) that brings about a concentration of stress. A screw hole may to some degree act as a weak spot.

stress shielding Bone deprived of functional stimulation by having its functional load reduced may react in the long-term by becoming less dense or strong.

subluxation A displacement of a joint but with partial contact between the two articular surfaces.

tension band The principle by which an implant, attached to the tension side of a fracture, converts the tensile force into a compressive force at the cortex opposite the implant. While wires, cables, and sutures are often used for tension band fixation, plates and external fixators, when appropriately placed, can also function as tension bands.

thread hole Discussed in conjunction with pilot hole.

toggling Slight movement at the couple between a screw and a plate or nail. Implants may be designed to allow toggle, eg, intramedullary nails where the tolerances of the assembly do not permit exact fit. Toggle between plates and screws may occur during plate failure with loosening of the implant.

torque The moment produced by a turning or twisting force. As an example: torque is applied to drive home and tighten a screw. The moment is equal to the product of the lever arm (in meters) and force (in Newtons), producing torsion and rotation about an axis (the unit of torque in Nm).

translation Displacement of one bone fragment in relation to another, usually at right angles to the long axis of the bone—see displacement.

union The bone has united and regained its normal stiffness and strength. In clinical terms, this means there is no movement or tenderness at the fracture site and no pain on stressing the fracture site. Radiologically, there should be evidence of bone trabeculae bridging the fracture site.

valgus Deviation away from the midline in the anatomical position.

varus Deviation toward the midline in the anatomical position.

wave plate The central section of a plate is contoured to stand off the near cortex over a distance of several holes. This leaves a gap between the plate and the bone, which (a) preserves the biology of the underlying bone, (b) provides a space for the insertion of a bone graft, and (c) increases the stability because of the distance of the "waved" portion of the implant from the neutral axis of the shaft. Such plating is useful in nonunion treatment.

wedge fracture Fracture complex with a third fragment in which, after reduction, there is some direct contact between the two main fragments—see butterfly fragment.

working length The distance between the two points of implant fixation (one on either side of the fracture) between an implant, usually an intramedullary nail, and the bone.

xenograft Bone or tissue transplanted from one species to another.

zone of injury The entire volume of bone and soft tissue damaged by energy transfer during trauma.